# Care of Adults with Chronic Childhood Conditions

Alice A. Kuo • Mariecel Pilapil
David E. DeLaet • Cynthia Peacock
Niraj Sharma
Editors

# Care of Adults with Chronic Childhood Conditions

## A Practical Guide

Second Edition

Springer

*Editors*
Alice A. Kuo
Division of Medicine-Pediatrics and Preventive Medicine
University of California
Los Angeles, CA, USA

David E. DeLaet
Medicine
University of Cincinnati College of Medicine
Cincinnati, OH, USA

Niraj Sharma
Department of Medicine, Brigham and Women's Hospital
Boston, MA, USA

Department of Pediatrics
Boston Children's Hospital
Boston, MA, USA

Harvard Medical School
Boston, MA, USA

Mariecel Pilapil
Medicine and Pediatrics
Northwell Health
Lake Success, NY, USA

Cynthia Peacock
Dept of Medicine and Pediatrics
Baylor College of Medicine
Houston, TX, USA

ISBN 978-3-031-54280-0 ISBN 978-3-031-54281-7 (eBook)
https://doi.org/10.1007/978-3-031-54281-7



This Springer imprint is published by the registered company Springer Nature Switzerland AG
The registered company address is: Gewerbestrasse 11, 6330 Cham, Switzerland

Paper in this product is recyclable.

*The editors would like to dedicate this book to the young adults with chronic childhood conditions who bridge the gap from pediatric to adult health care every day.*

# Preface

## Why a Second Edition?

Much has changed in the world since the first edition of this book was published in 2016—we have endured a global pandemic; society has become increasingly politically polarized; and structural determinants of health, in addition to social ones, are more recognized as having great impact on health outcomes for certain populations. In just a few years, the entire landscape in which children become adults has shifted and is entirely different. As a result, in this edition, we have new sections on telehealth, mental health, substance use and public health, among others. We also have a new section on hospital medicine, recognizing that healthcare transition issues are not only addressed in the outpatient setting. Given the tremendous positive feedback we received about the first edition, we hope that this version will continue to be helpful and relevant to clinicians caring for these patient populations.

## A Note on Terminology

Since the first edition, it has been even more apparent in many different situations that terminology and language matter tremendously when referring to groups of people. For this edition, we have attempted to follow the guidelines set forth in the first edition when it comes to referring to this target population by age, namely, "adolescents" refer to individuals age 14–18 years, "emerging adults" to individuals age 19–25 years, and "young adults" to individuals age 26–30 years.

For the expanded sections on gender identity exploration and transgender health and gender-diverse people, identifying one's pronouns has become a widespread practice in academic medicine and health care, even as it has become a target for polarization in mainstream society.

Finally, we have attempted not to use ableist language in sections describing disabilities. In particular, we have avoided using person-first language when describing autistic individuals, recognizing the growing preference from persons with lived experience for identity-first language (i.e., autistic individuals as opposed to individuals with autism). We have also tried to avoid using the term "autism spectrum disorder" as it is growing out of favor with increasing recognition of autism as an identity rather than as a disease or disorder.

This book is about adults with chronic childhood-onset conditions because we recognize that they have unique needs. As children, they are often termed children or youth with "special health care needs" (CYSHCN). CYSHCN are defined by the U.S. Health Resources and Services Administration (HRSA)'s Maternal and Child Health Bureau (MCHB) as "children who have or are at increased risk for a chronic physical, developmental, behavioral, or emotional condition and who also require more than routine health and related services" [1]. While the federal government and subsequently academic researchers continue to use the term "special health care needs," disability rights advocates have objected to the use of being called "special," as it is often used pejoratively and often will comment, "there's nothing special about having a disability." As a result, we have attempted to avoid using this designation whenever possible.

## Audience

This book is for the practicing adult healthcare provider—either generalist or specialist. For primary care physicians, this book provides a new framework for thinking about care of young adults and identifying opportunities to impact patient health outcomes over a life trajectory. For others, this book serves as a reference with approaches for caring for young adults with specific conditions acquired in childhood. While we understand that we have not presented every chronic childhood condition, we chose the most common conditions based on data from the U.S. Department of Health and Human Services that are illustrative of broader approaches.

This book also discusses the challenges facing this population of patients as they transition from the pediatric healthcare system to the adult healthcare system and highlights why this period is often associated with poor outcomes. Ultimately, we provide some strategies to improve health outcomes for young adults with chronic conditions and assist adult health providers in better understanding the challenges they face.

In a recent publication, the following questions were articulated regarding healthcare transitions: "Who most needs a deliberate transition plan, at what age should transition planning begin, how should the transfer of medical care occur, what preparation is required, and in what manner should the actual transfer of care take place?" Also, one of the most basic questions remains: "What are the effective strategies to engage the adult healthcare system in the care of these young people?" Targeting this book to adult healthcare providers will hopefully help bridge the gap that exists between the pediatric and adult healthcare systems.

## Understanding and Responding to Emerging Adulthood

This book is grounded in several guiding principles: patients live in the context of their families and communities, social determinants of health influence health outcomes and quality of life, and preventive measures and interventions applied in young adulthood can have a tremendous impact on an individual's life trajectory. The practice of internal medicine has been to date very medically focused, particularly in approaching chronic diseases of middle age and geriatrics. In order to take advantage of the opportunities to change the health trajectories of adults, both without and with chronic childhood conditions, the practice of internal medicine needs to shift towards a preventive paradigm in which the primary care physician provides anticipatory guidance to help patients change health behaviors that could be detrimental.

In this book, we present a model of primary and secondary prevention for emerging adulthood—primary prevention in which all young adults are screened for high-risk behaviors and health needs and secondary prevention in which young adults with chronic childhood conditions are optimized through coordinated care, connections to community resources, and social/family support. The second part of this book details the new developmental period of emerging adulthood and the opportunities for primary care physicians to optimize health during this time.

## Structure of this Book

This book is organized in nine parts. Part I provides a detailed overview of the healthcare transition from pediatrics to adult medicine from both a policy and practice perspective. We review the literature on healthcare transition and describe the efforts of the Maternal and Child Health Bureau (MCHB)-funded Center for Health Care Transition Improvement (Got Transition). In Part II, we introduce the concept of emerging adulthood as a developmental period and provide strategies to the adult primary care provider for providing improved comprehensive care for this age group. Part III is a new chapter addressing sexual health, including reproductive health, gender identity exploration, LGBTQ+ issues, and care for transgender and gender-diverse people. Part IV addresses public health and population considerations, and Part V examines mental health and substance use issues facing emerging and young adults. Part VI is divided into condition-specific chapters, each of which details a specific chronic childhood condition, starting with a clinical case and ending with summary reports that can be used as a quick guide. Part VII ties very closely to Part VI and reviews additional clinical considerations that are not necessarily condition-specific but are highly relevant to the care of many young adults with chronic childhood conditions. Part VIII is a new and extensive chapter addressing healthcare transition issues occurring in hospital medicine. Finally, Part IX describes certain socio-legal issues adult providers should be aware of when caring for this population.

Most of what is recommended in this book is based on pediatric literature and the care of children or youth who have the disease. Much of the information is derived from consensus statements among experts who have cared for young adults but not from randomized treatment control trials or blinded studies for this specific population of patients. Some inroads are being made to identify the appropriate care for young adults surviving with childhood conditions, but much more needs to be done.

Much more discussion needs to take place on how we care for a generation of individuals who are just recently having their healthcare needs recognized as a national issue. For more information and to use as a resource, we recommend investing in the Health and Well-Being of Young Adults, authored by the Committee on Improving the Health, Safety, and Well-Being of Young Adults; Board on Children, Youth, and Families with the Institute of Medicine and the National Research Council. Arguably, this is a population in whom the U.S. healthcare system needs to invest as the returns to this nation could be not only a healthy workforce but also a much healthier economy.

## Reference

1. Newacheck PW, Strickland B, Shonkoff JP, Perrin JM, McPherson M, McManus M, Lauver C, Fox H, Arango P. An epidemiology profile of children with special health care needs. Pediatrics. 1998;102:117–23.

Los Angeles, CA, USA — Alice A. Kuo
Houston, TX, USA — Cynthia Peacock
Cincinnati, OH, USA — David E. DeLaet
Hempstead, NY, USA — Mariecel Pilapil
Boston, MA, USA — Niraj Sharma

# Acknowledgments

Of all the lessons I learned from the COVID-19 pandemic, the most important one was about connections with people. We usually thank our families last, but given how much I relied on my husband, John, and two sons, Matthew (age 16) and Noah (age 12), during the pandemic, I have to acknowledge first and foremost that I could not be successful in anything at work without the stability at home that they provide me every day.

I have been at UCLA for over 30 years, and I continue to marvel at the amazing trainees and colleagues that I have the fortune to work with. As Division Chief of Medicine-Pediatrics and Preventive Medicine, I oversee a growing group of over 40 clinicians, seven research faculty and over 20 research and administrative staff who help us take on projects that have tremendous impact on the healthcare experience of patients. Our division's tagline is "to care for patients of all ages with a lifespan focus and addressing structural and social determinants of health." I come to work energized each day to be collaborating on such meaningful projects with outstanding people: Priyanka Fernandes, Candace Gragnani, Denise Nunez, Hannah Kwak, Emily Hotez, Kashia Rosenau, Gino Melillo, Zenith Khan, Amie Patel, Marco Hidalgo, Eric Curcio, Cecily Gallup, Julian Martinez, Rujuta Wilson, Judith Perrigo, Blanche Berzamin, Madeline Haley, Teresa Roth, Linelle Libang, Hillary Layer, Samantha Steffin, Lauren Jones, Francisco Flores, Alexandra Bowen, Adam Landeros, Marisol Macedo, Mariam Karapetyan, Moira Desphy, Juan Zelayandia, Charlene Choi, Dominic Do and Chris Nagel.

Every Tuesday morning and Friday afternoon, I am a primary care provider working in our med-peds clinics alongside my clinical faculty. My patient population is about 90% with neurodevelopmental conditions and the rest without, and I learn from them with each patient encounter. I am grateful for the privilege to be on the journey with my patients as together we navigate schools and developmental and social services. My patients inspire me to do research that will improve the quality of their lives and improve the problem of pediatric to adult transition.

**Alice A. Kuo**

A lot has happened in the world and especially in medicine since our first edition of this textbook. A pandemic has complicated our lives and for those in health care, the job has become harder. Some of us have witnessed more deaths in 1 year than in our whole career of practicing medicine. Many vulnerable patient populations have suffered tremendously including adults with chronic childhood conditions (ACCC). An article in Annals of Internal Medicine, April 2021, estimated a four-fold increased risk for COVID-19-related hospitalization and a 10-fold increased risk for COVID-19-related death in persons with Down syndrome. Many extremely vulnerable individuals found themselves self-isolating for months due to fears of getting the virus even after vaccines became readily available, ultimately causing significant mental health issues. The editors in this edition have included a section on mental health for ACCC to address some of these concerns.

What hasn't changed is the growing need for more healthcare providers to understand and champion the healthcare needs of ACCC which was the impetus behind the first edition of this book. As editors we were excited to see the reception for the first edition and with the second edition going to press, the editors are aware of a growing wave of physicians seeking medical knowledge to help become more inclusive of a growing population of ACCC patients in their clinical practice. I have told many of my colleagues, "if I get hit by a bus tomorrow, who will take over the clinical responsibilities caring for ACCC at our institution?" In the last decade, I have been overjoyed with the number of medical students and residents who are committed and dedicated to the healthcare needs of ACCC. My clinical team is training medical students, dental students, residents, fellows, social workers, and nurses how to care for adult patients with intellectual and developmental disabilities (I/DD). Some days, there are more students than patients in clinic. I sleep better knowing that the proverbial bus is now carrying the next generation of compassionate healthcare providers dedicated to providing the necessary and appropriate healthcare for adults with IDD. Here is hoping 2023 is a better year for all of us in the healthcare field.

**Cynthia Peacock, MD**

I want to begin by expressing gratitude to all of my adolescent and young adult patients. The relationships that I have developed with them over the years have inspired me to advocate on their behalf.

I also want to recognize my mentors and colleagues who have helped to guide me in my journey. The support that I received from my premedical advisor David F. Wilson and other members of the faculty and staff while an undergraduate at Miami University was instrumental in my gaining acceptance into the University of Cincinnati College of Medicine. As a medical student, I chose to pursue training in internal medicine and pediatrics in no small part because of the example set by stellar residents such as Chad Brands and Tom Webb. While a resident and junior faculty member at the University of Cincinnati and Cincinnati Children's Hospital Medical Center, I could always rely on mentors such as Joe Barrocas, Frank Biro, Phuong Le, and Caroline Mueller for sound advice. Similarly, the guidance I received from Olveen Carrasquillo and Steven Shea during my time as a fellow in the Division of General Medicine at the Columbia University College of Physicians and Surgeons has proven invaluable. I will be forever grateful to Eva Waite for giving me the opportunity to join the internal medicine-pediatrics faculty at the Icahn School of Medicine at Mount Sinai, and working with her, Ine Leus, Joe Truglio, and Jen Koestler and our many residents in caring for our patients has truly been one of the highlights of my career.

I further want to acknowledge my co-editors Alice, Cynthia, Niraj, and Mariecel. It has been such a pleasure working with each of them over the last nearly 8 years since we first conceived of this project and have developed now two editions of this text. The dedication each of them have for the care of their patients continues to spark their passion for work in this area of critical need. Having the opportunity to work over this period with my former medical student and resident Mariecel has been particularly special to me. I additionally want to thank Samantha Steffin, Sheilly Carpio, and Madeline Haley, without whose help this effort would have been immeasurably more difficult.

Lastly, I want to thank my family: my late father Jack and my mother Sandra, for always supporting my goals; my wife, Rebecca, whose dedication to and passion for her professional pursuits inspires me to be similarly committed to my own and who, along with our children Jack and Allison, helps me to maintain balance in my life.

**David E. DeLaet**

The task of putting this book together began in 2014 and has stood the test of time as a "labor of love." It is a love for our patients, their families, and all the providers involved in their care that has been the central motivation in developing this book. What began first as a casual conversation with my co-editors David, Alice, Cynthia, and Niraj has now evolved into our second edition. I am truly grateful for having had the opportunity to continue to work with and learn from them in this process.

Thank you to my division chiefs Sophia Jan and Joseph Conigliaro, who support and mentor me in my professional life and continue to be role models in their dedication to academic medicine.

A heartfelt thank you to my family: my parents Lillian and Alfredo, and my brother Brian who have supported me throughout my journey through medicine and are my rock. Lastly, none of this would be possible without the love and support of my husband Matthew and my children James and Kevin, who bring me joy every day and encourage me to live life to its fullest.

**Mariecel Pilapil, MD, MPH**

I would like to begin by thanking my co-editors. Having the opportunity to work with Alice, Cynthia, David, and Mariecel has been an absolute honor. I have learned so much from each of you. I am also so appreciative of the work and coordination that Samantha Steffin, Madeline Haley, and Sheilly Carpio have put into the ultimate production of this book.

I am so grateful to all my primary care patients who have inspired me over the years. Each has motivated me to be a better physician and to work towards improving transition care.

I have been honored to serve as a residency training director for over 22 years. The residents and medical students I have taught during this time are constantly pushing me to be a better teacher and doctor. I must also include all of my colleagues in the Medicine-Pediatrics Program Directors Association for their friendship.

There are three leaders in particular who have been meaningful in my career. Charles Christianson, MD, was my mentor in medical school who taught me what it means to be an ideal primary care physician. Charles

Pegelow, MD, served as my residency Program Director and inspired me to pursue a career in medical education. Gwendolyn Scott, MD, first taught me about youth born with HIV who transition to adulthood and motivated me to research ways to improve their care and that of others with chronic conditions of childhood origin.

I would like to thank my parents, Dr. Dharmendra and Santosh Sharma for their love and for raising me with the values to be the man I am today. Most importantly, I would like to thank my wife, Tanvi Sharma, MD, MPH, and our two brilliant daughters, Amari and Aesha, who truly give me inspiration, love, energy, and happiness on a daily basis.

**Niraj Sharma**

**To our staff:**

We the editors would like to give tremendous thanks to our assistants and staff without whom we could not have completed this revised edition. We know that it is not easy to corral busy physicians and get them to meet deadlines for submissions and revisions, but our staff did so with a smile and never a crossword. We owe a huge debt of gratitude to Samantha Steffin, Sheilly Carpio, and Madeline Haley as project managers who oversaw all of the administrative aspects of the book; and Asal Bastani and Andrew M. Smith who were student copyeditors who helped authors with formatting and reference checks. We could not have pulled this herculean task off without the help of this dedicated crew of individuals.

# Contents

# About the Editors

**Alice A. Kuo, MD, PhD** is Professor and Chief of Medicine-Pediatrics and Preventive Medicine at the David Geffen School of Medicine at UCLA and Professor of Health Policy and Management in the UCLA Fielding School of Public Health. Her research interests include access to and delivery of developmental services, cognitive and language development in young minority children, and services for children and adults with autism and other neurodevelopmental disabilities. She has published over 80 peer-reviewed articles and 15 book chapters and edited two books on these topics.

Since 2020, Dr. Kuo has been the Principal Investigator of the Autism Intervention Research Network on Physical Health (AIR-P, www.airpnetwork.ucla.edu). In addition to her research, Dr. Kuo has been involved in educational programs at several levels, including the Maternal and Child Health Bureau (MCHB)-funded University of California Leadership Education in Neurodevelopmental Disabilities (UC-LEND) program (www.uc-lend.med.ucla.edu) and the UCLA Maternal and Child Health Center of Excellence (www.mch.ucla.edu). At the post-graduate level, Dr. Kuo was the founding Director of the UCLA Combined Internal Medicine and Pediatrics Residency Program and led the program for 19 years, and she continues to be Director of the combined Internal Medicine/Preventive Medicine residency program at UCLA.

**Cynthia Peacock, MD** is Associate Professor of Medicine and Pediatrics at Baylor College of Medicine in Houston, Texas. Dr. Peacock is the founder of the Texas Children's Hospital-Baylor College of Medicine Transition Medicine Clinic and currently one of its Medical Directors. She is also Section Chief of Adult Developmental Medicine in the Medicine Department at Baylor College of Medicine. In addition, Dr. Peacock is Director of Adult Transition Medicine Program for Texas Children's Hospital. Her expertise is on the care of adults with chronic conditions of childhood and the use of the medical home model to deliver transition health care needs.

**David E. DeLaet, MD, MPH** is Associate Professor in the Department of Medicine, Division of General Internal Medicine at the University of Cincinnati College of Medicine in Cincinnati, Ohio. He also is Adjunct Associate Professor of Clinical Medicine at the Icahn School of Medicine in New York. Additionally, he is Associate Professor in the College of Arts and Sciences and Medical Director for the Physician Associate Studies Program at Miami University in Oxford, Ohio. He is a Fellow of the American College of Physicians and Fellow of the American Academy of Pediatrics.

**Mariecel Pilapil, MD, MPH** is Associate Professor of Medicine and Pediatrics at the Zucker School of Medicine at Hofstra/Northwell. She is a primary care physician in the Divisions of General Internal Medicine and General Pediatrics and cares for patients with chronic childhood conditions across the life spectrum. She is also a Co-Director of the Complex Care Clinic in General Pediatrics at Cohen Children's Medical Center, which is a program that cares for children with medical complexity.

**Niraj Sharma, MD, MPH** is an Assistant Professor of Internal Medicine and Pediatrics at Harvard Medical School. He is the Director of the Medicine-Pediatrics Unit in the Brigham and Women's Hospital (BWH) Department of Internal Medicine, Division of General Medicine. He is also Co-Director of the BWH Transition Care Team and is the Associate Director of the Bridges Adult Transition Program at Boston Children's Hospital (BCH). He is also the Director Emeritus of the Internal Medicine-Pediatrics Residency Training Program at BWH/BCH. He is a national leader in the field of transition medicine with numerous peer-reviewed publications, presentations, and grants in the field. He has built clinical programs to improve the transition process at BWH, BCH, and Mass General Brigham Health Care. He has also held a number of national positions, including former Co-Site Director and Cabinet Member of the Got Transition National Learning Collaborative and Director of the Medicine-Pediatrics Program Directors Association Transition Committee.

# Part I

# Facilitating the Transition from Pediatric-Oriented to Adult-Oriented Primary Care

# Defining Healthcare Transition 1

Patience H. White and Margaret A. McManus

## Defining Pediatric to Adult Transition

The process of moving from pediatric to adult care is referred to as "health care transition" or HCT. "HCT is the purposeful, planned movement of adolescents and emerging adults with and without chronic physical, behavioral and developmental conditions from child-centered to adult-oriented health care systems" [1]. It represents not only the passage from one developmental stage to another (dependence to independence to interdependence) but also the passage from one type of care (pediatric/family-centered care to adult/patient-centered care) and often the change to a different healthcare setting. Although all youth transit to adult-focused care, usually between the ages of 18 and 21, youth with special healthcare needs (YSHCN) typically require an expanded process of transition planning and integration into adult health care to address the exchange of more complex health information, competencies for self-care, transfer of primary and specialty care, and issues related to public program eligibility, decision-making supports, and coordination with community services.

The goal of HCT includes aiming for high-quality care through utilizing the quadruple aim approach: maximizing a positive youth/emerging adult and family/caregiver experience, improving overall health outcomes, improving healthcare utilization and reducing healthcare costs, and ensuring that patients, clinicians, and families can have a positive experience in the efforts to improve the transition process for YSHCN [2] .

Healthcare transition from pediatric to adult health care refers to a set of actions designed to ensure continuity of care between pediatric and adult healthcare settings and improve health literacy so that youth and emerging adults understand and manage their own health needs and navigate the healthcare system. Transition should include three components—planning, transfer, and integration into adult health care, which take place over time, beginning in early adolescence in a pediatric approach to care and continuing into emerging adulthood in an adult approach to care. It is a predictable life-course change that affects all youth, especially those with chronic conditions. Even if a youth remains with the same provider into adulthood, preparation for

P. H. White (✉)
Department of Medicine and Pediatrics, George Washington University School of Medicine and Health Sciences, Washington, DC, USA

The National Alliance to Advance Adolescent Health, Washington, DC, USA
e-mail: PWhite@thenationalalliance.org

M. A. McManus
The National Alliance to Advance Adolescent Health, Washington, DC, USA
e-mail: mmcmanus@thenationalalliance.org


A. A. Kuo et al. (eds.), *Care of Adults with Chronic Childhood Conditions*,
https://doi.org/10.1007/978-3-031-54281-7_1

adult-focused care is necessary. Because of the mobility of youth and emerging adults, the likelihood that they will change providers is almost certain, and thus the need to establish a structured transition process consistently available to improve outcomes from youth and emerging adults.

Taken together, these defining characteristics underscore the size and diversity of the population as well as the extent of their chronic and disabling conditions. Further, their higher poverty and uninsurance rates along with their higher rates of gaps in care underscore the complexity and volatility of this transition-aged population.

## Who Are Transition-Aged Adolescents and Emerging Adults?

The transition-aged population, ages 12–26, totals 65 million individuals or almost 20% of the US population [3], with nearly half identified as a racial or ethnic minority in 2019 [4]. Among this population between 25% and 35% are estimated to have one or more chronic conditions [5, 6], and an estimated 6.3% have a disability [7]. Those with a cognitive disability—an estimated 4.6% represent the most common disability type [8].

The population of adolescents and emerging adults (AEA) with chronic conditions and disability has been increasing substantially over the past several decades as has their survival rates [9]. Much of this increase in chronic conditions is due to greater prevalence of obesity/overweight, asthma, mental health/behavioral health conditions, learning disorders, and autism spectrum disorder. The increase in physical disability has actually declined over time, but disability due to neurodevelopmental or mental health condition has increased dramatically [10].

Several other characteristics are distinctive of the transition-aged population—notably changing age gradients between early (ages 10–14) and late adolescence (15–18) and emerging adulthood (19–25) in terms of selected characteristics pertaining to sociodemographic, health status, insurance coverage, and access to care [11]. National data reveal that a higher proportion of emerging adults compared to their younger peers are more likely to be poor (with incomes <200% of the federal poverty level), in fair or poor health, without insurance, with less reliance on public coverage, and with fewer having a usual source of care and making a doctor visit in the past year.

## What Is Known About Receipt of Transition Services?

The United States conducts a National Survey of Children's Health (NSCH) every year [12]. This nationally representative survey asks parents of 12–17 year olds if their youth received a set of transition preparation services, as follows:

- Youth had time alone with their doctor or other healthcare provider (HCP) at last visit.
- Doctors or other HCPs worked with youth to gain skills or understand changes in health care.
- Doctors or other HCPs discussed shift to adult provider.

The 2020–2021 NSCH found that only 20.5% of YSHCN and 16.0% of those without SHCN received all of these preparation services. These estimates reveal significant gaps in youths' receipt of recommended HCT planning services.

## What HCT Barriers Exist?

YSHCN and their parents/caregivers face many challenges in navigating the transition from pediatric to adult care, including gaining skills to manage their own health and learning to effectively utilize the healthcare system. These barriers have been well documented in the literature [1]. For youth and families, they cite negative beliefs and fears of the new adult care system, inadequate preparation, lack of communication between clinicians, few available adult primary care and specialty care clinicians, and loss or changes to their health insurance coverage. These challenges have resulted in poor health outcomes, with numerous studies showing increased morbidity and mortality for those who are often lost to follow-up or cannot find the services they need [13].

The literature has also documented transitional care issues that pediatric and adult clinicians find difficult [1]. These include communication gaps between pediatric and adult clinicians/systems, youth and emerging adult lack of knowledge and engagement in their own health, limited training for adult providers in emerging adult health and pediatric-onset conditions, and limited infrastructure for care coordination and staff support particularly in the adult healthcare system.

## What Are the Professional Recommendations for HCT?

Many professional societies in the United States, Europe, England, and Canada have put forward professional recommendations as have many professional societies and disease conditions [14]. In this section, the US recommendations put forward by the American Academy of Pediatrics (AAP), the American Association of Family Practice (AAFP), and the American College of Physicians (ACP) will be discussed as many other professional groups have adopted the HCT process recommended in this joint 2018 Clinical Report developed with pediatric and adult medical and nursing clinicians, and family and emerging adult experts.

The July 2023 reaffirmed 2018 Clinical Report with updated references and data [14] presented guiding principles around HCT, building on an earlier Clinical Report from 2011, where the focus centered on the pediatric responsibility for HCT preparation. The 2018 Clinical Report recognized the critical role of adult clinicians in accepting and partnering with emerging adults and their pediatric colleagues. Also discussed in the Clinical Report are positive outcomes associated with having a structured process (described later in this chapter). The Clinical Report outlines a structured process called the Six Core Elements of HCT, tested in several learning collaboratives using quality improvement methodologies [15, 16]. The Six Core Elements is not a model of care, but rather a pathway or approach that can be customized to improve the structured approach to HCT in many different types of primary or specialty care practices and can be customized to the complexity of youth involved and practice resources.

There are three Six Core Element packages for (1) pediatric practices where the youth is moving to an adult healthcare clinician [16], (2) family medicine and Med-peds practices that will care for the youth through the life span [17], and (3) internal medicine/family medicine/med-peds clinicians to assist in integrating the emerging adult into their adult practice [16]. Each package outlines in six steps what clinicians can do to create a structured approach, with sample tools in English and Spanish that can be customized.

For example, in Fig. 1.1, the Six Core Elements for the pediatric practice are shown and include (1) a **transition and care policy/guide** for youth and families that describe the process and what to expect; (2) a **tracking and monitoring** to be sure the youth gets the HCT services in the Six Core elements; (3) a **transition readiness assessment** repeated throughout the transition process to learn what skills the youth need to address to better prepare them for managing their own health; (4) **transition planning** with a plan of care that details the needed steps to attain the goals that the youth identifies and a medical summary; (5) **transfer of care** activities include a transfer package, with the final transition readiness assessment, plan of care, medical summary, and, if needed, legal documents and other clinical records that will be shared with the new adult clinician; and (6) **transfer completion** that includes confirmation of attendance at the initial adult visit and feedback to the practice by the emerging adult and family about the HCT process and if they felt prepared to transition to adult care. The Six Core Elements also have been outlined for adult clinicians who are integrating emerging adults into their practice. Figure 1.2 shows a summary of Six Core Elements approach for both pediatric and adult practices.

The Six Core Elements has been adapted for use in various models of care and practice set-

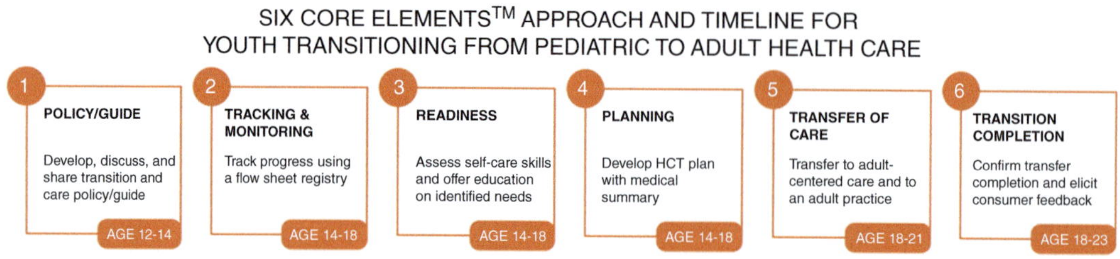


**Fig. 1.1** Steps of the Six Core Elements of Health Care Transition™. © 2020 Got Transition® (www.GotTransition.org) [17]

| Practice or provider | #1 Transition and/or care policy | #2 Tracking and monitoring | #3 Transition readiness and/or orientation to adult practice | #4 Transition planning and/or integration into adult approach to care or practice | #5 Transfer of care and/or initial visit | #6 Transition completion or ongoing care |
|---|---|---|---|---|---|---|
| **Pediatric**[a] | Create and discuss with youth and/or family | Track progress of youth and/or family transition preparation and transfer | Conduct transition readiness assessments | Develop transition plan, including needed readiness assessment skills and medical summary, prepare youth for adult approach to care, and communicate with new clinician | Transfer of care with information and communication including residual pediatric clinician's responsibility | Obtain feedback on the transition process and confirm young adult has been seen by the new clincian |
| **Adult**[a] | Create and discuss with young adult and guardian, if needed | Track progress of young adult's integration into adult care | Share and discuss welcome and FAQs with young adult and guardian, if needed | Communicate with previous clinician, ensure receipt of transfer package | Review transfer package, address young adult's needs and concerns at initial visit, update self-care assessment and medical summary | Confirm transfer completion with previous clinician, provide ongoing care with self-care skill building and link to needed specialists |

**Fig. 1.2** Summary of Six Core Elements approach for pediatric and adult practices. [a]Providers that care for youth and/or young adults throughout the life span can use both the pediatric and adult sets of core elements without the transfer process componentsSix Core Elements of Health Care Transition™. © 2020 Got Transition® (www.GotTransition.org) [17]

tings, such as transition clinics, transition consult services, and school-based health and mental health clinics. They have also been used for a broad population of youth and emerging adults with and without SHCN, including those with medically complex conditions, I/DD, and mental health conditions [18–24].

## Telehealth and HCT

Since the Pandemic in 2020, telehealth has become an integral part of health care. Past studies have shown that telehealth improves care coordination for youth with medical complexity and results in a decrease of unplanned visits [25, 26]. Though there is little literature available, telehealth also is an excellent way to offer healthcare transition services. Assessing readiness skills to learn about self-management and offering education and planning to move to an adult provider can easily be offered through telehealth. One area of HCT where telehealth can be especially helpful is in a joint telehealth visit. Joint visits where the pediatric and adult providers have a warm hand-off have been shown to improve outcomes for HCT [27–29]. When there is no clinic space available or the pediatric and adult provider clinics are not near each other, having a joint telehealth visit can be an excellent solution. A joint telehealth visit is not intended as a substitute for the initial adult visit and offers:

- Shared communication that strengthens continuity of care

- Improves the comfort and confidence the emerging adult and their parent/caregiver with their new clinician
- Allows the emerging adult and their parent/caregiver to convey their preferences and ask questions

To assist in providing a joint telehealth visit, Got Transition in conjunction with Children's Hospital of Philadelphia's medically complex care clinic developed a "Telehealth Tool Kit for a Joint Visit with Pediatric and Adult Health Care Clinicians and the Transferring Young Adult." The tool kit was reviewed by youth/emerging adults and parents and providers [30]. The tool kit includes two tip sheets:

- One for primary care teams with steps to follow to assist emerging adults with their parents and/or support persons to join a joint telehealth visit and includes sample content for the joint healthcare transition telehealth visit.
- One for emerging adults and their parents and/or support persons with information and questions to consider when they are joining a joint telehealth visit with their pediatric and future adult healthcare providers.

Got Transition conducted a pilot study within a specialty Medicaid managed care organization (HSCSN) in Washington, DC, around transitioning emerging adults with intellectual and developmental disabilities to adult health care. With local pediatric and adult primary care providers (HCPs), the HCT intervention included: a final pediatric visit, a medical summary, a joint HCT telehealth visit, and an initial adult visit. The feasibility of the joint telehealth visit was assessed via emerging adult and parent feedback surveys and interviews with participating HCPs. All six youth and families who participated in the joint telehealth visits responded it was very helpful to the question, "How helpful was the joint telehealth visit in making you more comfortable for this move to an adult doctor?" HCP perspective was gathered through a focus group of two pediatric and two adult providers who participated in the pilot. All HCPs found the joint telehealth visits very helpful and important to continue in future HCT work, especially for more complex patients. Scheduling the joint visits, however, was a challenge in the pilot [15]. In the future having a standing joint telehealth visit time available will assist with the scheduling issue.

## What HCT Quality Improvement Processes Are Available?

Key to implementing a structured HCT approach is utilizing quality improvement/implementation science methodology to make the process one that moves forward within the clinic/system with the clinician champion and results in improved process outcomes (see sect. VII for measurement strategies). The Six Core Elements have companion Implementation Guides available [31].

The Implementation Guides are intended to help clinicians/practices/systems support HCT improvements using the Six Core Elements of HCT for their youth and emerging adults transitioning to adult-centered care with or without changing their clinician. There are several free guides available:

- "How to Implement the Six Core Elements of Health Care Transition" [17] is an overview of the process designed by experience from several healthcare systems who implemented the Six Core Elements. It outlines nine steps with suggested strategies and tips:
  - Secure senior leadership support
  - Form an HCT QI improvement team that includes both pediatric and adult clinicians and youths/families
  - Outline an HCT improvement plan beginning with what success looks like and what changes one can make that results in improvement
  - Raise awareness about your HCT activities
  - Implement the Six Core Elements using the model of improvement
  - Plan for sustainability

- Plan for spread
- Communicate successes
- Tips for successes

- Each core element in the three packages has its own Implementation Guide, which contains practical guidance, resources, and examples for conducting HCT quality improvement (QI) in a range of healthcare settings. Each core element guide includes the purpose and objectives of the core element, a list of considerations in creating the core element tool, such as a policy [31] and incorporating the core element into a practice process. Also, there are tools, such as run charts, to assist with steps in the model of improvement approach and measures for each core element. In addition, each core element guide offers examples from available QI primary and specialty programs.
- The "Quality Improvement Primer" [32] is designed to be a companion piece to help with the understanding of QI and how to apply it to your transition work. All of the examples of tools for improvement are from HCT making it easier to utilize them in changing the clinic HCT process.

## What Are Measurement Options for Assessing HCT Performance?

A 2020 systematic review of outcomes of pediatric-to-adult HCT interventions identified transition measures used in published studies with rigorous evaluation designs [33]. Among the 19 studies included in this systematic review, all studied youth and emerging adults with one or more chronic conditions, and 16 studies (84%) reported a significant positive outcome consistent with the triple aim domains of population health, patient experience of care, and utilization and cost of care. With respect to population health, measures fell into four categories—adherence to care monitoring, disease-specific measures (e.g., A1c levels), patient-reported health and quality of life, and self-care. With respect to patient experience, a mix of measures were reported, including overall quality of care, care coordination, patient activation, problem solving, and receipt of needed services. With respect to utilization of care, there were three categories examined—utilization, processes of care, and costs of care. The utilization measures included hospital admissions/readmissions and length of stay, lapses in care, time interval between last pediatric and initial adult visit, and attendance at initial adult visit. The process of care measures included communication between pediatric and adult providers and increased referrals to adult care. No articles were found measuring the costs of care.

To help guide consideration of future HCT quality measures, Suris and Akre completed a Delphi study with an international panel of experts [34]. The following eight HCT indicators were identified as essential and very important: (1) patient not lost to follow-up, (2) patient attending scheduled visits in adult care, (3) patient building a trusting relationship with adult provider, (4) continuing attention by patient for self-management, (5) patient's first visit in adult care no later than 3–6 months after transfer, (6) number of ER visits for regular care in past year, (7) patient and family satisfaction with transfer of care, and (8) maintenance/improvement of standard for disease control evaluation.

Another set of suggested structure, process, and outcome measures—many similar to those listed above—were presented in *A Guide for Designing a Value-Based Payment Initiative for Pediatric-to-Adult Transitional Care* [35]. The first suggestion was to measure whether an organized HCT structure is in place since research finds that having an organized approach for transition planning, transfer of care, and integration into adult care is associated with positive outcomes for youth and emerging adults with chronic conditions [33]. Measurement tools that can be used to examine implementation of Got Transition's Six Core Elements include the Current Assessment of HCT Activities and the HCT Process Measurement Tool. Alternatively, it would be possible to use an EHR registry to examine the availability of a structured process as well as receipt of recommended HCT services. These measurement tools and sample registry tools are available in the Six Core Elements packages, links to which can be found in the implementation guide [31].

Also, referenced in the *VBP Guide* are process measures that examine utilization of care, such as:

- % of individuals, ages 18 and older, who made their initial adult primary care visit within 6 months of the last pediatric visit
- % of pediatric practices transferring their patients with a summary of care record using certified EHR technology and completing electronic exchange of summary of care record to new adult practice
- % of adult practices receiving summary of care record referral and who conduct clinical information reconciliation for medication, medication allergy, and current problem list
- % of individuals, ages 18 and older, who transferred to adult care with access to their current medical summary and emergency care plan
- % of individuals, ages 18 and older, who kept their second appointment with their adult PCP

The *VBP Guide* also suggests measuring consumer experience with HCT, using survey questions from the National Survey of Children's Health [36], which are intended to determine the extent to which youth ages 12–17 receive transition preparation assistance from their healthcare providers. Another consumer experience instrument, the "Mind the Gap Scale," has been used in transition studies for youth with arthritis [37]. Still another option is to use the Youth/Emerging Adult/Family Transition Feedback Surveys available in the Six Core Elements packages, links to which can be found in the implementation guides [31]. Got Transition also has a set of Clinician HCT Feedback Surveys, as well. Later in 2022, The National Alliance/Got Transition team, with a national advisory committee, will be publishing a quality measurement article that includes a set of guiding principles, an HCT measurement framework, a review of existing measures related to transition from national quality measure databases, and a comprehensive identification of quality measure gaps.

## What Are Payment Options for HCT?

Payment for the added time, training, and infrastructure necessary to provide recommended HCT services is typically cited as a significant barrier by pediatric and adult clinicians. Costs associated with providing a variety of HCT-related services are typically not recognized by Medicaid and commercial payers. Take, for example, the added time to conduct a transition readiness assessment and offer education and counselling on needed self-care skills or putting together a medical summary and emergency care plan or communicating between pediatric and adult clinicians. Just as important, infrastructure investments for HCT are woefully absent. These include pediatric and adult HCT training and QI, quality improvement support, workforce development (especially on the adult side to care for emerging adults with medical, social, behavioral, developmental complexity), and EMR functionality to document structure, process, and outcomes of HCT.

Before specific payment efforts can be considered, it is critical that clinicians with family advocates make a compelling case for needed changes, using data on the size and characteristics of transition-aged youth and emerging adults served in their practice, the scope of HCT services offered, and an estimate of lost revenue resulting from inadequate payment. These data can be supplemented with stories from parents and emerging adults about their concerns and experiences around HCT as well as from state-specific HCT data from the National Survey of Children's Health, available at www.gottranstion.org, which show that the vast majority of youth with and without SHCN are not receiving needed HCT preparation.

Using a combination of fee-for-service (FFS) and value-based payment (VBP) strategies makes best sense given the nascent HCT infrastructure available in most pediatric and adult care delivery systems. Though FFS continues to be the predominant form of payment, both Medicaid and commercial payers are moving forward to introduce and expand new financial incentives aligned with specific quality performance measures.

With respect to FFS options, there are a few key services/codes important to pursue [35]. Keep in mind that more options are available for youth and emerging adults with SHCN. Office visit codes can be used for established and new patients to provide transition education and counselling since these codes can now be reported based solely on either medical decision-making or total time spent on the date of the service. Preparation of a medical summary, transition plan, or transfer package can be coded either as non-face-to-face prolonged services or care management services. However, these codes often go unrecognized by payers. Communication/consultation between pediatric and adult clinicians can be coded using interprofessional consultation codes. Transition readiness assessment can be coded using the health risk assessment code.

With respect to VBP options, there are various methods that can be considered [35]. An enhanced FFS can be used to incentivize specific improvements—for example, paying a higher fee for the preparation of a medical summary, recognizing how important this information is for continuity of care between pediatric and adult clinicians. An infrastructure investment, typically a one-time only payment, can be used to update EMR functionality for HCT or support an HCT quality improvement pilot. A pay-for-performance payment can be used to reward pediatric and adult sites if certain utilization markers are met, including the exchange of medical information. A per-member-per-month payment can be used, for example, for pediatric practices who have emerging adults ages 22 and older to help expedite a planned transfer to adult care. An episode of care or bundled payment can be used to cover a set of recommended services for the year before and after transfer, with expectations of completed transfer, exchange of medical information, and retention in care. A direct payment to the consumer, in the form of a gift card, can also be an important incentive for ensuring that youth and emerging adults attend the last pediatric and initial appointments.

A detailed explanation of FFS options for HCT can be found in 2021 Coding and Payment Tip Sheet for Transition from Pediatric to Adult Care, which is updated every year by Got Transition and AAP. A detailed explanation of VBP options for HCT can be found in Recommendations for Value-Based Transition Payment for Pediatric and Adult Health Care Systems: A Leadership Roundtable Report.

## Future HCT Recommendations

There is a growing interest in clinical research to better understand what part of the structured process is essential and to outline a core set of outcome measurers. The 2018 Clinical Report also outlined HCT recommendations on needs for infrastructure supports especially in the adult health system, education and training, payment, and research [1]. Recently, a research agenda was put forward by the Children and Youth with Special Health Care Needs National Research Network called CYSHCNet [38] that recommended:

- Using implementations sciences methods, develop, and rigorously evaluate HCT models of care (e.g., RCTs or quasi-experimental designs) [38].
- Ensure that families and patients work with researchers to co-create new evidence-based HCT research.
- Develop process and outcome measures that reliably measure and predict transition success.
- Develop and evaluate fiscal and policy models that would support successful HCT.

## Conclusion

This initial chapter gives the reader an overview of healthcare transition, a key issue for all youth but especially youth with special healthcare needs. Adult providers have an essential role to play in integrating emerging adults into the adult approach to care and assisting them in their journey to health literacy and learning how to manage their own health and navigate the healthcare system.

## References

1. Cooley WC, Sagerman PJ. American Academy of Pediatrics American Academy of Family Physicians, American College of Physicians TCRAG. Supporting the health care transition from adolescence to adulthood in the medical home. Pediatrics. American Academy of Pediatrics Elk Grove Village, IL, USA. 2011;128:182–200.
2. Sikka R, Morath JM, Leape L. The quadruple aim: care, health, cost and meaning in work. BMJ Qual Saf. BMJ Publishing Group Ltd. 2015;24:608–10.
3. US Census Bureau. Annual estimates of the resident population by single year of age and sex for the United States: April 1, 2010 to July 1, 2019 (NC-EST2019-SYASEXN). Washington, DC: US Census Bureau, Population Division; 2022.
4. US Census Bureau USCB. Annual estimates of the resident population by sex, age, race alone or in combination, and Hispanic origin for the United States: April 1, 2010 to July 1, 2019 (NC-EST2019-ASR5H). Washington, DC: US Census Bureau, Population Division; 2020.
5. Child and Adolescent Health Measurement Initiative. National Survey of Children's Health 2016–2017 [Internet]. Data Resource Center for Child and Adolescent Health supported by the U.S. Department of Health and Human Services, Health Resources and Services Administration (HRSA), Maternal and Child Health Bureau (MCHB); [cited 2022 Sep 28]. www.childhealthdata.org
6. Centers for Disease Control and Prevention (CDC). Behavioral risk factor surveillance system survey data. Atlanta, GA: U.S. Department of Health and Human Services, Centers for Disease Control and Prevention; 2017.
7. Cheng L, Shaewitz D. The 2021 youth transition report: outcomes for youth and young adults with disabilities. Inst Educ Leadersh. 2021;
8. U.S Census Bureau ACS. ACS 1-year estimates public use microdata sample. Table generated by William Erickson; 2022.
9. Perrin JM, Anderson LE, Van Cleave J. The rise in chronic conditions among infants, children, and youth can be met with continued health system innovations. Health Aff (Millwood). 2014;33(12):2099–105.
10. Houtrow AJ, Larson K, Olson LM, Newacheck PW, Halfon N. Changing trends of childhood disability, 2001–2011. Pediatrics. 2014;134(3):530–8.
11. Spencer DL, McManus M, Call KT, Turner J, Harwood C, White P, et al. Health care coverage and access among children, adolescents, and young adults, 2010–2016: implications for future health reforms. J Adolesc Health. 2018;62(6):667–73.
12. Child and Adolescent Health Measurement Initiative. National Survey of Children's Health 2019–2020 [Internet]. Data Resource Center for Child and Adolescent Health supported by the U.S. Department of Health and Human Services, Health Resources and Services Administration (HRSA), Maternal and Child Health Bureau (MCHB); [cited 2022 Sep 28]. www.childhealthdata.org
13. Hart LC, Pollock M, Brown A, Shah N, Chung RJ, Sloane R, et al. Where did they go? Tracking young adult follow-up during the transition from pediatric to adult-oriented care. Clin Pediatr (Phila). 2019;58(11–12):1277–83.
14. White PH, Ardoin S. Transitioning wisely: improving the connection from pediatric to adult health care. Arthritis Rheumatol. 2016;68(4):789–94.
15. McManus M, White P, Barbour A, Downing B, Hawkins K, Quion N, et al. Pediatric to adult transition: a quality improvement model for primary care. J Adolesc Health. 2015;56(1):73–8.
16. White P, Schmidt A, Shorr J, Ilango S, Beck D, McManus M. Six core elements of health care transition 3.0. Washington, DC: Got Transition, The National Alliance to Advance Adolescent Health; 2020.
17. White P, Schmidt A, Shorr J, Ilango S, Beck D, McManus M. Six Core elements of health care transition™ 3.0. Washington, DC: Got Transition, The National Alliance to Advance Adolescent Health; July 2020.
18. McManus M, White P. Transition to adult health care services for young adults with chronic medical illness and psychiatric comorbidity. Child Adolesc Psychiatr Clin. 2017;26(2):367–80.
19. Osunkwo II, Cheryl C, Patterson C, Laura N, Cornette J, McManus P, et al. Implementing a structured health care transition (HCT) process for sickle cell disease (SCD) using quality improvement (QI): early results of a SCD HCT learning collaorative. Blood. 2019;134:5787.
20. White PH, Ilango SM, Caskin AM, la Guardia MGA, de, McManus MA. Health care transition in school-based health centers: a pilot study. J Sch Nurs. 2020:1059840520975745.
21. Lestishock L, Nova S, Disabato J. Improving adolescent and young adult engagement in the process of transitioning to adult care. J Adolesc Health. 2021;69(3):424–31.
22. Ames JL, Massolo ML, Davignon MN, Qian Y, Cerros HJ, Croen LA. Transitioning youth with autism spectrum disorders and other special health care needs into adult primary care: a provider survey. Autism. 2021;25(3):731–43.
23. Li L, Polanski A, Lim A, Strachan PH. Transition to adult care for youth with medical complexity: assessing needs and setting priorities for a health care improvement initiative. J Pediatr Nurs. 2022;62:144–54.
24. Jones MR, Hooper TJ, Cuomo C, Crouch G, Hickam T, Lestishock L, et al. Evaluation of a health care transition improvement process in seven large health care systems. J Pediatr Nurs. 2019;47:44–50.
25. Looman WS, Antolick M, Cady RG, Lunos SA, Garwick AE, Finkelstein SM. Effects of a telehealth care coordination intervention on perceptions of

health care by caregivers of children with medical complexity: a randomized controlled trial. J Pediatr Health Care. 2015;29(4):352–63.

26. McKissick HD, Cady RG, Looman WS, Finkelstein SM. The impact of telehealth and care coordination on the number and type of clinical visits for children with medical complexity. J Pediatr Health Care. 2017;31(4):452–8.
27. Eros A, Soós A, Hegyi P, Szakács Z, Eross B, Párniczky A, et al. Spotlight on transition in patients with inflammatory bowel disease: a systematic review. Inflamm Bowel Dis. 2020;26(3):331–46.
28. Cole R, Ashok D, Razack A, Azaz A, Sebastian S. Evaluation of outcomes in adolescent inflammatory bowel disease patients following transfer from pediatric to adult health care services: case for transition. J Adolesc Health. 2015;57(2):212–7.
29. McQuillan RF, Toulany A, Kaufman M, Schiff JR. Benefits of a transfer clinic in adolescent and young adult kidney transplant patients. Can J Kidney Health Dis. 2015;2(1):1–8.
30. White PH, Greenberg A. Telehealth toolkit for a joint visit with pediatric and adult health care clinicians and transferring young adults. Wash DC Got Transit Natl Alliance Adv Adolesc Health July 2020; 2022 Jun.
31. White PH, Schmidt A, Shorr J, Ilango SM, Beck D, McManus M. Six Core elements of health care transition 3.0: an implementation guide. Wash DC Got Transit Natl Alliance Adv Adolesc Health July 2020; 2020 Jul.
32. Noonan L, Mabus S, Ilango SM, Schmidt A, McManus M, Shorr J, et al. QI primer: using quality improvement to improve the health care transition process. Wash DC Got Transit Natl Alliance Adv Adolesc Health July 2020; 2020 Jul.
33. Schmidt A, Ilango SM, McManus MA, Rogers KK, White PH. Outcomes of pediatric to adult health care transition interventions: an updated systematic review. J Pediatr Nurs. 2020;51:92–107.
34. Suris JC, Akre C. Key elements for, and indicators of, a successful transition: an international Delphi study. J Adolesc Health. 2015;56(6):612–8.
35. McManus M, White P, Schmidt A. A guide for designing a value-based payment initiative for pediatric-to-adult transitional care; 2022.
36. Ilango SM, Lebrun-Harris LA, Jones JR, McManus MA, Cyr M, Mann MY, et al. Associations between health care transition preparation among youth in the US and other components of a well-functioning system of services. J Adolesc Health. 2021;69(3):414–23.
37. Shaw K, Southwood T, McDonagh J, Paediatric BS, of, Rheumatology A. Development and preliminary validation of the 'Mind the Gap'scale to assess satisfaction with transitional health care among adolescents with juvenile idiopathic arthritis. Child Care Health Dev. 2007;33(4):380–8.
38. Okumura MJ, Kuo DZ, Ware AN, Cyr MH, White PH. Improving health care transitions for children and youth with special health care needs. Acad Pediatr. 2022;22(2):S7–13.

# Part II

# Care of the Emerging Adult

# 2 Emerging Adulthood as a Developmental Stage

Emily Hotez, Julianna Rava, and Stacey Weinstein

## Case Study

Sam, a 25-year-old male, graduated from college 4 years ago. After college, he moved back in with his mother as he applied for jobs and tried to figure out the next step in his professional development. After transitioning through a series of short-term positions—and waffling on a decision to apply to graduate school—he never ended up saving enough money to live independently. He still lives with his mother, although she works the night shift as a nurse, so is often sleeping when Sam is awake. He would like to live with his friends from college, but his mother doesn't think it's a good idea. This is partially due to his frequent depressive episodes, during which he retreats to his bedroom for long stretches of time, often spending entire days playing video games or passively scrolling through social media.

## Chapter Overview

Sam is one of many in the "in-between" stage of life between adolescence and adulthood. Emerging adulthood (ages 18–26) is a developmental period in the life course characterized by transitions and instability in healthcare, education, employment, and interpersonal domains. Med-Peds providers are uniquely tasked with playing a leading role in both primary and secondary prevention efforts for this population. In particular, their roles include facilitating their healthcare transitions from pediatric to adult systems, addressing their pronounced mental and physical health challenges, and promoting their well-being across the myriad transitions characteristic of emerging adulthood [1].

The current chapter is written from our interdisciplinary perspectives as researchers and clinicians and thus is informed by both contemporary developmental science and real-world patient case studies. We seek to lay the foundation for prioritizing emerging adulthood in primary care; describe the developmental period of emerging adulthood as a period of both risk and opportunity; and suggest general approaches for addressing emerging adult patient needs and leveraging innovations in healthcare. Subsequent chapters will delineate more specific healthcare priorities and strategies for emerging adults with and without chronic conditions.

E. Hotez (✉) · S. Weinstein
Division of Medicine-Pediatrics and Preventive Medicine, University of California, Los Angeles, CA, USA
e-mail: ehotez@mednet.ucla.edu; sweinstein@mednet.ucla.edu

J. Rava
University of California, Los Angeles (UCLA), Fielding School of Public Health, Los Angeles, CA, USA
e-mail: JRava@mednet.ucla.edu


A. A. Kuo et al. (eds.), *Care of Adults with Chronic Childhood Conditions*,
https://doi.org/10.1007/978-3-031-54281-7_2

## Background and Context

Broadly, emerging adulthood is a unique developmental period, typically occurring between ages 18 and 26, but can span 14–29 by other definitions and across cultures. Indeed, research suggests that this period is becoming increasingly lengthened on a population level [2]. Generally speaking, emerging adulthood is characterized by instability and transitions across developmental domains [2]. Research shows that emerging adults experience changes in their overall worldviews; that is, their fundamental perspectives on social and metaphysical reality [3]. Emerging adults begin to prioritize the meaning-making of their lives and circumstances [4]. They also develop new conceptions of their identity and personality and construct new narratives about themselves [5].

In the context of these broad developmental changes, emerging adults also develop a meaningful sense of sexual orientation and identity [6]. They begin to take on new responsibilities in terms of finances, education, and employment [7, 8]. In addition, emerging adulthood is often characterized by changes in romantic relationships [9], shifts in family contact and relationship quality [10, 11], and other relational changes. All of these factors are inter-related and play a role in life satisfaction, well-being, and emerging adults' developmental trajectories more broadly [12].

There are, of course, numerous factors that can alter the course of emerging adults' developmental trajectories, including the two previous life stages of childhood and adolescence, which have a considerable impact on emerging adulthood outcomes [13]; these include sociodemographic characteristics, including socioeconomic status, race and ethnicity, gender, parental education, neighborhood, and other factors [14–16]. Myriad risk (e.g., adverse childhood experiences) [17] and protective factors, e.g., social support and resilience) [18–20] can further impact trajectories.

In addition, emerging adulthood is heterogeneous across individuals and groups. In many ways, emerging adults are actually in various life stages. Some pursue secondary and graduate level education, others enter the workforce, while others join the military. There are emerging adults who decide to get married, live with partners, or have children, while others live independently or in their parents' homes. Some might experience all of these milestones within emerging adulthood, while others might stay consistently in one or two stages throughout emerging adulthood. The flux of life transitions for the emerging adult population can have a significant effect on their general well-being.

Each of these societal and systemic contextual factors has shaped the developmental experiences of contemporary emerging adults. Med-Peds providers must consider these contextual factors as they pursue efforts to promote the health and well-being of emerging adults.

## Emerging Adulthood Today

Emerging adult development cannot be understood without recognizing the extent to which this developmental period is embedded within the broader social-historical context. Since the publication of the last version of this textbook in 2016, we have witnessed marked shifts in emerging adults' social landscape. In 2022, emerging adults in the United States are the most racially and ethnically diverse generation, with one in four emerging adults identifying as Latinx [21]. They are also more likely to have a college education and college-educated parents than prior generations [21]. Further, nearly one in five young adults identify as part of the LGBTQ+ community [22] and most emerging adults have positive views of have positive views of diverse gender identity options [21]. However, emerging adults are least likely to have healthcare coverage compared to other age groups [23]. While emerging adults have historically been an underserved group in the healthcare sphere, these shifts suggest that it is now more important than ever to promote health and well-being in this population.

First, it is critical to recognize the increasing pervasiveness of social media and its role in the daily lives of emerging adults. Evidence indicates that emerging adults are using social media now more than ever, even going so far as to categorize social media scrolling as "pathological" [24]. Social media has been linked to many mental and behavioral health indicators in this population, including anxiety and depression, delinquency, substance use empathy, and even suicide risk [25–27]. Although social media presents numerous risks, it also spurs potential intervention opportunities for a range of health outcomes [28]. Indeed, social media has served as a highly relevant and feasible tool for delivering a number of health-promoting interventions for emerging adults in the domains of nutrition, substance use, and others [29]. Generally speaking, it can be difficult to pinpoint the exact role of social media due to the dynamic nature of available technology and usage patterns; nonetheless, its positive and negative impacts on emerging adult development cannot be ignored [30].

A second—and highly potent—contextual factor to consider is the COVID-19 pandemic and its collateral consequences on the lives of emerging adults today. Indeed, Med-Peds providers seeking to serve emerging adults must also recognize the acute and potentially long-term effects of the COVID-19 pandemic and simultaneous events related to racial and ethnic discrimination and xenophobia, social and political conflicts, and myriad others. Research has already identified significant short-term mental and physical health challenges as a result of the pandemic [31]. These challenges stem from the direct impacts of the virus itself, as well as the indirect effects of co-occurring discrimination and stigma; healthcare fragmentation; and educational, vocational, and financial upheaval. Future research is required to understand its longer-term impact.

Third, the proportion of emerging adults enrolled in higher education is higher than at any time in US history, particularly among women [32]. The majority of research on emerging adulthood tends to focus on college student samples due to the convenience of recruitment for researchers. Although the college student body is increasingly diversifying, it still reflects a distinct population of emerging adults; that is, a population that is disproportionately White, female, and from higher socioeconomic statuses. These factors are important to consider when interpreting trends, as emerging adults who did not pursue higher education are often excluded from the literature, despite higher support needs [32].

Finally, greater societal awareness and attention toward health disparities have promoted greater disclosure and identification among those with multiple marginalized conditions. Over the past few years, emerging adults with certain chronic conditions—including intellectual and/or developmental disabilities (I/DD)—have increasingly disclosed or reported their disability, relative to previous years. Equivalent trends have also been documented for groups with other marginalized identities, including gender-diverse populations. Although visibility for these populations may be higher, stigma and other barriers to health persist.

## Health and Well-being of Emerging Adults

Emerging adults experience a range of distinct health challenges, relative to adolescent and older adult populations. First and foremost, this population shows increased vulnerability to mental health issues [6], demonstrating increased rates of depression, anxiety, eating-related disorders, substance use, nonsuicidal self-injury, suicidal ideation, and suicide attempts [7]. Over the last decade, we have seen increased rates of suicide among emerging adults; as of 2020, suicide is the second leading cause of death behind unintentional injury for young adults [33]. Further, a looming mental health crisis among this age group was exacerbated by the COVID-19 pandemic [34]. Of particular concern is that most who require mental health services, support, or treatments do not receive them, which further worsens mental health.

Mental health challenges are often accompanied by physical health issues as well [35]. For example, emerging adults have the highest likelihood of unintended pregnancy and sexually transmitted infections, making emerging adulthood the time of greatest sexual and reproductive health risk [36]. In addition, many emerging adults—particularly racial and ethnic minority emerging adults—grapple with obesity, hypertension, and pre-diabetes [37].

Many of these health disparities are partially linked to fragmented healthcare services characterized by gaps in healthcare transitions. Healthcare transitions refer to the processes required for moving from a child to an adult model of healthcare with or without a transfer to a new clinician [38]. It is well established in the research that in the United States, emerging adults are not receiving adequate transition preparation. There are multiple cascading effects of this shortcoming, including fragmented and lower quality healthcare, resulting in untreated or unaddressed health issues [38].

These disparities are further exacerbated by emerging adults' challenges in implementing health-promoting lifestyle behaviors. Emerging adults often experience a poor diet [39], casual sexual relationships [40], and physical inactivity [41]. Compounding these factors are low treatment adherence and access [35, 39, 40]. Health disparities are pronounced for minoritized emerging adult populations. In alignment with the minority stress model, minoritized populations experience more stressful interpersonal conflicts and have higher chronic cortisol, which further exacerbates health challenges [42]. Minoritized populations have an even higher likelihood of delaying care, relative to the general emerging adult population. They also experience negative effects of disclosure of minoritized status to their provider [43]. Socioeconomic factors such as residing in food deserts are also predictive of emerging adult physical health outcomes [44].

## Emerging Adulthood as an Opportunity

Although emerging adulthood can—for many reasons—represent a developmental period of risk, it also represents a key opportunity for health-promoting interventions. The majority of research on "sensitive periods" in development focuses efforts earlier in the lifespan (e.g., early childhood). The dynamic nature of emerging adulthood, however, makes this developmental period a ripe opportunity for health promotion through individual, family, and systemic-level interventions. Indeed, researchers have recently identified emerging adulthood as a key period for prevention [45]. For example, researchers have suggested that college students are uniquely situated for behavior change, as their environment and life stage provide the ideal opportunity to reform negative and develop health-promoting behaviors that will reduce their risk for health issues [41].

Opportunities for prevention can occur across multiple levels, systems, and sectors that interact and contribute to health promotion or health disparities. In the following section, we draw from clinical guidelines [38], empirical research, and insights from the field to outline general opportunities for Med-Peds providers to promote the health and well-being of their emerging adult patients. This list is not meant to be exhaustive and will be expounded upon in subsequent chapters.

### Prioritize Individual Differences and Tailor Interactions and Care Accordingly

As with all the patient interactions, ensuring patient-centered care is critical. In practice, this entails tailoring assessments and treatment protocols based on the needs, experiences, and preferences of the patients. A comprehensive literature review of 35 research publications revealed that emerging adults want providers who will listen and be sensitive to their needs, which are often different from others receiving healthcare at the same facility [46]. This is particularly important for individuals with I/DD and/or other marginalized groups. Acknowledging that each of these groups is not a monolith is critical [47]. Med-Peds providers can utilize a range of strategies to make their work more patient-centered and tailored, including concerted efforts to better understand their patients' preferences, engaging in community outreach efforts, and collaborating with other service sectors that serve this population.

## Seek to Foster Self-Determination and Self-Advocacy

The majority of research on fostering self-advocacy, perceived health competence, and self-efficacy focuses on emerging adults with chronic conditions [48, 49]. Over the past decade, however, it has become abundantly clear that these skills and capacities are health promoting for all emerging adults. In practice, supporting emerging adults in cultivating self-advocacy skills includes adapting approaches according to patient's readiness to change, collaborating with patients in their goal-setting efforts, and helping patients to break down individual health goals into small achievable actions [50].

## Integrate a Strength-Based Approach in Clinical Interactions

Med-Peds providers have the opportunity to promote or enhance their emerging adult patients' strengths, rather than focus exclusively on responding to problems. This can be accomplished in the context of taking a psychosocial history by integrating questions such as "What do you like doing?" "How would you describe yourself?" and "What are you most proud of?" The purpose of a strength-based approach is to mitigate the extent to which healthcare interactions contribute to stigma, which can, in turn, marginalize patients and discourage them from seeking care [51].

## Work Toward a Population-Health Approach for Emerging Adults

A significant impediment to creating scalable health-promoting approaches for emerging adults has been that this work has, to date, largely been siloed by disciplines. This, in turn, has resulted in the development of strategies and approaches that treat discrete vulnerabilities, rather than promote the overall population-level health of diverse emerging adults more broadly. In practice, addressing this gap in the field may entail Med-Ped providers collaborating or maintaining open dialogue with interdisciplinary healthcare providers, researchers, and community members [52]. These partnerships may take place in the context of quality improvement efforts; equity, diversity, and inclusion initiatives; or other clinic-wide activities.

## Cultivate an Early and Ongoing Transition-Focused Model of Care

Med-Peds providers have the opportunity to prepare emerging adults for adult care to facilitate a more seamless transition. This entails the assessment of transition readiness, discussion of a transition policy, initiation of a transition plan, and continuous updates of the transition plan [38]. A systematic review of over 200 articles focusing on models of transition-related care identified key components that facilitate care coordination between systems. These include the integration of a patient navigator or coordinator who is embedded within a health system to connect patients, families, providers, and community resources.

Care coordination can be facilitated through adopting models of transition care that are based on socioecological frameworks. These models consider sociodemographics and culture, healthcare access, and patient characteristics and highlight potential targets of intervention in a medical setting. It is recommended that these factors be integrated into transition readiness assessments as well as at all other points along the transition continuum [53]. Models that can synergize health, education, and social service sectors are also critical in preventing healthcare fragmentation [54].

## Pursue Health Equity in Clinics

While there are many potential avenues to pursue health equity in healthcare for emerging adults—as well as numerous potential outcomes—quality improvement has been cited as an important tool for equity-related efforts. Recommendations to ensure the effectiveness of quality improvement efforts include understanding existing disparities and subsequently utilizing community engagement to ensure that the initiative enhances health equity [55].

## Include Parents, Caregivers, and Other Family Members in Transition-Related Healthcare

Families express frustration about the lack of adequate transition-related support from their healthcare provider [56]. Many parents desire greater involvement in the transition process with some perceiving a lack of recognition of the importance of their role. Providers are tasked with parental responsibilities while also promoting the active participation of their emerging adult patients. In practice, this may require one-on-one time with emerging adults during the medical visit without the caregiver as well as joint visits during the transition process [57].

## Additional Considerations for Med-Peds Providers

Opportunities for emerging adult health promotion in the clinic level must begin in medical school and residency. Given the many competing priorities of medical training, a barrier in the field has been identifying opportunities for dedicated practice and education about emerging adulthood. Recent research suggests that the emergence of Med-Peds electives can strengthen medical students' interest in the combined specialty and foster greater transition-related skills and knowledge among future providers [58]. Future research should seek to pilot-test and evaluate medical curriculum enhancements that speak to the needs of emerging adults.

## Conclusion

Med-Peds providers have the opportunity to play a pivotal role in this critical life course transition. Let's return to Sam. What if his provider sought to understand his multidimensional strengths and weaknesses and tailor care accordingly? What if they were able to help Sam foster key self-advocacy skills to navigate mental health, employment, and other challenges? What if his provider coordinated with interdisciplinary services and support systems—as well as Sam's caregivers and family members—to ensure he experienced seamless, quality healthcare during the transition to adulthood? The goal of the current chapter was to guide Med-Peds providers in promoting the health and well-being of their emerging adult populations. We look forward to continued developments in the field of emerging adulthood that can promote thriving and lifelong health for this population.

## References

1. Gardner SE, Gonzaga AM, Kolarik RC. New program requirements present challenges and inspire innovations in med-Peds programs. Acad Pediatr. 2014;14(6):556–8.
2. Arnett JJ, Žukauskienė R, Sugimura K. The new life stage of emerging adulthood at ages 18–29 years: implications for mental health. Lancet Psychiatry. 2014;1(7):569–76.
3. Gutierrez IA, Park CL. Emerging adulthood, evolving worldviews: how life events impact college students' developing belief systems. Emerg Adulthood. 2015;3(2):85–97.
4. Mayseless O, Keren E. Finding a meaningful life as a developmental task in emerging adulthood: the domains of love and work across cultures. Emerg Adulthood. 2014;2(1):63–73.
5. Waters TEA, Fivush R. Relations between narrative coherence, identity, and psychological wellbeing in emerging adulthood: coherence identity and well-being. J Pers. 2015;83(4):441–51.
6. Morgan EM. Contemporary issues in sexual orientation and identity development in emerging adulthood. Emerg Adulthood. 2013;1(1):52–66.

7. Chatterjee S, Kim J, Chung S. Emerging adulthood milestones, perceived capability, and psychological Well-being while transitioning to adulthood: evidence from a national study. Financial Planning Rev [Internet]. 2021;4(4) [cited 2022 Sep 24]. https://onlinelibrary.wiley.com/doi/10.1002/cfp2.1132
8. Bosch LA, Serido J, Card NA, Shim S, Barber B. Predictors of financial identity development in emerging adulthood. Emerg Adulthood. 2016;4(6):417–26.
9. Gala J, Kapadia S. Romantic relationships in emerging adulthood: a developmental perspective. Psychol Stud. 2013;58(4):406–18.
10. Sneed JR, Johnson JG, Cohen P, Gilligan C, Chen H, Crawford TN, et al. Gender differences in the age-changing relationship between instrumentality and family contact in emerging adulthood. Dev Psychol. 2006;42(5):787–97.
11. Chopik WJ, Nuttall AK, Oh J. Relationship-specific satisfaction and adjustment in emerging adulthood: the moderating role of adult attachment orientation. J Adult Dev. 2022;29(1):40–52.
12. Sneed JR, Hamagami F, McArdle JJ, Cohen P, Chen H. The dynamic interdependence of developmental domains across emerging adulthood. J Youth Adolesc. 2007;36(3):351–62.
13. Halfon N, Larson K, Lu M, Tullis E, Russ S. Lifecourse health development: past, present and future. Matern Child Health J. 2014;18(2):344–65.
14. Daw J, Margolis R, Wright L. Emerging adulthood, emergent health lifestyles: sociodemographic determinants of trajectories of smoking, binge drinking, obesity, and sedentary behavior. J Health Soc Behav. 2017;58(2):181–97.
15. Perreira KM, Allen CD. The health of Hispanic children from birth to emerging adulthood. Ann Am Acad Pol Soc Sci. 2021;696(1):200–22.
16. Mello D, Wiebe D, Baker AC, Butner J, Berg C. Neighborhood disadvantage, parent-adolescent relationship quality, and type 1 diabetes in late adolescents transitioning to early emerging adulthood. Soc Sci Med. 2020;255:113010.
17. Davis JP, Dumas TM, Roberts BW. Adverse childhood experiences and development in emerging adulthood. Emerg Adulthood. 2018;6(4):223–34.
18. Szkody E, McKinney C. Indirect effects of social support on psychological health through self-esteem in emerging adulthood. J Fam Issues. 2019;40(17):2439–55.
19. Matud M, Díaz A, Bethencourt J, Ibáñez I. Stress and psychological distress in emerging adulthood: a gender analysis. JCM. 2020;9(9):2859.
20. Madewell A, Ponce-Garcia E. Assessing resilience in emerging adulthood: the resilience scale (RS), Connor–Davidson resilience scale (CD-RISC), and scale of protective factors (SPF). Personal Individ Differ. 2016;97:249–55.
21. Fry R, Parker K. Early benchmarks show 'post-millennials' on track to be most diverse, besteducated generation yet [internet]. Pew Research Center's Social & Demographic Trends Project; 2018. [cited 2022 Sep 28]. https://www.pewresearch.org/social-trends/2018/11/15/early-benchmarks-show-post-millennials-on-track-to-be-most-diverse-best-educatedgeneration-yet/
22. LGBT identification in U.S. Ticks up to 7.1% [Internet]. [cited 2022 Sep 28]. https://news.gallup.com/poll/389792/lgbt-identification-ticks-up.aspx
23. Bureau UC. Health insurance coverage among young adults aged 19 to 34 years: 2018 & 2019 [Internet]. Census.gov. [cited 2022 Sep 28]. https://www.census.gov/library/publications/2020/acs/acsbr20-02.html
24. Holmgren HG, Coyne SM. Can't stop scrolling!: pathological use of social networking sites in emerging adulthood. Addict Res Theory. 2017;25(5):375–82.
25. Stockdale LA, Coyne SM. Bored and online: reasons for using social media, problematic social networking site use, and behavioral outcomes across the transition from adolescence to emerging adulthood. J Adolesc. 2020;79(1):173–83.
26. Coyne SM, Hurst JL, Dyer WJ, Hunt Q, Schvanaveldt E, Brown S, et al. Suicide risk in emerging adulthood: associations with screen time over 10 years. J Youth Adoles. 2021;50(12):2324–38.
27. Vannucci A, Ohannessian CM, Gagnon S. Use of multiple social media platforms in relation to psychological functioning in emerging adults. Emerg Adulthood. 2019;7(6):501–6.
28. Inhae C, Jiwon K. Effects of mHealth intervention on sexual and reproductive health in emerging adulthood: a systematic review and meta-analysis of randomized controlled trials. Int J Nurs Stud. 2021;119:103949.
29. Chau MM, Burgermaster M, Mamykina L. The use of social media in nutrition interventions for adolescents and young adults—a systematic review. Int J Med Inform. 2018;120:77–91.
30. Davis K, Charmaraman L, Weinstein E. Introduction to special issue: adolescent and emerging adult development in an age of social media. J Adolesc Res. 2020;35(1):3–15.
31. Harriger JA, Joseph NT, Trammell J. Detrimental associations of cumulative trauma, COVID-19 infection indicators, avoidance, and loneliness with sleep and negative emotionality in emerging adulthood during the pandemic. Emerg Adulthood. 2021;9(5):479–91.
32. Arnett JJ. College students as emerging adults: the developmental implications of the college context. Emerg Adulthood. 2016;4(3):219–22.
33. Leading Causes of Death and Injury—PDFs|Injury Center|CDC [Internet]. 2022 [cited 2022 Sep 28]. https://www.cdc.gov/injury/wisqars/LeadingCauses.html
34. Liu CH, Zhang E, Wong GTF, Hyun S, Hahm H. "Chris." Factors associated with depression, anxiety, and PTSD symptomatology during the COVID-19 pandemic: clinical implications for U.S. young adult mental health. Psychiatry Res. 2020;290:113172.
35. Barlett CP, Barlett ND, Chalk HM. Transitioning through emerging adulthood and physical health implications. Emerg Adulthood. 2020;8(4):297–305.

36. Schlegel EC, Smith LH. Improving research, policy, and practice to address women's sexual and reproductive health care needs during emerging adulthood. Nurs Womens Health. 2021;25(1):10–20.
37. Urena-Bogarin EL, Martinez-Ramirez HR, Torres-Sanchez JR, Hernandez-Herrera A, CortesSanabria L, Cueto-Manzano AM. Prevalence of pre-diabetes in young Mexican adults in primary health care. Fam Pract. 2015;32(2):159–64.
38. White PH, Cooley WC, Transitions Clinical Report Authoring Group, American Academy of Pediatrics, American Academy of Family Physicians, American College of Physicians, et al. Supporting the health care transition from adolescence to adulthood in the medical home. Pediatrics. 2018;142(5):e20182587.
39. Collins S, Dash S, Allender S, Jacka F, Hoare E. Diet and mental health during emerging adulthood: a systematic review. Emerg Adulthood. 2022;10(3):645–59.
40. Sandberg-Thoma SE, Kamp Dush CM. Casual sexual relationships and mental health in adolescence and emerging adulthood. J Sex Res. 2014;51(2):121–30.
41. Goldstein CM, Xie SS, Hawkins MAW, Hughes JW. Reducing risk for cardiovascular disease: negative health behaviors in college students. Emerg Adulthood. 2015;3(1):24–36.
42. Parra LA, Benibgui M, Helm JL, Hastings PD. Minority stress predicts depression in lesbian, gay, and bisexual emerging adults via elevated diurnal cortisol. Emerg Adulthood. 2016;4(5):365–72.
43. Macapagal K, Bhatia R, Greene GJ. Differences in healthcare access, use, and experiences within a community sample of racially diverse lesbian, gay, bisexual, transgender, and questioning emerging adults. LGBT Health. 2016;3(6):434–42.
44. Testa A, Jackson DB, Semenza DC, Vaughn MG. Food deserts and cardiovascular health among young adults. Public Health Nutr. 2021;24(1):117–24.
45. Cleveland MJ, Goldstein AL. Opportunities and challenges for prevention and intervention in emerging adulthood: introduction to the special issue. Prev Sci. 2019;20(3):301–4.
46. Betz CL, Lobo ML, Nehring WM, Bui K. Voices not heard: a systematic review of adolescents' and emerging adults' perspectives of health care transition. Nurs Outlook. 2013;61(5):311–36.
47. Halkitis PN, Maiolatesi AJ, Krause KD. The health challenges of emerging adult gay men. Pediatr Clin N Am. 2020;67(2):293–308.
48. Lang AC, Greenley RN, Davies WH. Impact of perceived health competence on the quality of life of emerging adults with chronic health conditions. Emerg Adulthood. 2022;10(3):702–11.
49. Allen D, Scarinci N, Hickson L. Effects of patient- and family-centered care for young adults with chronic health conditions and their family members: a systematic review. Emerg Adulthood. 2022;10(3):689–701.
50. Dineen-Griffin S, Garcia-Cardenas V, Williams K, Benrimoj SI. Helping patients help themselves: a systematic review of self-management support strategies in primary health care practice. PLoS One. 2019;14(8):e0220116. Leroyer C, editor.
51. Klein DA, Paradise SL, Landis CA. Screening and counseling adolescents and young adults: a framework for comprehensive care. Am Fam Physician. 2020;101(3):147–58.
52. Bonnie RJ, Stroud C, Breiner H, Committee on Improving the Health S, Board on Children Y, Medicine I of, et al. Public health [Internet]. Investing in the health and well-being of young adults. National Academies Press; 2015. [cited 2022 Sep 28]. https://www.ncbi.nlm.nih.gov/books/NBK284781/
53. Schwartz LA, Tuchman LK, Hobbie WL, Ginsberg JP. A social-ecological model of readiness for transition to adult-oriented care for adolescents and young adults with chronic health conditions: transition readiness. Child Care Health Dev. 2011;37(6):883–95.
54. Wright C, Steinway C, Jan S. The genesis of systems of care for transition to adulthood services: emerging models in primary and subspecialty care. Curr Opin Pediatr. 2018;30(2):303–10.
55. Lion KC, Faro EZ, Coker TR. All quality improvement is health equity work: designing improvement to reduce disparities. Pediatrics. 2022;149(Supplement 3):e2020045948E.
56. Roy S, Valdez AMD, Trejo B, Bakewell T, Gallarde-Kim S, Martin AJ. "All circuits ended": family experiences of transitioning from pediatric to adult healthcare for young adults with medical complexity in Oregon. J Pediatr Nurs. 2022;62:171–6.
57. Coyne I, Sheehan A, Heery E, While AE. Healthcare transition for adolescents and young adults with long-term conditions: qualitative study of patients, parents and healthcare professionals' experiences. J Clin Nurs. 2019;28(21–22):4062–76.
58. Divatia H, Friedland AR. Virtual Med-Peds: description of the first virtual Med-Peds student elective during COVID-19. Cureus [Internet]. 2020 Dec 8 [cited 2022 Sep 28]. https://www.cureus.com/articles/40069-virtual-med-peds-description-of-the-first-virtual-med-pedsstudent-elective-during-covid-19

# 3 Health Care of Emerging Adults

Janet M. Ma, Susan H. Duan, Abigail R. Arons, Patrick J. Holman, Jessica L. Lucier, Rebecca K. Tsevat, Alice A. Kuo, Stacey Weinstein, Paul Bixenstine, Daniel Karlin, Faysal Saab, Linnaea Schuttner, and Angelica Zen

*Dylan is a 22-year-old young man presenting to your clinic for a well visit. He has just gotten a new job in health care and needs his immunization records and a tuberculosis test. He has no prior medical conditions or surgeries and takes no medications. He followed with a pediatrician throughout childhood and is up to date on his vaccines. He declines sexually transmitted infection (STI) screening or lab work today, stating that he has not been sexually active since his last testing. He is a never smoker and a social drinker. He is normotensive, his BMI is 22, and his physical exam is unremarkable. You print his immunization records, order a tuberculosis screen, and advise him to return in a year.*

When was the last time you saw a 22-year-old patient in your clinic? How long was the visit, and what issues were addressed? Internists may often consider visits with young adults to be brief, "easy" visits. After managing a schedule full of middle-aged and elderly patients with multiple chronic medical conditions, internists may find that there is not much to discuss in their visits with young adults and may even view these visits as opportunities to catch up or get ahead in their schedules. Most young adults are healthy, and these patients are sent on their way after a brief exam and a few routine labs. In fact, the United States Preventive Services Task Force (USPSTF) guidelines for a 22-year-old male can be summarized in a few words: check blood pressure and screen for tobacco use and sexually transmitted infections (STIs). It should not be surprising, then, that young adults have lower utilization of preventive care than other age groups [1].

But fast forward several years, and this 22-year-old young man becomes a 50-year-old obese man who develops diabetes, hypertension, and cardiovascular disease, and who ends up on dialysis because of diabetic nephropathy and needs a 3-vessel coronary artery bypass graft (CABG) from severe coronary artery disease (CAD). What was missed during those routine

J. M. Ma (✉) · S. H. Duan · P. J. Holman · J. L. Lucier · R. K. Tsevat · A. A. Kuo · S. Weinstein · P. Bixenstine · D. Karlin · F. Saab · A. Zen
Division of Medicine-Pediatrics and Preventive Medicine, University of California, Los Angeles, CA, USA
e-mail: JanetMa@mednet.ucla.edu; sduan@mednet.ucla.edu; pholman@mednet.ucla.edu; jlucier@mednet.ucla.edu; rtsevat@mednet.ucla.edu

A. R. Arons
Department of Internal Medicine, University of California, San Francisco, San Francisco, CA, USA

Division of Medicine-Pediatrics and Preventive Medicine, University of California, Los Angeles, CA, USA
e-mail: abigail.arons2@ucsf.edu

L. Schuttner
VA Puget Sound Healthcare System, Health Services Research & Development, Seattle, USA

Department of Internal Medicine, University of Washington, Seattle, USA


A. A. Kuo et al. (eds.), *Care of Adults with Chronic Childhood Conditions*,
https://doi.org/10.1007/978-3-031-54281-7_3

"easy" visits with him when he was younger and healthy? Was there anything that could have been prevented?

As it turns out, the answer is yes. During the young adult years, there are many opportunities for early intervention that can alter a patient's life course. These opportunities might not be so apparent to internists, who primarily see older adult patients who have already developed fixed habits and lifestyles and who suffer from several chronic medical conditions. In fact, many adult health conditions originate in childhood and adolescence during critical periods of development [1]. Combined internal medicine and pediatric (Med-Peds) physicians and family medicine physicians are more familiar with these childhood and adolescent antecedents to chronic disease, as they often witness firsthand the evolution of these conditions as their patients grow older and transition into adulthood. All primary care providers have an obligation to help minimize risk factors that can cause cardiovascular disease, cancer, and other adult chronic conditions, as well as to help maximize health-promoting protective factors that can facilitate development along optimal health trajectories.

## Addressing Emerging Adulthood During a Visit

The period of transition to adulthood between 18 and 25 years of age, now commonly referred to as "emerging adulthood," is a distinct phase in life that was first described originally by J.J. Arnett in 2000 and is a unique period involving a transition to independence [2]. This phase is wrought with challenges and changes that can impact the health of a patient for years to come. As described by Arnett, emerging adulthood can be defined as an age of identity exploration, instability, self-focus, feeling in between, and possibilities [2]. It is a state of flux and transition, and one in which medical providers can play a pivotal role in navigating young adults toward their future paths.

In this section, we will explore this state of flux and transition, as well as its possible health implications, using representative patient examples. We will end this section by exploring a helpful framework for providers to address these topics during their visits with emerging adults.

*Lisette is a 24-year-old young woman presenting to establish care. You start to flip through her chart, asking the occasional clarifying question about her past medical history, which seems relatively benign. She does not seem to have any alcohol, substance use, or mood problems; however, when you ask about sexual history, she tells you that she is monogamous with her boyfriend and gives you a little smile when admitting that she met him on Tinder. On physical exam, her body mass index (BMI) is 30, but her vital signs are within normal limits, and she has no focal abnormalities. Given her elevated BMI, you discuss ordering diabetes and cholesterol screening labs. She states that she knows she wants to lose weight and is planning to exercise more. You also offer STI screening, which she agrees to do. You review her vaccine records, let her know she is due for her flu shot, and complete her pap smear. At the end of the visit, you say "Nice to meet you, see you next year!" You quickly finish your charting and then look at your schedule and smile. You are pleased with yourself that you were able to do all her healthcare maintenance and catch up on some time so that you are no longer running 10 min behind schedule!*

Does this example seem representative to you? You addressed many topics including cervical cancer screening, immunizations, diabetes screening, hypercholesterolemia screening, anxiety/depression screening, alcohol/substance use screening, health histories, and sexually transmitted infection (STI) screening. That's a lot! However, this approach and plan of care may not be adequate for emerging adults like Lisette, as you did not fully address the developmental milestones and health behaviors that are crucial for this age group.

## Living Situation

We ask almost all of our pediatric and elderly patients about their living situation to evaluate for home safety and independence of Activities of Daily Living (ADLs). *Where do you live? Who do you live with at home? Do you need any help with your ADLs or instrumental ADLs?* But how often do you ask your emerging adults about their living situations?

It is commonly understood that most teenagers live with their parents through the end of high school and that most 30-year-olds live independently. However, emerging adulthood is characterized by more demographic heterogeneity. In fact, more than half of emerging adults in 2016 were living in their parents' homes, which is a significantly higher proportion than in the past [3]; this demographic shift is likely due to a variety of factors resulting in lower rates of financial independence by age 25. Emerging adults living at home are more likely to be in school and/or unemployed [3]. Additionally, a cultural shift has occurred such that only one-quarter of Americans now think that moving out of the parent's home is a "very important" part of adulthood [3].

If we had asked Lisette about her living situation, we would have learned more about her life. *Perhaps she lives at home to take care of her grandmother with dementia. Perhaps she lives with her parents because she is still in school. Perhaps she lives with a few roommates because she can't afford to live alone but feels unsafe in her current living situation. Perhaps she just moved to the city and is staying on her friend's couch as she searches for a job. Or, perhaps, she lives alone and is financially independent.*

Housing and social support during these transformative years can lay the foundation for adulthood. Furthermore, as healthcare providers, asking about housing can allow us to learn about our patients' social dynamics and assess potential needs and interventions related to housing insecurity, food insecurity, or safety concerns at home.

## Financial Independence: Education, Employment, and Insurance

The landscapes of education and early career employment have changed dramatically over the past several decades, which has major implications for the financial independence of this population. Surveys show that most Americans expect that young adults should complete schooling and have full-time jobs by the age of 22 [3]. However, the reality is that only 52% of 22-year-olds have completed school and only 37% are employed full time [3]. One contributing factor is the higher societal emphasis on collegiate and advanced education, demonstrated by the increasing percentage of people with at least a bachelor's degree from 23% in 1975 to 37% in 2016 [3]. Emerging adults also have higher rates of unemployment and lower income levels than in prior decades; in 2015, only 10% of emerging adults made over $30,000 per year, and only 1% made over $60,000 per year [3]. These trends are important to understand because there are potential health implications for emerging adults who have not yet achieved financial independence, including access to stable housing, food sources, routine medical care, and health insurance.

If we asked Lisette about these topics, we would have learned: *She recently graduated college. She is currently working part-time in a restaurant while looking for a full-time job related to her major. She thinks she is on her parents' insurance plan but states she hasn't really paid attention to her coverage. Nor does she know when she will stop being eligible for coverage on her parents' plan.*

Health insurance coverage for emerging adults has historically been a complex issue. Qualitative studies suggest that young adults do not feel at risk for health problems; accordingly, they have low levels of health insurance literacy and place little value on their health insurance [4]. The passage of the Affordable Care Act in 2010 allowed emerging adults to remain covered on their parent's insurance plans until the age of

26. After this law was passed, rates of uninsurance in this population decreased from 30% in 2011 to 16% in 2018 [5]. Additionally, up to 60% of this population reported having primary care physicians and completing annual exams by 2018 [5]. Though access to health insurance has improved, there are lingering barriers for this age group: some emerging adults do not have access to parental plans, and those who age out may not consider a need for health insurance or may opt for high-deductible catastrophic insurance.

Adult studies have shown that the presence of health insurance leads to many benefits, including increased access to healthcare and preventive visits as well as improved diagnosis and treatment of chronic health conditions [6]. It is reasonable to extrapolate those outcomes to the emerging adult population. These data highlight the urgency of reviewing insurance status with emerging adults during their preventive visits and discussing an insurance transition plan for those who will be aging out of parental coverage. While necessary for all emerging adults, continuity of insurance is particularly important for those with special health care needs, who often have gaps in insurance coverage during the transitional years [7] and who may have worse outcomes as a result.

## Sexual Health

The period of emerging adulthood often houses the developmental milestone of sexual exploration. While this topic will be explored in more detail in a later chapter, we will introduce the basic concepts here.

*Lisette mentioned that she had a boyfriend whom she met on* Tinder. *If we had asked about her relationship and thoughts on family planning, she would have shared that she has been dating her partner for 6 months. She does not want to get married or to have children for at least a few years, as she is focusing on finding a full-time job and pursuing financial independence. She states that she uses condoms most of the time, but they often get placed mid-way through the intercourse act. She also states she had Chlamydia once with a prior partner for which she was treated. She has never used other forms of birth control but would be interested in learning more about them.*

This vignette highlights the importance of targeted questions geared toward sexual health. With this information, we see that Lisette's current state reflects the average emerging adult in terms of sexual activity, marriage, and family planning. According to CDC data from 2017, roughly 50% of adolescents become sexually active by the age of 17 [8]. One study using survey data from the 2000–2018 General Social Survey showed that most emerging adults reported having sexual activity weekly or monthly and having one or more new sexual partners in the prior year [9]. Additionally, although adolescents and young adults between the ages of 15 and 24 years represent only 25% of the overall population, they account for nearly half of all new cases of STIs each year [10].

As we did for Lisette, it is important to inquire about sexual practices and offer screening for STIs when appropriate. With a thorough sexual history, we can properly assess safety during sexual encounters, identify patients who would be good candidates for HIV Pre-Exposure Prophylaxis (PrEP), and discuss other strategies to reduce sexual risks.

For all patients, we recommend using standardized, nonjudgement questions that will provide the necessary information to properly assess their sexual health. Some examples of standardized questions are as follows: *In order for me to understand you and how I can best help you, it's important that I ask several questions about your sexual health. How would you describe your gender identity and what are your preferred pronouns? Do you have sex with men, women, or both? How many different sexual partners have you had in the past 6 months? What methods of contraception do you use? How often do you use them? We can screen for Gonorrhea and Chlamydia in different locations based on the types of sex that you practice: using a urine test for those who practice insertive or vaginal sex, a throat swab for those who perform oral sex, and a rectal swab for those who practice receptive anal sex. Where should we screen you today?*

Lastly, Lisette's brief mention of the social media application *Tinder* requires the modern provider to have at least a rudimentary grasp of the habits and knowledge of this demographic. Social media has become a primary means to meet new romantic partners discretely and quickly and is a mainstay of this generation. In 2013, 1 in 5 adults between the ages of 25 and 34 and 1 in 10 adults greater than 18 years of age endorsed participating in online dating, either through cell phone applications or dating websites [11]. While some smartphone or Internet applications have respectable reputations, others are known for providing quick access to a one-night stand. People who seek partners online have reported higher risk sexual behaviors including more unprotected sex, more sexual partners, and more STIs [12–15]. Knowledge of these modalities can help tailor a provider's questions to screen for high-risk sexual behaviors accordingly.

## Family Planning

A separate developmental milestone related to sexual health is reproductive planning. In reviewing Lisette's answers, we may notice that her desire to avoid having children for several years and her suboptimal condom use are incongruent and place her at risk of unintended pregnancy. Family planning is highly relevant to this population but is rarely addressed during preventive visits. One study showed that only 18% of women between the ages of 18 and 44 who delivered a live infant in 2009 reported receiving preconception counseling, although 66% of women in this age group had an annual routine check-up [16].

According to CDC data from 2010, 37% of pregnancies were unintended (either unwanted or mistimed) among women who had ever been married [10]. For women like Lisette, between 15 and 24 years of age and not married or cohabitating, a full 79% of live births were unintended. Among married women between the ages of 25 and 44, almost 1 in 5 births were unintended [17].

When considering the factors leading up to unintended pregnancy, Lisette is not unique in her sporadic condom use. Sixty-one percent of all women using condoms do so inconsistently [18], and 95% of unintended pregnancies occur among women who use contraception incorrectly or inconsistently [19]. For patients like Lisette who want to avoid pregnancy for several years, it is imperative that providers discuss contraceptive options, including Long-Acting Reversible Contraception (LARC) methods, and use shared decision-making to find a method that is consistent with their goals. If Lisette's approach to pregnancy changes or if she continues to have sporadic use of contraception, it may be beneficial to suggest that she begin taking prenatal vitamins on a routine basis or use emergency contraception.

While initial conversations may target pregnancy prevention, it is also important to address future desires for pregnancy. In an age of relentless pursuit of higher education and ambitious careers, fertility may either be purposefully delayed or not considered. Unfortunately, as is well known to many doctors but less commonly known to patients, biology is rarely forgiving. According to data from the CDC's 2012 report on Assisted Reproductive Technology (ART), women are less likely to become pregnant and to carry a pregnancy to term as they age, with a drop-off that occurs in the mid- to late-30 s [20]. While about 40% of ART cycles for women at age 30 will result in a live birth, this number is closer to 30% by age 36 and only 12% by age 41 [20]. For those who successfully deliver, the risk of birth defects increases with age. Compared to babies born to women between 25 and 29 years of age, those born to women over the age of 40 have a higher risk of genetic abnormalities such as Down syndrome, cardiac defects, esophageal atresia, hypospadias, and craniosynostosis [21]. Discussing these statistics with young women should not function as a scare tactic but rather as a means for obtaining medically accurate information to plan their futures.

## Obesity

Another aspect of Lisette's history that should be addressed is her BMI of 30, which gives her the diagnosis of obesity. We partially addressed this diagnosis by screening for obesity-associated comorbidities including hypertension, diabetes, and hypercholesterolemia. However, we neglected to thoroughly discuss her weight, her current diet and exercise habits, and the possible implications for her future health. It is well known that young adulthood is the time period during which people experience the greatest amount of weight gain, which places them at increased risk of being overweight or obese in the future [22]. In fact rates of obesity at age 25 haveincreased by 30% in recent cohorts [23].

The comorbidities associated with elevated BMI may be well known to providers but are less well known to patients and include hypertension, hyperlipidemia, obstructive sleep apnea, metabolic syndrome, obesity hypoventilation syndrome, joint pain, depression, anxiety, fatty liver disease, gallstones, gastro-esophageal reflux, polycystic ovarian syndrome (PCOS), and adverse outcomes in pregnancy.

Given the possible future health implications, it is important to explore the possible effects of a higher BMI, so that patients understand their potential health trajectories. While doing so, it is crucial to use nonjudgmental language and a preventive health framework to avoid the perception of "fat shaming" and thereby jeopardize the patient–physician alliance. Examples of nonjudgmental approaches are as follows: *A few topics I address with all my patients during their annual physical are their typical diet, exercise habits, and weight. The reason I talk about weight is because it's my job to keep you as healthy as you are now for as long as possible by trying to prevent future disease. What did you eat in the past 24 h? What do you do on an average week for exercise? Is it okay if we spend a few minutes talking about your weight? How do you feel about your current weight? Are you familiar with the ways that a high BMI can affect your body and future health?*

With neutral and targeted open-ended questions as demonstrated above, we as healthcare providers can assess our patients' understanding of the potential sequelae of an unhealthy weight and start to fill in their knowledge gaps. We can then transition toward motivational interviewing strategies focused on promoting healthier lifestyles.

Lisette's case provides an illustration of many of the key preventive concerns in emerging adulthood. She is generally healthy but presents multiple issues that have serious implications for her future health and quality of life. Her choice and pattern of contraception, obesity, use of a social media application for dating, and her tenuous financial situation each offer a thread that, if followed, leads to highly relevant health topics that are frequently overlooked by the busy provider.

## Mental Health

*Recall Dylan, the 22-year-old healthy male you saw for a preventive visit. Six months later, he presents to your urgent care clinic with a complaint of palpitations. His heart rate is 92, and he appears to be in no acute distress in your office. As you begin your questioning, he describes occasional moments where he feels his heart racing, flushing of the face, and a wave of nausea. He also notes that his older brother has recently been diagnosed with bipolar disorder. After a benign cardiac exam, you obtain an electrocardiogram (EKG), which demonstrates normal sinus rhythm without abnormalities. Reassured, you diagnose him with panic disorder and prescribe an as-needed short-acting benzodiazepine. As you are about to leave, he asks if it is all right to continue using marijuana when he takes the benzodiazepine. Inquiring further, he reveals that he has begun to use marijuana nightly to help "calm his nerves."*

Dylan's case reflects many themes that are pertinent to the care of emerging adults. Mental health concerns, which are often preceded by a family history of psychiatric illness, often present as mild physical complaints and may be self-treated with illicit substances. Moreover, depression and anxiety may represent difficulty adjusting to new degrees of independence or lack thereof. Mental health disorders frequently present in early adulthood, with 74% of all psychiatric illnesses presenting before age 25 and 46% of all college-age adults reporting a psychiatric diagnosis within the past year [24]. Given the prevalence and significance of mental health concerns in this population, we will explore this topic in more detail in later chapter.

## Substance Use

Another major health concern inherent to emerging adulthood is substance use. Substance use often commences with exploratory behaviors in adolescence but peaks during young adulthood and can predict future habits. For example, regular alcohol consumption at a younger age is associated with increased problem drinking in adolescence and alcohol use disorder in adulthood [25, 26]. Substance use may often serve as a means of self-medication, as evidenced by frequent presentations of "dual diagnoses." Alcohol can be used to temper the symptomatology associated with the extremes of mania or depression, just as marijuana is often used for anti-anxiety purposes, such as in Dylan's case.

Additionally, tobacco consumption has been extremely common in this population with the increased social use of vaping over the past decade. In 2020, CDC and FDA data showed that at least 3.6 million youths used e-cigarettes, including about 1 in 5 high school students [27]. If asked "do you smoke cigarettes or use dipping tobacco?", many teenagers who vape answer "no"; thus, it is important to specifically use language about vaping and e-cigarettes. While more long-term data on vaping is needed, the CDC does discuss adverse outcomes on the developing brain—specifically to areas that control attention, learning, mood, and impulse control [27]. Given the high amounts of nicotine in these devices, many patients become addicted to nicotine and require significant planning and nicotine replacement therapies to successfully abstain.

Primary care providers should incorporate screening for substance use including vaping/e-cigarettes into all visits with emerging adults; screening should include questions about use patterns, dependence, effects on quality of life, and the presence of concomitant mental health issues. This broad and important topic will also be further discussed in a later chapter.

## Using the HEADDSS Assessment

As illustrated in the prior patient examples, providers may miss crucial opportunities for prevention and intervention in emerging adults if they adhere exclusively to the typical healthcare maintenance topics outlined by the USPSTF. These omissions may partly result from the fact that patients often do not view these topics as healthcare issues or may feel too embarrassed to bring them to the attention of their providers. To identify possible risk behaviors, we encourage the use of a standard set of questions targeted at the developmental milestones and lifestyle habits that are characteristic of the emerging adult population.

One common framework that is well known to pediatric providers is the HEADDSS (home, education, employment, activities, drugs, diet, sexual health, suicide) assessment (Table 3.1). Although more commonly used in adolescents, we believe that it can be instrumental in identifying key sociodemographic features of emerging adulthood as well. The HEADDSS assessment can facilitate questions about drug addiction, risky sexual practices, unhealthy diet and exercise habits, housing or food insecurity, and mental health symptoms, all of which are important issues that can impact future health.

**Table 3.1** Adapting the HEADDSS for use with emerging adults

| | | |
|---|---|---|
| **H**<br>Home, family, community environment | Assess housing security, home safety, and independence of ADL and instrumental ADLs | – Can you tell me about your home environment?<br>– Where do you live and with whom?<br>– Do you have any safety concerns at home?<br>– Do you have any difficulties taking care of yourself or your family? |
| **E**<br>Education plans, employment goals | Assess factors that promote financial independence | – Are you currently employed or in school?<br>– Are you having any trouble at school or at work? |
| **A**<br>Activities, hobbies, exercise | Assess exercise habits, social support, and healthy habits | – What do you like to do in your free time?<br>– What do you do for exercise in a typical week? |
| **D**<br>Diet | Assess current diet and patient literacy of healthy foods | – Can you tell me about your typical diet?<br>– What did you eat and drink yesterday for each meal and snack? |
| **D**<br>Drug exposure or use habits | Assess risk factors for and current addiction behaviors | – Do you use any tobacco products including vaping?<br>– Do you drink alcohol?<br>– Do you use any substances or drugs not prescribed to you?<br>– If yes to the above, how much, how frequent, and what route of administration? How do these substances affect your life? Do you have cravings or withdrawal symptoms? |
| **S**<br>Sex practices, contraception, relationships, reproductive planning and preconception care | Assess risk for STIs, unwanted pregnancies, sexual abuse, and intimate partner violence. | – How would you describe your gender identity, and what are your preferred pronouns?<br>– Are you in a relationship with anyone? Do you feel safe in your relationships?<br>– Do you have sex with men, women, or both? How many different sexual partners have you had in the past 6 months?<br>– What methods of contraception do you use and how often do you use them?. |
| **S**<br>Suicide, mental health | Assess mental health concerns including suicidal ideation, thoughts, and/or self-harming behaviors before they have permanent consequences | – Over the last 2 weeks, how often have you been bothered by having little interest or pleasure in doing things?<br>– Over the last 2 weeks, how often have you been bothered by feeling down, depressed, or hopeless?<br>– Have you had any thoughts of self-harm or committing suicide?<br>– Have you been feeling anxious?<br>– How have your anxiety and/or depressive symptoms affected your life? |

## A Paradigm Shift for the Preventive Visit

As discussed above, it is paramount that internists approach the care of young adults with the same eye toward preventive health as they do for adults of all ages, while simultaneously recognizing the developmental milestones and life circumstances that are unique to this population. Reframing the approach of young adult care to focus on chronic diseases that emerge before, during, and after this critical time period can lead to more comprehensive and effective care for a group of individuals whose health needs may otherwise go unnoticed or unaddressed. This paradigm shift can be challenging and time-consuming to adopt and requires collaboration and buy-in from all who provide primary care to young adults: pediatricians, family medicine physicians, obstetrician-gynecologists, general internists, and in some cases, other specialty providers. However, physicians cannot bear this responsibility alone and should rely on the support of all members of the healthcare team, including dieticians, pharmacists, behavioral health specialists, social workers, case managers, and peer health coaches. Each care team, in turn, should be customized to the needs of the patient population within and the environment surrounding an individual primary care practice.

The patient-centered medical home (PCMH) is one model for healthcare delivery that may enable this collective paradigm shift amongst all team members. While commonly considered in the context of children with special healthcare needs (SCHN), the coordinated and comprehensive care promoted through this model can be useful for those with and without chronic medical conditions. The National Committee for Quality Assurance (NCQA), which offers PCMH accreditation, requires six standards for certified PCMHs: (1) patient-centered access, (2) team-based care, (3) population health management, (4) care management and support, (5) care coordination and care transitions, and (6) performance measurement and quality improvement. According to the 2011 American Academy of Pediatrics (AAP), American Academy of Family Physicians (AAFP), and American College of Physicians (ACP) Transitions Clinical Report Authoring Group, "planned care, as the product of a partnership among health care professionals, youth, and families, has become an essential characteristic of the primary care medical home" [28].

Other models for healthcare delivery, initially designed for those with chronic diseases, can also be applied to the care of all young adults within a primary care setting. These include the Chronic Care Model, sponsored by the Robert Wood Johnson Foundation [29]; the Care for Chronic Conditions (ICCC) model published by the World Health Organization (WHO) [30]; and the Expanded Chronic Care Model proposed by Barr and colleagues [31]. These models also recognize and incorporate prevention efforts, social determinants of health, and enhanced community participation as core components of effective healthcare [29].

Common to these models is the recognition that patient care exists within larger communities and healthcare systems. *Recall Lisette, whose BMI of 30 places her in the obese category. A thorough history might elucidate challenges to achieving sustainable weight loss, such as a dearth of affordable produce in her local grocery stores or safe space in her neighborhood that is suitable for exercise.* Thus, in addition to focusing on the individual illnesses experienced by or preventable in young adults, clinicians should attend to population-level factors that influence the health of their patients, including their social determinants of health. The social determinants of health are the conditions in the environments where people are born, live, learn, work, play, worship, and age that affect a wide range of health, functioning, and quality-of-life outcomes and risks [32]. These social determinants can be grouped into five domains, including economic stability, education access and quality, healthcare access and quality, neighborhood and built environment, and social and community context [32]. To address these social determinants, physicians should not only inquire about aspects such as income, housing, education, and access to food as discussed in the vignette above but also connect patients to resources in their communities—often with the help of social workers and other members of the clinical care team.

Additionally, the routine preventive and disease-specific screening discussed earlier in this chapter should be supplemented with a population health management approach—that is, an understanding of "the health outcomes of a group of individuals, including the distribution of such outcomes within the group" [33]. The healthcare team should monitor measures related to disease burden, prevention, and social determinants of health for specific groups of patients as well as the entire clinic population on an ongoing basis. They should also ensure that their clinic or healthcare system incorporates quality improvement methodology such as Plan-Do-Study-Act (PDSA) cycles in order to continually improve health outcomes in the community.

While we have argued that chronic conditions in young adults exist on a continuum and that lessons obtained from caring for this population can be applied to all patients, there are special considerations for those with childhood-onset conditions. These general and disease-specific considerations will be addressed further in subsequent chapters, but it is worth mentioning that young adults with chronic conditions of childhood have increased medical and psychosocial needs that, if not addressed, can lead to negative health outcomes. Of note, emerging adults with complex medical conditions are at greater risk for developmental and psychosocial delays as well as worse general health, life satisfaction, and psychological well-being than their peers [34–36]. This population has also been shown to have lower educational achievement, lower incomes, higher odds of receiving public assistance, and more limited work experience than their counterparts without chronic conditions [35, 37, 38]. Special attention to the individual and population-level factors influencing their health, as well as coordinated care management between primary care providers and other specialists and multi-disciplinary team members, are of the utmost importance to advance the health and well-being of those with chronic childhood conditions. Additionally, as previously discussed in Chap. 1, a successful transition from pediatric to adult-centered health care may help mitigate the disparities they experience by increasing personal responsibility, enhancing autonomy, and facilitating self-reliance [34].

## Conclusion

Emerging adulthood is a distinct phase of life characterized by unique challenges and life circumstances, which have the potential to alter a patient's future health trajectory. As such, special attention must be paid to modifiable risk factors during this critical time period. A comprehensive approach to patient care that considers developmental, psychosocial, and socioeconomic contexts should be used for emerging adults with and without special health care needs. The HEADSS assessment, typically employed in adolescent medicine, can be incorporated into this comprehensive approach to identify targets for intervention. By implementing these steps, providers will be better equipped to prevent the development or exacerbation of chronic disease and thereby improve health outcomes for all young adults, regardless of their existing health conditions.

## References


1. Lau JS, Adams SH, Boscardin WJ, Irwin CE Jr. Young adults' health care utilization and expenditures prior to the affordable care act. J Adolesc Health. 2014;54(6):663–71.
2. Arnett JJ. Emerging adulthood: a theory of development from the late teens through the twenties. Am Psychol. 2000;55(5):469.
3. Vespa J. The changing economics and demographics of young adulthood: 1975–2016. www.census.gov/content/dam/Census/library/publications/2017/demo/p20-579.pdf
4. Dauner KN, Thompson J. Young adult's perspectives on being uninsured and implications for health reform. Qual Rep. 2014;19(4):1.
5. Gangopadhyaya A, Johnston EM. Impacts of the ACA's Medicaid expansion on health insurance coverage and health care access among young adults. Urban Institute; 2021, www.urban.org/research/publication/impacts-acas-medicaid-expansion-health-insurance-coverage-and-health-care-access-among-young-adults
6. Sommers BD, et al. Health insurance coverage and health—what the recent evidence tells us. N Engl J Med. 2017;377(6):586–93.
7. Lotstein DS, Inkelas M, Hays RD, Halfon N, Brook R. Access to care for youth with special health care needs in the transition to adulthood. J Adolesc Health. 2008 Jul;43(1):23–9.
8. Martinez GM, Abma JC. Sexual activity and contraceptive use among teenagers aged 15–19 in the United States, 2015–2017. NCHS Data Brief, no 366. Hyattsville, MD: National Center for Health Statistics. p. 2020.
9. Ueda P, Mercer CH, Ghaznavi C, Herbenick D. Trends in frequency of sexual activity and number of sexual partners among adults aged 18 to 44 years in the US, 2000-2018. JAMA Netw Open. 2020;3(6):e203833.
10. Centers for Disease Control and Prevention (CDC). Sexual risk behaviors: HIV, STD, & teen pregnancy prevention. Last updated April 15, 2016. http://www.cdc.gov/healthyyouth/sexualbehaviors/. Accessed 15 June 2016
11. Smith A, Duggan M. Online dating & relationships. Washington, DC: Pew Research Center's Internet and American Life Project; 2013. http://www.pewinternet.org/files/old-media//Files/Reports/2013/PIP_Online%20Dating%202013.pdf. Accessed 9 June 2016.
12. Bull SS, McFarlane M. Soliciting sex on the internet: what are the risks for sexually transmitted diseases and HIV? Sex Transm Dis. 2000;27(9):545–50.

13. Grov C, DeBusk JA, Bimbi DS, Golub SA, Nanin JE, Parsons JT. Barebacking, the internet, and harm reduction: an intercept survey with gay and bisexual men in Los Angeles and New York City. AIDS Behav. 2007;11(4):527–36.
14. McFarlane M, Bull SS, Rietmeijer CA. The internet as a newly emerging risk environment for sexually transmitted diseases. JAMA. 2000;284(4):443–6.
15. McFarlane M, Bull SS, Rietmeijer CA. Young adults on the internet: risk behaviors for sexually transmitted diseases and HIV. J Adolesc Health. 2002;31(1):11–6.
16. Robbins CL, Zapata LB, Farr SL, Kroelinger CD, Morrow B, Ahluwalia I, et al. Core state preconception health indicators-pregnancy risk assessment monitoring system and behavioral risk factor surveillance system, 2009. Morb Mortal Wkly Rep. 2014;63(3):1–62.
17. Mosher WD, Jones J, Abma JC. National Center for Health Statistics (US). Intended and unintended births in the United States: 1982-2010. National Health Statistics Reports, Number 55, July 24, 2012. http://www.cdc.gov/nchs/data/nhsr/nhsr055.pdf. Accessed June 15, 2016.
18. Frost JJ, Darroch JE. Factors associated with contraceptive choice and inconsistent method use, United States, 2004. Perspect Sex Reprod Health. 2008;40(2):94–104.
19. Gold RB, Sonfield A, Richards CL, Frost JJ. Next steps for America's family planning program: leveraging the potential of Medicaid and title X in an evolving health care system. Guttmacher Institute; 2009. https://www.guttmacher.org/sites/default/files/pdfs/pubs/summaries/NextStepsExec.pdf. Accessed 15 June 2016.
20. Centers for Disease Control and Prevention, American Society for Reproductive Medicine, Society for Assisted Reproductive Technology. 2012 Assisted Reproductive Technology National Summary Report. Atlanta, GA: US Department of Health and Human Services; 2014. https://www.cdc.gov/art/pdf/2012-report/national-summary/art_2012_national_summary_report.pdf. Accessed 15 June 2016.
21. Gill SK, Broussard C, Devine O, Green RF, Rasmussen SA, Reefhuis J, et al. Association between maternal age and birth defects of unknown etiology: United States, 1997-2007. Birt Defects Res A Clin Mol Teratol. 2012;94(12):1010–8.
22. Dummer TJ, Kirk SF, Penney TL, Dodds L, Parker L. Targeting policy for obesity prevention: identifying the critical age for weight gain in women. J Obes. 2012;2012:934895.
23. Reither EN, Hauser RM, Yang Y. Do birth cohorts matter? Age-period-cohort analyses of the obesity epidemic in the United States. Soc Sci Med. 2009;69(10):1439–48.
24. Blanco C, Okuda M, Wright C, Hasin DS, Grant BF, Liu S-M, et al. Mental health of college students and their non–college-attending peers: results from the National Epidemiologic Study on alcohol and related conditions. Arch Gen Psychiatry. 2008;65(12):1429–37.
25. Hingson RW, Heeren T, Winter MR. Age at drinking onset and alcohol dependence: age at onset, duration, and severity. Arch Pediatr Adolesc Med. 2006;160(7):739–46.
26. Pitkänen T, Lyyra A, Pulkkinen L. Age of onset of drinking and the use of alcohol in adulthood: a follow-up study from age 8–42 for females and males. Addiction. 2005;100(5):652–61.
27. "Quick facts on the risks of e-cigarettes for kids, teens, and young adults." Centers for Disease Control and Prevention, Centers for Disease Control and Prevention, 30 Sept. 2021, https://www.cdc.gov/tobacco/basic_information/e-cigarettes/Quick-Facts-on-the-Risks-of-E-cigarettes-for-Kids-Teens-and-Young-Adults.html
28. Cooley WC, Sagerman PJ. Supporting the health care transition from adolescence to adulthood in the medical home. Pediatrics. 2011;128(1):182–200.
29. Stellefson M, Dipnarine K, Stopka C. The chronic care model and diabetes management in US primary care settings: a systematic review. Prev Chronic Dis. 2013;10:E26.
30. World Health Organization. Innovative care for chronic conditions: building blocks for actions: global report; 2002. http://www.who.int/chp/knowledge/publications/icccglobalreport.pdf. Accessed 15 June 2016.
31. Barr VJ, Robinson S, Marin-Link B, Underhill L, Dotts A, Ravensdale D, et al. The expanded chronic care model: an integration of concepts and strategies from population health promotion and the chronic care model. Healthc Q. 2003;7(1):73.
32. Healthy people 2030, U.S. Department of Health and Human Services, Office of Disease Prevention and Health Promotion. https://health.gov/healthypeople/objectives-and-data/social-determinants-health. Accessed 6 Sep 2021.
33. Kindig D, Stoddart G. What is population health? Am J Public Health. 2003;93(3):380–3.
34. Rosen DS, Blum RW, Britto M, Sawyer SM, Siegel DM. Transition to adult health care for adolescents and young adults with chronic conditions: position paper of the Society for Adolescent Medicine. J Adolesc Health. 2003;33(4):309–11.
35. Wisk LE, Weitzman ER. Expectancy and achievement gaps in educational attainment and subsequent adverse health effects among adolescents with and without chronic medical conditions. J Adolesc Health. 2017;61(4):461–70.
36. Sawyer SM, Drew S, Yeo MS, Britto MT. Adolescents with a chronic condition: challenges living, challenges treating. Lancet. 2007;369(9571):1481–9.
37. Bloom SR, Kuhlthau K, Van Cleave J, Knapp AA, Newacheck P, Perrin JM. Health care transition for youth with special health care needs. J Adolesc Health. 2012 Sep;51(3):213–9.
38. Maslow GR, Haydon A, McRee AL, Ford CA, Halpern CT. Growing up with a chronic illness: social success, educational/vocational distress. J Adolesc Health. 2011;49(2):206–12.

# 4 Well Care of the Emerging and Young Adult

Susan H. Duan, Aditi Mhaskar, Nupur Agrawal, Carlie Stein, Janet M. Ma, Abigail R. Arons, Patrick J. Holman, Jessica L. Lucier, and Rebecca K. Tsevat

"Transition care" in the realm of academic medicine typically refers to the process of transitioning care from pediatric to adult providers. It often is associated with youth with special healthcare needs (YSHCN)/and patients with childhood conditions. This population acutely experiences the multiple challenges in our healthcare system in transitioning from pediatric to adult care. Concurrently, these patients are often undergoing major personal transitions—gaining more autonomy, leaving home, entering relationships, and pushing boundaries—which may challenge the management of their medical conditions and lead to poor outcomes. Significant work has taken place within the medical community to understand this period with the hopes of better serving this population [1]. Research suggests that this process goes more smoothly when it occurs gradually over time and is assisted by a multidisciplinary, team-based approach with attention to the patient's and family's broader context [2].

Lisette and Dylan, the patients in our earlier vignettes in Chap. 3, are not typically considered youth with special healthcare needs. And yet, they do have healthcare needs and risk factors that predispose them to chronic health conditions and poor outcomes. Rather than addressing healthcare in this age range as occurring between two distinct groups (those patients with special healthcare needs versus those without), it may be

S. H. Duan (✉) · A. Mhaskar · N. Agrawal · J. M. Ma
Division of Medicine-Pediatrics and Preventive Medicine, University of California, Los Angeles, CA, USA
e-mail: sduan@mednet.ucla.edu; NupurAgrawal@mednet.ucla.edu; JanetMa@mednet.ucla.edu

C. Stein
Department of Medicine, UAB School of Medicine, Birmingham, AL, USA
e-mail: chstein@uabmc.edu

A. R. Arons
Department of Internal Medicine, University of California, San Francisco, San Francisco, CA, USA

Division of Medicine-Pediatrics and Preventive Medicine, University of California, Los Angeles, CA, USA
e-mail: abigail.arons2@ucsf.edu

P. J. Holman · J. L. Lucier · R. K. Tsevat
Department of Internal Medicine, University of California, San Francisco, San Francisco, CA, USA
e-mail: pholman@mednet.ucla.edu; jlucier@mednet.ucla.edu; rtsevat@mednet.ucla.edu


A. A. Kuo et al. (eds.), *Care of Adults with Chronic Childhood Conditions*,
https://doi.org/10.1007/978-3-031-54281-7_4

helpful to think of both groups of patients with a range of chronic illnesses. As discussed throughout this chapter, emerging adulthood is a life stage full of transition. Mental health, metabolic disease, and substance use are chronic conditions that can appear or worsen during this period and may end up causing significant morbidity and mortality in the future. It is beneficial to apply the lessons of transition care to the emerging adult population as a whole and to see this developmental stage as a critical window for future health outcomes that can be best served by multidisciplinary, longitudinal teams, with attention to patient contexts. Further, conceptualizing the health risk factors identified during this period (mental health, sexual health, and substance use) as chronic diseases may inspire closer attention to screening and interventions in this population.

## Care Management Skills

Emerging adults, those 19–25 years of age, access primary care the least when compared to members of all other age groups in the United States. Despite increased access to insurance coverage and the elimination of copayments for preventive visits after the implementation of the Affordable Care Act, the overall utilization of primary care services in young adults remains low although it has improved [3, 4]. This can be observed in Fig. 4.1.

Research looking into the behaviors of healthy young adults without chronic conditions has elucidated numerous factors that impact their engagement with primary care. Issues with trust and communication and difficulty navigating the healthcare system are associated with decreased utilization of primary care services [5]. Lack of continuity of care, confidentiality (especially if the provider cares for other members of the patient's family), perceived provider competence, and familiarity with their provider are also problematic [5, 6]. Patients with established pediatricians may perceive the adult care model to be intimidating or lower in quality and may consequently be hesitant to transition to an adult provider [7]. Pediatricians may hope to retain patients they have seen for years while adult providers may lack the time and resources necessary to care for young adults comprehensively [7]. Young adults belonging to marginalized and disadvantaged populations are more likely to be disconnected from primary care and are at higher risk for poorer health outcomes [3, 4, 7, 8]. Familial factors (e.g., low education level, limited English proficiency, low socioeconomic status, limited parental support) and personal factors (e.g., poverty, lack of stable housing) contribute to difficulty navigating the healthcare system and subsequent gaps in essential care [7].

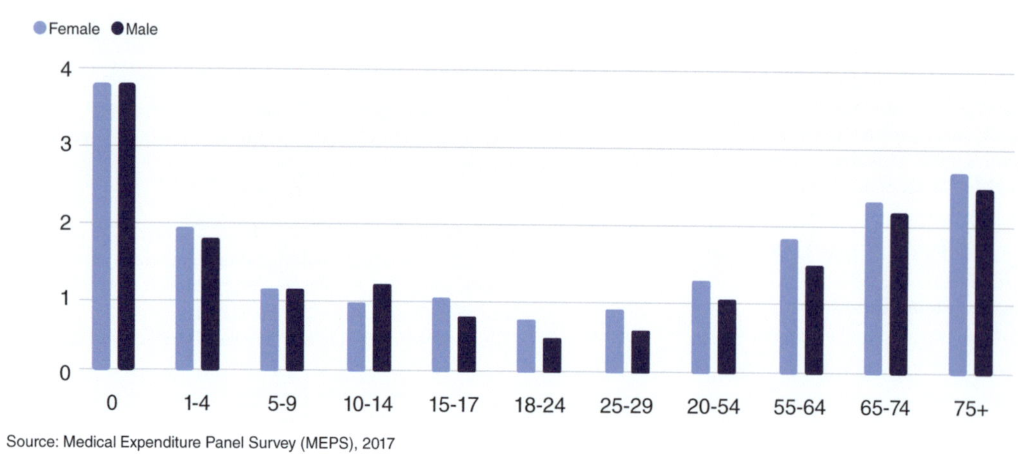


**Fig. 4.1** Primary care office visits by age and sex, 2017 [3]

## Skills and Strategies for the Adult Provider

Primary care providers who understand the unique healthcare needs of their young adult patients and show competence in caring for them can positively impact long-term engagement with the healthcare system [5, 8]. Providers should use a flexible, varied, and nonjudgmental approach when communicating with young adult patients in order to make them feel comfortable and heard [5]. Listening attentively and showing empathy are key [5]. Care decisions should involve the patient, and medical content should be explained clearly [5]. Anticipatory guidance should also be provided to guide patients on beneficial lifestyle modifications [9].

Increased access to the chosen primary care provider can provide opportunities to strengthen the patient–physician relationship. Patients in this age group may require more frequent visits to address urgent matters, such as contraception and sexual health [5, 6]. Strategies to improve care access, such as dedicating slots each day for same-day visits, expanding clinic hours, and using technology such as online portals and messaging systems, can improve continuity of care and patient likelihood to engage in ongoing care as well as decrease high costs associated with the use of emergency services [9]. The availability of integrated behavioral health systems in which primary care and mental health providers work alongside one another to address prevalent mental health issues, such as mood disorders, substance use, body image, trauma, and suicidality, can enhance economic, educational, and social well-being and improve primary care health outcomes [10, 11].

While transition of care models from pediatrics to adulthood has traditionally focused on adolescents and young adults with chronic conditions, there is evidence that implementing a transition protocol in the pediatric setting for patients without chronic illness is valuable [7, 12, 13] and increases the number of healthy young adults who complete a visit with an adult provider in a timely manner [7]. Teaching transition-focused skills to primary care residents can help train the next generation of providers on bridging care between adolescence and adulthood [12].

## USPSTF Recommendations for Emerging Adults

A chapter on the preventative healthcare of emerging adulthood would be lacking if it did not include a review of the guidelines for this age group as provided by the United States Preventative Task Force (USPSTF) [2]. The USPSTF, an independent panel of primary care and prevention experts, provides evidence-based recommendations for clinical preventative services. The panel reviews scientific evidence to determine whether primary care providers should offer screenings, counseling, or preventive medications and grade these recommendations. Grade A recommendations are ones that the panel deems, with high certainty, to have a substantial net benefit. Grade B recommendations are deemed to have a moderate net benefit with high certainty or a moderate to substantial benefit with moderate certainty. The USPSTF recommends clinical services that achieve an A or B grade.

Table 4.1 reviews the USPSTF recommendations for all patients within the emerging adult age group. Not surprisingly, a significant overlap can be seen between these guidelines and the characteristic domains of emerging adulthood discussed earlier. As such, these guidelines can serve as a roadmap for primary care providers in caring for this population.

The USPSTF provides additional screening recommendations for individuals who are determined to be at increased risk of morbidity and mortality from various conditions. These recommendations are noted in Table 4.2.

Healthcare providers should have a relatively low threshold to provide these screenings to emerging adults. The USPSTF guidelines do specify what factors would put an individual at increased risk for each health outcome in question. Often these factors are not rare. By way of example, the USPSTF notes that men who have

**Table 4.1** Summary of USPSTF Guidelines applicable to all patients ages 18–25

| For all patients 18–25 years of age | Recommendation | Grade | Release date |
|---|---|---|---|
| Risk Assessment and Referral to Genetic Counseling for BRCA-Related Cancers | Assess persons assigned female at birth with a personal or family history of breast, ovarian, tubal, or peritoneal cancer or who have an ancestry associated with breast cancer susceptibility 1 and 2 gene mutations with an appropriate brief familial risk assessment tool. Those with a positive result on the risk assessment tool should receive genetic counseling and, if indicated after counseling, genetic testing. | B | Aug 2019 |
| Cervical Cancer Screening | For individuals with a cervix aged 21–29: Screen for cervical cancer every 3 years with cervical cytology alone<br>Aged 30–65 years: Screen every 3 years with cervical cytology alone, every 5 years with high-risk human papillomavirus (hrHPV) testing alone, or every 5 years with hrHPV testing in combination with cytology (co-testing). | A | Aug 2018 |
| Chlamydia and Gonorrhea Screening[a] | Screen for gonorrhea in all sexually active persons assigned female at birth aged 24 years or younger and in those 25 years or older who are at increased risk for infection. | B | Sept 2021 |
| Depression Screening[a] | Screen for depression in the general adult population. Screening should be implemented with adequate systems in place to ensure accurate diagnosis, effective treatment, and appropriate follow-up. | B | Jan 2016 |
| Folic Acid for the Prevention of Neural Tube Defects | Use daily supplements containing 0.4–0.8 mg (400–800 μg) of folic acid for all persons who are planning or capable of pregnancy. | A | Jan 2017 |
| Hepatitis C Virus Infection | Screen for hepatitis C virus (HCV) infection in adults aged 18–79 years. | B | May 2020 |
| HIV Infection Screening | Screen for HIV infection in adolescents and adults aged 15–65 years. Younger adolescents and older adults who are at increased risk of infection should also be screened. | A | June 2019 |
| Hypertension Screening | Screen for hypertension with office blood pressure measurement (OBPM). Obtain blood pressure measurements outside of the clinical setting for diagnostic confirmation before starting treatment. | A | Apr 2021 |
| Intimate Partner Violence[a] | Screen for intimate partner violence (IPV) in those of reproductive age and provide or refer those who screen positive to ongoing support services. | B | Oct 2018 |
| Tobacco Smoking Cessation[a] | Ask all adults about tobacco use, advise them to stop using tobacco, and provide behavioral interventions and US Food and Drug Administration (FDA) approved pharmacotherapy for cessation to nonpregnant adults who use tobacco. | A | Jan 2021 |
| Unhealthy Alcohol Use[a] | Screen for unhealthy alcohol use and provide persons engaged in risky or hazardous drinking with brief behavioral counseling interventions to reduce unhealthy alcohol use. | B | Nov 2018 |
| Unhealthy Drug Use[a] | Screen by asking questions about unhealthy drug use. Screening should be implemented when services for accurate diagnosis, effective treatment, and appropriate care can be offered or referred. | B | June 2020 |

[a]Addressed in the HEADDSS assessment

sex with men (MSM) and those living with HIV are at the highest risk of syphilis, but also notes that being a male less than 29 years old is a risk factor.

As a note, the USPSTF also has a set of screening guidelines for pregnant persons, not included in this chapter.

**Table 4.2** Summary of USPSTF guidelines applicable to patients ages 18–25 with certain risk factors

| For persons at increased risk | Recommendation | Grade | Release date |
|---|---|---|---|
| Healthy Diet and Physical Activity for Cardiovascular Disease Prevention | Offer or refer adults with cardiovascular disease risk factors to behavioral counseling interventions to promote a healthy diet and physical activity. | B | Nov 2020 |
| Hepatitis B Virus Infection | Screen for hepatitis B virus (HBV) infection in adolescents and adults at increased risk for infection. | B | Dec 2020 |
| Latent Tuberculosis Infection Screening | Screen for latent tuberculosis infection (LTBI) in asymptomatic populations at increased risk | B | Sept 2016 |
| Prevention of HIV | Offer preexposure prophylaxis (PrEP) with effective antiretroviral therapy to persons who are at high risk of HIV acquisition. | A | June 2019 |
| Sexually Transmitted Infections | Counsel all sexually active adolescents and adults who are at increased risk for sexually transmitted infections (STIs). | B | Aug 2020 |
| Skin Cancer Prevention | Counsel about minimizing exposure to ultraviolet (UV) radiation for persons aged 6 months to 24 years with fair skin types to reduce their risk of skin cancer. | B | Mar 2018 |
| Syphilis Infection | Screen for syphilis infection in persons who are at increased risk of infection. | A | June 2016 |
| Weight Loss to Prevent Obesity-Related Morbidity and Mortality | Offer or refer adults with a body mass index (BMI) of 30 or higher (calculated as weight in kilograms divided by height in meters squared) to intensive, multicomponent behavioral interventions. | B | Sept 2018 |

## Immunizations

In addition to routine screenings, immunizations are a critical part of the healthcare maintenance of emerging adults. Table 4.3 lists the vaccines important for this age group, as designated by the CDC, assuming the completion of a childhood vaccination schedule [14].

In addition to the standard vaccinations above, additional vaccines should be considered. Hepatitis A and B vaccination should be provided to any patient who desires it, in addition to patients with specific risk factors and medical conditions. Haemophilus influenza B, meningococcal, and pneumococcal vaccines should be provided to those patients who are immunocompromised or functionally or anatomically asplenic. Specific details and further recommendations can be found on the CDC website.

Vaccine uptake is much lower in young adults than in childhood. The many transitional characteristics of emerging adulthood likely impact immunization uptake in this population: developing autonomy, inconsistent insurance and the lack of routine medical care, and frequent relocation may all contribute. Additionally, we know that the health behaviors and attitudes of young adults are powerfully influenced by the behaviors and attitudes of their peers (i.e., social norms) [15]. Research demonstrates that estimates of social norms are associated with young adults' intentions to receive the HPV vaccine [16]. The importance of immunization in this population has been underscored by the COVID-19 pandemic, not only for young adults but also for the promotion of general public health.

HPV vaccination deserves special attention in this population. A recent report noted that between 2010 and 2018 only 42% of females and 16% of males ages 18–21 had received at least 1 dose of HPV vaccine [17]. We are optimistic that these rates will improve as childhood HPV vaccination becomes more routine. Recent updates by the CDC's Advisory Committee on Immunization Practices (ACIP) suggest shared clinical decision-making about administering HPV vaccines to select populations between the ages of 27 and 45 [18]. Vaccination with the

**Table 4.3** Recommended vaccinations for all emerging adults

| Vaccine | Administration | Notes |
|---|---|---|
| Influenza | Annually | |
| Tetanus, diphtheria, pertussis (Tdap or Td) | One dose of Tdap after age 18 and then boosters with Tdap or Td every 10 years | Pregnant persons will also be offered during the third trimester of each pregnancy<br>1 dose of Td or Tdap for wound management as needed |
| Measles, mumps, rubella (MMR) | Once or two doses (4 weeks apart) for those without evidence of immunity | Contraindicated in pregnancy and the severely immunocompromised<br>Indications for two doses: Those with HIV, healthcare workers |
| Varicella | 2 doses 4–8 weeks apart for those without evidence of immunity | Contraindicated in pregnancy and the severely immunocompromised |
| Human Papilloma Virus (HPV) | 2 or 3 doses depending on age at the first dose | 3 doses for those who received the first dose after age 15 |
| COVID-19 | Dose administration depends on the vaccine type and booster schedule | |

nonavalent vaccine should be considered for those who have already received the quadrivalent vaccine, particularly those who are at elevated risk or who desire it.

For patients with certain disease states, additional screening and immunization guidelines exist. For example, both tuberous sclerosis and Down Syndrome have age-based guidance for healthcare maintenance in patients with these conditions. When appropriate, these guidelines will be addressed in later disease-specific chapters.

## Vaccines and Pregnancy

While pregnant women may receive most nonlive virus and bacterial vaccines as needed for routine immunizations, some vaccines are specifically recommended in pregnancy.

All pregnant women should receive Tdap, preferably in the third trimester, regardless of the timing of their prior dose. This facilitates the passive transmission of antibodies to the infant and reduces the infant's exposure to pertussis after birth. Pregnant women who have never been vaccinated or are only partially vaccinated against Td should receive a 3-dose series, one of which is Tdap.

Pregnant women should receive the inactivated influenza vaccine every October. The COVID-19 vaccine should be given for passive antibody transmission to the fetus and to reduce neonatal exposure to the virus.

Per current ACIP recommendations, live virus and bacterial vaccines are contraindicated during pregnancy. This includes measles-, mumps-, rubella-, and varicella-containing vaccines, live, attenuated influenza vaccine (FluMist), oral poliovirus vaccine (but not IPV), oral typhoid vaccine, and smallpox vaccines. It is recommended that women who receive a live vaccine should avoid pregnancy for 4 weeks afterwards, due to a theoretical risk of serious congenital disease from the organism in the vaccine. Of note, despite the lack of evidence of risk, ACIP does not recommend giving the HPV vaccine (a non-live vaccine) during pregnancy.

Women who are not immune to rubella or varicella should be vaccinated immediately in the post-partum period. A second varicella vaccine should be given 4–8 weeks later [19].

## Recent Immigrants with Vaccinations Outside the United States

If vaccine records of recent immigrants are not available, or standards for minimum age and intervals are not consistent with CDC recommendations, revaccination with routine vaccines is recommended. Verbal confirmation that a patient received the flu vaccine for that season is acceptable if records are not present.

Refugees are not required to receive vaccinations prior to arrival in the United States but may have received some doses through the Vaccination Program for US-Bound refugees. HIV screening is not routinely performed on recent immigrants or refugees but should be considered at the first visit. If a patient with HIV has severe immunosuppression (CD4 <200 cells/μL) or is immunosuppressed due to a different etiology, live virus vaccines such as MMR or varicella are contraindicated.

In cases where re-vaccination is not feasible or preferred, serologic testing is available for immunity to some organisms (Table 4.4). Serologic testing for varicella immunity may be preferred or more cost-effective than vaccination [19–21].

## Unknown Immune Status in Any Patient

If there is concern about whether a patient is immune or has a history of vaccination for a certain condition, some serologic tests are commonly available (Table 4.4). Revaccination is an option unless contraindicated (usually for a prior history of anaphylaxis with a specific vaccine, or live vaccines in a patient who is immunocompromised or pregnant). Extra doses of vaccines are usually not harmful. There may be a concern for a localized reaction at the injection site if appropriate intervals between the timing of vaccine doses are not maintained, but the risk of a life-threatening condition is rare [23].

**Table 4.4** Serologic testing for immunity [19]

| Vaccine | Tests |
|---|---|
| Hep A | IgG Ab for Hep A.<br>Patients coming from areas with endemic hepatitis A may have immunity from prior infection. |
| Hepatitis B | Revaccination with a 3-dose series followed by measuring HbsAg 4 weeks later is recommended.<br>Immunity may also be determined by negative Hep B core Ab, Hep B surface Ag, and positive Hep B surface Ab [22]. |
| MMR | Serologic testing for IgG antibodies to measles, mumps, and rubella |
| Varicella | IgG ELISA for Varicella establishes that a patient has antibodies from either previous vaccination or infection [21]. |

## Allergies

Patients with an egg allergy can receive most vaccines.

- Most influenza vaccines may have come into contact with an egg protein. If a patient has a confirmed egg allergy, they should receive the recombinant inactivated influenza vaccine or IIV.
- Measles and mumps vaccine development involves chick embryo fibroblast tissue culture. The resultant content of the egg protein in the vaccine is extremely low, and the MMR vaccine is still recommended.
- Patients who are traveling to destinations where yellow fever vaccines are recommended may develop hypersensitivity reactions to the yellow fever vaccine. If a person has severe egg allergies or is noted to have a positive skin test (scratch test or intradermal test) for the vaccine, desensitization can be performed prior to vaccination, per package insert recommendations.

It is more common that those with a severe allergic reaction to a vaccine have allergies to gelatin, neomycin, or a different component of that vaccine. It is recommended to refer the patient to an allergist if they have anaphylactic reactions to gelatin or neomycin, prior to receiving vaccines containing those components [24].

The current formulations of measles, mumps, rubella, or varicella-containing vaccines, live, attenuated influenza vaccine (Flumist), rabies vaccine, oral typhoid vaccines, and yellow fever vaccines contain gelatin. Patients with anaphylactic reactions to gelatin or gelatin-containing products should be referred to an allergist prior to receiving these immunizations [24, 25].

Natural rubber latex can be found in gloves, syringe plunger tips, and vial stoppers. If in the latter two, it will be noted on the vaccine manufacturer's inserts. The most common allergy to latex is delayed hypersensitivity, such as contact dermatitis. Vaccines may be administered to patients with this condition. If a patient has severe anaphylactic allergy to latex, these materials should be avoided. If administering vaccines that require latex-containing vials or syringes cannot be avoided in patients with severe allergies, the healthcare provider should be prepared to treat immediate reactions, such as anaphylaxis.

## Vaccine Adverse Event Reporting System and Vaccine Injury Compensation Program

The Vaccine Adverse Event Reporting System (VAERS) is a warning system to analyze reports of possible side effects from vaccination. It is co-administered by the CDC and FDA. Certain events are mandatorily reportable.

A table of reportable events following vaccination is available on the VAERS website at vaers.hhs.gov/faq.html. After COVID-19 vaccination, vaccine administration errors, serious adverse events, cases of multisystem inflammatory syndrome, or cases of COVID-19 resulting in hospitalization or death must be reported.

Other than mandatory reports, healthcare providers may report any adverse event of immunization to VAERS, even if they are unsure that the vaccine was the causative agent. Reports can also be given by patients and vaccine manufacturers. Due to the nature and sources of data collection, not all VAERS reports are indicative of a true adverse event of a vaccine. VAERS can "identify [if] unusual or unexpected patterns of reporting that might indicate possible safety problems" are noted [26]. The program will not offer medical advice or conclude whether a vaccine was the causative agent of an effect seen in the patient.

VAERS is not associated with the National Vaccine Injury Compensation Program (VICP), which is a Health Resources and Services Administration program that allows individuals to file a petition with the government for compensation for vaccine-associated injuries. Patients who are concerned that a vaccine covered by VICP resulted in an injury that lasted for more than 6 months, resulted in hospitalization and required surgical intervention, or resulted in death can be referred to the VICP website for more information on applying for compensation. A similar program, Countermeasures Injury Compensation Program (CICP), exists for the COVID-19 vaccine, which is not covered by the VICP [26, 27].

## Catch Up Vaccine Schedule

The most recent vaccine charts are available on the CDC website. The CDC Vaccine Schedules App for smartphones and tablets is recommended by the Advisory Committee on Immunization Practices and is available on the CDC website at https://www.cdc.gov/vaccines/schedules/hcp/schedule-app.html#download at the time of this writing.

Please see the appendix for vaccine recommendations and easy-to-read charts.

### Vaccine Hesitancy

No single best intervention exists to address this major public health concern. Having a conversation to understand the patients' concerns rather than a "top-down" approach has been helpful. The National Vaccine Advisory Committee has noted multiple studies showing that a provider's strong recommendation for a vaccine is more likely to improve vaccination rates among their patient population [28]. The CDC has patient handouts regarding common concerns and general hesitancy, as well as webinars, CME training, and quality improvement projects on immunizations for healthcare providers [29].

A common issue raised by vaccine-hesitant individuals has been the mercury content in vaccines. Thimerosal, a mercurial compound, has been used as an antimicrobial and antifungal preservative in vaccines since the 1930s. The elemental mercurial content in a thimerosal-containing vaccines is less than or equal to a 3 oz. can of tuna. There is no evidence that it causes harmful side effects or is retained in the human body. In 1999, thimerosal-free vaccines were developed for children less than 6 years old due to scientific concerns at that time.

Thimerosal-free single-dose vaccines are also available for adolescents and adults. Currently, FDA-approved vaccines that contain thimerosal are mainly multidose vials of influenza vaccine [24, 30].

Of note, even if patch or intradermal tests indicate hypersensitivity to thimerosal, positive results on these tests have not been associated with immediate reactions to thimerosal injected as part of a vaccine. These patients may still receive thimerosal-containing vaccines [24, 30].

## Telehealth

### Telehealth Considerations

The COVID-19 pandemic led to rapid changes in healthcare delivery with the growth of telemedicine as a way to prevent unnecessary exposures while maintaining access to medical care. Initially used as an effective platform to screen patients for COVID-19 symptoms, telemedicine quickly ramped up in medical centers throughout the country as a means to provide ongoing preventative and subspecialty care. With changes to telemedicine reimbursement and licensure regulations in 2020, providers were reimbursed at the same rate as in person visits [31, 32]. This included video and phone visits but also the use of remote monitoring to gather vital signs. These changes applied to physicians, nurse practitioners, and mental health and nutrition professionals, increasing opportunities for multidisciplinary care for patients while remaining in their homes. The US DEA also suspended the Ryan Haight Online Pharmacy Consumer Protection Act of 2008 allowing physicians to prescribe Schedule II–V medications with telemedicine, creating opportunities for medication management via telemedicine.

For many of our adults with complex conditions of childhood predisposing them to increased mortality and morbidity with COVID-19 infection, telemedicine became an important and effective means to access preventative care, urgent visits for COVID symptoms to addressing important issues including nutrition and mental health [33, 34].

Now that many hospitals and clinics throughout the country and around the globe have adapted to the world of telemedicine, many of the advantages are clear. For our most vulnerable patients with complex medical issues and need for caregiver support and transportation barriers, telemedicine adds convenience. Another added benefit is the ease of scheduling more frequent check-ins related to mental health, medication follow-ups, nutrition counseling, or discussion of social work resources. There are opportunities for more coordinated medical management without the cost of travel and time spent getting to doctors' offices or health centers. Patients and providers have reported satisfaction with telemedicine due to lesser waiting times, accessibility, convenience, and cost savings while maintaining communication and privacy [35].

Our patients with complex conditions of childhood are already at risk for mental health disorders such as anxiety and depression but with added psychosocial impacts of COVID-19-increased isolation, fear related to illness, and closing in-person school, work, and other social outlets—there is a concern for greater impacts on mental health for this population. Previous studies have shown effective management of these disorders with the use of telemedicine platforms and in October 2020, it was estimated as many as 41% of mental health visits were conducted via telemedicine [36, 37]. With CDC estimates of anywhere between 30 and 42% of adults over 18 endorsing symptoms of anxiety or depression during 2020–2022, compared to 10.8% in 2019, access to mental health resources on a grander scale has become a necessity [38, 39]. This includes national counseling platforms aimed at individual or group therapies, support groups for specific diseases, mental health screening, and medication management. There is also national work on the creation of telepsychiatry toolkits and resources for best practices in providing "telemental health" [40, 41].

While the advantages are clear, it is crucial we consider potential for health inequities in telemedicine. As many of our patients have comorbidities including intellectual disability, hearing/vision issues, technology dependence, or require caregiver support, this can add another layer of complexity. Successful use of telemedicine requires access to and skills needed for the use of digital technology. It is also important to consider insurance status, lack of privacy, language barriers, and the need for adaptive equipment which can create added barriers to effective healthcare visits. Difficulties with Internet connection have been shown to negatively impact communication in telehealth visits [42]. While in-home Internet service continues to increase, there is a disparity in use amongst the elderly, racial minorities, and adults with lower income or education highlighting the importance of continued improvements targeted at patient populations with increased risk of access issues to healthcare and telemedicine [43]. Office and technology checklists have been created to help screen patients appropriate for telemedicine given potential barriers to technology [44].

By enhancing efforts to improve telehealth access, we can continue to improve the care of our most vulnerable patients. For patients and families with complex conditions who live long distances from academic medical centers, telemedicine can provide the opportunity for consultation with unique specialty and multidisciplinary resources that they otherwise may not access at all including transition resources. With attention to the need for assistive devices and improved access to the Internet and technology, services for patients/families who need translator services or with low health literacy, we can continue to build on and improve outcomes for patients. Telemedicine advancements should include expansion and considerations for all of our patients, especially our adults with complex diseases of childhood.

## Appendix: CDC Schedule Attached

### Recommended Adult Immunization Schedule for ages 19 years or older

UNITED STATES **2022**

#### How to use the adult immunization schedule

1 Determine recommended vaccinations by age (**Table 1**)

2 Assess need for additional recommended vaccinations by medical condition or other indication (**Table 2**)

3 Review vaccine types, frequencies, intervals, and considerations for special situations (**Notes**)

4 Review contraindications and precautions for vaccine types (**Appendix**)

**Vaccines in the Adult Immunization Schedule***

| Vaccine | Abbreviation(s) | Trade name(s) |
|---|---|---|
| *Haemophilus influenzae* type b vaccine | Hib | ActHIB®<br>Hiberix®<br>PedvaxHIB® |
| Hepatitis A vaccine | HepA | Havrix®<br>Vaqta® |
| Hepatitis A and hepatitis B vaccine | HepA-HepB | Twinrix® |
| Hepatitis B vaccine | HepB | Engerix-B®<br>Recombivax HB®<br>Heplisav-B® |
| Human papillomavirus vaccine | HPV | Gardasil 9® |
| Influenza vaccine (inactivated) | IIV4 | Many brands |
| Influenza vaccine (live, attenuated) | LAIV4 | FluMist® Quadrivalent |
| Influenza vaccine (recombinant) | RIV4 | Flublok® Quadrivalent |
| Measles, mumps, and rubella vaccine | MMR | M-M-R II® |
| Meningococcal serogroups A, C, W, Y vaccine | MenACWY-D<br>MenACWY-CRM<br>MenACWY-TT | Menactra®<br>Menveo®<br>MenQuadfi® |
| Meningococcal serogroup B vaccine | MenB-4C<br>MenB-FHbp | Bexsero®<br>Trumenba® |
| Pneumococcal 15-valent conjugate vaccine | PCV15 | Vaxneuvance™ |
| Pneumococcal 20-valent conjugate vaccine | PCV20 | Prevnar 20™ |
| Pneumococcal 23-valent polysaccharide vaccine | PPSV23 | Pneumovax 23® |
| Tetanus and diphtheria toxoids | Td | Tenivac®<br>Tdvax™ |
| Tetanus and diphtheria toxoids and acellular pertussis vaccine | Tdap | Adacel®<br>Boostrix® |
| Varicella vaccine | VAR | Varivax® |
| Zoster vaccine, recombinant | RZV | Shingrix |

*Administer recommended vaccines if vaccination history is incomplete or unknown. Do not restart or add doses to vaccine series if there are extended intervals between doses. The use of trade names is for identification purposes only and does not imply endorsement by the ACIP or CDC.

Recommended by the Advisory Committee on Immunization Practices (www.cdc.gov/vaccines/acip) and approved by the Centers for Disease Control and Prevention (www.cdc.gov), American College of Physicians (www.acponline.org), American Academy of Family Physicians (www.aafp.org), American College of Obstetricians and Gynecologists (www.acog.org), American College of Nurse-Midwives (www.midwife.org), and American Academy of Physician Associates (www.aapa.org), and Society for Healthcare Epidemiology of America (www.shea-online.org).

**Report**

- Suspected cases of reportable vaccine-preventable diseases or outbreaks to the local or state health department
- Clinically significant postvaccination reactions to the Vaccine Adverse Event Reporting System at www.vaers.hhs.gov or 800-822-7967

**Injury claims**

All vaccines included in the adult immunization schedule except pneumococcal 23-valent polysaccharide (PPSV23) and zoster (RZV) vaccines are covered by the Vaccine Injury Compensation Program. Information on how to file a vaccine injury claim is available at www.hrsa.gov/vaccinecompensation.

**Questions or comments**

Contact www.cdc.gov/cdc-info or 800-CDC-INFO (800-232-4636), in English or Spanish, 8 a.m.–8 p.m. ET, Monday through Friday, excluding holidays.

Download the CDC Vaccine Schedules app for providers at www.cdc.gov/vaccines/schedules/hcp/schedule-app.html.

**Helpful information**

- Complete Advisory Committee on Immunization Practices (ACIP) recommendations: www.cdc.gov/vaccines/hcp/acip-recs/index.html
- *General Best Practice Guidelines for Immunization* (including contraindications and precautions): www.cdc.gov/vaccines/hcp/acip-recs/general-recs/index.html
- Vaccine information statements: www.cdc.gov/vaccines/hcp/vis/index.html
- Manual for the Surveillance of Vaccine-Preventable Diseases (including case identification and outbreak response): www.cdc.gov/vaccines/pubs/surv-manual
- Travel vaccine recommendations: www.cdc.gov/travel
- Recommended Child and Adolescent Immunization Schedule, United States, 2022: www.cdc.gov/vaccines/schedules/hcp/child-adolescent.html
- ACIP Shared Clinical Decision-Making Recommendations: www.cdc.gov/vaccines/acip/acip-scdm-faqs.html

U.S. Department of Health and Human Services
Centers for Disease Control and Prevention

Scan QR code for access to online schedule

CS310021-A

**Table 1** Recommended Adult Immunization Schedule by Age Group, United States, 2022

| Vaccine | 19–26 years | 27–49 years | 50–64 years | ≥65 years |
|---|---|---|---|---|
| **Influenza inactivated** (IIV4) or **Influenza recombinant** (RIV4) | 1 dose annually | | | |
| or **Influenza live, attenuated** (LAIV4) | 1 dose annually | | | |
| **Tetanus, diphtheria, pertussis** (Tdap or Td) | 1 dose Tdap each pregnancy; 1 dose Td/Tdap for wound management (see notes)<br>1 dose Tdap, then Td or Tdap booster every 10 years | | | |
| **Measles, mumps, rubella** (MMR) | 1 or 2 doses depending on indication (if born in 1957 or later) | | | |
| **Varicella** (VAR) | 2 doses (if born in 1980 or later) | 2 doses | | |
| **Zoster recombinant** (RZV) | 2 doses for immunocompromising conditions (see notes) | | 2 doses | |
| **Human papillomavirus** (HPV) | 2 or 3 doses depending on age at initial vaccination or condition | 27 through 45 years | | |
| **Pneumococcal** (PCV15, PCV20, PPSV23) | 1 dose PCV15 followed by PPSV23 OR 1 dose PCV20 (see notes) | | | 1 dose PCV15 followed by PPSV23 OR 1 dose PCV20 |
| **Hepatitis A** (HepA) | 2 or 3 doses depending on vaccine | | | |
| **Hepatitis B** (HepB) | 2, 3, or 4 doses depending on vaccine or condition | | | |
| **Meningococcal A, C, W, Y** (MenACWY) | 1 or 2 doses depending on indication, see notes for booster recommendations | | | |
| **Meningococcal B** (MenB) | 2 or 3 doses depending on vaccine and indication, see notes for booster recommendations<br>19 through 23 years | | | |
| ***Haemophilus influenzae* type b** (Hib) | 1 or 3 doses depending on indication | | | |

Recommended vaccination for adults who meet age requirement, lack documentation of vaccination, or lack evidence of past infection; Recommended vaccination for adults with an additional risk factor or another indication; Recommended vaccination based on shared clinical decision-making; No recommendation/Not applicable

**Table 2** Recommended Adult Immunization Schedule by Medical Condition or Other Indication, United States, 2022

| Vaccine | Pregnancy | Immuno-compromised (excluding HIV infection) | HIV infection CD4 percentage and count: <15% or <200 mm³ | HIV infection CD4 percentage and count: ≥15% and ≥200 mm³ | Asplenia, complement deficiencies | End-stage renal disease, or on hemodialysis | Heart or lung disease; alcoholism[1] | Chronic liver disease | Diabetes | Health care personnel[2] | Men who have sex with men |
|---|---|---|---|---|---|---|---|---|---|---|---|
| IIV4 or RIV4 | 1 dose annually | | | | | | | | | | |
| or LAIV4 | Contraindicated | | | | | Precaution | | | | 1 dose annually | |
| Tdap or Td | 1 dose Tdap each pregnancy | 1 dose Tdap, then Td or Tdap booster every 10 years | | | | | | | | | |
| MMR | Contraindicated* | Contraindicated | | 1 or 2 doses depending on indication | | | | | | | |
| VAR | Contraindicated* | Contraindicated | | | 2 doses | | | | | | |
| RZV | | 2 doses at age ≥19 years | | | 2 doses at age ≥50 years | | | | | | |
| HPV | Not Recommended* | 3 doses through age 26 years | | | 2 or 3 doses through age 26 years depending on age at initial vaccination or condition | | | | | | |
| Pneumococcal (PCV15, PCV20, PPSV23) | | 1 dose PCV15 followed by PPSV23 OR 1 dose PCV20 (see notes) | | | | | | | | | |
| HepA | 2 or 3 doses depending on vaccine | | | | | | | | | | |
| HepB | 3 doses (see notes) | 2, 3, or 4 doses depending on vaccine or condition | | | | | | | | | |
| MenACWY | 1 or 2 doses depending on indication, see notes for booster recommendations | | | | | | | | | | |
| MenB | Precaution | 2 or 3 doses depending on vaccine and indication, see notes for booster recommendations | | | | | | | | | |
| Hib | | 3 doses HSCT[3] recipients only | | | 1 dose | | | | | | |

Recommended vaccination for adults who meet age requirement, lack documentation of vaccination, or lack evidence of past infection; Recommended vaccination for adults with an additional risk factor or another indication; Recommended vaccination based on shared clinical decision-making; Precaution—vaccination might be indicated if benefit of protection outweighs risk of adverse reaction; Contraindicated or not recommended—vaccine should not be administered. *Vaccinate after pregnancy.; No recommendation/Not applicable

**1.** Precaution for LAIV4 does not apply to alcoholism. **2.** See notes for influenza; hepatitis B; measles, mumps, and rubella; and varicella vaccinations. **3.** Hematopoietic stem cell transplant.

## Notes Recommended Adult Immunization Schedule for ages 19 years or older, United States, 2022

**For vaccine recommendations for persons 18 years of age or younger, see the Recommended Child and Adolescent Immunization Schedule.**

**COVID-19 Vaccination**

**COVID-19 vaccines are recommended within the scope of the Emergency Use Authorization or Biologics License Application for the particular vaccine. ACIP recommendations for the use of COVID-19 vaccines can be found at** www.cdc.gov/vaccines/hcp/acip-recs/vacc-specific/covid-19.html.

**CDC's interim clinical considerations for use of COVID-19 vaccines can be found at** www.cdc.gov/vaccines/covid-19/clinical-considerations/covid-19-vaccines-us.html.

### *Haemophilus influenzae* type b vaccination

**Special situations**

- **Anatomical or functional asplenia (including sickle cell disease):** 1 dose if previously did not receive Hib; if elective splenectomy, 1 dose, preferably at least 14 days before splenectomy
- **Hematopoietic stem cell transplant (HSCT):** 3-dose series 4 weeks apart starting 6–12 months after successful transplant, regardless of Hib vaccination history

### Hepatitis A vaccination

**Routine vaccination**

- **Not at risk but want protection from hepatitis A** (identification of risk factor not required): 2-dose series HepA (Havrix 6–12 months apart or Vaqta 6–18 months apart [minimum interval: 6 months]) or 3-dose series HepA-HepB (Twinrix at 0, 1, 6 months [minimum intervals: dose 1 to dose 2: 4 weeks / dose 2 to dose 3: 5 months])

**Special situations**

- **At risk for hepatitis A virus infection:** 2-dose series HepA or 3-dose series HepA-HepB as above
  - **Chronic liver disease** (e.g., persons with hepatitis B, hepatitis C, cirrhosis, fatty liver disease, alcoholic liver disease, autoimmune hepatitis, alanine aminotransferase [ALT] or aspartate aminotransferase [AST] level greater than twice the upper limit of normal)
  - **HIV infection**
  - **Men who have sex with men**
  - **Injection or noninjection drug use**
  - **Persons experiencing homelessness**
  - **Work with hepatitis A virus** in research laboratory or with nonhuman primates with hepatitis A virus infection
  - **Travel in countries with high or intermediate endemic hepatitis A** (HepA-HepB [Twinrix] may be administered on an accelerated schedule of 3 doses at 0, 7, and 21–30 days, followed by a booster dose at 12 months)
  - **Close, personal contact with international adoptee** (e.g., household or regular babysitting) in first 60 days after arrival from country with high or intermediate endemic hepatitis A (administer dose 1 as soon as adoption is planned, at least 2 weeks before adoptee's arrival)
  - **Pregnancy** if at risk for infection or severe outcome from infection during pregnancy
  - **Settings for exposure, including** health care settings targeting services to injection or noninjection drug users or group homes and nonresidential day care facilities for developmentally disabled persons (individual risk factor screening not required)

### Hepatitis B vaccination

**Routine vaccination**

- **Age 19 through 59 years:** complete a 2- or 3-, or 4-dose series
  - 2-dose series only applies when 2 doses of Heplisav-B* are used at least 4 weeks apart
  - 3-dose series Engerix-B or Recombivax HB at 0, 1, 6 months [minimum intervals: dose 1 to dose 2: 4 weeks / dose 2 to dose 3: 8 weeks / dose 1 to dose 3: 16 weeks])
  - 3-dose series HepA-HepB (Twinrix at 0, 1, 6 months [minimum intervals: dose 1 to dose 2: 4 weeks / dose 2 to dose 3: 5 months])
  - 4-dose series HepA-HepB (Twinrix) accelerated schedule of 3 doses at 0, 7, and 21–30 days, followed by a booster dose at 12 months
  - 4-dose series Engerix-B at 0, 1, 2, and 6 months for persons on adult hemodialysis (note: each dosage is double that of normal adult dose, i.e., 2 mL instead of 1 mL)

***Note:** Heplisav-B not recommended in pregnancy due to lack of safety data in pregnant women

**Special situations**

- **Age 60 years or older* and at risk for hepatitis B virus infection:** 2-dose (Heplisav-B) or 3-dose (Engerix-B, Recombivax HB) series or 3-dose series HepA-HepB (Twinrix) as above
  - **Chronic liver disease** (e.g., persons with hepatitis C, cirrhosis, fatty liver disease, alcoholic liver disease, autoimmune hepatitis, alanine aminotransferase [ALT] or aspartate aminotransferase [AST] level greater than twice upper limit of normal)
  - **HIV infection**
  - **Sexual exposure risk** (e.g., sex partners of hepatitis B surface antigen [HBsAg]-positive persons; sexually active persons not in mutually monogamous relationships; persons seeking evaluation or treatment for a sexually transmitted infection; men who have sex with men)
  - **Current or recent injection drug use**
  - **Percutaneous or mucosal risk for exposure to blood** (e.g., household contacts of HBsAg-positive persons; residents and staff of facilities for developmentally disabled persons; health care and public safety personnel with reasonably anticipated risk for exposure to blood or blood-contaminated body fluids; hemodialysis, peritoneal dialysis, home dialysis, and predialysis patients; patients with diabetes)
  - **Incarcerated persons**
  - **Travel in countries with high or intermediate endemic hepatitis B**

***Note:** Anyone age 60 years or older who does not meet risk-based recommendations may still receive Hepatitis B vaccination.

### Human papillomavirus vaccination

**Routine vaccination**

- **HPV vaccination recommended for all persons through age 26 years:** 2- or 3-dose series depending on age at initial vaccination or condition:
  - **Age 15 years or older at initial vaccination:** 3-dose series at 0, 1–2 months, 6 months (minimum intervals: dose 1 to dose 2: 4 weeks / dose 2 to dose 3: 12 weeks / dose 1 to dose 3: 5 months; repeat dose if administered too soon)
  - **Age 9–14 years at initial vaccination and received 1 dose or 2 doses less than 5 months apart:** 1 additional dose
  - **Age 9–14 years at initial vaccination and received 2 doses at least 5 months apart:** HPV vaccination series complete, no additional dose needed

## Notes Recommended Adult Immunization Schedule, United States, 2022

- **Interrupted schedules:** If vaccination schedule is interrupted, the series does not need to be restarted
- **No additional dose recommended when any HPV vaccine series has been completed using the recommended dosing intervals.**

**Shared clinical decision-making**

- **Some adults age 27–45 years: Based on shared clinical decision-making,** 2- or 3-dose series as above

**Special situations**

- **Age ranges recommended above for routine and catch-up vaccination or shared clinical decision-making also apply in special situations**
  - **Immunocompromising conditions, including HIV infection:** 3-dose series, even for those who initiate vaccination at age 9 through 14 years.
  - **Pregnancy:** Pregnancy testing is not needed before vaccination; HPV vaccination is not recommended until after pregnancy; no intervention needed if inadvertently vaccinated while pregnant

### Influenza vaccination

**Routine vaccination**

- **Age 19 years or older:** 1 dose any influenza vaccine appropriate for age and health status annually
- For the 2021–2022 season, see www.cdc.gov/mmwr/volumes/70/rr/rr7005a1.htm
- For the 2022–23 season, see the 2022–23 ACIP influenza vaccine recommendations.

**Special situations**

- **Egg allergy, hives only:** any influenza vaccine appropriate for age and health status annually
- **Egg allergy–any symptom other than hives** (e.g., angioedema, respiratory distress) or required epinephrine or another emergency medical intervention: see Appendix listing contraindications and precautions
- **Severe allergic reaction (e.g., anaphylaxis) to a vaccine component or a previous dose of any influenza vaccine:** see Appendix listing contraindications and precautions
- **History of Guillain-Barré syndrome within 6 weeks after previous dose of influenza vaccine:** Generally, should not be vaccinated unless vaccination benefits outweigh risks for those at higher risk for severe complications from influenza

### Measles, mumps, and rubella vaccination

**Routine vaccination**

- **No evidence of immunity to measles, mumps, or rubella:** 1 dose
  - **Evidence of immunity:** Born before 1957 (health care personnel, see below), documentation of receipt of MMR vaccine, laboratory evidence of immunity or disease (diagnosis of disease without laboratory confirmation is not evidence of immunity)

**Special situations**

- **Pregnancy with no evidence of immunity to rubella:** MMR contraindicated during pregnancy; after pregnancy (before discharge from health care facility), 1 dose
- **Nonpregnant women of childbearing age with no evidence of immunity to rubella:** 1 dose
- **HIV infection with CD4 percentages ≥15% and CD4 count ≥200 cells/mm³ for at least 6 months and no evidence of immunity to measles, mumps, or rubella:** 2-dose series at least 4 weeks apart; MMR contraindicated for HIV infection with CD4 percentage <15% or CD4 count <200 cells/mm³
- **Severe immunocompromising conditions:** MMR contraindicated
- **Students in postsecondary educational institutions, international travelers, and household or close, personal contacts of immunocompromised persons with no evidence of immunity to measles, mumps, or rubella:** 2-dose series at least 4 weeks apart if previously did not receive any doses of MMR or 1 dose if previously received 1 dose MMR
- **Health care personnel:**
  - **Born before 1957 with no evidence of immunity to measles, mumps, or rubella:** Consider 2-dose series at least 4 weeks apart for measles or mumps or 1 dose for rubella
  - **Born in 1957 or later with no evidence of immunity to measles, mumps, or rubella:** 2-dose series at least 4 weeks apart for measles or mumps or at least 1 dose for rubella

### Meningococcal vaccination

**Special situations for MenACWY**

- **Anatomical or functional asplenia (including sickle cell disease), HIV infection, persistent complement component deficiency, complement inhibitor (e.g., eculizumab, ravulizumab) use:** 2-dose series MenACWY-D (Menactra, Menveo, or MenQuadfi) at least 8 weeks apart and revaccinate every 5 years if risk remains
- **Travel in countries with hyperendemic or epidemic meningococcal disease, or microbiologists routinely exposed to *Neisseria meningitidis*:** 1 dose MenACWY (Menactra, Menveo, or MenQuadfi) and revaccinate every 5 years if risk remains
- **First-year college students who live in residential housing (if not previously vaccinated at age 16 years or older) or military recruits:** 1 dose MenACWY (Menactra, Menveo, or MenQuadfi)
- For MenACWY **booster dose recommendations** for groups listed under "Special situations" and in an outbreak setting (e.g., in community or organizational settings and among men who have sex with men) and additional meningococcal vaccination information, see www.cdc.gov/mmwr/volumes/69/rr/rr6909a1.htm

**Shared clinical decision-making for MenB**

- **Adolescents and young adults age 16–23 years (age 16–18 years preferred) not at increased risk for meningococcal disease:** Based on shared clinical decision-making, 2-dose series MenB-4C (Bexsero) at least 1 month apart or 2-dose series MenB-FHbp (Trumenba) at 0, 6 months (if dose 2 was administered less than 6 months after dose 1, administer dose 3 at least 4 months after dose 2); MenB-4C and MenB-FHbp are not interchangeable (use same product for all doses in series)

**Special situations for MenB**

- **Anatomical or functional asplenia (including sickle cell disease), persistent complement component deficiency, complement inhibitor (e.g., eculizumab, ravulizumab) use, or microbiologists routinely exposed to *Neisseria meningitidis*:**
- 2-dose primary series MenB-4C (Bexsero) at least 1 month apart or 3-dose primary series MenB-FHbp (Trumenba) at 0, 1–2, 6 months (if dose 2 was administered at least 6 months after dose 1, dose 3 not needed); MenB-4C and MenB-FHbp are not interchangeable (use same product for all doses in series); 1 dose MenB booster 1 year after primary series and revaccinate every 2–3 years if risk remains

## Notes Recommended Adult Immunization Schedule, United States, 2022

- **Pregnancy:** Delay MenB until after pregnancy unless at increased risk and vaccination benefits outweigh potential risks
- For MenB **booster dose recommendations** for groups listed under "Special situations" and in an outbreak setting (e.g., in community or organizational settings and among men who have sex with men) and additional meningococcal vaccination information, see www.cdc.gov/mmwr/volumes/69/rr/rr6909a1.htm

**Note:** MenB vaccines may be administered simultaneously with MenACWY vaccines if indicated, but at a different anatomic site, if feasible.

### Pneumococcal vaccination

#### Routine vaccination

- **Age 65 years or older** who have not previously received a pneumococcal conjugate vaccine or whose previous vaccination history is unknown: 1 dose PCV15 or 1 dose PCV20. If PCV15 is used, this should be followed by a dose of PPSV23 given at least 1 year after the PCV15 dose. A minimum interval of 8 weeks between PCV15 and PPSV23 can be considered for adults with an immunocompromising condition,* cochlear implant, or cerebrospinal fluid leak to minimize the risk of invasive pneumococcal disease caused by serotypes unique to PPSV23 in these vulnerable groups.
- For guidance for patients who have already received a previous dose of PCV13 and/or PPSV23, see www.cdc.gov/mmwr/volumes/71/wr/mm7104a1.htm.

#### Special situations

- **Age 19–64 years** with certain underlying medical conditions or other risk factors** who have not previously received a pneumococcal conjugate vaccine or whose previous vaccination history is unknown: 1 dose PCV15 or 1 dose PCV20. If PCV15 is used, this should be followed by a dose of PPSV23 given at least 1 year after the PCV15 dose. A minimum interval of 8 weeks between PCV15 and PPSV23 can be considered for adults with an immunocompromising condition,* cochlear implant, or cerebrospinal fluid leak to minimize the risk of invasive pneumococcal disease caused by serotypes unique to PPSV23 in these vulnerable groups.
- For guidance for patients who have already received a previous dose of PCV13 and/or PPSV23, see www.cdc.gov/mmwr/volumes/71/wr/mm7104a1.htm.

***Note:** Immunocompromising conditions include chronic renal failure, nephrotic syndrome, immunodeficiency, iatrogenic immunosuppression, generalized malignancy, human immunodeficiency virus, Hodgkin disease, leukemia, lymphoma, multiple myeloma, solid organ transplants, congenital or acquired asplenia, sickle cell disease, or other hemoglobinopathies.

****Note:** Underlying medical conditions or other risk factors include alcoholism, chronic heart/liver/lung disease, chronic renal failure, cigarette smoking, cochlear implant, congenital or acquired asplenia, CSF leak, diabetes mellitus, generalized malignancy, HIV, Hodgkin disease, immunodeficiency, iatrogenic immunosuppression, leukemia, lymphoma, multiple myeloma, nephrotic syndrome, solid organ transplants, or sickle cell disease or other hemoglobinopathies.

### Tetanus, diphtheria, and pertussis vaccination

#### Routine vaccination

- **Previously did not receive Tdap at or after age 11 years:** 1 dose Tdap, then Td or Tdap every 10 years

#### Special situations

- **Previously did not receive primary vaccination series for tetanus, diphtheria, or pertussis:** 1 dose Tdap followed by 1 dose Td or Tdap at least 4 weeks after Tdap and another dose Td or Tdap 6–12 months after last Td or Tdap (Tdap can be substituted for any Td dose, but preferred as first dose), Td or Tdap every 10 years thereafter
- **Pregnancy:** 1 dose Tdap during each pregnancy, preferably in early part of gestational weeks 27–36
- **Wound management:** Persons with 3 or more doses of tetanus-toxoid-containing vaccine: For clean and minor wounds, administer Tdap or Td if more than 10 years since last dose of tetanus-toxoid-containing vaccine; for all other wounds, administer Tdap or Td if more than 5 years since last dose of tetanus-toxoid-containing vaccine. Tdap is preferred for persons who have not previously received Tdap or whose Tdap history is unknown. If a tetanus-toxoid-containing vaccine is indicated for a pregnant woman, use Tdap. For detailed information, see www.cdc.gov/mmwr/volumes/69/wr/mm6903a5.htm

### Varicella vaccination

#### Routine vaccination

- **No evidence of immunity to varicella:** 2-dose series 4–8 weeks apart if previously did not receive varicella-containing vaccine (VAR or MMRV [measles-mumps-rubella-varicella vaccine] for children); if previously received 1 dose varicella-containing vaccine, 1 dose at least 4 weeks after first dose
  - Evidence of immunity: U.S.-born before 1980 (except for pregnant women and health care personnel [see below]), documentation of 2 doses varicella-containing vaccine at least 4 weeks apart, diagnosis or verification of history of varicella or herpes zoster by a health care provider, laboratory evidence of immunity or disease

#### Special situations

- **Pregnancy with no evidence of immunity to varicella:** VAR contraindicated during pregnancy; after pregnancy (before discharge from health care facility), 1 dose if previously received 1 dose varicella-containing vaccine or dose 1 of 2-dose series (dose 2: 4–8 weeks later) if previously did not receive any varicella-containing vaccine, regardless of whether U.S.-born before 1980
- **Health care personnel with no evidence of immunity to varicella:** 1 dose if previously received 1 dose varicella-containing vaccine; 2-dose series 4–8 weeks apart if previously did not receive any varicella-containing vaccine, regardless of whether U.S.-born before 1980
- **HIV infection with CD4 percentages ≥15% and CD4 count ≥200 cells/mm³ with no evidence of immunity:** Vaccination may be considered (2 doses 3 months apart); VAR contraindicated for HIV infection with CD4 percentage <15% or CD4 count <200 cells/mm³
- **Severe immunocompromising conditions:** VAR contraindicated

### Zoster vaccination

#### Routine vaccination

- **Age 50 years or older:** 2-dose series RZV (Shingrix) 2–6 months apart (minimum interval: 4 weeks; repeat dose if administered too soon), regardless of previous herpes zoster or history of zoster vaccine live (ZVL, Zostavax) vaccination (administer RZV at least 2 months after ZVL)

#### Special situations

- **Pregnancy:** There is currently no ACIP recommendation for RZV use in pregnancy. Consider delaying RZV until after pregnancy.
- **Immunocompromising conditions (including HIV):** RZV recommended for use in persons age 19 years or older who are or will be immunodeficient or immunosuppressed because of disease or therapy. For detailed information, see www.cdc.gov/mmwr/volumes/71/wr/mm7103a2.htm.

2/17/2022 Centers for Disease Control and Prevention | Recommended Adult Immunization Schedule, United States, 2022

## Appendix Recommended Adult Immunization Schedule, United States, 2022

### Guide to Contraindications and Precautions to Commonly Used Vaccines

*Adapted from Table 4-1 in Advisory Committee on Immunization Practices (ACIP) General Best Practice Guidelines for Immunization: Contraindication and Precautions available at* www.cdc.gov/vaccines/hcp/acip-recs/general-recs/contraindications.html *and ACIP's Recommendations for the Prevention and Control of 2021-22 Seasonal Influenza with Vaccines available at www.cdc.gov/mmwr/volumes/70/rr/rr7005a1.htm*

**Interim clinical considerations for use of COVID-19 vaccines including contraindications and precautions can be found at**
www.cdc.gov/vaccines/covid-19/clinical-considerations/covid-19-vaccines-us.html

| Vaccine | Contraindications[1] | Precautions[2] |
|---|---|---|
| Influenza, egg-based, inactivated injectable (IIV4) | • Severe allergic reaction (e.g., anaphylaxis) after previous dose of any influenza vaccine (i.e., any egg-based IIV, ccIIV, RIV, or LAIV of any valency)<br>• Severe allergic reaction (e.g., anaphylaxis) to any vaccine component[3] (excluding egg) | • Guillain-Barré syndrome (GBS) within 6 weeks after a previous dose of any type of influenza vaccine<br>• Persons with egg allergy with symptoms other than hives (e.g., angioedema, respiratory distress) or required epinephrine or another emergency medical intervention: Any influenza vaccine appropriate for age and health status may be administered. If using egg-based IIV4, administer in medical setting under supervision of health care provider who can recognize and manage severe allergic reactions. May consult an allergist.<br>• Moderate or severe acute illness with or without fever |
| Influenza, cell culture-based inactivated injectable [(ccIIV4), Flucelvax® Quadrivalent] | • Severe allergic reaction (e.g., anaphylaxis) to any ccIIV of any valency, or to any component[3] of ccIIV4 | • Guillain-Barré syndrome (GBS) within 6 weeks after a previous dose of any type of influenza vaccine<br>• Persons with a history of severe allergic reaction (e.g., anaphylaxis) after a previous dose of any egg-based IIV, RIV, or LAIV of any valency. If using ccIV4, administer in medical setting under supervision of health care provider who can recognize and manage severe allergic reactions. May consult an allergist.<br>• Moderate or severe acute illness with or without fever |
| Influenza, recombinant injectable [(RIV4), Flublok® Quadrivalent] | • Severe allergic reaction (e.g., anaphylaxis) to any RIV of any valency, or to any component[3] of RIV4 | • Guillain-Barré syndrome (GBS) within 6 weeks after a previous dose of any type of influenza vaccine<br>• Persons with a history of severe allergic reaction (e.g., anaphylaxis) after a previous dose of any egg-based IIV, ccIIV, or LAIV of any valency. If using RIV4, administer in medical setting under supervision of health care provider who can recognize and manage severe allergic reactions. May consult an allergist.<br>• Moderate or severe acute illness with or without fever |
| Influenza, live attenuated [LAIV4, Flumist® Quadrivalent] | • Severe allergic reaction (e.g., anaphylaxis) after previous dose of any influenza vaccine (i.e., any egg-based IIV, ccIIV, RIV, or LAIV of any valency)<br>• Severe allergic reaction (e.g., anaphylaxis) to any vaccine component[3] (excluding egg)<br>• Adults age 50 years or older<br>• Anatomic or functional asplenia<br>• Immunocompromised due to any cause including, but not limited to, medications and HIV infection<br>• Close contacts or caregivers of severely immunosuppressed persons who require a protected environment<br>• Pregnancy<br>• Cochlear implant<br>• Active communication between the cerebrospinal fluid (CSF) and the oropharynx, nasopharynx, nose, ear, or any other cranial CSF leak<br>• Received influenza antiviral medications oseltamivir or zanamivir within the previous 48 hours, peramivir within the previous 5 days, or baloxavir within the previous 17 days. | • Guillain-Barré syndrome (GBS) within 6 weeks after a previous dose of any type of influenza vaccine<br>• Asthma in persons aged 5 years old or older<br>• Persons with egg allergy with symptoms other than hives (e.g., angioedema, respiratory distress) or required epinephrine or another emergency medical intervention: Any influenza vaccine appropriate for age and health status may be administered. If using LAIV4 (which is egg based), administer in medical setting under supervision of health care provider who can recognize and manage severe allergic reactions. May consult an allergist.<br>• Persons with underlying medical conditions (other than those listed under contraindications) that might predispose to complications after wild-type influenza virus infection [e.g., chronic pulmonary, cardiovascular (except isolated hypertension), renal, hepatic, neurologic, hematologic, or metabolic disorders (including diabetes mellitus)]<br>• Moderate or severe acute illness with or without fever |

1. When a contraindication is present, a vaccine should NOT be administered. Kroger A, Bahta L, Hunter P. ACIP General Best Practice Guidelines for Immunization. www.cdc.gov/vaccines/hcp/acip-recs/general-recs/contraindications.html
2. When a precaution is present, vaccination should generally be deferred but might be indicated if the benefit of protection from the vaccine outweighs the risk for an adverse reaction. Kroger A, Bahta L, Hunter P. ACIP General Best Practice Guidelines for Immunization. www.cdc.gov/vaccines/hcp/acip-recs/general-recs/contraindications.html
3. Vaccination providers should check FDA-approved prescribing information for the most complete and updated information, including contraindications, warnings, and precautions. Package inserts for U.S.-licensed vaccines are available at www.fda.gov/vaccines-blood-biologics/approved-products/vaccines-licensed-use-united-states.

## Appendix Recommended Adult Immunization Schedule, United States, 2022

| Vaccine | Contraindications[1] | Precautions[2] |
|---|---|---|
| *Haemophilus influenzae* type b (Hib) | • Severe allergic reaction (e.g., anaphylaxis) after a previous dose or to a vaccine component[3]<br>• For Hiberix, ActHib, and PedvaxHIB only: History of severe allergic reaction to dry natural latex | • Moderate or severe acute illness with or without fever |
| Hepatitis A (HepA) | • Severe allergic reaction (e.g., anaphylaxis) after a previous dose or to a vaccine component[3] including neomycin | • Moderate or severe acute illness with or without fever |
| Hepatitis B (HepB) | • Severe allergic reaction (e.g., anaphylaxis) after a previous dose or to a vaccine component[3] including yeast<br>• For Heplisav-B only: Pregnancy | • Moderate or severe acute illness with or without fever |
| Hepatitis A- Hepatitis B vaccine [HepA-HepB, (Twinrix®)] | • Severe allergic reaction (e.g., anaphylaxis) after a previous dose or to a vaccine component[3] including neomycin and yeast | • Moderate or severe acute illness with or without fever |
| Human papillomavirus (HPV) | • Severe allergic reaction (e.g., anaphylaxis) after a previous dose or to a vaccine component[3] | • Moderate or severe acute illness with or without fever |
| Measles, mumps, rubella (MMR) | • Severe allergic reaction (e.g., anaphylaxis) after a previous dose or to a vaccine component[3]<br>• Severe immunodeficiency (e.g., hematologic and solid tumors, receipt of chemotherapy, congenital immunodeficiency, long-term immunosuppressive therapy or patients with HIV infection who are severely immunocompromised)<br>• Pregnancy<br>• Family history of altered immunocompetence, unless verified clinically or by laboratory testing as immunocompetent | • Recent (≤11 months) receipt of antibody-containing blood product (specific interval depends on product)<br>• History of thrombocytopenia or thrombocytopenic purpura<br>• Need for tuberculin skin testing or interferon-gamma release assay (IGRA) testing<br>• Moderate or severe acute illness with or without fever |
| Meningococcal ACWY (MenACWY) [MenACWY-CRM (Menveo®); MenACWY-D (Menactra®); MenACWY-TT (MenQuadfi®)] | • Severe allergic reaction (e.g., anaphylaxis) after a previous dose or to a vaccine component[3]<br>• For MenACWY-D and Men ACWY-CRM only: severe allergic reaction to any diphtheria toxoid– or CRM197–containing vaccine<br>• For MenACWY-TT only: severe allergic reaction to a tetanus toxoid-containing vaccine | • Moderate or severe acute illness with or without fever |
| Meningococcal B (MenB) [MenB-4C (Bexsero); MenB-FHbp (Trumenba)] | • Severe allergic reaction (e.g., anaphylaxis) after a previous dose or to a vaccine component[3] | • Pregnancy<br>• For MenB-4C only: Latex sensitivity<br>• Moderate or severe acute illness with or without fever |
| Pneumococcal conjugate (PCV15) | • Severe allergic reaction (e.g., anaphylaxis) after a previous dose or to a vaccine component[3]<br>• Severe allergic reaction (e.g., anaphylaxis) to any diphtheria-toxoid–containing vaccine or to its vaccine component[3] | • Moderate or severe acute illness with or without fever |
| Pneumococcal conjugate (PCV20) | • Severe allergic reaction (e.g., anaphylaxis) after a previous dose or to a vaccine component[3]<br>• Severe allergic reaction (e.g., anaphylaxis) to any diphtheria-toxoid– containing vaccine or to its vaccine component[3] | • Moderate or severe acute illness with or without fever |
| Pneumococcal polysaccharide (PPSV23) | • Severe allergic reaction (e.g., anaphylaxis) after a previous dose or to a vaccine component[3] | • Moderate or severe acute illness with or without fever |
| Tetanus, diphtheria, and acellular pertussis (Tdap)<br>Tetanus, diphtheria (Td) | • Severe allergic reaction (e.g., anaphylaxis) after a previous dose or to a vaccine component[3]<br>• For Tdap only: Encephalopathy (e.g., coma, decreased level of consciousness, prolonged seizures), not attributable to another identifiable cause, within 7 days of administration of previous dose of DTP, DTaP, or Tdap | • Guillain-Barré syndrome (GBS) within 6 weeks after a previous dose of tetanus-toxoid–containing vaccine<br>• History of Arthus-type hypersensitivity reactions after a previous dose of diphtheria-toxoid—containing or tetanus-toxoid– containing vaccine; defer vaccination until at least 10 years have elapsed since the last tetanus-toxoid–containing vaccine<br>• Moderate or severe acute illness with or without fever<br>• For Tdap only: Progressive or unstable neurological disorder, uncontrolled seizures, or progressive encephalopathy until a treatment regimen has been established and the condition has stabilized |
| Varicella (VAR) | • Severe allergic reaction (e.g., anaphylaxis) after a previous dose or to a vaccine component[3]<br>• Severe immunodeficiency (e.g., hematologic and solid tumors, receipt of chemotherapy, congenital immunodeficiency, long- term immunosuppressive therapy or patients with HIV infection who are severely immunocompromised)<br>• Pregnancy<br>• Family history of altered immunocompetence, unless verified clinically or by laboratory testing as immunocompetent | • Recent (≤11 months) receipt of antibody-containing blood product (specific interval depends on product)<br>• Receipt of specific antiviral drugs (acyclovir, famciclovir, or valacyclovir) 24 hours before vaccination (avoid use of these antiviral drugs for 14 days after vaccination)<br>• Use of aspirin or aspirin-containing products<br>• Moderate or severe acute illness with or without fever |
| Zoster recombinant vaccine (RZV) | • Severe allergic reaction (e.g., anaphylaxis) after a previous dose or to a vaccine component[3] | • Moderate or severe acute illness with or without fever<br>• Current herpes zoster infection |

1. When a contraindication is present, a vaccine should NOT be administered. Kroger A, Bahta L, Hunter P. ACIP General Best Practice Guidelines for Immunization. www.cdc.gov/vaccines/hcp/acip-recs/general-recs/contraindications.html
2. When a precaution is present, vaccination should generally be deferred but might be indicated if the benefit of protection from the vaccine outweighs the risk for an adverse reaction. Kroger A, Bahta L, Hunter P. ACIP General Best Practice Guidelines for Immunization. www.cdc.gov/vaccines/hcp/acip-recs/general-recs/contraindications.html
3. Vaccination providers should check FDA-approved prescribing information for the most complete and updated information, including contraindications, warnings, and precautions. Package inserts for U.S.-licensed vaccines are available at www.fda.gov/vaccines-blood-biologics/approved-products/vaccines-licensed-use-united-states.

## References


1. Davis AM, Brown RF, Taylor JL, Epstein RA, McPheeters ML. Transition Care for Children with Special Health Care Needs. Pediatrics. 2014;134(5):900–8.
2. US Preventative services task force. Home page | United States Preventive Services Taskforce [Internet] [cited 2022 Oct 9]. https://www.uspreventiveservicestaskforce.org/uspstf/
3. Adams SH, Park MJ, Twietmeyer L, Brindis CD, Irwin CE Jr. Young adult preventive healthcare: changes in receipt of care pre- to post-affordable care act. J Adolesc Health. 2019;64(6):763–9.
4. Wong CA, Ford CA, French B, Rubin DM. Changes in young adult primary care under the affordable care act. Am J Public Health. 2015;105(Suppl 5):S680–5.
5. Davey A, Asprey A, Carter M, Campbell JL. Trust, negotiation, and communication: young adults' experiences of primary care services. BMC Fam Pract. 2013;14:202.
6. Davey A, Carter M, Campbell JL. Priorities for young adults when accessing UK primary care: literature review. Prim Health Care Res Dev. 2013;14(4):341–9.
7. Guzman A, Bring R, Master S, Rosenthal SL, Soren K. Improving the transition of adolescents from disadvantaged backgrounds from pediatric to adult primary care providers. J Pediatr Nurs. 2021;61:269–74.
8. Clark BA, Veale JF, Greyson D, Saewyc E. Primary care access and foregone care: a survey of transgender adolescents and young adults. Fam Pract. 2018;35(3):302–6.
9. Graves L, Leung S, Raghavendran P, Mennito S. Transitions of care for healthy young adults: promoting primary care and preventive health. South Med J. 2019;112(9):497–9.
10. Medicine SfAHa. Improving integration of behavioral health into primary care for adolescents and young adults. J Adolesc Health. 2020;67(2):302–6.
11. Richardson LP, McCarty CA, Radovic A, Suleiman AB. Research in the integration of behavioral health for adolescents and young adults in primary care settings: a systematic review. J Adolesc Health. 2017;60(3):261–9.
12. Kuo AA, Ciccarelli MR, Sharma N, Lotstein DS. A health care transition curriculum for primary care residents: identifying goals and objectives. Pediatrics. 2018;141(Suppl 4):S346–s54.
13. McManus M, White P, Barbour A, Downing B, Hawkins K, Quion N, et al. Pediatric to adult transi-

tion: a quality improvement model for primary care. J Adolesc Health. 2015;56(1):73–8.
14. Center for Disease Control. Adult immunization schedule by vaccine and age group | CDC [Internet]. 2022 [cited 2022 Oct 20]. https://www.cdc.gov/vaccines/schedules/hcp/imz/adult.html
15. Berkowitz AD. The social norms approach: theory, research and annotated bibliography. Higher Education Center for Alcohol and Other Drug Abuse and Violence Prevention, US Department of Education; 2004.
16. Stout ME, Christy SM, Winger JG, Vadaparampil ST, Mosher CE. Self-efficacy and HPV vaccine attitudes mediate the relationship between social norms and intentions to receive the HPV vaccine among college students. J Community Health. 2020;45:1187–95.
17. Chen MM, Mott N, Clark SJ, et al. HPV vaccination among young adults in the US. JAMA. 2021;325(16):1673–4.
18. Meites E, Szilagyi PG, Chesson HW, Unger ER, Romero JR, Markowitz LE. Human papillomavirus vaccination for adults: updated recommendations of the advisory committee on immunization practices. MMWR Morb Mortal Wkly Rep. 2019;68:698–702.
19. Center for Disease Control. ACIP vaccine information sources guidelines for immunization | CDC [Internet]. 2022 [cited 2022 Oct 9]. https://www.cdc.gov/vaccines/hcp/acip-recs/general-recs/special-situations.html
20. Center for Disease Control. Guidance for evaluating and updating immunizations during the domestic medical examination for newly arrived refugees | immigrant and refugee health | CDC [Internet]. 2022 [cited 2022 Oct 20]. https://www.cdc.gov/immigrantrefugeehealth/guidelines/domestic/immunizations-guidelines.html
21. Center for Disease Control. Chickenpox (Varicella) | Interpreting laboratory tests | CDC [Internet]. 2022 [cited 2022 Oct 20]. https://www.cdc.gov/chickenpox/lab-testing/lab-tests.html
22. Center for Disease Control. Hepatitis B virus resources for health professionals | CDC [Internet]. 2022 [cited 2022 Oct 20]. https://www.cdc.gov/hepatitis/hbv/profresourcesb.htm
23. Center for Disease Control. Ask CDC—vaccines & immunizations | CDC-INFO | CDC [Internet]. 2022 [cited 2022 Oct 9]. https://www.cdc.gov/cdc-info/vaccines-immunizations.html
24. Center for Disease Control. ACIP adverse reactions guidelines for immunization | CDC [Internet]. 2022 [cited 2022 Oct 9]. https://www.cdc.gov/vaccines/hcp/acip-recs/general-recs/adverse-reactions.html
25. Philadelphia TCH of. Vaccine ingredients—gelatin [internet]. The Children's Hospital of Philadelphia; 2014 [cited 2022 Oct 9]. https://www.chop.edu/centers-programs/vaccine-education-center/vaccine-ingredients/gelatin
26. Vaccine Adverse Event Report System. VAERS—FAQs [Internet]. [cited 2022 Oct 9]. https://vaers.hhs.gov/faq.html
27. Health Resources and Service Administration. National Vaccine Injury Compensation Program | HRSA [Internet]. [cited 2022 Oct 9]. https://www.hrsa.gov/vaccine-compensation
28. Recommendations from the National Vaccine Advisory Committee. Standards for adult immunization practice. Public Health Rep. 2014;129(2):115–23.
29. Center for Disease Control. Vaccine Education and Training for Healthcare Professionals | CDC [Internet]. 2022 [cited 2022 Oct 9]. https://www.cdc.gov/vaccines/ed/index.html
30. Center for Biologics Evaluation and Research. Thimerosal and vaccines. FDA [Internet] 2022 Sep 22 [cited 2022 Oct 20]. https://www.fda.gov/vaccines-blood-biologics/safety-availability-biologics/thimerosal-and-vaccines
31. Hollander JE, Carr BG. Virtually perfect? Telemedicine for covid-19. N Engl J Med. 2020;382:1679–81.
32. Centers for Medicare & Medicaid Services. Medicare telemedicine health care provider fact sheet | CMS [Internet]. [cited 2022 Oct 9]. https://www.cms.gov/newsroom/fact-sheets/medicare-telemedicine-health-care-provider-fact-sheet
33. Telehealth HHS. Telehealth and COVID-19 | [Internet]. [cited 2022 Oct 9]. https://telehealth.hhs.gov/patients/telehealth-and-covid/
34. Center for Disease Control. COVID-19: Telemedicine—what does it mean and why should you care? | CDC [Internet]. [cited 2022 Oct 9]. https://www.cdc.gov/coronavirus/2019-ncov/global-covid-19/telemedicine.html
35. Nanda M, Rajesh S. A review of patient satisfaction and experience with telemedicine: a virtual solution during and beyond COVID-19 pandemic. Telemed J E Health. 2021;27(12):1325–31.
36. Drago A, Winding TN, Antypa N. Videoconferencing in psychiatry, a meta-analysis of assessment and treatment. Eur Psychiatry. 2016;36:29–37.
37. Mehrotra A, Chernew M, Linetsky D, Hatch H, Cutler D, Schneider EC. The impact of the COVID-19 pandemic on outpatient care: visits return to prepandemic levels, but not for all providers and patients. 2020. Commonwealth Fund.
38. Center for Disease Control. Mental health—household pulse survey—COVID-19 [Internet]. [cited 2022 Oct 9]. https://www.cdc.gov/nchs/covid19/pulse/mental-health.html
39. Center for Disease Control. Estimates of mental health symptomatology, by month of interview: United States, 2019. 2019;1.
40. American Psychiatric Association. Psychiatry.org—Telepsychiatry toolkit [Internet]. [cited 2022 Oct 20]. https://www.psychiatry.org:443/psychiatrists/practice/telepsychiatry/toolkit
41. Shore J, Yellowlees P, Caudill R, Johnston B, Turvey C, Mishkind M, Krupinski E, Myers K, Shore P, Kaftarian E, Hilty D. Best Practices in Videoconferencing-Based Telemental Health April 2018. Telemed J E Health. 2018;24(11):827–32.

42. Almathami HKY, Win KT, Vlahu-Gjorgievska E. Barriers and facilitators that influence telemedicine-based, real-time, online consultation at patients' homes: systematic literature review. J Med Internet Res. 2020;22(2):e16407.
43. PEW Research Center. Demographics of Internet and Home Broadband Usage in the United States | Pew Research Center [Internet]. 2021 [cited 2022 Oct 9]. https://www.pewresearch.org/internet/fact-sheet/internet-broadband/
44. American Psychological Association. Office and technology checklist for telepsychological services [Internet]. [cited 2022 Oct 9]. https://www.apa.org/practice/programs/dmhi/research-information/telepsychological-services-checklist

# Considerations for Emerging and Young Adults with Chronic Childhood Conditions

5

Nabil Abou Baker, Janet M. Ma, and Susan H. Duan

Emerging adults with chronic childhood conditions have increased medical and psychosocial needs, and without additional support, they may experience worse outcomes compared with other young adults. Emerging adults with complex medical conditions, in general, have lower educational achievement and incomes, and more limited work experience than their peers [1]. Emerging adults with chronic conditions are also at higher risk for developmental difficulties, unnecessary dependency, and psychosocial delay [2]. However, a successful transition to adult health care may help prevent this inequality in outcomes by increasing a sense of personal responsibility, enhancing autonomy, and facilitating self-reliance [2].

Despite the benefit of excellent transition care for these emerging adults, studies have shown that their transition to adult health care is often poor. In one study, only about 20% of young adults were found to have made a successful transition to adult health care. In another, less than 25% of young adults reported that they had received appropriate transition counseling [3]. Rates of these discussions may be even lower among minorities [4]. In general, racial/ethnic minorities and those with problems with access to care or gaps in health insurance may have poorer transition outcomes.

## Patient-Centered Medical Home and Billing

The patient-centered medical home (PCMH) has been promoted as a promising model for care delivery for all patients, in particular adults with chronic childhood-onset conditions. The Maternal and Child Health Bureau (MCHB) core outcome explicitly specifies that children with special health-care needs (SHCN) should "receive services needed for transition to adulthood." [5] The PCMH is a model of primary care transformation that seeks to meet the health-care needs of patients and to improve patient and staff experiences, outcomes, safety, and system efficiency—in other words, to achieve the "Triple Aim" [6]. Health-care transitions have been associated with a well-functioning medical home [7].

The National Committee for Quality Assurance (NCQA), which offers PCMH accreditation, requires six standards for certified PCMHs: (1)

N. Abou Baker (✉)
Department of Medicine, Section of General Internal Medicine, University of Chicago, Chicago, IL, USA
e-mail: naboubaker@bsd.uchicago.edu

J. M. Ma · S. H. Duan
Division of Medicine-Pediatrics and Preventive Medicine, University of California, Los Angeles, CA, USA
e-mail: JanetMa@mednet.ucla.edu; sduan@mednet.ucla.edu


A. A. Kuo et al. (eds.), *Care of Adults with Chronic Childhood Conditions*,
https://doi.org/10.1007/978-3-031-54281-7_5

patient-centered access, (2) team-based care, (3) population health management, (4) care management and support, (5) care coordination and care transitions, and (6) performance measurement and quality improvement. According to the 2011 American Academy of Pediatrics (AAP), American Academy of Family Physicians (AAFP), and American College of Physicians (ACP) Transitions Clinical Report Authoring Group, "planned care, as the product of a partnership among health care professionals, youth, and families, has become an essential characteristic of the primary care medical home" [8].

Creating comprehensive care for patients with chronic diseases often worries physicians regarding billing and payment for services rendered. In the history of the authors of this chapter, they have not experienced any insurance claims denials for transitions of care. Got Transition and the American Academy of Pediatrics have created a billing and coding guide to help physicians accurately document and bill for these essential services [9]. This guide is based on the billing practices of 2021, which may change in the future.

## Chronic Care Model and Other Models of Chronic Disease Care

The chronic care model was developed in Seattle by the Improving Chronic Illness Care program, sponsored by the Robert Wood Johnson Foundation. It is one of the most popular models for comprehensive care of chronic illnesses. It uses a systematic approach to restructure medical care to create partnerships between health systems and communities with the goal of improving interactions between providers and patients, and, in turn, health-care outcomes. There are six areas of emphasis: (1) organization of health care (e.g., removing barriers to care and mobilizing sufficient care resources); (2) community linkages (e.g., creating partnerships with community-based resources and public health agencies); (3) self-management support (e.g., facilitating patient empowerment and skill-based learning); (4) delivery system design (e.g., coordinating and streamlining care processes and workflows); (5) decision support (e.g., providing guidance for providers through the electronic medical records (EMR) and other means to provide evidence- and value-based care); and (6) clinical information systems (e.g., tracking meaningful outcomes and providing feedback to both patients and providers) [10].

Other models have broadened the definition of comprehensive care for chronic conditions. These include the innovative care for chronic conditions (ICCC) model published by the World Health Organization (WHO) [11] and the expanded chronic care model proposed by Barr et al. [12]. These models also incorporate prevention efforts, social determinants of health, and enhanced community participation as core components of chronic disease care [10]. The ICCC also has a larger focus on supporting "positive policy environments" (e.g., partnerships, legislative frameworks, human resource allocation, leadership, and financing) in community and health-care organizations [11].

## Steps for Caring for Adults with Chronic Childhood-Onset Conditions

We here present our interpretation of the ten essential steps for adult primary care physicians (PCPs) accepting care for young adults with chronic childhood-onset conditions to provide them with the excellent, comprehensive care they deserve ("Appendix"). We assume that care takes place in the context of a PCMH that embraces comprehensive chronic disease management as defined by the chronic care model and other models. These steps have been adapted for adult practices from steps for children's practices that serve children with SHCN, such as those created by the national "Got Transition?" campaign.

### Step 1: Health-Care Policy Statement

The first step for a practice that will be caring for adults with a chronic childhood-onset condition is developing a written health-care policy statement for the transition and future care of the young adult. Attention to care transitions is an explicit part of the National Committee for Quality Assurance (NCQA) PCMH designation. This health-care policy should be developed with input from young adults transitioning to adulthood. Ideally, it may also be developed jointly with children's practices from which the adult practice often accepts transitioning patients. The policy should explicitly state the practice's expectations of the young transitioning adults and their families and describe the practice's transition and future care process.

After the policy is developed, all practice staff should be educated and trained regarding its implementation, including the specific roles of the patient, the family, and the health-care team members. The policy should be prominently displayed and readily available to patients and their families. A sample policy statement is available at the www.gottransition.org.

## Step 2: Tracking and Monitoring: Utilizing Clinical Information Systems

As specified in the chronic care model, practices should use clinical information systems to improve their practice [10]. Performance measurement and quality improvement are also part of NCQA PCMH accreditation. All transitioning young adults should be entered into a registry with tracking of data related to the achievement of a successful transition. Each pediatric and adult practice should develop its own measures to define success, such as completion of each step of the transition process and improvement in relevant patient disease outcomes. It should also include measures addressing social determinants of the patient's health (see Step 8).

For each patient, the registry should be used to track the young adults' progress and health status. If possible, this registry data should be incorporated into the EMR. This registry will enable the "empanelment" of patients. This means linking each patient to a care team and PCP [13]. In turn, this enables each physician and team to later engage in population health management (see Step 10). With the use of population health management systems, the care team will be able to better track patients as they progress through the transition. This will, in turn, empower practices to easily establish Plan, Do, Study, and Act cycles to improve care.

## Step 3: Transition Readiness Assessment and Goal-Setting

A transition readiness assessment should be conducted before the young adult transitions from the children's practice to the adult practice. Ideally, these assessments would have been performed at least yearly beginning no later than age 14 (www.gottransition.org), but this may not be within the practice's control. For a child whose illness began after the age of 14, catch-up will be needed to ensure a smooth transition of care.

The assessment should include an evaluation of competencies for self-care; insurance status with regard to eligibility for adult services; entitlements and guardianship; cultural and religious preferences; and young adult's ability to perform self-care management tasks, such as manage medications, keep appointments, track health issues, discuss their care with providers, manage their lifestyle choices, and perform other transition-related activities. There are several validated transition tools available, such as the Transition Readiness Assessment Questionnaire (TRAQ). It is imperative to assess social determinants of health and barriers that may impact the child's readiness [14, 15]. It is also important to tailor this care to the appropriate dependence and ability level of the patient.

Perhaps, the most important part of the transition process is the development of goals for successful health care. These goals should be developed collaboratively between the health-care team, young adult, and family. These goals again will ideally be created by the young adult's pediatric practice but regardless will need to be (re-) addressed by the accepting adult practice. These goals should be individualized based on factors identified during the readiness assessment, such as the young adult's medical status, intellectual ability, independence and future functioning goals, and guardianship status [8]. Goals should be set with regard to future functional status, employment, romantic relationships, and end-of-life care [8].

This time is also an opportunity to encourage the young adult to begin to assume more responsibility for his/her health care if he or she has not already [16]. The physician should attempt to ensure that the young adult understands his/her condition and medications, and, if parents are still closely involved, work with them to gradually release responsibility to their young adult. If the young adult is with his or her parents at the initial visit, physicians should also meet privately with the young adult, with the goal of encouraging their independence, if developmentally appropriate.

## Step 4: Written Health-Care Plan

For each young adult transitioning to adult care, a written health-care plan should be developed. The basic structure and elements of this plan should be standardized by each practice. However, every plan should be customized and adapted to each patient's unique needs [8]. Like the readiness assessment, this plan should ideally be initiated by the pediatric practice no later than age 14; [17] however, it again will need to be (re-)addressed and customized by the adult practice. Once transition goals have been created (see Step 3), the written plan should contain a list of prioritized actions to achieve these goals. Each action should have a process and time deadline for completion. Actions will need to be taken in many areas, including but not limited to the following categories.

### Creation of Health-Care Team

Team-based care is an essential element of the PCMH (see Step 6). Health-care team members need to be explicitly identified, including, most importantly, a point person for the young adult's care. The ideal point person is located in the accepting adult PCP's practice and can work closely with this physician. This person should act as an advocate and primary contact for the young adult and his/her family in navigating the transition process [2].

The point person and the physician cannot care for the patient alone. Advanced PCMH practices involve many others, particularly in the care of complex patients such as young adults with chronic childhood-onset conditions. These might include nutritionists/dieticians, pharmacists, behavioral health workers or psychiatrists, social workers, care managers, and even peer health coaches. Each care team will need to be customized to the needs of the patient and the environment and resources of the primary care practice.

Adult specialty physicians will also likely need to be identified and plans made to coordinate with these physicians and their practices (see Step 7). A plan should be made as well for where to receive same-day/urgent care, emergency care, and any inpatient tertiary care. It is helpful to review with the young adult or caregiver which medical situations merit emergency room visitation versus clinic phone calls or appointments.

### Insurance

The patient's insurance status should be scrutinized to ensure that care with all planned adult providers as well as any emergency care will be covered. If not, new providers may need to be selected or new insurance obtained. Patients and their families may need assistance in this process from a social worker or other community resources. Ideally, this insurance would also reimburse the new adult providers for transition planning and care coordination [17]. If applicable, care teams should check with state insurance providers (for example, Medicaid insurers) regarding changes in eligibility at ages 18–21 to ensure ongoing coverage as well as changes at age 26 for those patients utilizing parental insurance.

### Guardianship

For families of young adults with intellectual disabilities, it is important to plan early to address guardianship issues. The legal age of majority in most states is 18 years. The Health Insurance

Portability and Accountability Act (HIPAA) dictates that a physician cannot release information about a patient over 18 without the patient's express consent, regardless of the intellectual level or communication abilities of the patient [16]. Therefore, parents should be informed that when their young adult becomes 18, they will not be able to be given health information about their adult child without his or her consent or legal guardianship. There are less restrictive forms of guardianship that can provide specific decision-making support while not completely denying the young adult's participation in that decision. Families will need assistance deciding which form of guardianship best meets their needs and then pursuing it. Planning for decision-making support is best started at least by age 17 and resulting changes need to be documented in the medical record and communicated to new adult team members. For more details, please see Chap. 60 of this book.

### Culturally and Religiously Appropriate

Great care should be taken to ensure that the health-care goals, and corresponding actions are sensitive to cultural and religious practices and beliefs. For example, the emergency care plan may need to specify certain measures that are not to be taken, e.g., blood transfusions. Patient or family beliefs or preferences, such as preferred degree of involvement in decision-making and method and frequency of contact, and characteristics, such as their health-care literacy and level of understanding of the child's chronic condition(s), should be considered, and accommodations written into the health-care plan.

Social complexity, either alone or in combination with chronic medical conditions, is the source of many disparities in care for minority populations including those with cultural and language differences, immigrant and refugee populations, lesbian, gay, bisexual, transgender, and queer (LGBTQ+) youth, and families as well as youth affected by poverty and housing insecurity. Specific resources such as engagement of culturally similar peers, use of family navigators and community health workers, and involvement of local schools and community centers may help enhance the transition process for these young adults [18].

### Update Process

With each interaction, and no less than yearly, the young adult's primary care provider and the remainder of the health-care team should reevaluate the healthcare plan. Considering potential changes in the child's medical and social status, the plan should be updated as appropriate [17]. Any patient or family concerns may also warrant revision of the health-care plan.

## Step 5: Transfer of Care

Transition to adult care should occur when appropriate based upon a young adult's developmental level, medical status, and relevant policy/licensing requirements, e.g., age of transition from pediatric practices. Youth with special health-care needs often experience multiple transitions from pediatric care to less resource-rich adult health systems, for instance, with a variety of specialist physicians and with care coordination and social services which may be less available in an adult care setting. This necessitates flexibility in the age of transfer to adult care, possible delayed scheduling of specialist physician transfers, condition-specific protocols, and greater care coordination support [18]. Whenever possible, patients should only be transferred when medically stable, and the adult primary care provider should confirm acceptance of care of the young adult with the childhood primary care provider's team. A pretransfer visit to the adult practice may also be advised in the year before the transfer of care [8].

The accepting adult practice should ensure that they have all relevant previous medical information to assume care of the young adult. This should include the child's complete medical records, which may require obtaining a release of medical information, as well as an updated medical summary prepared by the childhood provider's health-care team. This medical summary should include all information relevant to the patient's present medical care and social situation. A copy should also be given to the family. There should also be a direct handoff of care between the childhood primary care provider and the accepting adult PCP, either in person or by phone [8] A similar handoff between present and future point persons, if not the PCPs, should also occur.

The adult practice should ensure that there is an emergency care plan, and if needed a condition fact sheet and appropriate legal documents, such as those detailing guardianship. The adult primary care provider should share this information with any adult specialists as well. Examples of a transition action plan, portable medical summary, and emergency care plan are available at www.gottransition.org.

Someone from the accepting adult primary care practice health-care team should contact the childhood primary care provider within 3 months of the transition to confirm that the transition of care has been successful. Feedback should also be elicited from the pediatric practice on the transfer process to improve and streamline this transition process for subsequent patients. Ideally, ongoing collaborative partnerships may be forged between childhood and adult providers. Practices should also ask patients and their families for feedback on their experience with the transfer process. The health-care team, both pediatric and adult, should engage in quality improvement processes to improve this transfer process for patients (see Step 10).

## Step 6: Team-Based Care

Once the health-care team has been created and the transition of care made, great attention should be paid to providing excellent, organized team-based care going forward. Clear roles for team members (physicians, nurses or medical assistants, administrative assistants, care coordinators, social workers, etc.) should be established. Ideally, roles should be constructed such that each individual is practicing "at the top of his/her license." All team members should be able to coordinate with each other. Optimally, this will involve frequent communication, both in person and via the EMR. Huddles—that is quick in-person meetings at the beginning/end of the day or even before/after individual patient visits—are one common excellent practice to make sure that all team members are on the same page. All members should also be empowered to do their jobs individually. This may include standing orders from physicians to enable nonphysician staff to complete tasks such as ordering routine labs or changing medications/dosages [13]. There will need to be frequent reflection to ensure workflows are optimized among team members. This is a key part of delivery system design under the chronic care model [10].

## Step 7: Care Coordination

In particular for young adults with chronic childhood-onset conditions, attention should be paid to the process of continued seamless coordination with specialists, who may also be transitioning from pediatric to adult providers. Care plans or patient data registries may need to be developed to share among these providers, and there may need to be planning for coordinated visits with multiple specialists and other activities of "chronic condition management" [8]. For patients with multiple adult providers, the medical summary should be shared (digitally if possible) among them to aid in the coordination of care [17]. A shared document in the EMR may be the ideal mechanism for this if all providers have access [19]. Otherwise, more traditional means such as faxing records and phone calls may be needed to coordinate care.

Communication is crucial between all care team members, including the primary care physician and specialty physicians. It is ideal to keep a list of available adult primary care and specialty care physicians familiar with complex transition patients, in line with recommendations by the Six Core Elements from Got Transition [20].

While traditionally primary care physicians referred to specialists, specialty physicians may also want to refer any of their patients without current primary care physicians to a trusted adult PCP with experience taking care of young adults with chronic childhood-onset conditions to help optimize their healthcare.

The PCP and his/her health-care team should put forethought into what situations necessitate consultation or referral to specialty providers. Ideally, the PCP should obtain relevant diagnostic studies before referral, preventing the need for unnecessary repeat specialty visits. With the rise of telemedicine (TM) visits, TM visits may be much easier for patients with chronic conditions and their families to attend. However, certain types of visits may necessitate physical exams or in-office procedures. Similar thought should be put into referral to tertiary or emergency care. If such care is necessary, the adult practice should be sure to provide extra support upon discharge to prevent readmission. Some academic centers have Evaluation and Treatment Centers, and high acuity urgent care that help prevent unnecessary ED visits and hospitalizations. It would be ideal to work closely with a case manager in the practice whose main function is managing this care coordination.

## Step 8: Address the Social Determinants of Health

The social determinants of health are everything that affects a person's health besides their actual disease process, i.e., where he/she lives, works, eats, and plays. These social determinants may have up to five times greater impact on health outcomes than medical care alone.

To address the social determinants of health, practices need to assess patient's needs with regard to income, housing, education, access to food, etc. Then, when issues are identified, patients need to be connected to resources to address these issues. Just as important as a connection to resources within the health-care system is the connection to resources in the community. Recall that the foundation of the chronic care model is the partnership between health systems and communities [10]. As more recent models for comprehensive management of chronic disease, such as the ICCC, have noted, community participation is essential to address the social determinants of health. Studies have shown that the biggest determinants of health for adolescents globally are national wealth, income inequality, and access to education [21]. Other important factors include safe and supportive families, safe and supportive schools, as well as positive and supportive peers [21].

Each practice will need to identify relevant community resources in their community. These may include such varied resources as job training programs, legal resources, insurance assistance offices, food kitchens, goodwill stores, etc. A social worker may be a good person to start with to help patients connect to these resources; however, all members of the health-care team should see it as their job to address these issues. A shared digital list/map of resources may be an ideal way to track these services, and each team member can contribute to this list as they learn about new resources. This may involve a substantial culture shift within the PCP's practice.

## Step 9: Self-Management Support

Young adult patients should be empowered to become managers of their own health. To do so requires support and education in self-care. Diabetes is an excellent example. Research has shown that diabetes self-management education (DSME) that teaches patients how to manage their diabetes can dramatically improve diabetes control. There are now national standards for DSME, including skill-based education on using medications safely and effectively; preventing, detecting, and treating acute and chronic complications; physical activity and nutrition; and personal strategies to address psychosocial issues. While there may not be national standards for all chronic childhood-onset conditions, the same principles should be expanded to help aging young adults successfully manage their own health. This may take many forms, including group classes, online modules, videos, or one-on-one tutorials. Doing regular transition assessment questionnaires would help identify the gaps for each patient, and the care team can then provide age-appropriate resources for each patient. The

Got Transition website has many helpful tools and resources to help adolescents take charge of their own health [20].

## Step 10: Population Health Management & Continuous Improvement

The final step of successful care for adults with childhood-onset chronic conditions is population health management. This is again an essential element of the PCMH as well as a core element of the Triple Aim. Population health was initially defined by Kindig and Stoddart [22] as "the health outcomes of a group of individuals, including the distribution of such outcomes within the group." Now, though, it has come to mean much more, including (1) addressing not only health but social determinants of health, (2) focusing not just on treatment but on prevention, and (3) assuming shared responsibility as a health-care team for patient outcomes [23]. Population health management is enabled by clinical information systems (See Step 3).

Using the patient data established in Step 3, the health-care team should periodically and continually reflect on the performance of all of their patients, regardless of whether or not these patients have scheduled visits upcoming. As mentioned, data should include disease measures as well as measures of social determinants of health. Data should be relevant to both providers and patients and, therefore, include both process and outcome measures. Practices should reflect on their performance and seek to improve it. This improvement should happen continuously using quality improvement methodologies, such as plan–do–study–act cycles. Quality improvement is the final necessary element of a PCMH. To improve performance, practices will need to work on improving all aspects of their practice, including steps 6–9. A few examples of such Healthcare Transition-related Quality Improvement projects and collaboration are found in these references [24, 25].

## Conclusions

Young adults with childhood-onset chronic conditions are at increased risk for poor developmental and health outcomes, and, therefore, ensuring that they receive excellent transition services, and then, excellent adult care is even more important than for other young adults. Excellent care for such patients requires (1) developing a health-care policy statement; (2) utilizing clinical information systems to track and monitor patient outcomes; (3) conducting transition readiness assessments and goal-setting; (4) written, comprehensive health-care planning; (5) transferring of care; (6) team-based care; (7) care coordination; (8) addressing social determinants of health; (9) self-management support; and (10) population health management and quality improvement. By implementing these steps, adult providers can achieve better, more equitable outcomes for young adults with childhood-onset chronic conditions.

## Appendix

| 10 Steps for caring for adults with chronic childhood-onset conditions |
|---|
| 1. Health-care policy statement<br>• written, posted, and readily available<br>• developed with the input of young adults and their families<br>• educate and train all health-care staff<br>• discuss with all entering young adults |
| 2. Tracking and monitoring<br>• data on all patients, including the detailed status of each individual<br>• measures of disease status and social determinants<br>• use for iterative improvement<br>• ideally integrate into the EMR |
| 3. Readiness assessment/goal-setting<br>• use a validated questionnaire<br>• address: Self-care, insurance, guardianship, culture/religion, self-management, etc.<br>• develop goals for functional status, employment, romantic relationships, end-of-life care |

| 10 Steps for caring for adults with chronic childhood-onset conditions |
|---|
| 4. Written health-care plan includes:<br>• creation of health-care team<br>• insurance<br>• guardianship<br>• cultural/religious beliefs<br>• update process |
| 5. Transfer of care<br>• time when appropriate<br>• obtain all relevant medical info<br>• obtain direct handoff |
| 6. Team-based care<br>• clear roles, top of license<br>• empowered<br>• frequent communication and reflection |
| 7. Care coordination<br>• criteria for referral and escalation or care<br>• communication, especially via EMR<br>• consider case manager |
| 8. Address social determinants of health<br>• screen for income, food, housing, etc.<br>• connect with internal and community-based resources |
| 9. Self-management support<br>• educate patients for self-care |
| 10. Population health management and quality improvement<br>• monitor performance measures on all patients<br>• use quality improvement strategies to continually improve |

## References


1. Bloom SR, Kuhlthau K, Van Cleave J, Knapp AA, Newacheck P, Perrin JM. Health care transition for youth with special health care needs. J Adolesc Health. 2012;51(3):213–9.
2. Rosen DS, Blum RW, Britto M, Sawyer SM, Siegel DM. Transition to adult health care for adolescents and young adults with chronic conditions. J Adolesc Health. 2003;33(4):309–11.
3. Sawicki GS, Lukens-Bull K, Yin X, Demars N, Huang IC, Livingood W, et al. Measuring the transition readiness of youth with special healthcare needs: validation of the TRAQ—transition readiness assessment questionnaire. J Pediatr Psychol. 2011;36(2):160–71.
4. Eilenberg JS, Paff M, Harrison AJ, Long KA. Disparities based on race, ethnicity, and socioeconomic status over the transition to adulthood among adolescents and young adults on the autism Spectrum: a systematic review. Curr Psychiatry Rep. 2019;21(5):32.
5. Center DR. Data Sheet: Maternal and Child Health Bureau's Core Outcomes for CSHCN [Internet]. cahmi.org: The Child and Adolescent Health Measurement Initiative. [cited 2022 Oct 1]. https://cahmi.org
6. Jackson GL, Powers BJ, Chatterjee R, Prvu Bettger J, Kemper AR, Hasselblad V, et al. The patient-centered medical home: a systematic review. Ann Intern Med. 2013;158(3):169.
7. Ilango SM, Lebrun-Harris LA, Jones JR, McManus MA, Cyr M, Mann MY, et al. Associations between health care transition preparation among youth in the U.S. and other components of a well-functioning system of services. J Adolesc Health. 2021;69(3):414–23.
8. Cooley WC, Sagerman PJ, American Academy of Pediatrics, American Academy of Family Physicians, American College of Physicians, Transitions Clinical Report Authoring Group. Supporting the health care transition from adolescence to adulthood in the medical home. Pediatrics. 2011;128(1):182–200.
9. McManus M, White P, Schmidt A, Slade R, Salus T, Bradley J. Coding and payment tip sheet for transition from pediatric to adult. Health Care. 2021;2021(2):33.
10. Stellefson M, Dipnarine K, Stopka C. The chronic care model and diabetes management in US primary care settings: a systematic review. Prev Chronic Dis. 2013;10:120180.
11. World Health Organization, editor. Innovative care for chronic conditions: building blocks for action: global report. Geneva: World Health Organization; 2002. 112 p.
12. Barr V, Robinson S, Marin-Link B, Underhill L, Dotts A, Ravensdale D, et al. The expanded chronic care model: an integration of concepts and strategies from population health promotion and the chronic care model. hcq. 2003;7(1):73–82.
13. Bodenheimer T, Ghorob A, Willard-Grace R, Grumbach K. The 10 building blocks of high-performing primary care. Ann Fam Med. 2014;12(2):166–71.
14. Gray WN, Schaefer MR, Resmini-Rawlinson A, Wagoner ST. Barriers to transition from pediatric to adult care: a systematic review. J Pediatr Psychol. 2018;43(5):488–502.
15. Jones C, Ritchwood TD, Taggart T. Barriers and facilitators to the successful transition of adolescents living with HIV from pediatric to adult care in low and middle-income countries: a systematic review and policy analysis. AIDS Behav. 2019;23(9):2498–513.
16. Lemly DC, Weitzman ER, O'Hare K. Advancing healthcare transitions in the medical home: tools for providers, families and adolescents with special healthcare needs. Curr Opin Pediatr. 2013;25(4):439–46.
17. American Academy of Pediatrics, American Academy of Family Physicians, American College of Physicians-American Society of Internal Medicine. A consensus statement on health care transitions for young adults with special health care needs. Pediatrics. 2002;110(6 Pt 2):1304–6.

18. White PH, Cooley WC, Transitions Clinical Report Authoring Group, American Academy of Pediatrics, American Academy of Family Physicians, American College of Physicians, et al. Supporting the health care transition from adolescence to adulthood in the medical home. Pediatrics. 2018;142(5):e20182587.
19. Chouteau WA, Allen SR. Implementation of a portable medical summary for adolescents and young adults with medical complexity in transition to adult health care. J Pediatr Nurs. 2019;48:35–41.
20. White P, Schmidt A, Shorr J, Ilango S, Beck D, McManus M, et al. Six core elements of health care transition 3.0.; 2020.
21. Viner RM, Ozer EM, Denny S, Marmot M, Resnick M, Fatusi A, et al. Adolescence and the social determinants of health. Lancet. 2012;379(9826):1641–52.
22. Kindig D, Stoddart G. What is population health? Am J Public Health. 2003;93(3):380–3.
23. Bostic RW, Thornton RLJ, Rudd EC, Sternthal MJ. Health in all policies: the role of the US Department of Housing And Urban Development and present and future challenges. Health Aff. 2012;31(9):2130–7.
24. Jones MR, Hooper TJ, Cuomo C, Crouch G, Hickam T, Lestishock L, et al. Evaluation of a health care transition improvement process in seven large health care systems. J Pediatr Nurs. 2019;47:44–50.
25. McManus M, White P, Barbour A, Downing B, Hawkins K, Quion N, et al. Pediatric to adult transition: a quality improvement model for primary care. J Adolesc Health. 2015;56(1):73–8.

# Part III

# Sexual Health

# Sexual and Reproductive Health 6

Tara Harris, Elizabeth Harper, and Jennifer M. LeComte

## Abbreviations

| | |
|---|---|
| ACIP | Advisory Committee on Immunization Practices |
| ACOG | American College of Obstetricians and Gynecologists |
| ACP | American College of Physicians |
| ACS | American Cancer Society |
| AED | Antiepileptic drug |
| ASCCP | American Society of Colposcopy and Cervical Pathology |
| CDC | Centers for Disease Control and Prevention |
| CIN | Cervical intraepithelial neoplasia |
| DES | Diethylstilbestrol |
| DMPA | Depot medroxyprogesterone acetate |
| HCV | Hepatitis C virus |
| HIV | Human immunodeficiency virus |
| HPV | Human papillomavirus |
| IUD | Intrauterine device |
| NTD | Neural tube defects |
| PSA | Prostate-specific antigen |
| SGO | Society of Gynecologic Oncology |
| STI | Sexually transmitted infection |
| USPSTF | United States Preventative Services Task Force |
| VTE | Venous thromboembolism |

T. Harris (✉)
Department of Obstetrics and Gynecology, Baylor College of Medicine, Houston, TX, USA
e-mail: tjharris@bcm.edu

E. Harper
Baylor College of Medicine, Houston, TX, USA
e-mail: elizabeth.harper@bcm.edu

J. M. LeComte
Philadelphia College of Osteopathic Medicine, Philadelphia, PA, USA
e-mail: lecomte@rowan.edu

## Sexual Health and Education

Comprehensive reproductive health-care and sexual education are essential components in the proper care and well-being of all persons. Unfortunately, standards of care are often unmet, and counseling on these subjects is withheld from patients with physical and intellectual disabilities. All persons are equally entitled to the full spectrum of reproductive healthcare and education as their individual needs require. Providers should approach every reproductive health visit, whether it is for routine screening or for specific concerns, with respect for patients' maturity, autonomy, dignity, and sexual identity. Patients with disabilities may present with frustrating histories of feeling dismissed, infantilized, or uninformed about their reproductive health. Their concerns and experiences should be treated seriously, and they should be addressed factually and respectfully. Although all patients should be given the opportunity to be interviewed alone if caregivers or others are present, the clinician can


A. A. Kuo et al. (eds.), *Care of Adults with Chronic Childhood Conditions*,
https://doi.org/10.1007/978-3-031-54281-7_6

also provide an appropriate framework for addressing these concerns in a mature and normalizing manner.

Any combination of a variety of distractions and misconceptions can hinder patients' access to standard reproductive healthcare and education. For patients with complex medical needs, focusing on more immediate concerns may lead to a prolonged delay of reproductive anticipatory guidance and screening. Among both the general public and many health-care professionals, assumptions abound regarding the sexuality of persons with disabilities, ranging from asexual and childlike to overly touchy and hypersexual. The initial reproductive health-focused visit may, therefore, reveal an assortment of perceptions, experiences, and questions regarding sexuality among patients with chronic conditions. Discrepancies between perceived intellectual levels and chronological age may hinder discussions regarding the complex development of sexuality. Neglect of these topics and denial of a patient's sexual desires and practices does not prevent their exploration but rather impedes the safety of such.

Patients with physical disabilities may particularly feel a long history of dismissal and frustration regarding sexual concerns. They may present with questions over an array of topics that some providers do not commonly encounter, such as sexual positioning, the ability to achieve orgasm, or management of incontinence during sexual activity. Providers and patients should speak collaboratively about what practices work and do not work for individual patients and address these concerns comprehensively and concretely.

The standard of care is also often unmet for basic reproductive health exams and screening in this population. These exams are by nature sensitive, invasive, and uncomfortable for all patients, and the additional reluctance to invade the personal boundaries of a patient with a variable range of understanding and ability to consent may hinder care. Providers and caregivers may erroneously believe that these patients are sheltered from both consensual and nonconsensual sexual activity, and subsequently disregard standard screening practices. Therefore, regardless of a patient's history of frequent or complex medical visits, providers should neither assume nor take for granted that routine reproductive healthcare and guidance have been addressed.

## Well-Woman Visits and Pelvic Examinations

Traditionally, the well-woman visit is an annual appointment with a primary care provider that is devoted to screening, counseling, and prevention of disease. Although any type of primary care provider can provide this care, visits with obstetricians/gynecologists typically focus more on reproductive health topics rather than the wider range of preventative health services [1, 2]. Women with disabilities are entitled to the same services at the same intervals as the general population; however, they often encounter barriers when seeking reproductive healthcare. Due to a fundamental lack of understanding or inaccessibility, patients may be turned away from providers who are ill-equipped to accommodate the different challenges that women with disabilities face. Clinicians may make assumptions about a patient's sexual needs and practices based on their disabilities and, therefore, not offer the same level of screening and counseling customarily provided at these visits. It befits clinicians, patients, and caregivers to recognize the unique obstacles to reproductive healthcare faced by women with disabilities and proactively address them.

Mobility issues may impede proper reproductive healthcare and examination. Facilities may be unable to accommodate patients needing assistance with transfer onto examination tables, or they may not have equipment that allows for such. Most reproductive health-care providers are also used to performing pelvic examinations in the traditional dorsal lithotomy position using stirrups; however, some women with disabilities are physically unable to be in that position, may be unable to support their legs on stirrups, or dorsal lithotomy might even increase a patient's spasticity. Common alternative positions include supine with knees opened to the side in a diamond-shaped or "frog leg" position; laying on one's side with hips and knees flexed as able in a version of the fetal position; and a modified pike position, where the patient lies supine and she or an assistant holds the legs upwards as tolerated. The latter two modified positions allow for examination without leg abduction and may be specifically useful for patients with spasticity, such as those with cerebral palsy.

During a gynecological exam or procedure, women with acquired or congenital spinal cord lesions (e.g., spina bifida) may experience autonomic dysreflexia. This occurs when the nervous system attempts to communicate painful stimuli up the spinal cord, is blocked by the lesion, and then triggers a reflex response of drastically increased blood pressure. While the patient does not detect the pain, the uncoordinated response by their sympathetic nervous system can lead to a sudden and potentially lethal situation. Signs and symptoms of autonomic dysreflexia include severe headache, hypertension, diaphoresis, arrhythmia, nausea, skin flushing, piloerection, congestion, and restlessness [3]. If a patient with a spinal cord lesion develops vital sign changes or any signs of discomfort during pelvic exams or procedures, the stimulus should be withdrawn gently but rapidly, and attention directed to patient stabilization.

## Cervical Cancer Screening

With proper screening, cervical cancer is the easiest female cancer to prevent or detect early. Cervical cancer screening, also known as the "Pap smear," is a critical component of the well-woman visit. Although women with disabilities are just as likely as the general population to get cervical cancer, there is evidence that they are less likely to receive the recommended screening [4]. Screening guidelines are regularly updated based on emerging evidence, and numerous stakeholder organizations contribute to the process. Different organizations may endorse different guidelines, and it is fundamental for providers to understand the goals of the involved organizations when determining which guidelines to follow. The current guidelines for cervical cancer screenings (Table 6.1) as established by the United States Preventative Services Task Force (USPSTF) have been endorsed by the American Society of Colposcopy and Cervical Pathology (ASCCP), the American College of Obstetricians and Gynecologists (ACOG), and the Society of Gynecologic Oncology (SGO). These guidelines apply to all persons with a cervix regardless of sexual activity or previous human papillomavirus (HPV) vaccination. The screening guidelines do not apply to persons with signs or symptoms of cervical cancer or to those with a higher-than-average risk of cervical cancer, specifically persons with a previous history of high-grade dysplasia, immunocompromised individuals, and those who were exposed in utero to diethylstilbestrol (DES) [5].

For patients at an average risk of cervical cancer, the USPSTF does not recommend cervical cancer screenings prior to age 21. For patients aged 21–29 years without previous

**Table 6.1** USPTFS cervical cancer screening guidelines

| Population | Recommendation |
|---|---|
| Age <21 | No screening |
| Age 21–29 | Cytology alone every 3 years |
| Age 30–65 | Cytology alone every 3 years<br>or<br>FDA-approved primary high-risk HPV screening every 5 years<br>or<br>Cytology and high-risk HPV co-testing every 5 years |
| Age >65 | Discontinue screening following adequate negative prior results[a] |
| Status post hysterectomy with removal of cervix | Discontinue screening in patients with no history of high-grade dysplasia |

[a]Defined as three negative cytology results, two negative cytology and high-risk HPV co-testing results, or two negative high-risk HPV screenings with appropriate intervals within the 10 years preceding screening discontinuation

abnormal screenings, cytology alone every 3 years is sufficient. As of this writing, the USPSTF does not recommend initial screening of patients aged 21–29 via high-risk HPV (hrHPV) testing due to the risk of unnecessary intervention, as it will most likely resolve spontaneously without long-term adverse effects. For patients aged 30–65 years with no history of abnormal Pap tests, any of the three following options are acceptable: cytology alone every 3 years, FDA-approved hrHPV testing every 5 years, or cytology plus hrHPV co-testing every 5 years. Cervical cancer screening is not recommended for patients older than 65 if they have adequate prior negative screenings and are at average risk of cervical cancer. Screening pap smears are also not recommended for patients who have undergone hysterectomy with removal of the cervix without a history of high-grade dysplasia.

## Management of Abnormal Cervical Cancer Screening

Abnormal test results prompt further investigation depending on a patient's age, results, and history. The recommendations for the management of abnormal cervical cancer screenings were set by the ASCCP in conjunction with other stakeholder organizations. Published in 2019, the most current iteration of recommendations is based on an individualized assessment of the immediate risk of CIN 3+ as determined by a patient's history, any previous testing, and current results. This is a departure from the prior recommendations which considered the results in isolation and were more algorithm based. As stated in the executive summary of the 2019 guidelines, "With a more nuanced understanding of how previous results affect risk, and more variables to consider," the 2019 guidelines further align management recommendations with the current understanding of HPV natural history and cervical carcinogenesis [6]. The ASCCP guidelines for risk-based management of abnormal cervical screening results can be found through their website, www.asccp.org [7].

## HPV Vaccination

Vaccination against HPV remains one of the most effective methods to prevent cervical and other HPV-associated cancers. Since the introduction of the HPV vaccine into the US population in 2006, the rates of HPV-related infection and cervical precancers have dropped significantly, including an estimated 81% reduction in infections with the HPV types that cause most HPV-related cancers and genital warts among young adult women [8]. Although the vaccine is ideally administered at 11–12 years of age, it is approved in the USA for persons aged 9–45. Vaccination is recommended for patients aged 9–26 regardless of sexual activity or prior HPV exposure. For patients aged 9–14, the recommendations are two doses spaced 6–12 months apart. Patients with weakened immune systems or those who start the series at age 15 or later should receive three doses at 1–2 then 6 months after the first dose. If a dose is given early, it will need to be repeated to achieve optimum immunogenicity; however, doses do not need to be repeated should the vaccine series be interrupted. For persons aged 27–45 years, health-care professionals should discuss an individual's risk of new HPV infection and employ shared decision-making regarding the protection offered by the vaccine.

Since 2006, three forms of the HPV vaccine have been approved in the USA: a bivalent (Cervarix), a quadrivalent (Gardasil), and a 9-valent (Gardasil 9). Since 2016, only the 9-valent has been distributed in the USA. All three of these vaccines protect against HPV 16 and 18, which are the most common causes of HPV-related cancers in the USA [9]. In cases where the vaccine series was interrupted, any licensed form of the HPV vaccine is acceptable for series completion in female patients. The bivalent vaccine was never approved for use in males in the USA; thus, if there is suspicion that a male received the bivalent vaccine, then the series needs to be restarted with either the quadrivalent or 9-valent vaccine [9]. Outside of that specific circumstance, neither ACOG nor the Advisory Committee on Immunization

Practices (ACIP) routinely recommends revaccination with the 9-valent vaccine for patients who received the other versions of the HPV vaccine [9, 10].

## Sexually Transmitted Infection Screening

Recommendations for routine sexually transmitted infection (STI) screening are based on patient age, history, and risk factors. STIs may present with symptoms, or patients may be completely asymptomatic until advanced disease or severe complications have developed. Patients with sensory deficits and intellectual disabilities may face additional challenges in detecting symptoms that might otherwise be alarming in the general population.

The Centers for Disease Control and Prevention (CDC) recommends annual screening for gonorrhea and chlamydia in all sexually active women up to age 25 [11]. For men and women aged 25 and older, providers should assess STI risk factors and employ shared decision-making regarding testing for chlamydia and gonorrhea. Screening for trichomoniasis is based on a patient's history and risk factors. Testing for gonorrhea, chlamydia, and trichomoniasis is done either via urine testing or a vaginal swab. The swab is small, widely well-tolerated, and can be collected by patients or caregivers if preferred.

Screening for the human immunodeficiency virus (HIV), hepatitis B, hepatitis C, and syphilis is done through blood testing. The CDC endorses a minimum of at least one lifetime HIV screening for patients between ages 13 and 64 [11]. They also recommend at least one lifetime screening for hepatitis C for adults aged 18 and older except in settings where the prevalence of HCV infection is less than 0.1% [11]. Patients with additional risk factors should have more frequent testing for these conditions as indicated. Additional screening for hepatitis B and syphilis is based on patient preference, risk factors, history, and concurrent conditions, such as pregnancy or immunosuppression.

## Breast Cancer Screening

Breast cancer education and screening are also critical components of the annual well-woman exam. For women in the United States, breast cancer is the most commonly diagnosed cancer and the second-leading cause of cancer deaths [12]. The rates of breast cancer do not differ between women with disabilities and those without. Importantly, several risk factors for breast cancer have increased prominence among women with disabilities, including nulliparity, obesity, decreased physical activity, higher than average exposure to chest radiation, and use of some forms of menstrual suppression therapy. Despite these considerations, women with disabilities are less likely than the general population to receive screening via mammogram at the recommended intervals. They are also more likely to have an advanced tumor at diagnosis and have a higher mortality rate from breast cancer than women without disabilities even when they are diagnosed at the same stage. Women with disabilities are also less likely to receive breast-conserving therapy than the general population.

For women with disabilities seeking mammography, some of the major obstacles include inaccessible facilities and equipment, as well as the physical requirements of typical mammography testing sites, which require standing and/or remaining still long enough for imaging. The CDC identified other barriers to breast cancer screening for this population, including provider knowledge and attitudes, lack of perceived risk, and focus on other health problems [13]. Their campaign "Breast Cancer Screening: The Right to Know" aims to promote breast cancer screening in women with disabilities. As part of this effort, they have published a tip sheet with examples of questions to ask and information to give when scheduling mammograms [14]. Clinicians referring patients for mammography should also contact their local sites to enquire about accommodations for their patient's individual needs.

Breast cancer screening options include breast self-examination, breast self-awareness, clinical breast examination, and mammography. Although regular self-exams, clinical exams, and mammography have led to earlier detection and improved survival rates, they have also been associated with increased rates of unnecessary intervention for indolent lesions. Public health efforts to optimize breast cancer screening between improved outcomes and reduced harm are ongoing, and, to that end, various stakeholder organizations have major differences in their recommendations for average-risk individuals. Organizations such as ACOG, the USPSTF, the American Cancer Society (ACS), and the American College of Physicians (ACP) have disparate recommendations on the ages to start and stop mammogram screening, appropriate screening intervals, appropriate combination of screening modalities, and the utility of clinical breast exams. Understandably, these variations can serve as a source of confusion for health-care providers and patients alike. Screening decisions should, therefore, be discussed via shared decision-making with the patient and incorporate the patient's values regarding the relative risks, harms, and benefits of the different modalities.

## Menstruation and Suppression

Menstruation can cause difficulties for all women including painful cycles, heavy bleeding, menstrual migraines, and mood changes. Patients with disabilities may have additional concerns related to their menses, including increased challenges with hygiene and subsequent skin irritation or infections. Patients and their caregivers may have anxiety about the potential problems that can accompany menstruation, and ideally, the conversation about menstrual concerns begins well before menarche. Clinicians must be comprehensive and sympathetic when providing guidance and treatment surrounding menstrual concerns. Patients with menstruation abnormalities should be carefully evaluated for hormonal, coagulopathic, or structural causes. Postmenopausal bleeding also requires a thorough assessment but, in many cases, is not pathologic.

Patients and caregivers requesting menstrual suppression should be carefully counseled to determine the best option given their individual circumstances as well as to set realistic expectations. Complete amenorrhea may not be achieved; the goal is the reduction of menstruation to manageable levels for improved quality of life. Of note, menstrual suppression therapy also has the potential benefit of serving as contraception. Menstrual suppression typically consists of hormonal therapy with either combined estrogen and progestin medications or those with progestin only. Surgical management options, including endometrial ablation or hysterectomy, are not considered as first-line for menstrual suppression or contraception alone due to the risks associated. Hysterectomy, in particular, should be considered only after the alternatives have been exhausted and should only be performed for cases meeting standard indications. Laws regarding sterilization of minors or persons under guardianship vary by state and should be checked.

## Hormonal and Nonhormonal Options

Hormonal options for menstrual suppression and/or contraception that combine estrogen and progestin include an oral contraceptive pill, the contraceptive patch, and the vaginal ring. These methods are all approximately 91% effective at preventing pregnancy with typical use. With combined estrogen and progestin methods, menstrual bleeding will occur predictably after a few days of nonuse. Depending on the formulation used, these "withdrawal weeks" can be scheduled monthly, every 3 months, or potentially even longer with extended cycling. Oral contraceptive pills are taken daily and are available in chewable or crushable options for patients with difficulty swallowing pills. Insertion of the vaginal ring may pose a challenge for patients with certain mobility limitations or may be considered invasive for others.

Estrogen-containing therapies are not appropriate for all patients due to the associated increased risk for venous thromboembolism

(VTE). This association precludes the use of estrogen-containing contraception in patients with specific medical issues, including but not limited to chronic hypertension, migraines with aura, and persons with multiple risk factors for atherosclerotic cardiovascular disease. Although it has not been well studied, there is also a theoretical concern for patients whose limited mobility also increases VTE risk. Although estrogen-containing medications are not contraindicated in patients with limited mobility, clinicians may prefer to limit the use of the patch specifically because it provides the highest estrogen exposure among the combined methods [15].

Progestin-only methods, in general, do not have the same VTE concerns as the estrogen-containing methods, and there are few contraindications to progestin therapy. The progestin-only options include oral progestin contraceptive pills, intramuscular depot medroxyprogesterone acetate (DMPA), the levonorgestrel-releasing intrauterine device (IUD), and the progestin subdermal implant. The most common side effect of progestin-only medications is irregular and unpredictable bleeding, which typically improves over time, though it can become an issue for some patients.

Progestin-only oral contraceptive pills are 91% effective as contraception with typical use. They must be taken at the same time daily, and higher doses may be required to achieve amenorrhea. As contraception, DMPA is approximately 94% effective with typical use. DMPA is a reliable method for menstrual suppression, achieving the highest established rate of amenorrhea at approximately 90% by the fourth dose [16]. DMPA is typically well-tolerated; however, weight gain is a common side effect and may specifically impact patients with limited mobility by making transfers more challenging. Prolonged use of DMPA is also associated with decreased bone density, although there is some evidence of recovery after discontinuation of use [17].

The levonorgestrel-releasing IUD is 99% effective as contraception and is approved for 3–7 years of use depending on the specific device. Although irregular bleeding is common, these devices provide a reduction in overall blood loss. A 2018 meta-analysis indicated amenorrhea rates around 20% in the first year of use of the 20 μg/day levonorgestrel-releasing IUD [18]. Although IUD insertion is quick and straightforward, it is also invasive and potentially quite painful. Placement of an IUD under sedation is an option for patients who are not good candidates for a routine office procedure. Additionally, patients with decreased sensation or spinal cord lesions such as spina bifida may have difficulty detecting issues with the IUD such as migration or infection and thus should be considered as candidates for this method on a case-by-case basis. Professionals should also be aware of the risk of autonomic dysreflexia during placement in these patients.

Despite being an excellent contraceptive method (99% effective with typical use), the subdermal progestin implant is unpredictable for menstrual suppression. Amenorrhea is achieved in approximately 20% of patients, and it has an up to 40% rate of unscheduled or prolonged bleeding in the first months of use [15]. Implant insertion may also require sedation in some patients.

Nonhormonal contraceptive options do not function as menstrual suppressants but may be considered for pregnancy prevention. The copper IUD is currently approved for up to 10 years and is 99% effective as contraception. It is associated with increased menstrual bleeding as well as the potential for increased cramping. Condoms are the only way to prevent STIs, and their use should be emphasized for that purpose. Assuming typical use, male condoms are 82% effective as contraception, and female condoms are 79% effective. Patients with spina bifida are at high risk for latex allergies and may require latex-free condoms; however, these may be less effective at preventing both pregnancy and STIs as they have a looser fit and decreased elasticity. Other barrier methods, such as the diaphragm, the cervical cap, and the sponge, are still available, although they have decreased in popularity in the United States. Spermicides may be used alone or in conjunction with barrier methods for additional protection.

Surgical permanent sterilization is also an option for individuals who are certain that they no longer desire to retain fertility. Although it is a highly effective contraception option (99%) for both males and females, sterilization should only be considered after extensive counseling given the surgical risks, the permanence of the procedure, and the ethical considerations involved.

Options for menstrual suppression and contraceptives are extensive and individual responses and experiences vary. Clinicians should have carefully shared decision-making-based discussions with patients and caregivers emphasizing benefits, risks, and flexibility. If a patient does not tolerate a chosen option for any reason, it should be discontinued and an alternative selected.

## Men's Health Screening

Routine men's reproductive healthcare should include discussions regarding the screening for prostate and testicular cancer as well as STI counseling and testing as indicated. Recommendations regarding prostate-specific antigen (PSA) and digital rectal exam screening in asymptomatic patients differ by stakeholder organization with the goal of balancing early detection versus potentially unnecessary intervention. Therefore, these screenings should be conducted on the basis of shared decision-making with patients regarding the benefits, risks, and individual risk factors.

Testicular cancer is one of the most common cancers among men. There is no widely accepted standard or routine screening recommendation for testicular cancer, although some clinicians advocate for testicular self-exams and/or clinical exams for screening. The USPSTF recommends against these exams as routine screening due to inadequate evidence that they offer benefits [19]. Given the disparate recommendations, clinicians should again employ a shared decision-making model and educate patients and/or their caregivers on examination techniques if indicated.

## Populations with Special Considerations

### Spina Bifida

Patients with spina bifida have a significantly increased risk of latex allergies. This must be considered when discussing different barrier methods of contraception and when choosing examination equipment and supplies.

Women with spina bifida seeking pregnancy should undergo preconception counseling regarding both general risks as well as those specific to their condition. Pregnant women with spina bifida may have a slightly increased risk of offspring with neural tube defects (NTDs) despite standard folate supplementation. The mechanism behind this is unclear and may involve complex genetic variances in folate metabolism. Although there have been debates regarding the ideal dosage of folic acid needed to prevent recurrent NTDs, currently ACOG recommends starting 4 mg/day 3 months prior to pregnancy and continuing at least through the 12th week of pregnancy [20].

During pregnancy, patients with spina bifida are at increased risk of nearly all adverse maternal outcomes, notably including unplanned Cesarean delivery, respiratory complications, and renal morbidities [21]. Spinal cord anatomical variations may complicate or preclude the use of regional anesthesia. Physicians performing Cesarean deliveries on spina bifida patients should be cognizant of potential altered urinary and digestive tract anatomy due to population-wide common surgical procedures, such as bladder augmentation, Mitrofanoff, and cecostomy. Given the potential complexities of managing these pregnancies and deliveries, pregnant patients with spina bifida should, in general, be considered high-risk. They benefit from the early involvement of a maternal-fetal medicine specialist as well as an anesthesia provider; pending the patient's specific issues, they may warrant a multidisciplinary team including urology, neurosurgery, and general surgery. As previously described, patients with spinal cord lesions including spina bifida are at risk of autonomic dysreflexia during any potentially painful procedures regardless of the patient's perception of pain. Providers should be aware of this potentially life-threatening response, particularly during major events such as vaginal or Cesarean delivery.

Men with spina bifida may experience decreased sexual function and infertility, though the rates have not been well established [22]. Medications such as sildenafil and tadalafil are frequently successful in treating erectile dysfunction in this population. Patients should be cautioned on the potential for orthostatic hypotension and priapism while using these medications, with emergency room precautions for erections lasting longer than 4 h.

All persons with spina bifida may experience neurogenic bladder or bowel incontinence, which may present embarrassment or discomfort during sexual activity. If desired, patients can perform their routine bladder and bowel regimens before intimacy.

## Down Syndrome

Women with down syndrome experience menopause on average 4–6 years earlier than the general population, putting them at increased risk for post-menopausal health conditions. While men with down syndrome are at significantly increased risk for infertility, females with down syndrome have fertility rates up to 30% by some estimates, and thus, contraception needs should be assessed and addressed.

## Seizure Disorders

Compared with the general population, patients with epilepsy are more likely to experience menstrual irregularities, regardless of the use of antiepileptic drugs (AEDs) [23]. AEDs may affect the efficacy of hormonal therapy for either contraception or menstrual suppression, as hormonal therapy may have a bidirectional interaction with enzyme-inducing antiepileptic medications [23]. Some AEDs are potential teratogens and may need to be changed for patients considering pregnancy.

Catamenial epilepsy refers to the exacerbation of seizure patterns in relation to the menstrual cycle and can occur independently or in conjunction with other seizure patterns. Understanding of the mechanisms behind this phenomenon continues to evolve, but the most basic and general principle identifies estrogen as a proconvulsant and progesterone as an anticonvulsant [24]. The natural changes in the levels and ratios of these hormones throughout the menstrual cycle may then potentially affect seizure patterns.

Catamenial epilepsy can frequently cause frustration in patients for several reasons: (a) diagnosis can be difficult, particularly with anovulatory patterns, requiring a careful record of seizures and menses; (b) catamenial epilepsy is often refractory to common antiepileptic treatments; and (c) uncoordinated management between neurologists and gynecologists may result in unclear messaging. The current mainstay treatment of catamenial epilepsy is an antiepileptic medication regimen along with menstrual suppression. Various combinations of AEDs and hormonal treatments have been trialed, but no studies are large or statistically significant enough thus far to suggest a standard therapy.

## Sickle Cell Anemia

Up to 89% of men with sickle cell anemia will experience priapism by age 20 [25]. Adolescents and their families must be counseled on the common and emergent nature of this condition to encourage prompt care.

## Cystic Fibrosis

Virtually all men with cystic fibrosis have a congenital bilateral absence of the vas deferens, resulting in infertility. Cystic fibrosis is not associated with changes in fertility in women. However, as the presence of cystic fibrosis significantly increases risks of diabetes mellitus, pulmonary infection, and malnutrition, pregnant women with cystic fibrosis should be referred to maternal-fetal medicine for high-risk obstetric management.

## Conclusions

Standards for the reproductive and sexual health of persons with disabilities or chronic conditions align entirely with those of the general population, yet the care they receive can be remarkably divergent. Clinicians, patients, and caregivers should be aware of these potential differences, including discrepancies in counseling and education, potential need for accommodations during the examination, and concerns unique to persons with specific conditions. Patients presenting for reproductive health-care visits will display a wide range of experiences, perceptions, and concerns, and visits must be tailored to the individual patient without biases or assumptions.

## References

1. ACOG Committee Opinion No. 755: well-woman visit. Obstet Gynecol. 2018;132(4):e181–6.
2. Stormo AR, Saraiya M, Hing E, Henderson JT, Sawaya GF. Women's clinical preventive services in the United States: who is doing what? JAMA Intern Med. 2014;174:1512–4.
3. Allen KJ, Leslie SW. Autonomic Dysreflexia—StatPearls—NCBI Bookshelf [Internet]. https://www.ncbi.nlm.nih.gov/books/NBK482434/. Accessed 2022 Apr 15.
4. Armour BS, Thierry JM, Wolf LA. State-level differences in breast and cervical cancer, 2008. Womens Health Issues. 2009;19(6):406–14.
5. ACOG Practice Advisory: Updated cervical cancer screening guidelines. Obstetrics & Gynecology; 2021.
6. Perkins RB, Guido RS, Castle PE, et al. 2019 ASCCP risk-based management consensus guidelines for abnormal cervical cancer screening tests and cancer precursors. J Low Genit Tract Dis. 2020;24(2):102–31.
7. ASCCP; 2022. https://www.asccp.org/. Accessed 15 Apr 2022.
8. Meites E, Szilagyi PG, Chesson HW, Unger ER, Romero JR, Markowitz LE. Human papillomavirus vaccination for adults: updated recommendations of the advisory committee on immunization practices. MMWR Morb Mortal Wkly Rep. 2019;68(32):698–702.
9. Petrosky E, Bocchini JA Jr, Hariri S, Chesson H, Curtis CR, Saraiya M, Unger ER, Markowitz LE, Centers for Disease Control and Prevention (CDC). Use of 9-valent human papillomavirus (HPV) vaccine: updated HPV vaccination recommendations of the advisory committee on immunization practices. MMWR Morb Mortal Wkly Rep. 2015;64(11):300–4.
10. American College of Obstetricians and Gynecologists. Human papillomavirus vaccination. ACOG Committee Opinion No. 809. Obstet Gynecol. 2020;136:e15–21.
11. Centers for Disease Control and Prevention (CDC). STI screening recommendations [internet]. Centers for Disease Control and Prevention. Centers for Disease Control and Prevention; 2021 [cited 2022Apr15]. https://www.cdc.gov/std/treatment-guidelines/screening-recommendations.htm
12. Howlader N, Noone AM, Krapcho M, Miller D, Bishop K, Altekruse SF, Kosary CL, Yu M, Ruhl J, Tatalovich Z, Mariotto A, Lewis DR, Chen HS, Feuer EJ, Cronin KA, editors. SEER cancer statistics review, 1975–2013, National Cancer Institute. MD: Bethesda.
13. Centers for Disease Control and Prevention. The right to know health promotion campaign; 2008. https://www.cdc.gov/ncbddd/disabilityandhealth/righttoknow/overview.html. Accessed 15 Apr 2022.
14. Centers for Disease Control and Prevention. The right to know health promotion campaign; 2008. https://www.cdc.gov/ncbddd/disabilityandhealth/righttoknow/documents/new/RTK%20Tip%20Sheet_English_508.pdf. Accessed 15 Apr 2022.
15. American College of Obstetricians and Gynecologists. Menstrual manipulation for adolescents with physical and developmental disabilities. Committee Opinion No. 668. Obstet Gynecol. 2016;128:e20–5.
16. Fritz MA, Speroff L. Long-acting methods of contraception. In: Fritz MA, Speroff L, editors. Clinical gynecologic endocrinology and infertility. 8th ed. Philadelphia: Wolters Kluwer/Lippincott Williams & Wilkins; 2011. p. 1059–93.
17. American College of Obstetricians and Gynecologists. Depot medroxyprogesterone acetate and bone effects. Committee Opinion No. 602. Obstet Gynecol. 2014;123:1398–402.
18. Sergison and Maldonado. Amenorrhea associated with LNG-IUS use. Am J Obstet Gynecol. 2019;
19. Screening for Testicular Cancer: U.S. Preventive Services Task Force Reaffirmation Recommendation Statement. Ann Intern Med. 2011;154(7):483.
20. American College of Obstetricians and Gynecologists. Neural tube defects. Practice Bulletin No. 187. Obstet Gynecol. 2017;130:e279–90.

21. Auger N, Arbour L, Schnitzer ME, Healy-Profitós J, Nadeau G, Fraser WD. Pregnancy outcomes of women with spina bifida. Disabil Rehabil. 2019;41(12):1403–9.
22. Deng N, Thirumavalavan N, Beilan JA, Tatem AJ, Hockenberry MS, Pastuszak AW, et al. Sexual dysfunction and infertility in the male spina bifida patient. Transl Androl Urol. 2018;7(6):941–9.
23. American College of Obstetricians and Gynecologists. Gynecologic management of adolescents and young women with seizure disorders. ACOG Committee Opinion No. 806. Obstet Gynecol. 2020;135:e213–20.
24. Verrotti A, D'Egidio C, Agostinelli S, Verrotti C, Pavone P. Diagnosis and management of catamenial seizures: a review. IJWH 2012;535, 4.
25. Mantadakis E, Cavender JD, Rogers ZR, Ewalt DH, Buchanan GR. Prevalence of priapism in children and adolescents with sickle cell anaemia. J Paediatr Hematol Oncol. 1999;21(6):518–22.

# 7 Gender Identity and Related Health Considerations

Nupur Agrawal and Jessica Abramowitz

Exploration of gender identity is a uniquely individual and sensitive process that has meaningful implications for how people navigate all aspects of life, including healthcare. It is imperative for health-care providers caring for adults to understand the multifaceted and nuanced nature of gender identity and to develop a comprehensive set of tools to guide patients of all identities in living healthy, fulfilled lives. Primary care providers have an especially powerful opportunity to facilitate gender-affirming care for their patients. By creating a safe environment for patients to be themselves and explore their gender-related goals, providers remove stigma, normalize gender diversity, build rapport, and promote equitable healthcare for this vulnerable population.

In this chapter, we discuss the process of gender identity development in children, adolescents, and adults; the difference between sex assigned at birth, gender identity, gender expression, and gender norms; gender diversity in adolescence and adulthood; the myriad challenges experienced by patients who are gender-diverse; social support and mental health considerations; and ongoing political and legal issues. We provide guidance on building safe spaces and forming strong patient–provider relationships with gender-diverse patients.

## Gender Identity Development

### Sex Assigned at Birth Versus Gender Identity

In human society, infants are assigned the sex of female, male, or intersex at birth primarily based on the appearance of external genitalia [1]. This designation puts individuals into groups defined by predictable lifelong physiological and biological patterns. What is ultimately unpredictable is how much this designation—an individual's sex assigned at birth—will overlap with gender identity—an individual's intimate experience of their own gender. For cis-gender people, there is a significant or complete alignment of sex assigned at birth and gender identity. For transgender people, there is a significant or complete misalignment of sex assigned at birth and gender identity. For gender-diverse people, there are variable levels of alignment and misalignment between the two constructs. Understanding this difference in sex

N. Agrawal (✉)
Division of Medicine-Pediatrics and Preventive Medicine, University of California, Los Angeles, CA, USA
e-mail: nupuragrawal@mednet.ucla.edu

J. Abramowitz
Department of Internal Medicine, Division of Endocrinology, UT Southwestern Medical Center, Dallas, TX, USA
e-mail: Jessica.Abramowitz@UTSouthwestern.edu


A. A. Kuo et al. (eds.), *Care of Adults with Chronic Childhood Conditions*,
https://doi.org/10.1007/978-3-031-54281-7_7

assigned at birth and gender identity is key in safely and productively guiding patients who are exploring their gender identity.

## Gender Identity Development in Childhood

The process of understanding gender identity development starts in childhood and can continue across an individual's lifespan. By age 2, children develop an awareness of physical differences between males and females; by 3, they can tell others whether they consider themselves to be a boy or a girl; and by 4, most children have a stable perception of their gender identity although this process can be delayed in children with gender incongruence [1].

## Gender Norms, Gender Expression, Gender Incongruence, and Gender Dysphoria

Observation of childhood behavior beautifully illustrates the differences between gender norms, gender expression, gender incongruence, and gender dysphoria. Gender norms are societal constructs—both explicit and implicit—that define what behaviors are considered appropriate based on one's gender. These expectations vary across families and societies and begin influencing attitudes and behaviors at an early age [2]. They determine acceptable forms of gender expression—the unique set of characteristics, including but not limited to name, pronouns, dressing style, hair, and behaviors, where people use to communicate their experienced gender to themselves and others. Gender nonconforming behaviors are often seen as deviations from normal and consequently reprimanded, which can create fear of punishment, isolation, and discrimination and suppress the process of self-exploration.

People can have variable gender expression without experiencing gender incongruence. For example, a cis-gender female may choose to wear a button-down shirt, pants, and men's work boots and to carry a wallet instead of a purse, but this does not mean that she identifies as a man. Gender incongruence is when a person identifies as a gender different than their sex assigned at birth. Some people experience significant discomfort with the misalignment between their physical body and lived gender experience; this is termed gender dysphoria. Others embrace their gender incongruence as the natural diversity that is innate to our species and do not necessarily experience distress; we define this as gender incongruence without dysphoria.

## Persistence of Gender Dysphoria into Adolescence and Adulthood

The age of initial feelings of gender dysphoria differs greatly among transgender and gender-diverse (TGD) individuals, but one study published in 2020 found that, for most transgender adults seeking surgical treatment, initial dysphoria had occurred by age 7 [3]. While many patients report that they have had feelings of gender dysphoria or a sense that "something was wrong," for as long as they can remember, others experience an onset of dysphoria in adolescence with changes of puberty. There are people who may not experience dysphoria until well into adulthood, and, for others, gender identity is a fluid concept that continues to evolve across their lifespan.

The following excerpt from *Kotch's Maternal and Child Health: Problems, Programs, and Policy in Public Health* provides insight into gender identity development and guidance for parents with gender-diverse children and adolescents:

> *Parents of school-age children exhibiting variable gender expression often seek professional advice on whether their child's gender-diverse behavior will persist into adulthood. The question is often phrased as: Is this just a phase that my child will outgrow, or is this truly forever? The answer is complex, and the data on this issue are mixed. Current data on lifelong persistence of gender incongruence in*

*children who present early show rates varying from 2% to 27%; these rates may be underestimates given that studies looking at persistence have historically been overly inclusive of all gender-nonconforming behaviors in childhood that are concerning to parents. Consistence, insistence, and intensity of gender-nonconforming behavior are often predictive factors of persistence into adulthood. Other factors associated with persistence include being assigned female at birth, older age at presentation, moving forward with social transition (living openly in experienced gender roles, which may include changing appearance, telling others, changing pronouns, and other actions), and persistent body dissatisfaction. Children whose gender dysphoria intensifies during puberty often experience agonizing feelings related to their bodily changes and may even develop body aversion. Of course, some adolescents show no signs of cross-gender behaviors in childhood and present in adolescence—a development that is often met with surprise by family members. Desistance, the process of a gender-nonconforming child's gender identity evolving to be more in line with the sex assigned at birth, often occurs around ages 10–13. Again, puberty is frequently the clarifying factor.*

While current data show that many children who express feelings of discomfort with their sex assigned at birth will not have persistent gender dysphoria into adolescence [2] and adulthood, children should not be forced to embrace their natal sex [4, 5]. In fact, affirmation of their diverse, and often fluid, expressions is the healthiest way to support children as they explore their gender identity [4].

Children and adolescents are encouraged to see trained medical and mental health professionals before the physical changes of puberty occur and/or before starting medical treatment to delineate their long-term goals [4–6]. Another tool that can help children and adolescents safely explore their gender identity is the use of medications, such as gonadotropin-releasing hormone (GnRH) analogs, to suppress puberty. The medical utilization of GnRH analogs is discussed in detail in Chap. 10, but it is important to generally understand that these medications provide patients with time to understand their gender identity by putting a fully reversible pause on the development of potentially undesirable and irreversible secondary sex characteristics. GnRH analogs can be initiated as early as Tanner Stage 2 [5, 6] and have been linked to improved psychosocial functioning [7, 8]. They afford better long-term cosmetic outcomes for those who choose to proceed with gender-affirming hormone therapy (GAHT). Not all TGD adolescents will choose to undergo pubertal blockade, and some may present too far into puberty for blockade to provide any significant benefit in which case initiation of GAHT would be the next step.

## Continued Exploration into Adulthood and Late Adulthood

There are unique aspects to caring for TGD patients in early and late adulthood. Many adults experience dysphoria for years prior to seeking GAHT. A study of transgender adults seeking gender-affirming genital surgery found that transgender men lived for a mean of 22.9 years and transgender women for a mean of 27.1 years before starting their gender transition [3]. Some older adults establishing care may have transitioned medically and/or surgically earlier in life, while others may be seeking GAHT for the first time in their later adult years. Initiation and continuation of GAHT in geriatric patients often require a more in-depth discussion regarding the risks versus benefits of GAHT in helping patients achieve their gender-related goals; this may include considering hormonal and physiological changes in age-matched cis-gender peers (see Chap. 10 for more details on GAHT in geriatric patients).

## Reasons for Gender Diversity

Studies seeking to understand why individuals are gender-diverse have found some possible contributing factors, including genetic causes and changes in the intrauterine hormonal environment during pregnancy. There is no evidence, though, to support that "social influences, parental differences, peer pressure, adverse childhood experiences, or other external factors" are the cause of gender incongruence or dysphoria [1].

## Prevalence of Gender Diversity

Data in this field is rapidly evolving, but studies suggest that currently 0.5–1.3% of humans identify as gender-diverse [9]. Research from the Williams Institute published in 2017 found that, in the United States, 0.7% of adolescents ages 13–17 (approximately 150,000 youth in total) and 0.6% of adults over the age of 18 (approximately 1.4 million adults in total) identify as transgender. California, Texas, New York, and Florida are home to the largest populations of transgender adolescents and adults [10]. An increasing number of patients are seeking gender-affirming care, so understanding the unique challenges faced by this population and having the tools to build an inclusive and safe environment in medical settings for all patients is more relevant than ever.

## Supporting Gender Identity Exploration in an Inclusive and Safe Environment for All Patients

### Uniqueness of Every Gender Journey

Perhaps the most important thing for an affirming provider to understand is that every gender journey is different. Every patient has a unique set of goals they are hoping to achieve with their health-care provider. Nonbinary and other gender-diverse patients may have very different goals than transgender male and female patients [11], but, even within subsets of patients, no two patients are the same. Inaccurate assumptions can be avoided by engaging patients in regular, comprehensive discussions regarding their goals of care.

### Understanding Patients' Lived Experiences and Goals

Having a gender identity that differs from a person's biological sex has a tremendous impact on many facets of life. Health-care providers who care for gender-diverse patients can best provide support by learning open-mindedly about patients' lived experiences and seeking to understand patients' individual goals. Providers are encouraged to start conversations with all patients by introducing themselves with their names and pronouns. This communicates to patients that they are in a safe environment to discuss potential gender-related health-care needs.

The following guide provides a list of questions health-care providers can ask to learn more about a patient's gender journey and transition-related goals in a sensitive, appropriate, and affirming manner:

- What name would you like me to use during our visits together?
- What pronouns do you use?
- Would you like me to update our electronic medical record to reflect your name and pronouns?*
- Is there anyone else who accompanied you to your visit today who you would like to include at some point in our conversation?
- Tell me about when you first started thinking about your gender and what the journey of exploring your gender has been like for you.
- What is your gender identity?
- What parts of your body cause you discomfort, or are there any body parts you wish you could change in some way?
- I'll provide a list of various body parts, and you can tell me whether they cause you any discomfort. Do you have any particular terms you would like me to use that will make it more comfortable for you to have this discussion with me?
  - Chest
  - Voice
  - Scalp hair
  - Menses (if applicable)
  - Genitalia

- Social presentation
- Body shape
- Other parts I haven't mentioned

- What changes would help you feel most comfortable in your body?
- What physical and emotional changes are you seeking with gender-affirming hormone therapy?
- How do you picture yourself 10 years from now?
- What can I do to best support you along your journey?

*Previously, the terminologies preferred name and preferred pronouns were appropriate. However, many TGD people feel that the names and pronouns they use are not preferences but rather an integral part of their identity. Thus, people should be asked what name and pronouns they use rather than what name and pronouns they prefer.

Familiarity with foundational terminology used in the gender health space is critical to initiating and continuing rich conversations with patients. Table 7.1, from *Kotch's Maternal and Child Health: Problems, Programs, and Policy in Public Health*, provides a detailed list of frequently used terms. It is important to note that terminology related to gender diversity is constantly evolving, and providers may not always have the words that individual patients find most comfortable. The best tool to address this issue is to ask: what terminology can I use to help you feel most comfortable in discussing your health?

**Table 7.1** Frequently used medical and colloquial terms for gender transition [1]

| Term | Definition |
|---|---|
| Cisgender (cis) | Person whose gender identity aligns with their sex assigned at birth. |
| Transgender (trans) | Person whose gender identity differs from their sex assigned at birth. |
| Transgender male (transmasculine) | Person assigned female at birth who identifies as a male. |
| Transgender female (transfeminine) | Person assigned male at birth who identifies as a female. |
| Gender diverse | Person whose gender identity differs from their sex assigned at birth but not necessarily limited to binary designations of male/female. |
| Gender nonbinary | Person who does not identify exclusively as male or female and whose gender identity falls somewhere on the spectrum between male and female. |
| Genderqueer | Another term for gender nonbinary; more commonly used by youth. |
| Gender fluid | Person whose gender fluctuates between more than one gender designation. |
| Agender | Person who does have or experience gender. |
| Intersex | Person whose combination of chromosomes, gonads, hormones, internal sex organs, and/or genitals differs from one of two expected patterns. |
| Gender dysphoria or dysphoria | Distress or impairment associated with experiencing a gender different than that assigned at birth. |
| Transition(ing) | Process that TGD people undergo to alter their social presentation and physical appearance to better align with their gender identity and gender expression. |
| Preferred name or name | Name by which an individual would like to be addressed. It may be the name assigned at birth or a chosen name. |
| Dead name | Name assigned at birth that an individual no longer chooses to use. It can be highly disturbing for a TGD individual to be referred to by their dead name. |
| Preferred pronouns or pronouns | Pronouns by which an individual would like to be addressed. Most commonly used are masculine pronouns (he/him/his), feminine pronouns (she/her/hers), and gender-neutral pronouns (they/them/theirs; now an acceptable singular pronoun). |
| Assigned female at birth (AFAB) | Colloquial short form is pronounced "a-fab"; occasionally may be used to discuss the birth-assigned sex of female without evoking feelings of dysphoria. |
| Assigned male at birth (AMAB) | Colloquial short form is pronounced "a-mab"; occasionally may be used to discuss the birth-assigned sex of male without evoking feelings of dysphoria. |

(continued)

**Table 7.1** (continued)

| Term | Definition |
|---|---|
| Male-to-female (MtF) | Colloquial short form is pronounced "em to eff"; occasionally may be used to discuss the direction of transition without evoking feelings of dysphoria. |
| Female-to-male (FtM) | Colloquial short form is pronounced "eff to em"; occasionally may be used to discuss the direction of transition without evoking feelings of dysphoria. |
| Hormone replacement therapy (HRT) or hormones | Use of testosterone or estrogen by an individual to achieve masculinizing or feminizing effects, respectively. |
| Testosterone (T) | Hormone used to achieve masculinizing effects on the body. Colloquially referred as T (short term testosterone), pronounced "tee." |
| Estrogen (E) | Hormone used to achieve feminizing effects on the body. Colloquially referred as E (short term testosterone), pronounced "ee." |
| Coming out | Process of disclosing TGD identity to others. |
| Stealth | Presenting as a member of the assigned gender, often in public areas; may occur by choice or secondary to fear of discrimination by others. |
| Passing | Ability to navigate life circumstances while being identified as a member of the experienced gender without being labeled as trans person. This cam enhance safety, job security, relationship building, housing status, and so on. It can also be gender-affirming. |
| Gender affirmation or reassignment surgery | Any surgical intervention that helps affirm a person's gender identity. |
| Chest reconstruction surgery | Colloquially referred to as top surgery. For transmasculine patients, this usually refers to bilateral mastectomy with chest contouring. For transfeminine patients, it refers to breast augmentation surgery. |
| Genital reconstruction or reproductive tract surgery | Colloquially referred to as bottom surgery. For transmasculine patients, this can refer to either metoidioplasty (using existing genital tissue to form a neophallus), phalloplasty (surgical creation of a penis) hysterectomy (removal of uterus), and/pr oophorectomy (removal of ovaries). For transfeminine patients, it can refer to orchiectomy (removal of testicles) or vaginoplasty (surgical creation of a vaginal canal). |
| Genital reconstruction or reproductive tract surgery | Colloquially referred to as bottom surgery. For transmasculine patients, this usually refers to bilateral mastectomy with chest contouring. For transfeminine patients, it refers to breast augmentation surgery. |
| Facial feminization surgery (FFS) | Surgery done to feminize the face of transfeminine patients. Colloquially short form is pronounced "eff-eff-ess". |

*Note that the terms, transgendered, tranny, transsexual, transsexualism, and gender identity disorder are outdated and can be considered offensive*

*There are generational, cultural, and personal difference in terminology used. Always ask an individual's preference rather than assuming*

## Eliminating the Concern for Gatekeeping

There has been increasing recognition of gender-diverse identities in society, and more people now are seeking gender-affirming care than ever before. Many people struggle with their feelings before finding the terminology to describe their experiences. Access to the Internet and consequently to online support groups and networks [12] is a popular way for patients to get health information and find communities where they can feel affirmed, especially when there is a lack of affirmation in their physical community. Many patients come to providers after having read about other people's journeys and comparing their own journeys to those of others. Some patients may feel that they have to provide a certain story to providers to gain access to gender-affirming medical care, especially if their story doesn't match more commonly experienced journeys [13]. This is because patients have long experienced discrimination in health-care settings, and providers are often viewed as gatekeepers of affirming care. Properly caring for TGD patients means creating a safe space where they can honestly discuss their journeys without fear of being denied access to care.

**Table 7.2** DSM-5 criteria for gender dysphoria in adolescents and adults

1. A marked incongruence between one's experienced/expressed gender and natal gender of at least 6 mo in duration, as manifested by at least two of the following:
   (a) A marked incongruence between one's experienced/expressed gender and primary and/or secondary sex characteristics (or in young adolescents, the anticipated secondary sex characteristics)
   (b) A strong desire to be rid of one's primary and/or secondary sex characteristics because of a marked incongruence with one's experienced/ expressed gender (or in young adolescents, a desire to prevent the development of the anticipated secondar sex characteristics)
   (c) A strong desire for the primary and/or secondary sex characteristics of the other gender
   (d) A strong desire to be of the other gender (or some alternative gender different from one's designated gender)
   (e) A strong desire to be treated as the other gender (or some alternative gender different from one's designated gender)
   (f) A strong conviction that one has the typical feelings and reactions of the other gender (or some alternative gender different from one's designated gender)
2. The condition is associated with clinically significant distress or impairment in social, occupational, or other important areas of functioning.
   Specify if:
   (a) The condition exists with disorder of sex development.
   (b) The condition is posttranslational, in that the individual has transitioned to full-time living in the desired gender (with or without legalization of gender change) and has undergone (or is preparing to have) at least one sex-related medical procedure or treatment regimen—namely, regular sex hormone treatment or gender reassignment surgery confirming the desired gender (e.g., penectomy, vaginoplasty in natal males; mastectomy or phalloplasty in natal females.

## Confirming Gender Incongruence and Dysphoria in Patients Seeking Care

As discussed earlier in this chapter, patients with gender incongruence may or may not experience distress, or dysphoria, related to their unique gender identity. However, in the current health-care infrastructure in the United States, a diagnosis of "gender dysphoria" is recognized as a medical condition for which care is approved by health insurance companies and is often required to get patients access to gender-affirming medical and surgical care. It is important to note that, while the diagnosis "gender dysphoria" is included in the Diagnostic and Statistical Manual-5 (DSM-5), the Manual specifically states that gender nonconformity is not a mental disorder [14]. It is the distress associated with gender nonconformity that allows "gender dysphoria" to be included in the DSM-5 and treatment to be offered [5].

Transgender and gender-diverse patients do not have a mental disorder, and a diagnosis of gender dysphoria should not be used for "stigmatization or for deprivation of civil and human rights" [6, 14]. Still, the use of a "diagnosis" can be viewed as pathologizing a normal and recognized phenomenon in human diversity, and providers in this sphere anticipate that, over time, the presence of gender incongruence alone will be sufficient to grant people access to the care they need (Table 7.2).

## Understanding and Addressing Challenges Faced by Transgender and Gender-Diverse Patients

### Overarching Barriers to Care

Connection to ongoing, supportive primary and mental healthcare is critically important for TGD adults, but, unfortunately, patients in this population frequently have difficulties accessing proper medical care. Discrepancies in care may arise from socioeconomic barriers, difficulty in finding a culturally competent health-care provider who understands the unique needs of TGD patients, and blatant discrimination [15, 16]. In a survey of 923 Canadian TGD adolescents and young adults, half of the respondents reported that their primary care physician was not aware of their transgender identity [17]. The same survey found that comfort with their doctor and having a doctor aware of their gender identity was positively correlated with improved general and mental health [17]. This highlights the need for an inclusive and informed care environment where patients can feel comfortable exploring their gender and discussing their needs with their health-care provider. There have been increasing calls to incorporate education on gender-inclusive care for all health-care providers [18–20], not just in the United States but across the world [21]. Even when a provider does not have the proper background to comprehensively care for a TGD patient, humility on the part of the health-care provider [22] can still provide the safe environment needed for patients to continue engaging in care and have positive long-term health outcomes. The goal is to ultimately increase the number of providers skilled in delivering comprehensive gender-affirming care in order to improve overall access to care, which unfortunately is limited and often restricted at this point.

## Challenges in Young Adulthood

Emerging adulthood, initially defined by Dr. Jeffrey Arnett and discussed in greater detail earlier in this textbook, describes the time in life when young adults ages 18–25 experience multiple life changes— moving from home, graduating from educational settings and trying to find employment, changes in relationships with family and parents—that can lead to a time period of relative instability [23]. For young TGD adults, this time period may be especially challenging as the process of gender identity exploration may coincide with other life stressors. The challenges of emerging adulthood have been associated with increased substance use and mental health issues [24], and the young TGD adult population has specifically been found to experience an increased risk of substance use, incarceration [25, 26], high-risk sexual behaviors, sex work, homelessness, mental health disorders, violence, discrimination, suicide, and worse health outcomes [1].

## Challenges in Older Adulthood

There may be generational differences in the general experiences and challenges faced by transitioning adults. Many adults, especially older adults, have established families, careers, and social aspects of their lives, which can sometimes create an additional layer of fear and vulnerability in coming out and living their authentic identities. In addition, older patients may have comorbid medical conditions that have to be considered when navigating initiation and management of GAHT, which is discussed in detail in Chap. 10.

## Supportive Mental Healthcare

As discussed previously, gender incongruence and gender dysphoria are not pathologic diagnoses that require mental healthcare. Even when a diagnosis of gender dysphoria is necessary to help patients gain access to essential healthcare, a visit with a mental health professional is not required for the diagnosis to be made or for treatment to be initiated.

However, mental healthcare is still a highly valuable tool and can be extremely useful for:

- Exploring gender identity in an effort to determine what it is, accept it and embrace it, and learn how it may be expressed
- Social transitioning, coming out to others, and presenting in a more gender-congruent manner
- Addressing chronic mental health issues, including, but not limited to, depression, anxiety, post-traumatic stress disorder, attention deficit-hyperactivity disorder, etc. [27]

Mental health professionals should be familiar with gender incongruence and the diagnostic criteria for gender dysphoria, and they should be culturally competent in the care of TGD individuals [5, 6]. There are unique approaches to gender-affirming psychotherapy and exploration that are tailored to an individual patient's developmental stage and allow for discussion of pertinent themes such as gender literacy, resilience, and sexuality [28]. These tools are routinely employed by experienced professionals in this field. Of course, like many other aspects of gender-affirming care, access to high-quality mental healthcare is often limited [29]. This may be related to insurance issues and a lack of available culturally competent providers. Providers and programs caring for TGD patients are encouraged to curate a list of gender-affirming therapists and psychiatrists in the community who accept different insurance plans or provide low-cost care to those without insurance in order to match patients with the best mental health providers for them.

When patients access care first through the mental health route, mental health providers are encouraged to connect patients with clinicians who can provide GAHT [6]. When patients access care first through their primary care or specialist providers, the treating clinician, if comfortable, can work with the patient to explore their needs and determine whether the patient will benefit from treatment without referral to a mental health provider [5]. Many patients may actually feel most comfortable discussing their mental health concerns with their primary care provider [27] who is likely to be familiar with all aspects of their care.

It is recommended that mental health concerns be addressed and relatively controlled prior to initiation of GAHT [5] regardless of whether this is done by a dedicated mental health provider or the patient's primary care provider. In practice, we often see that comorbid mental health conditions, especially anxiety and depression, improve significantly with initiation and maintenance of gender-affirming care. It is still critical to note though that many TGD individuals experience intense dysphoria, and the associated depression can be severe and co-occur with active or passive suicidality that may need to be addressed prior to or in parallel with GAHT. Studies have shown that rates of suicidal thoughts and attempts in this vulnerable population are significantly higher than in the general population [30]. Additional studies have shown increased rates of suicide attempts and success [31, 32]. Health-care providers should routinely screen for past and current suicidal and self-injurious behaviors, and clinics should have a suicide response plan in place [27]. The Trans Lifeline (1-877-565-8860), Trevor Lifeline (1-866-488-7386), and National Suicide Prevention Hotline (1-800-273-8255) are resources for patients considering suicide.

## Concurrent Neurodiversity

Transgender and gender-diverse individuals may have higher rates of neurodiversity, including autism spectrum disorders and other neurodevelopmental disorders [33–35], than in the general population. A systematic review of the literature found that 4.7–13.3% of children diagnosed with gender dysphoria had a diagnosis of autism spectrum disorder as well [36]. Clinicians should adapt their practice to accommodate the needs of neurodiverse patients, including, but not limited to, how assessments are performed, how providers speak to and engage with patients, and how appointments are scheduled and conducted [37].

## Pervasive Discrimination and Disparities

Transgender and gender-diverse patients are at high risk for pervasive discrimination and social disconnection [38]. The 2015 U.S. Transgender Survey, which collected data from 27,715 people and is the largest survey to date dissecting the trans experience in America, found "disturbing patterns of mistreatment and discrimination and startling disparities [...] when it comes to the most basic elements of life, such as finding a job, having a place to live, accessing medical care, and enjoying the support of family and community" with respondents also reporting "high levels of mistreatment, harassment, and violence in every aspect of life." People of ethnic minorities, people with disabilities, and people with undocumented immigration status experience the greatest health-care disparities across all parameters (see Table 7.3 for details). Discussion of these

**Table 7.3** Percentage of transgender and gender-diverse respondents reporting specific forms of disparities and discrimination based on the report of the 2015 US transgender Survey

| Health-care disparities | |
|---|---|
| 39% | Experienced serious psychological distress in month prior (versus 5% in the general population) |
| 59% | Disabled respondents who experienced serious psychological distress in the month prior |
| 40% | Attempted suicide in their lifetime (versus 4.6% of the general population) |
| 54% | Disabled respondents who attempted suicide in their lifetime |
| 33% | Reported at least one negative experience (e.g., verbal harassment and refusal of treatment) related to being transgender in a health-care setting in the year prior |
| 23% | Did not seek healthcare in the year prior due to fear of being mistreated |
| 42% | Disabled respondents who reported being mistreated by a health-care provider in their lifetime |
| 33% | Did not go to a health-care provider when needed because unable to afford it |
| 1.4% | Total percentage of respondents living with HIV (versus 0.3% of the general population) |
| 6.7% | Black respondents living with HIV |
| 19% | Black transgender women respondents living with HIV |
| 25% | Experienced a problem in year prior with insurance related to TGD identity |
| 55% | Denied coverage for transition-related surgery in the year prior |
| **Verbal, physical, and sexual violence and harassment** | |
| 10% | Experienced physical violence from immediate family members |
| 54% | Verbally harassed between grades K-12 |
| 46% | Verbally harassed in the year prior |
| 24% | Physically attacked between grades K-12 |
| 9% | Physically attacked in the year prior |
| 24% | Undocumented respondents physically attacked in the year prior |
| 13% | Sexually assaulted for being transgender in grades K-12 |
| 10% | Sexually assaulted for being transgender in the year prior |
| 59% | Avoided using restrooms in public, at work, or at school sometimes due to fear of confrontation in the year prior (and 11% avoided using restrooms in public at all times) |
| **Economic barriers and hardships** | |
| 30% | Fired, denied promotion, or experienced other discrimination at their job in the year prior |
| 29% | Total percentage of respondents living in poverty (versus 12% of the general population) |
| 43% | Latinx respondents living in poverty |
| 41% | Native American respondents living in poverty |
| 40% | Multiracial respondents living in poverty |
| 38% | Black respondents living in poverty |
| 45% | Disabled respondents living in poverty |
| 15% | Total percentage of respondents unemployed in 2015 (versus 5% in the general population) |
| 20% | Total percentage of respondents of color unemployed in 2015 |
| 24% | Respondents with disabilities who were unemployed |
| **Lack of stable housing and homelessness** | |
| 8% | Kicked out of their childhood home for their gender identity |
| 30% | Total percentage of respondents who experienced homelessness at some point in their lives |
| 50% | Undocumented respondents who experienced homelessness at some point in their lives |
| 12% | Total percentage of respondents who experienced homelessness in the year prior |
| 16% | Homeowners (versus 63% of the general population) |

differences of experience across demographics and the fact that one-third of the respondents of the survey identified as nonbinary make the findings inclusive and more relevant to extrapolation in clinical settings where we care for diverse patients.

## Legal Influence on Access to Care

As people of TGD identities gain increasing visibility in society, there has been a parallel increase in the debate surrounding the rights of this vulnerable population. Many states have introduced legislation that bans access to gender-affirming care for adolescents and criminalizes health-care providers who attempt to provide potentially life-saving medical and surgical care [39]. The rationale for the proposed restrictions often relies on misinterpretation and misrepresentation of concerns associated with the initiation of medical treatment at a young age, such as fertility issues. There are recognized benefits and risks of any medical intervention, and Chap. 10 discusses how providers can navigate these benefits and risks with individual patients in ultimately deciding the best treatment options for them.

In its Sustainable Development Goals, the United Nations identifies gender equality as a fundamental human right that is a prerequisite to ensuring all humans are able to live healthy and productive lives [2]. The political climate surrounding transgender rights is constantly evolving, and providers caring for TGD patients should utilize available resources to provide continued care to patients. Of course, legal constraints on the extent of care providers are able to offer may be present depending on the provider's location of practice. Affirming providers are encouraged to collaborate with local institutions and advocacy groups to identify the best way to address access of care issues for patients moving forward.

## Next Steps for the Affirming Provider

### Cultural Competence and Humility

It is important for health-care providers to be culturally competent and aware that not all of a TGD person's concerns are related to their gender identity [40]. Current literature primarily elucidates the experiences of White/Caucasian TGD patients and may not consider the social, cultural, and religious practices that influence the identities of patients from other demographic groups [1]. Patients with disabilities, undocumented status, and a primary language other than English may experience additional barriers to accessing life-saving, gender-affirming care [1, 38]. There are similar rates of common mental health disorders in the TGD population, but still, the prevalence of depression and anxiety may be greater in those experiencing compounded minority stress [41]. Trauma-informed training can also be beneficial. Anything providers can do to better understand and address the complex needs of their patients can improve the health-care experience of TGD individuals; providing the best care may sometimes mean connecting patients with other providers who are more experienced, skilled, or versed in meeting patients' needs.

### Ensuring Strong Social Support

Despite widespread discrimination and numerous disparities, research shows that strong social support can help TGD patients address the challenges associated with gender diversity. In The Report of the 2015 US Transgender Survey, 60% of respondents reported that their families supported them after finding out about their gender identity, and these respondents were consequently less likely to experience economic instability, homelessness, suicidality, and general health-care disparities [38]. Exploration of gender identity can span across an individual's lifespan, and robust social support during this process can minimize negative outcomes. Providers play a critical role in helping patients identify and possibly build the social support networks they need to thrive.

Question guide for health-care providers:

- Who do you consider to be your support system?
- Who do you reach out to when you need support?
- How can we work together to help you build the support system you need?

### Supporting Medical and Surgical Transition

There are social, medical, and surgical ways to help a patient's physical and emotional state align more with their experienced gender identity. Guidelines for GAHT are based on the use of hormones for decades in caring for TGD patients, but there is no clear consensus, except in adolescents, on whether GAHT should mimic the experiences of age-matched cis-gender peers. Conversations with patients in understanding their goals are the most important tool in determining the next steps.

Affirming providers may or may not feel comfortable initiating and maintaining patients on GAHT or guiding them through surgical decisions. It is still essential to understand the medical and surgical tools available to patients and be aware of general health-care maintenance requirements that can be fulfilled in any primary care setting. As a next step, providers are encouraged to read Chap. 10 in this textbook for a comprehensive overview of medical and surgical care for TGD patients.

## References

1. Gragnani CAN, Duan S, Lewis Hunter A, Kuo AA. School-age children. In: Kirby RSVS, editor. Maternal and child health: problems, programs, and policy in public health. 4th ed. Burlington, MA: Jones and Bartlett Learning; 2022. p. 255–95.
2. Weber AM, Cislaghi B, Meausoone V, Abdalla S, Mejia-Guevara I, Loftus P, et al. Gender norms and health: insights from global survey data. Lancet. 2019;393(10189):2455–68.
3. Zaliznyak M, Bresee C, Garcia MM. Age at first experience of gender dysphoria among transgender adults seeking gender-affirming surgery. JAMA Netw Open. 2020;3(3):e201236.
4. Rosenthal SM. Approach to the patient: transgender youth: endocrine considerations. J Clin Endocrinol Metab. 2014;99(12):4379–89.
5. Hembree WC, Cohen-Kettenis PT, Gooren L, Hannema SE, Meyer WJ, Murad MH, et al. Endocrine treatment of gender-dysphoric/gender-incongruent persons: an endocrine society* clinical practice guideline. J Clin Endocrinol Metab. 2017;
6. Coleman E, Bockting W, Botzer M, et al. Standards of care for the health of transsexual, transgender and gender-nonconforming people version 7. Int J Transgend. 2012;13:165–232.
7. Cohen-Kettenis PT, van Goozen SH. Pubertal delay as an aid in diagnosis and treatment of a transsexual adolescent. Eur Child Adolesc Psychiatry. 1998;7(4):246–8.
8. de Vries AL, Steensma TD, Doreleijers TA, Cohen-Kettenis PT. Puberty suppression in adolescents with gender identity disorder: a prospective follow-up study. J Sex Med. 2011;8(8):2276–83.
9. Cooper K, Russell A, Mandy W, Butler C. The phenomenology of gender dysphoria in adults: a systematic review and meta-synthesis. Clin Psychol Rev. 2020;80:101875.
10. Flores A, Herman J, Brown T, Wilson B, Conron K. Age of individuals who identify as transgender in the United States 2017. https://williamsinstitute.law.ucla.edu/research/transgender-issues/new-estimates--show-that-150000-youth-ages-13-to-17-identify-as-transgender-in-the-us/
11. Galupo MP, Pulice-Farrow L, Pehl E. "There Is Nothing to Do About It": nonbinary individuals' experience of gender dysphoria. Transgend Health. 2021;6(2):101–10.
12. Bretherton I, Thrower E, Zwickl S, Wong A, Chetcuti D, Grossmann M, et al. The health and well-being of transgender Australians: a national community survey. LGBT Health. 2021;8(1):42–9.
13. Liamputtong P, Noack-Lundberg K, Dune T, Marjadi B, Schmied V, Ussher J, et al. Embodying transgender: an analysis of trans women in online forums. Int J Environ Res Public Health. 2020;17(18)
14. American Psychiatric Association. Diagnostic and statistical manual of mental disorders. 5th ed. Washington, DC; 2013.
15. Sanchez NF, Sanchez JP, Danoff A. Health care utilization, barriers to care, and hormone usage among male-to-female transgender persons in New York City. Am J Public Health. 2009;99(4):713–9.
16. Safer JD, Coleman E, Feldman J, Garofalo R, Hembree W, Radix A, et al. Barriers to healthcare for transgender individuals. Curr Opin Endocrinol Diabetes Obes. 2016;23(2):168–71.
17. Clark BA, Veale JF, Greyson D, Saewyc E. Primary care access and foregone care: a survey of transgender adolescents and young adults. Fam Pract. 2018;35(3):302–6.
18. Hana T, Butler K, Young LT, Zamora G, Lam JSH. Transgender health in medical education. Bull World Health Organ. 2021;99(4):296–303.
19. Click IA, Mann AK, Buda M, Rahimi-Saber A, Schultz A, Shelton KM, et al. Transgender health education for medical students. Clin Teach. 2020;17(2):190–4.
20. Korpaisarn S, Safer JD. Gaps in transgender medical education among healthcare providers: a major barrier to care for transgender persons. Rev Endocr Metab Disord. 2018;19(3):271–5.
21. Martins RS, Saleh R, Kamal H, Gillani M, Merchant AAH, Munir MM, et al. The need for transgender healthcare medical education in a developing country. Adv Med Educ Pract. 2020;11:405–13.
22. Sallans RK. Lessons from a transgender patient for health care professionals. AMA J Ethics 2016. https://journalofethics.ama-assn.org/article/lessons-transgender-patient-health-care--professionals/2016-11.

23. Arnett JJ. Emerging adulthood: the winding road from the late teens through the twenties. 2nd ed. New York: Oxford University Press; 2015.
24. Arnett JJ, Schwab J. The Clark University poll of emerging adults: thriving, struggling, and hopeful; 2012.clark-university-poll-emerging-adults-findings.pdf
25. De Pedro KT, Gilreath TD, Jackson C, Esqueda MC. Substance use among transgender students in California Public Middle and High Schools. J Sch Health. 2017;87(5):303–9.
26. Hughto JMW, Reisner SL, Kershaw TS, Altice FL, Biello KB, Mimiaga MJ, et al. A multisite, longitudinal study of risk factors for incarceration and impact on mental health and substance use among young transgender women in the USA. J Public Health (Oxf). 2019;41:100–9.
27. Guidelines for the primary and gender-affirming care of transgender and gender nonbinary people; 2016. transcare.ucsf.edu/guidelines
28. Spencer KG, Berg DR, Bradford NJ, Vencill JA, Tellawi G, Rider GN. The gender-affirmative life span approach: a developmental model for clinical work with transgender and gender-diverse children, adolescents, and adults. Psychotherapy (Chic). 2021;58(1):37–49.
29. Snow A, Cerel J, Loeffler DN, Flaherty C. Barriers to mental health care for transgender and gender-nonconforming adults: a systematic literature review. Health Soc Work. 2019;44(3):149–55.
30. Herman JLBT, Haas AP. Suicide thoughts and attempts among transgender adults: findings from the 2015 U.S. transgender survey. UCLA School of Law Williams Institute; 2019.
31. Dickey LM, Budge SL. Suicide and the transgender experience: a public health crisis. Am Psychol. 2020;75(3):380–90.
32. Blosnich JR, Boyer TL, Brown GR, Kauth MR, Shipherd JC. Differences in methods of suicide death among transgender and nontransgender patients in the veterans health administration, 1999–2016. Med Care. 2021;59:S31–S5.
33. Strang JF, Kenworthy L, Dominska A, Sokoloff J, Kenealy LE, Berl M, et al. Increased gender variance in autism spectrum disorders and attention deficit hyperactivity disorder. Arch Sex Behav. 2014;43(8):1525–33.
34. Heylens G, Aspeslagh L, Dierickx J, Baetens K, Van Hoorde B, De Cuypere G, et al. The co-occurrence of gender dysphoria and autism spectrum disorder in adults: an analysis of cross-sectional and clinical chart data. J Autism Dev Disord. 2018;48:2217–23.
35. Hilton MN, Boulton KA, Kozlowska K, McClure G, Guastella AJ. The co-occurrence of neurodevelopmental disorders in gender dysphoria: Characteristics within a paediatric treatment-seeking cohort and factors that predict distress pertaining to gender. J Psychiatr Res. 2022;149:281–6.
36. Herrmann L, Bindt C, Schweizer K, Micheel J, Nieder TO, Haass J, et al. Autism spectrum disorders and gender dysphoria among children and adolescents: systematic review on the co-occurrence. Psychiatr Prax. 2020;47(6):300–7.
37. Cooper K, Mandy W, Russell A, Butler C. Healthcare clinician perspectives on the intersection of autism and gender dysphoria. Autism. 2022;13623613221080315
38. James SE, Herman JL, Rankin S, Keisling M, Mottet L, Anafi M. The report of the 2015 U.S. transgender survey. Washington, DC: National Center for Transgender Equality; 2016.
39. Conron KJ, O'Neill K, Vasquez LA, Mallory C. Prohibiting gender-affirming medical care for youth. UCLA School of Law Williams Institute; 2022.
40. American Psychological Association. Guidelines for psychological practice with transgender and gender nonconforming people. Am Psychol. 2015;70(9):832–64.
41. Bockting WO, Miner MH, Swinburne Romine RE, Hamilton A, Coleman E. Stigma, mental health, and resilience in an online sample of the US transgender population. Am J Public Health. 2013;103(5):943–51.

# 8 Sexual Abuse in Individuals with Intellectual Disability

Michelle Cornacchia

## Prevalence, Risk Factors, and Background

The World Health Organization (WHO) (2002) defines sexual abuse (SA) as "any sexual act, attempt to obtain a sexual act, unwanted sexual comments or advances, or acts to traffic or otherwise directed against person's sexuality using coercion, by any person regardless of their relationship to the victim, in any setting, including but not limited to home and work" [1]. For individuals with intellectual disabilities (ID) there have been additional definitions given the concern regarding capacity and ability to consent to sexual acts. An example of one definition seen in the literature is, "any situation involving any kind of sexual activity (i.e., unwanted sexual touching, being forced to touch someone, exposure to sexual contents, or sexual intercourse) that the individual does not want or consent to or is unable to understand due to his or her cognitive (i.e., intellectual) level" [2]. The differences in defining SA in this population have made it more difficult to study this issue. This among other factors that will be explored later in this chapter has also made it difficult to get an accurate prevalence of SA in individuals with disabilities.

M. Cornacchia (✉)
Geisinger Internal Medicine, Danville, PA, USA
e-mail: mcornacchia@geisinger.edu

In the literature, differing information was seen regarding prevalence and risk factors. However, one consistent statistic was that individuals with ID were at increased risk for SA compared to the general population [3]. The prevalence of SA among adults with ID ranged from 7% to 50% compared to the general population which ranged from 5% to 17% [3, 4]. Individuals with mild ID are at higher risk for SA than individuals with profound ID [4, 5]. This is likely because individuals with mild ID are more visible in society with school, work, and activities. Often women are at higher risk than men with ID for SA (Byrne 2017). One study reported 39–60% of women with ID were at risk of being sexually abused vs 16–30% of men [2]. However, the literature does report men with disabilities are more likely than men without disability to report a lifetime of sexual violence [6]. There is also a higher prevalence in institutionalized individuals with ID than individuals living in the community [5]. Lastly, prevalence was higher in individuals who had a range of impairments such as hearing loss or other sensory impairment [7].

There are multiple other risk factors that put individuals with ID at higher risk for abuse. Gil-Llario et al. organized these factors into three categories that included risk factors related to the individual, perceptions of risk of SA, and reporting the abuse [2]. Risk factors related to an individual include poor social and communication skills, myths and false beliefs regarding sex, lim-


A. A. Kuo et al. (eds.), *Care of Adults with Chronic Childhood Conditions*,
https://doi.org/10.1007/978-3-031-54281-7_8

ited ability to distinguish between appropriate–inappropriate sexual encounters, lack of positive sexual experiences, low self-esteem, need for help with personal body care, and inability to defend themselves. Increased tolerance of physical manipulation and trained compliance are unique risk factors of some individuals with disabilities given their dependence on others for personal care. Factors related to the perception of the risk of SA included denial of the risk of SA associated with relatives, friends, and caregivers. This can be a significant risk factor given family and/or acquaintances are often the perpetrators in sexual abuse cases involving individuals with ID. Another view that SA does not occur in familiar places can be misleading given abuse usually occurs in the home, neighborhood, or familiar public place such as residential care or day program [2]. The third category looks at barriers individuals with ID have in reporting abuse which may be related to fear of being punished, judged, or not believed in. They may have a sense of guilt or may have fears of being abandoned by family. Finally, they may not know how to report the abuse or who to report it to.

## Physiological and Physical Effects of SA

There are multiple psychological, physiological, and behavioral consequences seen in individuals with ID who have undergone SA. Like the general population, depression, anxiety, and PTSD have been seen [4]. Other emotional and psychological findings seen in individuals with ID include an increase in aggression, self-talk, inappropriate sexualized talk, and a higher risk of developing conduct disorder [4, 8]. Some physical effects seen in individuals with ID who have undergone SA include changes in bowel/bladder patterns, appetite, and sleep as well as unwanted pregnancies and sexually transmitted infections [8, 9]. Challenging behaviors such as crying, agitation, and temper outbursts have been reported as well as sexualized behaviors such as being preoccupied with sexual issues, wearing provocative clothing, or exposing unusual sexual interests. It is important to identify these effects of SA to allow for early recognition of SA in individuals with ID especially given there are multiple factors limiting their disclosure of abuse. Therefore, having providers aware of these red flags may help them further investigate if there has been a history of SA. Also, knowing these characteristics can help develop and implement treatment programs to help reduce challenging behaviors, care for psychological concerns, prevent re-victimization, and improve quality of life.

## Early Detection

Understanding and utilizing screening tools for individuals with ID is important to help identify SA. In one study of those who were abused in the past year, 40% reported little or no knowledge of abuse-related resources, and only 27% reported the incident (Houtrow et al. 2021). Barriers to reporting include deficiencies in communication and collaboration among agencies, lack of appropriate legislation, and lack of specific training and educational programs [10].

There are limited resources to help screen for SA as well as detect the risk of SA in individuals with ID. One risk assessment tool was developed by Liou in 2014, but some considered it not user-friendly and not reliable [2, 11]. Therefore, Gil-Llario et al. developed the Development and Psychometric Properties of the Detection of Sexual Abuse Risk Screening Scale (DSARss) in 2020. This screening tool is used to detect the risk of SA in individuals with ID. The DSARss divides the assessment into four categories looking at acceptance of the abuse due to affection, denial of the risk associated with places, risk of factors and self-protection skills, and lack of awareness of intimacy rules. Example questions include, "My father takes care of me, so it is okay to have sexual relationships with him," "It is impossible to be sexually abused in my home," "If someone tries to abuse me, I must cry 'Stop!' 'Help!'," and "It is okay if someone I know touches my butt," respectively [2].

Of note, the Sexual Experience Survey (SES) has been noted as one of the most widely used measures of unwanted sexual experiences, however, is not specifically for the ID population [12].

There are various models of screening for SA such as paper and pencil questionnaires or computer-assisted questionnaires; however, this may not be possible depending on the individuals' literacy. Though there are interview-conducted questionnaires that may help overcome this barrier, this is still limited given the scarce questionnaires geared toward individuals with ID. Lastly, face-to-face interviews have been reported as the most successful mode of screening for the general population, however, challenges include limited provider training as well as lack of time during a clinic visit to explore these concerns [13].

Given informal face-to-face interviews have been successful. Some screening questions could include:

1. Some people have had sex or been touched sexually when it wasn't their choice, has that ever happened to you? [8].
2. Have you ever been touched in areas covered by a bathing suit by someone other than your parents or your doctor? Can you tell me about that? [8].

Originated for individuals with a physical disability, the Abuse Assessment Screen-Disability (AAS-D) asks the following questions to screen for abuse/neglect:

1. Within the last year, have you been hit, slapped, kicked, pushed, shoved, or otherwise physically hurt by someone?
2. Within the last year, has anyone forced you to have sexual activities?
3. Within the last year, has anyone prevented you from using a wheelchair, cane, respirator, or other assistive devices?
4. Within the last year, has anyone you depended on refused to help you with an important personal need, such as taking your medicine, getting to the bathroom, getting out of bed, bathing, getting dressed, or getting food or drink?

## Prevention and Intervention

The prevalence of sexual abuse is higher in individuals who lack sexual education [7]. Therefore, sexual education is an important tool to reduce risk. However, some cultural and social beliefs limit the sexuality of individuals with intellectual disability. Some believe individuals with ID are asexual while others may view them as hypersexual. As a result, many adolescents with disabilities do not receive sex education in school or at home [8]. Even neurotypical individuals receive limited sexual education in the pediatrics office [8]. This prevents the necessary skills needed to make informed choices. This can also lead to various sexual problems such as inappropriate masturbation and/or discussing sexual desires in public as well as problems with reporting sexual abuse.

Education can be given in various settings. This can include the medical provider's office including but not limited to pediatric, internal medicine-pediatrics, and/or family medicine offices. They can provide anticipatory guidance that can help with a better understanding of their changing bodies and feelings. They can develop skills for navigating sexual desire and sexuality. Other topics to discuss could include gender identity, appropriate "private" vs "public" behaviors, prevention of sexually transmitted infections (STIs), and correct terminology to be able to advocate for themselves or report sexual violence. Providers can also provide contraceptives, screen for sexually transmitted infections, and/or place appropriate referrals [8, 14].

Questions you could consider exploring sexuality more could include:

1. Do you know what sex is? [8]
2. Is it ok if I ask you questions about your body and about sex? [8]
3. Many people have a hard time figuring out their sex. Is this an issue for you? [8]
4. Are you in a relationship? With whom? [8]

Education can also occur at school. Individuals can work with schools through their individualized education program (IEP) to include sexuality as part of their services/education. There are additional resources for schools such as *Sexuality and Disabilities: A Guide for Professionals* and *Seattle and King County Sexual Health Education Curriculum.* There have been educational programs studied and developed to help reduce SA and include resources like storybooks and support resources such as dolls, booklets, and explanatory videos.

Besides providers and academic educators, educating families/caregivers on sexual development and how to support it is important. There are disorder-specific resources such as *AAP Autism Toolkit: Sexuality of Children and Youth with Autism Spectrum Disorder*, *Children and Youth with Complex Cerebral Palsy: Care and Management,* the Spina Bifida Association, *and The Guide to Good Health for Teens and Adults with Down Syndrome.* There is also general information at http://amaze.org that can include videos about sexual education aimed at preteens. Organizations like Autism Speaks and Pacer Center have created helpful resources such as *Sexuality Education for Children and Adolescents with Developmental Disabilities: An Instructional Manual for Parents of and Individuals with Developmental Disabilities* and training centers in Minneapolis for parents of children with disabilities called *The Journey to Adulthood: What Parents Need to Know (Sexuality*), respectively.

In uncovering sexual abuse, there needs to be improved culture of acceptance in the medical provider's office. The atmosphere needs to promote disclosure as the norm. The medical staff needs training and support on how to recognize and care for victims of sexual abuse. There needs to be collaboration between the provider's office and community resources. These community resources could include a women's center, behavioral health, adult-protected services, and/or a criminal justice system.

Other medical/psychological resources could include Rape Crisis Centers (RCC) programs and/or sexual assault nurse examiner (SANE) programs. RCCs were created in the 1970s and offer crisis intervention support, counseling, and advocacy. The SANE program started around the late 1990s providing similar services. They also can include medical forensic evidence collection, trauma-informed crisis counseling, and safety planning. An online resource, if sexual abuse is suspected, is the Disability and Abuse Project: http://www.disability-abuse.com.

More attention is being brought to trauma-informed care as an effective intervention for victims of SA. Trauma-informed care uses strategies to minimize potential re-traumatization and provides multidisciplinary care [15]. For individuals with ID, it can include therapeutic medical play with games, toys, books, and role playing. It can help with facilitating the expression of feelings as well as enhance coping. It provides individualized accommodations based on an individual's needs. Examples would include reducing stimuli if the individual is sensitive to sensory input and accommodating with preferred communication techniques.

## Limitations

There are multiple limitations to understanding sexual abuse in individuals with ID given the questionable ability to consent to sexual acts for some individuals. Also, many times sexual abuse is underreported for various reasons. This can include limited communication, poor understanding of the difference between appropriate touch and inappropriate touch, memory issues, and fear of removal from home. Another challenge is there is not a standard method of collecting this information. Lastly, there are barriers to identifying SA in this population given that there are different presentations of post-traumatic stress disorder or other mental health needs in individuals with ID.

## Conclusion

In summary, individuals with disabilities are at increased risk for sexual abuse. The community needs to take a multidisciplinary approach with caregivers, school, and medical providers to help prevent abuse as well as identify and intervene when appropriate if abuse has occurred.

## References

1. World Health Organization (WHO). Violence Info—Sexual violence— Sexual Violence [Internet]. [cited 2022 Sep 30]. http://apps.who.int/violence-info/sexual-violence
2. Gil-Llario MD, Ballester-Arnal R, Morell-Mengual V, Caballero-Gascón L, Castro-Calvo J. Development and psychometric properties of the detection of sexual abuse risk screening scale (DSARSS). Sex Abus. 2019;32(7):850–77.
3. Basile KC, Breiding MJ, Smith SG. Disability and risk of recent sexual violence in the United States. Am J Public Health. 2016;106(5):928–33.
4. Smit MJ, Scheffers M, Emck C, van Busschbach JT, Beek PJ. Clinical characteristics of individuals with intellectual disability who have experienced sexual abuse. An overview of the literature. Res Dev Disabil. 2019;95:103513.
5. Tomsa R, Gutu S, Cojocaru D, Gutiérrez-Bermejo B, Flores N, Jenaro C. Prevalence of sexual abuse in adults with intellectual disability: systematic review and meta-analysis. Int J Environ Res Public Health. 2021;18(4):1980.
6. Mitra M, Mouradian VE, Fox MH, Pratt C. Prevalence and characteristics of sexual violence against men with disabilities. Am J Prev Med. 2016;50(3):311–7.
7. Byrne G. Prevalence and psychological sequelae of sexual abuse among individuals with an intellectual disability: a review of the recent literature. J Intellect Disabil. 2017;22(3):294–310.
8. Walters FP, Gray SH. Addressing sexual and reproductive health in adolescents and young adults with intellectual and developmental disabilities. Curr Opin Pediatr. 2018;30(4):451–8.
9. Goli S, Noroozi M, Salehi M. A comprehensive sexual health care program for educable intellectually disabled adolescent girls: protocol for a mixed methods study. Reprod Health. 2018;15(1):141.
10. McGilloway C, Smith D, Galvin R. Barriers faced by adults with intellectual disabilities who experience sexual assault: a systematic review and meta-synthesis. J Appl Res Intellect Disabil. 2018;33(1):51–66.
11. Liou W-Y. An illustrated scale measuring the sexual-abuse prevention knowledge of female high school students with intellectual disabilities in Taiwan. Sex Disabil. 2013;32(2):135–51.
12. Johnson SM, Murphy MJ, Gidycz CA. Reliability and validity of the sexual experiences survey–short forms victimization and perpetration. Violence Vict. 2017;32(1):78–92.
13. Diaz A, Peake K, Nucci-Sack A, Shankar V. Comparison of modes of administration of screens to identify a history of childhood physical abuse in an adolescent and young adult population. Ann Glob Health. 2017;83(5–6):726.
14. Houtrow A, Elias ER, Davis BE, Kuo DZ, Agrawal R, Davidson LF, Ellerbeck KA, Foster J, Fremion E, Leppert M, Saunders BS, Stille C, Vargus-Adams J, Yin L, Norwoood K Jr, Coleman C, Mann MY, Simpser E, Poon J, Yeargin-Allsopp M, Kuznetsov A. Promoting healthy sexuality for children and adolescents with disabilities. Pediatrics. 2021;148(1):1–14.
15. Reese S, Deutsch SA. Sexual assault victimization among children and youth with developmental disabilities. J Forensic Nurs. 2020;16(1):55–60.

# Care of Sexual and Gender Minority Patients

# 9

Gifty-Maria Ntim and Rebecca Rada

## Case Discussion

Jamie is a 22-year-old patient who uses she/they pronouns. She identifies as queer, nonbinary, and is currently in a monogamous relationship with a trans female partner who uses she/her pronouns. They were assigned female at birth. Their BMI is 33, they have never had a pap smear because they don't think they need one, and they recently got insurance through their job, which is why they are establishing care today. They have a history of anxiety, depression, and IBS (irritable bowel syndrome). They endorse social alcohol use, smoke cigarettes (½ pack per day), and endorse marijuana use socially as well. They are not currently on any medications. As a primary care physician, what are some of the topics you want to address during your visit with Jamie?

A lot of times when new patients establish care, the first steps into an office can give a clear message if they will feel welcome. There are a variety of ways LGBTQ+ individuals can feel welcomed into a medical clinic, ranging from bathroom signage indicating all genders can use facilities, pamphlets, and media with LGBTQ+ representation, front desk staff who ask for chosen pronouns, or intake forms with gender identity and sexual minorities clearly identified. These small changes can provide an environment of support, compassion, and equity. Ensuring intake forms have areas for pronouns, gender identity, and sexual minorities can ensure patients feel included and respected. In addition to creating an inviting office environment for LGBTQ+ patients, there are myriad other ways to instill rapport with patients, in particular, by using correct pronouns and chosen names for gender-diverse patients. One recent study showed that when transgender youth had their chosen name and correct pronouns used, they had decreased rates of depression and suicidal ideation [1].

In regard to primary care discussions with Jamie, tobacco cessation should be discussed. There is a known increased risk of tobacco use in the LGBTQ+ community, in particular with gay, lesbian, and bisexual individuals [2]. Talking through the options of tobacco cessation can be time consuming, but motivational interviewing has been found to be effective in tobacco cessation [3]. Also, for anyone who uses tobacco, a pneumonia vaccine is recommended as patients who use tobacco are at higher risk of pneumonia [4].

Gifty-Maria Ntim and Rebecca Rada contributed equally to the development of this chapter.

G.-M. Ntim (✉) · R. Rada
Division of Medicine-Pediatrics, University of California, Los Angeles, CA, USA
e-mail: gntim@mednet.ucla.edu; rrada@mednet.ucla.edu


A. A. Kuo et al. (eds.), *Care of Adults with Chronic Childhood Conditions*,
https://doi.org/10.1007/978-3-031-54281-7_9

Jamie states that they don't think they need a pap smear, which can be a common misconception for patients who are LGBTQ+ or who are not engaging in penile penetrative vaginal intercourse. It is important to have discussions revolving around sexual health, preventative health measures (HPV Vaccines, PrEP for those who have indications), and STI testing. For Jamie, it is advisable they receive a pap since they are over the age of 21, but as many LGBTQ+ patients have experienced trauma in their lifetime, it is okay to defer a pap until after rapport is built with the patient. There is also an option of doing a self-pap or referring to Ob/Gyn if it is something they are not able to tolerate.

Getting a detailed sexual history is essential for LGBTQ+ populations to better understand if pregnancy is a risk and if there are additional STI testing sites that need to be collected. It is important to consider the available organs for inventory for LGBTQ+ patients and also discuss the parts that are used for sex. For example, it is important to find out more about Jamie's partner who is a trans female. It is not known whether her partner has had gender-affirming bottom surgery, so she could still produce viable sperm, especially if she still has erectile function and uses that organ for sex. In this scenario, if Jamie is having receptive vaginal intercourse and does not want to get pregnant, contraception needs to also be discussed.

Dietary changes and exercise counseling should also occur during the visit or at a future visit as time permits. Jamie's BMI is 33 and falls within the obesity range. With that, they have an increased risk for chronic health issues in the future, including diabetes mellitus, cancer, heart disease, and obstructive sleep apnea [5]. Given her history of anxiety and depression, GAD7 and PHQ9 can also be obtained to determine if her symptoms are well managed or if she would benefit from counseling, medications, or both. There are increased rates of mental health issues within the LGBTQ+ community, so depression and anxiety should be addressed routinely [6]. Suicidal ideation and suicide completion are also increased in this population, especially in transgender individuals, in which 82% of transgender individuals have considered killing themselves and 40% have attempted suicide in their lifetime [7].

Providing care to LGBTQ+ individuals is incredibly rewarding and they comprise a group who has historically been discriminated against in the healthcare setting. Providing affirming, holistic, and patient-centered care is essential for the well-being of sexual and gender minority individuals and can be implemented into every practice.

## Introduction

It is known that LGBTQIA+ (lesbian, gay, bisexual, transgender, and queer/questioning, intersex, and asexual) individuals face disparities within society as well as within the healthcare system. While there have been many advancements in acceptance and protective measures for LGBTQ+ individuals, disparities still exist and are becoming even more polarizing. Many times, a healthcare provider can be the first person LGBTQ+ adolescents come out to, which has an impact on how they perceive healthcare providers from then on. Having an understanding, empathetic, compassionate, and supportive approach to these discussions can create rapport for LGBTQ+ individuals and their relationship with the healthcare system for the rest of their lives. Approximately 3.5% of adults in the United States identify as LGB and an estimated 0.3% of adults are transgender [8]. In the United States, youth aged 13–17 represent 0.7% identify as transgender [9]. There are many reasons for the increase in openly LGBTQ+ individuals now compared to prior years, with exposure and increase in acceptance, and transgender visibility accounting for major reasons.

Historically, LGBTQ+ individuals faced extreme hostility and discrimination within the medical system, whether it was from physicians, nurses, support staff, or inability to access insurance or care. According to the 2015 Transgender Survey, approximately 19% of transgender individuals were refused medical care at a physician's office, which often leads them to delay or opt out of care; 28% of transgender people ended up postponing medical care due to discrimination [9]. Often, LGBTQ+ adults have worse health outcomes ranging from preventative care, cancer outcomes, and substance use. The causes of these health outcomes are complex and have myriad different modalities. It is essential to treat LGBTQ+ patients with dignity, respect, and compassion as they continue to access and engage in the healthcare system. The increase in LGBTQ+ identifying youth proves a need for diverse, empathic, and affirming healthcare providers for these individuals as they age into the adult population.

LGBTQ+ patients should be treated as any other patient in the medical setting, but there are certain areas that need to be further explored in regard to their health. In particular, appropriate STI screenings and assessments, screening for Hepatitis B, screening for depression/anxiety, substance use screenings, discussion of PrEP for patients who may benefit, and appropriate preventative care measures need to be routinely brought up. These assessments will be further discussed later in the chapter.

## Terminology

**Glossary of Terms**

| | |
|---|---|
| **LGBTQ+** | An acronym for "lesbian, gay, bisexual, transgender and queer" with a "+" sign to recognize the limitless sexual orientations and gender identities. LGBTQ+ can be used interchangeably with sexual and gender minorities. |
| **Sexual orientation** | An inherent or immutable enduring emotional, romantic, or sexual attraction to other people. Note: an individual's sexual orientation is independent of their gender identity. |
| **Gender identity** | One's innermost concept of self as male, female, or a blend of both or neither—how individuals perceive themselves and what they call themselves. One's gender identity can be the same or different from the sex assigned at birth. |
| **Queer** | A term people often use to express a spectrum of identities and orientations that are counter to the mainstream. Queer is often used as a catch-all to include many people, including those who do not identify as exclusively straight and/or folks who have nonbinary or gender-expansive identities. This term was previously used as a slur but has been reclaimed by many parts of the LGBTQ+ movement. |
| **Gay** | A person who is emotionally, romantically, or sexually attracted to members of the same gender. Men, women, and nonbinary people may use this term to describe themselves. |
| **Non-binary** | An adjective describing a person who does not identify exclusively as a man or a woman. Nonbinary people may identify as being both a man and a woman, somewhere in between, or as falling completely outside these categories. While many also identify as transgender, not all nonbinary people do. Nonbinary can also be used as an umbrella term encompassing identities such as agender, bigender, genderqueer, or gender-fluid. |
| **Gender Dysphoria** | Clinically significant distress is caused when a person's assigned birth gender is not the same as the one with which they identify. |
| **Gender Expression** | External appearance of one's gender identity, usually expressed through behavior, clothing, body characteristics, or voice, and which may or may not conform to socially defined behaviors and characteristics typically associated with being either masculine or feminine. |
| **Sex Assigned at Birth** | The sex, male, female, or intersex, that a doctor or midwife uses to describe a child at birth based on their external anatomy. |

| | |
|---|---|
| **Transitioning** | A series of processes that some transgender people may undergo in order to live more fully as their true gender. This typically includes social transition, such as changing name and pronouns, medical transition, which may include hormone therapy or gender-affirming surgeries, and legal transition, which may include changing legal name and sex on government identity documents. Transgender people may choose to undergo some, all, or none of these processes. |
| **Transgender and Gender Diverse** | An umbrella term for people whose gender identity and/or expression is different from cultural expectations based on the sex they were assigned at birth. Being transgender does not imply any specific sexual orientation. Therefore, transgender people may identify as straight, gay, lesbian, bisexual, etc. |
| **Cisgender** | A term used to describe a person whose gender identity aligns with those typically associated with the sex assigned to them at birth. |

https://www.hrc.org/resources/glossary-of-terms

HRC Foundation Professional Resources, All Children All Families. Glossary of Terms.

Gender identity and sexual minorities are distinct entities that youth, adolescents, and adults explore throughout their lives. Gender identity is an individual's personal sense of gender [10]. Examples of gender identity include cis-gender, transgender, nonbinary, agender, and gender fluid. The table above provides definitions to terms that will be used throughout this chapter. Gender identity exploration is fluid and on a spectrum. Gender can become evident as young as 4–5, can become more pronounced around the time of puberty, or can happen later in life [11]. Sexual minorities are defined as the gender or genders in which someone is sexually attracted. Examples of sexual minorities include homosexual (gay, lesbian), bisexual, queer, pansexual, and asexual. Sexual minorities tend to become more pronounced around puberty, but can change and evolve over time.

More young people today identify as a part of the LGBTQ+ community than ever before, indicating the shift in how kids identify and how society and culture play a role in acceptance and fluidity [12]. While young people are becoming more open about gender identity and sexual minorities, there still exist myriad disparities in regard to mental health, substance use, health outcomes, and preventative care. While there are studies that detail the disparities that exist, many are in the context of LGBTQ+ individuals as an entire group and not narrowed down within specific entities. More literature and research is needed to explore the differences within these groups.

Transgender and gender diverse is defined as an umbrella term that encompasses the population of individuals whose gender identity does not match with their sex assigned at birth. In the healthcare field, gender dysphoria is a diagnosis given to individuals who are gender diverse, but the term will likely eventually be replaced by gender incongruence, which does not have a negative connotation related to it. A variety of treatment options are available for transgender patients, which can be provided by primary care (Family Medicine, Internal Medicine, Medicine/Pediatrics) as well as endocrinology. The informed consent model is an appropriate method to assess gender dysphoria and in moving forward with treatment. Previously, psychological evaluation was required prior to medical management, but as gender dysphoria and transgender are no longer designated as mental health pathologies, informed consent is a more holistic way to ensure transgender individuals receive appropriate care.

There are a variety of organizations with educational resources in regard to transgender care, many of which can be accessed for free. Hormone management of transgender patients can be a routine part of care and does not necessarily need to be managed by a specialist if adequate learning has been achieved. According to the 2015 Transgender Survey, 50% of transgender patients had to teach their physician about some aspect of their health needs [10]. While the field of LGBTQ+ healthcare is continuing to expand and evolve, transgender patients should be able to access care from affirming providers who are educated and knowledgeable about LGBTQ+ healthcare.

## Coming Out

Coming out as LGBTQIA+ can be nerve wracking and a cause for significant distress, whether it is an adolescent, young adult, or adult. The ramifications of coming out and having a family who is not supportive can be devastating. There are known increased rates of homelessness among LGBTQIA+ youth, especially people of color [13]. Social acceptance for LGBTQ+ youth involves family support, support from peers and at school, within the healthcare setting, and with affirming behavioral health as indicated. As discussed earlier, healthcare providers may be the first or only person someone has come out to. As young adults transition care from pediatricians to primary care providers, it can be difficult for LGBTQ+ patients to find an affirming provider. Ensuring that patients transition to an adult primary care physician in a comfortable, holistic, and compassionate way can ease the stress that comes with meeting a new physician, especially for LGBTQ+ patients.

## Disparities, Why They Exist

Many disparities exist within the LGBTQ+ community, ranging from access to healthcare, worsened health outcomes, increased risk for substance use, and decreased completion of preventative health measures. Studies have looked at these disparities and many can be divided into specific groups. For example, lesbian women have an increased risk of obesity and gay men have decreased rates of obesity. There can be a variety of reasons for this, in particular, given the unrealistic cultural expectations for gay men to be slim, fit, and youthful. The prevalence of these disparities indicates the need for providers who are affirming, who are aware of these disparities, and will address them within these specific groups.

In the healthcare setting, access to healthcare can be difficult for LGBTQ+ patients. Patients want to find a provider who is affirming and who will treat them with respect and dignity, so many postpone or delay care due to fear of discrimination. For patients who are in a rural area in particular, finding an affirming provider may result in them having to drive to a larger city, which isn't always feasible. Therefore, they may either not seek out care or will get care locally and may end up being mistreated.

Disease outcomes for the LGBTQ+ community are poorer compared to cis-gender counterparts in many areas. In particular, patients who are cis-gender and identify as lesbians have higher rates of breast cancer, cervical cancer, ovarian cancer, and cancers related to alcohol, smoking, and obesity. Reasons for increased rates can be attributed to poor access to cancer prevention and preventative health screenings, lack of insurance, many women may not choose to have a child or get pregnant (pregnancy was found to decrease the risk of ovarian cancer), and if they are diagnosed with cancer, may not have all of the available resources and care compared to their cis-gender counterparts.

Gay men are at significantly higher risk of contracting HIV and with that, have increased risk for certain cancers, including Kaposi sarcoma, non-Hodgkin lymphoma, and squamous cell cancers related to HPV [14]. In order to mitigate these disparities, access to preventative healthcare measures is essential. Whether that be encouraging patients to get a pap smear, mammogram, or colonoscopy, engaging the LGBTQ+ community in getting these screenings will help prevent progression of disease in many cases. The other social factors also play a role in cancer risk, including smoking, alcohol use, and obesity. Having discussions surrounding diet, exercise, weight loss, tobacco cessation, and alcohol use are additional ways to try and prevent disease progression.

## Minority Stress Theory

Minority stress is the psychosocial stress derived from having a minority status [15]. With the societal norms of heterosexuality, those who identify as LGBTQ+ can experience chronic distress, ultimately leading to adverse health outcomes. For a minority person in a stigmatizing and discriminating society, the conflict between them and the dominant culture can be onerous, and the resultant minority stress is significant [16]. Myriad studies have looked at how minority stress impacts physical and mental health outcomes, trying to mitigate those disparities and address them accordingly. While being LGBTQ+ can result in minority stress, there can also be compounding factors, including race, gender identity, especially for those who are transgender, and socioeconomic status that can be applied. The factors that play a role in minority stress include internalized homophobia, internalized transphobia, perceived stigma, hate incidents, and hate crimes.

Mental health outcomes related to LGBTQ+ individuals are known to be worse compared to their cisgender, heterosexual counterparts; minority stress theory has implications in these findings. Studies have found there is strong support for the impact of minority stress on mental health and substance use among sexual minority women, mediated by social–psychological resources [17]. Among gay men, Meyer's study found that minority stress is associated with a two to threefold increase in the risk for high levels of distress [16]. Minority stress may implicate a greater likelihood of risk-taking behaviors as well. Whether that includes sexual risk-taking and contraction of HIV/AIDS, polysubstance use, or intimate partner violence, more research needs to be done surrounding LGBTQ+ populations and the health implications of minority stress.

As a group, LGBTQ+ youth experience high rates of emotional, physical, and sexual abuse [18] and are significantly more likely to lack stable housing and family support and enter social service systems. LGBTQ+ youth have been noted to have increased adverse health outcomes, including rates or suicidal thoughts, suicide attempts, and depressive symptoms [19]. We know from data on adverse childhood experiences (ACEs) that people adapt to stressors. With this in mind, it is important to approach care of LGBTQ+ youth from a trauma informed care perspective and conceptualize the patient's presenting symptoms and behaviors as their responses to surviving.

## Resilience

Resilience refers to the ability to overcome significant stress or adversity. It is a dynamic process encompassing positive adaptation within the context of significant adversity [20]. A stress response can promote adaptation when turned on/off efficiently or pathophysiological responses when overused or dysregulated [21]. In order to provide whole-person, patient-centered care to LGBTQ youth and shift from a pathology mindset, an approach to care from a strength rather than deficit perspective is helpful [22]. Known factors that promote resilience include access to material resources, experiences of power and control, supportive relationships with significant others, having a sense of identity that fuels a sense of satisfaction, pride and purpose, a sense that things are fair and equitable, having cultural/community connection as well as a sense of social cohesion found through community connections [20, 22]. A child's development is influenced directly by the environment. Bronfenbrenner's ecological systems model provides a framework to target resilience at various social levels for LGBTQ youth [23].

- **Individual:** At the individual level, targeting self-efficacy, coping skills, health-promoting behaviors, social skills, social support networks, extracurricular/community activities as well as the ability to define/describe own identities with individual therapy, group therapy, and skilling training activities.
- **Micro:** Provide positive parent–child attachment/warmth, family cohesion and encour-

agement/support—provider sensitivity training, family/peer support/rejection, messaging at church, harassment/assault at school.
- **Meso:** relationships between groups from the first system (e.g., parent–teacher).
- **Exo:** greater social environment not directly touching children, safe affordable housing, queer people on TV.
- **Macro:** dominant cultural values, religious—antigay laws, lack of housing and employment protections, legalization of gay marriage.

Trauma-informed care (TIC) is an approach to care that assumes that an individual is more likely than not to have a history of trauma. TIC recognizes the presence of trauma symptoms and acknowledges the role trauma may play in an individual's life. TIC understands and considers the pervasive nature of trauma and promotes environments of healing and recovery rather than practices and services that may inadvertently retraumatize [24]. An important tenet of providing TIC to sexual and gender minority youth is to be open and supportive and not assume to know someone's identities or experiences. Key aspects of practicing Trauma Informed Care for LGBTQ-identified youth include the use of:

1. Affirmative language (chosen name, pronouns, etc.)
2. Gender-inclusive language to describe patients and their partners, friends, and family.
3. Open-ended questions to ask about patient's experience.

## Special Topics Impacting Sexual and Gender Minority Youth

Special consideration should be given to key issues that contribute to the health disparities seen in sexual and gender minority youth. These include:

1. Considerations around sexual debut and sexual activity—as previously mentioned, healthcare professionals and systems can play a key role in ensuring that sexual and gender minority individuals feel welcome and safe and can set the course for these individuals in terms of future engagement with health care. Creating a nonjudgmental, welcoming space for LGBTQ+ patients is key to alleviating stress and breaking down barriers that fuel some of the disparities seen in LGBTQ+ youth. It is important that healthcare professionals and their teams do not make assumptions about individuals and ask open-ended questions which allows them to get to know their patients better and assess any behaviors that may put them at risk for adverse health outcomes. It is important that patient's pronouns are elicited and used appropriately. Information from the Trevor project states that transgender and nonbinary youth whose pronouns were respected by all or most of the people in their lives attempted suicide at half the rate of those who did not have their pronouns respected [25].
2. STI prevention—approaching care from a holistic lens is important. As such, as with all youth who are sexually active, taking a comprehensive sexual history in LGBTQ+ patients is important. This needs to be done using a TIC approach. It is important to use open-ended questions when asking about sexual practices and assessing risk for various STIs. Examples of questions to consider asking are:
   (a) Tell me about your sex life
   (b) What body parts do you use for sex?
   (c) Who are your sexual partners, if any?
3. PrEP—in its 2021 update of Clinical Practice Guidelines for Preexposure Prophylaxis for the Prevention of HIV infection, the CDC recommends that all sexually active adults and adolescents should be informed about PrEP so as to decrease the stigma and help patients to overcome embarrassment of being open with medical providers about practices that may put them at risk for HIV [26].
4. Homelessness—homeless is a crisis in LGBTQ-identified youth with nearly one-third of these youth reporting lifetime experiences of homelessness or housing instability,

e.g., couch-surfing [27]. Parental rejection because of being LGBTQ plays a big role in this and these individuals report higher rates of lifetime homelessness which are associated with reporting more symptoms of several mental health disorders and higher levels of suicidality [27]. It is important to assess for homelessness and have LGBTQ-focused services for impacted individuals.

5. Eating disorders—eating disorders and disordered eating have been shown to happen at higher rates in sexual and gender minority individuals and this has been linked to the minority stress model as a result of the stigma and discrimination this group faces [28]. Research also suggests that sexual minority communities can have a detrimental effect on body image and eating behaviors. It is important to note that the US Preventive Services Task Force has found insufficient evidence to assess the balance of benefits and harms of screening for eating disorders in adolescents and adults; [29], however due to the known increased incidence of eating disorders in LGBTQ+ youth, being aware of this issue and assessing for risk of disordered or unhealthy eating or exercise practices in LGBTQ+ youth is important in the primary care setting.
6. Mental health and substance use—the effect of stigma and discrimination causing minority stress and impacting mental well-being in LGBTQ+ youth cannot be understated [15, 16]. As medical providers, being aware of the impact of minority stress on the mental well-being of sexual and gender minority individuals is important. Using validated screeners in primary care settings and developing safety plans and providing resources have been shown to have a positive impact on patients [30]. Providing a welcoming and positive environment is crucial to LGBTQ+ youth seeking and remaining in care.
7. Preventative health—it is important to educate sexual and gender minority individuals on age and organ-appropriate cancer screening so as to decrease the cancer disparities seen in LGBTQ+ patients.

## References


1. Russell ST, Pollitt AM, Li G, Grossman AH. Chosen name use is linked to reduced depressive symptoms, suicidal ideation, and suicidal behavior among transgender youth. J Adolesc Health. 2018;63(4):503–5.
2. Jamal A, Phillips E, Gentzke AS, et al. Current cigarette smoking among adults—United States, 2016. Morb Mortal Wkly Rep. 2018;67(2):53.
3. Heckman CJ, Egleston BL. Hofmann MTEfficacy of motivational interviewing for smoking cessation: a systematic review and meta-analysis. Tob Control. 2010;19:410–6.
4. Woodhead M. Guidelines for the management of adult lower respiratory tract infections. Eur Respir J. 2005;26(6):1138–80.
5. Fruh SM. Obesity: risk factors, complications, and strategies for sustainable long-term weight management. J Am Assoc Nurse Pract. 2017;29(S1):S3–S14.
6. McCabe SE, Hughes TL, Bostwick WB, West BT, Boyd CJ. Sexual orientation, substance use behaviors and substance dependence in the United States. Addiction. 2009;104(8):1333–45.
7. Austin A, Craig SL, D'Souza S, McInroy LB. Suicidality among transgender youth: elucidating the role of interpersonal risk factors. J Interpers Violence. 2022;37(5–6):NP2696–718.
8. Gates GJ. How many people are lesbian, gay, bisexual, and transgender? [Internet]. Williams Institute. [cited 2022 Oct 1]. https://williamsinstitute.law.ucla.edu/publications/how-many-people-lgbt/
9. Herman JL, Flores AR, O'Neill KK. How many adults and youth identify as transgender in the United States?—Williams Institute [Internet]. [cited 2022 Oct 1]. https://williamsinstitute.law.ucla.edu/publications/trans-adults-united-states/
10. Grant JM, Mottet LA, Tanis J, Harrison J, Herman JL, Keisling M. Injustice at every turn: a report of the national transgender discrimination survey. Washington: National Center for Transgender Equality and National Gay and Lesbian Task Force; 2011.
11. Kerr BA, Multon KD. The development of gender identity, gender roles, and gender relations in gifted students. J Couns Dev. 2015;93(2):183–91.
12. Andrew Adesman, MD, chief, developmental and behavioral pediatrics, Cohen Children's Medical Center, New York City; Amy Green, PhD, vice president, research, The Trevor Project, West Hollywood, Calif.; Joseph Kosciw, PhD, director, GLSEN Research Institute, GLSEN, New York City; JAMA Pediatrics, June 14, 2021, online.
13. Rapport E, Athanasian CE, Adesman A. Prevalence of Nonheterosexual Identity and Same-Sex Sexual Contact Among High School Students in the US From 2015 to 2019. JAMA Pediatrics 2021;175(9):970–72.
14. Dubrow R, et al. HIV infection, aging, and immune function: implications for cancer risk and prevention. Curr Opin Oncol. 2012;24(5):506.

15. Brooks VR. Minority stress and lesbian women. Lexington, MA: Lexington Books, D.C. Health and Co; 1981.
16. Meyer IH. Minority stress and mental health in gay men. J Health Soc Behav. 1995;36(1):38.
17. Lehavot K, Simoni JM. The impact of minority stress on mental health and substance use among sexual minority women. J Consult Clin Psychol. 2011;79(2):159–70.
18. Kosciw JG, Bartkiewicz M, Greytak EA. Promising strategies for prevention of the bullying of lesbian, gay, bisexual and transgender youth. Prevent Res. 2012;19(3)
19. Human Rights Campaign. 2018 LGBTQ Youth Report [Internet]; 2018. https://assets2.hrc.org/files/assets/resources/2018-YouthReport-0514-Final.pdf
20. Colpitts E, Gahagan J. The utility of resilience as a conceptual framework for understanding and measuring LGBTQ health. Int J Equity Health. 2016;15(1):60.
21. McEwen BS. Stress, adaptation, and disease. Allostasis and allostatic load. Ann N Y Acad Sci. 1998;840:33–44.
22. Johns MM, Poteat VP, Horn SS, Kosciw J. Strengthening our schools to promote resilience and health among LGBTQ youth: emerging evidence and research priorities from *the state of LGBTQ youth health and wellbeing* symposium. LGBT Health. 2019;6(4):146–55.
23. Hong JS, Espelage DL, Kral MJ. Understanding suicide among sexual minority youth in America: an ecological systems analysis. J Adolesc. 2011;34(5):885–94.
24. McCormick A, Scheyd K, Terrazas. Trauma-informed care and LGBTQ youth: considerations for advancing practice with youth with trauma experience. J Contemp Social Serv. 2018;99(2):160–9.
25. The Trevor Project. Pronouns usage among LGBTQ youth [Internet]. [cited 2022 Oct 1]. https://www.thetrevorproject.org/research-briefs/pronouns-usage-among-lgbtq-youth/
26. US Public Health Service. Preexposure prophylaxis for the prevention of HIV infection in the United States—2021 update, a clinical practice guideline. 2021;108.
27. Rhoades H, Rusow JA, Bond D, Lanteigne A, Fulginiti A, Goldbach JT. Homelessness, mental health and suicidality among LGBTQ youth accessing crisis services. Child Psychiatry Hum Dev. 2018;48:643–51.
28. Parker LL, Harriger JA. Eating disorders and disordered eating behaviors in the LGBT population: a review of the literature. J Eat Disord. 2020 Dec;8(1):51.
29. US Preventive Services Task Force, Davidson KW, Barry MJ, Mangione CM, Cabana M, Chelmow D, et al. Screening for eating disorders in adolescents and adults: US preventive services task force recommendation statement. JAMA. 2022;327(11):1061.
30. Batchelder AW, Stanton AM, Kirakosian N, King D, Grasso C, Potter J, et al. Mental health and substance use diagnoses and treatment disparities by sexual orientation and gender in a community health center sample. LGBT Health. 2021;8(4):290–9.

# Medical Care for Transgender and Gender-Diverse People

# 10

Jessica Abramowitz and Nupur Agrawal

Transgender and gender-diverse (TGD) patients undergoing transition have unique medical and healthcare needs that have historically been unmet due to a paucity of gender-affirming providers knowledgeable in their care. As increasing numbers of TGD members of the community seek both transition-related and general healthcare, providers have an opportunity and a responsibility to learn strategies for delivering comprehensive, compassionate, affirming, and safe care to members of this marginalized population.

In this chapter, we provide general guidance on initiating and maintaining gender-affirming hormone therapy (GAHT), an outline of options available to patients for surgical transition, and a comprehensive review of additional health considerations that are important in caring for TGD patients. Excellent guidelines already exist that provide more comprehensive information on the topics we discuss, and we will reference these guidelines throughout the chapter for further reading. We do attempt to provide a unique perspective on gender-focused healthcare through discussion of the evolving needs TGD individuals experience across their lifespan.

This chapter is founded upon the principles discussed in Chap. 7: Gender Identity and Related Health Considerations. Because understanding gender identity is foundational to providing medical care to TGD patients, we highly recommend reading Chap. 7 before reading this chapter on medical care.

## Foundational Steps in Initiating Medical Care for Transgender and Gender-Diverse Patients

### Gender-Inclusive Clinics and Environments

The patient's experience with the clinic begins as early as the scheduling of the patient appointment. It is important to consider all of the touch points where a patient may encounter clinic or scheduling staff and ensure that all staff has had basic training to enhance cultural competency and respect. Many health system portals allow patients to enter their chosen names and pronouns into the chart before the appointment. Staff should use these names and pronouns at all times to establish an affirming environment for all patients.

J. Abramowitz (✉)
Division of Endocrinology, Department of Internal Medicine, UT Southwestern Medical Center, Dallas, TX, USA
e-mail: Jessica.Abramowitz@UTSouthwestern.edu

N. Agrawal
Division of Medicine-Pediatrics and Preventive Medicine, University of California, Los Angeles, CA, USA
e-mail: nupuragrawal@mednet.ucla.edu


A. A. Kuo et al. (eds.), *Care of Adults with Chronic Childhood Conditions*,
https://doi.org/10.1007/978-3-031-54281-7_10

Staff and clinicians should avoid outing patients in a public setting [*outing*: revealing an aspect of someone's identity, such as gender identity or sexuality that they have not revealed to others or themselves]. If there are additional questions regarding the legal name or gender marker, then these are best addressed quietly away from other patients or families who may overhear these conversations. Staff and clinicians should also avoid invasive or unnecessary questioning that only serves to satisfy their curiosity.

For the safety and comfort of patients, it is best to have a designated gender-neutral bathroom. For clinics that have predominantly gendered environments (such as mammography centers, gynecology clinics, and urology clinics), patients can be offered first or last appointments of the day to avoid patient discomfort. Many institutions have ways of designating LGBTQ allies and champions on their websites. This allows patients to view this information before their appointment and know in advance that their provider will be culturally competent and sensitive. See the following example from the UCLA website *https://www.uclahealth.org/gender-health/programs-services*.

Comprehensive attempts should be made to affirm patients at every opportunity, but errors will eventually be made. If a provider recognizes that they have misgendered the patient, then the provider should immediately recognize the mistake, apologize to the patient, and then move on with the conversation. Dwelling on the mistake creates discomfort for both the patient and the provider. If a provider observes another person misgendering the patient, then they should gently correct the person in a constructive manner. In this way, people can improve sensitivity in practice.

## Assessment of Individual Patient Journey and Goals

Providers should build an understanding of each patient's gender exploration journey in order to best guide the next steps in treatment. This process begins with a detailed exploration of gender identity, which is discussed at length in Chap. 7. From a treatment standpoint, providers should additionally inquire about steps patients have taken to better align their outward gender expression with their gender identity. Questions to help guide this conversation:

- When did you start socially transitioning?
- When did you start using your name?
- When did you first ask others to use your pronouns?
- How has your social presentation evolved over time?
- Have you come out to anyone?
- Who has been supportive of your transition?
- What challenges have you had to face?

There are known healthcare disparities for TGD individuals, and difficulty finding a culturally competent provider is chief among them [1, 2]. Patients may have seen other providers in the past who discriminated against them or refused gender-affirming care. In this context, some patients may have never had access to GAHT, and other patients may have resorted to self-treatment as a means to move forward with their transition. Understanding a patient's history of treatment with hormone therapy is important to developing an ideal treatment plan moving forward.

The gender dysphoria experienced by different individuals may require different approaches to treatment and gender affirmation. For some TGD individuals, social transition may be adequate to alleviate dysphoria while for others treatment with GAHT is needed to aid with the feminization or masculinization of the body. Medical providers treating TGD patients should assess both the degree of dysphoria and the patient's specific goals for treatment. Nonbinary individuals may require varying degrees of feminization or masculinization to relieve dysphoria.

Questions to help guide this conversation:

- Have you ever used hormonal therapy?
- Have hormones been prescribed to you or have you taken them on your own?

- What forms (injections, pills, and patches) of hormone therapy have you used?
- What physical features are currently causing you the greatest dysphoria?
- What are your goals for treatment with hormone therapy?
- Are you comfortable administering your hormones, or is there someone who can help you?

## Importance of Passing

For many TGD individuals, a key component of transitioning and living comfortably in their affirmed gender is "passing" in all settings. Passing, more formally known as visual conformity with the affirmed gender, is when others perceive TGD individuals to be their true gender identity. People who successfully pass may choose to share their transition with others or to be stealthy—meaning they live in their desired gender without others knowing about their transition.

A study published in 2020 that surveyed 620 respondents in the United States found that greater acceptance, greater pride in their TGD identity, and transmasculine gender-affirming surgeries were associated with higher rates of passing and lower rates of depression and anxiety [3]. A survey of 54 transgender women in Japan found that GAHT, gender-affirming surgery, and living as a woman helped them pass, but there were limited resources to help them address other factors (e.g., voice training) that would facilitate access to women-only services [4]. Low rates of passing routinely correlate with gender-based victimization and associated nonaffirmation microaggressions, violence, discrimination, and rejection [5] although a recent study from Brazil showed that higher rates of passing, while protective from these factors, actually led to increased risk of suffering violence at home from family members [6]. Nonbinary patients have described passing as an often unattainable goal and feel satisfied when people recognize them as having an identity other than their sex assigned at birth [7].

These studies highlight the complexity of passing as well as the key role of gender-affirming treatment in supporting patients' physical and emotional safety. Similar to gender identity and gender expression, passing can mean different things for different people, so goals related to passing should be discussed on an individual basis.

## Shared Decision-Making

Patients now have access to numerous online resources, including forums, support groups, and videos, that provide a wealth of information regarding medical and surgical transition; patients routinely utilize this information to understand their gender journeys as well as the next steps in treatment. At the time of initial contact with providers, patients often have a sense of their path forward. Clinicians play a critical role in providing patients with evidence-based information about hormone therapy and treatment options, which may include differentiating between consensus-based guidelines used in medical practice versus anecdotal approaches that may be discussed in community settings but are not founded in evidence. Clinicians can also answer any questions patients may have and discuss the risks and benefits of various treatment options. In this setting, a shared decision-making model works best where the practitioner and the patient decide on the best plan of care for the patient based on the available evidence and the patient's goals [8]. While the database of evidence-based practices in the field of gender-affirming care is rapidly evolving and growing, there are still areas of care in which clear data are not available. In these situations, providers should feel comfortable discussing data that may be extrapolated from other populations as well as topics that have not been studied rigorously and systematically.

## Informed Consent Model

In the past, patients seeking care with gender-affirming hormones were required to present a letter from a mental health provider confirming the diagnosis of gender dysphoria before initiating GAHT. Currently, both the World Professional Association for Transgender Health (WPATH) eighth edition guidelines and the Endocrine Society Guidelines allow providers who feel comfortable in assessing and confirming the presence of gender dysphoria to make the diagnosis and initiate treatment without a referral letter from a mental health provider [9, 10]. This approach has been noted to favor patient autonomy and avoids paternalism by the medical professional [11]. A review of clinics using this approach found low rates of patient regret and no concerns about malpractice [12].

Informed consent involves a discussion of risks, benefits, and alternatives of treatment, and documentation of this discussion between patients and providers suffices for moving forward with care. This consent is received from parents and/or legal guardians for minor children and adolescents although youth should be involved in the decision-making process as the care impacts them directly.

Informed consent models may vary across clinics, but the general consensus in the field is that verbal consent to initiate GAHT is sufficient to start treatment (versus written consent, which is perceived to be another barrier for patients to overcome in gaining access to gender-affirming care). Providers should be familiar with these various consent models and work cooperatively with patients to help ease the initiation of hormone therapy and avoid medical "gatekeeping" (see Chap. 7 for further discussion).

## Principles of Medical Transition

### Overview

Treatment options available to patients depend on the age at which they present for gender-affirming care. Figure 10.1 provides a visual timeline of gender-affirming care across the continuum of life (please refer to the section titled "Gender Identity Development" in Chap. 7 for foundational information on the evolution of gender identity across the lifespan).

### Social Transition

Presenting in public as one's true gender identity can be an important part of transitioning for many TGD patients. This process, called social transition, refers to the many facets people adjust in

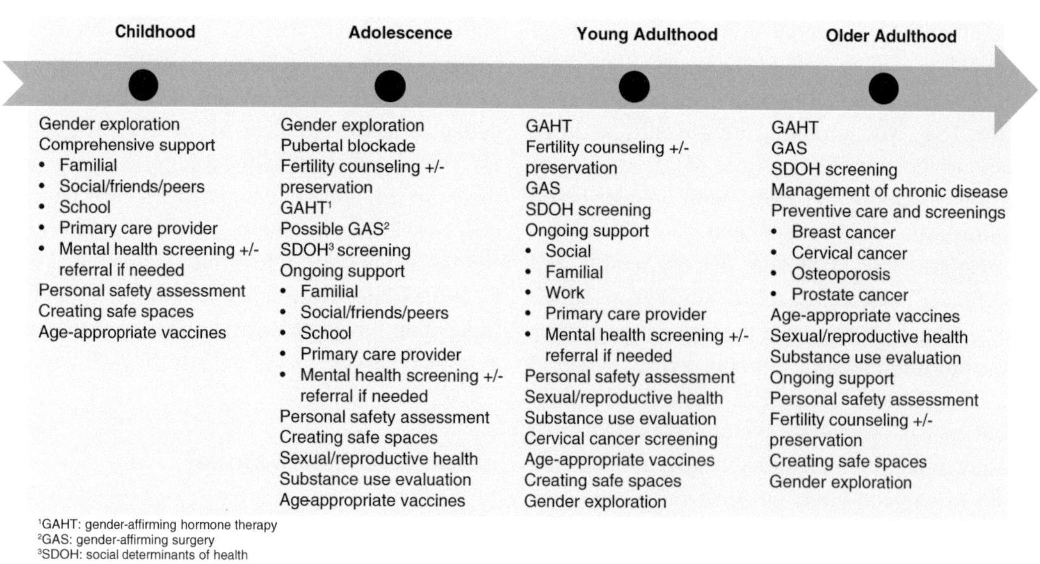


**Fig. 10.1** Healthcare considerations for transgender and gender-diverse patients across the lifespan

social settings to present as their authentic selves, including, but not limited to, name, pronouns, dressing style, hairstyle, and use of additional equipment (e.g., penile prosthetics, gaffs, binders) [13]. Many people incorporate some or all of the aforementioned changes into their lives before starting GAHT in order to facilitate coming out to family, friends, coworkers, and community members; experimenting with different ways of presenting to clarify long-term presentation goals; etc. Other patients may choose to hold off on changing how they present socially until after the initiation of GAHT. Hormones impact physical appearance and can make it emotionally easier for some people to come out to loved ones, ask others to use their name and pronouns, and pass as members of their experienced gender. Historically, patients were asked to spend at least 1 year living full-time in their gender identity to make sure they wanted to transition; doing so would eventually give them access to GAHT. We now know that forcing individuals to socially transition before they are ready can be harmful, and there is no prescribed timeline for social and medical transition.

Affirming providers should seek to understand the patient's individual goals related to social transition. The following is a question guide to facilitate this conversation:

1. What steps, if any, have you taken so far to socially transition?
2. What has your social transition looked like?
3. What tools have you used to present your gender identity?
4. What additional resources will help you successfully present publicly in the way you feel most comfortable?

## Treatment Options and Fertility Preservation for Young Adolescents

Gender identity development begins in childhood and can continue throughout one's lifetime. As discussed in Chap. 7, there are TGD patients who know as early as age two that they are gender incongruent. For many other patients though, puberty is the time of rapid physical and emotional growth that often elucidates underlying gender dysphoria. Patients in early adolescence who are questioning and exploring their gender identity can benefit from additional time to better understand their identity and related long-term goals. Gonadotropin-releasing hormone (GnRH) analogs—known colloquially as puberty blockers, pubertal blockers, or just blockers—form the cornerstone of gender-affirming treatment in this age group (Table 10.1). As the name suggests, blockers are used to halt puberty and put a pause on the often irreversible physical changes that accompany the evolving hormonal milieu during this time. Patients have to be at least at Tanner Stage 2 prior to qualifying for blockers. The pause is fully reversible. For patients who ultimately feel their gender identity is congruent with their sex assigned at birth, which is the rarer outcome, blockers can easily be discontinued, and natal puberty will resume without impact on long-term physical development. For patients who decide to continue with their transition, which happens the majority of the time, GAHT is introduced and titrated in a manner that allows TGD adolescents to experience desired pubertal changes contemporaneously with their age-matched cis-gender peers.

Given that most adolescents who pursue initiation of blockers eventually decide to move forward in their transition, one of the most important considerations to discuss with patients and parents is the desire for fertility preservation. Pubertal blockers halt the maturation of gametes, and data are not clear on the impact of long-term hormone exposure on the quality of gametes over time. For this reason, the discussion of options for fertility preservation becomes important. Fertility preservation in children and adolescents has more extensively been studied in oncology where patients have to make decisions regarding fertility at a young age [14]. Many pediatric cancer survivors feel that fertility is linked with the ultimate quality of life, and guidelines recommend that physicians counsel all patients on fertility preservation options and future reproduction before initiating treatment. Still, data show that only 60% of providers document providing fertil-

**Table 10.1** Gonadotropin-Releasing Hormone (GnRH) analogs for pubertal blockade

| GnRH analog | Brand name | Typical dosing | Frequency | Benefits | Risks |
|---|---|---|---|---|---|
| Histrelin | Supprelin LA | 50 mg | Subdermal implant exchanged annually[a] | Although FDA approved for 1 year placement, implant can remain effective for up to 18–24 months, which significantly minimizes need for routine office visits for injections. | Requires invasive procedure; implant can get embedded in scar tissue over time and may complicate removal; fertility considerations and potential bone density changes associated with all GnRH analogs |
| Leuprolide | Lupron | 3.75 mg IM[b] | Every month[c] | Does not require implant placement; easy to adjust or discontinue if needed | Injections can be painful; require monthly or quarterly visits to provider office; breakthrough bleeding for transmasculine patients if delay in injection; fertility considerations and potential bone density changes associated with all GnRH analogs |
| | | 11.25 mg IM<br>30 mg IM | Every 3 months | | |
| | Eligard | 7.5 mg SQ[d] | Every month[c] | | |
| | | 22.5 mg SQ | Every 3 months | | |

[a]Measuring luteinizing hormone (LH) levels can determine whether the histrelin implant is still effective, and the implant can be used up to 18–24 months if LH levels remain suppressed
[b]Intramuscular
[c]Monthly dosing can create barriers to accessing care in a timely manner and should be avoided unless there are medication shortages or other challenges involving insurance formulary
[d]Subcutaneous

ity counseling, <50% of patients recall getting this counseling, and < 30% of patients undergo fertility preservation. The largest barriers to pursuing fertility preservation in pediatric oncology patients are concern about treatment delay, the high cost of fertility preservation procedures, limited access to fertility specialists, and limited recall regarding reproductive options during overwhelming initial oncology visits.

The TGD youth population is unique from the pediatric oncology population, but the need for early counseling and barriers to fertility preservation overlap. Because GnRH analog use followed by the introduction of GAHT may impact fertility options for patients interested in having biological children in the future, it is imperative that providers initiate a conversation regarding options for fertility preservation at the first point of contact if possible. For many TGD youth, the discussion of fertility preservation can invoke significant dysphoria as even the thought of natal gametes can trigger discomfort. These conversations should, therefore, be held sensitively. In minors, legal guardians have to consent to move forward with gender-affirming treatments with or without fertility preservation, so engaging parents and other guardians on this topic is critical for comprehensive patient care. Providers should be able to provide referrals to reproductive endocrinologists as well as cryobanks where interested patients can pursue fertility preservation options. More is discussed on this topic in the "Additional Supportive Therapies" section that comes later in this chapter.

## Overview of Hormone Therapy in Post-pubertal Adolescents and Young Adults

For adults and adolescents (who present in late puberty, Tanner 4 and 5), testosterone and estradiol can be prescribed to help increase the hormone level of the affirmed gender [10]. Weight-based dosing allows for effective dosing as adolescents grow in size. These doses may be similar to adult doses depending on the size of the adolescent. The table below from the Endocrine Society Guidelines delineates the stepwise induction of desired puberty inP adolescents.

**Table 8. Protocol Induction of Puberty**

| |
|---|
| Induction of female puberty with oral 17β-estradiol, increasing the dose every 6 mo: |
| 5 μg/kg/d |
| 10 μg/kg/d |
| 15 μg/kg/d |
| 20 μg/kg/d |
| Adult dose = 2–6 mg/d |
| *In postpubertal transgender female adolescents, the dose of 17β-estradiol can be increased more rapidly:* |
| 1 mg/d for 6 mo |
| 2 mg/d |
| Induction of female puberty with transdermal 17β-estradiol, increasing the dose every 6 mo (new patch is placed every 3.5 d): |
| 6.25–12.5 μg/24 h (cut 25-μg patch into quarters, then halves) |
| 25 μg/24 h |
| 37.5 μg/24 h |
| Adult dose = 50–200 μg/24 h |
| *For alternatives once at adult dose, see Table 11.* |
| *Adjust maintenance dose to mimic physiological estradiol levels (see Table 15).* |
| Induction of male puberty with testosterone esters increasing the dose every 6 mo (IM or SC): |
| 25 mg/m²/2 wk (or alternatively, half this dose weekly, or double the dose every 4 wk) |
| 50 mg/m²/2 wk |
| 75 mg/m²/2 wk |
| 100 mg/m²/2 wk |
| Adult dose = 100–200 mg every 2 wk |
| *In postpubertal transgender male adolescents the dose of testosterone esters can be increased more rapidly:* |
| 75 mg/2 wk for 6 mo |
| 125 mg/2 wk |
| *For alternatives once at adult dose, see Table 11.* |
| *Adjust maintenance dose to mimic physiological testosterone levels (see Table 14).* |

Adapted from Hembree *et al.* (118).

Abbreviations: IM, intramuscularly; SC, subcutaneously.

## Masculinizing Hormone Therapy

Testosterone is the hormone used to masculinize the body and can be given in multiple formulations and at varying doses (Table 10.2). Providers should work with patients to determine the ideal formulation of testosterone administration. Patients who have fears of using needles themselves for injections can have caregivers learn to administer the injections. Subcutaneous testosterone is often easier to administer and has been found to be equivalent in efficacy to intramuscular testosterone [15, 16]. For other patients who do not want to use testosterone injections at all, there are gel formulations that are readily available options but may be cost-prohibitive depending on insurance coverage. Given the need for frequent dosing of testosterone (daily to weekly) regardless of formulation, patients should be taught to administer testosterone at home, so they do not need to come to the clinic for administration. The effects of testosterone begin in the first few months of treatment (Fig. 10.2), but changes continue for 3–5 years after the introduction of GAHT.

## Feminizing Hormone Therapy

Estradiol is the hormone used to feminize the body and can be given in multiple formulations and at varying doses (Table 10.3). In the setting of gender-affirming care, estradiol is administered in its 17β form to allow for the monitoring of hormone levels in the blood and decreased likelihood of thromboembolic phenomena and cardiovascular events compared to ethinyl estradiol [13, 17]. Oral is often the least expensive form of estradiol, but it has been shown to be associated with a higher risk of thromboembo-

**Table 10.2** Masculinizing hormone therapy

| Testosterone formulation | Typical Dosing | Frequency | Benefits | Risks |
|---|---|---|---|---|
| Parenteral (cypionate or enanthate)[a] | 40–100 mg SQ[b] or IM[c] | Weekly (every 2 weeks if not tolerated weekly) | More readily covered by insurance; weekly dosing (versus daily); better menstrual suppression | Peaks and troughs of levels can cause cyclical symptoms; low but present risk of pain, bleeding, infection at injection site; formation of scar tissue with IM use |
| | 1–8 mg | Daily | Avoids injections for those with needle phobia | Skin reactions to adhesive; visible to others; difficult to achieve therapeutic levels, may not be available |
| Transdermal gel (1.62% or 1%) | 40.5–81 mg | Daily | Avoids injections for those with needle phobia | Inadvertent medication exposure to others; difficult to achieve therapeutic levels |
| Oral pill[d] | 237 mg PO[e] | Twice daily | Option for patients with contraindications, adverse reactions, or treatment failure with other formulations; no hepatotoxicity as with prior oral formulations | Minimal to no side effects |

[a]Cypionate and enanthate are the two suspensions available for testosterone injections. Patients who have an allergic reaction to testosterone injections are likely reacting to the oil in the suspension. They can trial the alternate suspension to see if they tolerate it without reaction
[b]Subcutaneous
[c]Intramuscular
[d]Brand name Jatenzo
[e]Oral

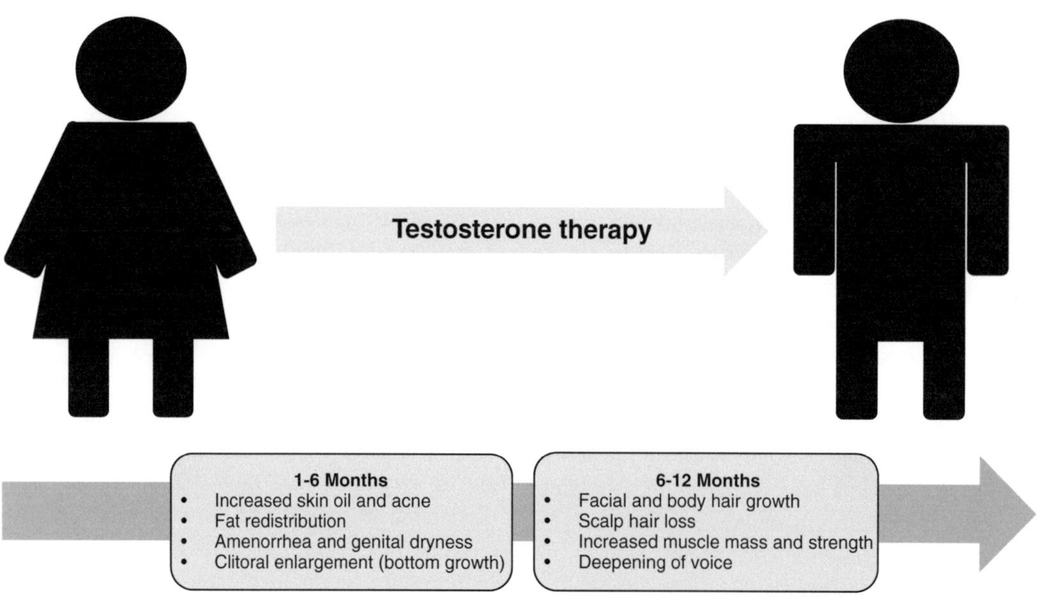


**Fig. 10.2** Onset of masculinizing changes with testosterone therapy over time

lism compared to the other forms of estradiol as it undergoes the first pass metabolism in the liver [10], but sublingual dosing may decrease this risk. Parenteral injections and patches, bypass liver metabolism, and, extrapolating from studies of postmenopausal cisgender women, these

**Table 10.3** Feminizing hormone therapy

| Estradiol formulation | Typical Dosing | Frequency | Benefits | Risks |
|---|---|---|---|---|
| Oral pill | 2–8 mg PO[a] or SL[b] | Twice daily (can be daily if desired) | Often least expensive and most readily covered by insurance | Metabolized by liver and may have increased risk of thrombosis if PO; takes time to dissolve SL since not manufactured for SL use |
| Transdermal patch | 0.025–0.3 mg | Patch is changed twice weekly | Reduced risk of thrombosis | Skin reactions to adhesive; visible to others; difficult to achieve therapeutic levels |
| Parenteral (valerate or cypionate)[c] | 2–5 mg (up to 10 mg) SQ[d] or IM[e] | Weekly (every 2 weeks if desired) | Reduced risk of thrombosis | There can be peak and troughs of levels causing cyclical symptoms. Low but present risk of pain, bleeding infection. Formation of scar tissue especially with IM injections. |

[a]Oral
[b]Sublingual
[c]Valerate and cypionate are the two suspensions available for estradiol injections. Patients who have an allergic reaction to estradiol injections are likely reacting to the oil in the suspension. They can trial the alternate suspension to see if they tolerate it without reaction
[d]Subcutaneous
[e]Intramuscular

forms of estradiol are less likely to cause thromboembolism [17]. There is a risk of supratherapeutic levels when using injectable estradiol [18], so levels should be monitored closely as discussed below. The effects of estradiol begin in the first few months of treatment (Fig. 10.3), but changes continue for 3–5 years after the introduction of GAHT.

When estradiol alone is insufficient in suppressing testosterone levels, antiandrogens are added to the medication regimen to help lower testosterone to undetectable levels (Table 10.4). The most commonly used antiandrogen in the United States is spironolactone. Spironolactone is a diuretic medication, an aldosterone antagonist, which also acts as an androgen antagonist in peripheral tissues [19]. In contrast to other diuretic medications, there is no renal loss of potassium with spironolactone, so monitoring for hyperkalemia with treatment is recommended. Cyproterone acetate, an androgen receptor antagonist, is not readily available in the United States but is frequently used in Europe and other parts of the world. Bicalutamide is an alternative androgen blocker with an increased risk of liver toxicity, and larger studies are needed to better understand its safety profile [20]. Alternate antiandrogen medications may also include 5-alpha-reductase inhibitors such as finasteride and dutasteride. Neither one of these medications blocks the effect of testosterone nor the amount of testosterone that is produced but instead blocks the conversion of testosterone to dihydrotestosterone; studies to better understand the efficacy of this class of medication as part of a feminizing regimen are needed [13, 21].

## Lab Monitoring

Routine monitoring of patients on GAHT includes measuring serum hormone levels to guide dosing adjustments. For individuals using testosterone for full masculinization, the goal range for testosterone is the midpoint of the normal testosterone range of approximately 400–700 ng/dL [10, 22]. In this setting, it is recommended to monitor total testosterone levels [10]. For injectable testosterone, levels can be measured mid-administration cycle (i.e., approximately 3 days after weekly injections or 1 week after biweekly injections). Providers can stop measuring estradiol levels in these patients once the cessation of menses is achieved, which typically happens within 6–12 months of initiation of testosterone therapy.

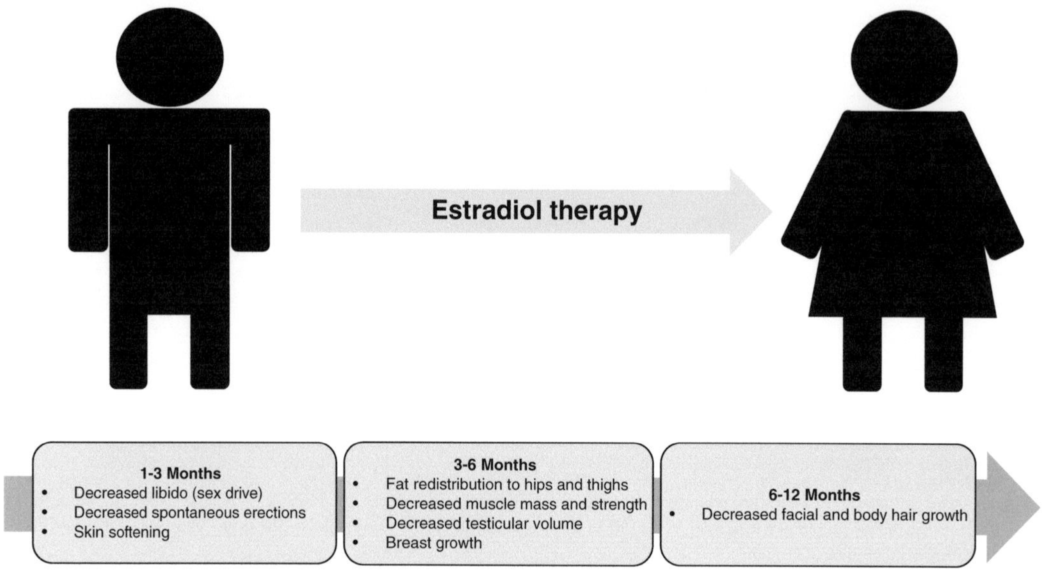


**Fig. 10.3** Onset of feminizing changes with estradiol therapy over time

**Table 10.4** Antiandrogen therapy to facilitate feminization

| Medication | Typical Dosing | Frequency | Benefits | Risks |
|---|---|---|---|---|
| Spironolactone | 50–200 mg PO[a] | Twice daily (can be daily if desired) | Inexpensive; readily available and covered by insurance | Hyperkalemia; dehydration |
| Cyproterone acetate | 25–50 mg PO | Daily | Potent antiandrogen | Not available in the US; can cause fulminant hepatitis |
| Finasteride<br>Dutasteride | 1–5 mg PO<br>0.5 mg PO | Daily | Adjunct or alternate agents for patients unable to tolerate spironolactone; more potent hair and skin effects; low side effect profile | Less potent; not well studied in context of gender-affirming therapy |
| Bicalutamide | 50 mg PO | Daily | Potent antiandrogen | Liver toxicity |
| GnRH analogues | Varies based on formulation | Varies based on formulation | Potent antiandrogen; see Table 11.1 for details of use | |

[a]Oral

For patients on estradiol, it is necessary to monitor both estradiol and testosterone levels. The target estradiol level for patients desiring full feminization is in the physiologic range of 100–200 pg/mL, and the goal for testosterone is total testosterone <55 ng/dL [10]. Providers can stop measuring testosterone levels if patients undergo orchiectomy as testosterone levels after the removal of testes will be undetectable.

While these are the target therapeutic hormone levels based on physiology, it is important to individualize hormone dosing to the patients' specific transition goals while ensuring safety based on age and comorbid conditions. Typically, hormone levels are checked every 3 months in the first year and then every 6–12 months after that. Hemoglobin and hematocrit levels should be monitored every 3 months in the first year for people on testosterone [10]. For patients taking spironolactone as an antiandrogen, potassium levels should also be monitored every 3 months. Guidelines recommend occasional monitoring of prolactin levels as well, though more recently published data suggest that prolactin levels do not increase during treatment with estradiol [23].

## Adverse Effects of Hormone Therapy

There are potential adverse effects associated with GAHT, which should be discussed with patients as part of the informed consent model before initiation of hormone therapy.

Adverse effects that may be associated with testosterone use include [10]:

- Erythrocytosis
- Severe liver dysfunction
- Coronary artery disease
- Cerebrovascular disease
- Hypertension
- Breast or uterine cancer
- Obstructive sleep apnea
- Mood changes [10]

Possible adverse effects associated with estradiol include:

- Thromboembolic disease
- Macroprolactinoma
- Breast cancer
- Coronary artery disease
- Cerebrovascular disease
- Cholelithiasis
- Hypertriglyceridemia
- Nausea, vomiting
- Mood changes

## Special Considerations

Young Adults: For young adults who began gender-affirming treatment earlier in adolescence, it is important to evaluate their ability to self-manage medication administration at the time of transition of care from the pediatric to the adult setting [24]. The understanding of self-administration as well as proper storage of medications is especially important for young adults who may be going to college and living independently for the first time.

Older adults: There are no specific guidelines regarding hormone dosing or adjustment in older adults. As in the case of all age groups, the individual's transition journey and goals of care should be discussed in detail to create a treatment plan that is both safe and effective. Specific strategies that may enhance the safety of hormone therapy in older adults include using the lowest effective doses of hormones as well as using formulations that minimize risk. A thorough medical history, including active or past venous thromboembolism, coronary artery disease, breast cancer, or erythrocytosis, can guide the discussion of the risks versus benefits of hormone therapy [25]. The care of the older adult also necessitates collaboration between different care providers, including primary care, internal medicine subspecialists, and mental health providers to safely care for this age group while aiding and supporting their gender transition.

## People with Nonbinary Identities

The gender transition for nonbinary individuals may be different than for people with binary feminine or masculine gender identities. For individuals who identify as more masculine, a low dose of testosterone may assist with physical masculinization. Higher doses of testosterone though are typically required for menstrual suppression [13]. If menses are causing dysphoria but additional masculinization is not needed, then alternative means to suppress menses may be used (see Table 10.5) [13]. For nonbinary feminine individuals, an antiandrogen alone or a low dose of estradiol can be considered [13]. It is also possible for surgical transition to be made without full masculinization or feminization; this includes top surgery (i.e., bilateral mastectomy with masculine chest reconstruction), breast augmentation, and other potentially modified gender-affirming surgeries.

**Table 10.5** Medications to induce secondary amenorrhea

| Medication | Brand name | Typical dosing | Frequency | Benefits | Risks |
|---|---|---|---|---|---|
| Norethindrone | Errin | 0.35 mg PO[a] | Daily | Readily available and covered by insurance | Not always successful in inducing secondary amenorrhea; breakthrough bleeding if pills skipped; potential increase in thrombogenicity; bone density issues long-term |
| Norethindrone acetate | Aygestin | 5 mg PO; can increase by 2.5 mg every 2 weeks for max daily dose of 15 mg PO | Daily | Readily available and covered by insurance | Breakthrough bleeding if pills skipped; potential increase in thrombogenicity; bone density issues long-term |
| Combined estrogen-progesterone oral contraceptive pills | Varies | Varies | Daily; skip placebo pills and take continuously | Readily available and covered by insurance | Breakthrough bleeding if pills skipped; potential increase in thrombogenicity |
| Etonogestrel subdermal implant | Nexplanon | 68 mg | Continuous; must be exchanged every 3 years | Good option for those desiring long-term contraception; radiopaque and can be easily located on X-ray if needed | Requires procedural placement; risk of pain, bleeding, infection with placement; variable bleeding (patients may not achieve amenorrhea especially if not using testosterone concurrently) |
| Intrauterine device | Varies | Varies | Continuous; must be exchanged every 3–10 years depending on type and brand used | Good option for those desiring long-term contraception | Requires procedural placement; risk of pain, bleeding, infection with placement |

[a]Oral

## Principles of Surgical Transition

### Overview of Gender-Affirming Surgeries

There are masculinizing (Fig. 10.4) and feminizing (Fig. 10.5) surgical procedures that TGD individuals may choose to pursue as a part of their gender-affirming care. Patients can be referred to surgical specialists for consultation regarding options for gender-affirming surgeries. Not all geographic parts of the country have surgeons trained in gender-affirming procedures, so patients often have to travel to receive the care they need. Additional barriers to surgery include insurance coverage, the age at which surgeons feel comfortable performing certain procedures as well as the age at which insurance companies are willing to cover procedures, access to hair removal services if needed, and a supportive environment needed for recovery [26, 27].

### Preoperative Clearance

As in the case of other surgeries, it may be necessary for primary care providers to write a surgical clearance or optimization letter before the gender-affirming surgery. There are guidelines to help assist with this, but in general, they follow similar considerations to other preoperative clearance guidelines [28].

### Chest Reconstruction Surgery

Transgender men or nonbinary masculine individuals may seek top surgery, which typically involves bilateral mastectomy with the creation of a masculine-appearing chest and the definition of the pectoralis muscle. Varying surgical techniques may be used to accomplish this [13]. Patients may be required to have drains in place as well as a compressive dressing postoperatively [13].

Early complications may include:

- Infections
- Hematoma
- Seroma
- Nipple-related complications (e.g., discoloration, aberrant shape)

Late complications may include:

- Scarring
- Poor healing
- Contour issues

**Fig. 10.4** Masculinizing surgical procedures

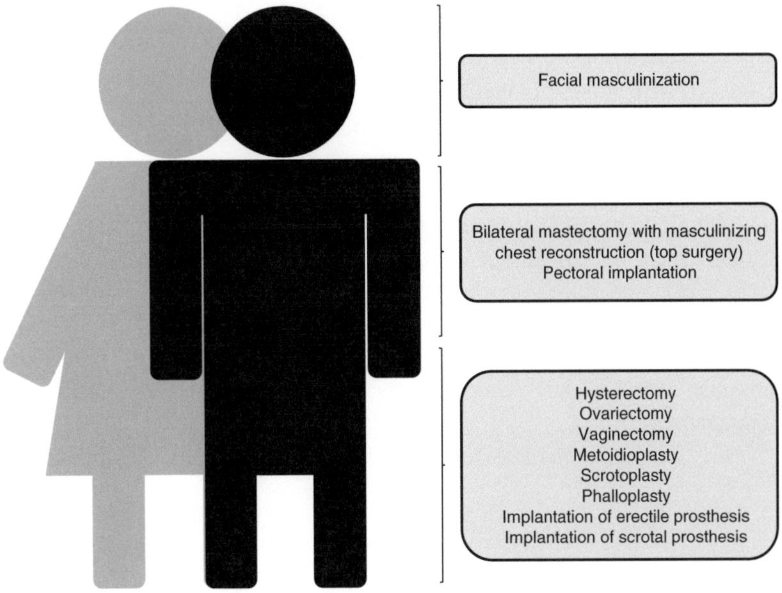

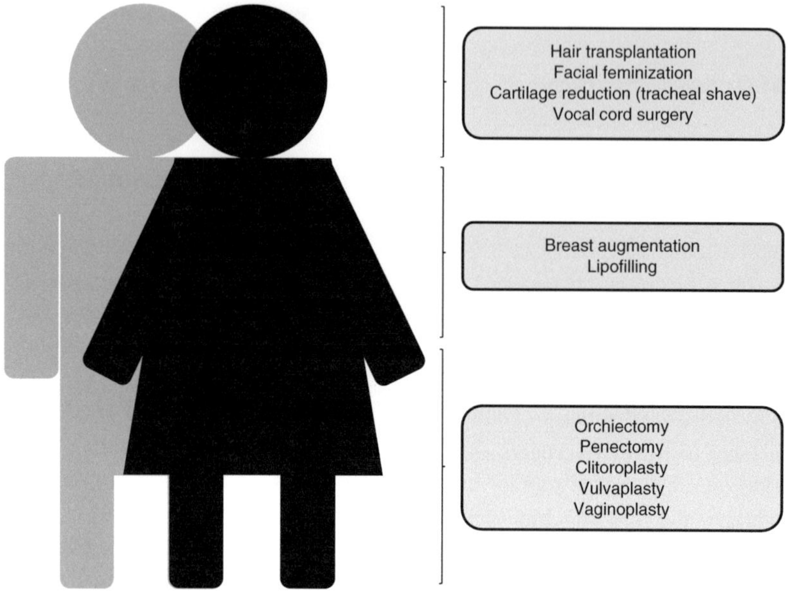


**Fig. 10.5** Feminizing surgical procedures

- Nipple-related complications (e.g., discoloration, aberrant shape)
- Neuropathic pain

Patients should be referred back to their surgeon in a timely manner for management of these complications [13]. Another potential complication may be persistent pain following mastectomy. A review of 90 transgender men who underwent top surgery over a 5-year period found that 27.4% reported ongoing pain either unilaterally or bilaterally [29]. This pain can typically be managed with nonopioid medications.

Breast growth for transgender women or nonbinary feminine individuals is variable on hormone therapy and some may decide to proceed with breast augmentation procedures. These procedures are done via implants using a silicone shell filled with saline or silicone placed under the breast tissue or pectoralis muscle [13]. Though complications overall are rare, there are possible early and late complications of breast augmentation.

Early complications may include:

- Hematoma
- Seroma
- Infections

Late complications may include:

- Incisional scarring
- Implant rupture
- Implant malposition
- Inadequate size and other esthetic complications

Referral to an experienced surgeon is recommended for further management and may require breast revision surgery [13].

## Genital Reconstructive Surgeries

Surgical reconstructive procedures can be performed to create a penis in transgender men via phalloplasty using radial forearm or anterior lateral thigh skin, and typically this is done after a hysterectomy and vaginectomy [13]. This is a complicated procedure typically done in stages. There are potential complications after this surgery.

Early complications may include:

- Wound infections
- Wound dehiscence
- Urinary catheter issues

- Flap loss
- Hematomas
- Rectal Injury

Late complications may include:

- Urethral strictures
- Wound scarring issues
- Granulation tissue

Patients should be followed by either their surgeon or, after discharge from care, by their primary care provider to monitor and assess for any complications [13].

Another procedure that may be performed is metoidioplasty to create a phallus utilizing the local tissue that has hypertrophied after treatment with testosterone and does not involve a grafting procedure. This surgery is shorter in duration and less complicated than phalloplasty [30]. The small phallus resulting from this procedure is not useable for penetrative intercourse [30]. This surgery can also integrate a vaginectomy and the creation of a scrotum using the labia majora [13]. Complications are similar to complications that may arise after a phalloplasty. The decision regarding which procedure to undergo is based on the patient's values and goals. If a patient desires to urinate while standing up, a metoidioplasty may be adequate, then but for transgender men interested in the use of the phallus for penetrative intercourse, a phalloplasty with a penile implant may be optimal [31].

Surgery can be performed to create a vaginal vault between the urethra and rectum in transgender women. The most common technique used for this procedure is the penile inversion technique. Postoperatively patients will need to dilate the vaginal canal to maintain vaginal depth. The patient's surgeon will provide instructions regarding the dilation technique and frequency, but typically dilation practices must be maintained for 1-year postoperatively. A zero-depth vagina or vulvoplasty may be offered to patients with a higher risk of surgical complications, inability or the lack of desire to dilate, and those not seeking penetrative vaginal intercourse [32]. Again there are possible complications following surgery [13].

Early complications may include:

- Bleeding
- Infection
- Skin or clitoral necrosis
- Suture dehiscence
- Urinary retention
- Vaginal prolapse
- Fistula formation

Late complications may include:

- Loss of vaginal depth or width
- Vaginal odor or discharge
- Granulation tissue.
- Fistula formation

## Face and Neck Surgical Procedures

Facial procedures are available to masculinize the face or thyroid cartilage. Masculinization of the thyroid cartilage can be performed by linking the rib cartilage present over the thyroid cartilage with the strap muscles of the body [33, 34]. Other procedures may include altering the forehead, chin, and hairline to enhance the masculinization of the face [34]. Feminization of the face may be performed with hairline lowering, forehead modification, rhinoplasty, or thyroid cartilage minimization (i.e., tracheal shave) [34].

## Letters of Support for Surgical Transition

Surgeons performing gender-affirming surgeries should understand the patient's gender journey, reasons for pursuing surgery, and anticipated surgical outcomes [9]. Surgeons can collaborate closely with the patient's interdisciplinary care team for a comprehensive assessment of the patient's surgical goals as well as an overarching care plan for addressing gender incongruence. Mental health evaluation remains an active part of the presurgical assessment of patients, and its role has evolved from a tool to confirm gender dysphoria to an assessment that provides an overall picture of the individual's mental health and social support systems; a well-done mental health evaluation ensures that mental health concerns are controlled and optimized before surgery and that patients have access to the support system they need to recover fully from the procedures. Breast augmentation and mastectomy typically require only one mental health assessment and letter while gonadectomy, hysterectomy, vaginoplasty, metoidioplasty, and phalloplasty may require two though updates guidelines recommend considering a single letter adequate [9, 13, 22].

## Additional Supportive Therapies

### Fertility Preservation

Treatment with estradiol or testosterone can affect natal gonadal function and the future fertility of TGD individuals. Estradiol can decrease testicular size as well as sperm production. Testosterone can lead to amenorrhea and anovulation that is possibly reversible [10, 13]. Fertility preservation should be discussed with all patients before treatment with pubertal suppression or GAHT [10]. For individuals assigned at male at birth (AMAB), this may involve sperm or embryo cryopreservation. For individual's assigned female at birth (AFAB), this may involve oocyte or embryo cryopreservation [35]. There are multiple considerations involved in fertility preservation including cost and access to care [36]. Additional considerations may be the dysphoria associated with the process of fertility preservation itself (e.g., producing a semen sample via masturbation may worsen dysphoria; administration of high doses of estrogen to stimulate follicle enlargement prior to egg retrieval may worsen dysphoria as well). Multiple studies have found that many TGD patients are either not interested in having children at all or may prefer adoption over having biological children when building their family [37, 38].

Open discussions can help providers better understand the patients' knowledge of fertility preservation options as well as the patients' family planning goals. Patients may need time to reflect on these options and discuss them with loved ones before making final decisions regarding whether or not to pursue fertility preservation. Guardians of minors pursuing gender-affirming care have to consent to the patient's final decision. Referrals should be made in a timely manner to specialty clinics to expedite preservation and avoid unnecessary delays in the initiation of hormone therapy.

Data on the impact of long-term GAHT exposure on gametes are sparse, and ideally, patients interested in having biological children would have the opportunity to pursue fertility preservation before initiating GAHT. However, this is not always feasible, and, for the reasons discussed above, patients may choose to defer fertility preservation after starting GAHT. Options for fertility preservation after being on gender-affirming treatments are constantly evolving; one medical team was able to facilitate oocyte cryopreservation in a Tanner stage 2 patient after treatment with pubertal blockers [39].

### Vocal Therapy

Communication and voice are an essential part of one's gender and gender expression [10]. Having a voice that does not lead to misgendering may be critical for "passability." For patients on testosterone, deepening of the voice typically begins after 6–12 months of testosterone therapy and peaks at approximately 1–2 years [10]. For patients on estradiol and antiandrogen treatment, voice changes do not typically occur, and voice therapy with a speech pathologist is used instead to change the voice [10]. Voice therapy is critical for both safe and effective modulation of the voice and communication style [9]. It is important for the treating provider to be aware of the availability of vocal therapy locally and virtually and bring this option to the patients' attention to further enhance their care and transition.

## Hair Removal and Growth

A primary concern of many transfeminine patients is the removal of unwanted hair. Estradiol in combination with androgen blockade thins the hair but must be used in combination with hair removal techniques. Patients may choose to pursue self-guided hair removal strategies at home, including but not limited to, shaving, waxing, and the use of depilatory creams. However, these strategies do not lead to permanent hair removal. More permanent strategies include professional waxing, electrolysis, and laser hair removal [13]. The best technique for a patient is determined based on their complexion, hair color, and hair texture, and patients should work with their esthetician to decide which strategy to pursue.

Hair removal from body areas that will be involved in gender-affirming surgery or serve as surgical site grafts may require hair removal before surgery. A survey of TGD adults found that dermatologic procedures are the most frequently sought by TGD females, and 59.4% utilized electrolysis for hair removal compared to 9.1% who used laser hair removal [40]. Providers should feel comfortable discussing these options with patients to help achieve a more congruent appearance and decrease dysphoria. Many patients will seek recommendations or referrals for culturally competent technicians and centers. The greatest barriers to accessing these services are high out-of-pocket costs and difficulty obtaining insurance coverage. Larger institutions may have the opportunity to collaborate with their dermatology departments to provide this medically necessary service to patients especially when required for surgery.

For transmasculine patients, there are multiple hair-related considerations as well: (1) prevention of androgenetic alopecia and loss of scalp hair, (2) stimulation of facial hair growth, and (3) management of changes associated with diffuse hair growth over the body. Testosterone dosing can be adjusted to prevent scalp hair loss, but for patients who are interested in continuing testosterone at the same dose, providers can utilize tools used for the treatment of androgenetic alopecia in cisgender men to treat the hair loss including finasteride and topical minoxidil. Topical minoxidil can also be applied to areas where patients desire increased hair growth, such as the beard area, when testosterone alone is not sufficient in stimulating full hair growth. Some patients may experience increased moisture in areas where there is excessive hair growth, especially in the genital area, which can predispose patients to fungal infections. The use of cornstarch-based powders can help manage sweating in these areas and prevent infections.

## Esthetics

Transfeminine patients often utilize hair and makeup to present more femme in social spaces and to pass as members of their true gender identity. Esthetics are more than just cosmetics in this population and can be lifesaving. Doing hair and makeup appropriately and in a way that accentuates feminine features is an acquired skill that may require guidance from a professional. Some estheticians specialize in hair and makeup for TGD people. Gender-affirming providers and programs are encouraged to collaborate with local estheticians who can assist patients in achieving their desired esthetic.

## Induction of Secondary Amenorrhea

Many AFAB patients experience dysphoria with ongoing menstruation and consequently desire induction of secondary amenorrhea to feel affirmed in their gender. There are contraceptive medications that can reliably help with the cessation of menses (Table 10.5). These options, when used consistently and as prescribed, can also function as contraception for patients having sex in a way that can result in pregnancy. Most of these medications can be prescribed and monitored by primary care providers, and all can be managed by physicians specializing in obstetrics and gynecology.

## Induction of Lactation

Breastfeeding offers many benefits for both the child and mother. Transgender women may be interested in being the primary or secondary breastfeeding parent. There have been several reports in the literature describing the induction of lactation in transgender women [41–45]. The same protocols used for lactation induction in cisgender women can be used in transgender women as well. Medications that can be used to induce lactation may include progesterone and domperidone. Manual milk expression using a breast pump can help increase breast milk production. Of note, these protocols are in the early stages of development and remain experimental, and milk supply may be low and not sufficient to meet the infant's caloric needs [44].

## Treatment of Acne Vulgaris

Acne is a potential side effect of treatment with testosterone. A large cohort study found that patients treated with testosterone were more likely to have acne than cisgender women, cisgender men, and TGD men and women not treated with hormones [46]. There are no specific guidelines for the treatment of acne in TGD patients, and evidence is extrapolated from the treatment of hormonal acne in cisgender individuals. Acne may be treated based on severity as follows [47]:

Mild acne

- Retinoids
- Benzoyl peroxide and topical antibiotics
- Topical antiandrogens

Moderate to severe acne

- Oral antibiotics
- Spironolactone (may not be optimal for use in this patient population)
- Hormonal contraceptives (may not be optimal for use in this patient population)

Severe acne

- Oral isotretinoin may be considered

# Management of Comorbid Conditions

## Addressing Mental Health Conditions

The mental health care and support of TGD individuals are described in detail in Chap. 7. It is most important to note that ongoing mental healthcare can offer additional support to individual patients and their families throughout the gender transition process and beyond. While not required to obtain GAHT or surgical treatment, psychotherapy can help patients navigate social and personal changes as well as issues that may arise in educational or work settings [9].

## Tobacco Use Disorders

There is an increased risk of venous thromboembolism (VTE) associated with concurrent use of estradiol and tobacco. Patients should be counseled about this risk and assisted with quitting tobacco as needed. The inability to attain tobacco cessation is not a contraindication to starting or continuing estradiol; informed consent should be used in these situations to ensure that patients understand the continued risk. Risk mitigation strategies include using transdermal estradiol as well as the possible addition of low-dose aspirin to prevent clots [13].

## Use of Alcohol and Other Drugs

A large meta-analysis published in 2022 found that TGD people are more likely to use tobacco and other substances, but they do not have increased rates of substance use disorders or alcohol use when compared to the cisgender population [48]. It is possible that increased use of tobacco and other substances may be related to trauma, minority stress, and maladaptive coping due to experiencing adverse events. Providers should work with patients to understand the underlying reasons for substance use, and abuse if present. This strategy avoids stigmatization and allows for the creation of a more appropriate and comprehensive treatment plan to address unhealthy substance use if one is needed.

## Pre-Existing Clotting Disorders

Venous thromboembolism is a potential adverse effect associated with estradiol use. Routine screening for hypercoagulable conditions is not recommended before initiation of GAHT [10]. Estradiol use in patients who have had a personal history of VTE depends on their medical history, cause of VTE, and risk of recurrence.

For patients with a personal history of VTE and known provoking cause, standard estradiol therapy can be started once the risk is removed. For patients with a personal history of VTE who have hypercoagulable disorders or other hypercoagulable states (e.g., underlying malignancy) and are at risk of clot recurrence, anticoagulation should be started, and informed consent should be used before initiation of transdermal estradiol [13]. For patients with a personal history of unprovoked VTE, a risk-benefit analysis and discussion should be done to determine whether patients require anticoagulation and the use of transdermal estradiol [13].

For patients with a family history of VTE but no personal history, evaluation for underlying hypercoagulable disorders with genetic testing can be considered. Patients with negative genetic testing can be treated with standard estradiol therapy. For patients with gene mutations, such as prothrombin gene mutation, treatment with anticoagulation should be started using guidelines for cisgender patients, and treatment with transdermal estradiol should be considered [13].

## Cardiovascular Disease

A systematic review of studies examining cardiovascular risk factors in TGD individuals found that testosterone use is associated with an increase in triglyceride and low-density lipoprotein (LDL) levels and a decrease in high-density lipoprotein (HDL). Estradiol use is associated with an increase in triglyceride levels. While there were few reported episodes of cardiovascular and thromboembolic events, these occurred more frequently in transfeminine patients [10, 49]. Overall studies that have been performed are retrospective, small, and short in duration and do not adjust for the presence of additional cardiovascular risk factors.

When calculating cardiovascular risk using the American Heart Association or other calculators using gender as a risk factor, in the absence of specific evidence, it is recommended to select the gender of the longest hormone exposure. This means that, if an individual has had an estrogen-predominant hormonal milieu during their lives, then select the gender of female in the calculator. If an individual has had a testosterone-predominant hormonal milieu during their lives, then select the gender of male in the calculator. As patients are on GAHT for longer periods of time, the gender used in the calculators may change.

In the setting of higher cardiovascular risk, it is recommended to consider the use of transdermal estradiol to lower the risk of VTE [13]. Patients should be counseled on other modes of risk reduction including tobacco cessation, weight loss, diet, and exercise [13]. This counseling is important to incorporate into the wellness care of all TGD patients. The specific guidance and need for intervention will vary based on the patient's age and associated risk factors.

## Neurodiversity, ADHD, and Autism Spectrum

Newer research is evaluating the co-occurrence of and interplay between autism spectrum identity, ADHD, anxiety, depression, and gender dysphoria. Clinicians should be aware of the potential co-occurrence of these entities when assessing, treating, and caring for neurodiverse individuals. Patients on the autism spectrum may show more rigidity of thought and express their feelings regarding their gender identities differently than neurotypical patients [50]. Tools that provide space and opportunity for patients to discuss their journeys in their own unique and preferred way can be very helpful in guiding the next steps in treatment (e.g., patients who do not feel comfortable verbally expressing their feelings may benefit from the opportunity to write their provider a letter in which they share their journey and goals). This topic is also discussed in Chap. 7.

### Geriatric Patients

Older adults who present for gender-affirming care may be seeking initiation or maintenance of GAHT as well as referrals for surgical services. The management of hormone therapy needs to be balanced with a known concern for polypharmacy and comorbid health conditions [25, 51]. It is recommended to use the lowest effective dose of GAHT as well as lower-risk formulations if possible [25]. Androgen blockers may not be needed in elderly patients given the natural decrease in testosterone production with age and should generally be avoided to prevent hyperkalemia and renal complications.

Additional topics to consider discussing in this population include assessment of neurological and psychiatric function including the presence of cognitive impairment, depression, and substance use; overall nutrition, food security, and management of weight-related conditions (e.g., hypertension, diabetes, hyperlipidemia); duration and quality of sleep; ability to manage medications and GAHT; urological function; general safety and screening for elder abuse; vision and hearing screenings; gait, stability, mobility, and fall risk; age-appropriate cancer screenings; and goals of care [25].

## Disease Prevention and Health-Care Maintenance

### Breast Cancer Screening

There are few cases of breast cancer reported in TGD patients on estradiol [52]. Retrospective data from studies done in the Netherlands and the United States did not find an increased risk of breast cancer [13, 53, 54]. It is recommended that TGD patients on estradiol undergo breast cancer screening with a mammogram every 2 years starting at age 50 if there has been at least 5 years of GAHT use [13]. AFAB patients who have not undergone top surgery should be screened according to guidelines for cisgender women [13]. There is no data currently available on the risk of cancer in AFAB patients who have undergone top surgery. For patients who have residual chest tissue after top surgery, annual chest wall examinations in combination with cancer screening modalities, such as ultrasound or MRI, can be considered [55].

### Osteoporosis Screening

Studies have found that transfeminine patients may be at increased risk of osteoporosis at baseline even before starting pubertal blockers and hormone therapy [56]. Most studies have found that bone density increases or is unchanged on estradiol [57]. The guidelines regarding when to start osteoporosis screening and the frequency of monitoring are not clear. For transmasculine patients, osteoporosis screening is recommended for those who stop testosterone treatment, are not consistent with testosterone use, or develop risk factors for osteoporosis [10]. This may include nonbinary patients who have neither therapeutic levels of estrogen nor testosterone as part of their hormonal milieu.

Endocrine Society guidelines recommend a baseline dual-energy X-ray absorptiometry (DEXA) scan for all adolescents before starting pubertal blockers as well as follow-up DEXA scans every 1–2 years until therapeutic hormone levels are established with GAHT [10]. DEXA scans should also be done for all transfeminine patients starting at age 60, and earlier in those who are not using estradiol regularly [10]. In the absence of additional evidence, bone density should be checked beginning at age 65 for all transgender people and should be considered between age 50 and 64 for those with risk factors [13]. The most recent position from the International Society of Clinical Densitometry recommends calculating the Z score using the normative database that matches the individual's gender identity, not their natal sex [58].

## Prostate Cancer Screening

The risk of prostate cancer in transfeminine patients is overall low, but there are reported cases [59]. Long-term use of estradiol typically leads to prostate atrophy [10] but does not eliminate the risk for prostate cancer. It is possible for transfeminine patients to develop prostate cancer even after gonadectomy [13]. Examination of the prostate may differ depending on anatomy: the prostate can be reached via a transrectal approach for patients with natal anatomy and via a neovaginal approach in patients who have undergone vaginoplasty [13]. Providers should consider patient comfort and potential dysphoria with this exam and prostate-specific antigen (PSA) lab monitoring. There have not been specific studies done to assess the effect of estradiol on PSA levels, but, in the setting of lower testosterone levels on treatment with estradiol, PSA levels are expected to be lower [60]. It may be more valuable to trend PSA levels over time rather than using single values to determine prostate cancer risk.

## Contraception and Prevention of Undesired Pregnancies

Hormone therapy alone is not adequate contraception for TGD individuals who are sexually active in a manner that could result in pregnancy [13]. Discussing the patients' sexual practices as well as their desire for pregnancy is critical. It is important to counsel patients and discuss options for contraception accordingly. Providers must provide education that changes in ejaculation on estradiol therapy and cessation of menses on testosterone therapy are not indicators of infertility. Patients with these changes can definitely get pregnant. In addition, patients who inconsistently use testosterone may be more likely to ovulate and get pregnant [10]. If patients are having sex in a way that can result in pregnancy, then they are encouraged to use contraception if pregnancy is undesired. Options in Table 10.5 can be used for contraception, but patients should be educated that all contraceptive pills, especially progesterone-only contraceptive pills, must be taken at the same time daily to prevent pregnancy.

For patients who are using testosterone and actively pursuing fertility, it is recommended that testosterone actually be discontinued to prevent fetal exposure and potential physical and developmental harm. In the setting of amenorrhea on testosterone, there may be delayed recognition of pregnancy in transmasculine patients, which can limit options for pregnancy discontinuation for the patient and also lead to inadvertent in-utero androgen exposure to the fetus.

Transfeminine patients may desire to carry a pregnancy, but uterine transplantation remains experimental. There are barriers to its use in the TGD population and requires further research [61].

## Prevention of HIV

Transgender and gender-diverse patients are at higher risk of HIV acquisition than their cis-gender counterparts. As highlighted in Chap. 7, there are data to show that TGD people in the United States are five times more likely to be living with HIV compared to the general population [62]. Minorities are disproportionately impacted. Forty-six percent of all transgender women in the United States and 41% of all transgender men in the United States are Black [63]. Latinx patients are the second most affected in both subgroups. However, these populations remain underrepresented in research [64]. There are geographic disparities as well: 43% of new HIV diagnoses in transgender people were in the southern part of the United States [63].

Transgender women are at the highest risk of getting HIV; worldwide transgender women are 49 times more likely to acquire HIV compared to the general population [65]. Most of the current literature on HIV is on men who have sex with men, but transgender women are a different population—they often have lower education and income levels, engage in sex work at higher rates, and value feminizing hormone therapy more than HIV care.

Pre-exposure prophylaxis (PrEP) involves the use of Truvada (emtricitabine and tenofovir disoproxil fumarate) or Descovy (emtricitabine and tenofovir alafenamide) to prevent HIV infection in patients who are at increased risk of acquiring HIV. These medications are taken once daily ahead of sexual activity to prevent HIV acquisition. Multiple trials have been done looking at PrEP in transgender populations. The iPrEx trial showed no efficacy of PrEP in preventing HIV infection in transgender women and showed that transgender women are more likely to have undetectable drug levels compared to nontransgender women participants [66]. None of the transgender women who seroconverted had detectable levels of tenofovir. The iFACT trial showed that PrEP does not impact the levels of estradiol in the body, but estradiol and cyproterone can diminish levels of tenofovir, which can impact the efficacy of PrEP in preventing HIV in this population [65]. The study sample size was small, so more research is needed. PrEP and post-exposure prophylaxis (PEP) should be offered to at-risk TGD patients for HIV prevention.

## Prevention of Other Sexually Transmitted Infections

It is recommended that providers screen for sexually transmitted infections (STIs) in TGD individuals using anatomy and sexual practices to guide relevant physical exams and testing. Common STIs to screen for include HIV, syphilis, gonorrhea, chlamydia, and hepatitis B and C. In terms of anatomy, patients who have undergone vaginoplasty do not have a cervix, so cervical pap smears and human papillomavirus (HPV) testing are not indicated [13]. Routine examination of the neovagina in patients who have undergone vaginoplasty is not indicated, but some patients may prefer this examination and find it affirming. The neovagina may be more posterior, and an anoscope may be more useful for examination than a standard speculum [13]. Asking about sexual practices can guide gonorrhea and chlamydia testing modality; triple site testing, which includes a urine sample, throat swab, and rectal swab, is indicated for penetrative genital, oral, and anal sex.

An anatomic survey can serve as a guide when determining which organs need to be screened for disease or symptoms. For example, the differential diagnosis of dysuria in an AMAB patient may include prostatitis if the prostate is still present and pelvic inflammatory disease in an AMAB patient with an intact uterus and fallopian tubes [13].

Using gender-neutral language when referring to body parts can help clinicians obtain a comprehensive sexual history in an affirming and sensitive manner. The Fenway Center in Boston has a helpful guideline for questions to ask [67]; their mnemonic uses the 8 P's:

1. **Preferences**: Do you have a preferred language that you use to refer to your body (i.e., genitals)? Are you currently sexually active? What kinds of sex do you engage in?
2. **Partners**: Are you sexually active with one partner or more than one? Are you dating anyone or sexually active? Do you have any outside partners? How would your partners identify themselves in terms of gender?
3. **Practices**: Do you use toys inside your [insert preferred language for genitals] or anus, or do you use them on your partners? Do you have any other types of sex that hasn't been asked about?
4. **Protection from STIs**: Are there some kinds of sex where you do not use barriers? Why?
5. **Past history of STIs**: If yes… Do you remember the site?
6. **Pregnancy**: Have you considered fertility preservation/banking gametes? Have you thought about having your own biological children, or carrying a pregnancy? When you are having sex, is there any exposure to sperm or chance of pregnancy? Have you considered contraceptive options?
7. **Pleasure**: Do you feel you are able to become physically aroused during sex? How satisfied are you with your ability to achieve orgasm? Do you have any pain or discomfort during or after orgasm? Is sex fun? Are you having sex for pleasure or are these other reasons (survival sex/transactional sex)

8. **Partner abuse**: Has anyone ever forced or compelled you to do anything sexually that you did not want to do? Is there any violence in any of your relationships? Do you feel safe at home?

## Providing Long-Term Comprehensive Care

### Closing the Disparities Gap

Members of the TGD community routinely encounter disproportionately high rates of healthcare disparities, insurance challenges, violence, harassment, rejection, socioeconomic barriers, homelessness, and substance use among other disparities [62]. These gaps, which are discussed in detail in Chap. 7, have strong implications for long-term health outcomes for patients. Providers caring for TGD patients must be acutely aware of the challenges their patients face and be equipped to connect patients with the resources necessary to address these barriers.

Providers are encouraged to (1) develop connections with affirming professionals and organizations in the local community and (2) curate and regularly update lists of these resources, so they can readily be shared with patients when needed. Resources should include support for legally changing name and gender markers, accessing public education, getting insurance coverage for GAHT and surgical procedures, preventing evictions and addressing shelter denials, using restrooms, protecting children from discrimination and harassment in school, and reaching economic stability. These protections ultimately promote safety, equality, and lifelong health and well-being for TGD patients.

### Evolving Care and Collaboration

The field of gender health is rapidly evolving, and there are more opportunities today than ever before to partner with people across the globe to provide much-needed, cutting-edge care to TGD patients. The collaboration will be key as professionals, patients, and community organizations team up to determine the best ways to address TGD healthcare needs and social determinants of health long-term. We encourage providers interested in caring for TGD patients to consider joining the World Professional Association for Transgender Health (WPATH), which sets the highest standards of care for TGD people across the world. Providers are also encouraged to reach out to the authors of this chapter to ask clarifying questions, seek guidance if interested in establishing centers of excellence at their institutions, and learn more about caring for their patients. We look forward to the collaboration.

## References


1. Sanchez NF, Sanchez JP, Danoff A. Health care utilization, barriers to care, and hormone usage among male-to-female transgender persons in New York City. Am J Public Health. 2009;99(4):713–9.
2. Safer JD, Coleman E, Feldman J, Garofalo R, Hembree W, Radix A, et al. Barriers to healthcare for transgender individuals. Curr Opin Endocrinol Diabetes Obes. 2016;23(2):168–71.
3. To M, Zhang Q, Bradlyn A, Getahun D, Giammattei S, Nash R, et al. Visual conformity with affirmed gender or "passing": its distribution and association with depression and anxiety in a cohort of transgender people. J Sex Med. 2020;17(10):2084–92.
4. Furutani M, Yu Z, Nakatsuka M. Gender expression among transgender women in Japan: support is needed to improve social passing as a woman. Acta Med Okayama. 2021;75(3):323–34.
5. Parr NJ, Howe BG. Factors associated with frequency of gender identity nonaffirmation microaggressions among transgender persons. Cult Health Sex. 2021;23(8):1094–110.
6. Peixoto EM, de Azevedo Oliveira Knupp VM, JRT S, Depret DG, de Oliveira Souza C, Messina MED, et al. Interpersonal violence and passing: results from a Brazilian trans-specific cross-sectional study. J Interpers Violence. 2021:8862605211005152.
7. Fiani CN, Han HJ. Navigating identity: experiences of binary and non-binary transgender and gender non-conforming (TGNC) adults. Int J Transgend. 2019;20(2–3):181–94.
8. Elwyn G, Frosch D, Thomson R, Joseph-Williams N, Lloyd A, Kinnersley P, et al. Shared decision making: a model for clinical practice. J Gen Intern Med. 2012;27(10):1361–7.

9. Coleman E, Radix AE et al. Standards of Care for the Health of Transgender and Gender Diverse People, Version 8. Int J Transgend Health. 2022 Sep 6;23(Suppl 1):S1-S259.
10. Hembree WC, Cohen-Kettenis PT, Gooren L, Hannema SE, Meyer WJ, Murad MH, et al. Endocrine treatment of gender-dysphoric/gender-incongruent persons: an Endocrine Society* clinical practice guideline. J Clin Endocrinol Metab. 2017;102:3869.
11. Ashley F, St Amand CM, Rider GN. The continuum of informed consent models in transgender health. Fam Pract. 2021;38(4):543–4.
12. Deutsch MB. Use of the informed consent model in the provision of cross-sex hormone therapy: a survey of the practices of selected clinics. Int J Transgend. 2012;13(3):140–6.
13. Guidelines for the primary and gender-affirming care of transgender and gender nonbinary people (2nd ed); June 2016. transcare.ucsf.edu/guidelines.
14. Appiah LC. Fertility preservation for adolescents receiving cancer therapies. Clin Obstet Gynecol. 2020;63(3):574–87.
15. Figueiredo MG, Gagliano-Juca T, Basaria S. Testosterone therapy with subcutaneous injections: a safe, practical, and reasonable option. J Clin Endocrinol Metab. 2022;107(3):614–26.
16. Spratt DI, Stewart II, Savage C, Craig W, Spack NP, Chandler DW, et al. Subcutaneous injection of testosterone is an effective and preferred alternative to intramuscular injection: demonstration in female-to-male transgender patients. J Clin Endocrinol Metab. 2017;102(7):2349–55.
17. Toorians AW, Thomassen MC, Zweegman S, Magdeleyns EJ, Tans G, Gooren LJ, et al. Venous thrombosis and changes of hemostatic variables during cross-sex hormone treatment in transsexual people. J Clin Endocrinol Metab. 2003;88(12):5723–9.
18. Tangpricha V, den Heijer M. Oestrogen and anti-androgen therapy for transgender women. Lancet Diabetes Endocrinol. 2017;5(4):291–300.
19. Corvol P, Michaud A, Menard J, Freifeld M, Mahoudeau J. Antiandrogenic effect of spirolactones: mechanism of action. Endocrinology. 1975;97(1):52–8.
20. Neyman A, Fuqua JS, Eugster EA. Bicalutamide as an androgen blocker with secondary effect of promoting feminization in male-to-female transgender adolescents. J Adolesc Health. 2019;64(4):544–6.
21. Irwig MS. Is there a role for 5alpha-reductase inhibitors in transgender individuals? Andrology. 2021;9(6):1729–31.
22. Deutsch MB. Gender-affirming surgeries in the era of insurance coverage: developing a framework for psychosocial support and care navigation in the perioperative period. J Health Care Poor Underserved. 2016;27(2):386–91.
23. Bisson JR, Chan KJ, Safer JD. Prolactin levels do not rise among transgender women treated with estradiol and spironolactone. Endocr Pract. 2018;24(7):646–51.
24. Society TE. Provider assessment of skill set 2020. https://www.endocrine.org/-/media/endocrine/files/practice/gender_provider_assessment_skill_set.pdf.
25. Gamble RM, Taylor SS, Huggins AD, Ehrenfeld JM. Trans-specific geriatric health assessment (TGHA): an inclusive clinical guideline for the geriatric transgender patient in a primary care setting. Maturitas. 2020;132:70–5.
26. Tabaac AR, Jolly D, Boskey ER, Ganor O. Barriers to gender-affirming surgery consultations in a sample of transmasculine patients in Boston, Mass. Plast Reconstr Surg Glob Open. 2020;8(8):e3008.
27. Cohen W, Maisner RS, Mansukhani PA, Keith J. Barriers to finding a gender affirming surgeon. Aesth Plast Surg. 2020;44(6):2300–7.
28. Shin SJ, Kumar A, Safer JD. Gender-affirming surgery: perioperative medical care. Endocr Pract. 2022;28(4):420–4.
29. Lang CL, Day DL, Klit A, Mejdahl MK, Holmgaard R. Low risk of persistent pain, sensory disturbances, and complications following mastectomy after gender-affirming surgery. Transgend Health. 2021;6(4):188–93.
30. Djinovic RP. Metoidioplasty. Clin Plast Surg. 2018;45(3):381–6.
31. Schechter LS, Safa B. Introduction to phalloplasty. Clin Plast Surg. 2018;45(3):387–9.
32. Salim A, Poh M. Gender-affirming penile inversion vaginoplasty. Clin Plast Surg. 2018;45(3):343–50.
33. Deschamps-Braly JC, Sacher CL, Fick J, Ousterhout DK. First female-to-male facial confirmation surgery with description of a new procedure for masculinization of the thyroid cartilage (Adam's Apple). Plast Reconstr Surg. 2017;139(4):883e–7e.
34. Deschamps-Braly JC. Facial gender confirmation surgery: facial feminization surgery and facial masculinization surgery. Clin Plast Surg. 2018;45(3):323–31.
35. Cheng PJ, Pastuszak AW, Myers JB, Goodwin IA, Hotaling JM. Fertility concerns of the transgender patient. Transl Androl Urol. 2019;8(3):209–18.
36. Boguszewski KE, Woods S, Ducar DM, Taylor JF. Transgender and gender diverse fertility choices: supporting the decision-making process for adolescents and young adults. J Pediatr. 2022;240:256–64. e1
37. Nahata L, Tishelman AC, Caltabellotta NM, Quinn GP. Low fertility preservation utilization among transgender youth. J Adolesc Health. 2017;61(1):40–4.
38. Chew D, Anderson J, Williams K, May T, Pang K. Hormonal treatment in young people with gender dysphoria: a systematic review. Pediatrics. 2018;141(4)
39. Martin CE, Lewis C, Omurtag K. Successful oocyte cryopreservation using letrozole as an adjunct to stimulation in a transgender adolescent after GnRH agonist suppression. Fertil Steril. 2021;116(2):522–7.
40. Ragmanauskaite L, Zhang Q, Kim J, Getahun D, Silverberg MJ, Goodman M, et al. Survey of dermato-

logic procedures in transgender adults. Dermatologic Surg. 2021;47(10):1379–83.

41. van Amesfoort JE, Van Mello NM, van Genugten R. Lactation induction in a transgender woman: case report and recommendations for clinical practice. Int Breastfeed J. 2024;19(1):18.
42. Delgado D, Stellwagen L, McCune S, Sejane K, Bode L. Experience of Induced Lactation in a Transgender Woman: Analysis of Human Milk and a Suggested Protocol. Breastfeed Med. 2023;18(11):888–93
43. Weimer AK. Lactation Induction in a Transgender Woman: Macronutrient Analysis and Patient Perspectives. J Hum Lact. 2023;39(3):488–94.
44. Wamboldt R, Shuster S, Sidhu BS. Lactation induction in a transgender woman wanting to breastfeed: case report. J Clin Endocrinol Metab. 2021;106(5):e2047–e52.
45. Reisman T, Goldstein Z. Case report: induced lactation in a transgender woman. Transgend Health. 2018;3(1):24–6.
46. Gao JL, King DS, Modest AM, Dommasch ED. Acne risk in transgender and gender diverse populations: a retrospective, comparative cohort study. J Am Acad Dermatol. 2022;87:1198.
47. Radi R, Gold S, Acosta JP, Barron J, Yeung H. Treating acne in transgender persons receiving testosterone: a practical guide. Am J Clin Dermatol. 2022;23(2):219–29.
48. Cotaina M, Peraire M, Bosca M, Echeverria I, Benito A, Haro G. Substance use in the transgender population: a meta-analysis. Brain Sci. 2022;12(3)
49. Maraka S, Singh Ospina N, Rodriguez-Gutierrez R, Davidge-Pitts CJ, Nippoldt TB, Prokop LJ, et al. Sex steroids and cardiovascular outcomes in transgender individuals: a systematic review and meta-analysis. J Clin Endocrinol Metab. 2017;102(11):3914–23.
50. de Vries AL, Noens IL, Cohen-Kettenis PT, van Berckelaer-Onnes IA, Doreleijers TA. Autism spectrum disorders in gender dysphoric children and adolescents. J Autism Dev Disord. 2010;40(8):930–6.
51. Masnoon N, Shakib S, Kalisch-Ellett L, Caughey GE. What is polypharmacy? A systematic review of definitions. BMC Geriatr. 2017;17(1):230.
52. Maglione KD, Margolies L, Jaffer S, Szabo J, Schmidt H, Weltz C, et al. Breast cancer in male-to-female transsexuals: use of breast imaging for detection. AJR Am J Roentgenol. 2014;203(6):W735–40.
53. Brown GR, Jones KT. Incidence of breast cancer in a cohort of 5,135 transgender veterans. Breast Cancer Res Treat. 2015;149(1):191–8.
54. Asscheman H, Giltay EJ, Megens JA, de Ronde WP, van Trotsenburg MA, Gooren LJ. A long-term follow-up study of mortality in transsexuals receiving treatment with cross-sex hormones. Eur J Endocrinol. 2011;164(4):635–42.
55. Sterling J, Garcia MM. Cancer screening in the transgender population: a review of current guidelines, best practices, and a proposed care model. Transl Androl Urol. 2020;9(6):2771–85.
56. Van Caenegem E, Taes Y, Wierckx K, Vandewalle S, Toye K, Kaufman JM, et al. Low bone mass is prevalent in male-to-female transsexual persons before the start of cross-sex hormonal therapy and gonadectomy. Bone. 2013;54(1):92–7.
57. Verroken C, Collet S, Lapauw B, T'Sjoen G. Osteoporosis and bone health in transgender individuals. Calcif Tissue Int. 2022;110(5):615–23.
58. The International Society for Clinical Densitometry. 2019 ISCD Official Positions 2019. https://iscd.org/wp-content/uploads/2021/09/2019-Official-Positions-Adult-1.pdf
59. Deebel NA, Morin JP, Autorino R, Vince R, Grob B, Hampton LJ. Prostate cancer in transgender women: incidence, etiopathogenesis, and management challenges. Urology. 2017;110:166.
60. Cheung AS, Lim HY, Cook T, Zwickl S, Ginger A, Chiang C, et al. Approach to interpreting common laboratory pathology tests in transgender individuals. J Clin Endocrinol Metab. 2021;106(3):893–901.
61. Jones BP, Williams NJ, Saso S, Thum MY, Quiroga I, Yazbek J, et al. Uterine transplantation in transgender women. BJOG. 2019;126(2):152–6.
62. James SE, Herman JL, Rankin S, Keisling M, Mottet L, Anafi M. The report of the 2015 U.S. transgender survey. Washington, DC: National Center for Transgender Equality; 2016.
63. Centers for Disease Control and Prevention. HIV and transgender people: HIV diagnoses; 2022. https://www.cdc.gov/hiv/pdf/group/gender/transgender/cdc-hiv-transgender-factsheet.pdf
64. Rosen JG, Malik M, Cooney EE, Wirtz AL, Yamanis T, Lujan M, et al. Antiretroviral treatment interruptions among black and Latina transgender women living with HIV: characterizing co-occurring, multilevel factors using the gender affirmation framework. AIDS Behav. 2019;23(9):2588–99.
65. Hiransuthikul A, Janamnuaysook R, Himmad K, Kerr SJ, Thammajaruk N, Pankam T, et al. Drug-drug interactions between feminizing hormone therapy and pre-exposure prophylaxis among transgender women: the iFACT study. J Int AIDS Soc. 2019;22(7):e25338.
66. Grant RM, Lama JR, Anderson PL, McMahan V, Liu AY, Vargas L, et al. Preexposure chemoprophylaxis for HIV prevention in men who have sex with men. N Engl J Med. 2010;363(27):2587–99.
67. Thompson J. Taking a sexual history with sexual and gender minority individuals; 2020. https://fenwayhealth.org/wp-content/uploads/6.-Taking-an-Affirming-Sexual-History.pdf

# Part IV

# Public Health and Population Considerations

# 11 Special Considerations for Emergency Preparedness

Denise M. Nunez

## Introduction

Emergency preparedness is a shared responsibility emerging from interactions between the individual, the individual's network of support, and the local and national governmental systems. Emergency preparedness refers to precautions taken prior to an emergency to reduce its impact and improve outcomes. Preparing for emergencies is essential to health and has greater influence in persons with chronic illnesses and/or special health care needs. According to FEMA's National Survey, Preparedness in America, approximately 20% of our population consists of adults with special health care needs. Data from the survey identified that 46% of persons with special health care needs have not thought of how to prepare for emergencies [1]. This lack of preparation is further complicated by the vulnerabilities of those with special health care needs, as lack of preparation will affect the response and outcome during an emergency. Data reviewed from the 2006–2012 Behavioral Risk Factor Surveillance System (BRFSS) found that individuals with special health care needs are more likely to state they are not prepared at all for emergency. They are also less likely to have emergency supplies and less likely to evacuate. Data from the survey also found that being female, non-White, with less education, less income, and uncoupled and living in an urban area increase the likelihood of being unprepared for an emergency. Lack of an emergency plan also was correlated with increased risk of injury and death [2]. Increased effort is needed in supporting our community of persons with chronic illness and special health care needs to improve outcomes and protect health during unexpected events. Physicians and the medical team are central to an individual with chronic illness' network of support. Physicians have a unique position of trust and opportunity to emphasize the importance of emergency preparedness and assist in creating a tailored plan to suit each patient's unique needs and the necessary considerations for a successful emergency plan.

D. M. Nunez (✉)
Division of Medicine-Pediatrics and Preventive Medicine, University of California, Los Angeles, CA, USA
e-mail: dmnunez@mednet.ucla.edu

## Emergency Preparedness Planning

Due to higher vulnerability, low preparedness in this group and higher potential need for specialized equipment, medication, and/or supplies, discussions on emergency preparedness are an influential component of a health plan and merits exploring by medical providers. There are various resources available to help create an emergency preparedness plan. One useful resource is the American Red Cross Disaster Safety plan, located at redcross.org.


A. A. Kuo et al. (eds.), *Care of Adults with Chronic Childhood Conditions*,
https://doi.org/10.1007/978-3-031-54281-7_11

## Steps to Emergency Preparedness

1. Create a Personal Support Network

   The first step in creating a successful plan is identifying individuals that provide care and may be available to assist an individual during emergencies. This group can consist of friends, family members, care givers, medical staff, and so on. This support network should be part of the plan, including potential roles/contributions, contact information, and resources they may provide. Discussions with the members of this network can help to provide more knowledge about useful resources and ways to optimize responding to a potential emergency.

2. Complete a Personal Assessment

   Individuals with chronic conditions, special health care needs, and disabilities benefit most from a personalized evaluation of daily needs, assistance required, and how they will be impacted during an emergency. This step can be further facilitated by physicians and the health care team. Physicians can set up a clinical visit to discuss recommendations that will best support health maintenance during an emergency. Completion of a personal assessment may include evaluation of activities of daily living (ADLs), review of medical equipment and medications necessary for health maintenance, and tools necessary for evacuation.

3. Gather Information

   Information about emergencies must be obtained to appropriately respond. An important step is to ensure connection to relevant alerts and notifications. Registration for alerts via email or text and identification of emergency alert systems should be explored and activated. Certain areas have a local emergency management office that can provide resources, and may have a registry of persons with special health care needs that may garner additional support during an emergency. Areas to evacuate with additional resources and personnel for those with special health care needs may be available and useful to identify. Information about insurance (health, life, and other emergency-related programs) should also be reviewed.

4. Create an Emergency Plan

   The outcome of preparation for emergencies is to create an emergency plan. A different plan should be created considering all potential emergencies related to the geographical location (e.g., earthquakes or hurricanes) and other possible hazards. The support network as discussed above should be involved in the creation and execution of the plan. Emergency escape routes and communication plans should be created. Alternative plans should also be created in case the original emergency plan cannot be executed. Methods of evacuation and meeting locations should be considered. A "grab and go bag," a portable toolkit with essential resources ready to take during evacuation, should be planned and created considering the relevant health conditions. A disaster supplies kit for sheltering-in-place should also be planned and stocked to support the relevant health conditions. The kit should contain at a minimum 3 days' worth of essentials, including clean water, non-perishable food items, a flashlight, first aid kit, 7-day supply of medications, sanitation and personal hygiene items, copies of personal documents, cell phone chargers, and cash. Additional items are highly recommended to support the individual needs as mentioned previously. Suggested items for various health care needs listed by category are listed in Table 11.1 and may be used to discuss emergency plans with patients [3].

Physicians may review a patient's medical conditions and special health care needs and discuss the importance of an emergency plan. Discussions with patients can help to prompt the development of a plan, considerations of essentials for health maintenance during and emergency, and may be used to discuss prevention of complications resulting from diagnoses and plan for improvement in a patient's quality of life [4, 5].

**Table 11.1** Special health care needs and resources to review in creating an emergency plan

| Special health care needs | Emergency resources to consider |
|---|---|
| Speech | Assistive devices<br>Laminated cards to communicate and communication plan |
| Sensory | Electronic device charger<br>Pop up tent<br>Noise canceling headphones/ear plugs<br>Soothing items |
| Vision | Braille labels for supplies<br>Audible list of supplies and contacts on USB/audio file<br>Communication supplies |
| Hearing | Hearing aid batteries<br>Pen and paper<br>Laminated cards to communicate and communication plan<br>Light source to assist with mouth reading |
| Mobility | Lightweight manual chair<br>Extra batteries<br>Patch kit for wheels<br>Portable air pump<br>Walker or cane<br>Team for assistance during evacuation |

## Pandemic Preparedness

Special consideration should be directed toward emergency preparedness for a pandemic. A COVID-19 disease resulting from the SARS-CoV-2 virus in 2019 caused an international crisis, testing the emergency preparedness of all national and domestic systems. Improvements to systems were essential to provide lifesaving interventions and supports and should be integrated into an individual's personal emergency plan. This is of utmost importance in preparing for the future, as the likelihood that another pandemic may occur in the next decade has been declared likely by the United States government [6].

Due to the obvious impact on health, physicians and the medical team are even more essential to creating a successful pandemic preparedness plan. A patient's medical conditions and special needs may be reviewed to discuss how various biological emergencies can affect their health to provide targeted advice. Additional protective resources may be discussed including personal protective equipment, specialized medications, vaccinations, and so on. Medical misinformation is a major problem and discussions on preparing for emergencies can be used to clarify questions and support decisions that will benefit a patient's health. Normalizing conversations with physicians on future planning is one helpful way to reduce the impact of medical misinformation.

Pandemic preparedness should include a discussion with the medical team and supportive medical staff as previously mentioned. Preparation guidance can be further derived from ready.gov/pandemic which includes detailed instructions on how to prepare for a pandemic, how to stay safe during a pandemic, and how to stay safe after a pandemic. A patient should also have an official source of information on surveillance and pandemic-related recommendations that will allow them to respond to updated information [7].

## Financial Considerations

In all categories of emergency preparedness (including pandemic preparedness), financial aspects are important to consider. Financial emergencies may also be considered as part of an emergency preparedness plan. Emergency preparedness plans should accommodate the resources and finances of the individual. Creation of a "grab and go bag" or kit should be done within the financial means of the person creating it, and fully stocking these tools may take a longer period if not financially feasible to do so. Emergency preparation is well suited to having economic reserves. Patients should be encouraged to have a savings account with approximately 3 months of financial needs available to cover. Insurance plans should also be reviewed and explored for optimal use. Additional insurance options may be added as needed and possible. Local resources should be explored for emergency needs, such as local food banks, pantries, and respite centers. National programs may also provide financial assistance, such as Temporary assistance for needy families program (TANF), which can be accessed for funds during emergencies.

## Mental Health Considerations

Emergency situations can be physically, emotionally, and mentally taxing. It is important to discuss the significant potential for mental health challenges during emergencies and plan accordingly. For individuals with mental health diagnoses, it is helpful to discuss the difficulties that emergencies may provide as part of their preparedness plan. For those who have never had a mental health diagnosis, potential for anxiety, depression, and adjustment disorder is very possible. Reviewing signs of emotional distress, such as difficulty concentrating, difficulty sleeping, and feelings of fear, anxiety, worry, numbness, or frustration, is supportive in creating a plan that considers management of mental wellness. Guidance may be to care for one's physical wellness, with exercise, healthy meals, and routines if possible. Connecting with others, taking breaks, and avoiding too much exposure to news while ensuring access to essential information are also helpful tips. If a mental health provider is an option, patients should be encouraged to seek support, as the impact of unexpected emergencies may have an unforeseeable end, with consequences experienced beyond the conclusion of the event [8].

## Websites for Emergency and Pandemic Preparedness

www.ready.gov/plan
www.ready.gov/pandemic
www.ready.gov/disability
www.emergency.cdc.gov
www.cdc.gov/disasters/chronic.html
www.redcross.org/get-help/how-to-prepare-for-emergencies/inclusive-preparedness-resources.html
https://www.cdc.gov/chronicdisease/pdf/infographics/emergency-H.pdf

## Conclusion

Physicians play a central role in management of chronic health conditions and for patients with special health care needs. They are well positioned to support patients in the development of successful emergency and pandemic preparedness plans. Patients with complex health conditions require support in creating appropriate considerations directed toward their unique needs during emergencies. Creating an emergency and pandemic preparedness plan is a significant tool for health and prevention that will reduce the impact of an emergency and will improve outcomes. Many resources exist to support adequate planning, but a simple conversation between patient and provider about emergencies in the setting of their health needs is enough to start the process and support the future, well-being, and survival of our patients during an emergency.

## References

1. Preparedness in America [Internet]. ready.gov. 2014 [cited 1 March 2022]. https://www.ready.gov/sites/default/files/2020-08/Preparedness_in_America_August_2014.pdf.
2. Smith D, Notaro S. Is emergency preparedness a 'disaster' for people with disabilities in the US? Results from the 2006–2012 Behavioral Risk Factor Surveillance System (BRFSS). Disabil Soc. 2015;30(3):401–18.
3. How to prepare for emergencies [Internet]. Red Cross. 2022 [cited 12 March 2022]. https://www.redcross.org/get-help/how-to-prepare-for-emergencies/types-of-emergencies/coronavirus-safety/preparing-for-disaster-during-covid-19.html.
4. Information for people with chronic conditions and disabilities [Internet]. Natural disasters and severe weather 2021 [cited 10 March 2022]. https://www.cdc.gov/disasters/chronic.html.
5. Morris J, Jones M. Emergency preparedness for people with disabilities. Arch Phys Med Rehabil. 2013;94(2):219–20.
6. American pandemic preparedness: transforming our capabilities [Internet]. Whitehouse.gov. 2022 [cited 16 April 2022]. https://www.whitehouse.gov/wp-content/uploads/2021/09/American-Pandemic-Preparedness-Transforming-Our-Capabilities-Final-For-Web.pdf.
7. Pandemics [Internet]. ready.gov/pandemic. 2022 [cited 16 April 2022]. https://www.ready.gov/pandemic.
8. Taking care of your emotional health [Internet]. https://emergency.cdc.gov/coping/selfcare.asp. 2022 [cited 16 April 2022]. https://emergency.cdc.gov/coping/selfcare.asp.

# Addressing Structural Racism 12

Maura E. Muñoz and Josephine A. Akingbulu

## Terms to Know to Better Understand Structural Racism

Informed and specific use of language for racial terms is important to understanding the root causes of the conditions and inequities that contribute to structural racism. Racism is a system of advantage based on race. It involves one group having the power to carry out systematic discrimination against other group or groups through the implementation of institutional policies and practices, and by shaping cultural beliefs and/or values that support racist practices within a society [1]. Racism exists in several levels, and breaking down these levels is helpful in better understanding how racism is perpetuated in society [2]. Refer to Table 12.1.

This provides a framework for understanding racial terms and the impact of racism on a micro (individual and interpersonal) and macro (institu-

**Table 12.1** Defining the levels of racism [2]

| | |
|---|---|
| Internalized racism | Occurs within individuals, a sense of inferiority or superiority based on one's race stemming from private beliefs, conscious or unconscious bias, larger social norms, and/or ideologies on race |
| Interpersonal racism | Is personally mediated and occurs between individuals involving differential treatment (discrimination), negative attitudes, or beliefs (prejudice) toward racial groups that influence interpersonal interactions between individuals and among groups |
| Institutional racism | Occurs within institutions and systems of power involving discriminatory institutional policies and/or practices that produce racial inequalities that advantage one racial group over other racial groups |
| Structural racism | Occurs among institutions and across societies, involves the cumulative effects of racism in history, culture, and ideologies within a society which effects policies, institutional practices, and laws that systematically advantage one racial group over other racial groups or defining them as "the norm" |

M. E. Muñoz (✉)
Department of Internal Medicine and Department of Pediatrics, Baystate Medical Center, UMass Chan Medical School, Springfield, MA, USA
e-mail: Maura.Munoz@Baystatehealth.org

J. A. Akingbulu
Division of Medicine-Pediatrics and Preventive Medicine, University of California, Los Angeles, CA, USA
e-mail: Josephine.akingbulu@cgu.edu


A. A. Kuo et al. (eds.), *Care of Adults with Chronic Childhood Conditions*,
https://doi.org/10.1007/978-3-031-54281-7_12

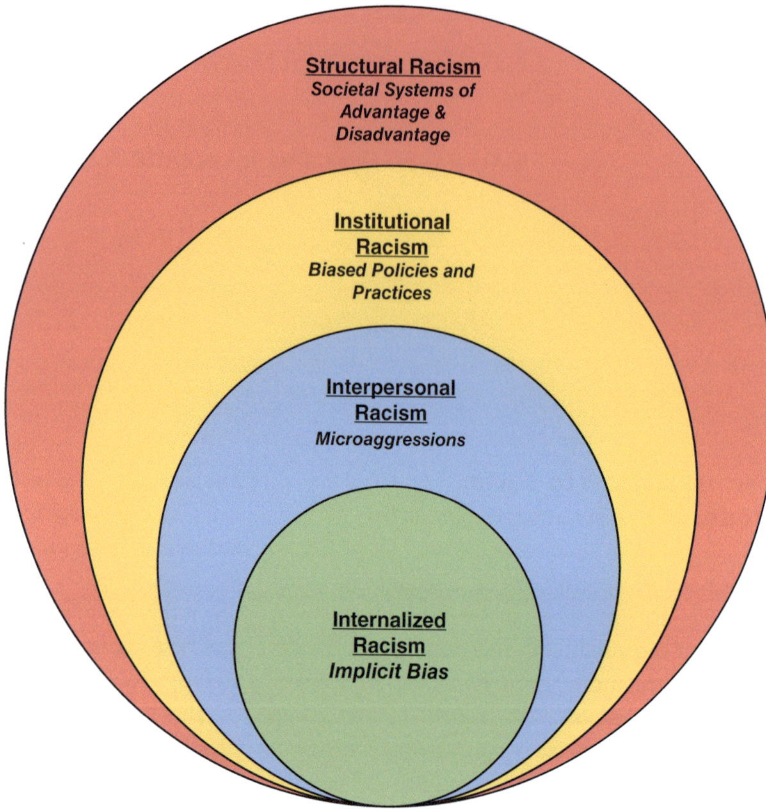


**Fig. 12.1** Conceptualizing the levels of racism from a micro and macro perspective

tional and structural) level within society. With an understanding of these levels of racism, other racial terms may be further conceptualized. Implicit bias is an example of individual racism. It is defined as unconscious or hidden bias. Implicit biases are negative associations against another racial group or groups that an individual unknowingly holds and expresses without conscious awareness [1]. Microaggressions are a form of interpersonal racism defined as everyday verbal and nonverbal insults, whether intentional or unintentional, that communicate hostile, derogatory, or negative messages to target individuals within a marginalized group [1]. Refer to Fig. 12.1.

Understanding and recognizing racism is an initial step in challenging individual thinking and the complex interactions of people, practices, institutions, and ideology that perpetuate inequity within society.

## Structural Racism in the United States

Acknowledging and understanding the history and current impacts of structural racism within society is a subsequent step in addressing structural racism. The history of structural racism and its ongoing propagation in the United States to establish and maintain power and privilege to White populations is deep. It involves the genocide and dispossession of Indigenous people in North America, the enslavement of Black people, and the racialization of immigration. It is important to recognize that structural racism within our country is significantly broader affecting many racial communities including Latinx, Asian American, Native Hawaiian, Pacific Islander, and racial communities targeted because of their religion (e.g., Muslim communities), which fully addressing is beyond the scope of this text. The following examples of structural racism involve housing access, political policies, and educational systems that contribute to health inequities affecting people of color.

## Redlining

Racialized residential segregation is a form of structural racism involving government, banking, credit institutions, private housing development institutions, and real-estate industries targeting Black homeowners and Black neighborhoods with generations of consequences upon these communities. To promote economic recovery during the Great Depression by expanding home ownership, the United States federal government established the Home Owners' Land Corporation (HOLC) in 1933. Home ownership programs were developed to offer government-insured mortgages as a form of federal aid. Part of the process of developing mortgage worthiness involved the HOLC creating maps of over 200 cities where red lines were drawn around communities with predominantly Black populations. These communities were designated as hazardous investment areas, resulting in residents within these communities not receiving HOLC loans. This was the origin of the term "redlining." Redlining made mortgages inaccessible to Black homeowners. This government-sanctioned process resulted in other restrictive practices that barred Blacks from home ownership such as undervaluing real estate in Black neighborhoods and legal agreements made by homeowners to block Black home buyers. In modern context, redlining has come to describe race-based exclusionary practices in real estate [2–4]. The Fair Housing Act of 1968 prohibits housing discrimination, and the Home Mortgage Disclosure Act of 1975 required the release of lending data. Despite this legislation, the impact of structural racism within the housing system has resulted in broad social disinvestment, disparities in neighborhood infrastructure, disparities in neighborhood services, and has deprived communities of intergenerational wealth transfer. Residential segregation has had associated health outcomes negatively impacting Black communities including poor birth outcomes, increased exposure to air pollutants, decreased longevity, and increased risk of chronic disease [5].

## Immigration

Exclusionary immigration policies within the United States represent another form of government-mediated structural racism. Historically, racialized immigration policies have served to propagate ideologies of national belonging along ethnic lines to diminish racialized immigrant groups as undesirable within society [6]. The racialization of immigration policies may be conceptualized within three pathways of policy implementation. First, immigration policies that limit or prohibit access to material and health resources, and from political and civic participation. Second, racialization propagated by disproportionate immigration criminalization and enforcement, including detention and deportation. The third pathway involves economic exploitation and disinvestment, for example, labor exploitation of migrant workers [7].

According to 2018 Department of Homeland Security data, 11.4 million unauthorized immigrants reside within the United States. Approximately 50% are from Mexico with a subsequent large percentage from El Salvador, Guatemala, and Honduras [8]. Under the administration of the 45th president, aggressive anti-immigration policies were instituted to reduce authorized and unauthorized immigration. A travel ban was instituted targeting predominantly Muslim and African countries (that also included Venezuela and North Korea). Entry of foreign nationals on H-1B and L-1 visas were suspended. This had an impact on the professional workforce, including healthcare professionals. Increased resources were allocated to fortifying the US–Mexico border, and Immigration and Customs Enforcement (ICE). This has contributed to immigrant community mistrust of institutions (including healthcare facilities) due to fear of detention or deportation. In 2018, a zero-tolerance immigration policy was implemented where the Department of Homeland Security referred unauthorized migrants to the Department of Justice for criminal prosecution. As a result of this policy, during the months of April to June of 2018, the government separated more than 2000 children from their parents at the US–Mexico border and housed these children in detention centers [9]. The long-term effects of this devastating adverse childhood event on the children affected by this policy remains to be seen. In 2020, Title 42 was evoked to empower federal authorities to prohibit migrants from entering the country at the US–Mexico border to prevent the spread of COVID-19. Along with restrictive policies, limiting access to health and social services negatively impact health outcomes for immigrants. Unauthorized immigrants are ineligible for healthcare subsidies under the Affordable Care Act (ACA) and are prohibited from purchasing health coverage on ACA exchanges. Many racial groups are impacted by racialized immigration policies, and these examples emphasize disproportionate impacts on Latinx immigrants.

## The American Medical Education System

Structural racism has influenced the infrastructure of the medical education system at multiple levels including racially restrictive admissions practices and discriminatory oversight of Black medical institutions. The first American medical school was the College of Philadelphia established in 1765. Admission policies were restrictive against students of color, and 82 years would pass before the first African American earned their medical degree from an American medical school. Due to this racism in admission policies, the first African American to earn his medical degree was Dr. James McCune Smith, he did so abroad at the University of Glasgow in 1837. In 1847, Dr. David Jones Peck became the first African American to graduate from a US medical school, earning his degree from Rush Medical College in Chicago. In 1864, Dr. Rebecca Lee Crumpler was the first African American woman to earn a medical degree from New England Female Medical College in Boston [10, 11]. Racism in medical school admissions was also pervasive against other communities of color. In 1880, Dr. José Celso Barbosa was the first Puerto Rican to graduate from an American medical school, earning his degree at the University of Michigan [12]. Dr. Charles Eastman in 1890 was the first Native American to graduate from an American medical school, and earned his degree at the Boston University School of Medicine [13]. This history of restrictive admissions policies has had long-term effects contributing to the under-representation of BIPOC medical students, faculty, and medical school leadership. From a community perspective, a lack of diversity within medical institutions has also contributed to a lack of racial representation of communities served.

The American Medical Association created the Council on Medical Education to evaluate medical education in 1904. Seven medical schools for Black students were established between 1868 and 1904 [10]. Abraham Flexner was an educator and reformer who was commissioned to study medical education in the United States and Canada [14]. In 1910, the Flexner report was published which examined medical college education and proposed reforms. Flexner's recommendations for the medical education of African Americans were to close five of the Black medical colleges, and encouraged resources be allocated toward the two remaining schools (Howard and Meharry). In 1923, only Meharry Medical College and Howard University Medical Department remained [15]. With the intention of medical school reform for improvement, this history of structural barriers targeting Black medical institutions is a factor that has also contributed to the gap of diversity within the medical education and health system. National statistics of the entering medical school class of 2021 showed that 11.3% of students are Black, 12.7% are Latinx origin, and 1% are American Indian or Alaskan Native [16].

## Structural Racism and Healthcare Inequities

The Institute of Medicine (IOM) published a report in 2003 titled “Unequal Treatment: Confronting Racial and Ethnic Disparities in Healthcare.” The IOM reviewed over 100 studies involving racial disparities in maternal and child heath, analgesia, diabetes, asthma, HIV/AIDS, renal transplantation, and cardiovascular disease. Their report stated that “Racial and ethnic disparities in healthcare exist. These disparities are consistent and extensive across a range of medical conditions and healthcare services, are associated with worse health outcomes, and occur independently of insurance status, income, and education, among other factors that influence access to healthcare. These disparities are unacceptable” [17]. Evidence continues to show the existence of racial disparities in healthcare. The Agency for Healthcare Research and Quality (AHRQ) reports on the progress for improving healthcare and reducing healthcare disparities. The U.S. Congress mandated that the report focuses on national trends in the quality of healthcare provided and disparities in healthcare delivery as it relates to racial and socioeconomic factors. At the time of the writing of this chapter, the most recent report looked at data from 2000 to 2017. The 2018 National Healthcare Quality and Disparities Report documented that Black, Native American, Alaska Native and Native Hawaiian, and Pacific Islander patients received worse care compared to White patients on 40% of the quality measures investigated with little or no improvement compared to past decades. Latinx patients were found to receive worse care compared to White patients for approximately 35% of quality measures. Quality measures included access to healthcare, quality of healthcare, processes of care, outcomes of care, and patient perceptions of care [18].

Seventeen years after the publication of the IOM report, the COVID-19 pandemic has brought racial health inequities to the forefront. Racial minorities in the United States have had higher rates of infection and death caused by COVID-19. During March–December 2020, racial and ethnic minority groups were found to have higher proportions of COVID-19-related hospitalization compared to White patients. The largest disparities in the proportion of patients hospitalized occurred early in the pandemic from April to July 2020. The disparities became less pronounced over time; however, in December 2020, the disparities persisted among racial/ethnic minority groups within all regions of the United States (most notably among Latinx patients in the Western United States). These disparities were driven by higher risk for COVID-19 exposure and higher risk for severe disease among racial and ethnic minority groups [19]. Age-standardized data from November 2020 showed that Latinx, Black, American Indian, and Alaskan Native people were almost 3 times as likely to die from COVID-19 and approximately 4 times as likely to be hospitalized as compared to White patients [20]. In May 2022, the United States tragically reached over one million deaths due to COVID-19. As of that time, the percentage of individuals within the United States who are partially vaccinated is 11.2% and those who are fully vaccinated is 66.5%. White Americans comprising 59% of the population are among 56% of the fully vaccinated. African Americans comprising 12% of the population are among only 10% the fully vaccinated [21].

The COVID-19 pandemic has demonstrated the interconnection of structural racism, social risk factors, and health [22]. Social determinants of health (SDOH) involve the conditions in which people are born, live, learn, work, and age that impact individual health and quality-of-life. SDOH may be conceptualized within five domains: economic stability, education access and quality, healthcare access and quality, neighborhood and built environment, and social and community context [23]. Racism is a social determinant that drives health inequities within all these domains. Racial inequities within each of these domains has contributed to disparities throughout the pandemic [24]. The examples of structural racism previously addressed are interconnecting factors. Residential segregation is a factor that impacts neighborhoods and built environments. Racialized immigration policies impact healthcare access and community context. The history of racialized medical school admission policies has also impacted healthcare access and quality. Understanding these interconnections are crucial to addressing the health equities revealed by the pandemic.

## Addressing Structural Racism

Decades of research has linked structural racism to healthcare inequities within the United States. The urgency of addressing this as a society has been propelled by the Black Lives Matter movement and the depth of healthcare disparities exposed by the COVID-19 pandemic among Black, Indigenous, and people of color. Racism is a public health crisis. What is our role as healthcare professionals? The depth and complexity of this crisis may feel overwhelming to confront. We hold a position of privilege providing essential services to treat and prevent disease, and to promote health to individuals, families, and communities. We also have opportunities to be involved in teaching, research, policy making, institutional leadership, and government. As there are levels to understanding modalities of racism, a tool for implementing change may also be broken down to micro and macro levels of interventions to dismantle structural racism. Refer to Table 12.2 [25, 26].

By naming and recognizing racism, by understanding the history of structural racism and its ongoing presence, and by learning the role of structural racism in propagating health inequities, we have opportunity to confront root causes of racism. Engagement within one or each of these levels of intervention is an act toward dismantling structural racism and confronting healthcare inequities. Given the complexity of structural racism and its multi-level implications, it is important to better understand how the social determinants of health perpetuate health inequities and disparities in the health field as they may foster racism via reinforcing systems such as those mentioned above. Racial/ethnic inequities are often rooted in social and structural determinants that impact the life of many [27]. Thus, in order to address structural racism, we must utilize a more interdisciplinary and scrupulous

**Table 12.2** Taking action to dismantle structural racism in healthcare (and may be applied generally). This table does not claim to behold all the answers for addressing structural racism. However, it is a tool for levels of engagement toward anti-racist work [5, 25, 26]

| | |
|---|---|
| Individual change | • Commitment to being anti-racist<br>• Identify and address personal implicit and explicit biases<br>• Being intentional with the use of anti-racist language<br>• Learn about racism |
| Interpersonal change | • Allyship to support a group or groups other than one's own<br>• Being an active bystander by calling out and addressing micro or macroaggressions when they occur<br>• Community engagement and involvement outside of the walls of the clinics and hospitals |
| Institutional change | • Institutional commitment to promoting and addressing anti-racist practices<br>• Development of community driven programs and engaging communities served (i.e., community needs assessments, board of advisors representative of communities served)<br>• Recruitment of diverse students, faculty, and staff within academic institutions<br>• Development of anti-racist and race-conscious academic curriculums<br>• Recruitment of diverse healthcare professionals and teams within healthcare settings<br>• Diversity in health administration and educational leadership<br>• Medical and public health research on racism and health |
| Structural change | • Advocating for policy reform<br>• Involvement with local, state, or national advocacy organizations to develop anti-racist policy reforms<br>• Involvement within national professional society or government organizations for policy development |

approach to addressing root issues and causes. Although there is not one comprehensive solution, there is a great need for enhancement highlighted by the COVID-19 pandemic. Leveraging culturally relevant tools and resources may serve as a starting point to operationalize current organizational initiatives that may be perfunctory in its pursuit of health equity.

## Community-Based Participatory Research

Research is an important component of addressing structural racism. Community-Based Participatory Research (CBPR) emphasizes the value and importance of conducting research and implementing interventions *with* disparaged communities instead of *to* them or *in* them [28]. Research questions or topics that originate for the community, are community-designed, and derive from lived experience may better inform social and health efforts to create better health outcomes for all. This form of research seeks to operationalize health equity by utilizing a more emic approach to healthcare.

## Implementation Science

Implementation science is another tool that can be helpful in bridging the gaps of inequity due to structural racism. This field allows practitioners and professionals to not only document and highlight the many racial/ethnic gaps and disparities, but it provides room to translate research to more equity-oriented practice and innovation. Data collection and analysis have emphasized and illuminated the gaps in access, intervention, and care between racial groups as seen during the COVID-19 pandemic. Implementation science uses theoretical and methodological approaches to create tangible objectives that have been informed by this research. It is also important to note that some theories and methodologies may also have racist foundations that need innovation in order to mitigate the perpetuation of racism in practice.

## Workforce Training and Education

Structural racism has developed over time and has been ingrained in the minds and behaviors of people. Therefore, it is important to examine the education and training of the social and health workforce. For example, health and medical schools often include conversations of race and its relevance to health outcomes; however, not much is discussed on the impacts of racism in these respective sectors. In order to advance health equity, we must work to include medical anthropologists, social scientists, social epidemiologists, historians, community voices, and leaders in the conversation and teaching of our workforce [29]. Educating practitioners on the impact of biases, stigma, discrimination, and racism is not an overnight process. However, it is a step in ensuring that diversity training has a more culturally responsive and self-analytical basis. It can also provide a platform for more self-reflection and critical analysis to better address and mitigate racism on an individual level as the accumulation of these individual actions can detrimentally impact communities.

In addition, conversations in this arena tend to be primarily focused on the need for health-equity instead of addressing the specific components such as structural racism that impede this effort altogether. It is important to note that conversations like these can also be perceived as controversial and may require discourse in the classroom to properly educate and sensitize health practitioners who will be leaders in the healthcare space. Just as there has been pushback to have these discussions in hopes of educating medical students, the medical education curriculum has also seen an increase in courses attempting to focus on health equity in general. For example, institutions have created coursework, fellowships, and programs to better educate trainees on the topic of health equity. Although this is an innovative first step that integrates public health into medical practice, it may also be remiss to not incorporate theories, history, and legislative components related to structural racism and its impact on health equity. Thus, highlighting the need to improve and make this space more relevant to the hindrances marginalized racial groups face in healthcare.

## Linguistic-Responsiveness and Cultural Humility

Rhetoric is essential to conveying any narrative. As such, it is important to use a community-centered approach to better understand health outcomes. For example, sickle cell disease (SCD) affects approximately 1 in every 400–500 African American newborns in the United States [30]; a topic that will be further explored in future chapters. Significant disparities exist in health outcomes for patients with SCD, with average life expectancy in California and George being 43 years for females and 41 years for males, compared to 54 years for the national average life expectancy for a person with SCD [31, 32]. This difference can be attributed to challenges accessing health services and systemic and institutional racism that many patients with SCD can face when attempting to access health services.

In addition, healthcare practitioners may inaccurately imply that there are genetic differences between races when things like social experience or ancestry may be a more accurate way to characterize health differences. Generalizations can further exacerbate stigma, discrimination, and medical racism in health [33]. Linguistic-responsiveness can be helpful in communicating with and about communities as epigenetics, the study of how behaviors and environment can cause changes in how genes function [34], can contribute to health disparities over time.

## Structural and Cultural Responsiveness

In sum, it is not enough to only acknowledge structural racism and the role it plays in health outcomes for impacted communities. The COVID-19 pandemic is yet another historical moment that has highlighted the need for innovative, relevant, and effective strategies to address this issue at its root. It has brought the need for structural competence and cultural responsiveness to the forefront of health practice, care, and social services for the population. Structural competence is the ability to understand how downstream clinical symptoms, problems, and diseases are influenced by upstream social determinants of health [35]. Although there are limitations to competency, a structurally responsive approach to discernment and identification of structural racism can be helpful in repudiating its effects.

Stigma is not merely produced in day-to-day, individual interactions; it is exacerbated by more structural causes. It is important to analyze organizational and institutionalized policies and practices, or the lack thereof, that may govern or guide individual actions resulting in large impact [36]. Structural competency goes beyond the practice, it seeks to address the underlying issues and pushes us to think of more integrative and interdisciplinary approaches for solutions. Our role as health practitioners is to continuously seek, develop, and utilize tools that may assist in dismantling structural racism and the role it plays in healthcare inequity or inform the work of others in areas where the change needs to occur.

## References

1. Mcleod J. Understanding Racial Terms and Differences. National Institutes of Health. 2021. https://www.edi.nih.gov/blog/communities/understanding-racial-terms-and-differences. Accessed 3 April 2022
2. Boynton-Jarrett R, Raj A, Inwards-Breland DJ. Structural integrity: recognizing, measuring, and addressing systemic racism and its health impacts. EClinicalMedicine. 2021;36:100921. https://doi.org/10.1016/j.eclinm.2021.100921. Accessed 3 April 2022.
3. Jackson C. What is Redlining? The New York Times. 2021. https://www.nytimes.com/2021/08/17/realestate/what-isredlining.html. Accessed 3 April 2022.
4. Bailey Z, Feldman J, Bassett M. How structural racism works-racist policies as a root cause of U.S. racial health inequities. N Engl J Med. 2021;384:768–73.

5. Bailey ZD, Krieger N, Agénor M, et al. Structural racism and health inequities in the USA: evidence and interventions. Lancet. 2017;389:1453–63.
6. Viruell-Fuentes EA, Miranda P, Abdulrahim S. More than culture: structural racism, intersectionality theory, and immigrant health. Soc Sci Med. 2012;75:2099–106.
7. Misra S, Kwon S, Abraído-Lanza AF, et al. Structural racism and immigrant health in the United States. Health Educ Behav. 2021;48(3):332–41.
8. Baker B. Estimates of the unauthorized immigrant population residing in the United States: January 2015–January 2018. p. 14.
9. American Bar Association. Family separation and detention [Internet]. [cited 2022 Oct 22]. https://www.americanbar.org/advocacy/governmental_legislative_work/priorities_policy/immigration/familyseparation/.
10. Murphy B. LibGuides: Black history month: a medical perspective: education [Internet]. [cited 2022 Oct 22]. https://guides.mclibrary.duke.edu/Blackhistorymonth/education.
11. Duke University Medical Center. Chronology of achievements—Black history month: a medical perspective—LibGuides at Duke University Medical Center [Internet]. [cited 2022 Oct 22]. https://guides.mclibrary.duke.edu/Blackhistorymonth/chronology.
12. Weiner S. Celebrating 10 Hispanic pioneers in medicine | AAMC [Internet]. Association of American Medical Colleges. [cited 2022 Oct 22]. https://www.aamc.org/news-insights/celebrating-10-hispanic-pioneers-medicine.
13. Crumpler RL. Standing room only crowd learns of BUSM Alum, first native American Graduate of U.S. Medical School | Chobanian & Avedisian School of Medicine [Internet]. [cited 2022 Oct 22]. https://www.bumc.bu.edu/busm/2014/03/19/standing-room-only-crowd-learns-of-busm-alum-first-native-american-graduate-of-u-s-medical-school/.
14. The Flexner Report | Perspectives of change [Internet]. [cited 2022 Oct 22]. https://perspectivesofchange.hms.harvard.edu/node/99.
15. Savitt T. Abraham Flexner and the Black medical schools. J Natl Med Assoc. 2006;98(9):1415–24.
16. Association of American Medical Colleges. Medical school enrollment more diverse in 2021 [Internet]. AAMC. [cited 2022 Oct 22]. https://www.aamc.org/news-insights/press-releases/medical-school-enrollment-more-diverse-2021.
17. Institute of Medicine. Unequal treatment: confronting racial and ethnic disparities in health care. Washington, DC: The National Academic Press; 2003.
18. Agency for Healthcare Research and Quality. 2018 National healthcare quality and disparities report [Internet]. [cited 2022 Oct 22]. https://www.ahrq.gov/research/findings/nhqrdr/nhqdr18/index.html.
19. Romano SD, Blackstock AJ, Taylor EV, et al. Trends in racial and ethnic disparities in COVID-19 hospitalizations, by region-United States, March-December 2020. MMWR Morb Mortal Wkly Rep. 2021;70:560–5.
20. Hill L, Artiga S. COVID-19 cases and deaths by race/ethnicity: current data and changes over time. Kaiser Family Foundation. 2022. https://www.kff.org/coronavirus-covid-19/issue-brief/covid-19-cases-and-deaths-by-race-ethnicity-current-data-and-changes-over-time/. Accessed 6 May 2022.
21. Emory University. COVID19 health equity report. [Internet]. 2022. [cited 2022 Oct 22]. https://covid19.emory.edu/national-report#resseg. Accessed 6 May 2022.
22. Egede LE, Walker RJ. Structural racism, social risk factors, and COVID-19—A dangerous convergence for Black Americans. N Engl J Med. 2020;383:e77.
23. Healthy People 2020. Social Determinants of Health. U.S. Department of Health and Human Services. [Internet]. [cited 2022 Oct 22]. https://health.gov/healthypeople/priority-areas/social-determinants-health.
24. Center for Disease Control and Prevention (2020). Introduction to COVID19 racial and ethnic health disparities. [Internet]. [cited 2022 Oct 22]. https://www.cdc.gov/coronavirus/2019-ncov/community/health-equity/racial-ethnic-disparities/index.html.
25. Evans MK, Rosenbaum L, Malina D, et al. Diagnosing and treating systemic racism. N Engl J Med. 2020;383:274–6.
26. Hardeman RR, Medina EM, Boyd RW. Stolen breaths. N Engl J Med. 2020;383:197–9.
27. Shelton RC, Adsul P, Oh A. Recommendations for addressing structural racism in implementation science: a call to the field [Internet]. Ethnicity & disease. Ethnicity & Disease; 2021. [Internet]. [cited 2022 Oct 22]. https://www.ncbi.nlm.nih.gov/pmc/articles/PMC8143847/.
28. Community-based participatory research for health [Internet]. Google Books. Google; [cited 2022 Sep 29]. https://books.google.com/books?hl=en&lr=&id=Gkk3DwAAQBAJ&oi=fnd&pg=PA13&dq=community-based%2Bparticipatory%2Bresearch%2Bhealth%2Bequity&ots=0SFDCHGB9i&sig=Umm8wktz16LFFvspEbZvTxeOzjk#v=onepage&q=community-based%20participatory%20research%20health%20equity&f=false.
29. Bailey ZD, Krieger N, Agénor M, Graves J, Linos N, Bassett MT. Structural racism and health inequities in the USA: evidence and interventions [Internet]. Lancet. Elsevier; 2017 [cited 2022 Sep 29]. https://www.sciencedirect.com/science/article/pii/S014067361730569X.
30. CDC. Sickle cell disease in California and Georgia: death rate estimates [Internet]. Centers for Disease Control and Prevention. 2020 [cited 2022 Oct 22]. https://www.cdc.gov/ncbddd/sicklecell/features/keyfindings-scd-death-rate-estimates-ca-ga.html.
31. Lubeck D, Agodoa I, Bhakta N, Danese M, Pappu K, Howard R, et al. Estimated life expectancy and income of patients with sickle cell disease compared

with those without sickle cell disease. JAMA Netw Open. 2019;2(11):e1915374.
32. APA PsycNet [Internet]. American Psychological Association. [cited 2022 Oct 3]. https://psycnet.apa.org/record/2010-06645-017.
33. Original Article. Community perceptions of genomic research [Internet]. [cited 2022 Oct 3]. https://www.med.unc.edu/cher/wp-content/uploads/sites/1048/2013/09/Community-perceptions-of-genomic-research-implications-for-addressing-health-disparities.pdf.
34. What is epigenetics? [Internet]. Centers for Disease Control and Prevention. 2022 [cited 2022 Oct3]. https://www.cdc.gov/genomics/disease/epigenetics.htm#:~:text=Epigenetics%20is%20the%20study%20of,body%20reads%20a%20DNA%20sequence.
35. Shim RS, Search for more papers by this author, Psychiatry Dof, Send correspondence to Dr. Shim ([email protected])., S S-S, JS S, et al. Dismantling structural racism in psychiatry: a path to mental health equity [Internet]. American Journal of Psychiatry. 2021 [cited 2022 Sep 29]. https://ajp.psychiatryonline.org/doi/full/10.1176/appi.ajp.2021.21060558.
36. Stigma, prejudice and discrimination against people with mental illness [Internet]. Psychiatry.org—Stigma, prejudice and discrimination against people with mental illness. [cited 2022 Oct 3]. https://www.psychiatry.org/patients-families/stigma-and-discrimination.

# Integrating Neurodiversity and Disability Rights into Primary Care Practices

# 13

Emily Hotez, Julianna Rava, Zachary Williams, Patrick Dwyer, Kashia A. Rosenau, and Morénike Giwa Onaiwu

## Background

The following chapter focuses on creating neurodiversity-oriented healthcare practices and policies in primary care clinics. We begin with a case study of "Ari," a neurodivergent patient that exemplifies the role of primary care providers in promoting the health, well-being, and thriving of neurodivergent people. This chapter was inspired by Ari and others like her. We begin this chapter describing Ari, defining neurodiversity and other key terminology, and providing an overview of the neurodiversity landscape. Subsequently, we outline the interpersonal, educational, clinical, research, and policy barriers to integrating neurodiversity-oriented care into healthcare clinics. These are barriers that—if addressed—can more effectively support patients with diverse needs and preferences, including but not limited to those who identify as neurodivergent. We then highlight several emerging promising practices and approaches that can potentially address the previously described barriers. We close the chapter by providing actionable recommendations and resources for primary care providers, such as those caring for patients such as Ari.

## Presentation of a Case Study

The following case study was reported to us by a primary care provider.

Ari came to me for primary care when she was 13 years old. She was finishing up eighth grade and going into high school. Although she was still in middle school, she had already received many diagnoses. These included diagnoses of schizoaffective disorder, obsessive-compulsive disorder, bipolar disorder, anxiety, depression, and attention-deficit/hyperactivity disorder (ADHD). Additionally, she was simultaneously taking six different psychotropic medications.

Over the course of our interactions together, I came to question her myriad diagnoses and medications. To be sure, she had substantial anxiety about the future. Throughout our interactions, however, I learned that it was the constraints and rigidity within her environment that were creating and exacerbating her struggles. Rather than try "fix" her with medication, I brainstormed

E. Hotez (✉) · J. Rava · K. A. Rosenau
Division of Medicine-Pediatrics and Preventive Medicine, University of California, Los Angeles, CA, USA
e-mail: ehotez@mednet.ucla.edu; juliannarava@g.ucla.edu; krosenau@mednet.ucla.edu

Z. Williams
Vanderbilt University School of Medicine, Nashville, TN, USA
e-mail: Zachary.j.williams@vanderbilt.edu

P. Dwyer
Olga Tennison Autism Research Centre, School of Psychology and Public Health, La Trobe University, Bundoora, VIC, Australia

M. G. Onaiwu
Rice University, Houston, TX, USA


A. A. Kuo et al. (eds.), *Care of Adults with Chronic Childhood Conditions*,
https://doi.org/10.1007/978-3-031-54281-7_13

with her possible strategies for augmenting her environment to better meet her needs. Ultimately, I diagnosed her exclusively with autism and significantly pared down her medication utilization.

She remained my patient throughout her high school years. During this time, she learned more about autism and neurodiversity and her art abilities completely blossomed. I will never forget the visit in which she showed me her Instagram page with all of her incredible art and also taught me about TikTok. I remember fondly how she would bounce both hands on her thighs with the palms facing upwards when she got excited or anxious while talking about these topics.

After working together for a while, it was clear that she was increasingly accepting who she was and becoming aware of her strengths and challenges. I witnessed her father also learning more about who she was, truly embracing her identity development, and continuously acknowledging her strengths. Their evolving relationship was amazing to see. After completing 2 years of community college, she was accepted to a prestigious art school."

Tragically, Ari passed away in July of 2020. In her legacy, the authors of the current chapter see the immense role of healthcare providers and others who support and care for neurodivergent individuals in promoting health, well-being, and thriving.

## Defining Neurodiversity

The current chapter was co-authored by both autistic and non-autistic researchers and advocates, brought together via our work on the Autistic Researcher Review Board of the Autism Intervention Research Network on Physical Health (ARRB, AIR-P). In the context of this work, the autistic researchers among us co-authored a published commentary outlining principles of neurodiversity and our vision for supporting neurodivergent individuals in healthcare, research, and policy spheres [1]. In this chapter, we define neurodiversity and other key terminology relevant to the provision of neurodiversity-oriented care. An overview of these definitions is provided in Table 13.1, but we encourage healthcare providers to read this chapter to better understand the tenets of neurodiversity.

"Neurodiversity" can be a slightly ambiguous term. Indeed, Walker distinguishes between three different meanings of "neurodiversity." The first meaning is the simplest. "Neurodiversity" can simply refer to the existence of diversity in minds and brains. Diversity of minds and brains is found throughout humanity, including the "neurotypical" population, as well as "neurodivergent" groups or "neurominorities" such as autistic and ADHD people [2]. Soon after the term was first developed in discussions within the Independent

**Table 13.1** Neurodiversity terminology

| Terminology | Definition |
|---|---|
| Neurodiversity | The existence of diversity in minds and brains |
| Neurodiversity movement | An advocacy movement supporting neurodiversity approaches<br>Opposes attempts to find a "cure" for neurodivergent individuals, along with interventions that promote "indistinguishability from peers"<br>Advocates for greater acceptance and support of neurologic differences and adoption of more person-centered goals consistent with the preferences of neurodivergent people |
| Neurodivergent/ Neurominority | A neurotype whose members' minds or brains differ from what is socioculturally typical and normative in ways that are associated with disability. Autism is only one example (others are intellectual disability, ADHD, etc.) |
| A Neurodiversity approach to health & Well-being | A neurodiversity approach to well-being is in alignment with Seligman's Positive Emotions, Engagement, Relationships, Meaning, and Accomplishment (PERMA) theory of well-being<br>According to this theory, healthcare providers seeking to improve the well-being of neurodivergent individuals should promote their (1) Positive emotions or subjective sense of well-being; (2) Engagement; (3) Relationships with others; (4) Meaning and purpose in life; and (5) Accomplishments |

Living on the Autism Specrum (InLv) email listserve, Singer compared "neurodiversity" to "biodiversity," suggesting that just as diversity of species can be good for ecosystems, so might diversity of minds and brains be beneficial for human societies [3]. In this first sense, "neurodiversity" simply describes the reality of human neurocognitive diversity, although it may not be value-neutral: [4] the positive connotation of the term suggests this diversity is a good thing.

The other two meanings of neurodiversity can be harder to pin down. Walker speaks of a neurodiversity "paradigm," alternatively described as a "framework" [5] or as multiple "approaches" [2, 6]. These neurodiversity approaches represent certain ways of conceptualizing and addressing human neurocognitive diversity. They represent a set of prescriptions, such as the idea that neurodivergent people should be respected and accepted as they are, and not be subjected to attempts to "cure" or "normalize" them. These neurodiversity approaches are closely intertwined with the neurodiversity "movement," an advocacy movement supporting neurodiversity approaches.

But what exactly does it mean to follow a neurodiversity approach? Different sources can give different answers, which is one reason for speaking of multiple "approaches" rather than a single monolithic "paradigm." For example, some say that a neurodiversity approach is aligned with the social model of disability (at least insofar as autism is concerned, e.g., [7, 8]); this model suggests that disability is caused by societal barriers, not the inherent characteristics of disabled people. This would in turn imply that intervention should focus on changing society, not the neurodivergent person. Other understandings of a neurodiversity approach recognize both individual and societal contributions to disability, [9] which might allow intervention to address either. For example, someone could try to teach useful skills to a neurodivergent person without suggesting there is something inherently pathological about who they are. This diversity of views arises from the evolving, leaderless nature of the neurodiversity movement: advocates have been free to reinterpret and reinvent ideas [3, 10]. Nevertheless, it is possible to identify some common themes within neurodiversity approaches.

Neurodiversity advocates almost invariably question assumptions that the challenges neurodivergent people face always are due to their "deficits." While neurodiversity advocates do recognize that neurodivergent people face very real challenges and are disabled [11], they direct attention to ways in which our society can create or exacerbate many of these challenges. For example, although autistic people are officially regarded as having social and communication "deficits," research suggests there are two sides to this story, and that neurotypical people often struggle to understand and communicate with autistic people [12, 13]. Moreover, autistic people's social differences can elicit rapid negative judgements [14] and these negative judgements can lead to discrimination against autistic people in contexts such as job interviews [15]. Difficulties communicating with, and biases against, neurodivergent people are clearly relevant to healthcare settings. As discussed later in this chapter, there are many ways in which contemporary practices in healthcare settings can create barriers to care for autistic people.

Unfortunately, attributing neurodivergent people's challenges to their own "deficits" is just one of many examples of problematic discourse that are widespread today. It seems reasonable to assume that describing someone as having deficiencies could damage their self-esteem, and perhaps exacerbate the high rates of co-occurring mental health challenges among neurodivergent people [16, 17]. Furthermore, as we have seen, the accuracy of terms like "deficit" is often questionable. It can be unclear whether a neurodivergent person's challenges are due to their shortcomings, or whether society contributes to the problems they face. Thus, these traditional language choices are not only derogatory and potentially harmful, but also far from objective [18]. For additional information, we also encourage providers review our AIR-P "inclusive language guide," which we developed as a resource for healthcare providers serving neurodivergent individuals [18].

Protecting neurodivergent people from discrimination and from violations of their rights is another priority for neurodiversity advocates. This too is relevant to healthcare. In situations when resources are scarce, as with organ transplants or the COVID-19 pandemic, neurodivergent people—especially those with intellectual disabilities—can face explicit discrimination even in official processes, [19, 20] over and above unconscious discrimination in particular cases.

Many neurodiversity advocates are also concerned about neurodivergent people's opportunities to exercise autonomy, or rather, the lack thereof. Autistic children tend to show lower levels of self-determination than non-disabled people [21]. Autistic young adults can have complex relationships with parents, in which they might both rely on their parents for advocacy support, yet also desire to have greater independence [22]. Guardianship or conservatorship of neurodivergent adults represents an extreme of low self-determination and loss of legal rights, and many neurodiversity advocates therefore oppose guardianship and advocate for supported decision-making as an alternative [8, 23]. These dynamics can create complex dilemmas for healthcare providers: in many matters, providers can be legally required to defer to the wishes of guardians of children or conserved adults, yet providers should strive to encourage the involvement of neurodivergent people in decisions about their healthcare as much as feasible based on relevant laws and neurodivergent people's communicative abilities.

Despite neurodiversity advocates' efforts to direct attention to societal issues impacting neurodivergent people, it is important to clarify that neurodiversity advocates are *not* opposed to medical, cure-oriented interventions for medical issues, such as epilepsy or gastrointestinal problems [9, 24]. However, this is quite different from attempting to cure an individual's neurodivergence (e.g., autism or ADHD). Taken together, the neurodiversity movement is multi-faceted. In the preceding section, we aimed to emphasize its complexities in order to illustrate the importance of individualized approaches to healthcare that are responsive to the heterogenous needs of neurodiverse individuals. In the following sections, we provide background on how the field arrived at this nuanced understanding of neurodiversity and how the unfolding of the neurodiversity landscape informs healthcare today.

## Disability Policy: Shaping the Neurodiversity Landscape

Table 13.2 provides an overview of U.S. laws and policies that have been enacted in order to improve the quality of life for neurodivergent individuals. Much of the progress for neurodivergent people has been associated with greater acceptance of disabled people in society and with the triumphs of disability advocacy movements.

There are three federal laws fundamental to increasing accessibility in the education and employment of neurodivergent people, which we define here.

1. *The Americans with Disabilities Act (ADA; Pub.L. 101–336)*: The ADA prohibits discrimination and promotes equal opportunity for disabled people. Although enforcement of the ADA can be difficult, the passage of the ADA was a defining triumph for disability advocates.
2. *The Individuals with Disabilities Education Act (IDEA; Pub.L. 101–476):* The IDEA, which replaced the Education for All Handicapped Children Act (Public Law [Pub.L.] 94–142) [25], requires school systems and classrooms to adapt their environments for integration of students with disabilities, including neurodivergent children. Under the IDEA, educational supports and services are provided to school-age children with disabilities and early intervention is available to infants and toddlers with disabilities.
3. *The Workforce Innovation and Opportunity Act (WIOA; Pub.L. 113–128)*: The WIOA, a reauthorization of the 1998 Workforce Investment Act (Pub.L. 105–220), provides new job training and employment services focused on transition-age youth and adults

**Table 13.2** Neurodiversity milestones and contributions to the neurodiversity and neurodivergence landscape

| Neurodiversity milestone | Contribution to the neurodiversity landscape |
|---|---|
| Americans with Disabilities Act (ADA, Pub.L. 101–336) signed into law in 1990 | Prohibited discrimination and promoted equal opportunity for disabled people. The ADA is divided into five titles: Employment, Public Services, Public Accommodations, Telecommunications, Miscellaneous |
| Education for All Handicapped Children Act passed in 1975 (Now known as the Individuals with Disabilities Education Act [IDEA, Pub.L. 101–476]) | Makes educational support and services available to children with disabilities and their families. Part B statute ensures a "free appropriate public education" from age three through 21. The Part C statute provides early intervention services to infants and toddlers |
| Health Insurance Portability and Accountability Act of 1996 (HIPAA, Pub.L. 104–191) | Created national standards to protect the privacy rights of patients and their health information<br>For neurodivergent individuals, this provided a layer of protection in employment and education and enforced discretion of medical information among family members |
| Centers for Medicaid and Medicare (CMS) updated guidelines (2014) | Under the "early and periodic screening, diagnostic and treatment services" (EPSDT) section of the guidelines, children and young adults up to age 21 can access necessary autism services<br>Required the HCBS 1915(c) waiver to provide living arrangements for disabled people in integrated community settings |
| Workforce Innovation and Opportunity Act (WIOA, Pub.L. 113–128) signed into law in 2015 | Provided new job training and employment services focused on transition-age youth and adults with disabilities |

with disabilities. Additionally, the law states that "competitive, integrated" employment is preferred for workers with and without disabilities.

Accessible employment and education are crucial to improving the well-being of neurodivergent children and adults. Access to educational support is associated with achieving postsecondary education and better quality of life in adulthood. Further, competitive employment is important for overall health–as majority of U.S. adults gain health insurance through their employer [26] and it is associated with positive mental health among disabled adults. Therefore, ADA, IDEA, and WIOA have created positive impacts on the general well-being of neurodivergent people throughout the life course.

Within the realm of health services, there are several pieces of legislation that support broad improvements in quality healthcare, but have significant implications for neurodivergent individuals.

1. *The Health Insurance Portability and Accountability Act of 1996 (HIPAA; Pub.L. 104–191)*: HIPAA was a federal law that created national standards to protect the privacy rights of patients and their health information [27]. For neurodivergent individuals, this provides a layer of protection in employment and education, among other rights.
2. *The Centers for Medicaid and Medicare (CMS)*: In 2014, CMS updated their guidelines for Medicaid coverage of autism services for children and adults. Under the "early and periodic screening, diagnostic and treatment services" (EPSDT) section of the guidelines, children and young adults up to age 21 can access necessary autism services. Establishing immediate access to services is a vital step in ensuring long-term quality of life for autistic people [28].
3. *CMS Health and Community-Based Settings (HCBS) guidelines*: That same year, CMS updated their HCBS guidelines; the new guidelines required the HCBS 1915(c) waiver to provide living arrangements for disabled people in integrated community settings. Prior to the updated HCBS 1915(c) waiver, one in five autistic adults had never lived independently and majority were living with their parents or caregivers [29]. Further, many autistic young adults were experiencing social

isolation and lack of community participation [30]. The new requirements of the HCBS 1915(c) waiver removed the financial burden of accommodating supports for community integrated living arrangements and created an opportunity to improve the well-being of autistic children, adults, and their families.

4. *The Social Security Administration (SSA)*: SSA offers two disability programs that assist neurodivergent people—Social Security Disability Insurance (SSDI) and Social Security Income (SSI). Both SSDI and SSI provide monthly income support to cover the service needs of disabled people, although reforms to SSI in particular are urgently demanded by many advocates [31]. Notably, even the maximum possible level of SSI payments ($841 USD per month for an individual as of January 2022) still falls well beneath the poverty line, which does not account for the additional expenses typically faced by disabled and neurodivergent people. Furthermore, access to SSI is conditional on a strict asset cap that prevents SSI recipients from saving more money than would be needed to live, if no emergency arose, for more than a handful of weeks [31].

Attempts to provide equal opportunities in education (IDEA), employment (WIOA), and health services (HIPAA, Medicaid) are central to improving the societal barriers for neurodivergent people. This emphasizes the need to maintain, expand, and improve the policy and legislative frameworks established to protect neurodivergent people in the United States and other countries. However, the medical establishment is still fixated in a deficit-based system. Many primary care providers understand neurodivergence as an abnormal trait that requires "fixing" the person, which is based in the medical model of disability. To challenge this assumption, the social model of disability reframes the argument—rather, society imposes restrictions on disabled individuals and the structural environment needs to be adapted to support full participation of disabled people in society. While the social model challenges the medical model's deficit-based approach, it notably does not fully encapsulate the needs of neurodivergent individuals [18].

A lack of guidance from medical organizations and societies in implementing neurodiversity principles leaves primary care providers to fend for themselves to learn new strategies or risk feeling incompetent in providing care to neurodivergent patients. It is important for the medical system and providers to understand neurodivergent people and also feel confident providing quality healthcare. As a provider, knowing the laws and federal policies that impact the overall well-being of neurodivergent people is necessary to supporting access to accommodations in education, employment, and health services.

## Barriers to Neurodiversity-Oriented Care

Despite the proliferating neurodiversity landscape and providers' increasing understanding of the intersection of disability rights and healthcare, there remain barriers to translating principles of neurodiversity into healthcare contexts by providing what we term "neurodiversity-oriented care." In the current chapter, we define neurodiversity-oriented care as healthcare that is responsive to the diverse needs, experiences, and preferences of neurodivergent individuals and is distinct from outdated "one-size-fits-all" practices. In practice, neurodiversity-oriented care entails providing healthcare and healthcare environments that are flexible and accommodating, individually and culturally tailored, and reflective of the perspectives of individuals with a wide range of lived experiences. To date, the barriers to implementing and scaling efforts toward neurodiversity-oriented healthcare occur across multiple systems and sectors.

### Interpersonal Barriers to Neurodiversity-Oriented Care

Interpersonal interactions between patients and healthcare providers are often characterized by patients' anticipation or experience of both implicit and explicit stigma, broadly defined as the social devaluation of individuals with certain characteristics, identities, or statuses through bias, prejudice, negative stereotyping, and discrimination [32]. Research shows that lifelong stigma toward marginalized groups—including neurodivergent individuals—begins to develop in early childhood (as early as elementary school) and continues to proliferate throughout adulthood [33–35]. It is therefore not surprising that healthcare providers hold stigmatizing perspectives of neurodivergent individuals well before they enter their healthcare professions. Stigmatizing attitudes often do not get corrected in medical education and training, as will be discussed in subsequent sections. As a result, healthcare providers often unconsciously and consciously stigmatize their patients in the healthcare interactions [36–39].

Stigma manifests in multiple ways in healthcare interactions. At the most basic level, providers often consider neurodivergent individuals—even children—too complex to treat, citing working with them as a "minefield" for example [40]. As a result, providers often choose not to provide care for this population. They may, in turn, refer them to specialists for even the most basic preventive treatments. This practice of automatically referring neurodivergent individuals to specialist care—on top of interminable wait times, lengthy commutes to see the few specialty doctors in the community, and lack of coordination between medical entities—can significantly delay treatment and worsen outcomes [41].

Stigma also manifests when providers preemptively assume that neurodivergent patients will not understand something and communicate exclusively with their caregiver [42]. This practice can prevent conversations that address the patient's specific concerns. Similarly, providers often gloss over important treatment details, presumed to be too complicated for the patient to comprehend [42]. Physicians may also attribute health concerns solely to the neurodivergent condition. This is often at the expense of making a veritable effort to investigate and treat the concern, resulting in treatable health conditions being overlooked or mismanaged [37]. Across both scenarios, neurodivergent patients are not getting their needs met.

A lifelong exposure to stigma—in healthcare interactions and otherwise—often results in neurodivergent individuals engaging in camouflaging, or using strategies to compensate for or hide traits associated with the neurodivergent condition [43, 44]. Camouflaging has been reported in some studies to create considerable stress and fatigue, potentially contributing to poor mental and physical health and compounding stigma-related health disparities [45].

Stigma also creates health disparities because it may prevent neurodivergent people from accessing appropriate services [46]. Difficulty communicating with medical professionals and not feeling understood by one's doctor are among the most common barriers to healthcare reported by autistic individuals in medical settings [47, 48], and these specific barriers have been associated with poorer health outcomes including untreated physical and mental health problems [49]. Though the pathways from stigma to health disparities in neurodivergent individuals have not been studied in depth, it is likely that neurodivergent individuals who feel stigmatized by their healthcare providers will be less willing to seek medical care or follow provider recommendations, subsequently leading to under-treatment of medical issues (see also [49]). Cumulatively, even seemingly insignificant details in interpersonal interactions may make the difference in whether a neurodivergent patient receives quality versus fragmented and insufficient healthcare.

## Medical Education and Training

Barriers to neurodiversity-oriented care are largely attributable to lack of quality neurodiversity-focused medical education and training. Indeed, there is well-established research that shows that medical students, residents, and current physicians do not receive adequate training in this area. Overall, physicians report stress, lack of confidence, fear, and anxiety in providing care for neurodivergent patients [36]. Fewer than half report high confidence that they can provide quality care to neurodivergent patients [50].

Lack of knowledge originates from shortcomings in medical education training worldwide [51]. For example, only half of U.S. medical school deans report having education curricula about biopsychosocial aspects of caring for patients with neurodiversity or chronic conditions in their schools [52]. Medical education competencies typically do not specifically identify neurodivergent conditions or disabilities [53] and in the instances where a disability-focused curriculum is available, content typically focuses on those with physical conditions [52]. It is therefore not surprising that there is a lack of adequate training on specific neurodivergent sub-groups who have particularly high support needs, such as neurodivergent pregnant women [54].

In the event that a disability-focused curriculum does exist in medical schools, much of the educational content frames neurodevelopmental conditions as pathology rather than considering them within the neurodiversity paradigm. In practice, this entails curricula that focus on neurodivergent characteristics as problems to be prevented or fixed. This, in turn, cements bias in providers and gives them reason to believe that being neurodivergent is inherently less desirable due to it being a disease state. Emerging research has found that medical education and training does not adequately support providers in training on providing ADA accommodations [55]. Indeed, physicians struggle with navigating key aspects of patient care for neurodivergent individuals, including ableism, self-determination, coordinating care, and offering accommodations [56].

These gaps in medical education are further compounded by the lack of neurodiversity-focused continuing medical education opportunities, which could ostensibly be leveraged to help established providers feel more comfortable providing care to their neurodivergent patients. Although short educational courses, such as the UK National Health Service's *Oliver McGowan Mandatory Training in Learning Disability and Autism* [57], are available to some providers, many providers are unaware of or unable to access such material, particularly in a continuing education context. Thus, there remains a much greater need for continuing medical education opportunities specifically related to neurodiversity and providing healthcare for neurodivergent individuals.

Training gaps are found in the United States and internationally, making it a global public health issue [58, 59]. Medical students overwhelmingly report that they desire more neurodiversity-specific training [60]. Taken together, a lack of sufficient medical education and training compromises provider confidence and self-efficacy in supporting their neurodivergent patients, impedes the quality of care they are able to provide, and further compounds health disparities for neurodivergent populations.

## Gaps in Clinical Practice

Efforts to propagate neurodiversity-oriented healthcare are thwarted by barriers that exist within clinical practice. Clinical practice guidelines are oftentimes outdated and there are limited efforts to update or correct them [61]. As a result, guidelines often do not align with theoretical models or frameworks that support principles of neurodiversity. These frameworks include the social and public health models of disability that emphasize the role of external factors and social determinants of health on quality of life [62, 63]. Even if clinical practice guidelines are updated, they are not always translated into clinical practice [64]. These limitations result in clinical practice that is not neurodiversity-oriented—that is, practice that is not attuned to the specific needs of neurodivergent individuals. This might entail rigid adherence to protocols that are not responsive to those with diverse abilities and preferences.

These limitations also result in built environmental characteristics within clinics that are not conducive to health-promotion for this population. A statewide review of California clinics, for example, found that less than 10% of clinics had height-adjustable examination tables, and only one-third of interior provider offices met accessibility criteria [65]. Further, even when accessible equipment is available to a physician, it is not always used during patient examinations [66]. Challenges also extend to telehealth, which is often inaccessible to neurodivergent patients [67].

Limitations in clinical practice are perpetuated by interdisciplinary siloes. Siloes exist between multiple fields, including medical education, research, clinical practice guidelines, and communities of neurodiversity advocates [68]. Indeed, researchers have cited lack of physician collaboration with other disciplines, including genetics and the medical humanities, as a barrier to integrating principles of neurodiversity into healthcare [69, 70]. Barriers to neurodiversity-oriented care in clinical practice lead to compromised care, lower treatment adherence and utilization, and fragmented services which indirectly create health disparities.

## The Role of Research in Impeding Neurodiversity-Oriented Care

Healthcare providers are limited in the extent to which they can provide neurodiversity-oriented care in their clinics due to a dearth of research that supports the inclusion of neurodiversity principles into clinic operations. It is well-established that there is a lack of research on the health of neurodivergent individuals. Indeed, a recent review of 300 randomized clinical trials published in high-impact medical journals found that neurodivergent individuals were represented in only 2% of trials and could have been included in others with relatively minor methodological adjustments [71]. As a result, research on healthcare practices and policies often do not focus on this population.

There is also a lack of research on existing approaches to integrating neurodiversity topics into medical and post-medical education [55]. Medical student-driven initiatives are beginning to spur innovation in medical curricula; however, there is a lack of standardization and evaluation of these efforts, which limits the extent to which educators are clear on what to integrate into curricula and the pedagogical approaches are most effective. Beyond this, there is limited qualitative research that seeks to meaningfully understand neurodivergent individuals' perspectives on healthcare services or accommodations. Participatory research approaches, in which researchers collaborate with neurodivergent individuals to co-design and develop supports and services (e.g., the AASPIRE Healthcare Toolkit [72]) are even less frequently utilized. This field is beginning to grow, but there is a substantial need for additional work in this area [37, 68]. Lack of research across all of these areas thwarts the development, implementation, and evaluation of promising practices and limits the scalability and sustainability of existing approaches that move the needle on neurodiversity-oriented care.

## Shortcomings in Policy for Neurodiversity-Oriented Care

A lack of research and evidence means that policymakers—particularly those who have a role in healthcare decisions—have limited evidence to rely on when making policy decisions. This, in turn, limits the extent to which neurodivergent populations are included in policy decisions. As an example, in December 2020, the Advisory Committee on Immunization Practices (ACIP) Coronavirus Disease 2019 (COVID-19) Vaccine Working Group issued recommendations for prioritizing and allocating vaccinations for the first available mRNA vaccines from Pfizer-BioNTech and Moderna. Almost all neurodivergent individuals were ineligible for vaccination based on the Phase 1 tiered guidelines. It is possible that robust data and evidence would have facilitated their inclusion into the guidelines [73].

Generally speaking, lifelong stigma and misinformation that does not get corrected means that many policymakers have a misunderstanding of the needs, experiences, and priorities of neurodivergent populations. In effect, stigma and misinformation—rather than research and evidence—may affect policy decisions overtime and continue to exclude these groups.

Myriad barriers exist in interpersonal interactions between providers and patients; education and training environments; clinical practice guidelines and recommendations; research and evaluation strategies; and policy decisions. While barriers to neurodiversity-oriented healthcare persist, the field can look toward emerging promising practices and approaches as a means to dismantle these barriers.

## Promising Practices and Approaches

In recent years, several promising practices and approaches for promoting neurodiversity-oriented care have emerged. These emerging efforts can—at least in part—combat the barriers to neurodiversity-oriented care discussed in the preceding section. Promising practices and approaches include improvements to the extent to which healthcare-related research aligns with the perspectives of neurodivergent individuals; initiatives to advance medical student and physician knowledge about neurodiversity; and increasing implementation of coordinated medical home models in primary care. The following examples discuss strategies and models for healthcare providers motivated to enhance care for neurodivergent populations.

### Research: Lived Experience and Participatory Research Methods

Lived experience and participatory research methods—in the form of both quantitative and qualitative studies—offer insight into the experiences of neurodivergent people. Quantitative research has demonstrated that many neurodivergent individuals do not receive adequate quality care and qualitative studies detail personal experiences explaining the *why* underlying these findings. This combination elucidates systemic gaps in care and, in turn, highlights opportunities for primary care intervention. As an example, quantitative lived experience research has identified low utilization rates of women's health services among autistic women, particularly OB/GYN healthcare [74]. To understand why autistic women are not accessing health services at the same rate as other adult women, Moseley et al. [75] attempted to describe the menopause experience for autistic women through qualitative lived experience research. Through qualitative interviews, autistic women explained menopause can be more difficult to navigate with pre-existing difficulties, such as communication and executive functioning.

Lived experience research also illuminates the mechanisms underlying health disparities among individuals with I/DD [76–78]. As an example, Nicolaidis et al. [37] conducted interviews with autistic adults and healthcare stakeholders to understand the patient-, provider-, and system-level experiences of providing healthcare to autistic people. Autistic individuals' delayed processing speed, non-verbal communication tools, and overstimulation of sensory inputs; providers' knowledge and assumptions of autism characteristics and openness to offering accommodations during patient visits; and systemic barriers to healthcare access were all identified as underlying mechanisms via this lived experience research.

In addition to lived experience research, providers can also look toward participatory research, a research strategy that prioritizes collaborations between researchers and individuals with lived experience. Participatory research practices are becoming more prominent within neurodiversity-related clinical research. Overall, there are different levels of participatory research and engagement that can be utilized in improving the healthcare experiences of neurodivergent people. Community-based participatory research (CBPR) [79] has garnered significant attention within neurodiversity-oriented research. CBPR requires researchers and community partners to be equally engaged throughout the entire process. An example of a CBPR approach to improving neurodiversity-oriented care is the Academic Autism Spectrum Partnership in Research and Education (AASPIRE) [80], which is comprised of members of the autistic community, the academic community, and the community of people who provide support and services to autistics. AASPIRE has utilized their model in multiple studies to improving interactions with healthcare providers and address systemic gaps in care [37].

Lived experience and participatory research approaches can inform providers' efforts to move beyond "tokenistic" practices (i.e., practices based on stigma or misinformation) and meaningfully engage with neurodivergent community members when improving clinical practices.

## Physician Training and Toolkits

Physicians do not feel confident or properly trained to care for neurodivergent people. Therefore, innovative training strategies are necessary to educate the current physician workforce. For example, the Extension for Community Healthcare Outcomes (ECHO) program developed a provider virtual training program to support the health service needs of neurodivergent individuals [81]. In a study of ECHO provider participation, satisfaction, learning, self-efficacy, and change in practice, the majority expressed expanding their knowledge and competency in providing care to individuals with I/DD, felt supported by a community of practice, often learning from one another, and shared resources with wider office teams–potentially influencing systemic changes.

Physician toolkits have been useful instruments in improving patient–provider interactions. Advocacy organizations, such as the Special Olympics and the Autistic Self Advocacy Network, have been essential in disseminating physician toolkits [82]. Similarly, the academic-community partnership, AASPIRE, created a toolkit for autistic individuals and their primary care providers [72]. These toolkits aim to inform physicians about the characteristics of neurodivergent patients, make them aware of relevant accommodations and supports, and provide best practice tools to improve the quality of healthcare for these individuals. A breakdown of the domains of each toolkit are provided in Table 13.3.

**Table 13.3** Primary care provider toolkit domains

| Toolkit name | Audience | Domains |
|---|---|---|
| AASPIRE Healthcare Toolkit | Patients and supports; healthcare providers | Patient and provider:<br>– Healthcare<br>– Staying healthy<br>– Your rights in healthcare<br>– Autism information<br>– Medical information<br>– Checklists and worksheets<br>Healthcare providers:<br>– Autism information, diagnosis, referrals<br>– Caring for patients on the autism spectrum<br>– Ethical and legal considerations<br>– Associated conditions<br>– Resources |
| Real talk: Provider toolkit—Improving quality of sexual health care for patients with disabilities | Healthcare Provider | – What do providers need to know<br>– Questions to ask yourself as a provider<br>– Questions to ask the patient<br>– Improving access and attitudes<br>– Resources |
| Healthcare for adults with I/DD, toolkit for primary care providers | Healthcare providers | – General issues (informed consent, communicating effectively, etc.)<br>– Physical health issues (preventive care checklist, etc.)<br>– Behavioral and mental health Issues (caregiver checklist, crisis management, medication checklist, etc.)<br>– Health watch tables (autism, down syndrome, etc.)<br>– Resources |

## Medical Student-Driven Neurodiversity Initiatives

While it is crucial to increase the competence of our current physician workforce, there is an additional need to prepare future doctors in treating neurodivergent people. Student-led initiatives to integrate disability care into the curriculum have sprung up across the country. At University of California, Los Angeles (UCLA), medical students started the Disability and Chronic Illness (DCI) group. In this group, they advocate for more time spent on understanding the characteristics of individuals with disabilities and the systemic issues that lead to low quality healthcare. Similar groups are proliferating across the country, including the Disability Advocacy Coalition in Medicine, focused on improving disability medical school curricula across campuses. Across all of these medical student advocacy efforts, many medical students self-identify as having a disability themselves.

In addition to education medical students, it is also necessary to create neurodiversity-oriented education for nurses and other healthcare professionals [83]. Therefore, next steps in these initiatives may consider improvements to healthcare education for nursing students, dentists, physician assistants, and other allied health professionals. Prior research suggests that disability-focused trainings are more effective when co-developed with neurodivergent people. In effect, these student-driven initiatives should strive to prioritize neurodivergent input [84].

## Patient-Centered Medical Home Models

Since the early 1990s, the Academy of American Pediatrics has supported utilization of a medical home model in children's healthcare [85]. The medical home aims to deliver primary care in a comprehensive, coordinated, family-centered system. Children with special healthcare needs without access to a medical home are more likely to experience poorer health outcomes than other children [86]. While much of the current research focuses on children, a medical home model remains critical for neurodivergent adults. Implementing the medical home model in primary care systems enables continuity of care and access to services that are necessary to improve health outcomes for neurodivergent people. Below are a few examples of medical home models that have been utilized in the clinical setting.

An example of a patient-centered medical home model that addresses the needs of neurodivergent individuals across the lifespan is the University of California's Leadership Education in Neurodevelopmental Disabilities (UC-LEND) at University of California, Los Angeles. The UC-LEND clinic involves an interdisciplinary team of healthcare providers (primary care, social work, psychology, neurology, occupational therapy, and public health) working together with individuals with ADHD, autism, and related neurodevelopmental disabilities and their families in navigating the healthcare system. Figure 13.1 provides an overview of the UC-LEND clinic medical home model. When the COVID-19 pandemic hit, the LEND clinic resorted to a telehealth format for appointments. This alternative structure has provided relief to families in reducing travel time, costs, and stress while still engaging with their clinical team. The UC-LEND clinic continues to adapt to meet the needs of its patients and provide care within preferred-settings.

In addition to UC-LEND, Kong et al. (2020) propose a medical home model called the, "Systematic Network of Autism Primary Care Services" (SYNAPSE) for neurodivergent individuals and their families [87]. The model synthesizes the healthcare coproduction framework, the medical neighborhood, and chronic healthcare management to create a model that supports the direct needs of the neurodivergent community. The novelty of the SYNAPSE model is that it creates a network of primary care providers across a geographic area founded in the values of the medical home model–as members, there are standardized protocols across the network. Figure 13.2 presents the framework of the SYNAPSE model.

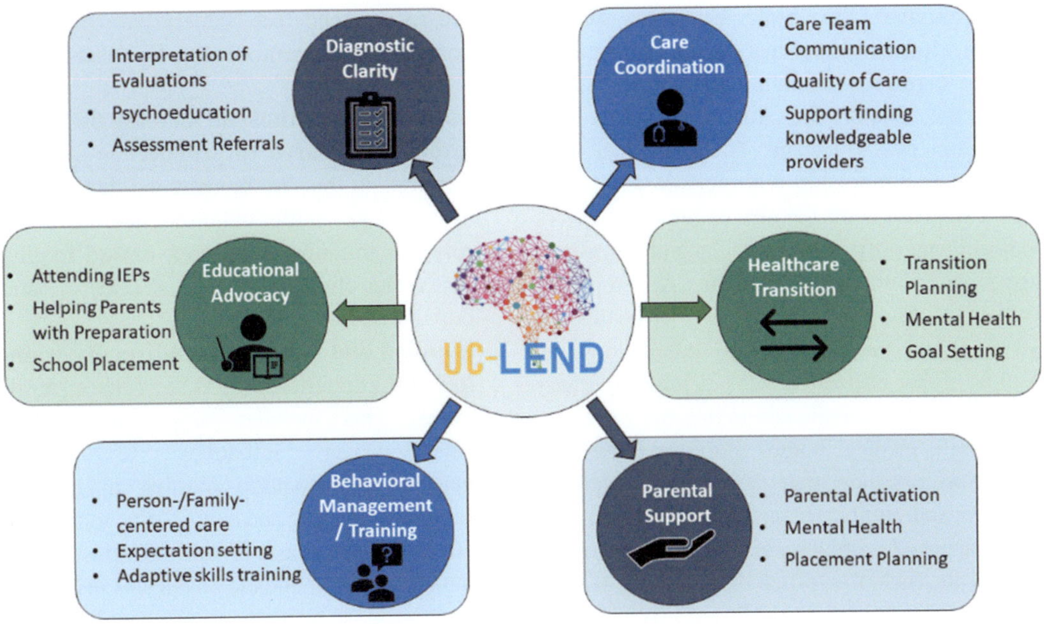


**Fig. 13.1** UC-LEND clinic model

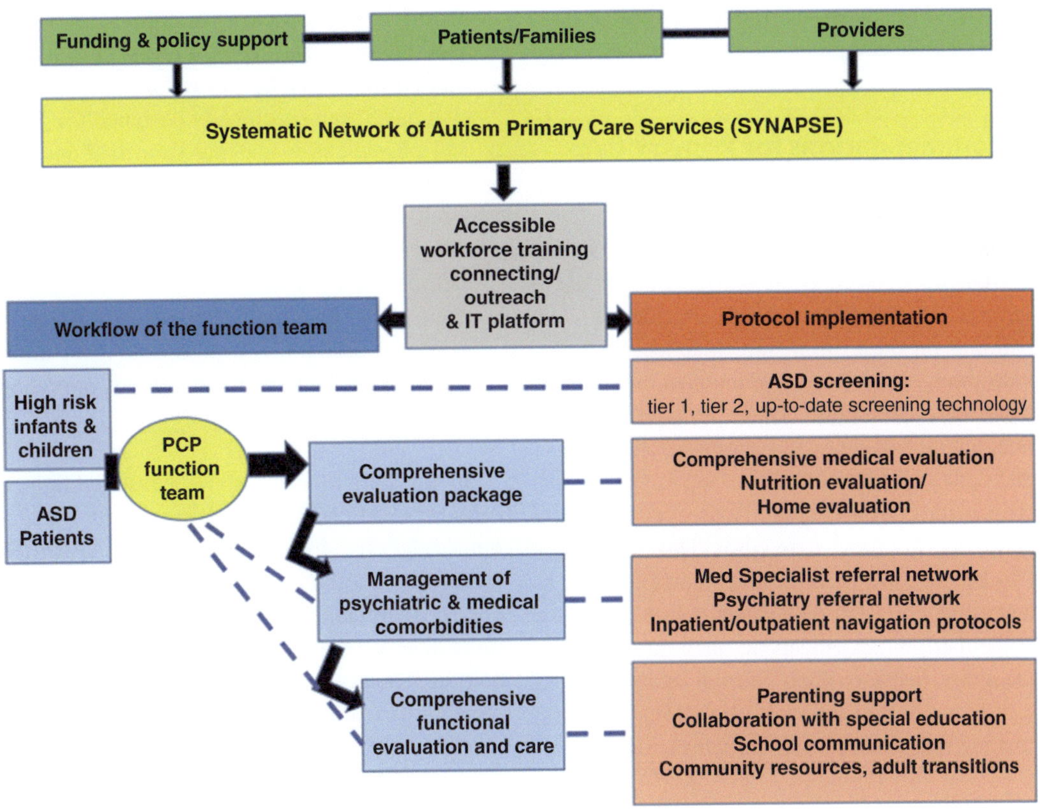


**Fig. 13.2** SYNAPSE model [87]

Finally, the Ohio State University (OSU) Wexner Medical Center has also implemented a primary care medical home for autistic adults called the Center for Autism Services and Transition (CAST). The CAST model was designed in partnership with autistic adults and their caregivers with the aim to remove barriers to healthcare [88]. Autistic adults and transition-age autistic youth that utilized the CAST reported greater satisfaction in the delivery of healthcare services and patient–provider interactions, as well as higher utilization rates of preventive services than other autistic adults [88, 89].

Overall, medical homes are considered supportive primary care strategies for neurodivergent children and adults. However, there are significant barriers to implementing the model on a large scale, including office restructuring of payments, time, and workflows. While the UC-LEND, SYNAPSE, and CAST models represent promising models of care, more research is needed to demonstrate their scalability, cost-effectiveness, and public health benefits.

## Recommendations for Primary Care Providers

In recognition of the burgeoning neurodiversity movement—as well as the barriers that persist in integrating neurodiversity in healthcare—and building on these promising practices, we provide three actionable recommendations for primary care providers. These recommendations integrate lessons learned from research, practice, and education. In addition to recommendations, we provide corresponding resources and concrete ways for primary care providers to engage (Table 13.4). We view these recommendations as a starting point for physicians seeking to make immediate enhancements to their practice, but recognize that providing neurodiversity-oriented care is predicated on establishing long-standing, trusting relationships with patients and families.

We recommend that primary care providers and others serving neurodivergent populations:

1. **Support efforts that can increase the translation of research to practice.** In order to accomplish this, we recommend that providers engage with ongoing neurodiversity research initiatives and work toward forging researcher-clinician partnerships and collaborations.
2. **Support and expand neurodiversity training and education efforts for future physicians.** This includes supporting medical student-driven initiatives to bolster neurodiversity-focused training in medical schools, attending and contributing to medical education conferences and symposia, and interfacing with autistic physicians and advocacy groups. Neurodivergent people should be given opportunities to shape these education programs.
3. **Improve clinical care via enhancements to patient–provider interactions.** Physicians can utilize virtual healthcare provider toolkits that have been specifically designed for guiding physicians in making sure their interactions with neurodivergent patients are health-promoting. They can also better understand emerging care models that facilitate neurodiversity-oriented care. Across all of their work, physicians can engage with self-advocate and affiliate groups to gain additional knowledge and skills about providing neurodiversity-oriented care.

In the current chapter, we have highlighted resources that can assist physicians with the recommendations listed above. The AASPIRE Healthcare Toolkit (Tables 13.3 and 13.4) clearly defines actionable items that can be implemented immediately by physicians and an additionally helpful resource physicians can recommend to patients for support navigating primary care services.

**Table 13.4** Multi-sector recommendations and resources for healthcare providers

| Resources | Descriptions | Ways to engage |
|---|---|---|
| **Recommendation**: Increase translation of research to practice in order to provide evidence-based neurodiversity-oriented care | | |
| The Autism Intervention Research Network on Physical Health (AIR-P) | The AIR-P establishes and maintains an interdisciplinary, multicenter research network for scientific collaboration focused on autism and physical health, particularly for underserved and vulnerable populations | *Scholars Pilot and Feasibility Funding Program*<br>– Apply for funds to facilitate primary data collection or secondary data analysis<br>*Infrastructure for Collaborative Research* (forthcoming)<br>– Submit proposals for circulation to create multi-site research studies or conduct secondary data analysis<br>*Join the AIR-P Network*<br>– Join the AIR-P Network newsletter and stay up to date on opportunities to engage |
| International Society for Autism Research (INSAR) | INSAR is a scientific and professional organization devoted to advancing knowledge about autism by promoting high-quality research | *INSAR Community Collaborator Request (ICCR)*<br>Autism researchers can connect with "community collaborators" (i.e., autistic people and their family members/caregivers) who are interested in partnering with autism researchers in designing, conducting, and disseminating research studies relevant to autism<br>*Join a Committee*<br>Connect with others through multiple committees and special interest groups that focus on a variety of topics related to autism research |
| **Recommendation:** Support and expand neurodiversity training and education efforts for future physicians | | |
| Medical Students with Disability and Chronic Illness (MSDCI) | The MSDCI is a national organization committed to increasing disability inclusion and representation in healthcare | *Explore Guides and Resources*<br>Valuable resources and up to date information on disability care are compiled on the MSDCI website<br>*Encourage Students to Start a Chapter*<br>A toolkit is provided on how to start a chapter in order to ease the process and empower students |
| Disability Advocacy Coalition in Medicine (DAC Med) | DAC Med seeks to create a culture of disability inclusion in medicine at the Feinberg School of Medicine at Northwestern University | *Attend a Conference*<br>Network with other providers and students focused on addressing ableism in medical care |
| Autistic Doctors International (ADI) | ADI is a peer-support and advocacy group for medical doctors who identify as autistic, or on the autistic spectrum. It was founded in April 2019 with seven members and, to date, has over 500 members, with an associated group for autistic medical students. Over half the members are in the UK, with others from the United States, Canada, Australia, and Europe | *Attend a Group*<br>– ADI is true to their peer-support group origins and hosts free private support groups with no required participation |

(continued)

**Table 13.4** (continued)

| Resources | Descriptions | Ways to engage |
|---|---|---|
| **Recommendation:** Improve clinical care via enhancements to patient–provider interactions | | |
| Academic-Autistic Spectrum Partnership in Research and Education (AASPIRE) | AASPIRE is a leader in community-based participatory research and focuses on improving the lives of autistic adults. In addition, AASPIRE created a Healthcare Toolkit that is a phenomenal resource for both clinicians and autistic patients alike to improve primary care delivery | *Utilize Autism Healthcare Accommodations Tool (AHAT)*<br>Encourage patients to complete the AHAT for customized accommodations report they can give to their primary care providers with specifics on their individualized needs and preferences<br>*Engage with the Healthcare Providers Toolkit*<br>The toolkit includes information on autism diagnosis, considerations when caring for autistic patients, legal and ethical information, patient worksheets, and patient resources |
| Autistic Self-Advocacy Network (ASAN) | ASAN follows the principle of Nothing About Us, Without Us! Members have a common goal of advancing the disability rights movement, especially regarding autism. ASAN focuses heavily on impacting policy and actively advocating for change | *Engage with Action Alerts*<br>ASAN provides up to date information on federal and state legislation and action items to effectively advocate for disability rights<br>*Engage with Affiliate Groups*<br>Join a state or local ASAN affiliate disability advocacy group |

## Conclusions

The current chapter discusses the importance of integrating principles and lessons learned from the neurodiversity movement into primary care. We introduced the term "neurodiversity-oriented care," defined as a non-stigmatizing healthcare approach that accepts disability as difference rather than pathology and accommodates the varied needs and preferences of patients. Although there have been myriad barriers to successfully implementing neurodiversity-oriented care within primary care clinics, we look forward to the continued expansion and adoption of the promising practices we describe in this chapter. Based on these barriers and promising practices, we delineate a brief list of recommendations for primary care providers. While these recommendations are by no means exhaustive—and cannot fully address all of the barriers we have outlined in this chapter—we believe these recommendations can be a starting point for implementing long-term, sustainable, scalable change in primary care clinics.

We look forward to continuing to support healthcare providers in quality improvement, training, and other initiatives that will further enhance neurodiversity-oriented care. Our hope is that lessons learned from patients like Ari—as well as the continued developments in the field we cited in this chapter—will inspire many advances in neurodiversity-oriented healthcare during the years to come.

## Appendix

## References

1. Brown HM, Dwyer PSR, Gassner DL, Onaiwu MG, Kapp SK, Ne'eman A, et al. The Autism Intervention Research Network on Physical Health Autistic Researcher Review Board. Pediatrics. 2022;149(Suppl 4):e2020049437F.
2. Walker N, Raymaker DM. Toward a neuroqueer future: an interview with Nick Walker. Autism Adulthood. 2021;3(1):5–10.
3. Singer J. Neurodiversity: the birth of an idea. Lexington; 2017. 82 p.
4. Ne'eman A, Pellicano E. Neurodiversity as politics. Hum Dev. 2022;66(2):149–57.
5. Kapp SK, editor. Autistic community and the neurodiversity movement: stories from the front-

line [Internet]. Singapore: Springer Singapore; 2020 [cited 2022 Sep 30]. http://link.springer.com/10.1007/978-981-13-8437-0

6. Dwyer P. The neurodiversity approach(es): what are they and what do they mean for researchers? Hum Dev. 2022;66(2):73–92.
7. den Houting J. Neurodiversity: an insider's perspective. Autism. 2019;23(2):271–3.
8. Help protect Californians with developmental disabilities [Internet]. [cited 2022 Sep 30]. https://thinkingautismguide.com/2022/03/action-alert-help-protect-californians-with-developmental-disabilities.html
9. Bailin A. Clearing up some misconceptions about neurodiversity [Internet]. Scientific American Blog Network. [cited 2022 Sep 30]. https://blogs.scientificamerican.com/observations/clearing-up-some-misconceptions-about-neurodiversity/.
10. Chapman R. Neurodiversity studies: a new critical paradigm [Internet]. Routledge and CRC Press. [cited 2022 Sep 30]. https://www.routledge.com/Neurodiversity-Studies-A-New-Critical-Paradigm/Rosqvist-Chown-Stenning/p/book/9780367503253.
11. Neurodiversity FAQ [Internet]. Thinking person's guide to autism. [cited 2022 Sep 30]. https://thinkingautismguide.com/so-youre-doing-story-about.
12. Crompton CJ, Ropar D, Evans-Williams CV, Flynn EG, Fletcher-Watson S. Autistic peer-to-peer information transfer is highly effective. Autism. 2020;24(7):1704–12.
13. Edey R, Cook J, Brewer R, Johnson MH, Bird G, Press C. Interaction takes two: typical adults exhibit mind-blindness towards those with autism spectrum disorder. J Abnorm Psychol. 2016;125(7):879–85.
14. Sasson NJ, Faso DJ, Nugent J, Lovell S, Kennedy DP, Grossman RB. Neurotypical peers are less willing to interact with those with autism based on thin slice judgments. Sci Rep. 2017;7(1):40700.
15. Whelpley CE, May CP. Seeing is disliking: evidence of bias against individuals with autism spectrum disorder in traditional job interviews. J Autism Dev Disord [Internet]. 2022 [cited 2022 Sep 30]. https://link.springer.com/10.1007/s10803-022-05432-2.
16. Hotez E, Rosenau KA, Fernandes P, Eagan K, Shea L, Kuo AA. A national cross-sectional study of the characteristics, strengths, and challenges of college students with attention deficit hyperactivity disorder. Cureus [Internet]. 2022 [cited 2022 Sep 30]. https://www.cureus.com/articles/81766-a-national-cross-sectional-study-of-the-characteristics-strengths-and-challenges-of-college-students-with-attention-deficit-hyperactivity-disorder.
17. Lai MC, Kassee C, Besney R, Bonato S, Hull L, Mandy W, et al. Prevalence of co-occurring mental health diagnoses in the autism population: a systematic review and meta-analysis. Lancet Psychiatry. 2019;6(10):819–29.
18. Dwyer P, Ryan JG, Williams ZJ, Gassner DL. First do no harm: suggestions regarding respectful autism language. Pediatrics. 2022;149(Suppl 4):e2020049437N.
19. Felt AB, Mitcham D, Hathcock M, Swienton R, Harris C. Discrimination and bias in state triage protocols toward populations with intellectual disabilities during the COVID-19 pandemic. Disaster Med Public Health Prep. 2022;16(5):1772–4.
20. Richards CT, Crawley LM, Magnus D. Use of neurodevelopmental delay in pediatric solid organ transplant listing decisions: inconsistencies in standards across major pediatric transplant centers. Pediatr Transplant. 2009;13(7):843–50.
21. Morán ML, Hagiwara M, Raley SK, Alsaeed AH, Shogren KA, Qian X, et al. Self-determination of students with autism spectrum disorder: a systematic review. J Dev Phys Disabil. 2021;33(6):887–908.
22. Van Hees V, Roeyers H, De Mol J. Students with autism spectrum disorder and their parents in the transition into higher education: impact on dynamics in the parent–child relationship. J Autism Dev Disord. 2018;48(10):3296–310.
23. Autistic Self Advocacy Network. Empowering leadership: a systems change guide for autistic college students and those with other disabilities—Autistic Self Advocacy Network [Internet]. https://autisticadvocacy.org/. 2014 [cited 2022 Sep 30]. https://autisticadvocacy.org/resources/books/empowering-leadership-a-systems-change-guide-for-autistic-college-students-and-those-with-other-disabilities/.
24. Rosa SDR. The self-advocate/parent dialogues, day one: zoe [Internet]. Thinking person's guide to autism. 2011 [cited 2022 Sep 30]. https://thinkingautismguide.com/2011/09/self-advocateparent-dialogues-day-one.html.
25. A History of the Individuals With Disabilities Education Act [Internet]. Individuals with Disabilities Education Act. [cited 2022 Sep 30]. https://sites.ed.gov/idea/IDEA-History/.
26. Health insurance coverage of the total population [Internet]. KFF. 2020 [cited 2022 Sep 30]. https://www.kff.org/other/state-indicator/total-population/.
27. Moore W, Frye S. Review of HIPAA, part 1: history, protected health information, and privacy and security rules. J Nucl Med Technol. 2019;47(4):269–72.
28. Towle PO, Patrick PA, Ridgard T, Pham S, Marrus J. Is earlier better? The relationship between age when starting early intervention and outcomes for children with autism spectrum disorder: a selective review. Autism Res Treat. 2020;2020:7605876.
29. Anderson DK, Liang JW, Lord C. Predicting young adult outcome among more and less cognitively able individuals with autism spectrum disorders. J Child Psychol Psychiatr. 2014;55(5):485–94.
30. Roux AM, Shattuck PT, Rast JE, Rava JA, Edwards AD, Wei X, et al. Characteristics of two-year college students on the autism spectrum and their support services experiences. Autism Res Treat. 2015;2015:391693.
31. Morris ZA, McGarity SV, Goodman N, Zaidi A. The extra costs associated with living with a disability in the United States. J Disabil Policy Stud. 2021:104420732110435.

32. Lee KM, Arriola-Sanchez L, Lumeng JC, Gearhardt A, Tomiyama AJ. Weight stigma by association among parents of children with obesity: a randomized trial. Acad Pediatr. 2022;22(5):754–60.
33. Bellanca FF, Pote H. Children's attitudes towards ADHD, depression and learning disabilities: children's attitudes towards ADHD, depression and learning disabilities. J Res Spec Educ Needs. 2013;13(4):234–41.
34. Siperstein GN, Parker RC, Bardon JN, Widaman KF. A national study of youth attitudes toward the inclusion of students with intellectual disabilities. Except Child. 2007;73(4):435–55.
35. Christensen LL, Fraynt RJ, Neece CL, Baker BL. Bullying adolescents with intellectual disability. J Ment Health Res Intellect Disabil. 2012;5(1):49–65.
36. Pelleboer-Gunnink HA, Van Oorsouw WMWJ, Van Weeghel J, Embregts PJCM. Mainstream health professionals' stigmatising attitudes towards people with intellectual disabilities: a systematic review. J Intellect Disabil Res. 2017;61(5):411–34.
37. Nicolaidis C, Raymaker DM, McDonald KE, Baggs WAEV, Dern S, Kapp SK, et al. "Respect the way I need to communicate with you": healthcare experiences of adults on the autism spectrum. Autism. 2015;19(7):824–31.
38. Malik-Soni N, Shaker A, Luck H, Mullin AE, Wiley RE, Lewis MES, et al. Tackling healthcare access barriers for individuals with autism from diagnosis to adulthood. Pediatr Res. 2022;91(5):1028–35.
39. VanPuymbrouck L, Friedman C, Feldner H. Explicit and implicit disability attitudes of healthcare providers. Rehabil Psychol. 2020;65(2):101–12.
40. Como DH, Floríndez LI, Tran CF, Cermak SA, Duker LIS. Examining unconscious bias embedded in provider language regarding children with autism. Nurs Health Sci. 2020;22(2):197–204.
41. Bourne MJ, Smeltzer SC, Kelly MM. Healthcare inequities among adults with developmental disability: an integrative review with implications for nursing education. Nurse Educ Pract. 2021;57:103225.
42. Agaronnik N, Campbell EG, Ressalam J, Iezzoni LI. Communicating with patients with disability: perspectives of practicing physicians. J Gen Intern Med. 2019;34(7):1139–45.
43. Hull L, Petrides KV, Allison C, Smith P, Baron-Cohen S, Lai MC, et al. "Putting on my best normal": social camouflaging in adults with autism spectrum conditions. J Autism Dev Disord. 2017;47(8):2519–34.
44. Perry E, Mandy W, Hull L, Cage E. Understanding camouflaging as a response to autism-related stigma: a social identity theory approach. J Autism Dev Disord. 2022;52(2):800–10.
45. Cook J, Hull L, Crane L, Mandy W. Camouflaging in autism: a systematic review. Clin Psychol Rev. 2021;89:102080.
46. Ali A, Hassiotis A, Strydom A, King M. Self stigma in people with intellectual disabilities and courtesy stigma in family carers: a systematic review. Res Dev Disabil. 2012;33(6):2122–40.
47. Mason D, Ingham B, Urbanowicz A, Michael C, Birtles H, Woodbury-Smith M, et al. A systematic review of what barriers and facilitators prevent and enable physical healthcare services access for autistic adults. J Autism Dev Disord. 2019;49(8):3387–400.
48. Walsh C, Lydon S, O'Dowd E, O'Connor P. Barriers to healthcare for persons with autism: a systematic review of the literature and development of a taxonomy. Dev Neurorehabil. 2020;23(7):413–30.
49. Doherty M, Neilson S, O'Sullivan J, Carravallah L, Johnson M, Cullen W, et al. Barriers to healthcare and self-reported adverse outcomes for autistic adults: a cross-sectional study. BMJ Open. 2022;12(2):e056904.
50. Iezzoni LI, Rao SR, Ressalam J, Bolcic-Jankovic D, Agaronnik ND, Donelan K, et al. Physicians' perceptions of people with disability and their health care: study reports the results of a survey of physicians' perceptions of people with disability. Health Aff. 2021;40(2):297–306.
51. Ajuwon PM, Afolabi Lesi FE, Odukoya O, Melia C. Attitudes of medical students toward disabilities in Nigeria. Int J Disabil Hum Dev [Internet]. 2015 [cited 2022 Sep 30];14(2). https://www.degruyter.com/document/doi/10.1515/ijdhd-2014-0017/html.
52. Seidel E, Crowe S. The state of disability awareness in American medical schools. Am J Phys Med Rehabil. 2017;96(9):673–6.
53. Association of American Medical Colleges. Core competencies for entering medical students [Internet]. AAMC. [cited 2022 Sep 30]. https://www.aamc.org/services/admissions-lifecycle/competencies-entering-medical-students.
54. Amir N, Smith LD, Valentine AM, Mitra M, Parish SL, Moore Simas TA. Clinician perspectives on the need for training on caring for pregnant women with intellectual and developmental disabilities. Disabil Health J. 2022;15(2):101262.
55. Adirim Z, Sockalingam S, Thakur A. Post-graduate medical training in intellectual and developmental disabilities: a systematic review. Acad Psychiatry. 2021;45(3):371–81.
56. Kuhlthau KA, Delahaye J, Erickson-Warfield M, Shui A, Crossman M, van der Weerd E. Health care transition services for youth with autism spectrum disorders: perspectives of caregivers. Pediatrics. 2016;137(Suppl 2):S158–66.
57. The Oliver McGowan mandatory training in learning disability and autism [Internet]. Health Education England. 2020 [cited 2022 Sep 30]. https://www.hee.nhs.uk/our-work/learning-disability/current-projects/oliver-mcgowan-mandatory-training-learning-disability-autism.
58. Trollor JN, Ruffell B, Tracy J, Torr JJ, Durvasula S, Iacono T, et al. Intellectual disability health content within medical curriculum: an audit of what our future doctors are taught. BMC Med Educ. 2016;16(1):105.
59. Burge P, Ouellette-Kuntz H, Isaacs B, Lunsky Y. Medical students' views on training in intellectual

disabilities. Can Fam Physician. 2008;54(4):568–571.e6.
60. Crane JM, Strickler JG, Lash AT, Macerollo A, Prokup JA, Rich KA, et al. Getting comfortable with disability: the short- and long-term effects of a clinical encounter. Disabil Health J. 2021;14(2):100993.
61. Novak I. Evidence-based diagnosis, health care, and rehabilitation for children with cerebral palsy. J Child Neurol. 2014;29(8):1141–56.
62. Kattari SK, Lavery A, Hasche L. Applying a social model of disability across the life span. J Hum Behav Soc Environ. 2017;27(8):865–80.
63. Schendel D, Roux AM, McGhee Hassrick E, Lyall K, Shea L, Vivanti G, et al. Applying a public health approach to autism research: a framework for action. Autism Res. 2022;15(4):592–601.
64. Rodby-Bousquet E. The gap between current knowledge and clinical practice in childhood disability. Dev Med Child Neurol. 2018;60(10):969–70.
65. Mudrick NR, Breslin ML, Liang M, Yee S. Physical accessibility in primary health care settings: results from California on-site reviews. Disabil Health J. 2012;5(3):159–67.
66. Agaronnik N, Campbell EG, Ressalam J, Iezzoni LI. Accessibility of medical diagnostic equipment for patients with disability: observations from physicians. Arch Phys Med Rehabil. 2019;100(11):2032–8.
67. Valdez RS, Rogers CC, Claypool H, Trieshmann L, Frye O, Wellbeloved-Stone C, et al. Ensuring full participation of people with disabilities in an era of telehealth. J Am Med Inform Assoc. 2021;28(2):389–92.
68. What can physicians learn from the neurodiversity movement? J Ethics | American Medical Association [Internet]. [cited 2022 Sep 30]. https://journalofethics.ama-assn.org/article/what-can-physicians-learn-neurodiversity-movement/2012-06.
69. Finucane BM, Ledbetter DH, Vorstman JA. Diagnostic genetic testing for neurodevelopmental psychiatric disorders: closing the gap between recommendation and clinical implementation. Curr Opin Genet Dev. 2021;68:1–8.
70. Wald HS, McFarland J, Markovina I. Medical humanities in medical education and practice. Med Teach. 2019;41(5):492–6.
71. Feldman MA, Bosett J, Collet C, Burnham-Riosa P. Where are persons with intellectual disabilities in medical research? A survey of published clinical trials: where are persons with intellectual disabilities? J Intellect Disabil Res. 2014;58(9):800–9.
72. Nicolaidis C, Raymaker D, McDonald K, Kapp S, Weiner M, Ashkenazy E, et al. The development and evaluation of an online healthcare toolkit for autistic adults and their primary care providers. J Gen Intern Med. 2016;31(10):1180–9.
73. Hotez E, Hotez PJ, Rosenau KA, Kuo AA. Prioritizing COVID-19 vaccinations for individuals with intellectual and developmental disabilities. EClinicalMedicine. 2021;32:100749.
74. Ames JL, Massolo ML, Davignon MN, Qian Y, Croen LA. Healthcare service utilization and cost among transition-age youth with autism spectrum disorder and other special healthcare needs. Autism. 2021;25(3):705–18.
75. Moseley RL, Druce T, Turner-Cobb JM. 'When my autism broke': a qualitative study spotlighting autistic voices on menopause. Autism. 2020;24(6):1423–37.
76. Morris R, Greenblatt A, Saini M. Healthcare providers' experiences with autism: a scoping review. J Autism Dev Disord. 2019;49(6):2374–88.
77. Mazurek MO, Harkins C, Menezes M, Chan J, Parker RA, Kuhlthau K, et al. Primary care providers' perceived barriers and needs for support in caring for children with autism. J Pediatr. 2020;221:240–245.e1.
78. Unigwe S, Buckley C, Crane L, Kenny L, Remington A, Pellicano E. GPs' confidence in caring for their patients on the autism spectrum: an online self-report study. Br J Gen Pract. 2017;67(659):e445–52.
79. Israel BA, Coombe CM, Cheezum RR, Schulz AJ, McGranaghan RJ, Lichtenstein R, et al. Community-based participatory research: a capacity-building approach for policy advocacy aimed at eliminating health disparities. Am J Public Health. 2010;100(11):2094–102.
80. Nicolaidis C, Raymaker D, McDonald K, Dern S, Ashkenazy E, Boisclair C, et al. Collaboration strategies in nontraditional community-based participatory research partnerships: lessons from an academic–community partnership with autistic self-advocates. Prog Community Health Partnersh. 2011;5(2):143–50.
81. Thakur A, Pereira C, Hardy J, Bobbette N, Sockalingam S, Lunsky Y. Virtual education program to support providers caring for people with intellectual and developmental disabilities during the COVID-19 pandemic: rapid development and evaluation study. JMIR Ment Health. 2021;8(10):e28933.
82. Cheetham T. An E-toolkit for primary health care of adults. In: Rubin IL, Merrick J, Greydanus DE, Patel DR, editors. Health care for people with intellectual and developmental disabilities across the lifespan [internet]. Cham: Springer International Publishing; 2016 [cited 2022 Sep 30]. p. 1795–1799. http://link.springer.com/10.1007/978-3-319-18096-0_139.
83. Hahn JE. Addressing the need for education: curriculum development for nurses about intellectual and developmental disabilities. Nurs Clin N Am. 2003;38(2):185–204.
84. Gillespie-Lynch K, Bisson JB, Saade S, Obeid R, Kofner B, Harrison AJ, et al. If you want to develop an effective autism training, ask autistic students to help you. Autism. 2022;26(5):1082–94.
85. Medical home initiatives for children with special needs project advisory committee. The medical home. Pediatrics. 2002;110(1):184–6.
86. Akobirshoev I, Parish S, Mitra M, Dembo R. Impact of medical home on health care of children with and without special health care needs: update from the 2016 National Survey of Children's Health. Matern Child Health J. 2019;23(11):1500–7.
87. Kong X, Liu J, Chien T, Batalden M, Hirsh DA. A systematic network of autism primary care services

(SYNAPSE): a model of coproduction for the management of autism spectrum disorder. J Autism Dev Disord. 2020;50(5):1847–53.
88. Hand BN, Coury DL, White S, Darragh AR, Moffatt-Bruce S, Harris L, et al. Specialized primary care medical home: a positive impact on continuity of care among autistic adults. Autism. 2021;25(1):258–65.
89. Alain G, Gilmore D, Krantz M, Hanks C, Coury DL, Moffatt-Bruce S, et al. Expenditures and healthcare utilization of patients receiving care at a specialized primary care clinic designed with and for autistic adults. J Gen Intern Med. 2022;37(10):2413–9.

# Part V

# Mental Health and Substance Use

# 14 Managing Stress as an Emerging Adult

David B. Riddle, Alyssa Hertz, and Eric A. Storch

## Introduction

Emerging adulthood is a period within the cycle of development noted for its numerous milestones and life transitions [1]. Previously characterized as a brief transition, the pathway into adulthood is now longer and complicated by social and economic burdens; therefore, emerging adulthood constitutes a unique life stage [2, 3]. This developmental period provides opportunities for positive changes in one's life course but is often associated with heightened instability, stress, and increased risk for behavioral and mental health problems [4]. Emerging adulthood entails development of autonomy, exploring romantic relationships, establishing their own identity, living arrangements, and pursuing career or higher education opportunities [2, 5]. In the midst of these novel life experiences, young adults are more likely to encounter situations that require critical decision-making skills and judgment. The transitions that are representative during this stage of life can generate high levels of stress that can significantly impact physical and mental health [5], making this a critical juncture for this specific demographic to connect to psychological and psychiatric services.

Given the sensitive nature of the emerging adulthood stage, it is critical to understand the role of stress and its impact on individual functioning within this population. While not all emerging adults will face debilitating levels of stress, the transitions experienced during this stage can lead to increased levels of distress, which if not addressed appropriately, could jeopardize the overall well-being of emerging adults. Heightened levels of distress can lead to the onset of mental health-related concerns such as anxiety, mood disorders, substance use, eating disorders, and increases in suicidal ideation and behavior [6]. The increased onset of higher-leveled demands and variety of stressors, including major transitions such as living alone, entering the workforce, or pursuing higher education, as well as daily, novel events, all have the potential to create stressors that impact emerging adults' mental health and well-being.

Equally as important as understanding stress, awareness and connection to appropriate stress management is also vital to emerging adults. Stress management may present itself in the form of healthy coping mechanisms such as exercising, healthy dieting, establishing and maintaining positive social and romantic relationships, and engaging in enjoyable activities. However, when levels of experienced stress lead to impairing levels of distress, it may become difficult for emerging adults to connect with appropriate tools and supports for managing their stress.

D. B. Riddle (✉) · A. Hertz · E. A. Storch
Department of Psychiatry and Behavioral Sciences, Baylor College of Medicine, Houston, TX, USA
e-mail: david.riddle@bcm.edu; Alyssa.hertz@bcm.edu; eric.storch@bcm.edu


A. A. Kuo et al. (eds.), *Care of Adults with Chronic Childhood Conditions*,
https://doi.org/10.1007/978-3-031-54281-7_14

## Understanding Stress

Stress is a normal and inevitable experience in life and can have a significant impact on one's physical and mental health. Stress is defined as a person's response to their internal or external environment that they perceive to be threatening and/or exceed available resources [7]. Consequently, stress can have a negative impact on both one's physical and mental health. For example, physical health complications may include stroke, heart disease, peptic ulcers, and a weakened immune system. Stress has been shown to negatively impact both mental and physical health [8] and inappropriate or unhealthy coping responses to this stress has the potential to further impact emerging adults' overall well-being. Repeated exposure to stress has also been linked to an increase in psychiatric disorders such as depression, anxiety, substance use, eating disorders, and suicidal ideation [6, 7]. Compared to other age groups, emerging adults tend to experience excessive and heightened levels of stress [9].

## Emerging Adulthood and Mental Health

The onset of mental health-related concerns in emerging adults may be due to several psychological factors such as dramatic shifts in psychosocial development, uncertainty, and less parental supervision, as well as a series of biological changes [10–12]. Relatedly, emerging adulthood can be broken down into five distinct characteristics including identity explorations, instability, self-focus, feeling in-between, and possibilities and optimism [13]. Within each of these characteristics or experiences within emerging adulthood, there lies potential for negative impacts on an individual's mental health. For example, when exploring one's identity, there comes a sense of fulfillment; yet, this can also come with feelings of uncertainty, Similarly, emerging adulthood is a developmental phase that comes with a variety of transitions (e.g., changing places of residence, transitions in employment, relationships). The concept of being self-focused is characterized by a lessened demand of obligations to others, and an increased focus on more individualized roles and needs. However, in living a more self-focused life, emerging adults may be at greater risk for forgoing social relationships and demonstrating depressive symptoms [13].

Approximately 8.9 million emerging adults are diagnosed with a mental illness. Broken down further, 40% have at least one psychiatric disorder, with anxiety, mood, and substance use disorders as the most common [4, 13]. Unfortunately, emerging adults often underutilize mental health services for reasons such as lack of resources, social stigma, logistical barriers (e.g., time, health insurance, transportation), and cultural beliefs and norms [12]. Despite the barriers experienced during this stage of development, it is imperative to identify means for emerging adults to learn stress management strategies and to manage aversive and negative emotions.

## Anxiety Disorders

Anxiety disorders are rampant within the emerging adulthood population, with an estimated 22.3% having met diagnostic criteria [14]. The most commonly diagnosed include generalized anxiety disorder (GAD), panic disorder (PD), and agoraphobia [15]. Some of these anxiety-related disorders have been linked to emotional neglect during childhood and adolescents [16]. Given the nature of anxiety-related disorders and the additional stress factors that may exacerbate anxiety-related symptoms in emerging adults, connecting this population to effective resources is crucial. Seeking treatment for anxiety-related disorders in childhood is often facilitated by the presence of a caring and trusting adult (e.g., parent and/or guardian) but the concept of seeking out mental health resources transitions into the responsibility of the newly emerged adult.

## Mood Disorders

The onset of emerging adulthood also comes with a variety of experiences including establishing identity, exploring one's role within society, and navigating additional education experiences, and the job market. The introduction of these new stressors can negatively impact mood. Studies have shown that mood disorders, such as depression, are fairly prevalent within the emerging adulthood population [17]. Studies have also shown that depressive symptoms in emerging adults are influenced by relationships, supports, and communication styles experienced during adolescence, suggesting that risk factors during teenage years may impact trajectory of depressive symptoms into adulthood [18]. Experiencing depressive symptoms as well as establishing appropriate coping mechanisms can prove difficult, especially for individuals who are exploring the concept of independence or unfamiliar with mental health services.

## Substance Use Disorders

The onset of substance use concerns and disorders occurs during adolescence, when teenagers begin to experiment with drugs and other substances. An in-depth review found that among the emerging adult population, males are more likely to experience substance use and substance use concerns than their female peers, and White young adults are more likely to develop substance use concerns related to alcohol [19]. Emerging adults also have a variety of risk factors that increase their chances of substance use disorders including socioeconomic status, parent education, family substance use history, and neighborhood instability [19]. This phase of increased use and experimentation with various substances includes significant increases in cigarette smoking, binge-drinking, and illicit drug use, and these increases in experimentation have been associated with increases in responsibilities, work life, and personal and romantic relationships [20].

## Eating Disorders

Eating disorders are debilitating psychiatric disorders that are characterized by disturbances in eating behavior and distorted views of one's own body [21]. The most commonly diagnosed eating disorders include anorexia nervosa (AN), bulimia nervosa (BN), and binge eating disorder (BED), with onset typically occurring during emerging adulthood [22]. Emerging adulthood, as previously stated, is a period that consists of a variety of life changes including development of role identity, exploring personal and professional relationships, and embracing higher levels of responsibility. While these factors may prove exciting for many individuals, they may also prove to be contributing variables that result in increased levels of stress for others. The stressful components of navigating emerging adulthood have some correlation to the trajectory and onset of eating disorders within this population [21] and evidence suggests that eating disorders may impact psychosocial functioning in later stages of adulthood [23].

## Suicidal Ideation

Suicide rates in the United States have drastically increased over the past decade, and is currently the tenth leading cause of death overall and second leading cause of death for individuals between the ages of 10 and 34 [24]. A recent study examined the effects of support on suicidal ideation in emerging adults and found that increased levels of familial support were associated with decreased levels of suicidal ideation [25]. Similarly, studies have shown that concerns related to self-efficacy, poor coping skills, and substance use are correlating factors for higher levels of suicidal ideation [26]. Considering the additional stressors of emerging adulthood, it would appear that in addition to seeking appropriate treatments for depressive symptoms, suicidal ideation, and self-harming behaviors, emerging adults would greatly benefit from establishing healthy coping skills, connecting to positive and supportive social groups, and maintaining any positive connections with family members and loved ones.

## Common Stressors

### Emerging Adulthood and Career Development

Deciding on a career path is one most important developmental task during emerging adulthood as it impacts well-being, self-esteem, and life satisfaction [27]. Emerging adults put time and effort into educational and/or training opportunities that will aid in optimal and desired career paths. Based on one's interests, skills, and competencies, the number of career opportunities is endless. In fact, it is not common for many individuals to undergo several changes in their career trajectories before choosing a stable career. Emerging adults who are more autonomous, aspire to maximize potential, and have higher levels of self-acceptance are more likely to transition into their career with greater ease [28]. Moreover, those reporting higher levels of psychological well-being display greater confidence when making career decisions [28, 29]. However, for some, the transition into the working world may be overwhelming and daunting as they navigate this new identity.

Entering into the modern-day workforce has become increasingly competitive as the job market continuously restructures itself and educational and training demands increase [30, 31]. Compared to previous generations where the transition into a career was more direct, emerging adults experience greater uncertainty and instability in their career choices, which can result in distress and concerns about one's future. It is also suggested challenges faced during this transition may be due to lack of preparedness and differing expectations. Emerging adults are expected to shift from one role to another with little to no preparation. For those who do secure employment, significant stressors such as less structure and feedback from colleagues and/or supervisors and difficulties establishing interpersonal relationships, often lead to dissatisfaction in their professional lives [32]. This may lead to "jumping around" to explore newer opportunities and delaying a full-time, secure career before 30 [33]. Consequently, career-related stressors are likely to contribute to the onset and maintenance of mental health disorders such as depression and burnout [34].

### Emerging Adulthood and Romantic Relationships

Interest in romantic relationships typically begins during adolescents and is characterized by intense expressions of affection and initiation of sexual encounters. As relationships progress into emerging adulthood, these relationships transition into companionship, love, and security, with emerging adults beginning to consider long-term commitment [35]. The development and maintenance of intimate relationships during emerging adulthood can lead to positive developmental outcomes such as higher self-esteem, greater quality of life, enhanced self-concept, and experience of positive emotions. Moreover, romantic relationships can foster in the formation of one's identity and promote higher psychological well-being [35]. In contrast to older cohorts, relationship patterns during emerging adulthood have shifted. Perhaps one of the most defining differences is delaying the pursuit of relationships or marriage [36].

Emerging adults are faced with a unique challenge of trying to balance many of life's demands outside of relationships (i.e., school, work), which may contribute to heightened levels of stress. Oftentimes, emerging adults lack adequate resources and therefore are faced with a dilemma of prioritizing relationships or other individual goals. When caught in this predicament, emerging adults have a tendency to pursue their personal goals before committing to a romantic relationship [36]. As a result, relationships within this age range are better characterized by involvement in several romantic, sexual encounters, and cohabitation that requires less commitment, which may lead to more frequent breakups [37]. Some studies found 46–82% of emerging adults reported a significant source of stress evolves from involvement in relationships [38]. Most notable is the negative impact daily minor external stressors have on the relationship. Research has found that increased stressors are strongly associated with decreased relationship satisfaction [39]. For example, work stressors (i.e., long hours, energy demands, conflicts) may interfere with one's ability to spend time with their partner and/or exacerbate arguments, which at times has been associated with domestic violence [33, 36].

## Emerging Adulthood and Social Relationships

Friendships play a critical role in helping to shape one's identity and psychological adjustment during transitional periods [38]. However, due to heightened instability and frequent transitions, friendships can also become a source of stress [40]. Perhaps one of the greatest stressors faced regarding friendships is the initiation, maintenance, and termination of friendships. For example, the transition from high school to college or switching jobs can lead to psychosocial and emotional stressors as friendships may naturally begin to fade. Individuals are likely to report feelings of loneliness, depression, and low self-esteem and they attempt to navigate new social groups [41]. Additionally, emerging adults often engage in comparison making to inform decision-making. This can lead to elevated stress levels if individuals are or perceive themselves as failing to achieve similar or desired milestones (e.g., career, marriage, moving out). Conversely, emerging adults who experience more stressors in their daily lives are more likely to disengage from social interactions which may contribute to poorer peer relationships [42]. Stress is also correlated with mental health disorders, such as depression and anxiety, which may exacerbate anti-social behaviors such as displaying less positive affect and participating less in conversation [43].

## Emerging Adults and Living Transitions

Achieving independence and leaving the parental home is a major milestone in emerging adulthood. Leaving the parental home can be perceived as exciting and hopeful, yet, others may evaluate the transition as unsettling and anxiety-provoking [44]. Stress accompanying living transitions can be categorized into non-normative/unexpected changes (i.e., moving back home with parents) and failing to make a transition that is normative for the respective age group (i.e., still living at home). After living independently, emerging adults view moving back home as unacceptable and/or as a failure to achieve appropriate milestones toward total independence. This transition may also be assumed to be related to problems in other domains of the individuals' life (e.g., work, relationship) [45]. For emerging adults who continue to live with their parents, stress is often linked to upward comparisons with similar aged peers. Those still living at home believe they are not progressing in normative developmental milestones [45]. Moreover, emerging adults living with their parents face the struggle of transforming the adult–child relationship into one that is mutual. Most emerging adults feel stuck in a "child" role which can constrain independence and trigger conflict [44]. For those who successfully leave the home, homesickness has been often cited as a common stressor among emerging adults. Homesickness is characterized by distress associated with anticipating or actually leaving the home. Often, emerging adults living on their own for the first time lack appropriate resources and coping skills which may exacerbate stress levels [46]. In some instances, homesickness has been linked to depressive and/or anxiety symptoms that can lead to marked impairment [47].

## Gender and Stress

The transition into adulthood is undoubtedly a stressful experience which can be influenced by one's gender [4]. Epidemiological research has supported men and women to react differently with stress, with women reporting higher levels of psychological distress and perceiving stressors to be more chronic and threatening [48]. Furthermore, the sources of stress differ among genders. Women have reported interpersonal and romantic relationships [49] contribute most to their stress whereas men identified financial and career-related situations as their greatest source of stress [50]. In addition to reacting to stress differently, researchers have also argued that men and women utilize different coping strategies to manage stress [51]. Women are more likely to seek out social supports whereas as men express an acute stress response to immediately react to a perceived threat or to run away from the threatening stimuli [52].

Gender role stress, characterized by difficulties in meeting societal imposed roles [53], may also contribute significantly to stress in emerging adults. This is particularly seen in females who are faced with additional pressures when making life decisions [45]. For example, women seeking out higher levels of education in pursuit of less-traditional career paths (e.g., doctor) may be seen as disrupting societal norms [54] which may play significant stress on women when deciding career paths. Additionally, women who decide to delay marriage and having children while engaging in self-exploration are perceived as selfish [55]. Although men and women experience stress during emerging adulthood, research supports gender differences in the experience of stress.

## Culture and Stress

Emerging adulthood is a time period in which the transition from adolescence to adulthood is prolonged; however, this is not a universal phenomenon. The transition into adulthood and adoption of responsibilities is subjective based on one's cultural affiliation [56]. Industrialized or postindustrial countries, which tend to adopt Westernized values, have deemed independence as a determining factor of achieving adulthood [57]. Countries such as the United States, Canada, and Germany are more likely to pursue higher levels of education and postpone marriage in pursuit of personal goals which allow for further exploration [58]. Conversely, collectivist cultures, such as China and India, place greater emphasis on marriage, responsibility, and financially supporting parents which leads to a brief transition from adolescence into adulthood [56]. Within these individualistic cultures, the construct of emerging adulthood is further influenced by minority culture practices. For example, within the United States, minority groups that emphasize commitment to family typically have a shortened or absent emerging adulthood period [56, 58].

Additional factors such as education, social class, and geographical location also impact transition into adulthood. Educational opportunities can be limited by external factors such as finances and early parenthood. These restricted opportunities are often found in minority rather than in the majority culture and therefore these individuals may have a shortened or absent exploration period [58]. Research has also called into question whether emerging adulthood exists across socioeconomic status [59]. It is argued that adolescents belonging to upper middle class and the middle class can be afforded with financial flexibility to explore educational, occupation, and personal interests before taking on the responsibilities of adulthood [59]. Alternatively, adolescents from lower socioeconomic backgrounds are perceived to have less opportunity for self-exploration [60, 61]. Lastly, in developing countries, residing in urban compared to rural areas has influenced emerging adulthood [58]. Individuals living in rural areas were more likely to focus on marriage and financially supporting family compared to their urban counterparts [62].

## Skills for Managing Stressors

Understanding how to cope with stressors is a vital component to navigating emerging adulthood. Using a variety of healthy coping skills such as proper sleep hygiene, maintaining a healthy diet, establishing work–life balance, and fostering positive relationships with friends, family, and romantic interests, can help emerging adults cope with the transitions they experience as well as stressors they may face. There are additional skills that have been proven to be effective for managing stress, that are accessible and do not require prolonged involvement from a trained professional, such as deep breathing, progressive muscle relaxation (PMR), and guided imagery [63]. Additionally, connecting with other trusted others, including emerging adult peers and establishing healthy and positive social relationships, can present as a protective factor against potential distress and mental health-related concerns. However, there are times when emerging adults may experience levels of distress that lead to additional mental health concerns that require them to connect to higher levels of care, such as psychotherapy.

## Sleep Hygiene

Sleep is a biological process that is crucial for physical and mental health functioning [64]. However, it is estimated that approximately 70 million Americans suffer from a sleep disorder [65] which can directly impact stress levels. Insufficient sleep activates the autonomic nervous system and the HPA-axis, which are the body's two main stress systems [66]. Sleep hygiene is behavioral and environmental changes that are designed to promote sleep quantity and quality [67]. Sleep hygiene includes psychoeducation about sleep, maintaining a regular sleep and wake routine, in addition to avoiding/reducing caffeine, nicotine, and alcohol intake before bed, minimizing daytime naps, and using the bed for activities outside of sleep and sex [68]. Getting quality sleep promotes the ability to tolerate and manage fluctuating stress levels [69]. Moreover, it can be hypothesized incorporating sleep hygiene practices into one's daily routine enhances self-regulatory energy, which aids in managing stressors [70]. Therefore, adopting and practicing appropriate sleep hygiene can be a valuable stress management technique.

## Healthy Diet

Stress can serve as a catalyst for unhealthy eating patterns. When faced with actual or perceived stressors, the body craves "comfort foods," which are foods that have higher fat and sugar content [71]. Although comfort foods boost serotonin levels and induce feelings of comfort, adopting a healthy and balanced nutritional diet can positively impact stress levels.

## Social Support

Supportive friendships are pivotal during emerging adulthood due to numerous and rapid transitions that occur. As emerging adults begin to explore their identity and rely less on parents/caregivers, friendship begins to fulfill that "parental" role by providing support, companionship, security, validation, and advice regarding important decisions. Positive friendships are associated with a plethora of physical and mental health benefits, increased life satisfaction, and positive affect [72]. Furthermore, these positive relationships foster prosocial behaviors that help to enhance and deepen social networks [73]. Studies have found that positive social support fosters resilience to manage daily and chronic stressors. Moreover, resilient individuals are more likely to use active coping skills (e.g., problem solving, seeking support) when under stress [74]. Conversely, few or negative social supports have been linked to increased heart rate and blood pressure, which play a major role in elevated stress levels. It may be theorized that social support may act as a buffer against the physiological repercussions of stress. In sum, having healthy and positive social supports aid in the use of effective coping skills which protect against stress.

## Progressive-Muscle Relaxation

Muscle tension is a reflexive response to stress. When endured for long period of time, muscle tension can trigger and maintain stress-related disorders [75]. Progressive-muscle relaxation (PMR) is a mindfulness-based intervention that involves intentionally tensing and relaxing all of the body's muscle groups, from head to toe. Individuals are instructed to tense specific muscles for 5–7 followed by a 20–30 s period of relaxing the muscle [76]. PMR teaches individuals to differentiate between states of tensions versus relaxation. Research has supported the use of PMR as an inexpensive and effective way to manage stress [77]. Furthermore, PMR has been associated with reductions in negative affect as seen in depression and anxiety disorders [78]. Aside from tension relief, PMR allows for disengagement from one's own thoughts and stressors and ability to focus on relaxing the body's muscles [79]. Overall, PMR is an effective stress management tool as it aids in the reduction of physiological indicators of stress (e.g., cortisol) and may help to regulate homeostasis in the body [79].

## Diaphragmatic Breathing

Diaphragmatic breathing or "deep breathing" [80] is an intervention that has been demonstrated to be effective in managing stress levels [81]. When an individual is under stress, a new breathing pattern emerges, which consists of small and shallow breaths that stems from the chest and shoulders. Inadvertently, this type of breathing exacerbates stress [82]. Diaphragmatic breathing involves intentionally focusing on the inhalation and exhalation of one's breath. This technique involves expanding the lungs into the diaphragm, which allows the individual to slow breathing and decrease respiratory rate [83]. Researchers have argued that breathing techniques help to improve negative affect [84] and mental health diagnoses such as PTSD and major depressive disorder [85].

## Guided Imagery

Guided imagery is another effective strategy that has been documented to manage stress [86]. Guided imagery is a focused meditation technique that guides the individual to imagine a relaxing, comfortable, and safe place [87]. It typically begins by instructing the individual to engage in diaphragmatic breathing which helps to release tension in the body. Following, the individual then begins to visualize a pleasant image or scene [86]. Guided imagery is often conducted via audio or video recording or by the provider [88]. Researchers purport guided imagery aids in the management of stress by distracting the individual from the intrusive thoughts that are eliciting negative affect [89]. Furthermore, studies have found guided imagery is effective in reducing cortisol levels and releasing endorphins (hormones that help the nervous system manage stress) [87]. Guided imagery allows individuals to conjure up pleasurable imagery within their minds that can have a profound impact on stress levels [86].

## Cognitive Behavioral Therapy

Cognitive behavioral therapy (CBT) is an evidence-based psychotherapeutic treatment that targets and changes maladaptive thinking and behavioral patterns that negatively impact emotions [90]. CBT for stress management includes providing psychoeducation about stress in addition to various techniques. The main intervention utilized is cognitive restructuring which entails replacing destructive thoughts with more adaptive ones and restructuring of behavioral patterns that further influence negative emotions [91]. CBT proposes that unhelpful thoughts trigger negative affect, which can deplete an individuals' ability to effectively manage stressors. Therefore, it is hypothesized that challenging faulty thinking patterns will promote the ability to manage stressors [92]. CBT as an approach to therapy has been proven to have both short-term and long-term effects, with studies indicating that individuals who saw reduction in symptoms continued to do so, even after one-year posttreatment [93]. Additional strategies include time-management and/or problem-solving skills, developing and establishing a daily routine, communication skills, and relaxation strategies (e.g., diaphragmatic breathing, PMR, guided imagery) and these techniques have been proven to help alleviate distressing and repetitive negative thinking patterns [94].

## Barriers and Facilitators to Stress Management

Emerging adults have mixed experiences with engaging in the workforce. Many individuals are unemployed, work low-wage jobs, or are in pursuit of higher education, all of which impact their access to health insurance plans and sufficient income to cover the cost of mental health services [95, 96]. Although there are current efforts to improve access to effective and appropriate mental healthcare services, financial strain and burden still prove a critical barrier to engaging in psychotherapy. Similarly, a lack of education and understanding of mental health and relevant services serves as an additional barrier to connecting with appropriate mental healthcare. In addition to the more logistical barriers to receiving appropriate services for stress management, there still exists a stigma around mental health disorders, lack of awareness of available resources, and fear of negative consequences on career trajectory [97].

Although emerging adulthood in and of itself can be a challenging time for individuals, especially those who experience heightened states of stress, there are facilitators to accessing treatment and support. Studies have demonstrated that connecting with a mentor or caring and trusting adult may be a key factor in helping emerging adults navigate this stage of life [98]. Additionally, connecting emerging adults to resources such as housing, career preparation, vocational training, and independent-living skills can also promote overall positive well-being. The utilization of a mentor and/or appropriate resources may help emerging adults navigate their newfound responsibilities, the workforce, and societal expectations that come with this developmental stage [99]. Exploring these methods of resources and identifying other potential facilitators to stress management may help emerging adults journey through the various changes that occur during the transition from adolescence into adulthood. While there are many stressors that come with emerging adulthood, some of these experiences can be exciting as they signal growth and opportunity.

## Conclusion

The transition from adolescence into emerging adulthood consists of a variety of changes and new experiences. Within this developmental stage, individuals begin to solidify their identity both internally and within their communities. Emerging adulthood is a stage that consists of a multitude of opportunities including pursuing career interests, seeking post-secondary education, developing and strengthening familial and kindred relationships, as well as pursuing romantic interests. However, this is also a time in which individuals may experience a variety of stressors as a result of their newfound independence, increased responsibilities, and shifts in relationships. Stress, when compounded and untreated, can result in detrimental outcomes to one's mental and physical health. There are a variety of methods for coping with stress that are both evidence-based and accessible for this population. Utilizing tools such as diaphragmatic breathing and progressive muscle relaxation may help to alleviate stress in vivo, whereas building healthy habits such as diet, exercise, and engaging in positive social support may provide more preventative measures. However, emerging adulthood presents several barriers to connecting with appropriate services and coping skills, including financial burdens, lack of education, and stigma around mental health-related services. Yet, there is hope for this population as the field of psychology begins to better understand and explore emerging adulthood as a concept. Connecting emerging adults to appropriate resources and individuals who can serve as mentors may help alleviate some of their experienced stressors in order to better navigate their journey into adulthood.

## References


1. Rosemond MM, Owens D. Exploring career development in emerging adult collegians. Education. 2018;138(4):337–51.
2. Côté JE. The dangerous myth of emerging adulthood: an evidence-based critique of a flawed developmental theory. Appl Dev Sci. 2014;18(4):177–88.
3. Wood D, Crapnell T, Lau L, Bennett A, Lotstein D, Ferris M, Kuo A. Emerging adulthood as a critical stage in the life course. In: Halfon N, Forrest C, Lerner R, Faustman E, editors. Handbook of life course health development. Cham: Springer; 2018. p. 2018.
4. Matud M, Díaz A, Bethencourt J, Ibáñez I. Stress and psychological distress in emerging adulthood: a gender analysis. J Clin Med. 2020;9(9):2859.
5. Nelson LJ. The theory of emerging adulthood 20 years later: a look at where it has taken us, what we know now, and where we need to go. Emerg Adulthood. 2021;9(3):179–88.
6. Larzelere MM, Jones GN. Stress and health. Prim Care. 2008;35(4):839–56.
7. Asberg KK, Bowers C, Renk K, McKinney C. A structural equation modeling approach to the study of stress and psychological adjustment in emerging adults. Child Psychiatry Hum Dev. 2008;39:481–501.
8. Howland M, Armeli S, Feinn R, Tennen H. Daily emotional stress reactivity in emerging adulthood: temporal stability and its predictors. Anxiety Stress Coping. 2017;30(2):121–32.
9. Deckro GR, Ballinger KM, Hoyt M, Wilcher M, Dusek J, Myers P, et al. The evaluation of a mind/body intervention to reduce psychological distress and perceived stress in college students. J Am Coll Health. 2002;50(6):281–7.
10. Fuhrmann D, Knoll LJ, Blakemore SJ. Adolescence as a sensitive period of brain development. Trends Cogn Sci. 2015;19(10):558–66.
11. Johnson SB, Blum RW, Giedd JN. Adolescent maturity and the brain: the promise and pitfalls of neuroscience research in adolescent health policy. J Adolesc Health. 2009;45(3):216–21.
12. Smriti D, Ambulkar S, Meng Q, Kaimal G, Ramotar K, Park SY, et al. Creative arts therapies for the mental health of emerging adults: a systematic review. Arts Psychother. 2022;77:101861.
13. Arnett JJ. Does emerging adulthood theory apply across social classes? National Data on a persistent question. Emerg Adulthood. 2016;4(4):227–35.
14. Cougle JR, Keough ME, Riccardi CJ, Sachs-Ericsson N. Anxiety disorders and suicidality in the National Comorbidity Survey-Replication. J Psychiatr Res. 2009;43(9):825–9.
15. Kranzler A, Elkins RM, Albano AM. Anxiety in emerging adulthood: a developmentally informed treatment model. In: Pediatric anxiety disorders [Internet]. Elsevier; 2019 [cited 2022 Oct 16]. p. 499–519. http://www.scopus.com/inward/record.url?scp=85081309535&partnerID=8YFLogxK.
16. Schimmenti A, Bifulco A. Linking lack of care in childhood to anxiety disorders in emerging adulthood: the role of attachment styles. Child Adolesc Mental Health. 2015;20:41–8.
17. Key substance use and mental health indicators in the United States: results from the 2020 National Survey on Drug Use and Health. 2020;156.
18. Finan LJ, Ohannessian CM, Gordon MS. Trajectories of depressive symptoms from adolescence to emerging adulthood: the influence of parents, peers, and siblings. Dev Psychol. 2018;54(8):1555.
19. Stone AL, Becker LG, Huber AM, Catalano RF. Review of risk and protective factors of substance use and problem use in emerging adulthood. Addict Behav. 2012;37(7):747–75.
20. Wood D, Crapnell T, Lau L, Bennett A, Lotstein D, Ferris M, Kuo A. Emerging adulthood as a critical stage in the life course. In: Handbook of life course health development. 2018. pp. 123–143.
21. Potterton R, Richards K, Allen K, Schmidt U. Eating disorders during emerging adulthood: a systematic scoping review. Front Psychol. 2020;10:3062.
22. Micali N, Hagberg KW, Petersen I, Treasure JL. The incidence of eating disorders in the UK in 2000–2009: findings from the general practice research database. BMJ Open. 2013;3(5):e002646.
23. Mason TB, Heron KE. Do depressive symptoms explain associations between binge eating symptoms and later psychosocial adjustment in young adulthood? Eat Behav. 2016;23:126–30.
24. Heron M. National vital statistics reports. Natl Vital Stat Rep. 2018;67(6).
25. Olatunji OA, Idemudia ES, Olawa BD. Family support, self-efficacy and suicidal ideation at emerging adulthood: a mediation analysis. Int J Adolesc Youth. 2020;25(1):920–31.
26. Gonzalez VM. Factors linking suicidal ideation with drinking to cope and alcohol problems in emerging adult college drinkers. Exp Clin Psychopharmacol. 2019;27(2):166.
27. Hlado'o P, Juhanak L, Hlouskova L, Lazarova B. Exploring the roles of career adaptability, self-esteem, and work values in life satisfaction among emerging adults during their career transition. Emerg Adulthood. 2022;10(1):135–48.
28. Viola MM, Musso P, Inguglia C, Coco AL. Psychological well-being and career indecision in emerging adulthood: the moderating role of hardiness. Career Dev Q. 2016;64(4):387–96.
29. Zhou M, Xu Y. University students' career choice and emotional well-being: its relation to work personality, vocational identity, and career thoughts. J Psychol. 2013;142:21–35.
30. Krahn HJ, Howard AL, Galambos NL. Exploring or floundering? The meaning of employment and educational fluctuations in emerging adulthood. Youth Soc. 2015;47(2):245–66.

31. Kwok CYN. Managing uncertainty in the career development of emerging adults: implications for undergraduate students. Aust J Career Dev. 2018;26(3):137–49.
32. Creed PA, Hughes T. Career development strategies as moderators between career compromise and career outcomes in emerging adults. J Career Dev. 2012;40(2):146–63.
33. Seiffge-Krenke I, Luyckx K. Competent in work and love? Emerging adults' trajectories in dealing with work-partnership conflicts and links to health functioning. Emerg Adulthood. 2014;2(1):48–58.
34. Baker TB, McFall RM, Shoham V. Current status and future prospects of clinical psychology: toward a scientifically principled approach to mental and behavioral health care. Psychol Sci Public Interest. 2008;9(2):67–103.
35. Gomez-Lopez M, Viedjo C, Ortega-Ruiz R. Well-being and romantic relationships: a systematic review in adolescence and emerging adulthood. Environ Res Public Health. 2019;16(13):2415.
36. Watkins NK, Beckmeyer JJ. Assessing young adults' beliefs regarding the importance of romantic relationships. J Fam Issues. 2020;41(2):158–82.
37. Fisher H. 2006. The drive to love: the neural mechanism for mate selection.
38. Chow CM, Ruhl H. Friendships and romantic stressors and depression in emerging adulthood: mediating and moderating roles of attachment representations. J Adult Dev. 2014;21(2):106–15.
39. Karney BR, Neff LA. Couples and stress: how demands outside a relationship affect intimacy within the relationship. 2013
40. Lapierre S, Poulin F. Friendship instability and depressive symptoms in emerging adulthood. J Am Coll Health. 2022;70(5):1306–10.
41. Paul EL, Brier S. Friend sickness in the transition to college: precollege predictors and college adjustment correlates. J Couns Dev. 2001;79(1):77–89.
42. Dissing AS, Jørgensen TB, Gerds TA, Rod NH, Lund R. High perceived stress and social interaction behaviour among young adults. A study based on objective measures of face-to-face and smartphone interactions. PLoS One. 2019;14(7):e0218429.
43. Kupferberg A, Bicks L, Hasler G. Social functioning in major depressive disorder. Neurosci Biobehav Rev. 2016;69:313–32.
44. Kins E, De Mol J, Beyers W. "Why should I leave?" Belgian emerging adults' departure from home. J Adolesc Res. 2014;29(1):89–119.
45. Bell S, Lee C. Transitions in emerging adulthood and stress among young Australian women. Int J Behav Med. 2008;15(4):280–8.
46. Stroebe M, Van Vliet T, Hewstone M, Willis H. Homesickness among students in two cultures: antecedents and consequences. Br J Psychol. 2002;93(2):147–68.
47. Thurber CA, Walton EA. Homesickness and adjustment in university students. J Am Coll Heal. 2012;60(5):415–9.
48. Lopez-Madrigal C, de la Fuente J, Garcia-Manglano I, Martinez-Vicente JM, Peralta-Sanchez FJ, Amate-Romera J. The role of gender and age in the emotional well-being outcomes of young adults. Int J Environ Res Public Health. 2020;18:1–20.
49. Hankin BL, Mermelstein R, Roesch L. Sex differences in adolescent depression: stress exposure and reactivity models. Child Dev. 2007;78(1):279–95.
50. Kneavel M. Relationship between gender, stress, and quality of social support. Psychol Rep. 2021;124(4):1481–501.
51. Anbumalar C, Agines D, Jaswanti VP, Priya D, Reniangelin D. Gender differences in perceived stress levels and coping strategies among college students. Int J Indian Psychol. 2017;4:22–33.
52. Taylor SE, Klein LC, Lewis BP, Gruenewald TL, Gurung RA, Updegraff JA. Biobehavioral responses to stress in females: tend-and-befriend, not fight-or-flight. Psychol Rev. 2000;107(3):411.
53. Kazmiercazk M. The feminine and masculine gender role stress—conclusions from polish studies. Pol Psychol Bull. 2010;41:20–30.
54. Yoder JD, Schleicher TL. Undergraduates regard deviation from occupational gender stereotypes as costly for women. Sex Roles. 1996;34(3):171–88.
55. Lampman C, Dowling-Guyer S. Attitudes toward voluntary and involuntary childlessness. Basic Appl Soc Psychol. 1995;17(1–2):213–22.
56. Nelson L, Badger S, Wu B. The influence of culture in emerging adulthood: perspectives of Chinese college students. Int J Behav Dev. 2004;28(1):26–36.
57. Arnett JJ. Conceptions of the transition to adulthood among emerging adults in American ethnic groups. New Dir Child Adolesc Dev. 2003;100:63–76.
58. Arnett JJ. Emerging adulthood: a theory of development from the late teens through the twenties. Am Psychol. 2000;55(5):469.
59. Arnett JJ. College students as emerging adults: the developmental implications of the college context. Emerg Adulthood. 2016;4(3):219–22.
60. Furstenberg FF. On a new schedule: transitions to adulthood and family change. Future Child. 2010;20:67–87.
61. Silva JM. Coming up short: working class adulthood in an age of uncertainty. New York: Oxford University Press; 2013.
62. Cheah CSL, Trinder KM, Gokavi TN. Urban/rural and gender differences among Canadian emerging adults. Int J Behav Dev. 2010;34:339–44.
63. Varvogli L, Darviri C. Stress management techniques: evidence-based procedures that reduce stress and promote health. Health Sci J. 2011;5(2):74.
64. Altena E, Baglioni C, Espie CA, Ellis J, Gavriloff D, Holzinger B, Schlarb A, Frase L, Jernelov S, Riemann D. Dealing with sleep problems during home confinement due to the covid-19 outbreak: practical recommendations from a task force of the European CBT-I academy. J Sleep Res. 2020;29:e13052.
65. Institute of Medicine, Committee on Sleep Medicine and Research, Board on Health Sciences Policy. Sleep

disorders and sleep deprivation: an unmet public health problem. Washington: National Academies Press; 2006.
66. McEwan BS, Karatsoreos IN. Sleep deprivation and circadian disruption: stress, allostasis, and allostatic load. Sleep Med Clin. 2015;10:1–10.
67. Irish LA, Kline CE, Gunn HE, Buysse DJ, Hall MH. The role of sleep hygiene in promoting public health: a review of empirical evidence. Sleep Med Rev. 2015;22:23–36.
68. Brick CA, Seely DL, Palermo TM. Associations between sleep hygiene and sleep quality in medical students. Behav Sleep Med. 2010;8:113–21.
69. Anderson C. The impact of sleep on dealing with daily stressors—a need for controlled laboratory evidence. Commentary on Barber, Munz, Bagsby & Powell (2009) 'Sleep consistency and sufficiency: are both necessary for less psychological strain?'. Stress Health. 2010;26(3):194–7.
70. Hamilton NA, Catley D, Karlson C. Sleep and the affective response to stress and pain. Health Psychol. 2007;2007(26):288–95.
71. Gonzalez MJ, Miranda-Massari JR. Diet and stress. Psychiatr Clin N Am. 2016;2016(37):579–89.
72. Padilla-Walker LM, Memmott-Elison MK, Nelson LJ. Positive relationships as an indicator of flourishing during emerging adulthood. Faculty Publications; 2017. pp. 4717.
73. Miething A, Almquist YB, Östberg V, Rostila M, Edling C, Rydgren J. Friendship networks and psychological well-being from late adolescence to young adulthood: a gender-specific structural equation modeling approach. BMC Psychol. 2016;4(1):1–11.
74. Ozbay F, Johnson DC, Dimoulas E, Morgan CA III, Charney D, Southwick S. Social support and resilience to stress: from neurobiology to clinical practice. Psychiatry (Edgmont). 2007;4(5):35.
75. American Psychiatric Association. Diagnostic and statistical manual of mental disorders, 5th ed. 2013.
76. Jacobson E. Progressive relaxation. Chicago: Chicago University Press; 1939.
77. Sundram BM, Dahlui M, Chinna K. Effectiveness of progressive muscle relaxation therapy as a worksite health promotion program in the automobile assembly line. Ind Health. 2016;54:204–14.
78. Gangadharan P, Madani AH. Effectiveness of progressive muscle relaxation techniques on depression, anxiety and stress among undergraduate nursing students. Int J Health Sci Res. 2018;8:155–63.
79. Dolbier CL, Rush TE. Efficacy of abbreviated progressive muscle relaxation in a high-stress college sample. Int J Stress Manag. 2012;19:48–68.
80. Forman JW, Myers D. The personal stress reduction program. Hoboken: Prentice Hall; 1987.
81. Hopper SI, Murray SL, Ferrara LR, Singleton JK. Effectiveness of diaphragmatic breathing for reducing physiological and psychological stress in adults: a quantitative systematic review. JBI Database System Rev Implement Rep. 2019;17(9):1855–76.
82. Consolo K, Fusner S, Staib S. Effects of diaphragmatic breathing on stress levels of nursing students. Teach Learn Nurs. 2008;3:67–71.
83. Toussaint L, Nguyen QA, Roettger C, Dixon K, Offenbächer M, Kohls N, et al. Effectiveness of progressive muscle relaxation, deep breathing, and guided imagery in promoting psychological and physiological states of relaxation. Evid Based Complement Alternat Med. 2021;2021:5924040.
84. Stromberg SE, Russell ME, Carlson CR. Diaphragmatic breathing and its effectiveness for the management of motion sickness. Aerospace Med Hum Perform. 2015;86:452–7.
85. Descilo T, Vedamurtachar A, Gerbarg PL, Nagaraja D, Gangadhar BN, Adelson B, Braslow LH, Marcus S, Brown RP. Effects of a yoga breath intervention alone and in combination with an exposure therapy for post-traumatic stress disorder and depression in survivors of the 2004 south-east Asia tsunami. Acta Psychiatr Scand. 2010;121:289–300.
86. Hart J. Guided imagery. Alternat Compliment Ther. 2008;14:295–9.
87. Bigham E, McDannel L, Luciano I, Salgado-Lopez G. Effects of a brief guided imagery on stress. Biofeedback. 2014;42:28–35.
88. Felix MMDS, Ferreira MBG, da Cruz LF, Barbosa MH. Relaxation therapy with guided imagery for postoperative pain management: an integrative review. Pain Manag Nurs. 2019;20:3–9.
89. Norelli SK, Long A, Krepps JM. Relaxation techniques. In: StatPearls. StatPearls Publishing; 2021.
90. Hofmann SG, Asnaani A, Vonk IJ, Sawyer AT, Fang A. The efficacy of cognitive behavioral therapy: a review of the meta-analysis. Cogn Ther Res. 2012;36:427–40.
91. Crum J. Understanding mental health and cognitive restructuring with ecological neuroscience. Front Psychiatry. 2021;12:697095.
92. Nakao M, Shirotsuki K, Sugaya N. Cognitive-behavioral therapy for management of mental health and stress-related disorders: recent advances in techniques and technologies. Biopsychosoc Med. 2021;15:16.
93. DiMauro J, Domingues J, Fernandez G, Tolin DF. Long-term effectiveness of CBT for anxiety disorders in an adult outpatient clinic sample: a follow-up study. Behav Res Ther. 2013;51(2):82–6.
94. Feldman G, Greeson J, Senville J. Differential effects of mindful breathing, progressive muscle relaxation, and loving-kindness meditation on decentering and negative reactions to repetitive thoughts. Behav Res Ther. 2010;48(10):1002–11.
95. Cadigan JM, Lee CM, Larimer ME. Young adult mental health: a prospective examination of service utilization, perceived unmet service needs, attitudes, and barriers to service use. Prev Sci. 2019;20(3):366–76.
96. Substance Abuse and Mental Health Services Administration (SAMSHA). Results from the 2013

National Survey on Drug Use and Health: Mental Health Findings. Rockville: 2013 National Survey on Drug Use and Health: mental health findings; 2014. NSDUH series H-49, HHS Publication No. (SMA). 14-4887.

97. Eisenberg D, Hunt J, Speer N, Zivin K. Mental health service utilization among college students in the United States. J Nerv Ment Dis. 2011;199(5):301–8.
98. Gilmer TP, Ojeda VD, Leich J, Heller R, Garcia P, Palinkas LA. Assessing needs for mental health and other services among transition-age youths, parents, and providers. Psychiatr Serv. 2012;63(4):338–42.
99. Schulenberg JE, Sameroff AJ, Cicchetti D. The transition to adulthood as a critical juncture in the course of psychopathology and mental health. Dev Psychopathol. 2004;16(4):799–806.

# 15 Adverse Childhood Events and Trauma-Informed Care

Karinne Van Groningen, Denise M. Nunez, and Candace Gragnani

## Introduction

Adverse childhood events (ACEs) are potentially traumatic events that are experienced by individuals before the age of 18 years. Examples of ACEs include experiencing violence, abuse, or neglect, witnessing violence in the home and/or community, and having a family member attempt or die by suicide [1]. The link between ACEs and long-term health outcomes was first established by the landmark CDC-Kaiser ACE study, published in the American Journal of Preventive Medicine in 1998 [2]. The study was conducted at Kaiser Permanent, a not-for-profit health maintenance organization (HMO) that currently operates in nine states and the District of Colombia, from 1995 to 1997. During the initial phase of the study, over 9000 Southern California Kaiser patients completed a standard questionnaire about childhood abuse and exposure and forms of household dysfunction after completing a standardized medical evaluation. The study questionnaire included three categories of abuse (psychological, physical, or sexual abuse) and household dysfunction during childhood (exposure to substance abuse, mental illness, violent treatment of mother or stepmother, and criminal behavior in the household). Respondents consisted mainly of White individuals, those over the age of 50 years, those considered middle/upper class, and those who at least attended some college or more. More than half of respondents reported at least one ACE and one-fourth reported experiencing two or more ACEs. Further, a graded relationship between the number of ACEs and adult health risk behaviors and diseases was observed. Individuals who had experienced four or more ACEs, as compared to those without any ACE, had a 4–12-fold increased risk for alcoholism, drug abuse, depression, and suicide attempts. Similarly, the number of ACEs an individual had experienced showed a graded relationship with the presence of adult diseases, including ischemic heart disease, cancer, and chronic lung disease. The second phase of the study, with over 17,000 participants, revealed additional links between ACEs and poor adult health outcomes, finding that 69.9% of participants had experienced at least one ACE [3].

K. Van Groningen (✉)
Division of Preventive Medicine, Department of Medicine, University of California, Los Angeles, Los Angeles, CA, USA

D. M. Nunez
Department of Medicine, University of California, Los Angeles, Los Angeles, CA, USA
e-mail: dmnunez@mednet.ucla.edu

C. Gragnani
Division of Internal Medicine-Pediatrics, General Internal Medicine and Health Services Research, Department of Medicine, UCLA, Los Angeles, CA, USA
e-mail: CGragnani@mednet.ucla.edu


A. A. Kuo et al. (eds.), *Care of Adults with Chronic Childhood Conditions*,
https://doi.org/10.1007/978-3-031-54281-7_15

After the landmark CDC-Kaiser ACE study, researchers expanded the definition of ACEs and assessed their impact on a myriad of adult health conditions. In the Philadelphia ACE Project, researchers expanded ACEs to include exposure to bullying, community violence, neighborhood safety, racism, and living in foster care to further assess for the impact of adverse experiences occurring outside of the home as well as study ACEs in a more racially diverse urban setting [4]. Using this expanded definition, the Philadelphia Urban ACE Survey found that 83.2% of respondents reported exposure to at least one ACE and notably, respondents reported higher exposure levels to Conventional ACEs than participants in the original CDC-Kaiser study with majority White participants, highlighting the disproportionate levels of adversity experienced by minority and lower-income populations. Lastly, numerous other studies have accumulated additional long-term negative sequalae associated with ACEs, including mental health conditions in adulthood such as anxiety, depression, antisocial personality, and substance dependence [5–8].

The profound impact of ACEs on lifelong health, opportunity, and overall well-being has influenced numerous policy guidelines. The American Academy of Pediatrics (AAP) released a policy statement calling for the prevention of childhood toxic stress, which is an extended activation of the stress response and result of ACEs [9, 10]. Additionally, the role of ACEs was central to the 2014 Substance Abuse Mental Health Services Administration (SAMHSA) treatment improvement protocol on trauma-informed care in behavioral health [11].

In recent years, surveillance of ACEs has become an important public health practice, both for assessing the burden of ACEs within our society and for encouraging the use of trauma-informed care practices. At both the national and state levels, ACEs screenings and trauma-informed care practices have become priorities to addressing longstanding health inequities. This chapter will review the pathophysiologic link between ACEs and adult health risks and conditions, ACEs screenings in practice and general considerations, trauma-informed care practices, and ongoing public health efforts to screen for ACEs and prevent their negative health sequalae (Fig. 15.1).

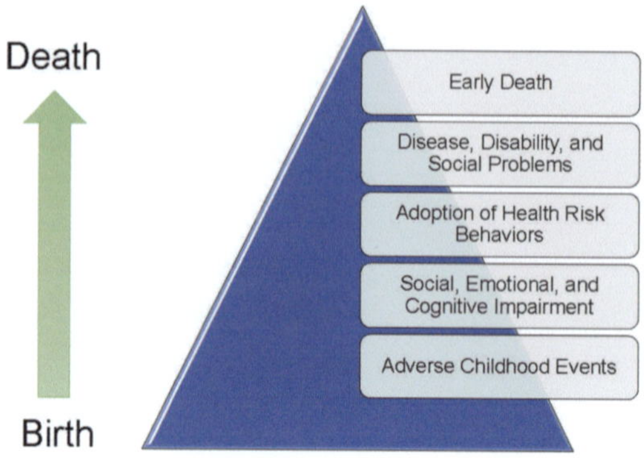


**Fig. 15.1** The ACE pyramid (Derived from CDC-Kaiser study). Link https://www.cdc.gov/violenceprevention/aces/about.html. [1]

## The Toxic Stress Response

The pathophysiologic mechanism linking ACEs to adult health risks and conditions is the toxic stress response—the extreme, frequent, or extended activation of the stress response without the support of an adult [10]. To date, extensive evidence suggests that early adversity catalyzes a myriad of biological pathways that alter the functioning of the brain, neuroendocrine stress response, and immune functioning, both independently and collectively. Preventing the toxic stress response occurs not at the molecular level, but rather at the level of social interaction and public health.

Fetuses, infants, and children are particularly at risk for the effects of toxic stress due to their rapid development and neural plasticity. Plasticity can be thought of as an intricate process where the brain responds to changes in the environment [12]. Early childhood is a critical period during which environmental changes have a disproportionately significant impact on development when compared to environmental changes that occur later in life [13].

In addition to brain plasticity, ACEs and subsequent toxic stress can alter the response of the neuroendocrine-immune (NEI) network. The NEI network plays a critical function in physical, cognitive, and socioemotional development by responding to stressful situations [10]. For example, when a child experiences stress, their level of cortisol rises, triggering the sympathetic nervous system's fight-or-flight response. When repeated stressful events occur, a child experiences chronically elevated levels of cortisol. This suppresses immune system functioning and alters inflammatory responses [14, 15]. Moreover, chronic elevations in cortisol are associated with hypertension, insulin resistance, obesity, type 2 diabetes, and cardiovascular disease [16, 17].

Empirical evidence has shown the broad impact of ACEs on the NEI network. Children exposed to risk factors for toxic stress including poverty, community violence, and a caregiver with a mental health disorder are more likely to develop and have more severe asthma, a condition with a known inflammatory/stress component [18–20]. In addition, a study examining the impact of early life stress on adult inflammation followed infants from birth to the age of 32 years and found that maltreated children showed a significant and graded increased risk for clinically relevant C-reactive protein levels in adulthood [21]. The effect of childhood maltreatment on adult inflammation was found to be independent of stress in adulthood and adult health and adult behaviors, highlighting the life-long health impacts of traumatic events in childhood.

Despite the profound negative effects of toxic stress, there is evidence to show that a stable and supportive caregiver environment can change toxic stress to "tolerable stress" and alter long-term health risks and outcomes [10, 22, 23]. Thus, with the evidence that changing a child's environment can mitigate toxic stress and its sequalae, the AAP has called for pediatric providers to "complement the early identification of developmental concerns with a greater focus on those interventions and community investments that reduce external threats to healthy brain growth [9]." Becoming aware of the effects of toxic stress is just the first step in mitigating its long-term effects. By advocating for policy that prevents the risk factors for toxic stress, we can promote lifelong health and improved well-being.

## ACEs Screening

In the landmark CDC-Kaiser ACE study, researchers asked adult patients to retrospectively report on experiences occurring prior to 19 years of age [2]. The screening tool used in the second wave ("wave II") of the original study measured 10 ACE categories comprising three overall domains: (1) Child abuse (physical, emotional, and sexual abuse), (2) Neglect (physical and emotional), and (3) Household challenges (mental illness in the household, substance abuse in the household, divorce/separation, parental incarceration, and mother treated violently) [3]. This wave II tool contained 28 questions, 10 requiring a dichotomous "yes/no" response, and 18 questions requiring responses using a 5-point Likert-type rating scale rating frequency from "never" to "very often."

After the original CDC-Kaiser ACE study, additional ACE screening tools were developed with various modifications. Holden et al. in 2019 found 20 different versions [24]. The CDC currently uses an 11-item screening tool for the Behavioral Risk Factor Surveillance Survey (BRFSS) [25]. While the original ACE screening tool and the BRFSS are used for adults, other tools are intended for pediatric populations, such as the 9-item screening tool called the National Survey of Children's Health-Adverse Childhood Experiences (NSCH-ACEs) [26]. The NSCH-ACEs leaves out questions about child abuse and neglect, however like the original CDC-Kaiser tool, includes questions about financial hardship, loss of a biological parent, household mental illness, substance abuse, and domestic violence. Further, the NSCH-ACEs expands into additional areas including racial discrimination and neighborhood violence.

In California, ACEs Aware, a statewide initiative to screen for ACEs, has a variety of tools for different patient populations including a pediatric screen for parents of children 0–11 years old, a pediatric screen for parents of adolescents 12–19 years old, a self-report tool for adolescents 12–19 years old, and an adult self-report tool.

Screening for ACEs does not reveal underlying health conditions, but rather identifies risk factors, i.e., having experienced child abuse or neglect, which are associated with increased risks of health problems [27]. As such, interventions aimed at targeting ACEs focus on social resources such as food and housing support and behavioral health services. Moreover, by understanding a patient's individual life experiences and trauma, providers can better practice evidence-based trauma-specific treatment approaches. Important considerations when screening for ACEs include: (1) Choosing which patient population to screen, (2) Ensuring that medical providers who conduct screens are educated on trauma-informed care practices, and (3) If a patient screens positive, there are evidence-based resources to provide.

There are varied opinions on whether ACEs screenings are appropriate. Opposers of screening argue that the process re-surfaces trauma and can, in fact, be harmful for patients. Further, clinics with patients who screen positive may not have sufficient resources to provide, thus surfacing trauma without providing needed intervention. Moreover, screenings may not be accurate as individuals are unlikely to truthfully disclose intimate and traumatic facts about their life. Alternatively, supporters of ACEs screenings note that by identifying patients' lived experiences, we can better provide individualized trauma-informed care. Further, a positive ACE screen can lead to connection to resources to address ongoing events such as behavioral health needs and/or food or housing insecurity. Nevertheless, ACEs screenings should be implemented thoughtfully and in clinics with appropriate resources to provide services to patients who screen positive. Clinics should also ensure that patients are not repeatedly screened—if a patient is screened in a primary care office, their results should be shared with social work and case management to eliminate repeat screenings in different settings (Fig. 15.2).

## Pediatric ACEs and Related Life Events Screener (PEARLS)

CHILD - To be completed by: **Caregiver**

At any point in time since your child was born, has your child seen or been present when the following experiences happened? Please include past and present experiences.

*Please note, some questions have more than one part separated by "OR." If any part of the question is answered "Yes," then the answer to the entire question is "Yes."*

**PART 1:**

1. Has your child ever lived with a parent/caregiver who went to jail/prison?
2. Do you think your child ever felt unsupported, unloved and/or unprotected?
3. Has your child ever lived with a parent/caregiver who had mental health issues? *(for example, depression, schizophrenia, bipolar disorder, PTSD, or an anxiety disorder)*
4. Has a parent/caregiver ever insulted, humiliated, or put down your child?
5. Has the child's biological parent or any caregiver ever had, or currently has a problem with too much alcohol, street drugs or prescription medications use?
6. Has your child ever lacked appropriate care by any caregiver? *(for example, not being protected from unsafe situations, or not cared for when sick or injured even when the resources were available)*
7. Has your child ever seen or heard a parent/caregiver being screamed at, sworn at, insulted or humiliated by another adult?

   Or has your child ever seen or heard a parent/caregiver being slapped, kicked, punched beaten up or hurt with a weapon?
8. Has any adult in the household often or very often pushed, grabbed, slapped or thrown something at your child?

   Or has any adult in the household ever hit your child so hard that your child had marks or was injured?

   Or has any adult in the household ever threatened your child or acted in a way that made your child afraid that they might be hurt?
9. Has your child ever experienced sexual abuse? *(for example, anyone touched your child or asked your child to touch that person in a way that was unwanted, or made your child feel uncomfortable, or anyone ever attempted or actually had oral, anal, or vaginal sex with your child)*
10. Have there ever been significant changes in the relationship status of the child's caregiver(s)? *(for example, a parent/caregiver got a divorce or separated, or a romantic partner moved in or out)*

CENTER for YOUTH WELLNESS | UCSF Benioff Children's Hospital Oakland

**Add up the "yes" answers for this first section:** ☐

*Please continue to the other side for the rest of questionnaire* →

This tool was created in partnership with UCSF School of Medicine.

Child (Parent/Caregiver Report) – Deidentified

**Fig. 15.2** ACEs aware screening tool for children ages 0–11. Link to include image (screener tool Part 1 and Part 2) to provide an example: https://www.acesaware.org/wp-content/uploads/2019/12/PEARLS-Tool-Child-Parent-Caregiver-Report-De-Identified-English.pdf. [2]

**PART 2:**

1. Has your child ever seen, heard, or been a victim of violence in your neighborhood, community or school?
*(for example, targeted bullying, assault or other violent actions, war or terrorism)*
2. Has your child experienced discrimination?
*(for example, being hassled or made to feel inferior or excluded because of their race, ethnicity, gender identity, sexual orientation, religion, learning differences, or disabilities)*
3. Has your child ever had problems with housing?
*(for example, being homeless, not having a stable place to live, moved more than two times in a six-month period, faced eviction or foreclosure, or had to live with multiple families or family members)*
4. Have you ever worried that your child did not have enough food to eat or that the food for your child would run out before you could buy more?
5. Has your child ever been separated from their parent or caregiver due to foster care, or immigration?
6. Has your child ever lived with a parent/caregiver who had a serious physical illness or disability?
7. Has your child ever lived with a parent or caregiver who died?

**Add up the "yes" answers for the second section:** ☐

CENTER for YOUTH WELLNESS | UCSF Benioff Children's Hospital Oakland

This tool was created in partnership with UCSF School of Medicine.

Child (Parent/Caregiver Report) – Deidentified

**Fig. 15.2** (continued)

## Trauma-Informed Care

Traumatic events can lead to long-term physical and emotional effects. In medicine, patients' past trauma may influence their relationship with the healthcare system and limit preventive care service utilization. Recently, trauma-informed care (TIC) practices have been used to create a patient-centered care delivery approach.

According to SAMHSA, trauma is defined as the "result of an event, series of events, or set of circumstances that is experienced by an individual as physically or emotionally harmful or life threatening and that has lasting adverse effects on the individual's functioning and mental, physical, social, emotional, or spiritual well-being [11]." Moreover, TIC is the delivery of healthcare services that includes an understanding of trauma and an awareness of how trauma can affect patient perceptions of the healthcare system [11]. TIC can be viewed in two main domains: universal trauma precautions and trauma-specific care [28].

Universal trauma precautions are simple changes healthcare providers can make when interacting with all patients. While it is not possible for providers to let patients take control of their entire visit, at the start of visits, providers can have patients list their goals for the appointment. In addition, providers can give choices to patients during the visit and specifically, the physical exam. For example, a provider may say, "I need to examine your heart and lungs, which would you like for me to examine fist?" This level of collaboration during the visit can allow patients to feel more in-control, something trauma survivors generally lack in medical settings [29]. Alternatively, trauma-specific care is employed when providers know that a patient has experienced a traumatic event. Thus, in addition to universal trauma precautions, a provider may be increasingly sensitive during parts of the visit, for example during a genitourinary exam on a survivor of sexual violence.

TIC employs patient-centered principles that have been shown to increase patient retention and engagement [30]. TIC has been widely accepted in fields such as addiction and mental health, child protection, and the penal system [31]. However, these principles can be incredibly effective in setting such as primary care, which is the first point of contact for many patients as they enter and navigate the healthcare system. Utilizing TIC practices can help patients feel they are in a safe place, feel empowered, and promote further engagement in their health.

## ACEs Screening in Practice: CDC BRFSS and California ACEs Aware

Numerous public health campaigns are exploring the prevalence of ACEs within our society and striving for methods by which to prevent toxic stress and improve health. The CDC employs the Behavioral Risk Factor Surveillance Survey (BRFSS), which is an annual, state-based, random-digital-dial telephone survey that collects data from non-institutionalized U.S. adults (18 yo and older) regarding health risk factors and conditions [32]. The BRFSS started in 2009 and has included, for at least 1 year, 48 states plus the District of Columbia. ACE questions are categorized into two categories: abuse and household challenges, with each category divided into multiple subcategories. Neglect items were added to the survey in 2019. Data from 2011 to 2014 included 214,157 individuals, which were 51.5% female, 68.1% White, 8.4% Black, and 15.6% Latinx [33]. The total number of individuals who experienced 1, 2, 3, and 4 or more ACEs was 23.5%, 13.4%, 8.8%, and 15.8%, respectively [33]. The prevalence of ACEs seen within the BRFSS is similar to what was observed in the original CDC-Kaiser ACE study, where almost two-thirds of surveyed adults reported at least one ACE and approximately one in four reported three or more ACEs. Moreover, ACEs were present across all populations; however, certain populations were more vulnerable to experiencing ACEs due to socioeconomic and racial factors.

In December 2019, California launched ACEs Aware, a first-in-the-nation effort to screen patients for ACEs [34]. The effort was led by California's first ever surgeon general and pediatrician, Dr. Nadine Burke Harris, an advocate for eliminating toxic stress and ACE exposure. ACEs Aware provides a variety of free online trainings for healthcare providers who conduct ACEs screenings [35]. As part of the initiative, California provides coverage for ACEs screenings for Medi-Cal patients and in 2021, significantly expanded coverage via state Senate Bill (SB) 428, the ACEs Equity Act, which requires all health insurance plan contracts that provide coverage for pediatric services and preventive care to include coverage for ACE screening. Between January 2020 and June 2021, 781,400 Medi-Cal providers conducted ACE screenings [36]. Of the 651,200 unique Medi-Cal beneficiaries screened for ACEs, 6% had an ACE score of 4 or more [36]. Further, of the healthcare providers who completed ACEs Aware training, two-thirds reported they planned to implement changes in their practice and 40% planned to change their management approach based on the patient's ACE score and toxic stress risk assessment [36].

At both the national and state levels, ACEs screening data highlights the profound prevalence of ACEs and toxic stress within our society. On the individual patient levels, ACEs screenings can help clinical teams provide more equitable, effective, and trauma-informed healthcare by individualizing care based on a patient's unique lived experiences.

## Summary and Future Considerations

The original CDC-Kaiser ACE study, published in 1998, established the dose–response relationship between ACE exposure and adult health risk behaviors and diseases. In subsequent years, scientific and empirical evidence linked ACE exposure to poor health outcomes via the toxic stress response. Toxic stress chronically turns on the sympathetic nervous system, elevating cortisol levels and driving the fight-or-flight response. This in turn impacts an individual's life-long health. Reassuringly, with interventions aimed at ACE exposure, toxic stress and long-term health sequalae can be mitigated.

ACE exposure is assessed via ACEs screenings, with numerous ongoing initiatives being led at the national, state, and community levels. Current population-based ACE screenings continue to show high levels of ACE exposure first witnessed in the original CDC-Kaiser ACE study, highlighting the chronic and profound levels of trauma within our society, particularly for racial minorities and socioeconomically marginalized populations. Moreover, understanding the level of ACE exposure within populations can promote trauma-informed care practices, which employs patient-centered principles that have been shown to increase patient retention and engagement.

The science of ACEs has led to numerous public health initiatives, most notably the CDC's BRFSS and California's ACEs Aware program. These policy initiatives are part of a greater shift within our healthcare system to focus on prevention and acknowledgement of the myriad of social factors and environments that affect health. Future initiatives and studies should be aimed at assessing the healthcare outcomes of individuals and communities when ACE exposures are addressed. Lastly, ACEs and TIC practices should be integrated into early medical education to further influence the next generation of healthcare professionals to tackle the social, root-causes of health and longstanding health inequities within our society.

## References


1. About the CDC-Kaiser ACE Study |Violence Prevention | Injury Center | CDC [Internet]. 2022. https://www.cdc.gov/violenceprevention/aces/about.html. Accessed 2 Oct 2022.
2. Felitti VJ, Anda RF, Nordenberg D, Williamson DF, Spitz AM, Edwards V, et al. Relationship of childhood abuse and household dysfunction to many of the leading causes of death in adults. The adverse childhood experiences (ACE) study. Am J Prev Med. 1998;14(4):245–58.
3. Dube SR, Williamson DF, Thompson T, Felitti VJ, Anda RF. Assessing the reliability of retrospective reports of adverse childhood experiences among adult HMO members attending a primary care clinic. Child Abuse Negl. 2004;28(7):729–37.
4. Cronholm PF, Forke CM, Wade R, Bair-Merritt MH, Davis M, Harkins-Schwarz M, et al. Adverse child-

hood experiences: expanding the concept of adversity. Am J Prev Med. 2015;49(3):354–61.
5. Afifi TO, Enns MW, Cox BJ, Asmundson GJG, Stein MB, Sareen J. Population attributable fractions of psychiatric disorders and suicide ideation and attempts associated with adverse childhood experiences. Am J Public Health. 2008;98(5):946–52.
6. Edwards VJ, Holden GW, Felitti VJ, Anda RF. Relationship between multiple forms of childhood maltreatment and adult mental health in community respondents: results from the adverse childhood experiences study. Am J Psychiatry. 2003;160(8):1453–60.
7. Unpacking the impact of adverse childhood experiences on adult mental health—PMC [Internet]. https://www.ncbi.nlm.nih.gov/pmc/articles/PMC6007802/. Accessed 2 Oct 2022.
8. Shonkoff JP, Garner AS, Committee on Psychosocial Aspects of Child and Family Health, Committee on Early Childhood, Adoption, and Dependent Care, Section on Developmental and Behavioral Pediatrics. The lifelong effects of early childhood adversity and toxic stress. Pediatrics. 2012;129(1):e232–46.
9. Garner AS, Shonkoff JP. Committee on psychosocial aspects of child and family health, committee on early childhood, adoption, and dependent care, section on developmental and behavioral pediatrics. Early childhood adversity, toxic stress, and the role of the pediatrician: translating developmental science into lifelong health. Pediatrics. 2012;129(1):e224–31.
10. TIP 57: Trauma-Informed Care in Behavioral Health Services | SAMHSA Publications and Digital Products [Internet]. https://store.samhsa.gov/product/TIP-57-Trauma-Informed-Care-in-Behavioral-Health-Services/SMA14-4816. Accessed 2 Oct 2022.
11. Substance Abuse and Mental Health Services Administration. Tip 57: trauma-informed care practices in behavioral health services. 2015.
12. Nelson CA. Neural plasticity and human development. Curr Dir Psychol Sci. 1999;8(2):42–5. https://doi.org/10.1111/1467-8721.00010.
13. Fox NA, Rutter M. Introduction to the special section on the effects of early experience on development. Child Dev. 2010;81(1):23–7.
14. Webster JI, Tonelli L, Sternberg EM. Neuroendocrine regulation of immunity. Annu Rev Immunol. 2002;20:125–63.
15. Tonelli L, Webster JI, Rapp KL, Sternberg E. Neuroendocrine responses regulating susceptibility and resistance to autoimmune/inflammatory disease in inbred rat strains. Immunol Rev. 2001;184:203–11.
16. Björntorp P, Rosmond R. The metabolic syndrome—a neuroendocrine disorder? Br J Nutr. 2000;83(Suppl 1):S49–57.
17. Hotamisligil GS. Inflammation and metabolic disorders. Nature. 2006;444(7121):860–7.
18. Chen E, Fisher EB, Bacharier LB, Strunk RC. Socioeconomic status, stress, and immune markers in adolescents with asthma. Psychosom Med. 2003;65(6):984–92.
19. Chen E, Chim LS, Strunk RC, Miller GE. The role of the social environment in children and adolescents with asthma. Am J Respir Crit Care Med. 2007;176(7):644–9.
20. Morillo-Vanegas D, Sanchez-Salcedo P, Sebastián Ariño AF. Relationship between pediatric asthma and psychosocial status of caregivers. Respir Med. 2020;174:106187.
21. Danese A, Pariante CM, Caspi A, Taylor A, Poulton R. Childhood maltreatment predicts adult inflammation in a life-course study. Proc Natl Acad Sci USA. 2007;104(4):1319–24.
22. Fisher PA, Stoolmiller M, Gunnar MR, Burraston BO. Effects of a therapeutic intervention for foster preschoolers on diurnal cortisol activity. Psychoneuroendocrinology. 2007;32(8–10):892–905.
23. Miller GE, Lachman ME, Chen E, Gruenewald TL, Karlamangla AS, Seeman TE. Pathways to resilience: maternal nurturance as a buffer against the effects of childhood poverty on metabolic syndrome at midlife. Psychol Sci. 2011;22(12):1591–9.
24. Holden GW, Gower T, Chmielewski M. Methodological considerations in ACEs research. In: Adverse childhood experiences: using evidence to advance research, practice, policy, and prevention. San Diego: Elsevier Academic Press; 2020. p. 161–82.
25. Ford DC, Merrick MT, Parks SE, Breiding MJ, Gilbert LK, Edwards VJ, et al. Examination of the factorial structure of adverse childhood experiences and recommendations for three subscale scores. Psychol Violence. 2014;4(4):432–44.
26. Bethell CD, Carle A, Hudziak J, Gombojav N, Powers K, Wade R, et al. Methods to assess adverse childhood experiences of children and families: toward approaches to promote child Well-being in policy and practice. Acad Pediatr. 2017;17(7S):S51–69.
27. Hughes K, Bellis MA, Hardcastle KA, Sethi D, Butchart A, Mikton C, et al. The effect of multiple adverse childhood experiences on health: a systematic review and meta-analysis. Lancet Public Health. 2017;2(8):e356–66.
28. Raja S, Hasnain M, Hoersch M, Gove-Yin S, Rajagopalan C. Trauma informed care in medicine: current knowledge and future research directions. Fam Community Health. 2015;38(3):216–26.
29. Katon W, Sullivan M, Walker E. Medical symptoms without identified pathology: relationship to psychiatric disorders, childhood and adult trauma, and personality traits. Ann Intern Med. 2001;134(9 Pt 2):917–25.
30. Rittenhouse DR, Shortell SM. The patient-centered medical home: will it stand the test of health reform? JAMA. 2009;301(19):2038–40.
31. Behavioral Risk Factor Surveillance System ACE Data |Violence Prevention|Injury Center|CDC [Internet]. 2022. https://www.cdc.gov/violenceprevention/aces/ace-brfss.html. Accessed 2 Oct 2022.
32. Purkey E, Patel R, Phillips SP. Trauma-informed care: better care for everyone. Can Fam Physician. 2018;64(3):170–2.

33. Merrick MT, Ford DC, Ports KA, Guinn AS. Prevalence of adverse childhood experiences from the 2011–2014 behavioral risk factor surveillance system in 23 states. JAMA Pediatr. 2018;172(11):1038–44.
34. Home [Internet]. ACEs Aware. https://www.acesaware.org/. Accessed 2 Oct 2022.
35. Training [Internet]. ACEs Aware. https://www.acesaware.org/learn-about-screening/training/. Accessed 2 Oct 2022.
36. ACEs Aware. Quarterly progress report: ACEs screening and provider training data. 2021;1.

# Transitions for Young Adults with Psychosis and Mania

16

Arya Shah, Matthew Baum, Andrew Pines, Rachel Conrad, and Zachary B. Millman

## Introduction

Psychosis and mania are serious psychiatric syndromes that are the source of tremendous personal, familial, and public health burdens worldwide. Historically, patients affected by these disorders have often only been treated and empirically studied after years of illness, limiting the long-term benefits of care and hindering our understanding of the early course of psychopathology. Recent decades, however, have witnessed an emergence of early detection and intervention work in psychosis and mania, substantially improving our understanding of the clinical features, risk factors, prognoses, and, critically, treatment of these illnesses. Intervention in the early course of the disorder is now widely recognized as the gold standard of care for people with psychosis and mania; nonetheless, given that these disorders tend to emerge during adolescence and young adulthood, many patients continue to experience significant barriers to accessing quality care.

Psychotic symptoms are characterized by hallucinations (auditory, visual, and/or tactile intrusions) and delusions (false beliefs about oneself or the environment that are held tenaciously despite disconfirming evidence) that cause significant distress and/or impairment. Mania, which occurs in the context of an underlying bipolar affective disorder (BPAD), often involves, among other symptoms, increased energy and excitability, and features of grandiosity, delusional thinking, increased risk-taking, and sleep disturbance. Psychosis and mania often co-occur and are usually associated with a range of other psychiatric symptoms including negative symptoms (a marked decline in typical expressive, motivational, or social functioning, as often seen in schizophrenia), depressive symptoms, and anxiety. The appropriate psychiatric diagnosis for individuals presenting with psychosis or mania depends on the specific combination and course of symptoms, which can be challenging or impossible to discern in the early course of these disorders. With this in mind, the first acute episodes can be more parsimoniously referred to as "first

A. Shah (✉) · M. Baum · A. Pines
Department of Psychiatry, Brigham and Women's Hospital, Boston, MA, USA
e-mail: arya.shah@ucsf.edu; mbaum@bwh.harvard.edu; apines@bwh.harvard.edu

R. Conrad
Department of Psychiatry, Brigham and Women's Hospital, Boston, MA, USA

Center for Bioethics, Harvard Medical School, Boston, USA
e-mail: rachel@rachelconradmd.com

Z. B. Millman
Psychotic Disorders Division, McLean Hospital, Belmont, MA, USA

Department of Psychiatry, Harvard Medical School, Boston, MA, USA
e-mail: zmillman@mclean.harvard.edu


A. A. Kuo et al. (eds.), *Care of Adults with Chronic Childhood Conditions*,
https://doi.org/10.1007/978-3-031-54281-7_16

episode psychosis" (FEP) and "first episode mania" (FEM).

Clinicians and researchers have also made attempts to characterize the preceding clinical risk states to FEP and FEM with hopes of supporting earlier identification and, possibly, prevention of the illnesses altogether. In psychotic disorders, this has been referred to as the "clinical high-risk" (CHR) framework. Individuals at CHR are within the age range of greatest risk for first psychosis (typically 12–25), are help-seeking due to mental distress and/or impairment, and present with one or more constellations of risk factors or psychosis-like syndromes. Although efforts are being made to develop an analogous framework for the mania prodrome, this work is considerably less developed than that of the CHR field.

In this chapter, we discuss the concepts of early-stage psychosis and mania, covering basic clinical and epidemiological findings, challenges to accessing care, and the critical role of comprehensive interventions that include both pharmacological and psychosocial components. Although the early course of serious mental illness is often insidious, we focus our discussion on the first acute, identifiable lifetime illness episodes, including FEP and FEM, as well as on more recent work focusing on the CHR or putatively prodromal stages of psychosis.

## Barriers to Care for Young Adults with Serious Mental Illness

Many adolescents and young adults face extensive barriers to establishing and maintaining mental health treatment due to a range of factors, including rapidly changing developmental needs, challenges inherent to youth psychopathology, and limitations of the healthcare system. For individuals with emerging serious mental illness—here referring to psychosis or mania—these barriers to care are often accentuated. Psychosis and mania often first develop between the ages of 12 and 25, disrupting important academic, occupational, and social milestones and requiring intensive treatments that may involve unwelcome lifestyle changes, side effects, and influences on identity and social functioning. Thus, at the point of transition from pediatric to adult mental health care, additional barriers to treatment uptake for youth with serious mental illness include disillusionment with the mental health care system and stigma related to illness and to meeting societal expectation [1], compounding the risk of falling through the cracks between pediatric medicine and adult medicine [2].

Young adults often struggle with the organizational skills, time management, and persistence needed to navigate complex healthcare systems [3]. These factors can be amplified by a patient's anosognosia (lack of insight into a disease), which is often associated with the acute stages of severe mental illness. Ambivalence about treatment and the system's limitations might further dissuade individuals from proactively seeking psychiatric treatment. Traditional screening and referral pathways rely on primary care, and many young adults who have an emerging severe mental illness are medically healthy and do not have routine encounters in primary care. Studies have shown that transitional-aged youth desire improved social and peer support, treatment flexibility, and opportunities to form strong therapeutic relationships [4]. Such care might be implemented by adapting an existing multidisciplinary model [5] for the treatment of early-stage psychosis and mania, including coordinated specialty care (CSC), discussed later in this chapter, to meet the unique needs of this population.

## Epidemiology and Risk

Both psychotic and bipolar disorders tend to present early in adulthood. While there is a small spike in the incidence of mania among middle-aged individuals, evidence indicates that FEM will present by age 20 in close to a fifth of cases, with rates increasing to over 50% for first-episode mania occurring before the age of 30 [6]. In comparison, there is a similar prevalence of schizophrenia onsetting before age 18 (0.5%) and after age 18 (~0.5–1%) [7, 8] though still with a peak onset age of 15–24 in the transition from adolescence to young adulthood. The prevalence of very early onset (before age 13) is very low (0.04%). The lifetime prevalence of psychotic disorders in general is ~3.5% [9]. The prevalence of schizophrenia in particular is much lower at ~0.5–1%; globally, the prevalence of pediatric/childhood BPAD is approximately 1 out of 200 (0.5%), with sub-diagnostic symptoms being significantly more prevalent (4.3%) [10]. BPAD disorder represents a common source of disability around the world [11].

Assessment of risk factors for and the epidemiology of CHR syndromes is less straightforward given evidence that the diagnostic criteria are less valid when applied to the general population than to individuals seeking clinical care for associated symptoms. However, community studies to date suggest a prevalence of 1–8% in youth and young adults [12, 13]. Notably, subtle psychosis-like experiences are endorsed among 5–10% of the general population and at greater rates among children and early adolescents, but in most cases they are transitory and not indicative of emerging psychosis [14]. Clinical concern may be warranted when such experiences persist over time and cause distress and/or impairment, thereby fulfilling the criteria for a CHR syndrome. The CHR literature is largely consistent with the FEP literature in that many of the same risk factors for FEP contribute to the risk of presenting with CHR psychopathology and subsequently a transition to psychosis, including environmental stressors and familial loading of psychosis. Interestingly, despite consistent clinical and epidemiological evidence that cannabis use increases the risk of FEP, CHR studies have generally found little effect of cannabis exposure on the transition to psychosis [15]. This is likely a product of sampling bias.

The prediction of FEP among individuals at CHR is a major area of research. Clinically, factors at baseline that are reliably associated with later transition include more severe positive and negative symptoms (as well as very brief psychotic episodes as described above), poorer social functioning, more impaired neurocognitive ability, and greater levels of lifetime exposure to maltreatment or other traumas [16–18]; importantly, however, it is likely that these clinical risk factors are predictive of broader clinical courses in this population (including the course of psychosocial functioning and affective disorders), not only the onset of psychosis [19]. Human genetics is increasingly building the case that the risk factors for major psychiatric disorders also cut across current diagnostic silos. For example, evidence from population studies finds that first-degree relatives of those with schizophrenia have nearly equivalently elevated risk of developing either bipolar disorder or schizophrenia, and vice versa [20]. Recent large-scale genomic studies have also found genome-wide significant risk loci shared between multiple diagnostic entities [21]. Family history and genetic predisposition are well-known risk factors for the development of early-onset bipolar disorder [22, 23].

The identification of factors contributing to the development of BPAD remains an area of significant research; studies have demonstrated the polygenicity of BPAD, which necessitates large-scale investigations in order to accurately understand the effects of specific gene loci and/or environmental influences in the development of illness [24]. Schizophrenia is a highly heritable condition in which risk is not determined by a few genetic variants of large effect, but by variations across at least 108 genetic regions [25]. It is highly polygenic. In the pediatric population, one notable exception is the 22q11.2 deletion syndrome (encompassing DiGeorge and velocardiofacial syndromes), where the prevalence of schizophrenia is very high (25%), though also influenced by polygenic risk [26]. There are several environmental risk factors that have been proposed, including cannabis use [27] and adverse events during pregnancy (e.g., severe maternal infections) [28] or birth (e.g., hypoxic insults) [29].

## Differential and Diagnosis

### Clinical High Risk

Several structured interviews have been developed for assessing and determining the presence of CHR syndromes [30]. Most commonly, a CHR designation is ascribed to patients who present with newly emerging or worsening "attenuated" symptoms of psychosis that are clinically relevant but of insufficient intensity to warrant a psychotic disorder diagnosis. The individual may feel compelled to act on unfounded suspiciousness, for example, but is perplexed by these suspicious thoughts and maintains reality-testing abilities. It is also ascribed to patients who present with psychotic symptoms that are of threshold intensity but insufficient duration (i.e., a number of minutes) to meet the criteria for a psychotic disorder, as well as those who present with a recent, marked decline in global functioning in the context of genetic risk of psychosis (e.g., a first-degree relative with a psychotic disorder).

Youth at CHR for psychosis usually meet the criteria for at least one other DSM diagnosis, largely depressive and anxiety disorders, although substance use, trauma-related, and attention-deficit/hyperactivity disorder (ADHD) are also common [31]. The co-presence of each of these common disorders can complicate diagnosis given their overlapping symptoms (e.g., suspiciousness can reflect a psychosis-related paranoia or a trauma-related fear; morbid ideation can reflect a psychosis-related nihilism or a depressive preoccupation with suicide). Furthermore, each of these commonly co-occurring disorders can be associated with transient psychotic experiences that do not necessarily indicate CHR psychopathology. The frequency, duration, and persistence of the symptoms in conjunction with the degree of distress and impairment are used to differentiate transient subclinical symptoms from those that represent a CHR syndrome.

It should be noted that diagnosis and disclosure of CHR status carry special clinical and ethical implications given that the CHR designation refers to risk for a future disorder versus presenting concerns at the time of assessment, even though the majority of individuals at CHR do not go on to develop psychosis. Undue fear, stigma, and shame may stem from disclosing CHR status to youth and their families; thus, the costs and benefits of doing so must be carefully weighed on a case-by-case basis [32].

## First-Episode Psychosis

In contrast to the attenuated symptoms we reviewed in CHR, symptoms of FEP are more intense, can quickly become a psychiatric emergency meriting acute hospitalization, and can cause prolonged, progressive cognitive impairments significantly interfering with the pursuit of a young person's prior life plans [33]. Psychosis is itself, however, merely a term to describe a type of symptom and, though can be present on its own, is often part of heterogeneous symptomatic presentations from depression to mania. The heterogeneity of psychosis is also profound at the biological level, with multiple etiologies including nutritional, endocrine, rheumatological, substance-induced, autoimmune, and idiopathic. Here, we focus on idiopathic or "primary" psychosis, while stressing the importance of considering the broad differential of reversible causes of psychosis in this population.

History and collateral are important, as an identifiable prodrome (as discussed in the CHR section) with a temporally extended history of declining school performance and social isolation increases the pretest probability for a primary psychotic disorder. Any acute changes should heighten concern for alternative and reversible causes of psychosis. Moreover, because psychotic symptoms and symptoms that resemble psychosis are much more prevalent than psychotic disorders, it is always important to keep in mind a broad differential when evaluating first-episode psychosis. In the pediatric and adolescent population, it is especially important to consider substance-induced psychoses, which notably can be seen with intoxication with anticholinergic (e.g., diphenhydramine), stimulant (e.g., ADHD medications), hallucinogenic, cannabinoid, or synthetic cannabinoid agents or blockers of the *N*-methyl-D-aspartate (NMDA) receptor (e.g., the cough syrup dextromethorphan or ketamine). They are usually peripheral signs of intoxication, and psychotic symptoms often resolve with the cessation of the offending agent. Sometimes, substance use can induce nutritional causes of psychosis, such as nitrous oxide "whippets," leading to rapid depletion of vitamin B12.

The range of many rare alternative causes includes Wilson's disease, neuropsychiatric lupus, and autoimmune encephalitis. Anti-NMDA receptor encephalitis, though thought to be present only in 0.5–3% of cases of FEP, is important to highlight here as it can present as a mimic of primary psychoses in this age group, but the proper treatment is immunomodulation; any young person with focal neurological deficits or seizures should strongly be considered for extensive work-up including consultations to neurology and psychiatry, electroencephalogram (EEG), brain magnetic resonance imaging (MRI), and lumbar puncture with auto-antibody testing in cerebrospinal fluid and serum. Other red flags include a viral-like prodrome, a history of cancer or ovarian teratoma, new-onset seizures in the last year especially treatment-refractory, autonomic instability, rapid (within 3 months) progression, and adverse reactions to antipsychotics [35, 36]. However, autoimmune encephalitis can appear even without any of these red-flag symptoms, and thus, there are some who advocate for EEG, MRI, and serum antibody testing in all cases [34].

In the pediatric and adolescent population, there are other primary psychiatric disorders other than schizophrenia that involve symptoms resembling psychosis, including trauma-related disorders and neurodevelopmental disorders such as autism. However, if psychotic features are prolonged and debilitating, the presence of a primary psychotic disorder should be considered as there can be comorbid disease.

### First-Episode Mania

The diagnosis of BPAD in a pediatric population continues to be an area of significant ambiguity, with discrepancies existing between research and clinical [7] criteria for bipolar disorders [37]. A "broad" phenotype of bipolar mania, which included prominent irritability, has been replaced by disruptive mood dysregulation disorder (DMDD) in DSM-5; in contrast, diagnostic guidelines recognize euphoria and episodic course as being more specific indicators of pediatric bipolar illness [38]. Additional subtypes, such as cyclothymia, BPAD–II, and BPAD not otherwise specified, have been shown to be less stable across the lifespan, often converting to a different diagnosis over the course of several years [39]. Currently, the opinion holds that an accurate diagnosis of bipolar disorder in a pediatric patient can be made utilizing DSM criteria [40].

The presence of comorbid illnesses, such as ADHD, substance use disorders, conduct disorder, obsessive-compulsive disorder, post-traumatic stress disorder, disruptive mood dysregulation disorder, oppositional defiant disorder, and anxiety disorders, can overlap with bipolar disorder in terms of symptomatology; this can contribute to an ambiguous clinical picture, which can further complicate the diagnosis of childhood bipolar illness. Patients may frequently present with symptoms and histories consistent with unipolar depression, with an underlying bipolar diathesis only being revealed at the time of the first manic or hypomanic episode [41].

## Prognosis and Course

### Clinical High Risk

Approximately 25% of help-seeking young people at CHR develop a formal FEP within 2.5 years after identification [42]. Approximately 73% of these diagnostic transitions are to schizophrenia spectrum disorders, but a nontrivial portion also develop affective psychosis (e.g., bipolar disorder) [43]; thus, despite the real clinical value offered by the CHR framework, it is critical to remember that most individuals with CHR syndromes do not transition to psychosis. Among this larger group, positive and negative symptoms tend to improve on average, with approximately 50% achieving remission from their initial CHR status [44]; however, persistence of baseline non-psychotic disorders or emergence of new nonpsychotic disorders is the norm, with approximately one-third experiencing significant ongoing psychosocial difficulty and/or psychiatric disorders, usually depressive and anxiety disorders [45, 46].

## First-Episode Psychosis

Schizophrenia onset before the age of 13 tends to come with more severe impairment relative to later adolescent or young adult onsets [47]. Though the positive symptoms of psychosis including hallucinations and delusions are often the focus of evaluations, there is increasing understanding that for some, progressive cognitive impairments are a core feature of disease and the cause of substantial functional impairment, representing an important unmet clinical need [33, 48, 49]. In terms of course, it was previously assumed that prognosis was very poor; however, more recent data show that there is considerable heterogeneity in the course and outcomes of those with a diagnosis of schizophrenia. A significant proportion of patients are maintain relative stability of symptoms, employment, and other markers of global recovery [50]. In general, the smaller the interval between the onset of psychotic symptoms and appropriate pharmacological and psychosocial interventions, the better the outcome.

## First-Episode Mania

Earlier onset of FEM has been associated with a family history of bipolar disorder and/or substance use, and it can be associated with more severe and/or atypical features at presentation [6]. Minimizing the incidence of recurrence during this year may significantly alter the overall illness trajectory [51]. Cognitive changes, including in overall processing speed, memory, and some aspects of executive functioning, can be seen within the first year following a first manic episode [52].

The course of illness following FEM is influenced by time to treatment following the initial presentation. There is evidence that early interventions in FEM can improve symptoms and treatment response and prevent illness recurrence and hospitalization. Despite this, significant delays in care exist, with individuals with manic symptoms with psychosis experiencing longer delays to treatment compared to individuals with FEP without manic symptoms [53]. Rates of recurrence are known to be high in the first year following FEM. Factors associated with poorer illness outcomes include early onset of symptoms, low socioeconomic status, and presence of family history of affective illness [39]. While many individuals experience symptomatic recovery in the year following their first manic episode, rates of functional recovery are much lower and have been motivators for the development of coordinated psychosocial intervention early in the course of illness [54].

## Intervention

For FEP, FEM, and CHR, treatment of underlying and/or comorbid illnesses, such as substance use disorder, anxiety, insomnia, or medical disorders, is an important aspect of the intervention. Furthermore, assessing imminent safety risks, such as risk of self-injury or suicide, is especially important given the significant risk of death by suicide in bipolar illness and in mixed states in particular.

Much of the study of treatment for bipolar illness in children and adolescents has focused on the management of acute mania and/or depression, without addressing longer-term risks and outcomes [55]. In general, mood stabilizers and atypical antipsychotics are considered first-line pharmacotherapy in pediatric bipolar disorder, though close attention should be given to the potential side effects and long-term metabolic risks associated with many of these agents; while monotherapy is ideal, combination treatment is often required [56].

In FEP, evidence-based treatment includes two adequate trials of an atypical antipsychotic, which should be maintained for at least 4–6 weeks with utilization of serum medication levels to settle any concern for adherence/proper plasma concentration, and if two adequate trials have failed, a move to clozapine monotherapy [57].

Because there is little evidence to suggest that one antipsychotic is superior to another for the two trials [58], medications with lesser risks of long-term metabolic derangements are favored. Though long-acting injectable formulations have traditionally been reserved for cases where adherence is an issue, recent data suggest that clinical and functional outcomes may improve the earlier a person is transitioned to a long-acting formulation [59].

Several approaches have been tested to prevent or delay the onset of psychosis among youth at CHR, including psychosocial treatments (e.g., cognitive behavioral therapy [CBT]), antipsychotic medication, omega-3 fatty acids, and cognitive remediation, among others. Best practice guidelines currently highlight the role of CBT and other psychosocial interventions for this population, which evidence suggests may reduce the risk of FEP by approximately 50% [60]. Low-dose antipsychotic medications may be appropriate in certain cases such as rapidly progressing positive symptoms, but given the considerable metabolic risks associated with these medications (particularly for youth) should generally be considered short-term interventions used to support primarily psychological interventions [61].

Gold standard care for individuals with first episodes of psychotic and bipolar illness typically involves "wrap-around services" covering several individual and contextual aspects of the disorder. Early treatment within a specialized clinic can enhance quality of life, protect against rehospitalization, and improve patients' experience with mental health care. A primary example of these services is coordinated specialty care (CSC), a recovery-oriented treatment that emphasizes shared decision-making between patient and provider and delivers a range of services including individual psychotherapy, family education, work and educational support, and medication management. Targets of psychosocial interventions might include supporting employment and education, with the utility of vocational training being increasingly highlighted. Psychological interventions such as family-focused therapy [62], psychoeducation [63], mindfulness-based cognitive therapy [64], and interpersonal/social rhythm therapy [65] are also being studied as potentially useful psychotherapeutic adjuncts to care for serious mental illness.

CSC models, such as in the National Institute of Mental Health Recovery After Initial Schizophrenia Episode (RAISE) early treatment program, are increasingly felt to be the gold standard of care [66]. Many states have specialized FEP clinics that adopt this approach, though they tend to be located near major academic medical centers, and primary pediatric providers can play an important role in helping to connect patients and families to these programs if they are not already referred. Despite limited data on FEM, evidence is increasingly showing that individuals experiencing first manic episodes might similarly benefit from early CSC. Interventions like family-focused therapies, CBT, and skills-based programming can improve outcomes and support psychosocial functioning.

## Conclusion

While early intervention remains a key aspect of care in FEM and FEP, there is increasing interest in understanding and identifying prodromal states and early indicators of illness [67] which can have important implications for early interventions. Additionally, while the CSC model is well-established for early intervention in FEP, clinical data have generally been limited to persons with non-affective psychosis [68]. Such restrictions have resulted in a significant lack of programs intended to meet the needs of children, adolescents, and young adults experiencing FEM and/or affective psychoses. This issue reflects the significant disparity in both research and access pertaining to early interventions for FEM in BPAD as compared to schizophrenia and first-episode psychosis (FEP). Future research might focus on identifying risk factors or sources of vulnerability that might predict populations at increased risk of developing bipolar illness [69] as well as strengthening data to support multidisciplinary intervention programs as the standard of care in FEM.

## References


1. Loos S, Walia N, Becker T, Puschner B. Lost in transition? Perceptions of health care among young people with mental health problems in Germany: a qualitative study. Child Adolesc Psychiatry Ment Health. 2018;12(1):41.
2. Reneses B, Escudero A, Tur N, Agüera-Ortiz L, Moreno DM, Saiz-Ruiz J, et al. The black hole of the transition process: dropout of care before transition age in adolescents. Eur Child Adolesc Psychiatry. 2022;32:1285.
3. Fogler JM, Burke D, Lynch J, Barbaresi WJ, Chan E. Topical review: transitional services for teens and young adults with attention-deficit hyperactivity disorder: a process map and proposed model to overcoming barriers to care. J Pediatr Psychol. 2017;42(10):1108–13.
4. Gilmer TP, Ojeda VD, Leich J, Heller R, Garcia P, Palinkas LA. Assessing needs for mental health and other services among transition-age youths, parents, and providers. Psychiatr Serv. 2012;63(4):338–42.
5. Kessler RC, Amminger GP, Aguilar-Gaxiola S, Alonso J, Lee S, Üstün TB. Age of onset of mental disorders: a review of recent literature. Curr Opin Psychiatry. 2007;20(4):359–64.
6. Kennedy N, Everitt B, Boydell J, van Os J, Jones PB, Murray RM. Incidence and distribution of first-episode mania by age: results from a 35-year study. Psychol Med. 2005;35(6):855–63.
7. American Psychiatric Association. Diagnostic and statistical manual of mental disorders. 5th ed. Washington, DC: American Psychiatry Publishing; 2013.
8. Hua LL, Committee on Adolescence. Collaborative care in the identification and management of psychosis in adolescents and young adults. Pediatrics. 2021;147(6):e2021051486.
9. Perälä J, Suvisaari J, Saarni SI, Kuoppasalmi K, Isometsä E, Pirkola S, et al. Lifetime prevalence of psychotic and bipolar I disorders in a general population. Arch Gen Psychiatry. 2007;64(1):19.
10. Kessler RC, Avenevoli S, Green J, Gruber MJ, Guyer M, He Y, et al. National Comorbidity Survey Replication Adolescent Supplement (NCS-A): III. Concordance of DSM-IV/CIDI diagnoses with clinical reassessments. J Am Acad Child Adolesc Psychiatry. 2009;48(4):386–99.
11. Ferrari AJ, Stockings E, Khoo JP, Erskine HE, Degenhardt L, Vos T, et al. The prevalence and burden of bipolar disorder: findings from the global burden of disease study 2013. Bipolar Disord. 2016;18(5):440–50.
12. Kelleher I, Murtagh A, Molloy C, Roddy S, Clarke MC, Harley M, et al. Identification and characterization of prodromal risk syndromes in young adolescents in the community: a population-based clinical interview study. Schizophr Bull. 2012;38(2):239–46.
13. Schimmelmann BG, Michel C, Martz-Irngartinger A, Linder C, Schultze-Lutter F. Age matters in the prevalence and clinical significance of ultra-high-risk for psychosis symptoms and criteria in the general population: findings from the BEAR and BEARS-kid studies. World Psychiatry. 2015;14(2):189–97.
14. van Os J, Linscott RJ, Myin-Germeys I, Delespaul P, Krabbendam L. A systematic review and meta-analysis of the psychosis continuum: evidence for a psychosis proneness–persistence–impairment model of psychotic disorder. Psychol Med. 2009;39(2):179–95.
15. Farris MS, Shakeel MK, Addington J. Cannabis use in individuals at clinical high-risk for psychosis: a comprehensive review. Soc Psychiatry Psychiatr Epidemiol. 2020;55(5):527–37.
16. Catalan A, Salazar de Pablo G, Aymerich C, Damiani S, Sordi V, Radua J, et al. Neurocognitive functioning in individuals at clinical high risk for psychosis. JAMA Psychiatry. 2021;78(8):859.
17. Fusar-Poli P, Salazar de Pablo G, Correll CU, Meyer-Lindenberg A, Millan MJ, Borgwardt S, et al. Prevention of psychosis. JAMA Psychiatry. 2020;77(7):755.
18. Kraan T, Velthorst E, Smit F, de Haan L, van der Gaag M. Trauma and recent life events in individuals at ultra high risk for psychosis: review and meta-analysis. Schizophr Res. 2015;161(2–3):143–9.
19. Hartmann JA, McGorry PD, Destree L, Amminger GP, Chanen AM, Davey CG, et al. Pluripotential risk and clinical staging: theoretical considerations and preliminary data from a transdiagnostic risk identification approach. Front Psychiatry. 2021;11:553578.
20. Lichtenstein P, Yip BH, Björk C, Pawitan Y, Cannon TD, Sullivan PF, et al. Common genetic determinants of schizophrenia and bipolar disorder in Swedish families: a population-based study. Lancet. 2009;373(9659):234–9.
21. Cross-Disorder Group of the Psychiatric Genomics Consortium. Identification of risk loci with shared effects on five major psychiatric disorders: a genome-wide analysis. Lancet. 2013;381(9875):1371–9.
22. Lapalme M, Hodgins S, LaRoche C. Children of parents with bipolar disorder: a metaanalysis of risk for mental disorders. Can J Psychiatry. 1997;42(6):623–31.
23. Carlson GA, Meyer SE. Bipolar disorder in youth. Curr Psychiatry Rep. 2000;2(2):90–4.
24. Barnett JH, Smoller JW. The genetics of bipolar disorder. Neuroscience. 2009;164(1):331–43.
25. Schizophrenia Working Group of the Psychiatric Genomics Consortium. Biological insights from 108 schizophrenia-associated genetic loci. Nature. 2014;511(7510):421–7.
26. Cleynen I, Engchuan W, Hestand MS, Heung T, Holleman AM, Johnston HR, et al. Genetic contributors to risk of schizophrenia in the presence of a 22q11.2 deletion. Mol Psychiatry. 2021;26(8):4496–510.
27. Cannon TD, Cadenhead K, Cornblatt B, Woods SW, Addington J, Walker E, et al. Prediction of psychosis

in youth at high clinical risk. Arch Gen Psychiatry. 2008;65(1):28.
28. Canetta S, Brown A. Prenatal infection, maternal immune activation, and risk for schizophrenia. Transl Neurosci. 2012;3(4):320–7.
29. Rosso IM. Obstetric risk factors for early-onset schizophrenia in a Finnish birth cohort. Am J Psychiatry. 2000;157(5):801–7.
30. Miller TJ, McGlashan TH, Rosen JL, Cadenhead K, Ventura J, McFarlane W, et al. Prodromal assessment with the structured interview for prodromal syndromes and the scale of prodromal symptoms: predictive validity, interrater reliability, and training to reliability. Schizophr Bull. 2003;29(4):703–15.
31. Addington J, Piskulic D, Liu L, Lockwood J, Cadenhead KS, Cannon TD, et al. Comorbid diagnoses for youth at clinical high risk of psychosis. Schizophr Res. 2017;190:90–5.
32. Mittal VA, Dean DJ, Mittal J, Saks ER. Ethical, legal, and clinical considerations when disclosing a high-risk syndrome for psychosis. Bioethics. 2015;29(8):543–56.
33. Elvevåg B, Goldberg TE. Cognitive impairment in schizophrenia is the core of the disorder. Crit Rev Neurobiol. 2000;14(1):1–21.
34. Guasp M, Giné-Servén E, Maudes E, Rosa-Justicia M, Martínez-Hernández E, Boix-Quintana E, et al. Clinical, neuroimmunologic, and CSF investigations in first episode psychosis. Neurology. 2021;97(1):e61–75.
35. Pollak TA, Vincent A, Iyegbe C, Coutinho E, Jacobson L, Rujescu D, et al. Relationship between serum NMDA receptor antibodies and response to antipsychotic treatment in first-episode psychosis. Biol Psychiatry. 2021;90(1):9–15.
36. Dubey D, Pittock SJ, McKeon A. Antibody prevalence in epilepsy and encephalopathy score: increased specificity and applicability. Epilepsia. 2019;60(2):367–9.
37. Shain BN. Pediatric bipolar disorder and mood dysregulation: diagnostic controversies. Adolesc Med State Art Rev. 2014;25(2):398–408.
38. NICE. Surveillance report 2017: bipolar disorder: assessment and management (2014) NICE guideline CG185. London: National Institute for Health and Care Excellence (NICE); 2017.
39. Birmaher B, Axelson D, Goldstein B, Strober M, Gill MK, Hunt J, et al. Four-year longitudinal course of children and adolescents with bipolar spectrum disorders: the course and outcome of bipolar youth (COBY) study. Am J Psychiatry. 2009;166(7):795–804.
40. Youngstrom EA, Birmaher B, Findling RL. Pediatric bipolar disorder: validity, phenomenology, and recommendations for diagnosis. Bipolar Disord. 2008;10(1p2):194–214.
41. Daveney J, Panagioti M, Waheed W, Esmail A. Unrecognized bipolar disorder in patients with depression managed in primary care: a systematic review and meta-analysis. Gen Hosp Psychiatry. 2019;58:71–6.
42. Salazar de Pablo G, Radua J, Pereira J, Bonoldi I, Arienti V, Besana F, et al. Probability of transition to psychosis in individuals at clinical high risk. JAMA Psychiatry. 2021;78(9):970.
43. Fusar-Poli P, Bechdolf A, Taylor MJ, Bonoldi I, Carpenter WT, Yung AR, et al. At risk for schizophrenic or affective psychoses? A meta-analysis of DSM/ICD diagnostic outcomes in individuals at high clinical risk. Schizophr Bull. 2013;39(4):923–32.
44. Addington J, Cornblatt BA, Cadenhead KS, Cannon TD, McGlashan TH, Perkins DO, et al. At clinical high risk for psychosis: outcome for nonconverters. Am J Psychiatry. 2011;168(8):800–5.
45. Lin A, Wood SJ, Nelson B, Beavan A, McGorry P, Yung AR. Outcomes of nontransitioned cases in a sample at ultra-high risk for psychosis. Am J Psychiatry. 2015;172(3):249–58.
46. Schlosser DA, Jacobson S, Chen Q, Sugar CA, Niendam TA, Li G, et al. Recovery from an at-risk state: clinical and functional outcomes of putatively prodromal youth who do not develop psychosis. Schizophr Bull. 2012;38(6):1225–33.
47. Vourdas A, Pipe R, Corrigall R, Frangou S. Increased developmental deviance and premorbid dysfunction in early onset schizophrenia. Schizophr Res. 2003;62(1–2):13–22.
48. Collins PY, Patel V, Joestl SS, March D, Insel TR, Daar AS, et al. Grand challenges in global mental health. Nature. 2011;475(7354):27–30.
49. McCarroll SA, Hyman SE. Progress in the genetics of polygenic brain disorders: significant new challenges for neurobiology. Neuron. 2013;80(3):578–87.
50. Harrison G, Hopper K, Craig T, Laska E, Siegel C, Wanderling J, et al. Recovery from psychotic illness: a 15- and 25-year international follow-up study. Br J Psychiatry. 2001;178(6):506–17.
51. Gignac A, McGirr A, Lam RW, Yatham LN. Course and outcome following a first episode of mania: 4-year prospective data from the systematic treatment optimization program (STOP-EM). J Affect Disord. 2015;175:411–7.
52. Daglas R, Allott K, Yücel M, Pantelis C, Macneil CA, Berk M, et al. The trajectory of cognitive functioning following first episode mania: a 12-month follow-up study. Austral N Z J Psychiatry. 2016;50(12):1186–97.
53. Marwaha S, Hett D, Johnson S, Fowler D, Hodgekins J, Freemantle N, et al. The impact of manic symptoms in first-episode psychosis: findings from the UK national EDEN study. Acta Psychiatr Scand. 2021;144(4):358–67.
54. McMurrich S, Sylvia LG, Dupuy JM, Peckham AD, Peters AT, Deckersbach T, et al. Course, outcomes, and psychosocial interventions for first-episode mania. Bipolar Disord. 2012;14(8):797–808.
55. Findling RL, Stepanova E, Youngstrom EA, Young AS. Progress in diagnosis and treatment of bipolar disorder among children and adolescents: an international perspective. Evid Based Mental Health. 2018;21(4):177–81.

56. McClellan J, Kowatch R, Findling RL. Practice parameter for the assessment and treatment of children and adolescents with bipolar disorder. J Am Acad Child Adolesc Psychiatry. 2007;46(1):107–25.
57. Osser DN, Roudsari MJ, Manschreck T. The psychopharmacology algorithm project at the Harvard south shore program. Harv Rev Psychiatry. 2013;21(1):18–40.
58. Lieberman JA, Stroup TS, McEvoy JP, Swartz MS, Rosenheck RA, Perkins DO, et al. Effectiveness of antipsychotic drugs in patients with chronic schizophrenia. N Engl J Med. 2005;353(12):1209–23.
59. Kim S, Kim S, Koh M, Choi G, Kim JJ, Paik IH, et al. Effects of long-acting injectable paliperidone palmitate on clinical and functional outcomes in patients with schizophrenia based on illness duration. J Clin Psychiatry. 2021;82(1):20m13446.
60. McGorry PD, Mei C, Hartmann J, Yung AR, Nelson B. Intervention strategies for ultra-high risk for psychosis: progress in delaying the onset and reducing the impact of first-episode psychosis. Schizophr Res. 2021;228:344–56.
61. Schmidt SJ, Schultze-Lutter F, Schimmelmann BG, Maric NP, Salokangas RKR, Riecher-Rössler A, et al. EPA guidance on the early intervention in clinical high risk states of psychoses. Eur Psychiatry. 2015;30(3):388–404.
62. Miklowitz DJ, Schneck CD, Singh MK, Taylor DO, George EL, Cosgrove VE, et al. Early intervention for symptomatic youth at risk for bipolar disorder: a randomized trial of family-focused therapy. J Am Acad Child Adolesc Psychiatry. 2013;52(2):121–31.
63. Rabelo JL, Cruz BF, Ferreira JDR, de Viana BM, Barbosa IG. Psychoeducation in bipolar disorder: a systematic review. World J Psychiatry. 2021;11(12):1407–24.
64. Perich T, Manicavasagar V, Mitchell PB, Ball JR, Hadzi-Pavlovic D. A randomized controlled trial of mindfulness-based cognitive therapy for bipolar disorder. Acta Psychiatr Scand. 2013;127(5):333–43.
65. Perich T, Mitchell PB. Psychological interventions for young people at risk for bipolar disorder: a systematic review. J Affect Disord. 2019;252:84–91.
66. Kane JM, Robinson DG, Schooler NR, Mueser KT, Penn DL, Rosenheck RA, et al. Comprehensive versus usual Community Care for First-Episode Psychosis: 2-year outcomes from the NIMH RAISE early treatment program. Am J Psychiatry. 2016;173(4):362–72.
67. Luby JL, Navsaria N. Pediatric bipolar disorder: evidence for prodromal states and early markers. J Child Psychol Psychiatry. 2010;51(4):459–71.
68. Jauhar S, Ratheesh A, Davey C, Yatham LN, McGorry PD, McGuire P, et al. The case for improved care and provision of treatment for people with first-episode mania. Lancet Psychiatry. 2019;6(10):869–76.
69. Conus P, Ward J, Hallam KT, Lucas N, Macneil C, McGorry PD, et al. The proximal prodrome to first episode mania a new target for early intervention. Bipolar Disord. 2008;10(5):555–65.

# Emerging Adulthood and Depression: An Overview of Chronic Illness and Treatment

17

David B. Riddle, Zachary S. Appenzeller, and Eric A. Storch

## Introduction

Depressive disorders are a common and debilitating set of mental conditions defined by far more than merely a transient experience of sadness. Depression is characterized by a variety of cognitive, behavioral, emotional, and physiological symptoms that have profound impacts on sufferers, their loved ones, and society more generally. Individuals with depression account for 60% of all documented suicides [1]. The most common depression diagnosis is major depressive disorder. Individuals with major depressive disorder exhibit symptoms including low mood, diminished interest in previously enjoyable activities, changes in weight and appetite, difficulty sleeping, fatigue, feelings of worthlessness, and thoughts of death [2]. Persistent depressive disorder (PDD) is a more chronic form of depression that can pose significant challenges for sufferers. Individuals with persistent depressive disorder struggle with chronic low, depressed mood for more days than not for a period of at least 2 years and may experience symptoms including changes in appetite, difficulty sleeping, fatigue, and low self-esteem [2].

Major depressive disorders (MDDs), when diagnosed during childhood or adolescence, can lead to functional impairments later on in life, making the transition for teenagers into emerging adulthood a rather difficult experience [3]. This is especially important to consider given the various significant life milestones that are met during emerging adulthood (i.e., enrolling in higher education, pursuing the workforce, and gaining independence). Adolescents who experience depressive symptoms may be at greater risk for functional impairment as they transition into emerging adulthood, especially if these symptoms go untreated [4].

## Prevalence of MDD

Approximately 20.6% of individuals in the USA will experience a major depressive episode at some point throughout their lives [5]. This estimate has substantially increased from 2005, where the lifetime prevalence of MDD was 16.6% [6]. Twelve-month prevalence rates for MDD in the USA are between 6.7 [6] and 10.4% [5]. A meta-analysis of data on major depressive disorder from 1994 to 2014 across 30 countries indicates a lifetime prevalence of 10.8%, a 1-year

D. B. Riddle · E. A. Storch (✉)
Department of Psychiatry and Behavioral Sciences, Baylor College of Medicine, Houston, TX, USA

Center for Anxiety and OCD, Alexian Brothers Behavioral Health Hospital, Hoffman, IL, USA
e-mail: david.riddle@bcm.edu; eric.storch@bcm.edu

Z. S. Appenzeller
Louis A. Faillace, MD, Department of Psychiatry and Behavioral Sciences, University of Texas Health Houston, Houston, TX, USA


A. A. Kuo et al. (eds.), *Care of Adults with Chronic Childhood Conditions*,
https://doi.org/10.1007/978-3-031-54281-7_17

prevalence of 7.2%, and a point prevalence of 12.9% [7]. MDD appears to disproportionately impact females, at a 2:1 ratio compared to males. In one international study, a 12-month prevalence of MDD was observed in 5.8% of females and 3.5% of males [8]. It is worth noting that the prevalence of MDD during the COVID-19 pandemic has increased considerably, with some estimates that there are an additional 53.2 million cases of MDD globally (a 25.6% increase from pre-pandemic estimates) [9].

## Prevalence of PDD

Estimates of lifetime prevalence of PDD in the USA are variable, ranging from 0.9 to 6.4% [6, 10–12]. Twelve-month estimates for PDD fall between 0.5 and 2.5%. Following similar demographic trends as MDD, PDD is twice as likely to occur in women than men [10]. Interestingly, rates of chronic depression are lower in developing countries than in developed countries [13].

## Epidemiology of MDD

The monoamine hypothesis proposes that individuals experience depression as a result of deficient receptor functioning or lower concentrations of norepinephrine, serotonin, and dopamine in the central nervous system [14]. There is strong evidence to support this claim, which provides the field with a theoretical framework for the use of specific psychopharmacological interventions for the treatment of MDD [15]. Differences in brain structure among depressed individuals can also help provide an explanation for MDD. Through the use of magnetic resonance imaging, individuals with depression display smaller hippocampal volume, decreased caudate nucleus size, and a higher level of pituitary volume. Positron emission tomography scans also show that individuals with depression have lower levels of activity in the frontal cortical areas and increased activity in the amygdala, subgenual cingulate cortex, and other limbic sites [16, 17]. An excess secretion of the primary stress hormone, cortisol, has also historically been noted in individuals with depression [18]. It is postulated that individuals with depression experience more persistent hyperactivation of the hypothalamic–pituitary–adrenal (HPA) axis, which results in the excess release of cortisol and subsequent depressive symptoms [19]. When individuals experience chronic activation of the HPA axis during childhood as a result of stressful, early life experiences, the resulting development of a more sensitive HPA axis provides a biologically driven explanation of a diathesis-stress model for depression [20]. MDD is a moderately heritable disorder, with estimates based on twin studies ranging from 31 to 42% [21, 22]. This indicates that while around one-third of MDD can be explained by genetics, environmental influences contribute significantly.

The behavioral model of depression proposes that depression results from behavioral inhibition and is maintained through negative reinforcement via avoidance and escape [23]. A chain reaction called the depressive spiral starts with an input from the environment that leads to a decrease in reward. As a result of this decrease in reward, the individual experiences a drop in mood. This drop in mood influences the individual to engage in fewer behaviors. By engaging in fewer behaviors, the individual experiences their environment as increasingly void of pleasure. This then perpetuates their already low mood, influencing them to engage in even fewer (potentially reinforcing) behaviors, helping to explain the low mood, anhedonia, amotivation, and avoidance noted in MDD.

Beck's cognitive theory of depression postulates that the thoughts, or perspective, one takes on a situation are critical to the development and maintenance of depression [24]. Individuals with depression are noted to have negative automatic thoughts about themselves, the world, and the future that are often distorted and inaccurate appraisals of their experiences. Automatic thoughts are thoughts that are spontaneous, require no effort, are usually accepted as truth, and logically implicate emotions. When automatic thoughts are distorted, as they often are for depressed individuals, their inaccurate and negatively biased interpretations go unchallenged and have negative impacts on their mood state. These automatic thoughts are believed to be influenced by an individual's core beliefs/schemas, which serve as a template for how the individual processes information in their world [25]. These maladaptive schemas or core beliefs develop early on in life and remain dormant until activated by current life stressors. Schemas have been shown to be highly stable and enduring constructs in depressed individuals [26].

## Epidemiology of PDD

Biological and neuroanatomical findings for PDD share a great deal of overlap with those of MDD. However, one unique finding is that a gene-environment correlation between the short allele of *5-HTTLPR* and childhood maltreatment is specifically observed in more chronic and persistent depression and not in episodic depression [27, 28]. Given the minimal differentiation in biological and neuroanatomical differences between PDD and MDD, the epidemiology specific to PDD is therefore best illuminated by an understanding of psychosocial factors that influence the presentation.

In one sample of individuals with PDD, upwards of 75.6% of participants experienced significant childhood trauma [29]. 61% of individuals reported childhood emotional abuse, and 25% reported childhood sexual abuse. Spinhoven and colleagues [30] also found emotional neglect to be a predictor of more chronic depression. While child abuse appears to be the relative constant among individuals with PDD, it is important to note that the presence of childhood trauma does not directly correlate with PDD; however, the frequency of childhood trauma experienced can be an independent determinant for the disorder [31]. When compared to those with MDD, individuals with PDD reported receiving less care from their parents and reported significantly worse early parental relationships [32].

Pervasive interpersonal fear avoidance is hypothesized to be at the core of PDD, developing as a result of this childhood maltreatment [33]. While this interpersonal style may have been adaptive for the individual to withstand their childhood, the resulting impairments in interpersonal processing and functioning seek to contribute to their dysfunction. This leads to a perceptual disconnection from the interpersonal environment, where the individual never learns to understand the behavioral feedback of others. As a result, they fail to understand that their behavior has consequences, and what they say and do can influence a desired outcome.

Cognitively, individuals with chronic depression reported higher levels of impaired autonomy and overvigilance, as well as higher levels of dysfunctional attitudes when compared to an MDD sample. As a result of years of unremitting depression, individuals with PDD often have little hope for the future and feel helpless that they can do anything about it [26]. Chronically depressed individuals, on average, have highly rigid internalized expectations. This perfectionism often gets in the way of individuals with PDD, as they hold onto inflexible beliefs about how they, others, and life ought to be [34]. When life inevitably does not go perfectly to plan, this reinforces their belief that life is hopeless, and they are helpless, which perpetuates their negative affect and passivity toward life, which would indicate a greater level of emotional inflexibility [35]. Poor social skills are hypothesized to be a result of their avoidant approach to life, which further appears to alienate the sufferer from others. When they do engage with others, they frequently struggle to adequately connect, reinforcing their beliefs that they are inadequate. Others may be highly conflict-avoidant in their interpersonal relationships. This is consistent with a carryover of interpersonal fear avoidance from childhood and the lack of insight that they have the agency to impact life's outcomes [33].

## Depression in Emerging Adulthood

A recent survey found that 21 million Americans above the age of 18 years experienced at least one major depressive episode in the year 2020 [36]. Among those surveyed, the highest prevalence rate of MDD was observed in individuals in emerging adulthood, between the ages of 18 and 25 years (17%). Depressive symptoms are often correlated with lower quality of life and increased health-related concerns and can lead to long-term consequences for recurrent depressive symptoms [37]. Additionally, emerging adults who experience depression may also be at greater risk for suicide, substance abuse disorders, adjustment disorders, lower self-esteem, and lower levels of life and career satisfaction [38]. Despite depression disproportionately impacting emerging adults, few studies have directly illuminated the variables that contribute to and maintain depression within this developmental stage.

Emerging adulthood is a fairly new stage within the development cycle, which encompasses the transition period to adulthood between the ages of 18 and 25 years [39]. Arnett theorized that emerging adulthood can be distinguished from late adolescents and young adulthood in three significant ways: demographically, subjectively, and pertaining to identity exploration. An awareness of the unique life stressors and changes that occur during this developmental period may provide further insight into risk factors for developing depression. For example, as individuals transition from adolescence to adulthood, there comes a natural shift in relationships between children and their parents and guardians. A shift in relationships may present as a stressor in and of itself as this change would also mean a shift toward greater levels of independence. Taking on a higher level of responsibility and building a sense of independence would also imply alterations in the way families and parents provide accommodations. Families of individuals with depressive-related disorders often accommodate depressive behaviors by stepping in and fulfilling various roles and tasks for the individual, which further reinforces depressive behaviors [40] and these accommodating behaviors often sustain and prolong depressive symptoms in emerging adults [41].

In addition to a shift in relationships, emerging adults also begin to explore opportunities to pursue avenues within the workforce or higher education institutions. However, this exploration of self and constructing one's identity as an individual also presents potential risk factors for the onset or prolonging of depressive symptoms. For example, the unemployment rate among emerging adults is roughly 8% [42], which presents some concerns from a public health standpoint. Additionally, studies have demonstrated that unemployed emerging adults are three times more likely to experience depressive symptoms than their employed peers [37].

## Assessing Depression in Emerging Adulthood

Numerous assessment approaches have been validated for use in emerging adults. Some examples of self-report assessments include the Beck Depression Inventory (BDI) [43] and the Patient Health Questionnaire (PHQ-9) [44], both of which demonstrated significant validity and reliability among emerging adults. The BDI-II across numerous studies has been proven to have significant internal consistency (0.9) and test–retest reliability (0.73–0.96; [45]). The PHQ-9 has also been demonstrated as valid and reliable, with an internal consistency of 0.86–0.89 [44]. In addition to self-report measures for depression, clinician-rated assessments can be used to determine symptoms' presentation and severity of MDD. For example, the Hamilton Depression Rating Scale (HAM-D) [46] is a clinician-rated tool used to assess patients' depressive symptoms prior to, during, and concluding psychotherapy. Similar to other measures used for MDD, the HAM-D has demonstrated strong interrater reliability (0.98) and test–retest reliability (0.81) and is a valid measure for assessment and progress monitoring of depressive symptoms [47]. Relying on such measures is vital not only to the identification of depressive-related concerns among the emerging adult population, but also such psychometrically sound measures can be used to help determine the best course of treatment, whether therapeutic or pharmacological, to implement with patients.

## Treating Depression in Emerging Adulthood

There are several evidence-based approaches to treating depressive disorders, including cognitive-behavioral therapy (CBT), behavioral activation, acceptance and commitment therapy (ACT), and interpersonal psychotherapy (IPT). Each of these modalities utilizes unique yet similar approaches to targeting depressive symptoms and has been proven to be an effective form of psychotherapy.

A widely used form of psychotherapy, CBT, focuses on the conceptualization of one's thoughts, feelings, and behaviors and how these three components are interrelated. Studies have demonstrated the effectiveness of CBT in treating adolescents with depressive symptoms; however, CBT alone may only result in a slight reduction of symptoms overall. A key component of the success of CBT in treating individuals with depression is the inclusion of behavioral activation and cognitive restructuring [47]. Additionally, CBT has been found to be a labor-intensive and costly form of intervention that often requires extensive involvement from patients [48]. Given the nature of the emerging adulthood developmental stage, finding the time and financial resources to engage in standard CBT may prove to be a challenge in and of itself.

Behavioral activation is a form of psychosocial treatment that targets depressive symptoms by directly influencing behavioral change and guiding patients to understand the relationship between their behavior and environment. The goal of this form of treatment is to help connect individuals with positive rewards within their environments and to break away from harmful behaviors such as avoidance or rumination [49]. Emerging adults who experience depressive symptoms experience a variety of changes and alterations to both their internal and external environments. At times, it can be difficult for emerging adults with depression to connect with enjoyable and fulfilling activities. Through behavioral activation, there is the potential to reconnect with, or discover, positive rewards within one's environment to help combat stressors and contributing factors to depressive symptoms.

Similar to behavioral activation, acceptance and commitment therapy (ACT) is a CBT-based approach to treatment for depressive symptoms. ACT relies on a more mindfulness-based approach to behavioral therapy, which emphasizes the concept of accepting one's lived experiences. ACT incorporates several processes such as acceptance, cognitive defusion, being present, value setting, and committed action [50]. Each of these core components interacts with one another to focus and improve upon an individual's psychological flexibility or their ability to be present in the moment in order to focus on behavioral change in order to maintain their chosen values. This shift from ruminating on more negative experiences and engaging in avoidance behaviors allows patients to re-engage with activities and hobbies that were once enjoyable.

Interpersonal psychotherapy (IPT) is an effective evidence-based treatment for reducing symptoms of major depressive disorder [51]. The goal of IPT is to help patients focus on the present, in order to reduce depressive symptoms and recognize how these symptoms impact social and interpersonal functioning [52]. IPT is typically broken down into three phases to help patients navigate their depression and related impairments. The first phase consists of assessing current impairment, gathering data on the history of symptoms, and focusing on an interpersonal area of concern that is being impacted by current symptoms. The next phase includes exploring relationships, interpersonal conflicts, and impairment in roles and transitions, with the goal of helping the patient make change within their lives. The final phase of IPT focuses on reflecting back on treatment progress, what it means to conclude therapy, and discussing the best responses for potential relapse of symptoms [53]. When compared to other approaches to treating depression, such as CBT, IPT has been demonstrated to provide similar results [54]. The process of engaging in IPT appears to be less burdensome on patients than its more cognitive-behavioral-focused counterparts, which could make this approach to treatment a bit more viable and meaningful for emerging adults. The phase of emerging adulthood often involves the evolution and development of a variety of interpersonal relationships. Individuals often see transitions within their familial relationships, begin to embark on new relationships, and even pursue romantic relationships. With such a heavy emphasis on change in relationships, IPT serves as an ideal approach to treating individuals with MDD in order to reduce symptomology and aid in maintaining and fostering healthy relationships.

In addition to treating depression with psychotherapeutic approaches, emerging adults may also be prescribed psychopharmacological treatments, such as antidepressants, to alleviate their symptoms. Medications such as serotonin reuptake inhibitors (SRIs), selective serotonin reuptake inhibitors (SSRIs), tricyclic antidepressants (TCAs), and monoamine oxidase inhibitors (MOIs) are often used to treat depressive symptoms [55]. Antidepressant medication has been demonstrated as an effective intervention for treating individuals with MDD, but studies have demonstrated that side effects of these medications may impact treatment adherence and more severe presentations of depression in addition to comorbid diagnoses may cause greater levels of side effects [56]. However, for individuals who experience MDD, medication alone may not be the sole solution to improved outcomes. Studies have demonstrated that adults who receive both psychotherapy and pharmacological treatments see greater levels of symptom reduction than those who receive antidepressant medication alone [51], suggesting that a more collaborative and integrated approach to treatment is needed for symptom reduction.

## Conclusion

MDD is a commonly experienced mental health disorder, especially among adolescents and those transitioning into adulthood. Experiencing feelings of hopelessness, lack of interest, and fatigue are just some of the symptoms that can negatively impact daily functioning. Emerging adulthood consists of a variety of opportunities for growth and development, but these exciting components of this developmental phase can be impacted by chronic depressive symptoms. Additionally, with the various changes and stressors among emerging adults, it is possible for negative experiences to further exacerbate presenting depressive symptoms. The potential risk factors at play emphasize the importance of screening and assessing for such symptoms. Therapeutic approaches that focus on cognitive restructuring, such as CBT, or more interpersonal-focused concerns, such as IPT, have been proven to be effective methods of treatment. Additionally, ACT has demonstrated significant results in symptom reduction by engaging and empowering individuals. There are also numerous pharmacological approaches that emerging adults may benefit from, but these approaches are better accompanied by psychological interventions. Given the fragile nature of the emerging adult phase of the development cycle, connecting to these systems of care is key.

## References


1. Gaynes BN, West SL, Ford CA, Frame P, Klein J, Lohr KN. Screening for suicide risk in adults: a summary of the evidence for the U.S. preventive services task force. Ann Intern Med. 2004;140(10):822.
2. American Psychiatric Association. Diagnostic and statistical manual of mental disorders. 5th ed. American Psychiatric Association; 2013. https://doi.org/10.1176/appi.books.9780890425596.
3. Peters AT, Jacobs RH, Feldhaus C, Henry DB, Albano AM, Langenecker SA, et al. Trajectories of functioning into emerging adulthood following treatment for adolescent depression. J Adolesc Health. 2016;58(3):253–9.
4. Copeland WE, Shanahan L, Davis M, Burns BJ, Angold A, Costello EJ. Increase in untreated cases of psychiatric disorders during the transition to adulthood. Psychiatr Serv. 2015;66(4):397–403.
5. Hasin DS, Sarvet AL, Meyers JL, Saha TD, Ruan WJ, Stohl M, et al. Epidemiology of adult *DSM-5* major depressive disorder and its specifiers in the United States. JAMA Psychiatry. 2018;75(4):336.
6. Kessler RC, Berglund P, Demler O, Jin R, Merikangas KR, Walters EE. Lifetime prevalence and age-of-onset distributions of DSM-IV disorders in the National Comorbidity Survey Replication. Arch Gen Psychiatry. 2005;62(6):593.

7. Lim GY, Tam WW, Lu Y, Ho CS, Zhang MW, Ho RC. Prevalence of depression in the community from 30 countries between 1994 and 2014. Sci Rep. 2018;8(1):2861.
8. Ferrari AJ, Somerville AJ, Baxter AJ, Norman R, Patten SB, Vos T, et al. Global variation in the prevalence and incidence of major depressive disorder: a systematic review of the epidemiological literature. Psychol Med. 2013;43(3):471–81.
9. Santomauro DF, Mantilla Herrera AM, Shadid J, Zheng P, Ashbaugh C, Pigott DM, et al. Global prevalence and burden of depressive and anxiety disorders in 204 countries and territories in 2020 due to the COVID-19 pandemic. Lancet. 2021;398(10312):1700–12.
10. Blanco C, Okuda M, Markowitz JC, Liu SM, Grant BF, Hasin DS. The epidemiology of chronic major depressive disorder and dysthymic disorder: results from the National Epidemiologic Survey on alcohol and related conditions. J Clin Psychiatry. 2010;71(12):1645–56.
11. Kessler RC. Lifetime and 12-month prevalence of DSM-III-R psychiatric disorders in the United States: results from the National Comorbidity Survey. Arch Gen Psychiatry. 1994;51(1):8.
12. Riolo SA, Nguyen TA, Greden JF, King CA. Prevalence of depression by race/ethnicity: findings from the National Health and nutrition examination survey III. Am J Public Health. 2005;95(6):998–1000.
13. Gureje O. Dysthymia in a cross-cultural perspective. Curr Opin Psychiatry. 2011;24(1):67–71.
14. Delgado PL. Depression: the case for a monoamine deficiency. J Clin Psychiatry. 2000;61(Suppl 6):7–11.
15. Saveanu RV, Nemeroff CB. Etiology of depression: genetic and environmental factors. Psychiatr Clin N Am. 2012;35(1):51–71.
16. Mayberg HS, Liotti M, Brannan SK, McGinnis S, Mahurin RK, Jerabek PA, et al. Reciprocal limbic-cortical function and negative mood: converging PET findings in depression and normal sadness. AJP. 1999;156(5):675–82.
17. Drevets WC, Frank E, Price JC, Kupfer DJ, Holt D, Greer PJ, et al. Pet imaging of serotonin 1A receptor binding in depression. Biol Psychiatry. 1999;46(10):1375–87.
18. Carpenter WT, Bunney WE. Adrenal cortical activity in depressive illness. AJP. 1971;128(1):31–40.
19. Beatriz Currier M, Nemeroff BC. Inflammation and mood disorders: proinflammatory cytokines and the pathogenesis of depression. AIAAMC. 2010;9(3):212–20.
20. Heim C, Shugart M, Craighead WE, Nemeroff CB. Neurobiological and psychiatric consequences of child abuse and neglect. Dev Psychobiol. 2010;52(7):671–90.
21. Sullivan PF, Neale MC, Kendler KS. Genetic epidemiology of major depression: review and meta-analysis. AJP. 2000;157(10):1552–62.
22. Kendler KS, Gatz M, Gardner CO, Pedersen NL. Personality and major depression: a Swedish longitudinal, population-based twin study. Arch Gen Psychiatry. 2006;63(10):1113.
23. Craighead WE, Miklowitz DJ, Craighead LW. Psychopathology: history, diagnosis, and empirical foundations. 3rd ed. Hoboken: Wiley; 2017. p. 668.
24. Beck AT. Cognitive therapy and the emotional disorders. Oxford: International Universities Press; 1976. p. 356.
25. Sacco WP, Beck AT. Cognitive theory and therapy. In: Handbook of depression. 2nd ed. New York: Guilford Press; 1995. p. 329–51.
26. Riso LP, Newman CF. Cognitive therapy for chronic depression. J Clin Psychol. 2003;59(8):817–31.
27. Brown GW, Harris TO. Depression and the serotonin transporter 5-HTTLPR polymorphism: a review and a hypothesis concerning gene–environment interaction. J Affect Disord. 2008;111(1):1–12.
28. Uher R, Caspi A, Houts R, Sugden K, Williams B, Poulton R, et al. Serotonin transporter gene moderates childhood maltreatment's effects on persistent but not single-episode depression: replications and implications for resolving inconsistent results. J Affect Disord. 2011;135(1–3):56–65.
29. Negele A, Kaufhold J, Kallenbach L, Leuzinger-Bohleber M. Childhood trauma and its relation to chronic depression in adulthood. Depress Res Treat. 2015;2015:1–11.
30. Spinhoven P, Elzinga BM, Hovens JGFM, Roelofs K, Zitman FG, van Oppen P, et al. The specificity of childhood adversities and negative life events across the life span to anxiety and depressive disorders. J Affect Disord. 2010;126(1–2):103–12.
31. Wiersma JE, Hovens JGFM, van Oppen P, Giltay EJ, van Schaik DJF, Beekman ATF, et al. The importance of childhood trauma and childhood life events for chronicity of depression in adults. J Clin Psychiatry. 2009;70(7):983–9.
32. Lizardi H, Klein DN, Ouimette PC, Riso LP, Anderson RL, Donaldson SK. Reports of the childhood home environment in early-onset dysthymia and episodic major depression. J Abnorm Psychol. 1995;104(1):132–9.
33. McCullough JP, Clark SW. Persistent depressive disorder (dysthymia) and its treatment. In: McKay D, Abramowitz JS, Storch EA, editors. Treatments for psychological problems and syndromes. Chichester: Wiley; 2017. p. 153–67. https://doi.org/10.1002/9781118877142.ch11.
34. Riso LP, du Toit PL, Blandino JA, Penna S, Dacey S, Duin JS, et al. Cognitive aspects of chronic depression. J Abnorm Psychol. 2003;112(1):72–80.
35. Schwartz J, Ordaz SJ, Kircanski K, Ho TC, Davis EG, Camacho MC, et al. Resting-state functional connectivity and inflexibility of daily emotions in major depression. J Affect Disord. 2019;249:26–34.
36. Substance Abuse and Mental Health Service Administration (SAMHSA). Key Substance Use and

Mental Health Indicators in the United States: results from the 2020 National Survey on Drug Use and Health. 2020;156.
37. McGee RE, Thompson NJ. Unemployment and depression among emerging adults in 12 states, behavioral risk factor surveillance system, 2010. Prev Chronic Dis. 2015;12:140451.
38. Martínez-Hernáez A, Carceller-Maicas N, DiGiacomo SM, Ariste S. Social support and gender differences in coping with depression among emerging adults: a mixed-methods study. Child Adolesc Psychiatry Ment Health. 2016;10(1):2.
39. Arnett JJ. Emerging adulthood: a theory of development from the late teens through the twenties. Am Psychol. 2000;55:469–80.
40. Leonard RC, Guastello A, Cooke D, Storch EA, Lebowitz ER, Riemann BC. An initial study of symptom accommodation in adults with depression. J Cogn Ther. 2021;14(3):537–51.
41. Kagan ER, Frank HE, Kendall PC. Accommodation in youths' mental health: evidence and issues. Curr Dir Psychol Sci. 2018;27(4):227–31.
42. US Bureau of Labor Statistics. Current Population Survey (CPS) [Internet]. https://www.bls.gov/cps/. Accessed 1 Oct 2022.
43. Beck AT, Steer RA, Brown G. Beck depression inventory-II. American Psychological Association; 2011. https://doi.org/10.1037/t00742-000.
44. Kroenke K, Spitzer RL, Williams JBW. The PHQ-9. J Gen Intern Med. 2001;16(9):606–13.
45. Hamilton M. A rating scale for depression. J Neurol Neurosurg Psychiatry. 1960;23(1):56–62.
46. Iannuzzo RW, Jaeger J, Goldberg JF, Kafantaris V, Sublette ME. Development and reliability of the HAM-D/MADRS interview: an integrated depression symptom rating scale. Psychiatry Res. 2006;145(1):21–37.
47. Oud M, de Winter L, Vermeulen-Smit E, Bodden D, Nauta M, Stone L, et al. Effectiveness of CBT for children and adolescents with depression: a systematic review and meta-regression analysis. Eur Psychiatry. 2019;57:33–45.
48. Lepping P, Whittington R, Sambhi RS, Lane S, Poole R, Leucht S, et al. Clinical relevance of findings in trials of CBT for depression. Eur Psychiatry. 2017;45:207–11.
49. Dimidjian S, Martell CR, Herman-Dunn R, Hubley S. Behavioral activation for depression. In: Clinical handbook of psychological disorders: a step-by-step treatment manual. 5th ed. New York: The Guilford Press; 2014. p. 353–93.
50. Hayes SC, Strosahl K, Wilson KG. Acceptance and commitment therapy: the process and practice of mindful change. 2nd ed. New York: Guilford Press; 2012. p. 402.
51. Cuijpers P, Sijbrandij M, Koole SL, Andersson G, Beekman AT, Reynolds CF. Adding psychotherapy to antidepressant medication in depression and anxiety disorders: a meta-analysis. World Psychiatry. 2014;13(1):56–67.
52. Weissman MM, Markowitz JC, Klerman G. Comprehensive guide to interpersonal psychotherapy [Internet]. 2017. https://www.basicbooks.com/titles/myrna-m-weissman/comprehensive-guide-to-interpersonal-psychotherapy/9780786722969/ Accessed 1 Oct 2022.
53. Ravitz P, Watson P, Lawson A, Constantino MJ, Bernecker S, Park J, et al. Interpersonal psychotherapy: a scoping review and historical perspective (1974–2017). Harv Rev Psychiatry. 2019;27(3):165–80.
54. Lemmens LHJM, Arntz A, Peeters F, Hollon SD, Roefs A, Huibers MJH. Clinical effectiveness of cognitive therapy vs interpersonal psychotherapy for depression: results of a randomized controlled trial. Psychol Med. 2015;45(10):2095–110.
55. Anderson HD, Pace WD, Libby AM, West DR, Valuck RJ. Rates of 5 common antidepressant side effects among new adult and adolescent cases of depression: a retrospective US claims study. Clin Ther. 2012;34(1):113–23.
56. Bet PM, Hugtenburg JG, Penninx BWJH, Hoogendijk WJG. Side effects of antidepressants during long-term use in a naturalistic setting. Eur Neuropsychopharmacol. 2013;23(11):1443–51.

# Managing OCD and Anxiety as Emerging Adults

# 18

David B. Riddle, Madeleine N. Fuselier, Julia Rose Iacono, Linda Wu, and Eric A. Storch

## Introduction

When youth and adolescents begin psychotherapy as a form of treatment for their presenting social, emotional, and behavioral concerns, they often have a parent or guardian who is involved in the process. The parent/guardian is most likely the one who sought out treatment for their child and takes on the responsibility for seeing that their child gets to and from therapy sessions. There are, however, some cases in which the child has a high level of insight into their presenting problems and initiates the process of seeking out treatment, but nonetheless, they still may be reliant on their parent to facilitate the process and handle the financial aspect of treatment. As these youth grow older, they may find themselves still receiving treatment or in the need to engage in therapy for additional or remerging mental health concerns. Their time in therapy as a minor allowed for greater levels of dependency on their parent or guardian, but as they emerge into young adulthood, there comes a greater desire for independency, which often requires taking on greater levels of responsibility for their own health care. This newly bestowed responsibility may prove challenging for individuals. Managing one's mental health care can be difficult as engaging in treatment requires a particular level of self-awareness and self-discipline.

However, entering the stage of emerging adulthood presents its own experiences and challenges. The emerging adulthood developmental stage consists of developing role identity, navigating the workforce, exploring post-secondary educational opportunities, building autonomy, and deepening social and romantic relationships. For individuals with chronic disorders, such as obsessive-compulsive disorder (OCD) and anxiety-related disorders, this stage of development may prove even more difficult. Understanding the intricacies of this developmental stage, how OCD and anxiety-related disorders influence individual functioning, and navigating treatment options (including barriers and facilitators to services) are vital to connecting emerging adults to evidence-based treatments and resources.

## Emerging Adulthood

The stage of development that is now referred to as emerging adulthood was developed fairly recently as societies and cultures began to progress and demonstrate socioeconomic changes. Previously, this stage was enveloped within the

D. B. Riddle · M. N. Fuselier · J. R. Iacono · L. Wu · E. A. Storch (✉)
Department of Psychiatry and Behavioral Sciences, Baylor College of Medicine, Houston, TX, USA
e-mail: david.riddle@bcm.edu; madeleine.fuselier@bcm.edu; llw2@rice.edu; eric.storch@bcm.edu


A. A. Kuo et al. (eds.), *Care of Adults with Chronic Childhood Conditions*,
https://doi.org/10.1007/978-3-031-54281-7_18

young adult phase of development, which consisted of individuals from the ages of 18–40. There has been a shift in the paradigm of industrialized societies since the twentieth century, where young adults are no longer immediately entering the workforce following secondary education, onset age of marriage occurs later on, and young adults have begun to engage in greater exploration during their 20s than in previous generations [1]. During emerging adulthood, individuals begin to explore job opportunities, explore their passions and interests, invest in post-secondary educational pursuits, and navigate their own identities. This is also a stage in which many natural transitions occur, including increases in responsibilities, shifts in familial relationships, and development of a greater sense of independence and autonomy.

Emerging from adolescence to adulthood also presents natural transitions in the makeup of psychopathology. Behaviors that one experiences in adolescence may attenuate as the individual emerges into adulthood [2]. Transitioning into young adulthood has been proven to be especially challenging for individuals with mental health disorders, as this is a period that includes a series of events that require young adults to adjust to shifts in relationships and navigate significant changes in physical and psychosocial development [3, 4]. This demographic often experiences lower rates of employment, higher rates of poverty, and increased risk of substance abuse concerns [5, 6]. These transitions prove to be more significant for youth within the foster care system, who may lack a mentor or caring adult in their life. Youth who are transitioning into adulthood while engaged in mental health services may be more likely to drop out of mental health services in comparison with their adult counterparts [7]. This potential threat to one's connection to mental health-related services could prove detrimental to long-term outcomes and further emphasizes the importance of understanding these chronic concerns within emerging adults.

Characteristics of obsessive-compulsive disorder (OCD) include obsessions; unwanted, intrusive, thoughts or images, and compulsions; and repetitive behaviors or mental rituals that one is compelled to complete [8]. Similarly, anxiety, which can present in several forms including generalized anxiety disorder (GAD), social anxiety disorder (SAD), panic disorder, and separation anxiety disorder, have overlapping characteristics including excessive worry and anxiety, with difficulty in controlling the level of worrying experienced, and physiological symptoms that coincide with worry including restlessness, fatigue, and irritability [8]. These two disorders share similar symptomology and may present either in isolation from each other or as comorbid diagnoses that impact individuals' daily functioning.

OCD and anxiety-related disorders may impact individuals who are emerging into adulthood and have proven to have significant prevalence rates among this population. Approximately 20% of adults suffer from some form of mental illness, with the majority suffering from an anxiety-related disorder. Additionally, studies show that the prevalence of anxiety-related disorders tends to increase from adolescence to adulthood and that these disorders are not novel but rather an extension of preexisting concerns experienced during childhood and adolescence [9]. When considering OCD and anxiety-related disorders within this demographic, it is important to examine how these symptomologies may impact daily functioning. Within the emerging adult population, individuals may choose to either pursue higher forms of education or pursue a variety of career paths.

## OCD and Anxiety-Related Disorders

Everyone experiences intrusive thoughts that cause some level of anxiety or worry to some degree in their day-to-day lives [10]. However, for some individuals, these intrusive thoughts can become excessive, unwanted, and impairing. Such thoughts may also lead to a series of behaviors that one may feel compelled to complete in order to alleviate the distress that coincides with these thoughts. Studies have found that roughly 1–2% of children and adolescents have some form of diagnosed OCD and approximately 40%

go on to experience some form of chronic OCD-related condition [11]. There are numerous ways in which OCD may present. Some of the more common presentations of OCD include obsessions related to contamination/germs and cleaning compulsions, intrusive thoughts regarding harm to one's self or others and compulsions to avoid events that would lead to harm, obsessions and compulsions related to symmetry and "just right" behaviors, and intrusive and unwanted sexual or religion/spirituality-oriented thoughts [12]. Regardless of its presentation, when individuals experience OCD, they face intrusive and unwanted thoughts that impair their daily functioning and also may experience a series of compulsive behaviors that can delay or extend typical tasks, such as leaving a room or sending an email, and in more severe cases, these compulsive behaviors may prohibit functioning entirely.

Given the nature of OCD-related disorders and how various externalizing symptoms may present themselves, it is pertinent to understand how emerging adults may navigate coping with their obsessive and compulsive behaviors. The stage of emerging adulthood is one that consists of several sources of stress and potential anxiety. As individuals navigate their identities, establish their roles and career trajectories, and explore social and romantic relationships, it is understandable how such experiences may exacerbate anxiety-related symptoms. Anxiety disorders have been documented as the most prevalent mental health disorder among adolescents and young adults and present a series of impairments including lower psychosocial functioning, lower life satisfaction, and chronic stress [13].

## Treatment for OCD and Anxiety-Related Disorders

### Exposure and Response Prevention (ERP)

Exposure and response prevention (ERP), a form of cognitive behavioral therapy (CBT), is the gold standard treatment for OCD [14] and other anxiety disorders [15]. Numerous studies have demonstrated the effectiveness of ERP across the lifespan and have also demonstrated that ERP is an effective, evidence-based approach to treatment, even across modalities (e.g., telehealth and in-person psychotherapy) [16] that has been proven to have positive results for patients, with roughly 70–85% responding to treatment [17]. Through ERP, patients are exposed to increasingly distress-provoking situations while refraining from compulsive responses and avoidance [18]. As patients face their obsessional fears without relying on compulsions to decrease their distress, they learn that the feared outcome is unlikely to occur and that they can cope in healthier ways. Treatment providers work with patients to develop a scaffolded sequence, often referred to as a fear hierarchy, of exposures so that each produces a challenging but manageable level of distress. Patients gain confidence, skills, and insight with each exposure that prepares them to advance to the next one in the sequence. Unfortunately, despite the overwhelming evidence demonstrating the efficacy of ERP, this treatment modality remains underutilized [19].

ERP is an intensive approach that requires considerable patient engagement. This is an important consideration for providers working with emerging adults. When children with OCD and anxiety-related disorders receive treatment, parents/guardians are likely to assume primary responsibility for arranging treatment and ensuring their child attends appointments and engages in therapist-assigned homework between sessions. However, as these children progress into adolescence and then emerging adulthood, they take on more responsibility for their own treatment. During this time, treatment attrition may become more likely, especially given the demanding nature of ERP. Motivational Enhancement Therapy for Treatment Attrition (MET-TA), a transdiagnostic intervention for emerging adults with mental health needs [20], can be employed alongside ERP to target barriers to treatment retention among emerging adults. This may prove a vital component to the engagement and maintenance of psychotherapy amid the numerous external factors that may influence an emerging adult's decisions to seek mental health resources.

## Cognitive Therapy Approaches

Cognitive therapy (CT) is an evidence-based treatment modality that has demonstrated efficacy for a variety of mental health diagnoses [21]. CT is based on the concept that thoughts, emotions, and behaviors are intricately connected and that changes in any one of these domains can lead to changes in the other two [22]. For example, negative thoughts can lead to negative emotions, which might then in turn lead to negative behaviors. The consequences of those behaviors might lead to more negative thoughts, and the cycle continues. CT rests on the notion that intervention at any stage of this cycle will have compounding effects. CT has been shown to be effective as a treatment for both OCD and anxiety-related disorders [23], though these results are less significant than OCD treated by ERP. More recent efforts to address anxiety-related disorders have examined the effects of Internet-based approaches to treatment, which would ideally allow for financially feasible, flexible, and individually tailored interventions. However, efforts in the field have struggled to develop generalizable findings, especially for individuals with comorbid diagnoses, including those who may be diagnosed with more than one anxiety-related disorder [24, 25]. This further emphasizes the significance of understanding anxiety within older adolescents as it impacts emerging adults in order to develop efficacious treatments that are also accessible.

## Pharmacological Approaches

In addition to psychotherapeutic approaches to treating OCD and anxiety-related disorders, there is also evidence to indicate the efficacy of pharmacological interventions. Common methods of pharmacological treatment include serotonin reuptake inhibitors (SRIs) and selective serotonin reuptake inhibitors (SSRIs), which in a recent meta-analysis demonstrated to have significant effects in the reduction of OCD and anxiety-related symptoms [26]. Overall, these medications have been proven to lead to a substantial reduction in symptoms (29–49%) and little evidence suggests that one SSRI yields greater effects than another [27]. Treating both OCD and anxiety-related disorders with these approaches may require prolonged prescription adherences in order to increase and maintain outcomes. However, providing pharmacological treatments in combination with psychotherapeutic approaches has been demonstrated to provide more desirable outcomes [28].

## Family Accommodation

High levels of parental and family accommodation are associated with worse treatment outcomes for individuals with OCD and anxiety-related disorders [29]. A recent study found that family accommodation has high prevalence rates among adolescents, especially those who may experience social anxiety symptoms; however, little to no understanding of the correlation between parental anxiety symptoms and adolescent symptoms was thoroughly examined [30]. This would suggest that ongoing investigation of the connection between parental anxiety and adolescent anxiety is crucial to better understanding the effects of family accommodation on the emerging adult population.

Emerging adults with OCD and anxiety-related disorders accustomed to high levels of parental and family accommodation find themselves at an interesting crossroads as they face transitions such as moving out of the childhood home and away from their parents for the first time. Not only do these individuals face the often-daunting task of learning how to function as adults in a new environment, but they may also face the added challenge of learning how to cope with OCD and anxiety-related symptoms in the absence of parental and family accommodation for the first time. It is important for treatment providers to consider the potential lingering impacts of parental and family accommodation that may be present in individuals who no longer experience regular accommodation and the possibility that the emerging adult population might still experience significant parental and family accommodation even when no longer residing in the family home. Social support systems are vital for emerging adults with OCD and anxiety-related disorders, and higher levels of social support have been found to predict treatment responses in OCD [31]. Emerging adults should be empowered to transfer knowledge to their support systems that allow family and loved ones to provide support in healthy ways.

## Facilitators and Barriers to Care

There are a number of general barriers to treatment for mental illness, especially in young adults. The first set of hurdles is a barrier to even seeking help to begin with. These include perceived stigma and embarrassment, poor mental health literacy, and a preference for self-reliance [32]. Additionally, many emerging adults believe that stress is normal in college, that they do not need treatment, that their symptoms will improve naturally, and that they do not have time for treatment. This perception can also prevent them from seeking treatment [33]. Better mental health literacy could combat this problem by changing these perceptions [32]. There are other barriers, though. For instance, emerging adults may have changing or unstable job situations. Some may be unemployed, work low-wage jobs, or be in pursuit of higher education. These job situations all impact access to health insurance plans and sufficient income to pay for mental health services and create another barrier that emerging adults face [34]. Moreover, as emerging adults leave home, their parents are no longer managing their mental health care. For many, this is the first time that they will have to seek mental health care themselves. As they take on other adult responsibilities, making and keeping mental health appointments may become overwhelming or impossible [7].

During emerging adulthood, there are also specific barriers to OCD and anxiety treatment that present given individuals' life context and changes. The first of these is simply a lack of OCD and anxiety treatment tailored to the population. There are treatments tailored to children and adults, but few promote age-related independent functioning and other important factors in emerging adulthood. In addition, overprotective and controlling parent behaviors can both hold emerging adults back from independence and hinder treatment [9]. Furthermore, this population is more likely to drop out the mental health treatments than adults and also has an increased risk of low treatment engagement [7, 33].

Though there are many barriers to well-being in emerging adulthood, there are protective factors and preemptive measures that can prevent the dropout of mental health treatment in this population. A focus group of emerging adults and parents of emerging adults found several key barriers that could be addressed to facilitate better care. Time constraints such as early morning meetings and long wait times at providers often interfered with jobs and were difficult to manage. Additionally, the short duration and low frequency of appointments with their provider as well as high provider turnover made this group of emerging adults feel like they had a weak patient-provider relationship. Providing more flexible meeting times with more punctual provider schedules as well as ensuring better provider-patient relationships through more frequent and longer meetings could decrease dropout in emerging adults with mental illness. This focus group also found that community-based services and more flexible, mobile services were perceived as facilitators of treatment attendance and efficacy [7]. This could include Internet-mediated treatments such as Web-based online CBT interventions, videoconferencing, and mobile application interventions [35].

During emerging adulthood, there are also many factors that can not only facilitate better treatment and increased treatment engagement but also boost overall well-being. Among these, mentorship is both a good predictor of success and a predictor of reduced symptoms for emerging adults with mental illness. Stable housing, employment support, education and vocational testing and training, age-specific housing, and an independent living skills program were also identified as potential factors in increasing the overall well-being of emerging adults [7]. These factors can help emerging adults manage the lack of structure that often comes with more independence. Additionally, they may be able to help emerging adults manage the changes in socioeconomic status, employment, and age-related expectations that come with more independence and may be debilitating without help [2]. There are many changes occurring as adolescents transition into adults, many of which can make it hard to maintain stable treatment and some of which can instigate more stress and anxiety. These changes, though, can be exciting and allow for growth if emerging adults with mental illness are given the tools they need to step into their new roles while still receiving the care they need.

## Conclusion

Emerging adulthood, as a developmental stage, comes with its own challenges and anxiety-provoking experiences, making this phase of life even more challenging for individuals with OCD and anxiety-related disorders. For those individuals with chronic or child/adolescent-onset OCD and anxiety, seeking mental health treatments can be challenging. As children and teenagers, individuals are often connected to mental health services through the guidance of a caring and trusting parent or guardian. However, transitioning into emerging adulthood requires a greater sense of independence and autonomy. This newfound sense of responsibility can make navigating appropriate mental health resources and consistently engaging in psychotherapy challenging for emerging adults. The gold standard of treatment, ERP, requires consistent involvement and willingness to engage both in and outside of therapeutic sessions. Although there are barriers to engaging in treatment and even accessing treatment, there is hope for emerging adults. Resources that focus on promoting skill development, navigating career and educational options, and promoting self-advocacy may help emerging adults connect with mental health services. Additionally, maintaining and strengthening strong family and social relationships may help curb accommodating behaviors that would otherwise maintain OCD and anxiety-related symptoms.

## References


1. Arnett JJ. Emerging adulthood: what is it, and what is it good for? Child Dev Perspect. 2007;1(2):68–73.
2. Schulenberg JE, Sameroff AJ, Cicchetti D. The transition to adulthood as a critical juncture in the course of psychopathology and mental health. Dev Psychopathol. 2004;16(4):799–806.
3. Fuhrmann D, Knoll LJ, Blakemore SJ. Adolescence as a sensitive period of brain development. Trends Cogn Sci. 2015;19(10):558–66.
4. Smriti D, Ambulkar S, Meng Q, Kaimal G, Ramotar K, Park SY, et al. Creative arts therapies for the mental health of emerging adults: a systematic review. Arts Psychother. 2022;77:101861.
5. Cadigan JM, Lee CM, Larimer ME. Young adult mental health: a prospective examination of service utilization, perceived unmet service needs, attitudes, and barriers to service use. Prev Sci. 2019;20(3):366–76.
6. Stone AL, Becker LG, Huber AM, Catalano RF. Review of risk and protective factors of substance use and problem use in emerging adulthood. Addict Behav. 2012;37(7):747–75.
7. Gilmer TP, Ojeda VD, Leich J, Heller R, Garcia P, Palinkas LA. Assessing needs for mental health and other services among transition-age youths, parents, and providers. Psychiatr Serv. 2012;63(4):338–42.
8. American Psychiatric Association. Diagnostic and statistical manual of mental disorders. 5th ed. American Psychiatric Association; 2013. https://doi.org/10.1176/appi.books.9780890425596.
9. Hoffman LJ, Guerry JD, Albano AM. Launching anxious young adults: a specialized cognitive-behavioral intervention for transitional aged youth. Curr Psychiatry Rep. 2018;20(4):25.
10. U.S. Department of Health and Human Services, National Institutes of Health, (Updated 2020). Obsessive-Compulsive Disorder: When Unwanted Thoughts or Repetitive Behaviors Take Over (NIH Publication No. 20-MH-4676). https://www.nimh.nih.gov/sites/default/files/documents/health/publications/obsessive-compulsive-disorder-when-unwanted-thoughts-take-over/20-mh-4676-ocd.pdf.
11. Nazeer A, Latif F, Mondal A, Azeem MW, Greydanus DE. Obsessive-compulsive disorder in children and adolescents: epidemiology, diagnosis and management. Transl Pediatr. 2020;9(Suppl 1):S76–93.
12. Abramowitz JS, Deacon BJ, Olatunji BO, Wheaton MG, Berman NC, Losardo D, et al. Assessment

of obsessive-compulsive symptom dimensions: development and evaluation of the dimensional obsessive-compulsive scale. Psychol Assess. 2010;22(1):180–98.

13. Asselmann E, Beesdo-Baum K. Predictors of the course of anxiety disorders in adolescents and young adults. Curr Psychiatry Rep. 2015;17(2):7.
14. Siffert V, Riahi C, Stanley MA, Fletcher TL. Exposure and response prevention for obsessive-compulsive disorder: a case study of a veteran with violent intrusive thoughts. J Cogn Psychother. 2019;33(1):71–81.
15. Sars D, van Minnen A. On the use of exposure therapy in the treatment of anxiety disorders: a survey among cognitive behavioural therapists in The Netherlands. BMC Psychol. 2015;3(1):26.
16. Harvey AM, et al. Management of OCD: focus on psychotherapy. Psychiatr Ann. 2022;52(4):138–42. https://doi.org/10.3928/00485713-20220308-01.
17. Foa EB, Liebowitz MR, Kozak MJ, Davies S, Campeas R, Franklin ME, et al. Randomized, placebo-controlled trial of exposure and ritual prevention, clomipramine, and their combination in the treatment of obsessive-compulsive disorder. Am J Psychiatry. 2005;162(1):151–61.
18. Abramowitz JS. Variants of exposure and response prevention in the treatment of obsessive-compulsive disorder: a meta-analysis. Behav Ther. 1996;27:583–600.
19. Scherr SR, Herbert JD, Forman EM. The role of therapist experiential avoidance in predicting therapist preference for exposure treatment for OCD. J Contextual Behav Sci. 2015;4:21–9.
20. Mistler LA, Sheidow AJ, Davis M. Transdiagnostic motivational enhancement therapy to reduce treatment attrition: use in emerging adults. Cogn Behav Pract. 2016;23(3):368–84.
21. Shafran R, Clark DM, Fairburn CG, Arntz A, Barlow DH, Ehlers A, et al. Mind the gap: improving the dissemination of CBT. Behav Res Ther. 2009;47(11):902–9.
22. Liese BM, Beck AT. Cognitive-behavioral therapy of addictive disorders. New York: The Guilford Press; 2022.
23. Carpenter JK, Andrews LA, Witcraft SM, Powers MB, Smits JAJ, Hofmann SG. Cognitive behavioral therapy for anxiety and related disorders: a meta-analysis of randomized placebo-controlled trials. Depress Anxiety. 2018;35(6):502–14.
24. Berger T, Boettcher J, Caspar F. Internet-based guided self-help for several anxiety disorders: a randomized controlled trial comparing a tailored with a standardized disorder-specific approach. Psychotherapy (Chic). 2014;51(2):207–19.
25. White SW, Albano AM, Johnson CR, Kasari C, Ollendick T, Klin A, et al. Development of a cognitive-behavioral intervention program to treat anxiety and social deficits in teens with high-functioning autism. Clin Child Fam Psychol Rev. 2010;13(1):77–90.
26. Del Casale A, Sorice S, Padovano A, Simmaco M, Ferracuti S, Lamis DA, et al. Psychopharmacological treatment of obsessive-compulsive disorder (OCD). Curr Neuropharmacol. 2019;17(8):710–36.
27. Krebs G, Heyman I. Obsessive-compulsive disorder in children and adolescents. Arch Dis Child. 2015;100(5):495–9.
28. Bandelow B, Sher L, Bunevicius R, Hollander E, Kasper S, Zohar J, et al. Guidelines for the pharmacological treatment of anxiety disorders, obsessive-compulsive disorder and posttraumatic stress disorder in primary care. Int J Psychiatry Clin Pract. 2012;16(2):77–84.
29. Palitz SA, Kendall PC. Anxiety disorders in children. In: Bui E, Charney ME, Baker AW, editors. Clinical handbook of anxiety disorders. Cham: Springer International Publishing; 2020. p. 141–56. https://doi.org/10.1007/978-3-030-30687-8_7.
30. Lebowitz ER, Woolston J, Bar-Haim Y, Calvocoressi L, Dauser C, Warnick E, et al. Family accommodation in pediatric anxiety disorders. Depress Anxiety. 2013;30(1):47–54.
31. Herzog P, Osen B, Stierle C, Middendorf T, Voderholzer U, Koch S, et al. Determining prognostic variables of treatment outcome in obsessive–compulsive disorder: effectiveness and its predictors in routine clinical care. Eur Arch Psychiatry Clin Neurosci. 2022;272(2):313–26.
32. Gulliver A, Griffiths KM, Christensen H. Perceived barriers and facilitators to mental health help-seeking in young people: a systematic review. BMC Psychiatry. 2010;10(1):113.
33. LeBlanc NJ, Brown M, Henin A. Anxiety disorders in emerging adulthood. In: Bui E, Charney ME, Baker AW, editors. Clinical handbook of anxiety disorders. Cham: Springer International Publishing; 2020. p. 157–73. https://doi.org/10.1007/978-3-030-30687-8_8.
34. McGorry P, Bates T, Birchwood M. Designing youth mental health services for the 21st century: examples from Australia, Ireland and the UK. Br J Psychiatry Suppl. 2013;54:s30–5.
35. Blackburn AM, Goetter EM. Treatment of anxiety disorders in the digital age. In: Bui E, Charney ME, Baker AW, editors. Clinical handbook of anxiety disorders. Cham: Springer International Publishing; 2020. p. 297–313. https://doi.org/10.1007/978-3-030-30687-8_16.

# Substance Use Disorders

# 19

James Powers, George Weyer, Rachel Conrad, Kevin M. Simon, and Oscar Bukstein

## Introduction

Substance use disorder treatment and management have improved over the past few years. However, substance use disorders (SUDs) among transitional-age youth (TAY) remain a significant concern, and it is essential that TAY providers be well-versed in their management. Opioid overdose deaths are increasing in TAY and account for a substantial share of mortality in this age group [1].

Between 2015 and 2019, over 21,000 young people (aged 10–24) died of an unintentional drug overdose, resulting in over 1.2 million years of life lost [2]. With recreational cannabis (marijuana) use being legal in more states (19 as of May 2022), rates of cannabis use across age groups and the concentration of THC in available products are both increasing [3, 4]. While there have been long-term reductions in tobacco use among adolescents since the 1990s, the introduction and rapid adoption of electronic cigarettes (e-cigarettes)—"vaping"—threaten this progress [5]. Dynamic factors such as racial inequality, geography, socio-political climate, and peers influence these trends. Without appropriate interventions, knowledgeable providers, and adequate resources, the population—especially those most disadvantaged—is at risk of the worst outcomes [6, 7].

Risk factors for SUDs include age of onset, familial history, comorbid psychiatric disorders, and experiencing trauma, along with social and environmental influences during childhood [8]. The onset of substance use is among the outcomes most strongly linked to prior adverse childhood experiences (events that occur during childhood that could be considered significantly negative or potentially traumatic such as child maltreatment or domestic violence) [9].

Generally, substance use disorders are best treated in a multidisciplinary fashion, combining medication treatment with behavioral or other psychosocial interventions [10, 11]. Goals can vary based on individual circumstances, but treatment aims at supporting affected persons to recover from their use disorder. Recovery, as defined by the Substance Abuse and Mental Health Administration (SAMHSA), is *"a process of change through which individuals improve their health and wellness, live a self-directed life, and strive to reach their full potential."* It emphasizes optimizing overall well-being along the four dimensions of health (typically including

J. Powers (✉) · R. Conrad · K. M. Simon · O. Bukstein
Harvard Medical School, Boston, MA, USA
e-mail: jpowers0@bwh.harvard.edu; rconrad@bwh.harvard.edu; kevin.simon@childrens.harvard.edu; oscar.bukstein@childrens.harvard.edu

G. Weyer
University of Chicago, Chicago, IL, USA
e-mail: ggweyer@bsd.uchicago.edu


A. A. Kuo et al. (eds.), *Care of Adults with Chronic Childhood Conditions*,
https://doi.org/10.1007/978-3-031-54281-7_19

abstinence or reduction in substance use), housing, sense of purpose, and social relationships [12]. Given that addiction is a chronic and relapsing condition, patients at any stage of recovery should be supported to remain engaged in treatment and encouraged to adopt harm reduction behaviors to reduce the negative consequences of substance use. Approaching patients with compassion, avoiding stigmatizing language, offering flexibility in treatment structure, and supporting re-engagement in care after relapse are critical components of substance treatment for TAY [6, 13, 14].

## Screening, Assessment, and Diagnosis

While effective care for substance use disorder requires the identification of affected persons, the evidence supporting the routine screening of adolescents is mixed, and similar to other mental health conditions, it is common for persons who develop substance use disorders in childhood to initially present for treatment in adulthood [15]. The US Preventive Services Task Force's 2020 guideline recommends screening for persons older than 18 (a grade B recommendation) but found the evidence for screening adolescents insufficient [16]. However, the American Academy of Pediatrics and the American Academy of Child and Adolescent Psychiatry recommend screening as part of routine care for adolescents [17, 18]. Pragmatically, clinicians already including an assessment of substance use could consider using validated screening instruments such as the CRAFFT, AUDIT, S2BI, or BSTAD, the latter two being available online [17]. Clinicians should also consider a focused assessment of substance use in patients presenting with potential medical or psychiatric complications of substance use [19, 20].

Confidentiality is a common concern when assessing substance use in the TAY population. Clinicians in general practice settings can approach this similarly to other sensitive topics (e.g., reproductive health or sexually transmitted infections) where adolescents have increased privacy rights. Clinicians working in specialized substance use settings must adhere to the Federal confidentiality regulations as detailed in 42 C.F.R. §2.12(e), which broadly prohibits all disclosures (including to parents) without an adolescent's written consent [21]. Knowledge of local law is important as many states allow adolescents under the age of 18 to consent to substance use treatment without parental consent [22].

Substance use disorders (e.g., "alcohol use disorder," "opioid use disorder," and "cannabis use disorder") are defined by the DSM-5 using a common approach (see text box). Generally, a person must meet two or more out of 11 criteria within 12 months and severity (mild, moderate, and severe) is by a number of positive criteria [23].

**DSM-5 Diagnostic Criteria for Substance Use Disorder**

Two or more criteria must be meet in the prior 12 months.

Use in larger amounts or for longer periods of time than intended.

Unsuccessful efforts to cut down or quit.

Excessive time spent getting, using, intoxicated, and recovering from effects.

Craving or intense desire/urge to use substance.

Failure to fulfill major obligations.

Continued use despite social/interpersonal problems.

Activities/hobbies reduced or given up.

Recurrent use in physically hazardous situations:

Recurrent use despite physical or psychological problems caused by or worsened by use.

Tolerance.

Withdrawal.

Severity is determined by the number of symptoms present:

2–3: Mild severity

4–5: Moderate severity

6 or More: Severe

After a substance use disorder is identified, treatment planning is guided by a comprehensive assessment that characterizes the severity of substance use (frequency, dose, administration method, etc.), identifies other substance use, screens for common comorbid mental health conditions (major depression, anxiety, ADHD), assesses social factors that may impact treatment (housing, family support, insurance, transportation), assesses use of harm reduction strategies, and, importantly, identifies the patient's motivations and goals [21].

## Behavioral Interventions for Substance Use

Behavioral approaches to substance use treatment have heightened importance in the management of adolescents owing to the limited access to some FDA-approved pharmacologic therapies. A 2020 systematic review of 118 randomized controlled trials evaluated seven common types of behavioral interventions including motivational interviewing, family-focused therapy, cognitive-behavioral therapy, psychoeducation, contingency management, peer group therapy, and intensive case management. Brief motivational interviewing (1–2 sessions) was found to be more effective than usual care for reducing alcohol use and improving legal outcomes but had no impact specifically on cannabis use. Among higher-intensity interventions, family-based interventions were found to be the most effective for a range of substance use outcomes, but, even for more intensive interventions, there was little evidence for a reduction in cannabis use [11]. In adults, cognitive behavioral therapy (CBT) is the most commonly available evidence-based behavioral treatment modality [10, 24].

Behavioral interventions for substance use can be accessed within different levels of care, as defined by the American Society of Addiction Medicine (ASAM), that range from outpatient treatment (Level 1.0: Episodic clinic visits for community-dwelling patients) to more intensive services such as intensive outpatient treatment (Level 2.0: Nine or more hours of treatment across 3–5 days per week) or residential treatment (Level 3.0: Weeks to months of live-in treatment). TAY patients can access treatment across this entire continuum and, in many cases, would be best served by treatment programs with expertise in the TAY population [25].

## Alcohol Use Disorder

In the United States, alcohol is the most commonly used and misused substance by both adolescents and adults. Over 50% of adults, 23% of children and adolescents younger than age 17 and 1% of children under age 12 endorse alcohol use during the past month [26]. Alcohol use beginning in adolescence is of particular importance as exposure during this critical neurodevelopmental period has been shown to increase the risk of alcohol use disorder (AUD) later in life and lead to persistent changes in neural activity and behavior. Studies have shown various neurobiological changes in adulthood related to alcohol misuse during adolescence, including thinning and decreased volume of the prefrontal cortex—the area of the brain associated with executive functioning [27]. Additionally, adolescents who already meet the criteria for AUD as compared to unaffected teens demonstrate worse cognitive performance, changes in gray and white matter brain structure, and differences in functional brain activation patterns [28].

Alcohol acts broadly on a number of different central nervous system (CNS) targets, primarily the GABAergic, dopaminergic, serotonergic, and glutamatergic systems. The acute neuropsychiatric effects of alcohol use vary based on the quantity consumed and may include mild anxiolytic effects, increased social disinhibition, speech impairment, balance and coordination impairment, sedation, and loss of consciousness [29]. Long-term use may lead to impaired cognitive function, hepatic inflammation, heart disease, cancer, and mood disorders [30]. Clinical signs of alcohol intoxication include respiratory depression, bradycardia, impaired mental status (confusion, stupor, etc.), hyporeflexia, vomiting, and seizures [31].

While patients with mild AUD may be treated successfully with behavioral interventions alone, more severe cases of AUD should be managed with behavioral and pharmacologic treatment [11]. Effective medications are available for AUD treatment but are underutilized. First-line medications with FDA-approval include naltrexone (daily oral or monthly intramuscular formulations) and acamprosate (three times daily oral medication). Second-line medications include disulfiram (daily oral medication but contraindicated in persons still consuming alcohol) and off-label use of topiramate (once or twice daily oral medication). Additionally, gabapentin (three times daily oral medication), while not FDA-approved, has efficacy for both alcohol withdrawal and ongoing treatment [32]. There are currently no FDA-approved medications for AUD in adolescence, though some studies have shown efficacy for naltrexone and disulfiram as well as questionable efficacy of ondansetron [33].

## Cannabis Use Disorder

Epidemiologically, rates of cannabis use are increasing across all age groups. In 2014, 3.9% of pregnancies were exposed to cannabis. Furthermore, 7.4% of adolescents 12–17 years old, 19.6% of young adults 18–25 years old, and 6.6% of adults over 26 years old reported using cannabis during the past month [34]. Cannabis can be consumed through different routes of administration, including smoking, vaping, dabbing, oral (edibles, capsules, whole plant, etc.), and topical. While it is difficult to estimate the prevalence of the different routes of administration, the literature demonstrates that in the United States and Canada, smoking continues to be most common among both adolescents and adults though rates of vaping appear to be increasing over time [35].

The cannabinoids delta-9-tetrahydrocannabinol (THC) and cannabidiol (CBD) act on endogenous cannabinoid receptors in the human body called the endocannabinoid system, of which there are two main receptor types—CB1 which is primarily concentrated in the nervous system and CB2 which is primarily concentrated in the immune system. THC acts as a partial agonist on CB1 and CB2, and its activation of CB1 leads to the psychoactive effects of cannabis. CBD has a low affinity for both CB1 and CB2, and it is thought to generate its (non-psychoactive) effects by acting as a ligand on non-endocannabinoid receptors [36].

Common physiologic effects of cannabis use include dose-dependent tachycardia, increased blood pressure, vasodilation leading to characteristic conjunctival injection, increased respiratory rate, dry mouth, and increased appetite. Neuropsychiatric effects range from pleasurable effects (e.g., decreased anxiety, increased sociability, and euphoria) to negative effects (e.g., worsened anxiety, dysphoria, paranoia, panic, and even acute psychosis). Despite common misperceptions, cannabis use can lead to dependence and cessation of use can lead to withdrawal symptoms [37]. As compared to adults, adolescents who use cannabis may demonstrate a higher degree of executive function impairment, may not experience the same decrease in post-intoxication cravings, and may not show the same lingering deficits in learning that adults may experience after a period of abstinence [38].

There are no FDA-approved medications for the treatment of CUD in any age group, although there are positive studies demonstrating the efficacy of medications and supplements such as n-acetylcysteine and topiramate [39]. Psychosocial interventions, such as addiction counseling, family-based therapy, cognitive-behavioral therapy, and motivational interviewing, are typically utilized although evidence of effectiveness is limited [11].

## Tobacco Use Disorder

Tobacco is the leading cause of preventable disease and death in the United States and a large majority of tobacco use starts in the TAY population. The Centers for Disease Control and Prevention (CDC) reports that in 2020, 23.6% (3.65 million) of high school and 6.7% (800,000) of middle school students reported current (past 30-day) use of any tobacco product [40]. In 2019, tobacco use accounted for 7.69 million deaths and 200 million disability-adjusted life-years internationally [41]. According to the CDC, current smokers in the United States include 8% of adults 18–24 years of age, 16.7% of adults 25–44 years of age, 17% of adults 45–64 years of age, and 8.2% of adults 65 years of age and older [42].

Tobacco can be consumed through a number of smoking and non-smoking means, including but not limited to cigarettes, e-cigarettes and vapes, cigars, hookahs, chewing tobacco, dip, and snuff. Dependence on tobacco products is mediated through the psychoactive drug nicotine. Nicotine binds to acetylcholine receptors in the CNS leading to dopamine release, which mediates its initially rewarding and addictive properties. Psychoactive effects include improved concentration, reduced stress and anxiety, appetite suppression, and pleasure, however as dependence develops, withdrawal from nicotine often leads to irritability, anxiety, worsened mood, increased appetite, difficulty with concentration, insomnia, and cravings [43]. Physiologic effects of nicotine include increased heart rate and blood pressure, increased respiratory rate, reduced coronary blood flow, increased skeletal muscle blood flow, hyperglycemia, blood hypercoagulability, nausea, vomiting, and diarrhea. The association of tobacco use with cancer is mediated primarily through numerous other carcinogenic substances contained within tobacco products [44].

First-line pharmacotherapy options for tobacco cessation in adults include varenicline, bupropion, and nicotine replacement (gum, lozenges, patch, etc.) [45]. While all three options have demonstrated efficacy in increasing tobacco cessation rates and decreasing withdrawal symptoms as compared to placebo, according to the Evaluating Adverse Events in Global Smoking Cessation Study (EAGLES) trial, varenicline may be slightly superior in quit rates [46]. It is reasonable to choose among these options based on patient preference, though one should consider side effect profiles and contraindications (e.g., bupropion is contraindicated in patients with seizure disorders). Nicotine replacement therapy can be offered as combination therapy of either a short-acting form of nicotine (e.g., lozenge) is used in conjunction with a longer-acting form (e.g., patch). The combination of nicotine replacement therapy with varenicline or bupropion may increase quit rates in some patients. Of note, the FDA *removed* its previously issued black-box warning for varenicline and bupropion leading to increased neuropsychiatric effects after it was determined that smoking cessation benefits notably outweighed any possible neuropsychiatric risks.

For children and adolescents, counseling interventions are recommended to help prevent the onset of tobacco use, but there is much less evidence to guide interventions for tobacco cessation in youth who are already smoking [47]. Pharmacotherapy options similar to those used in adults may be considered in the adolescent population with limited data showing improved cessation rates with the use of nicotine replacement and bupropion [48].

## Opioid Use Disorder

The United States has been experiencing a worsening crisis of opioid use disorder (OUD) and opioid overdose deaths since the 1990s with such deaths expected to total 80,816 in 2021 [49]. Since 2013, these trends have been driven by the rapid proliferation of potent synthetic opioids (fentanyl analogs), which are now responsible for the overwhelming majority of opioid overdose deaths [50]. Premature deaths from opioids are particularly burdensome for young adults—by 2016 opioids were responsible for 20% of all deaths among persons 24–30 years and 12.4% of all deaths among persons aged 15–24 years [51]. While heroin and synthetic opioids such as fentanyl are responsible for the overwhelming majority of overdose deaths among adults, prescription opioids are reported to be responsible for more overdoses than illicit opioids among adolescents ages 15–19 years, although illicit opioid use was increasing faster [52]. A 2015 sample of commercial claims showed that 12.9%

of patients ages 16–25 years were prescribed opioids and up to one-third of those prescriptions were by dental clinicians [53]. Rates of prescription opioid misuse range from 3.8% in adolescents to 7.8% in young adults with the source of misused opioids commonly being friends, family, or a single prescriber [54]. While patients under 18 years old have been excluded from national opioid prescribing guidelines, evidence suggests that pediatric clinicians can reduce the risk of harm from prescription opioids by implementing similar safeguards, namely using the lowest effective daily dose, limiting the duration of initial opioid prescriptions, avoiding opioid prescribing with concurrent benzodiazepine use, and relying on short-acting opioids [55–57].

"Opioids" broadly refer to substances that act on the endogenous opioid systems. Opioids can be consumed via a number of routes, including oral, intranasal, intravenous, subcutaneous, intramuscular, and smoking. Examples of opioids include heroin, fentanyl, morphine, codeine, oxycodone, hydrocodone, tramadol, methadone, and endorphins (e.g., enkephalins, dynorphins, and beta-endorphins). Mu-type opioid receptor activation in the CNS results in analgesia, euphoria, respiratory depression, and miosis, while activation outside of the CNS can lead to cough suppression and constipation. Clinically, opioid intoxication may present with slurred speech, sedation, miosis, decreased respirations, and decreased bowel activity. Mental status can range from euphoric to irritable to comatose. Chronic opioid use leads to an attenuation of response (tolerance) and physiologic dependence. Abrupt discontinuation can lead to multiple days of withdrawal symptoms including intense cravings, dysphoria, gastrointestinal discomfort (especially diarrhea and cramping), lacrimation, and rhinorrhea. Administration via intravenous or subcutaneous injection is associated with heightened overdose risk and risks of numerous infections (HIV, hepatitis C, bacterial endocarditis, etc.) and other injuries [31].

Treatment of adults with OUD should optimally include pharmacologic treatment and behavioral interventions. First-line medications for opioid use disorder (MOUD) include methadone (full mu-opioid agonist), buprenorphine–naloxone (suboxone and others; partial mu agonist/antagonist), and naltrexone (Vivitrol, ReVia; mu-opioid antagonist). Generally, agonist treatment (methadone or buprenorphine) is recommended by experts over antagonist treatment (naloxone), though it is reasonable to select among these options based on patient-specific factors [58]. While robust evidence supports the use of MOUD in adults, these treatments are underutilized even in patients presenting with non-fatal opioid overdose [19, 59, 60]. The evidence for the use of these medications specifically within TAY is more limited, but their use is encouraged [61, 62]. A 2022 systematic review found four randomized controlled trials in this population, all assessing a combination of buprenorphine and psychosocial or therapeutic treatments, found that buprenorphine was effective and that longer duration medication tapers were more effective than shorter tapers [63]. While more studies are needed, clinicians should work to increase access to known treatments as TAY face more difficulty accessing medications and demonstrate lower rates of treatment retention [64]. Psychosocial and psychotherapeutic interventions should be used to augment MOUD and include motivational interviewing, cognitive-behavioral therapy, and contingency management. Participation in such an intervention should not be a requirement for patients to receive MOUD. Contingency management has been shown to increase treatment retention, though generally, evidence is insufficient to promote one psychosocial intervention over another [65].

In addition to formal treatment, harm reduction services offer a substantial opportunity to diminish harm from OUD, including for persons who continue problematic use [66]. Evidence-based harm reduction strategies include dispensing the opioid antagonist naloxone to persons at risk of harm from opioids or individuals who may be in a position to act as a lay responder, including minors [67]. Additional harm reduction services include syringe exchange programs, fentanyl testing supplies, pre-exposure prophylaxis, and diagnostic services for common infections such as hepatitis C and HIV [66, 68, 69].

## Stimulant Use Disorder

According to the National Survey on Drug Use and Health, in 2018 it was estimated that 561,000 persons aged 12 or older met the criteria for stimulant use disorder in the past year in the United States—0.2% of adolescents (12–17 years of age), 0.5% of young adults (18–25 years of age), and 0.2% of adults 26 years of age and older [70]. There is a particularly complex association between stimulant use and psychosis and studies have shown that rates of stimulant use in people who experience psychosis are much higher than the general population [71].

"Stimulants" generally refer to a class of psychoactive substances that lead to increased feelings of awareness and activation usually by increasing dopamine availability in the CNS. A number of prescription and non-prescription substances fall under this category, including methylphenidate, dextroamphetamine/amphetamine, methamphetamine, and cocaine. The different substances may be consumed through various routes—orally ingested, snorted, smoked, or injected. Neuropsychiatric effects of stimulant use vary based on the degree of intoxication and the specific substance ingested. Generally, clinical neuropsychiatric manifestations include heightened attention/awareness, appetite suppression, insomnia, elevated mood, and bruxism. More severe presentations include symptoms such as euphoria, positive psychotic symptoms such as perceptual disturbances, illusions, auditory/visual/tactile hallucinations, or paranoia, psychomotor agitation, and aggression. Stimulant use can affect nearly all body systems, though notably affects the cardiovascular system, and can lead to elevated heart rate, elevated blood pressure, and increased systemic vascular resistance, all of which can lead to serious and sometimes unfortunately fatal complications of stimulant use [31].

Despite the need for pharmacologic treatment options, there are no approved medications for stimulant use disorder [72]. All persons with a stimulant use disorder should be offered psychosocial interventions. While the evidence is insufficient to recommend any single specific psychosocial or therapeutic intervention above others, research does show that these interventions likely lead to a decrease in drug use, a decrease in unsafe sexual behaviors, and that combining more than one intervention (e.g., contingency management, cognitive-behavioral therapy, motivational interviewing, and support groups) is likely more effective than offering a single intervention [73].

## Sedative, Hypnotic, or Anxiolytic Use Disorder

According to the National Survey on Drug Use and Health, in 2018, it is estimated that 751,000 persons aged 12 or older met criteria for sedative use disorder in the past year in the United States—0.3% of adolescents (12–17 years of age), 0.7% of young adults (18–25 years of age), and 0.2% of adults 26 years of age and older [70]. Most sedative-hypnotic substances are prescription medications. The three major subcategories are benzodiazepines (e.g., alprazolam, diazepam, and lorazepam), barbiturates (e.g., phenobarbital, secobarbital, and butobarbital), and the "Z-drugs" (e.g., zolpidem, zaleplon, and zopiclone). Sedative hypnotics all act as CNS depressants by increasing the activity of GABA (the nervous system's principal inhibitory neurotransmitter). Lower doses may lead to drowsiness, anxiolysis, and fatigue, though at higher doses/intoxication, effects include dizziness, impaired motor coordination, slurred speech, respiratory suppression, and over-sedation. Some people may experience a "paradoxical response," in which disinhibition leads to symptoms including confusion, activation, and aggression. Chronic use over time may lead to tolerance and dependence [74].

Pharmacologic treatment for these disorders most commonly involves a controlled taper off the medication, which is often safe to do in the outpatient setting. Benzodiazepine discontinuation has been more thoroughly studied than the discontinuation of barbiturates and Z-drugs [75]. There is little evidence to guide specific taper regimens, though for benzodiazepines it is commonly recommended to gradually reduce the dose by 25% every 1–2 weeks over a course of roughly 6 weeks [76, 77]. Generally, patients with longer histories of use have an increased likelihood of withdrawal symptoms and it is appropriate to modify the taper based on symptoms. More rapid tapers can be attempted in inpatient settings. Another common strategy for benzodiazepine tapers is to switch to a longer-acting medication than the one the patient is currently using to decrease the risk of withdrawal side effects (e.g., switch from lorazepam to chlordiazepoxide) [76, 77]. There does not seem to be enough evidence to recommend augmenting a taper with any additional medications [78]. Patients should also be offered psychosocial interventions that demonstrate improved outcomes when combined with medication tapers compared to tapers alone. Cognitive-behavioral therapy has the strongest evidence [79].

## Summary

In summary, it is vitally important that medical and behavioral health providers of children, adolescents, and adults of all ages remain up-to-date with the diagnosis and management of substance use disorders. Generally, treatment should include both medication and psychosocial interventions when available. Due to a lack of research and inadequate numbers of specialized substance use treatment programs, children and adolescents often do not have access to medications to treat substance use disorders, and psychosocial services available to children and adolescents may differ from those available to adults [80]. Healthcare providers should be aware of the barriers to treatment encountered by transitional-age youth with substance use disorders. While for some, abstinence or sobriety may be a goal, harm reduction approaches from compassionate and non-judgmental providers may provide some patients with the most optimal and realistic outcomes. Treatment should emphasize practical strategies to help decrease the negative social, financial, legal, and health-related consequences of substance use.

## References


1. Friedman J, Godvin M, Shover CL, Gone JP, Hansen H, Schriger DL. Trends in drug overdose deaths among US adolescents, January 2010 to June 2021 | Adolescent Medicine | JAMA | JAMA Network [Internet]. https://jamanetwork.com/journals/jama/fullarticle/2790949?widget=personalizedcontent&previousarticle=2790981. Accessed 3 Oct 2022.
2. Hall OT, Trimble C, Garcia S, Entrup P, Deaner M, Teater J. Unintentional drug overdose mortality in years of life lost among adolescents and young people in the US from 2015 to 2019. JAMA Pediatr. 2022;176(4):415–7.
3. Hasin DS, Shmulewitz D, Sarvet AL. Time trends in US cannabis use and cannabis use disorders overall and by sociodemographic subgroups: a narrative review and new findings. Am J Drug Alcohol Abuse. 2019;45(6):623–43.
4. Wilson J, Freeman TP, Mackie CJ. Effects of increasing cannabis potency on adolescent health. Lancet Child Adolesc Health. 2019;3(2):121–8.
5. Johnston LD, Miech RA, O'Malley PM, Bachman JG, Schulenberg JE, Patrick ME. Monitoring the future National Survey Results on drug use, 1975–2018: overview, key findings on adolescent drug use. Institute for Social Research. Institute for Social Research; 2019. https://eric.ed.gov/?id=ED594190. Accessed 3 Oct 2022.
6. Bukstein OG. Treating adolescents with substance use disorders. New York: The Guilford Press; 2019. p. 268.
7. Porche MV, Fortuna LR, Tolou-Shams M. Unpacking the layers: dismantling inequities in substance use services and outcomes for racially minoritized adolescents. Child Adolesc Psychiatr Clin N Am. 2022;31(2):223–36.
8. Morales AM, Jones SA, Kliamovich D, Harman G, Nagel BJ. Identifying early risk factors for addiction later in life: a review of prospective longitudinal studies. Curr Addict Rep. 2020;7(1):89–98.
9. Hughes K, Bellis MA, Hardcastle KA, Sethi D, Butchart A, Mikton C, et al. The effect of multiple adverse childhood experiences on health: a systematic review and meta-analysis. Lancet Public Health. 2017;2(8):e356–66.
10. Ray LA, Meredith LR, Kiluk BD, Walthers J, Carroll KM, Magill M. Combined pharmacotherapy and cognitive behavioral therapy for adults with alcohol or substance use disorders: a systematic review and meta-analysis. JAMA Netw Open. 2020;3(6):e208279.
11. Steele DW, Becker SJ, Danko KJ, Balk EM, Saldanha IJ, Adam GP, et al. Interventions for substance use disorders in adolescents: a systematic review. Rockville: Agency for Healthcare Research and Quality (US); 2020. http://www.ncbi.nlm.nih.gov/books/NBK557291/.
12. Nugent C. SAMHSA's working definition of recovery. 8.

13. Alinsky RH, Hadland SE, Quigley J, Patrick SW, Committee on Substance Use and Prevention. Recommended terminology for substance use disorders in the care of children, adolescents, young adults, and families. Pediatrics. 2022;149(6):e2022057529.
14. Bagley SM, Hadland SE, Schoenberger SF, Gai MJ, Topp D, Hallett E, et al. Integrating substance use care into primary care for adolescents and young adults: lessons learned. J Subst Abus Treat. 2021;129:108376.
15. McGorry PD, Purcell R, Goldstone S, Amminger GP. Age of onset and timing of treatment for mental and substance use disorders: implications for preventive intervention strategies and models of care. Curr Opin Psychiatry. 2011;24(4):301–6.
16. Krist AH, Davidson KW, Mangione CM, US Preventive Services Task Force, et al. Screening for unhealthy drug use: US preventive services task force recommendation statement. JAMA. 2020;323(22):2301–9.
17. Levy SJL, Williams JF, Committee on Substance Use and Prevention. Substance use screening, brief intervention, and referral to treatment. Pediatrics. 2016;138(1):e20161211.
18. Burkstein OG, Bernet W, Arnold V, Beitchman J, Shaw J, Benson S, et al. Practice parameter for the assessment and treatment of children and adolescents with substance use disorders. J Am Acad Child Adolesc Psychiatry. 2005;44:609–21.
19. Larochelle MR, Bernson D, Land T, Stopka TJ, Wang N, Xuan Z, et al. Medication for opioid use disorder after nonfatal opioid overdose and association with mortality: a cohort study. Ann Intern Med. 2018;169(3):137–45.
20. Esmaeelzadeh S, Moraros J, Thorpe L, Bird Y. Examining the association and directionality between mental health disorders and substance use among adolescents and young adults in the U.S. and Canada—a systematic review and meta-analysis. J Clin Med. 2018;7(12):E543.
21. SAMSHA. TIP 31: Screening and Assessing Adolescents for Substance Use Disorders | SAMHSA Publications and Digital Products [Internet]. https://www.store.samhsa.gov/product/TIP-31-Screening-and-Assessing-Adolescents-for-Substance-Use-Disorders/SMA12-4079. Accessed 3 Oct 2022.
22. Conrad R, Brumbaugh B. Respect for persons in the psychiatric treatment of children and adolescents. Psychiatr Clin N Am. 2021;44(4):613–25.
23. Hasin DS, O'Brien CP, Auriacombe M, Borges G, Bucholz K, Budney A, et al. DSM-5 criteria for substance use disorders: recommendations and rationale. Am J Psychiatry. 2013;170(8):834–51.
24. Wakeman SE, Larochelle MR, Ameli O, Chaisson CE, McPheeters JT, Crown WH, et al. Comparative effectiveness of different treatment pathways for opioid use disorder. JAMA Netw Open. 2020;3(2):e1920622.
25. Mee-Lee D. The New ASAM criteria for the treatment of addictive, substance-related, and co-occurring conditions—what you might need to re-form for healthcare reform. 10.
26. Cohen SM, Alexander RS, Holt SR. The spectrum of alcohol use: epidemiology, diagnosis, and treatment. Med Clin N Am. 2022;106(1):43–60.
27. Cservenka A, Brumback T. The burden of binge and heavy drinking on the brain: effects on adolescent and young adult neural structure and function. Front Psychol. 2017;8:1111.
28. Jacobus J, Tapert SF. Neurotoxic effects of alcohol in adolescence. Annu Rev Clin Psychol. 2013;9:703–21.
29. Maillard A, Cabé N, Viader F, Pitel AL. Neuropsychological deficits in alcohol use disorder; 2020. p. 103–28.
30. Spanagel R. Alcoholism: a systems approach from molecular physiology to addictive behavior. Physiol Rev. 2009;89(2):649–705.
31. Rastegar DA, Fingerhood MI. The American Society of Addiction Medicine handbook of addiction medicine. 2nd ed. New York: Oxford University Press; 2020.
32. Reus VI, Fochtmann LJ, Bukstein O, Eyler AE, Hilty DM, Horvitz-Lennon M, et al. The American Psychiatric Association practice guideline for the pharmacological treatment of patients with alcohol use disorder. Am J Psychiatry. 2018;175(1):86–90.
33. Hammond CJ, Gray KM. Pharmacotherapy for substance use disorders in youths. J Child Adolesc Subst Abuse. 2016;25(4):292–316.
34. Hasin DS. US epidemiology of cannabis use and associated problems. Neuropsychopharmacology. 2018;43(1):195–212.
35. Wadsworth E, Craft S, Calder R, Hammond D. Prevalence and use of cannabis products and routes of administration among youth and young adults in Canada and the United States: a systematic review. Addict Behav. 2022;129:107258.
36. Slawek DE, Curtis SA, Arnsten JH, Cunningham CO. Clinical approaches to cannabis: a narrative review. Med Clin N Am. 2022;106(1):131–52.
37. Ashton CH. Pharmacology and effects of cannabis: a brief review. Br J Psychiatry. 2001;178:101–6.
38. Gorey C, Kuhns L, Smaragdi E, Kroon E, Cousijn J. Age-related differences in the impact of cannabis use on the brain and cognition: a systematic review. Eur Arch Psychiatry Clin Neurosci. 2019;269(1):37–58.
39. Gray KM, Carpenter MJ, Baker NL, DeSantis SM, Kryway E, Hartwell KJ, et al. A double-blind randomized controlled trial of *N*-acetylcysteine in cannabis-dependent adolescents. Am J Psychiatry. 2012;169(8):805–12.
40. Gentzke AS. Tobacco product use among middle and high school students—United States, 2020. MMWR Morb Mortal Wkly Rep. 2020. https://www.cdc.gov/mmwr/volumes/69/wr/mm6950a1.htm.
41. Reitsma MB, Kendrick PJ, Ababneh E, Abbafati C, Abbasi-Kangevari M, Abdoli A, et al. Spatial, temporal, and demographic patterns in prevalence of smoking tobacco use and attributable disease burden in 204 countries and territories, 1990–2019: a systematic analysis from the Global Burden of Disease Study 2019. Lancet. 2021;397(10292):2337–60.

42. Cornelius ME. Tobacco product use among adults—United States, 2020. MMWR Morb Mortal Wkly Rep. 2022. https://www.cdc.gov/mmwr/volumes/71/wr/mm7111a1.htm.
43. Benowitz NL. Pharmacology of nicotine: addiction, smoking-induced disease, and therapeutics. Annu Rev Pharmacol Toxicol. 2009;49:57–71.
44. Mishra A, Chaturvedi P, Datta S, Sinukumar S, Joshi P, Garg A. Harmful effects of nicotine. Indian J Med Paediatr Oncol. 2015;36(1):24–31.
45. US Preventive Services Task Force, Owens DK, Davidson KW, Krist AH, Barry MJ, Cabana M, et al. Primary care interventions for prevention and cessation of tobacco use in children and adolescents: US preventive services task force recommendation statement. JAMA. 2020;323(16):1590–8.
46. Anthenelli RM, Benowitz NL, West R, St Aubin L, McRae T, Lawrence D, et al. Neuropsychiatric safety and efficacy of varenicline, bupropion, and nicotine patch in smokers with and without psychiatric disorders (EAGLES): a double-blind, randomised, placebo-controlled clinical trial. Lancet. 2016;387(10037):2507–20.
47. Owens DK, Davidson KW, Krist AH, US Preventive Services Task Force, et al. Interventions for tobacco smoking cessation in adults, including pregnant persons: US preventive services task force recommendation statement. JAMA. 2021;325(3):265–79.
48. Myung SK, Park JY. Efficacy of pharmacotherapy for smoking cessation in adolescent smokers: a meta-analysis of randomized controlled trials. Nicotine Tob Res. 2019;21(11):1473–9.
49. Ahmad F, Rossen L, Sutton P. Products—vital statistics rapid release—provisional drug overdose data [Internet]. 2022. https://www.cdc.gov/nchs/nvss/vsrr/drug-overdose-data.htm. Accessed 3 Oct 2022.
50. Baldwin GT, Seth P, Noonan RK. Continued increases in overdose deaths related to synthetic opioids: implications for clinical practice. JAMA. 2021;325(12):1151–2.
51. Gomes T, Tadrous M, Mamdani MM, Paterson JM, Juurlink DN. The burden of opioid-related mortality in the United States. JAMA Netw Open. 2018;1(2):e180217.
52. Gaither JR, Shabanova V, Leventhal JM. US National Trends in pediatric deaths from prescription and illicit opioids, 1999–2016. JAMA Netw Open. 2018;1(8):e186558.
53. Schroeder AR, Dehghan M, Newman TB, Bentley JP, Park KT. Association of Opioid Prescriptions from Dental Clinicians for US adolescents and young adults with subsequent opioid use and abuse. JAMA Intern Med. 2019;179(2):145–52.
54. Hudgins JD, Porter JJ, Monuteaux MC, Bourgeois FT. Prescription opioid use and misuse among adolescents and young adults in the United States: a national survey study. PLoS Med. 2019;16(11):e1002922.
55. Chua KP, Brummett CM, Conti RM, Bohnert A. Association of opioid prescribing patterns with prescription opioid overdose in adolescents and young adults. JAMA Pediatr. 2020;174(2):141–8.
56. Dowell D, Haegerich T, Chou R. No shortcuts to safer opioid prescribing. N Engl J Med. 2019;380(24):2285–7.
57. Brat GA, Agniel D, Beam A, Yorkgitis B, Bicket M, Homer M, et al. Postsurgical prescriptions for opioid naive patients and association with overdose and misuse: retrospective cohort study. BMJ. 2018;360:j5790.
58. Crotty K, Freedman KI, Kampman KM. Executive summary of the focused update of the ASAM National Practice Guideline for the treatment of opioid use disorder. J Addict Med. 2020;14(2):99–112.
59. Taylor JL, Samet JH. Opioid use disorder. Ann Intern Med. 2022;175(1):ITC1–16.
60. Volkow ND, Jones EB, Einstein EB, Wargo EM. Prevention and treatment of opioid misuse and addiction: a review. JAMA Psychiatry. 2019;76(2):208–16.
61. Hadland SE, Aalsma MC, Akgül S, Alinsky RH, Bruner A, Chadi N, Galagali PM, Kreida EC, Robinson CA, Wilson JD. Medication for adolescents and young adults with opioid use disorder. J Adolesc Health. 2021;68:632–6.
62. Committee on Substance Use and Prevention. Medication-assisted treatment of adolescents with opioid use disorders. Pediatrics. 2016;138(3):e20161893.
63. Becker SJ, Scott K, Helseth SA, Danko KJ, Balk EM, Saldanha IJ, et al. Effectiveness of medication for opioid use disorders in transition-age youth: a systematic review. J Subst Abuse Treat. 2022;132:108494. https://www.journalofsubstanceabusetreatment.com/article/S0740-5472(21)00220-8/fulltext.
64. Viera A, Bromberg DJ, Whittaker S, Refsland BM, Stanojlović M, Nyhan K, et al. Adherence to and retention in medications for opioid use disorder among adolescents and young adults. Epidemiol Rev. 2020;42(1):41–56.
65. Rice D, Corace K, Wolfe D, Esmaeilisaraji L, Michaud A, Grima A, et al. Evaluating comparative effectiveness of psychosocial interventions adjunctive to opioid agonist therapy for opioid use disorder: a systematic review with network meta-analyses. PLoS One. 2020;15(12):e0244401.
66. Taylor JL, Johnson S, Cruz R, Gray JR, Schiff D, Bagley SM. Integrating harm reduction into outpatient opioid use disorder treatment settings: harm reduction in outpatient addiction treatment. J Gen Intern Med. 2021;36(12):3810–9.
67. Stockings E, Hall WD, Lynskey M, Morley KI, Reavley N, Strang J, et al. Prevention, early intervention, harm reduction, and treatment of substance use in young people. Lancet Psychiatry. 2016;3(3):280–96.
68. Peiper NC, Clarke SD, Vincent LB, Ciccarone D, Kral AH, Zibbell JE. Fentanyl test strips as an opioid overdose prevention strategy: findings from a syringe services program in the southeastern United States. Int J Drug Policy. 2019;63:122–8.
69. Puzhko S, Eisenberg MJ, Filion KB, Windle SB, Hébert-Losier A, Gore G, et al. Effectiveness of

interventions for prevention of common infections among opioid users: a systematic review of systematic reviews. Front Public Health. 2022;10:749033. https://doi.org/10.3389/fpubh.2022.749033.
70. Lipari RN, Park-Lee E (2019) Key substance use and mental health indicators in the United States: results from the 2018 National Survey on Drug Use and Health
71. Sara GE, Large MM, Matheson SL, Burgess PM, Malhi GS, Whiteford HA, et al. Stimulant use disorders in people with psychosis: a meta-analysis of rate and factors affecting variation. Aust N Z J Psychiatry. 2015;49(2):106–17.
72. Ronsley C, Nolan S, Knight R, Hayashi K, Klimas J, Walley A, et al. Treatment of stimulant use disorder: a systematic review of reviews. PLoS One. 2020;15(6):e0234809.
73. Tran MTN, Luong QH, Le Minh G, Dunne MP, Baker P. Psychosocial interventions for amphetamine type stimulant use disorder: an overview of systematic reviews. Front Psychiatry. 2021;12:512076. https://doi.org/10.3389/fpsyt.2021.512076.
74. Griffin CE, Kaye AM, Bueno FR, Kaye AD. Benzodiazepine pharmacology and central nervous system-mediated effects. Ochsner J. 2013;13(2):214–23.
75. Pollmann AS, Murphy AL, Bergman JC, Gardner DM. Deprescribing benzodiazepines and Z-drugs in community-dwelling adults: a scoping review. BMC Pharmacol Toxicol. 2015;16(1):19.
76. National Center for PTSD Veterans Affairs (2013) Effective treatments for PTSD: helping patients taper from benzodiazepines.
77. Ogbonna CI, Lembke A. Tapering patients off of benzodiazepines. Am Fam Physician. 2017;96(9):606–10.
78. Baandrup L, Ebdrup BH, Rasmussen JØ, Lindschou J, Gluud C, Glenthøj BY. Pharmacological interventions for benzodiazepine discontinuation in chronic benzodiazepine users. Cochrane Database Syst Rev. 2018;2018:CD011481. https://doi.org/10.1002/14651858.CD011481.pub2/full.
79. Parr JM, Kavanagh DJ, Cahill L, Mitchell G, Young MR. Effectiveness of current treatment approaches for benzodiazepine discontinuation: a meta-analysis. Addiction. 2009;104(1):13–24.
80. Hendrickx G, De Roeck V, Maras A, Dieleman G, Gerritsen S, Purper-Ouakil D, et al. Challenges during the transition from child and adolescent mental health services to adult mental health services. BJPsych Bull. 2020;44(4):163–8.

# College Mental Health

# 20

Jessica Haddad, Meera Menon, and Rachel Conrad

## Introduction

U.S. college students are facing a mental health crisis. Over the last several decades, there have been steadily increasing rates of mental health problems at colleges and universities [1]. Depression, anxiety, and suicidal behaviors in particular have reached record highs at the collegiate level [1]. Potential explanations for these national trends include more students with preexisting psychiatric disorders pursuing postsecondary education [2] due to treatment advances, progressively increasing societal expectations for academic achievement, financial stressors, the pressure to succeed, and technological advancements [3, 4].

Exacerbating this trend, the novel coronavirus (SARS-CoV-2) and its corresponding disease (COVID-19) have had tremendous impacts on college students' mental health [5]. Rates of anxiety and depression in college-age individuals have skyrocketed during the pandemic [6, 7]. In addition, rates of low self-esteem, loneliness, stress, substance misuse, and suicidality have grown rapidly [8]. This may be because college students are encountering unique stressors including interruptions in their education, technological concerns about online learning, hindrance of physical activity and extracurricular activities, social isolation, lack of college belongingness, decreased family income, financial concerns threatening their future education, and uncertainty about future employment [9, 10].

There is an expanding need for mental health services on college campuses. According to the 2019–2020 Association of College Counseling Center Directors (AUCCCD) survey, which compared pre-pandemic data (July 1, 2019, through March 15, 2020) and pandemic data (March 16, 2020, through June 30, 2020), the COVID-19 pandemic has had dramatic impacts on service delivery [7]. Most notably, the utilization of telehealth services increased by 6811%. Although service demand was inconsistent across institutions, 81% of counseling centers reported utilizing at least one method to manage increased demand for services.

## Unique Developmental Needs and Challenges

### General Health Literacy

Emerging adulthood is a transitional period between adolescence and adulthood, usually defined as ages 18–25. This transition to adult-

J. Haddad · R. Conrad (✉)
Department of Psychiatry, Harvard Medical School and Brigham and Women's Hospital, Boston, MA, USA
e-mail: jhaddad@bwh.harvard.edu

M. Menon
The Ohio State University Medical Center, Columbus, OH, USA
e-mail: rconrad@bwh.harvard.edu


A. A. Kuo et al. (eds.), *Care of Adults with Chronic Childhood Conditions*,
https://doi.org/10.1007/978-3-031-54281-7_20

hood is a vulnerable time, especially for those individuals who choose to enroll in college [10]. College-related stressors include leaving and living away from home, academic pressures, social demands, and increased access to alcohol and drugs, which might impair medical decision-making. Furthermore, most college students lack the healthcare literacy, maturity, and organizational skills to effectively and independently manage their own medical care [10]. The Jed Foundation's "Set to Go" Initiative is an example of an online resource aimed at preparing students, families, and high school counselors for the transition to college [11].

Specific populations have additional barriers to health care when transitioning to college, often stemming from both personal and systemic deficits. For example, college students with ADHD struggle with time management, task prioritization, and efficient learning [12]. System-wise, there is a scarcity of ADHD-trained providers on college campuses [12]. To increase access to care for this population, prior to transitioning to college their providers should focus on developing a more personal provider-patient dynamic that slowly shifts the responsibility of care to patients while encouraging independence through trust and empathy [12]. Additionally, guiding patients on their educational future (e.g., slower transition with fewer courses and joining a 2-year or junior college) and care involvement (e.g., teaching how to access support and schedule appointments) is needed to tailor care. Utilizing technology that already captures patient attention may be a successful method of imparting these skills [12].

## Help-Seeking

Despite high rates of psychiatric symptoms, distress, and suicide in college students, most afflicted students are not utilizing treatment [13–16]. Approximately 40% and 34% of college students today report experiencing depressive symptoms and anxiety symptoms, respectively [1]. However, only 13% of students utilized campus counseling center services during the 2019–2020 academic year [7]. Help-seeking behaviors are largely influenced by an individual's attitude and knowledge about treatment [14]. Barriers to treatment include cultural and societal stigmas around mental illness and treatment. In fact, while only 6% of college students say they would think less of someone who received mental health treatment (personal stigma), 45% think that other people would (perceived public stigma) [14]. Some recent evidence suggests that many untreated students actually have positive attitudes and beliefs about treatment, which implies that solely addressing stigma is insufficient to address help-seeking [14]. Other potential barriers to treatment include lack of perceived need, reliance on non-professional services, social influences (e.g., whether close friends or family have used treatment), uncertainty about how to access services, concerns about cost and insurance coverage, and lack of diversity or cultural humility among providers [14].

## Sociopolitical Impacts on College Mental Health

Political and social climates have direct and indirect impacts on college students' mental health [17, 18]. In times of sociopolitical unrest, there is heightened stress among marginalized individuals and communities [18]. Not only do these groups face direct threats to their livelihood when policy changes occur, but they are also often targets of animosity and anger-fueled rhetoric from opposing parties [18, 19]. "Hot button issues" include college affordability, gun control, racial justice, immigration status, LGBTQ healthcare, and sexual assault. Political discord on campus has been shown to decrease the sense of unity and sense of belongingness on campus [19]. However, political activism among underrepresented minorities (URM) might mitigate race-related anxiety, particularly for Latinx students [17]. It should be noted that due in part to the algorithmic nature of social media programs, excessive social media use among college students has been shown to exacerbate political polarization and increase psychological distress [20].

The impact of social unrest during COVID-19 may have compounded the increased anxiety and depression among college students during the COVID-19 pandemic. After the highly publicized killing of unarmed Black men, many college students and young adults were engaged in social activism and protests against racism and police violence. More than half of young adults cite concerns with police violence toward minorities as a major stressor [21]. New research shows that concerns about the social climate during COVID-19 were significantly associated with increasing symptoms of generalized anxiety disorders among college students [22].

## Underrepresented Minorities

Historically underrepresented minorities (URMs) have been enrolling in college in progressively higher numbers over the last 25 years [23]. As such, today's colleges and universities serve a diverse student population in terms of age, race/ethnicity, socioeconomic status, and academic readiness [23]. College is a time when students often explore their racial/ethnic, gender, and sexual identities [15], which makes it imperative for colleges to implement culturally informed mental health programs and improve support for URM students. Currently, the majority of counseling center staff are White, heterosexual, or cisgender females [7].

Students from racial and ethnic minority backgrounds have increased rates of mental health problems but are less likely to utilize mental health services due to a variety of factors including discrimination, imposter syndrome, stigma, and limited availability of diverse and culturally competent mental health providers [13, 14, 24]. Asian college students tend to be least likely to utilize treatment despite having similar rates of psychiatric symptoms compared to White students [13, 15]. Mental health disparities are also quite stark in Black men [25]. These disparities are partially explained by issues of social injustice, systemic racism, and police brutality, as research has shown that exposure to the killing of unarmed Black people by police has been associated with worse mental health outcomes [18]. They might also be a consequence of underreporting or lack of reporting given treatment underutilization, educational disparities, low college enrollment, and higher dropout rates in this group [24]. Latinx young adults have also been enrolling in college at unprecedented rates over the last two decades [23]. Studies of this group have shown mental health symptoms to be positively associated with cultural stressors and negatively associated with familial values and religiosity [26].

Relatedly, lesbian, gay, bisexual, transgender, queer or questioning, and other sexual minorities (LGBTQ+) have higher rates of mental health symptomatology than their heterosexual counterparts. These students are also more likely to utilize mental health services [15]; however, they tend to seek off-campus services, likely due to perceived stigma on campus [27]. Transgender students have particularly high rates of mental health disorders, trauma, and suicidality [15, 28]. Compared to cisgender students, they experience more violence, have more sex partners and more sexually transmitted infections, use more alcohol and other substances, and report more barriers to academic success [28]. Increasing access to care for these students is imperative and campuses should emphasize hiring providers competent in sexual identity issues.

## Trends in Acuity

### Psychiatric Symptoms and Diagnosis in College Students

The acuity and volume of psychiatric symptoms on college campuses have steadily and dramatically increased over the last several decades. According to a recent Healthy Minds Study, which gathered data from 32,754 college students in the United States in 2020, 41% of college students have a lifetime diagnosis of at least one mental disorder [1]. More specifically, 39% of college students have major or moderate depression, 34% have an anxiety disorder, 11% have an eating disorder, 23% have engaged in non-suicidal self-injury within the past year, and 13% reported suicidal ideation within the past year. There were similar results from an Active Minds survey of 2086 college students from April 2020, in which 91% had stress or anxiety, 80% reported loneliness, and 55% did not know where to go if they needed mental health services [29].

The American College Health Association-National College Health Assessment (ACHA-NCHA) 2015 survey, which includes data on 93,034 students from 108 colleges or universities in the United States, found similarly high rates of psychiatric symptoms and diagnoses and also revealed complex relationships among racial-ethnic minority status, mental illness symptomatology, and psychiatric diagnoses [30]. College students who identify as Black, Indigenous, or People of Color (BIPOC) generally had lower rates of self-reported past-year psychiatric diagnosis and symptoms of mental illness compared to White students. However, compared to White students, Asian/Pacific Islander students were significantly more likely to endorse having felt hopeless, having felt so depressed that it was difficult to function, and having felt overwhelmed by anger and were also significantly more likely to have seriously considered or attempted suicide, all in the past year. Past-year suicide attempts among Black and Latinx students were significantly elevated compared with White students. Multiracial students were more likely to engage in intentional self-injury and attempt suicide compared to White students. American Indian, Native Alaskan, and Native Hawaiian students had strikingly higher rates of attempted suicide compared to Whites. Thus, there are blatant inconsistencies between psychiatric diagnoses and symptomatology in BIPOCs.

The lower rates of self-reported psychiatric diagnoses among BIPOC college students compared to Whites could represent a true difference in prevalence or could reflect disparities in mental health care [13]. Systemic bias has been shown to limit BIPOC students' access to mental health services. When this population does access care, a lack of culturally competent clinicians might result in the minimization or misinterpretation of their symptoms, or even misdiagnosis and mistreatment [15]. Evidence has shown that language and instruments for detecting psychiatric symptoms might be less sensitive for use among certain BIPOC [31]. Another possible explanation could be underreporting or lack of reporting in BIPOC due to stigma [13].

## Treatment Utilization

The number of students who visited campus counseling centers rose 30% from Fall 2009 to Spring 2015 [30], compared to an average 6% institutional enrollment increase [32]. Given this discrepancy, it is possible that counseling centers that receive funding based on student body size might be underfunded [32]. Although it appears that more students are seeking help, given the alarmingly high rates of distress, psychiatric symptoms, and suicide on college campuses, it can be argued that treatment utilization is still relatively low [13–16].

Bourdon and colleagues analyzed data from 3734 college sophomores at a large, urban university to explore which mental health concerns were associated with on-campus service utilization [33]. Information was collected on four college health services that are common at universities nationwide: (1) University Counseling Services (provides therapy services, professional training, consultation, and outreach); (2) University Health Services (provides outpatient primary care and refers students to counseling if indicated); (3) The Wellness Resource Center (disseminates resources about healthy and safe lifestyle); and (4) Disability Support Services (assists students with gaining access to all university programs, services, and events by providing disability services and helping the university comply with the ADA). The authors found that alcohol use disorder symptoms predicted the most overall and specific service utilization, followed by depression symptoms and stressful life events. Anxiety symptoms and antisocial behaviors were not significant predictors. More specifically, use of University Counseling Services was significantly associated with depression and being Black, use of University Health Services was positively associated with stressful life events and being female and was negatively associated with being Asian, and use of both the Wellness Resource Center and Disability Support Services was associated mainly with alcohol use disorder symptoms.

## Medications

Psychiatric medication use by U.S. college students has been trending upward according to the Center for Collegiate Mental Health [32]. In 2020, 24% of college students reported taking psychiatric medication within the past year [14]. More specifically, 6% used psychostimulants, 17% used antidepressants, 1% used antipsychotics, 7% used anxiolytics, 3% used mood stabilizers, and 4% used sleep medications [14]. These numbers were unanimously higher in students with positive depression or anxiety screens. Increased medication use might indicate a higher prevalence of psychiatric diagnoses requiring treatment, a lower threshold to offer medication among prescribers, or increased access to mental health care. Students living on campus are less likely to use psychotropic medications [14], although the reasons for this are uncertain.

## Suicide Among College Students

There has been a significant upward trend in suicide and non-suicidal self-injury behaviors, and suicide is currently the third leading cause of death among college students, after unintentional injury and homicide [34]. 15–20% of students today have considered suicide, with 9% reporting having attempted suicide and 20% reporting self-injury [30]. Self-harm and suicidality were elevated in transfer students and students with a history of psychological trauma [30]. Just like psychiatric symptoms and diagnoses in general, there were racial and ethnic discrepancies in suicidality. Asian students had higher rates of suicidal ideation and suicide attempts despite lower rates of psychiatric diagnoses compared to White students, which is concerning for under-detection and underdiagnosis in this group [15]. Multiracial students, similar to Asian students, had higher rates of suicidal ideation and attempts [15]. LGBTQ+ students also had elevated rates of suicidal thoughts and behaviors, with over two-thirds endorsing suicidal ideation, two-thirds reporting self-injury, and over one-third attempting suicide [30]. According to the WHO World Mental Health Surveys International College Student Project, which collected data from 13,984 first-year college students across 19 colleges in eight countries (Australia, Belgium, Germany, Mexico, Northern Ireland, South Africa, Spain, and the United States), sexual minority status was most strongly correlated with suicidal thoughts and behaviors, which was consistent cross-nationally [16].

Many colleges have historically responded to suicidal students by mandating a medical leave of absence to reduce their liability; however, the vast majority of students who experience suicidal ideation do not end up attempting it [3]. In fact, suicide rates in college students who live on campus are lower than those of similarly aged individuals not enrolled in college [7]. This indicates college campuses might inherently offer some layer of protection against suicide by offering a sense of community, fostering student independence, distance from intrafamilial conflict, barriers to obtaining weapons, and potentially more access to mental health services than in the community. As such, involuntary leave should function as a last resort and colleges should instead aim to make changes that will prevent suicide among their students.

The Jed Foundation (JED), which aims to prevent suicide and promote mental health among college students, was founded by Phil and Donna Satow in 1998 after their son died of suicide when he was a student in college. JED used the US Air Force's research about suicide prevention in the mid-1990s to develop the Comprehensive Approach to Mental Health Promotion and Suicide Prevention for Colleges and Universities. This strategic plan encompasses four thematic areas: (1) prevention and enhancing protective factors (develop life skills and promote social connectedness), (2) early intervention (identify students at risk and increase help-seeking behavior), (3) assuring access to a full range of clinical care and services (provide mental health and substance use services and follow crisis management procedures), and (4) restricting access to potentially lethal means [11].

JED Campus (https://www.jedcampus.org/) is a program JED launched in 2013 to guide schools through the comprehensive process of self-assessment and strategic planning around suicide prevention and mental health promotion [11]. JED works collaboratively with schools by assessing their policies, programs, and services and providing a feedback report and optional consultation with senior JED clinician consultants. As of April 2022, there are over 370 JED Campus schools, representing more than 4.8 million students. The program has resulted in increased gatekeeper training, increased screening for mental health problems during visits to health services, expanded access to 24/7 crisis support, expanded access to naloxone on campus, and increased environmental safety and means restriction protocols (e.g., securing building roofs, windows, chemistry laboratories, and firearm policies). Evidence is promising so far, with trends suggesting drops in rates of suicide, overdose deaths, psychiatric emergencies and hospitalizations, and dropout rates.

## Substance Use

There is mixed evidence regarding trends in collegiate substance use, but the general prevalence of substance use in the United States has dropped or remained relatively flat over the last couple of decades. However, the trends vary by substance, as data suggest that heavy alcohol use may be decreasing, while nicotine and marijuana use are rising. Furthermore, during the COVID-19 pandemic, 24.7% of young adults ages 18–24 years reported that they started or increased substance use to cope with pandemic-related stress or emotions [35].

According to data from the recent Healthy Minds Study, 2% of college students have been diagnosed with a substance use disorder (SUD) in their lifetime [14]. Alcohol and substance use among college students is positively associated with rates of depression, anxiety, suicidal ideation, and relationship violence and is negatively correlated with academic performance and overall well-being [11]. Thus, the education, prevention, and treatment of substance use disorders are in the best interest of the college [11]. According to the National Epidemiologic Survey on Alcohol and Related Conditions (NESARC) study, treatment utilization is currently and historically low among students with SUDs [36].

Alcohol use is prevalent in the college student population; however, rates of binge drinking among 18- to 22-year-olds have been decreasing in the past decade. According to the 2019 National Survey on Drug Use and Health (NSDUH), 27.7% of people in this age group who are not enrolled in college full-time and 33% of full-time college students in this age group reported binge drinking in the past month, in which binge drinking was defined as consuming 4–5 drinks in a row [37]. Rates of alcohol use disorder among emerging adults dropped from 17.7 to 10.9% from 2002 to 2015 [38].

Marijuana use is also high and rising among college students. According to NSDUH, rates of current marijuana users increased from 17.3% in 2002 to 19.9% in 2015. Rates have subsequently increased further, and a 2020 study revealed relatively stable prevalence rates of 30% [14]. The popularity of vaping tetrahydrocannabinol (THC) oil is on the rise according to the University of Michigan's annual U.S. National Monitoring the Future Panel Study. Between 2017 and 2019, the percentage of 19-to-22-year-old college students who vaped marijuana at least once in the past 30 days (30-day prevalence) increased from 5 to 14% [39]. One possible reason for increased marijuana use is the public decline in perceived risk of harm from regular marijuana use. In 2019, only 24% of those aged 19–22 perceived regular use of marijuana as carrying great risk of harm, which is among the lowest levels since 1980 when tracking of this age group began [39]. It is likely that rates of marijuana use will continue to increase as it becomes decriminalized and legalized across states.

Similarly, college students have been vaping nicotine at rapidly increasing rates. Between 2017 and 2019, the 30-day prevalence of vaping nicotine increased from 6 to 22% among college students and from 8 to 18% among 19-to-22-year-olds not in college [39]. However, cigarette use among young adults continues its long-term decline, with 30-day prevalence near the all-time low at 7.9% in 2019 for college students and at 16% for same-aged youth not in college [39]. Young adults believe that vaping e-cigarettes is less harmful than using combustible tobacco cigarettes [40]. However, studies by the U.S. Food and Drug Administration show that e-cigarette aerosol contains harmful substances including nicotine, heavy metals like lead, volatile organic compounds, and cancer-causing agents, and the long-term risk of vaping will not be known for several decades [40].

The prevalence of other illicit drug use has remained relatively low for the last two decades. In 2020, only 1% of college students used cocaine, 1% used stimulants (e.g., Ritalin and Adderall) without a prescription or more than prescribed, 1% used LSD, 2% used psilocybin, and <1% used heroin, opioid pain relievers, benzodiazepines, methamphetamines, MDMA, ketamine, kratom, or athletic performance enhancers within the last 30 days [14]. Of note, the data from the Healthy Minds Study are based on self-report, and so it is possible that surveyed college students did not accurately report use.

## System Barriers to Psychiatric Care for College Students

### Ethical and Legal Challenges Around Consent

Principle-based medical ethics serve as an analytic framework to resolve ethical issues and are broadly defined as respect for autonomy, beneficence, nonmaleficence, and justice [41]. These principles must be considered when balancing a student's personal rights with a university's duties [42]. Conflict arises when federal legislation and case law conflict with these ethical principles.

*Autonomy* refers to the idea that every individual has a unique viewpoint and has self-directing freedom in decision-making [41]. An autonomous individual should act with intent and understanding and without controlling influence [41]. Parental figures and university officials are examples of controlling influences that could challenge a college student's autonomy. Many students rely on their parents for basic resources (e.g., finances, transportation, and housing), resulting in a functional interdependence. As such, although at age 18 an individual in the United States has a legal right to autonomous medical decision-making, college students sometimes have no choice but to involve their parents in their medical care [42, 43].

Ideally, high-risk college students would collaborate with their families, mental health providers, and school administrators when making treatment decisions; however, the student might not grant permission for the school to contact their parents. There are two federal laws that regulate the sharing of student mental health records: the Family Educational Rights and Privacy Act (FERPA) of 1974 and the Health Insurance Portability and Accountability Act (HIPAA) Privacy Rule of 1996. FERPA protects the privacy of public students' personal education records, as well as certain student health records [44]. HIPAA protects sensitive health information and is especially relevant for off-campus treatment. Both FERPA and HIPAA have been amended to allow schools to break confidentiality in emergency situations (45 CFR § 164.512(j)(1)). Complicating matters further, state privacy laws regarding mental health supersede FERPA and HIPAA if they are more stringent, and several states require the college to break confidentiality if a student is considered a threat to themselves or others. School officials should review federal and state laws when considering talking to a parent without a student's consent.

*Beneficence* is defined as acting to produce or promote the well-being of others, which in the clinical setting dictates that the provider acts in good faith as an advocate for their patient [41]. A provider's personal perception of beneficent behavior should not violate a patient's autonomy.

Alternatively, *nonmaleficence* refers to the ethical and legal duty of medical providers to "do no harm" [41]. This principle is closely related to "duty to warn." In the case of *Tarasoff v. Regents of the University of California* (1976), graduate student, Prosenjit Poddar, disclosed to his psychotherapist that he was planning on killing a fellow student, Tatiana Tarasoff, who had rejected his advances [45]. The psychotherapist informed the police, but Poddar was deemed rational and immediately released from custody. There was no warning given to Tarasoff or her family, and months later, Tarasoff was brutally murdered by Poddar. Tarasoff's family sued the university and several of its employees. The California Supreme Court held that mental health workers have a duty to warn a third party of harm if there is a foreseeable risk of injury or death and an identifiable contact. The doctrine has since expanded to "duty to protect," which involves "whatever steps are reasonably necessary under the circumstances."

Finally, *justice* refers to distributing resources and treating people fairly and equitably [41]. Unfortunately, there are many injustices in college mental health. Recently, it has been brought to light that URMs are psychiatrically diagnosed and treated differently than non-URMs [43]. Healthcare disparities include access to care, resources, inappropriate prescribing, and discriminatory language and behavior.

Involuntary treatment enmeshes several ethical and legal principles. In situations where a student poses a serious risk of harm to self or others, beneficence and nonmaleficence may outweigh autonomy. These situations are not uncommon. In fact, about 17% of college students sent to the hospital for mental health concerns are done so on an involuntary basis [7]. Involuntary treatment can be distressing and potentially traumatic for patients, their families, and their providers [43]. In the long term, involuntary treatment might reduce an individual's willingness to voluntarily seek mental health treatment in the future due to the negative experience. Alternatively, some individuals might look back with gratitude on the experience and experience reduction of symptoms. College students are vulnerable to feelings of disempowerment; thus, before a decision is made about involuntary treatment providers should carefully consider all potential outcomes [43].

## Medical Leaves of Absence

A medical leave of absence (MLOA) is defined as a temporary interruption in a student's program of study based on a physical or mental health problem or problems that render the fulfillment of a student's academic responsibilities no longer possible (34 CFR 668.22). A MLOA may be indicated for a student when staying at school puts them or others at significant risk of harm, when they need a higher level of care, when academic performance is being adversely impacted by their health, or when being at college is causing significant distress. Students might be apprehensive to take a MLOA due to academic and employment concerns, financial concerns (e.g., financial aid, loans, or scholarships might be affected), and social concerns (e.g., stigma, losing social support, and living at home) [46]. Although ideally the school and the student work in conjunction to decide about leave, there are times when the college might mandate an involuntary MLOA if a student is deemed to pose a significant risk of harm to themselves or others. Many colleges have been criticized for using their conduct codes to remove all students deemed suicidal from campus in order to limit the colleges' liability, rather than making decisions in the student's best interest [46]. These involuntary leaves often progress quickly and result in students being evicted from campus housing, sometimes without time to gather their belongings [3].

According to federal anti-discrimination laws such as the Americans with Disabilities Act (ADA) [47] and Section 504 of the Rehabilitation Act of 1973 [48], students with disabilities, including psychiatric disabilities, are entitled to reasonable accommodations to assist them in staying in school and to protect them from punitive action if they require medical leave. However, colleges have a long history of violating these laws. For instance, in a class action lawsuit filed in 2018, a group of Stanford University students alleged that the university repeatedly violated state and federal anti-discrimination laws through its involuntary medical leave of absence policy that required students who posed a "significant risk" or whose behavior "severely" disrupted the campus to take leave [49]. Student plaintiffs alleged that the university coerced them into leaving and that they were banned from campus housing before even collecting their belongings. In 2019, Stanford University agreed to a historic settlement in which they agreed to the following: (1) The university would take additional steps to accommodate distressed students before pressuring them to leave, (2) the university would not discriminate against students with mental health disabilities regarding MLOA, (3) the university would make it easier for students to re-enroll, (4) the university would provide greater clarity and transparency about the implications of an involuntary medical leave, and (5) the opinion of the students' personal treatment providers would be given "significant weight" regarding their ability to function at school. The Disability Rights Advocates in San Francisco called the agreement "most comprehensive (settlement) ever to protect college students with mental health disabilities from unnecessary exclusion" [49].

More recently, the U.S. Attorney's Office for the District of Rhode Island and the Disability Rights Section of the Civil Rights Division of the U.S. Department of Justice (DOJ) investigated how Brown University treated undergraduate students seeking to return from a medical leave of absence taken for mental health reasons [50]. The investigation covered undergraduate students who tried to return to Brown between the Fall 2012 and Spring 2017 semesters. The DOJ claims that Brown violated the ADA by (1) denying some undergraduate students' applications to return to Brown following medical leaves of absence, when the students met all of the requirements for returning to school, and the students' doctors and therapists said they were ready to return; (2) failing to allow some students to return after fewer than two semesters of leave where the student requested an earlier return and the student met all of the other requirements for returning to school; and (3) imposing unnecessary eligibility criteria for readmission that screened out or tended to screen out students with mental health disabilities. Brown did not admit that this was true but entered into a settlement with the DOJ on August 10, 2021.

Colleges and universities are following suit. Going forward, medical leave and return policies should have parity between mental and physical health. Decisions about voluntary and involuntary MLOA should be made on a case-by-case basis, always considering the best interest of the student. We must also consider the role of the mental health clinician who is treating the student. For instance, mandating the treating clinician to weigh in on a student's eligibility to return to campus may represent a conflict of interest.

## Risk Assessment on College Campuses

Colleges have certain legal obligations to prevent student suicide and violence on campus. Several landmark legal cases have changed how institutions respond to high-risk students. The case of *Tarasoff v. Regents of the University of California*, discussed earlier, established that there are circumstances in which clinicians should violate the confidentiality of their patients with the assurance of public safety [45]. Then came the Virginia Tech shooting of 2007, the deadliest school shooting in U.S. history, in which student Seung Hui Cho killed 32 students and faculty members and injured an additional 17 people [51]. After this horrifying incident, colleges scrambled to flag students with mental health issues earlier by creating threat assessment teams, expanding on-campus psychiatric services, and improving communication between mental health clinicians and other university officials.

In 2009, a Massachusetts Institute of Technology (MIT) graduate student, Han Nguyen, completed suicide on campus (Dzung Duy Nguyen v Massachusetts Institute of Technology) [52]. His parents alleged that MIT's negligence led to their son's wrongful death. The Massachusetts Supreme Judicial Court avowed that the university no longer stands "in loco parentis" to its students but that it does have a duty to take reasonable measures to protect a student from suicide. In this case, the court found that the university did take adequate measures by repeatedly offering psychiatric recommendations and resources that the student declined. Around the same time, Katherine Rosen, a pre-med student in her junior year at the University of California, Los Angeles (UCLA), was stabbed in the neck and chest by a classmate (Regents of University of California v Superior Court) [53]. Damon Thompson, her assailant, had a history of paranoid delusions and auditory hallucinations, had been barred from campus housing, and had allegedly told a university official that Rosen had made derogatory comments about him. Rosen survived the attack and sued UCLA for negligence, alleging that the campus was aware of Thompson's "dangerous propensities" and failed to warn and protect her. The California Supreme Court recently overturned a lower court ruling and asserted that public colleges have a duty to protect students from foreseeable violence on campus.

Taken together, these legal cases have made clear that colleges and universities have certain duties, obligations, and liabilities. Institutions today have to be more proactive about identifying students who are potentially suicidal or violent and be more assertive about intervening before harm occurs [54]. Although certain standards of care have been established, legislation and guidelines regarding campus threat assessment are still needed.

## Systems and Models of Psychiatric Care

Systems and models of mental health care for college students have evolved over the years and often reflect societal, cultural, and economic shifts [2]. U.S. colleges began to recognize the influence of mental health on education after the mental hygiene movement formed in the early 1900s. After World War I, many young veterans enrolled in college and struggled to adjust to modern life. It was not until the late 1930s that colleges saw the emergence of the "clinical counselor." In the 1940s after World War II, again millions of young men returned from war and required extensive mental health services, such that colleges began to expand resources. The 1960s saw the emergence of the community mental health model, which emphasized integrative and collaborative care. Collaborative models of care are integrative programs that combine psychiatry, primary care, health promotion, and counseling that have the potential to provide comprehensive care to transitional-age youth [2]. In the 1970s and 1980s, campuses started becoming increasingly diverse due to URM enrolling in college at higher rates. Finally, in the mid-1990s, the Internet dramatically expanded self-help resources. There is very limited empirical research assessing the effectiveness of mental healthcare systems and models on college campuses, and the existing evidence is mixed [2].

Systems of mental health care include preventive services, acute treatment, rehabilitation, transitional treatment, and maintenance treatment [55]. Prevention tends to be non-clinical in the college setting and might include health education and health promotion. Acute and maintenance treatments, on the other hand, are clinical enterprises that tend to reside in student health centers, counseling centers, and community resources.

Models of mental health care vary by scope and structure. Currently, there are four main structural models of mental health care: (1) separate counseling centers and student health centers, (2) clinically integrated care, (3) administratively integrated care, and (4) clinically and administratively integrated care [2]. Clinical integration involves merging a transitional counseling center with a comprehensive student mental health unit at the student health center. Administrative integration refers to staffing, record-keeping, and certification requirements. According to the AUCCCD Annual Survey, most colleges today have no formal integration model [2].

These structural models are supplemented by additional programming such as gatekeeper training (GKT), in which individuals working closely with students (e.g., faculty, staff, and other students) are taught how to identify warning signs of a suicide crisis and how to respond. The first GKT program, Question, Persuade, and Refer, was launched in 2016, and since then, others have been developed such as Kognito and ASIST. Many institutions have also formed behavioral intervention teams, which are groups of campus professionals who meet regularly to identify students at risk and then intervene before a serious problem arises. Other programming includes case management services, hospital resources (emergency departments, inpatient units), residential programs, partial hospitalization programs, outpatient resources, and student health services [2].

### Targeted Outreach to Minority-Identified Populations

Culturally sensitive outreach to URM students is crucial to address the underutilization of collegiate mental healthcare services [13, 14, 24]. Ideally, students should be receiving messages that address mental health stigmas shortly after matriculation into college. In 2017, the Steve Fund and Jed Foundation partnered to create the Equity in Mental Health Framework, a set of evidence-based recommendations for institutions to work toward mental health equity for URMs [56]. Briefly, these recommendations are to:

1. Make the mental health and well-being of students of color a campus-wide priority through mission statements, funding, staffing, etc.
2. Engage students to provide guidance and feedback.
3. Recruit, train, and retain a diverse faculty and staff that represent the student body.
4. Create opportunities to reflect on current sociopolitical issues.
5. Create roles focused on the well-being and success of URM.
6. Maintain an effective response system to reported incidents or raising concerns.
7. Offer support in varied formats (e.g., mentor networks, discussion groups, transition programs, and workshops on common challenges).
8. Promote programs and services through multiple channels (e.g., in-person and social media).
9. Gauge the effectiveness of programs and practices via data collection on satisfaction and outcomes and refine offerings accordingly.
10. Share information and resources within and between institutions.

## Future Directions

### Flexible Treatment Models

The demand for college mental health services has been surging, resulting in longer wait times for appointments and increased caseloads for providers. The obvious solution is to hire more counseling staff; however, as demand continues to increase, this treatment model might not be sustainable [3]. Instead of directing all students to individual therapy, counseling centers should consider alternatives that are less time-intensive and less expensive. One alternative treatment model is known as "stepped care," in which students are offered the lowest levels of treatment first (i.e., peer support and online self-care modules) and then the services are intensified as needed. Another flexible-care model started at Brown University is known as "single session," in which students are offered brief, same-day appointments for immediate concerns (e.g., anxiety about an upcoming test) without entering continuing therapy [3]. One disadvantage of this model is that counseling center resources are devoted to rapid-access services, and students who require more longitudinal care might be negatively impacted. Other options include peer support, group therapy, and stress management workshops and seminars, all of which can serve multiple students at once [3]. Students might also be referred to community providers, although ideally institutions should follow up to ensure treatment is on track. Although most colleges and universities require students to have health insurance, this health insurance may provide coverage in their hometown but not in the area that surrounds their college. Parents should identify gaps in medical and mental health coverage and consider purchasing supplemental plans in the event that their student needs care when away from home. Telepsychiatry, discussed in the section "System Barriers to Psychiatric Care for College Students," is another flexible option that increases access to care considerably.

## Peer Support

Peer support programs have become increasingly popular on college campuses. Peer-to-peer communication reduces the stigma of mental illness and has been shown to promote help-seeking behavior [57]. Through peer counseling, students hear about the experiences of others with similar challenges, which allows them to gain insight and learn how to cope with the day-to-day stressors of college life. Other benefits include social connectedness, feelings of group belonging, personal empowerment, and hopefulness [57]. In the past, colleges and universities have had liability concerns about student involvement given their lack of expertise and treating such a vulnerable population. However, adequately trained peer counselors who are well-informed about resources can function as an added level of detection and support and might actually reduce liability for colleges [3]. More recently, peer support has been available through social media platforms, which reach a wider demographic but have many potential risks such as misinformation and hostile or derogatory interactions. However, recent evidence suggests that the benefits of online peer-to-peer support outweigh the potential risks [57].

## Destigmatization and Psychoeducation Campaigns

Psychoeducation and public campaigns are commonly used methods to increase help-seeking behaviors through destigmatization and increasing awareness of mental illness. For instance, Cornell Minds Matter is Cornell University's student mental health advocacy group that hosts a variety of events and social activities such as Feel Good Fridays, Dining with Diverse Minds, Random Acts of Kindness, Student Assembly Lift Your Spirits Event, and the Social Belonging Project. The number and frequency of these psychoeducation events make discussions about mental health ubiquitous on campus and thus raise awareness of student mental health concerns, destigmatize help-seeking, and encourage healthy self-care behaviors among students [11]. Active Minds is a national nonprofit organization with over 600 university-based chapters across the United States. This student organization holds greater than 4000 events annually to promote mental health advocacy and suicide prevention [58]. Although there is limited evidence about the effectiveness of psychoeducation campaigns [59], they show some promise when used in conjunction with other methods [11]. For instance, "Signs of Suicide" is a multimodal program that utilizes public campaigns, psychoeducation, GKTs, and crisis intervention procedures that have been shown in randomized control studies to reduce self-reported suicide attempts by 40–64% among youth [60].

## Telepsychiatry in the College Setting

Telemedicine is the process of providing health care from a distance through technology, often using videoconferencing [61]. Telemedicine has become an extraordinarily popular method of mental healthcare delivery [62]. Telehealth increases access and fills treatment gaps, especially in areas with limited resources. Even before the COVID-19 pandemic, colleges were expanding telehealth services for students unable or unwilling to come to the counseling center in person. However, after the COVID-19 pandemic resulted in millions of college students leaving campus to return home, many students had no choice but to receive counseling on a virtual platform [62]. During the pandemic, the utilization of telehealth services increased by 6811% [7].

Telepsychiatry is a subset of telemedicine that encompasses a variety of different services including mental health screenings, psychiatric evaluations, psychotherapy, psychoeducation, and psychopharmacology [61]. It can be used in a variety of different settings including private practice, outpatient clinics, hospitals, correctional facilities, schools, nursing homes, and military treatment facilities. Research into telepsychiatry has been encouraging thus far. Multiple studies have found satisfaction to be high among patients and psychiatrists alike [63]. Furthermore, evidence has found that telepsychiatry is equivalent to in-person care in diagnostic accuracy, treatment effectiveness, quality of care, and patient satisfaction [61]. In fact, telepsychiatry may even be preferable for certain populations such as individuals with autism or severe anxiety disorders [64].

There are several limitations to telepsychiatry. Firstly, it lacks the nuances of in-person communication. Second, cross-state licensure policy dictates that mental health providers must be licensed in the state where the patient is located, which is deemed the place where "the practice of medicine" occurs [61]. A survey of college psychiatrists conducted in May 2020 revealed that 87.8% of respondents reported facing the dilemma of choosing between providing psychiatric care to students across state lines without a waiver versus abandoning students during the immediate aftermath of the COVID-19 pandemic onset [65]. In the 2020–2021 school year, just over half of schools reported providing services to out-of-state students during the pandemic [7]. Third, there are data privacy and malpractice policy considerations, and telepsychiatry therefore should be done over a secure, HIPAA-compliant platform. Finally, financial reimbursement for telepsychiatry services must be requested from Medicare on the federal level and by Medicaid and private insurance companies on the state level. Despite these potential limitations, technology is growing at exponential rates and will undoubtedly play a role in mental healthcare delivery going forward.

## Cross-Campus Wellness Initiatives

As treatment demands continue to rise, campuses need to start shifting focus to preventive measures and targeting root causes of psychological distress. Promoting student well-being across campus might reduce demand by preventing psychological crises from developing in the first place. Colleges are building up infrastructure through wellness spaces, coaches, online tools, and noncredit courses [3]. Wellness spaces take various forms, but ultimately should serve as a reprieve from the day-to-day challenges of collegiate life. Certain institutions can afford massage chairs and spa services, but others might simply utilize existing campus spaces to designate a place where students can meditate or relax on comfortable chairs. Sensory elements, like light therapy, music therapy, or aroma diffusers, can particularly help students who struggle with seasonal affective disorder, autism spectrum disorder, or ADHD. Colleges might also hire wellness coaches to teach students about topics such as stress management and building resilience [3]. Colleges might consider hiring a chief wellness officer to oversee some of these efforts.

To truly change campus culture, wellness initiatives should occur at every level of the institution. For example, professors can invest in the academic and personal success of their students by making certain changes such as learning and using students' names, being conscientious of student schedules when assigning homework and examinations, modeling health habits and behavior (e.g., sending emails during the workday rather than the middle of the night), and simply making themselves available to talk [3]. Some institutions are even developing wellness courses. Carleton College offers a noncredit 10-week course known as "Happy Hour" that meets for an hour a week and focuses on finding purpose and optimism in life. At the University of Southern California, "Thrive: Foundations of Well-Being" is a one-credit course that will eventually be mandatory for all new students. Colleges can also consider running campus-wide wellness campaigns that promote healthy habits, like the Jed Foundation's "Seize the Awkward" campaign that encourages students to ask how their peers are doing to fill a moment of silence in a conversation. Campuses can also offer various forms of stress relief such as petting zoos on the quad, door decorating, or providing free late-night snacks.

## Conclusion

College is a vulnerable time as adolescents transition into adulthood, in which students must manage leaving and living away from home, academic pressures, social demands, and increased access to alcohol and drugs. Over the last couple of decades, there have been steadily increasing rates of depression, anxiety, suicidality, and other mental health problems among U.S. college students. Rates of anxiety and depression further skyrocketed during the COVID-19 pandemic due to unique stressors including interruptions in their education, technological concerns about online learning, hindrance of physical activity and extracurricular activities, social isolation, lack of college belongingness, decreased family income, financial concerns threatening their future education, and uncertainty about future employment. Although many students are not appropriately utilizing treatment, some of which is due to systemic barriers, there has overall been increased demand for services among most colleges and universities. As such, there is an expanding need for mental health services on college campuses. Flexible-care models (e.g., stepped care) and telepsychiatry are changing how colleges provide mental health care to their students.

## References

1. Healthy Minds Study—Healthy Minds Network. https://healthymindsnetwork.org/hms/.
2. Downs N, et al. Be true to our schools—models of care in college mental health. Curr Psychiatry Rep. 2018;20(9):72. https://doi.org/10.1007/s11920-018-0935-6.
3. Brown S. Overwhelmed: the real campus mental-health crisis and new models for well-being. The Chronical of Higher Education; 2020.
4. Karyotaki E, Cuijpers P, Albor Y, Alonso J, Auerbach RP, Bantjes J, et al. Sources of stress and their associations with mental disorders among college students: results of the World Health Organization world mental health surveys international college student initiative. Front Psychol. 2020;11:1759.
5. Aristovnik A, Keržič D, Ravšelj D, Tomaževič N, Umek L. Impacts of the COVID-19 pandemic on life of higher education students: a global perspective. Sustain For. 2020;12(20):8438.
6. Bureau UC. Household pulse survey data tables. Census.gov. https://www.census.gov/programs-surveys/household-pulse-survey/data.html.
7. Association for University and College Counseling Center Directors. Annual Survey. 2020.
8. Son C, Hegde S, Smith A, Wang X, Sasangohar F. Effects of COVID-19 on college students' mental health in the United States: interview survey study. J Med Internet Res. 2020;22(9):e21279.
9. Liu CH, Pinder-Amaker S, Hahm HC, Chen JA. Priorities for addressing the impact of the COVID-19 pandemic on college student mental health. J Am Coll Heal. 2022;70(5):1356–8.
10. Conrad RC, Hahm HC, Koire A, Pinder-Amaker S, Liu CH. College student mental health risks during the COVID-19 pandemic: implications of campus relocation. J Psychiatr Res. 2021;136:117–26.
11. MacPhee J, Modi K, Gorman S, Roy N, Riba E, Cusumano D, et al. A comprehensive approach to mental health promotion and suicide prevention for colleges and universities: insights from the JED Campus Program—National Academy of Medicine. https://nam.edu/a-comprehensive-approach-to-mental-health-promotion-and-suicide-prevention-for-colleges-and-universities-insights-from-the-jed-campus-program/.
12. Fogler JM, Burke D, Lynch J, Barbaresi WJ, Chan E. Topical review: transitional services for teens and young adults with attention-deficit hyperactivity disorder: a process map and proposed model to overcoming barriers to care. J Pediatr Psychol. 2017;42(10):1108–13. https://academic.oup.com/jpepsy/article/42/10/1108/4057690
13. Chen JA, Stevens C, Wong SH, Liu CH. Psychiatric symptoms and diagnoses among U.S. college students: a comparison by race and ethnicity. Psychiatr Serv. 2019;70(6):442–9. https://doi.org/10.1176/appi.ps.201800388.
14. Eisenberg D, Lipson SK, Heinze J, Zhou S. The healthy minds study. 26.
15. Liu CH, et al. The prevalence and predictors of mental health diagnoses and suicide among U.S. college students: implications for addressing disparities in service use. Depress Anxiety. 2019;36(1):8–17. https://doi.org/10.1002/da.22830.
16. Mortier P, et al. Suicidal thoughts and behaviors among first-year college students: results from the WMH-ICS project. J Am Acad Child Adolesc Psychiatry. 2018;57(4):263–273.e1. https://www.jaacap.org/article/S0890-8567(18)30057-1/fulltext.

17. Hope EC, Velez G, Offidani-Bertrand C, Keels M, Durkee MI. Political activism and mental health among black and Latinx college students. Cult Divers Ethn Minor Psychol. 2018;24(1):26–39.
18. Bor J, Venkataramani AS, Williams DR, Tsai AC. Police killings and their spillover effects on the mental health of black Americans: a population-based, quasi-experimental study. Lancet. 2018;392(10144):302–10.
19. Politics on the quad: students report on division and disagreement at five US universities. https://www.brandeis.edu/cmjs/noteworthy/ssri/politics-quad.html.
20. Haddad JM, Macenski C, Mosier-Mills A, Hibara A, Kester K, Schneider M, et al. The impact of social media on college mental health during the COVID-19 pandemic: a multinational review of the existing literature. Curr Psychiatry Rep. 2021;23(11):70.
21. Stress in America™ 2020: A National Mental Health Crisis. https://www.apa.org/news/press/releases/stress/2020/report-october.
22. Liu CH, Wong GTF, Hyun S, Hahm HC. Concerns about the social climate, finances, and COVID-19 risk on depression and anxiety: an analysis on U.S. young adults across two waves. J Psychiatr Res. 2022;148:286–92.
23. Race and ethnicity in higher education: a status report. Race and Ethnicity in Higher Education. https://www.equityinhighered.org/resources/report-downloads/race-and-ethnicity-in-higher-education-a-status-report/.
24. Williams KDA, Adkins A, Kuo SI, LaRose JG, Utsey SO, Guidry JPD, et al. Mental health disorder symptom prevalence and rates of help-seeking among university-enrolled, emerging adults. J Am Coll Heal. 2021;71(1):61–8.
25. Williams KDA, Adkins AE, Kuo SIC, LaRose JG, Utsey SO, Guidry JPD, et al. Risk, protective, and associated factors of anxiety and depressive symptoms and campus health services utilization among black men on a college campus. J Racial Ethn Health Disparities. 2022;9(2):505–18.
26. Corona R, Rodríguez VM, McDonald SE, Velazquez E, Rodríguez A, Fuentes VE. Associations between cultural stressors, cultural values, and Latina/o college students' mental health. J Youth Adolesc. 2017;46(1):63–77.
27. Dunbar MS, Sontag-Padilla L, Ramchand R, Seelam R, Stein BD. Mental health service utilization among lesbian, gay, bisexual, and questioning or queer college students. J Adolesc Health. 2017;61(3):294–301.
28. American College Health Association. American College Health Association-National College Health Assessment II: reference group executive summary spring 2015. 2015.
29. Ellis CG. Cross-cultural aspects of depression in general practice. S Afr Med J. 2003;93(5):342–5.
30. Xiao H, Carney DM, Youn SJ, Janis RA, Castonguay LG, Hayes JA, et al. Are we in crisis? National mental health and treatment trends in college counseling centers. Psychol Serv. 2017;14(4):407–15.
31. Bourdon JL, Moore AA, Long EC, Kendler KS, Dick DM. The relationship between on-campus service utilization and common mental health concerns in undergraduate college students. Psychol Serv. 2020;17(1):118–26.
32. Injury Data Visualization Tools | WISQARS | CDC. https://wisqars.cdc.gov/data/non-fatal/home.
33. Czeisler MÉ. Mental health, substance use, and suicidal ideation during the COVID-19 pandemic—United States, June 24–30, 2020. MMWR Morb Mortal Wkly Rep. 2020;69(32):1049–57. https://www.cdc.gov/mmwr/volumes/69/wr/mm6932a1.htm.
34. Grant BF, et al. Prevalence of 12-month alcohol use, high-risk drinking, and DSM-IV alcohol use disorder in the United States, 2001–2002 to 2012-2013: results from the National Epidemiologic Survey on Alcohol and Related Conditions. JAMA Psychiatry. 74(9):911–23. https://jamanetwork.com/journals/jamapsychiatry/fullarticle/2647079.
35. Section 6 PE tables—results from the 2019 National Survey on drug use and health: detailed tables, SAMHSA, CBHSQ. https://www.samhsa.gov/data/sites/default/files/reports/rpt29394/NSDUHDetailedTabs2019/NSDUHDetTabsSect6pe2019.htm#tab6-21b.
36. Bunnell RE, Agaku IT, Arrazola RA, Apelberg BJ, Caraballo RS, Corey CG, et al. Intentions to smoke cigarettes among never-smoking US middle and high school electronic cigarette users: National Youth Tobacco Survey, 2011–2013. Nicotine Tob Res. 2015;17(2):228–35.
37. Johnston LD, Miech RA, O'Malley PM, Bachman JG, Schulenberg JE, Patrick ME. Monitoring the future national survey results on drug use, 1975–2018: overview, key findings on adolescent drug use. Institute for Social Research. Institute for Social Research; 2019. https://eric.ed.gov/?id=ED594190.
38. E-cigarette use among youth and young adults: a report of the surgeon general. GA: U.S. Department of Health and Human Services, Centers for Disease Control and Prevention, National Center for Chronic Disease Prevention and Health Promotion, Office on Smoking and Health; 2016, p. 298.
39. Holm S. Principles of Biomedical Ethics, 5th edn.: Beauchamp T L, Childress J F. Oxford University Press, 2001, pound19.95, pp 454. ISBN 0-19-514332-9. J Med Ethics. 2002;28(5):332.
40. Conrad R. Legal and ethical challenges in the psychiatric treatment of college students. Curr Psychiatry Rep. 2020;22(9):50.
41. Conrad R, Brumbaugh B. Respect for persons in the psychiatric treatment of children and adolescents. Psychiatr Clin North Am. 2021;44(4):613–25. https://www.sciencedirect.com/science/article/abs/pii/S0193953X21000599?via%3Dihub.

42. Chapman K. A PREVENTABLE TRAGEDY AT VIRGINIA TECH: WHY CONFUSION OVER FERPA'S PROVISIONS PREVENTS SCHOOLS FROM ADDRESSING STUDENT VIOLENCE. Publ Interest Law J. 2009;18:38.
43. Tarasoff v. Regents of Univ. of Cal. | Case Brief for Law School | LexisNexis. Community. https://www.lexisnexis.com/community/casebrief/p/casebrief-tarasoff-v-regents-of-univ-of-cal.
44. Law & Psychiatry: "Depressed? Get Out!": Dealing With Suicidal Students on College Campuses | Psychiatric Services. https://ps.psychiatryonline.org/doi/full/10.1176/ps.2006.57.7.914.
45. Appelbaum PS. Law & Psychiatry: "depressed? Get out!": dealing with suicidal students on college campuses. PS. 2006;57(7):914–6.
46. Settlement Agreement between the United States and Brown University. https://www.ada.gov/brown_sa.html.
47. 34 C.F.R. Part 104. US Department of Education (ED). https://www2.ed.gov/policy/rights/reg/ocr/edlite-34cfr104.html.
48. Stanford and students with mental health disabilities reach landmark settlement. Disability Rights Advocates. 2019. https://dralegal.org/press/stanford-and-students-with-mental-health-disabilities-reach-landmark-settlement/.
49. Disability Rights Section CRD. Notice of Proposed Rulemaking Proposal to Revise Regulations under Title II and Title III of the Americans with Disabilities Act (ADA). https://www.ada.gov/regs2010/ADAregs2010.html.
50. Disability Rights Section CRD. Notice of Proposed Rulemaking Proposal to Revise Regulations under Title II and Title III of the Americans with Disabilities Act (ADA). https://www.ada.gov/regs2010/ADAregs2010.htm.
51. Virginia tech shooting leaves 33 dead. The New York Times. https://www.nytimes.com/2007/04/16/us/16cnd-shooting.html.
52. Nguyen v. Mass. Inst. of Tech., 479 Mass. 436 | Casetext Search + Citator. https://casetext.com/case/nguyen-v-mass-inst-tech-1.
53. Regents of University of California v Superior Court, 413 P 3d 656 (Cal2018).
54. Appelbaum PS. Responsibility for suicide or violence on campus. Psychiatr Serv. 2019;70(4):350–2. https://doi.org/10.1176/appi.ps.201900060.
55. Peng Q, Liang C, Ji W, De S. A first principles investigation of the mechanical properties of g-TlN. MNSMS. 2012;02(04):76–84.
56. The Equity in Mental Health Framework. The Steve Fund. https://www.stevefund.org/equity-mental-health-framework/.
57. Naslund JA, Aschbrenner KA, Marsch LA, Bartels SJ. The future of mental health care: peer-to-peer support and social media. Epidemiol Psychiatr Sci. 2016;25(2):113–22.
58. Mission and impact. Active Minds. https://www.activeminds.org/about-us/mission-and-impact/.
59. Klimes-Dougan B, Klingbeil DA, Meller SJ. The impact of universal suicide-prevention programs on the help-seeking attitudes and behaviors of youths. Crisis. 2013;34(2):82–97.
60. Psychiatry.org. What is telepsychiatry? https://psychiatry.org:443/patients-families/telepsychiatry.
61. Kichloo A, et al. Telemedicine, the current COVID-19 pandemic and the future: a narrative review and perspectives moving forward in the USA. Fam Med Community Health. 2020;8(3):e000530. https://fmch.bmj.com/content/8/3/e000530.
62. Shore J. What is telepsychiatry? American Psychiatric Association: APA Committee on Telepsychiatry; 2020. https://www.psychiatry.org/patients-families/what-is-telepsychiatry.
63. Schubert NJ, Backman PJ, Bhatla R, Corace KM. Telepsychiatry and patient–provider concordance. Can J Rural Med. 2019;24(3):75.
64. Neurodivergent people share their experience of the pandemic. Verywell Mind. 2023. https://www.verywellmind.com/how-neurodivergence-impacts-experiences-of-the-pandemic-5186107.
65. Treatment challenges for college psychiatrists and their patients. Psychiatric Times. 2020. https://www.psychiatrictimes.com/view/treatment-challenges-college-psychiatrists-patients.

# 21 Chronic Pain

Natasha Piracha and Kristin Wong

## Case

Ben is a 21-year-old man with a diagnosis of sickle cell disease who is transitioning to the adult primary care clinic. He describes long-standing pain that is both sharp and stabbing in his back and legs and burning in his fingertips. Outside of his crises, the sharp pain is generally controlled with as-needed morphine tablets. Throughout the last decade, he has had admissions for sickle cell-related pain crises, usually exacerbated by viral illness, dehydration after playing many days of football, or changes in the seasons, which generally lead to a 3- to 4-day hospital stay. He recently presented to the adult emergency department with pain that did not respond to his home medications and describes to you feeling judged and dismissed when he asked for the medications that typically worked for him in the pediatric emergency department. He hopes you can both help him navigate this new adult environment and treat his chronic pain so he can continue activities he loves, which include playing sports with his friends and attending all of his college classes.

## Pain Definitions and Pathophysiology

The International Association for the Study of Pain (IASP) redefined pain in 2020 as "An unpleasant sensory and emotional experience associated with, or resembling that associated with, actual or potential tissue damage" [1]. This definition is further expanded with the addition of six keynotes:

- Pain is always a personal experience that is influenced to varying degrees by biological, psychological, and social factors.
- Pain and nociception are different phenomena. Pain cannot be inferred solely from activity in sensory neurons.
- Through their life experiences, individuals learn the concept of pain.
- A person's report of an experience of pain should be respected.
- Although pain usually serves an adaptive role, it may have adverse effects on function and social and psychological well-being.

N. Piracha
Pediatric Palliative Care, Department of Pediatrics, Columbia University Vagelos College of Physicians and Surgeons and NewYork-Presbyterian, New York, NY, USA

Adult Palliative Care Service, Department of Medicine, Columbia University Vagelos College of Physicians and Surgeons and NewYork-Presbyterian, New York, NY, USA
e-mail: np2775@cumc.columbia.edu

K. Wong (✉)
Departments of Medicine and Pediatrics, Rutgers Health New Jersey Medical School, Newark, NJ, USA
e-mail: kgw22@njms.rutgers.edu


A. A. Kuo et al. (eds.), *Care of Adults with Chronic Childhood Conditions*,
https://doi.org/10.1007/978-3-031-54281-7_21

- Verbal description is only one of several behaviors to express pain; inability to communicate does not negate the possibility that a human or a nonhuman animal experiences pain.

Pain can be further categorized by duration and by type or etiology. Chronic pain, defined as pain lasting or recurring for more than 3 months, will be the focus of this chapter. Chronic pain can be divided into its etiologies, including but not limited to chronic primary pain, neuropathic pain, visceral pain, and musculoskeletal pain [2, 3].

Nociceptive pain, which includes visceral pain, arises from impending or active damage to non-neural tissue, activating nociceptors. Somatic nociceptive pain is generally well-localized and described as sharp or aching, while visceral somatic pain is poorly localized and dull in nature, related to capsular stretch or obstruction. Neuropathic pain is caused by a lesion or disease of the somatosensory nervous system, either centrally or peripherally. It is often described as burning, tingling, electric shock-like with or without associated numbness, or allodynia (pain secondary to a stimulus that would generally not induce pain).

## Total Pain

The term "total pain" highlights the complex relationship between a person's physical and existential pain, as seen in Fig. 21.1 [4]. In particular, for patients with life-limiting illness, pain outside of physical pain is often overlooked, which can lead to mismanagement of a patient's total suffering.

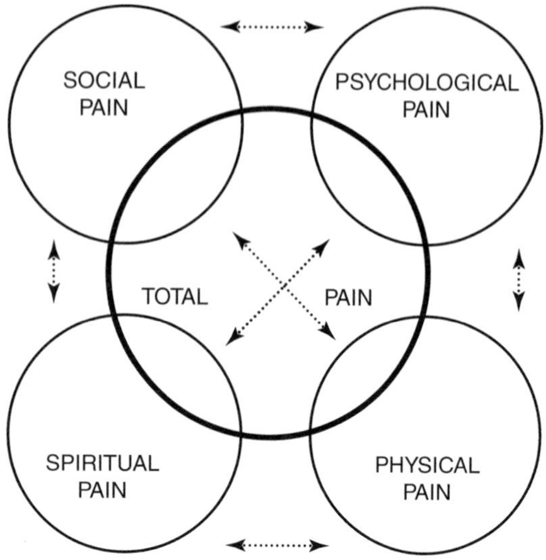


**Fig. 21.1** "Total Pain" conceptualizes the bidirectional influence of physical, psychological, social, and spiritual experiences on and from pain [4]

## Epidemiology of Chronic Pain

The prevalence of chronic pain in pediatrics and adolescents is estimated to be about 25%, with the true number of patients likely higher, secondary to misdiagnoses and/or diagnostic uncertainty. Many of these adolescent patients will continue to have chronic pain into adulthood. Depending on their type of pain, children and adolescents with chronic pain may present to adult providers with chronic opioid use and a higher tolerance for medications [5]. See the section on special considerations in transitional care for further discussion.

## Common Conditions in Adulthood

Many conditions in adolescence have associated chronic pain symptoms, requiring complex and multi-modal management. As a primary example, chronic pain in sickle cell disease has an increasing prevalence with age with upward of over 55% of adults experiencing pain on more than half their days [6]. The etiology of chronic pain in sickle cell disease is complicated and frequently a combination of different pain sites and pain types, from repetitive nociceptive pain due to vaso-occlusive crises to neuropathic pain due to opioid-induced hyperalgesia. Given the complexity of physiology and etiology of pain in sickle cell disease, it is often suboptimally treated with opioids and can be associated with other comorbid conditions like psychiatric illnesses, autoimmune disease, and impairments to quality of life [6].

Patients with progressive neuromuscular disorders also suffer from chronic pain that is amplified by the loss of function—some studies report 70% of patients with myotonic dystrophy type 1 and 90% of patients with facioscapulohumeral dystrophy report pain [7]. Experts in this area suggest that the assessment of chronic pain in these patients must include the number of pain sites and each site's pain intensity to fully comprehend a patient's pain experience [7]. In addition to the complex relationship between pain and function, long-term survivors of pediatric cancers also experience an interplay between their chronic pain and psychological well-being, presenting as increases in post-traumatic stress, anxiety, and poorer quality of life [8].

## Treatment Options

Prior to considering treatment options for chronic pain, it is important to perform a multi-dimensional assessment of the physical manifestations, etiologies, and impact of pain on the person's quality of life. This requires a comprehensive physical and neurologic examination and a psychosocial and functional assessment. Various tools exist for both verbal and non-verbal patients, one of which was developed by the American Academy of Family Physicians and provides a comprehensive kit for the assessment and management of chronic pain [9]. As chronic pain is life-long for many, setting goals focused on best improving one's quality of life, rather than setting expectations of complete elimination of pain, can empower the patient and help prevent medication misuse. This is accomplished by utilizing shared decision-making and formalized pain treatment plans, all rooted in a strong patient-provider relationship.

## Strategies in Prescribing Medications

Table 21.1 refers to many commonly used medications for chronic pain, depending on etiology. As a person's pain can have many etiologies, using a combination of pharmacologic agents early may be necessary. Additionally, for patients with a life-limiting illness, having a sense of prognosis can help guide pharmacologic decision-making. In general, it is also important to balance the risk of side effects of a particular medication with its overall benefits and be able to educate and guide patients when trialing different therapies to mitigate expectations and monitor for complications.

**Table 21.1** Pharmacotherapy for chronic pain

| Treatment | MOA | Role | Notes |
|---|---|---|---|
| Acetaminophen | Exact MOA unknown, thought to inhibit prostaglandin synthesis in CNS/blockage of peripheral pain receptors | Can be used as an initial non-opioid analgesic for mild pain or as adjuvant therapy | Dose adjustment/caution in patients with chronic liver dysfunction or acute liver failure |
| Non-steroidal anti-inflammatory (NSAIDs) | COX inhibition, clinical relevance of non-prostaglandin-mediated effects not completely understood | Pain secondary to musculoskeletal or inflammatory etiology | Significant adverse effects and drug–drug interactions, especially with chronic use Limit to the lowest dose with the lowest duration possible |
| Opioids | Inhibition of central and peripheral opioid receptors | Use in severe non-cancer or neuropathic pain when all other therapies have been exhausted | Dose adjustments necessary with increasing tolerance. Assess risk for misuse/abuse and dependence prior to and after initiation |
| Methadone | Binds to opioid receptors inhibiting ascending pain pathways. Also with NMDA receptor antagonism | Indications similar to opioids and generally used in opioid-tolerant patients. Also has benefits in neuropathic pain | In addition to pain, it can be used in medical-assisted therapy for opioid use disorder. Recommend collaboration with addiction medicine |
| Medicinal cannabis | Stimulates cannabinoid receptors, primarily CB1 and CB2, expressed throughout the body | Multiple therapeutic uses including pain control, antiemetic, and neuromodulation | Not federally approved. Legalized use varies from state to state. Limited data on therapeutic benefits and long-term effects |
| Neuropathic agents | | | |
| SNRI | Inhibition of serotonin and norepinephrine reuptake | Appropriate first-line therapy for neuropathic pain | Beneficial for patients with concomitant depressed mood. More favorable side effect profile compared to TCA |
| TCA | Inhibition of serotonin and norepinephrine reuptake | Appropriate first-line therapy for neuropathic pain, especially if comorbid depression | Many side effects |
| Gabapentinoids | Reduces excitability of neurons centrally | First line for neuropathic pain without comorbid depression. Has other non-pain uses | Dose reduce if renal impairment |

## Procedural Therapies

Procedural strategies in the management of chronic pain can offer highly effective and long-lasting relief. However, they tend to be site-specific therapies such as nerve blocks, joint injections, epidural injections, and ganglion blocks. Choosing the best candidate for these procedures takes collaboration with interventional colleagues, like pain management, anesthesia, radiology, and surgery. Advancements in these targeted therapies, as with ultrasound guidance, have led to improved safety, accuracy, and procedural effectiveness [10]. Other procedures include implantable drug-delivery pumps or surgical options to reduce nerve compression, contractures, or other causes of site-specific pain. The risks of such procedures including bleeding, infection, and postoperative pain must be weighed with the reduction in chronic pain or other potential benefits like gains in function.

## Physical Therapy and Exercise

Physical therapy and exercise are frequently included as the mainstay form of treatment for various types of pain and can be essential to the maintenance of function. However, the delivery of manual therapies can be just as complex as the pain itself, owing to varying operator techniques, patient expectations, and coexisting psychosocial factors [11]. Physiatrists have similar challenges in the approach to pain as general practitioners do—having to balance pharmacologic and non-pharmacologic treatment modalities, incorporating shared decision-making into clinical care, generating opportunities for education and development, etc. Thus, the positive effects of physical therapy can be heavily dependent on the patient-provider relationship, and failure of one technique may require subsequent trials and possibly alternative providers.

Likewise, different forms of exercise have also had variations in outcomes. In a review performed to establish new guidelines for the American College of Physicians (ACP), exercise and motor control exercise were found to reduce pain intensity and increase function in patients with chronic low back pain [12]. Activities like yoga and tai chi have also shown moderate improvements in pain, but more modest effects on function [12]. While these studies only addressed chronic pain of the lower back, many of these benefits can still be appreciated in other types and locations of chronic pain. It is also important to consider a patient's ability to fully participate and have access to these activities.

## Other Modalities

Many physicians have also incorporated other non-traditional treatment options such as transcutaneous electrical nerve stimulation (TENS), acupuncture, and mindfulness strategies. In a Cochrane systematic review, studies using TENS for the treatment of chronic pain have had modest outcomes, however, were frequently wrought with low-quality evidence and were at high risk for bias, limiting the ability to make strong recommendations for the risk or benefit of TENS therapy [13]. Studies looking at acupuncture in chronic low back pain also had limitations in evidence and outcomes; however, in another Cochrane review, studies suggest some short-term improvement in function and physical quality of life [14]. Mindfulness-based therapies, such as mindfulness-based stress reduction (MBSR), on the other hand, seem to have more reliable evidence and can be just as effective as cognitive behavioral therapies [12]. Acceptance and commitment therapy (ACT), another type of psychotherapy, can provide impactful reductions in depression and subsequently an improved quality of life [15]. However, these and various forms of psychotherapy are still being studied and their effectiveness in chronic pain management is not yet fully understood.

Additionally, like all other modalities, patients must be agreeable, be able to participate fully, and have ease of access to these therapies in order to gain maximal benefit. Patients may also provide their own methods of treatment, some of which are rooted in cultural or societal influences. Providers should remain open-minded and non-judgmental but also weigh the risks and benefits of recommending or discouraging non-evidence-based medicine. Being able to "compromise" and provide multi-modal care in some cases can strengthen a patient's trust and relationship with their provider.

## Special Considerations in Transitional Care to Adulthood

It is important to note that patients with verbal and/or cognitive deficits that affect their ability to communicate, experience chronic pain that is frequently underestimated and undertreated [16]. Disorders such as autism, cerebral palsy, and severe intellectual disabilities require a thorough review of their symptoms—paying close attention to non-verbal cues, changes in behavior, and a thoughtful interview of the patient's proxy—and are critical in understanding the pain needs of these patients [16]. Depending on a patient's ability to understand, cooperate with, or have access to a particular treatment modality, physicians may be limited to only a few options in the management of chronic pain. Thus, fully understanding and maximizing a patient's neurocognitive and physical capabilities can be helpful in deciding which options they will be able to achieve the greatest benefit from.

Complications of chronic pain include comorbid mental health conditions, dependency on pharmacologic and nonpharmacologic therapies, and the associated stigmas and added strain to family, caretaker, and provider relationships. Advancements in cognitive behavioral and psychological therapies can help to alleviate some of the mental health effects on involved parties, but continuing education and training must also address the external cultural, socioeconomic, and implicit or explicit biases toward patients with chronic pain within the healthcare community. Opioid management, though the standard of care for many pain conditions like sickle cell disease, has become saturated with the stigma associated with judgmental terms like "addict" and "drug-abuser" [17]. Stigma has resulted in patient and provider barriers to the treatment of opioid use disorders and the prevention of opioid-related overdoses. Consequently, it is extremely important for providers to avoid pejorative language when treating patients with chronic pain to stop the perpetuation of stigma and stereotypes [17]. Medication-assisted therapies and other treatment options now exist to assist patients with drug-use disorders and are referenced in Chap. 19: Substance Use Disorders.

It is also especially important to recognize that socioeconomically disadvantaged populations and underrepresented minorities (URMs) experience greater pain and have less access to treatment than others [18, 19]. For example, despite prior studies showing Blacks are less likely to abuse opioids than Whites, many studies show that Blacks are less likely to be prescribed opioids, yet are subjected to closer monitoring for misuse [19]. Other studies have also shown that URMs experience higher levels of pain, but are frequently undertreated [19]. These disparate outcomes are the result of multiple different barriers within the healthcare system and are still being investigated in order to provide meaningful change. Providers must also be vigilant in this endeavor, being conscious of their biases and proactive in the delivery of equitable care.

## References

1. Raja SN, Carr DB, Cohen M, Finnerup NB, Flor H, Gibson S, et al. The revised International Association for the Study of Pain definition of pain: concepts, challenges, and compromises. Pain. 2020;161(9):1976–82.
2. Treede RD, Rief W, Barke A, Aziz Q, Bennett MI, Benoliel R, et al. A classification of chronic pain for ICD-11. Pain. 2015;156(6):1003–7.
3. Loeser JD, Treede RD. The Kyoto protocol of IASP basic pain terminology. Pain. 2008;137(3):473–7.
4. Mehta A, Chan LS. Understanding of the concept of "total pain": a prerequisite for pain control. J Hosp Palliat Nurs. 2008;10(1):26–32.
5. Forgeron P, Higginson A, Truskoski C. Departure from pediatric care: transitioning of adolescents with chronic pain to adult care. Pain Manag Nurs. 2017;18(5):273–7.
6. Osunkwo I, O'Connor HF, Saah E. Optimizing the management of chronic pain in sickle cell disease. Hematology Am Soc Hematol Educ Program. 2020;2020(1):562–9.
7. Miró J, Gertz KJ, Carter GT, Jensen MP. Chronic pain in neuromuscular disease: pain site and intensity differentially impacts function. Phys Med Rehabil Clin N Am. 2012;23(4):895–902.
8. Patton M, Forster VJ, Forbes C, Stokoe M, Noel M, Carlson LE, et al. Characterizing pain in long-term survivors of childhood cancer. Support Care Cancer. 2022;30(1):295–303.
9. AAFP. Chronic pain toolkit. 2021.
10. Korbe S, Udoji EN, Ness TJ, Udoji MA. Ultrasound-guided interventional procedures for chronic pain management. Pain Management. 2015;5(6):466–82.
11. Coronado RA, Bialosky JE. Manual physical therapy for chronic pain: the complex whole is greater than the sum of its parts. J Man Manip Ther. 2017;25(3):115–7.
12. Chou R, Deyo R, Friedly J, Skelly A, Hashimoto R, Weimer M, et al. Nonpharmacologic therapies for low Back pain: a systematic review for an American College of Physicians Clinical Practice Guideline. Ann Intern Med. 2017;166(7):493.
13. Gibson W, Wand BM, Meads C, Catley MJ, O'Connell NE. Transcutaneous electrical nerve stimulation (TENS) for chronic pain—an overview of Cochrane reviews. Cochrane Database Syst Rev. 2019;2019(4):CD011890. https://doi.org/10.1002/14651858.CD011890.pub3.
14. Mu J, Furlan AD, Lam WY, Hsu MY, Ning Z, Lao L. Acupuncture for chronic nonspecific low back pain. Cochrane Database Syst Rev. 2020;12(12):CD013814. https://doi.org/10.1002/14651858.CD013814.

15. Veehof MM, Trompetter HR, Bohlmeijer ET, Schreurs KMG. Acceptance- and mindfulness-based interventions for the treatment of chronic pain: a meta-analytic review. Cogn Behav Ther. 2016;45(1):5–31.
16. Riquelme I, Pades Jiménez A, Montoya P. Parents and physiotherapists recognition of non-verbal communication of pain in individuals with cerebral palsy. Health Commun. 2018;33(12):1448–53.
17. Lyden J, Binswanger IA. The United States opioid epidemic. Semin Perinatol. 2019;43(3):123–31.
18. Nephew BC, Incollingo Rodriguez AC, Melican V, Polcari JJ, Nippert KE, Rashkovskii M, et al. Depression predicts chronic pain interference in racially diverse, income-disadvantaged patients. Pain Med. 2022;23(7):1239–48.
19. Morales ME, Yong RJ. Racial and ethnic disparities in the treatment of chronic pain. Pain Med. 2021;22(1):75–90.

## Resources

AAFP chronic pain toolkit [9]. https://www.aafp.org/dam/AAFP/documents/patient_care/pain_management/cpm-toolkit.pdf.

# 22 Eating Disorders

Meghna Raphael, Drusilla M. Rosales, Albert C. Hergenroeder, and Beth H. Garland

## Abbreviations

| | |
|---|---|
| AN | Anorexia nervosa |
| ARFID | Avoidant restrictive food intake disorder |
| BMI | Body mass index |
| BN | Bulimia nervosa |
| CBT | Cognitive-behavioral therapy |
| CEDS | Certified Eating Disorders Specialist |
| DSM-5 | Diagnostic and Statistical Manual of Mental Disorders, Fifth Edition |
| ED(s) | Eating disorders |
| FBT | Family-based therapy |
| IOP | Intensive Outpatient Program |
| IPT | Interpersonal therapy |
| MI | Motivational interviewing |
| OSFEDs | Other specified feeding and eating disorders |
| PHP | Partial Hospitalization Program |
| RD | Registered dietitian |
| RDN | Registered dietitian nutritionist |
| TGW | Treatment Goal Weight |

**Case Vignette**

*An 18-year-old college student comes for her first visit with her adult primary care provider with a complaint of dizziness. She reports having a diagnosis of anorexia nervosa. She runs 5–10 miles daily and is vague regarding her diet. Her last menstrual cycle was 6 months ago. She reports a past medical history of one hospitalization for bradycardia and severe malnutrition 2 years ago. She is taking no prescribed medications and takes over-the-counter vitamins, calcium carbonate, and occasional laxatives. She attends a university full-time and is not employed. She denies recent sexual intercourse and substance use. Physical examination is remarkable for the patient wearing several shirts and a sweater despite the visit occurring during the summer months. Her weight, in clothing, was 101 pounds; height was 5′7″; body mass index (BMI) was 15.8 kg/m$^2$; blood pressure was 88/50 mmHg; and pulse was 58 beats per minute. She looks pale. Her hair is thin and her is skin dry, especially her hands. Her hands and feet are cool with a mild violaceous hue. She has no lymphadenopathy; her thyroid is normal to palpation; her oral mucosa*

M. Raphael (✉) · D. M. Rosales · A. C. Hergenroeder · B. H. Garland
Texas Children's Hospital, Houston, TX, USA
e-mail: msebasti@bcm.edu; dmrosale@bcm.edu; achergen@texaschildrens.org; bhgarlan@texaschildrens.org


A. A. Kuo et al. (eds.), *Care of Adults with Chronic Childhood Conditions*,
https://doi.org/10.1007/978-3-031-54281-7_22

*appeared dry; her heart sounds are distant in the supine position and louder in the seated position; and her abdomen is scaphoid with no organomegaly. She has no peripheral edema.*

The goal of the chapter is for the adult primary care provider to understand the diagnosis and management of two common eating disorders (EDs), anorexia nervosa (AN), and bulimia nervosa (BN) and recognize avoidant restrictive food intake disorder (ARFID) and other specified feeding and eating disorders (OSFEDs) in a young adult who is transitioning into their adult practice.

Specific objectives are as follows. The reader will be able to:

1. Describe the epidemiology of eating disorders in adolescents and adults and identify the challenges associated with the transition of care into adult practice.
2. Apply diagnostic criteria for AN, BN, ARFID, and OSFED to re-evaluate a patient with a reported diagnosis of an eating disorder in adolescence or diagnose a young adult presenting to their adult provider.
3. Initiate a comprehensive assessment for a new patient with an eating disorder diagnosis, including staging malnutrition and identifying its medical complications.
4. Recognize the need for an interdisciplinary treatment team and recommend an appropriate level of care based on the severity of illness.

## Epidemiology

Eating disorders are a class of disorders that are characterized by psychological symptoms (e.g., fear of weight gain and overvaluation of body shape or size), leading to maladaptive behavioral changes in nutrition or eating, physical activity, and other compensatory behaviors. While the Diagnostic and Statistical Manual of Mental Disorders, Fifth Edition (DSM-5), lists multiple EDs, this chapter will focus on the diagnosis, treatment, and special considerations for young adults with AN, BN, ARFID, and OSFED [1].

The estimated lifetime prevalence of AN is 0.8%, and for BN, it is 0.28% [2]. The large majority of EDs are diagnosed in females, yet they occur in males. EDs can affect patients of all races, ethnicities, body sizes, and socioeconomic classes [3]. Patients with EDs are at significantly higher risk of premature mortality as compared to the general population, with death primarily occurring in adulthood due to suicide [4, 5]. The mean age at which patients with EDs present in adolescence is 12.5 years, though they can present for the first time in emerging adulthood, most commonly between the ages of 19 and 24 years [2, 6]. Nearly 30% of adolescent-onset eating disorders persist into adulthood [7]. At the time of transition to an adult care provider, these young adults are vulnerable to disruptions to care as they attempt to self-manage their condition while they navigate their legal and functional independence from parents, begin employment, or higher education [8].

## Diagnosis

When a patient is evaluated by the adult provider, the pediatric diagnosis should be reexamined as the eating disorder may evolve with time. For example, an individual who initially was diagnosed with AN may later meet the criteria for BN or another alternative diagnosis. The evolution of the disease may require different treatment strategies [9].

The DSM-5 provides criteria for the diagnosis of these disorders. Key features to differentiate between AN, BN, ARFID, and OSFED (including Atypical AN, purging disorder, and BN of low frequency and/or limited duration) are summarized in Table 22.1 [1].

**Table 22.1** Differentiating between types of eating disorders [1]

| | Anorexia nervosa | Bulimia nervosa | Avoidant restrictive food intake disorder |
|---|---|---|---|
| Behaviors | Lower than required energy intake and/or excessive exercise (restrictive subtype). May include binge eating and/or purging (binge–purge subtype). | Must include both binge eating and inappropriate compensatory behaviors (intentional vomiting, fasting, laxative abuse etc.).[a] | Food avoidance is typically due to sensory characteristics of food, fear of physical discomfort, or lack of interest in eating. |
| Weight trajectory/ nutritional status | Low weight for expected growth trajectory.[b] | Normal or above normal.[c] | Includes any of the following: weight loss, nutritional deficiency, dependence on nutritional supplements, issues with psychosocial functioning. |
| Frequency/ duration | Not defined | Behaviors occur at least once/week for 3 months. Severity defined by frequency.[d] | Not defined |
| Body image concerns/ fear of weight gain | Present | Present | Absent |
| Conditions to rule out | Another medical or mental health condition. | Anorexia nervosa, another medical or mental health condition. | Food availability concerns, culturally sanctioned practices, body image concerns, another medical or mental health condition. |

[a] If purging behaviors occur without binge eating, consider diagnosis of purging disorder
[b] If weight has decreased significantly, but is still at or above normal for age, sex, height, consider diagnosis atypical anorexia nervosa
[c] If weight is significantly low, consider the diagnosis of anorexia nervosa–binge/purge subtype
[d] If all other criteria for Bulimia Nervosa are met, except for the frequency and duration criteria, consider diagnosis of Bulimia Nervosa of low frequency and/or limited duration

## Assessment and Diagnosis

### Preparing for the Initial Visit

The initial visit with the adult provider will be facilitated by having the pediatric medical records at the time of the first visit, especially the growth chart, which ideally maps the premorbid trajectory of the weight and BMI so an estimate of the patient's treatment goal weight (TGW), can be made. In the authors' practice, growth records are requested from the referring provider when the referral is made.

In the authors' opinions, best practice includes weighing the patient in a gown, after voiding, on the same scale at each visit, to obtain an accurate and serially comparable measurement. If this is not feasible, effort should be made to remove outer layers of clothing prior to weighing the patient, as weights or other heavy objects may be kept in clothing to influence the weight measurement. The patient can be weighed with their back to the scale if the patient prefers not to see their weight. This is not a uniform practice, with some providers allowing the patient to see their weight. If this is done, the provider should be prepared to help the patient process the weight information during the clinic visit. The authors have found that knowing their weight can be a source of stress, particularly when the patient is struggling with an active eating disorder. The provider may tell the patient that their weight is up, down, or unchanged, or show them their plotted weight or BMI trajectory, without disclosing the absolute weight.

In the authors' clinical practice, the urine is assessed by dipstick for specific gravity and ketones at each clinic visit. Ketonuria is an indicator of acute starvation and can be an indicator for admission when other supportive criteria are present. A low urine specific gravity ($\leq$1.005) can be a sign of intentional excessive water consumption. The patient may do so in order to artificially elevate their weight prior to a medical assessment. If a low urine specific gravity is noted, the patient can be asked to void again, and the weight and specific gravity determination can be repeated until the specific gravity is >1.005. If there is a concern about water loading, the process of voiding and reweighing may need to be repeated several times within a clinic visit in order to obtain an accurate weight.

**Case Vignette**

*The patient described in the initial case vignette was asked to remove outer layers of clothing, void, and was reweighed. Her weight was determined to be 98 lbs. She had 2+ ketones on a dipstick urine analysis and her urine specific gravity was 1.010.*

## The Initial Meeting: Identifying Goals and Sources of Support

When meeting with a new patient, it is reasonable to ask the patient what their expectations are for the clinic visit: Is it to establish a medical home with the practice? What role do they see the adult provider playing in their care, and for their eating disorder specifically? The names, contact information, and release of information for other providers (dietitian, psychologist, and psychiatrist) involved in the patient's treatment team should be obtained. Sources of support such as caregivers should be identified. If the patient is ≥18 years of age, they may be seen alone. Some young adults do not know this and are accompanied by their parents or caregivers into the room.

**Key Tips for Providers: Preparatory Steps**

- Obtain pediatric or prior providers' records, if possible.
- Minimize errors in the measurement of weight and recognize that some patients may not benefit from knowing their weight. Decide how you want to provide weight information.
- Urine dipstick assessments can be a useful office tool.
- Identify the patient's goals for the visit.
- If accompanied by an adult caregiver, it is advised that the medical provider (1) spend some time with the patient alone to allow for responses that may be filtered by the presence of their parent and (2) ask permission from the young adult for a parent to remain for a portion of the assessment.

## History and Examination

The history should include details regarding dietary habits, exercise history, compensatory behaviors, prior weight or growth trajectory, goal weight or size, body image concerns, and past medical and family histories. Not all information can and will be obtained during the first visit. The patient may not be comfortable disclosing all aspects of the disorder during the interview, and gradual disclosure is common.

### Weight History

Having obtained growth charts or weight and height collected over time from previous medical providers is ideal and can help to determine the extent and rate of weight change. In the absence of prior weight and BMI data, a weight history from the patient, including highest and lowest weights, and a timeline of weight loss can help determine TGW. For patients with BN or ARFID, weight loss may not be present, and instead, weight fluctuations (in BN) or failure to grow as expected (in ARFID) may have occurred.

### Diet History

The goal is to obtain a crude estimate of the intake pattern and eating disorder behaviors to assess the risk for refeeding syndrome and/or the need for a higher level of care. Refeeding syndrome refers to a rare constellation of metabolic and clinical complications that arise from the rapid re-nourishment of a malnourished individual [3]. Once urgent concerns are addressed, a more detailed dietary history can be obtained at a later time by a dietitian. The provider can start by asking the patient what they ate and drank in the past 24 h, including caffeine and alcohol intake. Patients with eating disorders are not always forthcoming, so asking follow-up questions may be necessary.

For patients with restrictive eating behaviors, useful questions include:

- What percentage of the meal/snack did you complete?
- Are you choosing non-fat or sugar-free food items?
- Is this a typical day? (Patients will report good days when intake is higher than normal and bad days when intake is significantly lower. You can also ask “How many good days versus bad days do you have in a week?”)
- Does intake differ on the weekends? (Patients may sleep in late to skip meals.)
- Do you restrict or limit foods in order to drink alcoholic beverages later in the day? Do you eat differently the day after drinking?
- Do you have a calorie goal for the day or per meal? How do you track calories? How many days per week do you meet this goal? How many days per week are you under this goal? (Eating less than planned.)
- Have you ever gone a full day or more without eating?

Assessing for binge eating episodes may require questions to cover the full definition of binge eating (e.g., eating a large amount of food, in a specific time period, and feeling a loss of control during the episode).

- How often do you find yourself eating a meal, larger than a typical meal that others may eat? Please give me an example of what you ate the last time it occurred. Did you purge afterward?
- While you were eating that meal/snack, did you experience feeling out of control when you were eating (e.g., as if you may have wanted to stop but found you just could not stop eating, or continued to eat despite being uncomfortably full)? Do you ever black out or cannot remember portions of the binge/eating episode?
- Did you experience a sense of guilt or shame after a binge? Do you ever eat in secret? Do you wake up at night to binge?
- What foods or events might trigger a binge?
- Is alcohol involved with overeating/binge eating episodes?

For a patient with ARFID:

- Do fears of physical sensations of discomfort (e.g., choking, nausea, and abdominal pain) keep you from eating expected amounts of food?
- Do you see yourself as disinterested in food and eating?
- Are there certain textures, smells, or colors of foods that you avoid?
- Did you have any feeding difficulties as a child?

If time allows, the provider might ask more in-depth questions to identify safe and fearful foods, for example:

What foods have you cut out or do you avoid?

What foods feel safe and comfortable to eat?

Do you read food labels? What are you looking for or avoiding?

Do you have any food rules and where did these come from? (e.g., Internet sources.)

**Key Tips from the Dietitian When Doing a Dietary Recall**

- Ask the patient to start with the first time they eat or drink something, rather than asking to start with “breakfast.” Many patients have varied schedules, skip meals, or do not eat full meals, so categorizing in this way can lead them to provide inaccurate information.
- Ask for times of each eating occurrence to get an idea of restriction or binge patterns. Some patients will not eat until dinner, while others will not eat after 4 pm, for example.
- Ask about all sources of caffeine intake, not just coffee. Some patients will drink caffeinated water or sports drinks.

## Exercise History

The provider may ask questions in different ways to understand the frequency, duration, and intensity of exercise. For example,

- What types of exercise do you engage in and how often do you exercise?
- Do you engage in physical activities outside of formal exercise (e.g., do you count your steps; do you use a fitness app)?
- Do you take the long way to get to a destination?
- Do you stand to eat or work rather than sit?
- Do you have rules about exercise that you follow?
- If you are not able to meet that goal(s), how does that affect your mood/day? How much stress does it cause?
- How much do you skip out on other activities (e.g., time with friends or family) in order to complete exercise?

## Other Compensatory Behaviors

These can include self-induced vomiting, diuretic use, insulin misuse, diet pills use, and laxative use. Coffee, when consumed quickly, can be used as a laxative by patients. Some patients will also drink "digestive" teas or supplements, which contain laxatives or are advertised as a weight loss product. Questions to ask include:

- When you experience guilt after eating or drinking, what do you do?
- Do you purge after every meal, or are there certain foods, drinks, or events that will trigger a purge?
- How many times per day or per week do you purge?
- Have you ever taken any pills to aid in weight loss?
- If insulin-dependent: Have you ever skipped a dose or lowered your insulin dose to avoid weight gain?

**Key Tips for Asking About Other Eating Disorder Behaviors**

- Ask further clarifying questions to quantitate the extent and frequency of these behaviors.
- Patients may not be forthcoming, often due to guilt or worry that disclosure may lead to a higher level of care being recommended, and hence, non-judgmental tone and language should be adopted.
- Not every question can be asked on the first visit, and the interdisciplinary team and follow-up visits can complete the assessment.

## Body Image

Asking a patient if they have a goal weight helps determine whether they have a desire for further weight loss or a fear of weight gain. Sample questions include:

- "How would you feel if you gained 2–10 lbs.?" or "How much weight gain would be too much?" also help to assess for the presence of a fear of weight gain.
- Dissatisfaction with body size can be assessed by asking if they identify any areas of their body as problematic: "What areas about your body concern you most?" or "What parts of your body, if any, do you struggle to look at?"

The presence of behaviors such as body checking (which may include pinching, excessive weighing or mirror checking, and measuring different areas of the body) or body avoidance (e.g., wearing unusually large or warm clothes especially when the weather would not suggest it, avoiding photographs/reflections) also indicates concerns about body image. The percentage of their day that they spend thinking about food or body size can provide a gauge of the level of distress caused by body image concerns and can be followed over time.

**Key Tips for Asking About Other Body Image Concerns**

- Providing hypothetical scenarios to probe the patient's comfort with a change in body size can help gauge distress over body image or a fear of weight gain.
- Patients may state that they have no concerns about weight gain or they see themselves as too thin. They may be aware of what their providers/caregivers may prefer to hear. However, if their behaviors continue to interfere with weight gain (e.g., restriction despite advice to increase nutrition), this may indicate a functional fear of weight gain.

## Family History of Mental Health Issues and Eating Disorders

Ask about the family history of similar concerns (e.g., eating struggles and specific ED diagnoses).

**Case Vignette**

*With further questioning the patient described in the case vignette revealed that she often skipped breakfast and lunch. She typically eats at the end of the day, and her meal the day prior to her visit included a piece of chicken breast, a cup of carrots and peas, and half a cup of cooked brown rice. Besides the running, her exercise regimen included strength training activities 3 days/week. Her medical providers have told her that she was malnourished, but she continues to worry that her stomach and thighs are too big. While she is regularly dizzy with a change in position, she also experienced an episode where she briefly passed out after completing a run a few days ago. She stated that all the women in her family have never weighed over 110 lbs., and given that she is shorter than most of the female members of her family, she estimates she should easily weigh below that. She reported weighing herself each day before any intake to decide how she proceeds with food for the rest of the day.*

## Signs and Symptoms

A review of systems and physical examination will help recognize the manifestations of malnutrition. Common symptoms and physical examination findings are described in Table 22.2 [3, 10].

## Diagnosing Malnutrition

In order to diagnose malnutrition, a minimum of two of the indicators described in Table 22.3 must be met [11].

**Table 22.2** Review of systems and physical examination Findings in eating disorders [3, 10]

| Symptoms | Physical examination findings |
|---|---|
| Pallor or fatigue<br>Dizziness, pre-syncope, and syncope<br>Abdominal pain, bloating, and constipation<br>Hair loss, dry skin, and brittle nails<br>Poor concentration or sleep disruption<br>Chest pain or palpitations<br>Poor wound healing<br>Muscle cramps<br>Sexual dysfunction and decreased libido<br>Missed or light menstrual cycles | Cachexia and wasting<br>Cognitive slowing, lanugo, thinning of scalp hair. Pallor, skin discoloration due to hypercarotenemia, brittle nails, scarring/callouses along the knuckles from self-induced vomiting (Russel's sign), scars from prior cutting episodes, dental enamel erosion, parotid enlargement<br>Bradycardia, postural tachycardia or hypotension, peripheral edema, acrocyanosis<br>Abdominal discomfort with palpation, accumulated stool burden, scaphoid abdomen<br>Testicular atrophy, breast atrophy, vaginal dryness |

**Table 22.3** Diagnosing malnutrition [11]

| | Non-severe (moderate) malnutrition | Severe malnutrition |
|---|---|---|
| **Energy intake**<br>This is an estimate of recent intake compared to estimated energy needs | ≤75% of estimated energy needs for ≥3 months | ≤50% of estimated energy needs for ≥1 month |
| **Weight loss**<br>This is reported as % of total body weight (TBW) lost from baseline weight | 5% TBW in 1 month<br>7.5% TBW in 3 months<br>10% TBW in 6 months<br>20% TBW in 1 year | >5% TBW in 1 month<br>>7.5% TBW in 3 months<br>>10% TBW in 6 months<br>>20% TBW in 1 year |
| **Physical assessment**<br>Muscle loss, subcutaneous fat loss, and/or fluid accumulation | Mild | Severe |

## Determining Estimated Energy Needs

In order to determine a rough estimate of recent energy intake, you will first need to estimate daily energy requirements for your patient. For sedentary female patients >18 years old, their estimated energy needs are 34 kcal/kg/day. For sedentary male patients >18 years old, their estimated energy needs are 36 kcal/kg/day [12].

> **Case Vignette**
>
> *For the case vignette described, the patient weighs 44.5 kg, and the estimated energy needs are 44.5 × 34 = 1514 kcal/day. If she is eating 500 kcal/day that equates to consuming 32% of her estimated energy needs and would meet the severe malnutrition criterion in* Table 22.3.

## Determining Treatment Goal Weight (TGW)

We would expect most patients to return to their premorbid weight, rather than assume that a BMI > 18.5 is the goal [13]. Due to the change in the diagnostic criteria for AN in the DSM-5, there has been an increase in the subset of patients with higher BMIs that meet criteria for atypical AN or AN-restricting type. Research with respect to the energy adaptations in this subset of patients is minimal and presents mixed findings. We know from adult literature on weight loss that metabolic adaptation occurs and resting energy expenditure is reduced more than would be predicted (i.e., adaptive thermogenesis) in patients with premorbid overweight and obesity, making it easier for these patients to return to a BMI in the overweight or obese range [14]. The extent of weight gain required and refeeding protocols to resolve complications of malnutrition for these patients has not been determined. It is the authors' practice to norm patients with premorbid overweight and obesity to their premorbid weight initially, with a focus on the resolution of symptoms of malnutrition, dietary adequacy, and resolution of eating disorder thoughts and behaviors. It is possible that the patient's weight may stabilize lower than their premorbid weight and estimated TGW may need to be revised as the patient progresses through treatment—this should be an interdisciplinary team decision.

> **Case Vignette**
>
> *Growth charts for the patient in the case vignette above were obtained (*Fig. 22.1*). Based on her growth trajectory prior to the onset of her eating disorder between ages 14 and 16, the authors normed this patient to the 50*th *percentile BMI for age. Using the Centers for Disease Control and Prevention growth curve, the authors determine that the BMI at the 50*th *percentile for an 18-year, 6-month-old woman is 21.4 kg/m*$^2$*. Using her height, 169.3 cm (1.693 m), we calculate her TGW to be 61.3 kg, using the equation: TGW = BMI × Height (m) × Height (m).*

Other examples of determining TGW are described.

***Patient A*** This 18-year-old woman with premorbid obesity began losing weight rapidly

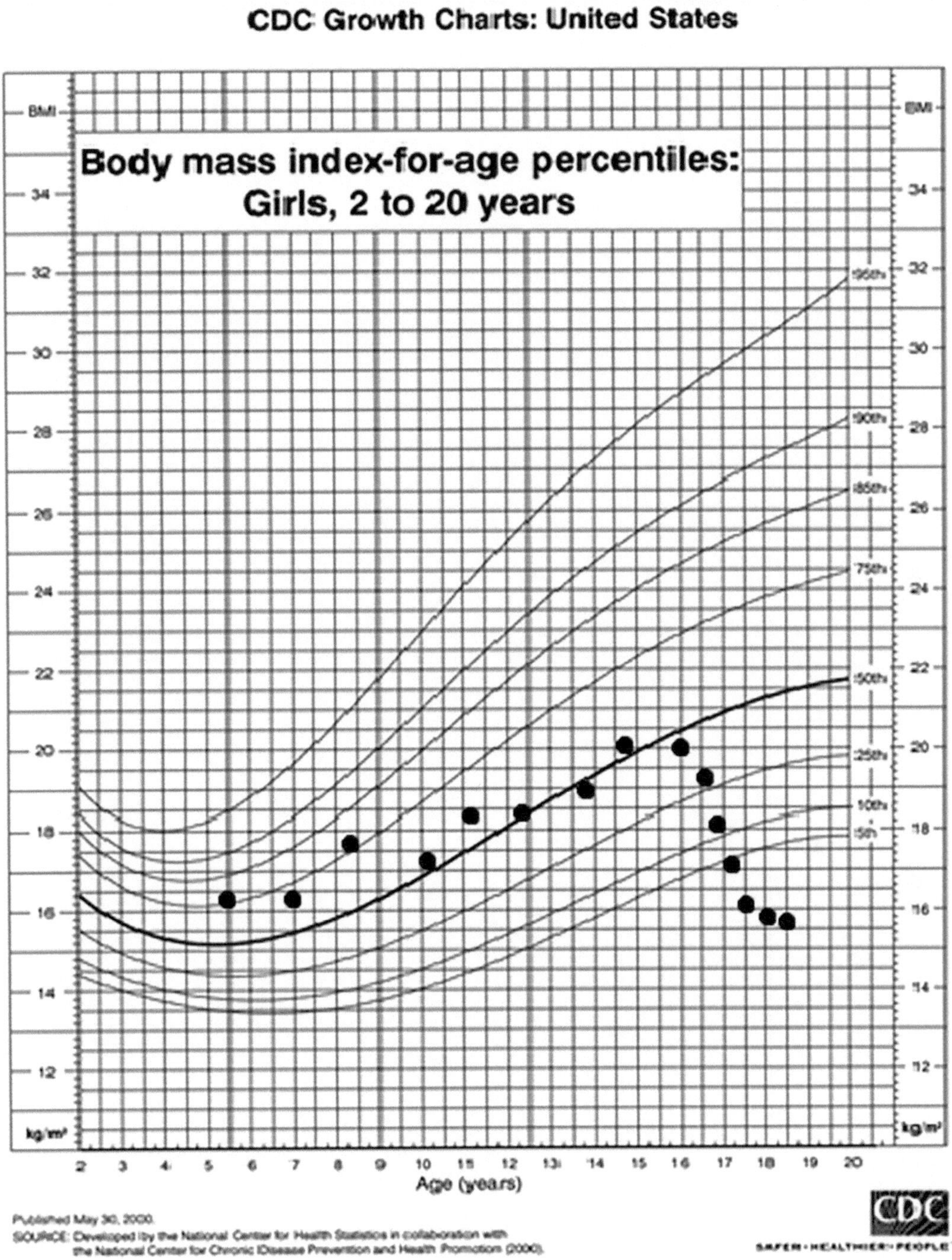


**Fig. 22.1** BMI-for-age growth chart of patient described in initial case vignette

when she joined the wrestling team at age 15 (Fig. 22.2). Though her BMI never reached what ostensibly might be seen as an unhealthy range, she was malnourished, manifested as bradycardic, fatigued, and had incurred multiple injuries. The authors' treatment goal was weight stabilization with a resolution of symptoms and improved eating behaviors to eventually support her desired level of physical activity.

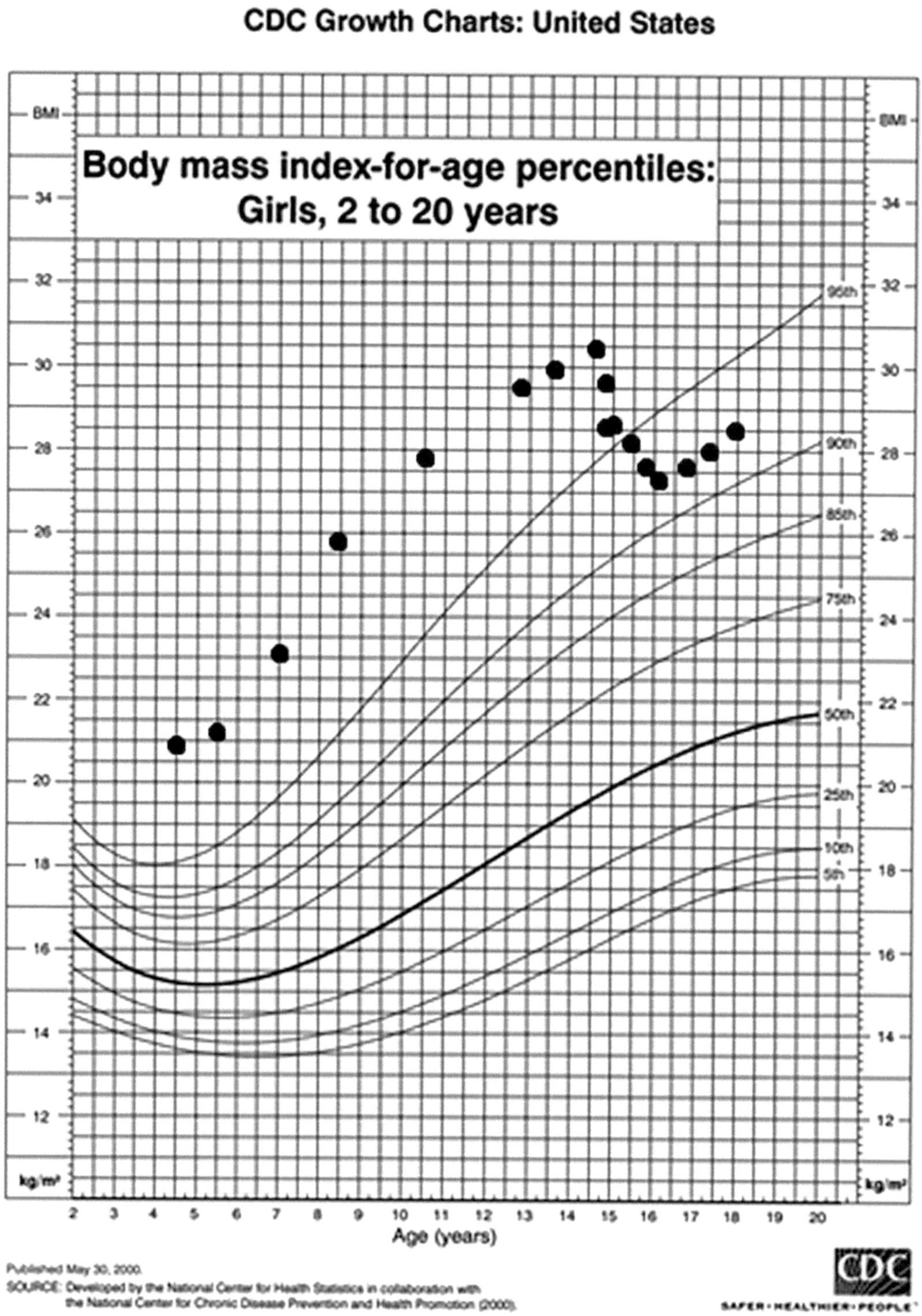


Fig. 22.2 BMI-for-age growth chart for Patient A

***Patient B*** This 17-year-old was normed by the authors to the 25th percentile BMI-for-age (Fig. 22.3).

If history is limited and previous growth data are not available, aim for a minimum BMI >18.5 with a resolution of signs and symptoms

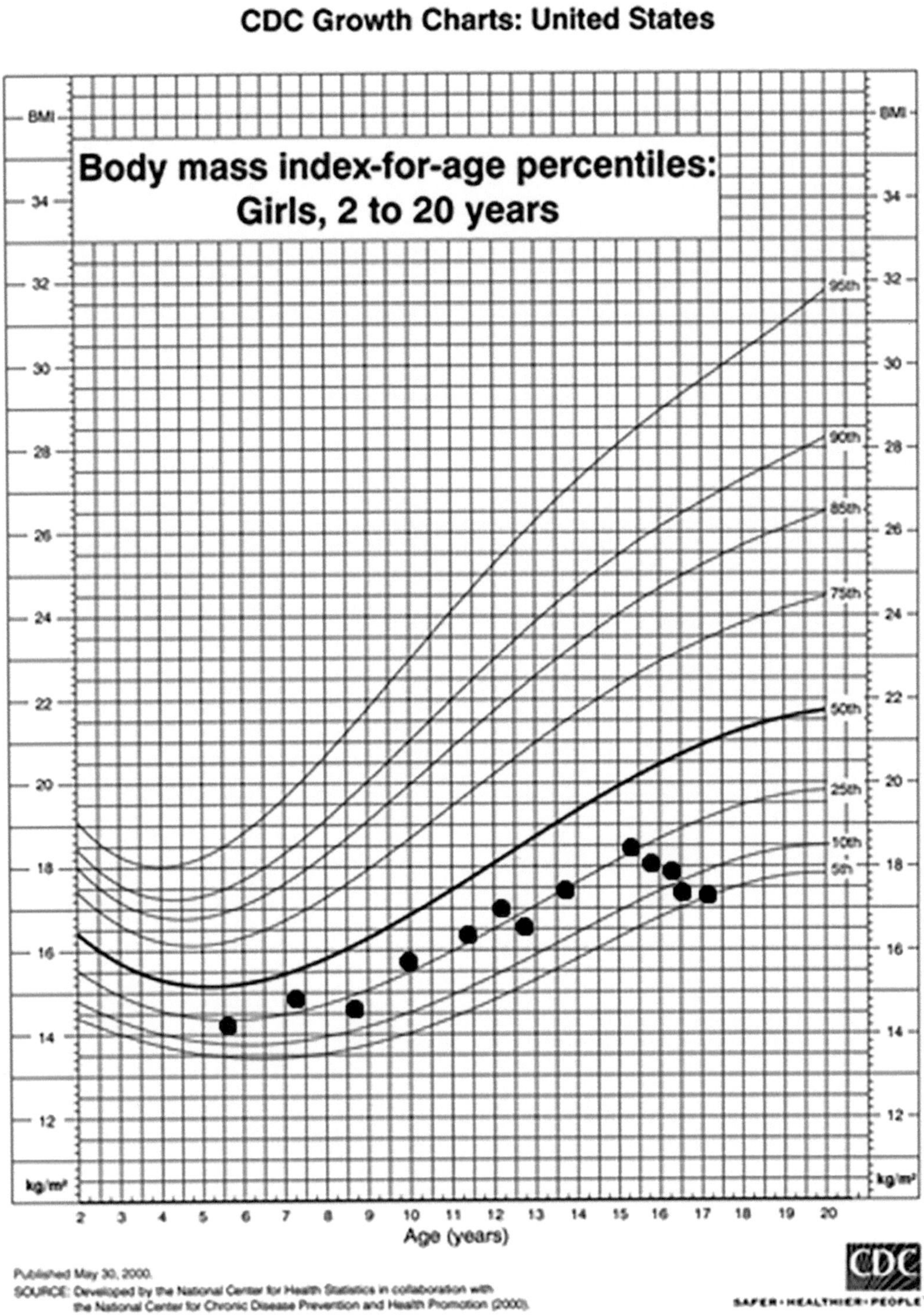


**Fig. 22.3** BMI-for-age growth chart for Patient B

(e.g., resumption of menses, normal vital signs, and no symptoms of malnutrition or energy deficit).

## Laboratory Evaluation

Laboratory evaluation for a patient with an eating disorder can include tests to identify medical complications from the eating disorder and to identify alternate diseases that may present with similar symptoms (Table 22.4) [3, 15].

## Treatment and Care

### Team Members and Level of Care

Once the assessment is complete and an ED diagnosis has been confirmed, the provider and

**Table 22.4** Laboratory evaluation [3, 15]

| |
|---|
| Complete blood count and serum ferritin<br>• Malnutrition-related bone marrow suppression and resultant pancytopenia.<br>• Abnormalities related to an underlying alternate illness such as cancer, inflammatory bowel disease, or rheumatological diseases that may present with weight loss. |
| Inflammatory markers (erythrocyte sedimentation rate or C-reactive protein)<br>• Elevated inflammatory markers can raise suspicion for an alternate reason for the weight loss. |
| Blood urea nitrogen and creatinine<br>• Acute kidney injury due to dehydration related to water restriction or purging.<br>• Underlying chronic kidney disease may present with poor growth and malnutrition. |
| Electrolytes (sodium, potassium, magnesium, calcium, and phosphorus)<br>• Low serum sodium levels due to excessive water consumption (to artificially elevate the weight prior to medical visits); increased sodium levels due to limited water consumption and dehydration (fear of any oral intake including water).<br>• Low serum potassium due to vomiting or laxative abuse.<br>• Along with serum potassium, levels of magnesium and phosphorus may decrease due to rapid calorie intake, leading to refeeding syndrome. |
| Serum liver transaminase levels<br>• Mildly elevated due to starvation-induced hepatocyte autophagy.<br>• Moderately elevated if the patient develops refeeding syndrome. |
| Urine analysis<br>• Urine specific gravity may provide insight into the patient's hydration status (limited water intake or excessive water intake).<br>• Ketonuria is often noted due to starvation. |
| Thyroid hormone tests<br>• Thorough review of systems can help determine whether malnutrition is better explained by an intrinsic thyroid disease.<br>• Without intrinsic thyroid disease, a euthyroid-sick pattern (normal or low TSH and T4, low T3) can be seen in patients with chronic malnutrition. |
| Specific vitamin and mineral levels<br>• Typically, not necessary.<br>• Maybe considered on a case-by-case basis depending on the nutrition history. |
| Cardiac testing<br>• Electrocardiogram: Bradycardia or a slow junctional rhythm; prolonged QT intervals, though this is not thought to be directly caused by anorexia nervosa; abnormalities in the setting of electrolyte disturbances.<br>• Echocardiography is not indicated unless prompted by clinical symptoms. |
| Evaluation for amenorrhea<br>• Hormonal testing and a pregnancy test if the review of systems indicates an alternate explanation for the missed menstrual cycles.<br>• Bone density measurement using dual X-ray absorptiometry in patients with amenorrhea for >6 months. |

patient should consider the most appropriate level of care. An interdisciplinary team is necessary for ED treatment [16, 17]. The team most often consists of a medical provider, a registered dietitian (RD) or registered dietitian nutritionist (RDN), and a psychotherapist. Additional team members may include a second therapist to assist with family therapy/intervention or to address specific comorbidity (e.g., obsessive-compulsive disorder), a psychiatrist for additional diagnostic clarity and medication management, and/or physical therapist, or sports medicine physician for a proper return to physical activity after medical nutritional rehabilitation manifests as cardiovascular stability. Ideally, each team member has expertise in managing eating disorders and has the ability and patient release of information to communicate between themselves. Some medical providers, dietitians, and psychotherapists may also be Certified Eating Disorders Specialist (CEDS), but many experts in eating disorder care are not CEDS.

Options of care range from most intensive (i.e., inpatient management) to least intensive (i.e., standard outpatient management). Table 22.5 describes different levels of care in treatment and patient factors and medical/health factors to consider for choosing a level of care. Which ED treatment programs are covered differs greatly by insurance and payer source. Patients and families may benefit from requesting a case manager or social worker affiliated with their insurance or provider's clinic office to help navigate the financial decision of care.

## Medical Hospitalization

This should be considered when there is a risk for refeeding syndrome (Table 22.6), significant abnormalities in vital signs, electrolyte disturbances, syncope, or need for nasogastric feeds.

## Partial Hospitalization Programs (PHPs)

These programs typically have a minimum programming of 5 days per week/20 h per week; some programs may be designed for more treatment up to 6–7 days per week [18]. At the PHP level and above, treatment is the primary focus for the young adult, often with little time or liberty to complete other activities regularly. The PHP level is the most intense level of treatment where an adult patient continues to reside at home or in independent living.

## Intensive Outpatient Programs (IOPs)

These programs are typically 3–4 h/day and 3–5 days per week [18]. Often, patients gradually step down in an IOP (e.g., move from 4 days a week to 3 days a week), which is one reason why different programs or different patients' experiences of programs may vary significantly. Starting at the IOP level, adults typically return to other activities of daily living (e.g., work and school); therefore, programming often occurs mostly during late afternoon/evening hours. It is important that a patient be able to demonstrate some independence and motivation with eating in order to enter an IOP, as most meals may be eaten outside of the program.

## Other Considerations

If there is a comorbid, acute psychiatric condition, appropriate levels of care should be decided with respect to safety and co-presenting symptomatology. Adults presenting with suicidal intention, active self-harm, or suicidal ideation without the ability to create and adhere to a safety plan without one-to-one supervision are not can-

**Table 22.5** Different levels of care defined with respect to program, patient, and health characteristics [10, 24, 40]

| Level of Care | Range of therapeutic days per week (hours per week) | Meal management/ supervision | Living arrangements | Engaged in typical daily activities for the majority of the day (e.g., school/ work) | Goals of the program | Patient medical status (% estimated health body weight) | Structure needed by the patient | Motivation to recover | Appropriate for young adults with comorbid active SI/ psychosis |
|---|---|---|---|---|---|---|---|---|---|
| Outpatient | 1–2 (<9 h) | Full independence | Independent living[a] | Yes | Independence | Medically stable (>85%) | Self-sufficient<br>Can greatly reduce incidents of purging<br>Can manage exercise | Fair to good | No |
| Intensive outpatient program (IOP) | 3–5 (≥9 h)[b] | 15–50% supervised | Independent living | Yes | Increase independence<br>Return to "real life" | Medically stable (>80%) | Needs some structure to gain weight<br>Can greatly reduce incidents of purging, with some independence<br>Needs mild structure around exercise | Fair | No |
| Partial hospitalization (PHP) | 5–7 (≥20 h) | 70–90% supervised | Independent living | No | Becoming more independent<br>Ability to eat on their own and tolerate distress | Medically stable (>80%) | Needs some structure to gain weight<br>Can greatly reduce incidents of purging<br>Needs structure around exercise | Fair cooperative | No |

| Level of Care | Range of therapeutic days per week (hours per week) | Meal management/ supervision | Living arrangements | Engaged in typical daily activities for the majority of the day (e.g., school/ work) | Goals of the program | Patient medical status (% estimated health body weight) | Structure needed by the patient | Motivation to recover | Appropriate for young adults with comorbid active SI/ psychosis |
|---|---|---|---|---|---|---|---|---|---|
| Residential | 7 (varies) | 100% supervised | Live on site | No | Weight restoration<br>Behavioral symptom management<br>Prepare for return to home | Not requiring tube feeds or daily laboratory tests (<85%, typically >75%) | Needs supervision during and after all meals<br>Can ask for support to inhibit purging<br>Needs structure around exercise | Poor to fair<br>Uncooperative with treatment at lower levels of care | Yes |
| Inpatient | 7 (varies) | 100% supervised | Live on site | No | Medical stabilization | HR <40 bpm<br>Orthostatic hypotension with symptoms.<br>Temp <96°<br>Significant ECG or electrolyte abnormality<br><75%, or acute weight decline with food refusal | Needs tube feeds<br>Needs supervision during and after all meals<br>Unable to control binge/ purge/exercise episodes | Very poor<br>Uncooperative with treatment at lower levels of care | Yes |

[a] Independent living may also be inclusive of a young adult living with a family member or roommate. Independent living indicates that the young adult is responsible for securing their own housing/living arrangement outside of the treatment program

[b] Between program variation is high for IOP and PHP with respect to number of hours of treatment and program structure (e.g., meal management). Within the program differences also occur, most often at the IOP level; as a patient makes progress, they may participate in fewer aspects of the program to allow for a gradual shift to outpatient management

**Table 22.6** Risk factors for refeeding syndrome [10]

| |
|---|
| • Severe malnutrition as defined in Table 22.3 and/ or BMI ≤ 15 |
| • Caloric intake of ≤500 kcal/day for 10+ days |
| • Weight loss >10–15% of total body weight in 3–6 months |
| • Patients with significant comorbid substance use: alcohol, diuretics, laxatives, and/or insulin misuse |
| • Electrolyte abnormalities |
| • Patients with a history of weight loss surgery |

If one or more of these risk factors are present, consider suitability for medical hospitalization. In the authors' opinion, allowing the patient to eat ad lib well beyond 40 kcal/kg body weight/d during the first week is a risk factor for refeeding syndrome

didates for a PHP or less intense program; residential or inpatient should be considered in these cases. For adults presenting with ED and active psychosis or schizophrenia diagnosis and/or differential monitoring, a consult with psychiatry is recommended and consideration of a level of care higher than PHP (e.g., residential or inpatient) is needed [18]. In the authors' opinion, substance abuse, misuse, or dependence is navigated on an individual basis for each patient and the presence of either complicates the recovery. If a short-term detoxification treatment is necessary and can be completed with medical safety, this would take precedence over longer-term eating disorder work. Once the initial detoxification program is complete, an ED intensive program with special consideration to not reinitiating substance use is the indicated treatment in the authors' opinion. Other common comorbidities (e.g., major depressive disorder, generalized anxiety disorder, and obsessive-compulsive disorder) must be co-treated in the level of care chosen if the patient is going to recover.

## Management

### Nutritional Management

#### Outpatient

Patients should be referred to an RD/RDN for individualized nutrition planning and management [10]. The authors ask the patient to set at least one specific/measurable/attainable goal to increase intake when they are in the clinic. Patients may be eating very little; therefore, setting a goal to increase intake incrementally from where they are at presentation, rather than starting with what might be considered normal intake for a patient of their size or age, is important both for avoiding refeeding syndrome and patient adherence to the plan.

**Tips from the RD for Creating Management Plans with Patients**

- Avoid discussing calories and using categorizing language such as "good/ healthy" versus "bad/unhealthy" foods.
- Avoid focusing on numbers, and this includes weight (have patients remove scale from home if they are willing).

For the patient with AN or ARFID (malnutrition), it is recommended to start increasing by 250–500 calories per day, which is equivalent to one to two high-calorie nutritional supplements per day. The provider should recommend specific brands and formulations based on local availability and cost. If specific guidance is not provided, the patient may choose to add a low-calorie supplement drink and limit their medical nutritional recovery. If time allows, using a motivational interviewing-informed approach to develop a plan with the patient can be beneficial [19]. For example:

- "Ideally, I'd suggest you increase your intake by adding two nutritional supplement drinks per day; what feels most doable this week to move closer to that goal?"

  For patients with BN or with binge episodes, a starting goal may center around the timing of meals, as patients with BN may report patterns of restriction, leading to binge/ purge episodes. Often, binge/purge episodes are tied to feelings of guilt and breaking this cycle of bingeing and purging is a welcomed first step for the patient.

- "Ideally, I recommend that people have 3 meals and 1 snack spread throughout the day, as regular eating times lead to less binge episodes. What change is most doable to try this week to help with eating a meal or snack every 3–5 h?"

  A person with BN and little to no treatment experience may be less aware of their pattern of eating. A first goal can also be to have patients track their eating, bingeing, and purging habits for 1 week to look for times of the day or events in the day that may represent a pattern. Once a pattern is recognized, setting goals to alter those maladaptive patterns may be easier.

  For patients who are purging through self-induced emesis, laxative abuse, or over-exercise, try to set a goal to reduce these behaviors. For example:
- "Ideally you would stop purging all together, but often patients find a more gradual process doable. What goal for this week would you set for yourself to reduce your purging?"

There are several strategies that can help with a reduction in binge/purge behaviors:

- The urge to purge typically passes within 20 min encourages patients to find distractions after meals until the urge passes: reading, journaling, playing with pets or children, meditation, art, listening to music, telephoning a loved one, etc.
- Avoid purchasing trigger foods or storing food on the counter/out in the open.
- Encourage bathroom use prior to a meal so that bathroom use after a meal will not be as necessary. Encourage showering earlier in the day to avoid body checking/purging while showering at the end of the day.
- Encourage appropriate use of laxatives for the promotion of bowel function.
- Set exercise limitations to avoid over-exercise.

For the patient with ARFID, often treatment goals with their psychotherapist may address anxiety management strategies and a reduction of avoidance behaviors to eating or certain types of foods. Communicating with their therapist may support ongoing goals such as food exposure and or increasing the variety of foods consumed.

- "Ideally, you are able to eat a variety of foods to support your nutrition. It takes practice to challenge yourself with eating new foods, and it is okay to start with a challenge that is not the absolute hardest. What is one food that you could try this week that you have been avoiding?"

Patients can benefit from starting a multivitamin, as well as calcium supplementation if dairy intake is less than three servings per day. It is also common that they will experience gastrointestinal discomfort, such as constipation, bloating, gas, and early satiety. Prepare the patient for these sensations, and normalize that they will improve with improved nutrition. Home remedies include herbal, decaffeinated, teas (mint, ginger, and chamomile), heating pads, soaking in a warm bath, simethicone, deep breathing, and/or meditation.

If the patient is at high risk for refeeding syndrome and refuses hospital admission, the authors recommend that the patient:

- Increase intake by approximately 100 calories every 2–3 days.
- Start a multivitamin.
- Have serum electrolytes and glucose monitored prior to increasing nutrition and 3 and 7 days later.
- Replete any electrolyte deficiencies through oral supplementation of potassium, phosphorus, or magnesium (if this can be safely done based on levels).
- Avoid fluid overload.

Weight restoration typically occurs more slowly on an outpatient basis, typically 0.5–1 pound per week. A trend of weight loss after three follow-up visits is an indicator that the patient would benefit from a higher level of care.

#### Inpatient

Refeeding can proceed more aggressively due to the ability to monitor vital signs and electrolytes more closely. In the authors' opinion, an inpatient plan could include:

- Starting the refeeding process at 40 kcal/kg/day. The typical malnourished patient loses weight in the first few days of admission [3, 10, 12].
- Advance by 250–300 calories every 1–3 days to promote a weight gain of 2–4 pounds per week. Most patients will require high caloric intake to promote sustained weight gain, often as high as 4000 kcal/day [3].
- Serum electrolytes and glucose should be monitored daily for a minimum of 5–7 days. The monitoring may need to be more frequent based on electrolyte levels.
- Start a multivitamin.
- Replete any electrolyte deficiencies if they develop. The authors' clinical practice is to prophylactically supplement electrolytes for the first 5 days after hospitalization (sodium phosphate and potassium phosphate powder to provide 8–16 mmol of elemental phosphate and 7–14 mmol of elemental potassium per day) [20, 21]. If prophylactic supplementation is done, electrolytes can be monitored every 48 h for 5–7 days.
- Avoid fluid overload and be vigilant to provide slow enteral fluids. For example, the authors limit daily fluid intake in the first days to 80% of estimated maintenance fluids and only use intravenous fluids when acute hemodynamic instability or significant acidosis exists.
- Diet composition should consist of 50% carbohydrates, 20% protein, and 30% fat, delivered through three meals and 1–3 snacks per day.
- Ideally, caloric values of foods and calorie targets would not be directly discussed with patients to minimize an unhealthy focus on caloric goals. An exchange-based system or the plate method for selecting foods is suitable to encourage balance and appropriate amounts of nutrients.
- Meal times should be limited to about 40–45 min, and snack times should be limited to about 20–25 min.
- The authors supplement with a liquid nutritional supplement for any incomplete meals to complete the prescribed calorie intake for the day; if the supplement is not completed, a nasogastric tube is placed for delivery of the supplement.

## Exercise Management

Exercise limitation should be recommended in patients who are at a low %TGW, have lost a significant amounts of weight, or have symptoms or vital sign abnormalities.

Sample exercise recommendations for outpatients with non-severe (moderate or mild) malnutrition:

For those >90% TGW
    Reduce training volume by 33–50%
If 85–90% TGW
    Reduce training volume by 50%
If <85% TGW
    In general, no exercise
    Exceptions: If they are menstruating normally, 80–85% TGW, have normal vital signs, and no symptoms, some exercise may be allowed while monitoring for weight gain.

## Psychological Interventions

Psychotherapists may differ in their treatment approach to a young adult with an ED. Encouraging your young adult patient to inquire with their therapist about the type of treatment they do is recommended. Cognitive-behavioral therapy (CBT) has empirical support for adults with AN and BN. Interpersonal therapy (IPT) has also shown effectiveness with persons with BN [17, 22–27]. Young adults with AN who live with their parents/caregivers or who have close, supportive connections to a family that lives close to them may benefit from an upward extension of family-based therapy (FBT), the treatment best supported for children and adolescents with EDs, especially AN [28]. Given that the evidence base of CBT for AN still has limitations and given that AN has significant malnutrition comorbidities that may impact treatment participation (e.g., weakness, poor concentration/attention, and psychomotor/cognitive slowing), derivations of FBT that include supporting the autonomy of the young adult may be appropriate [29–31]; however, this is understudied at this time.

One treatment consideration is that EDs, most notably AN, present in a young adult with varying degrees of motivation for recovery. For some who may be pre-contemplative or early contemplative of change, the eating disorder is often perceived to have more benefits than consequences to the individual. When ambivalence or even discord is present when attempting to support a young adult in starting treatment, MI may provide helpful communication tools and strategies to improve ambivalence and guide toward change but is not solely sufficient [19, 32–34]. Early research has indicated mixed findings, where MI interventions have impacted positively the patient's readiness for change and treatment completion rates. Current guidelines for adult psychotherapy are often available online such as those provided by the Society of Clinical Psychology [22].

## Pharmacotherapy

Several trials have examined the role of psychotropic medications for the treatment of AN; however, the benefit has not been seen for most. Olanzapine may have a limited role in promoting weight gain. Given the relative non-response, psychotropic medications are rarely utilized in patients with AN alone. Under specific circumstances, there may be a role of medications in the treatment of EDs. These include the following: (1) If there is a comorbid condition such as generalized anxiety disorder or major depressive disorder, treatment of the comorbid disorder may alleviate some symptoms of the eating disorder; (2) selective serotonin reuptake inhibitors, specifically high doses of fluoxetine (60 mg/day), have been found to be beneficial for the treatment of BN [35–37].

Hormone therapy, specifically estradiol patch therapy (0.1 mg/day patch changed twice weekly) with supplemental progesterone (medroxyprogesterone 2.5 mg daily for 10 days every month), may be continued in young adult women with amenorrhea who may still have the potential to accrue bone mineral density [37–39]. In the absence of clinically significant fractures, bisphosphonates are contraindicated in reproductive-age women due to their potential for teratogenicity and long half-life [39].

If the patient is on appetite-suppressing medications for other indications (e.g., stimulants for ADHD and topiramate for migraine headaches), it is appropriate to weigh the pros and cons of continuing therapy. Alternative treatment options can be considered, particularly if the patient has a severe ED. If the appetite-suppressing medicines are continued due to risks associated with inadequate treatment of the other disease process, the timing of medication should be considered and the patient should be advised to maintain a regular eating schedule despite a lack of hunger cues.

## Recovery

There is much focus and less consensus on what defines recovery in patients with EDs. Recovery literature focuses on four major areas of recovery: medical, behavioral (e.g., completion of meals), psychological (e.g., reduction of body image disturbance), and the patient's own definition of recovery/well-being. Individuals with AN who they have achieved weight restoration though still experience psychological symptoms, are considered to be partially recovered. Similarly, individuals with BN are partially recovered when some but not all diagnostic criteria are met. When no diagnostic criteria are met for a sustained period, an individual with an eating disorder is thought to be fully recovered [1].

## Resources for Providers

https://www.aedweb.org/publications—best for providers with some information for families.

https://www.nationaleatingdisorders.org/—best for families and patients.

**Case Vignette**

*The patient's history was reassessed to be consistent with her diagnosis of AN, restricting type. Based on the TGW calculations described, she was noted to be at ~72% of TGW. Due to her dizziness with recent syncope, low blood pressure, and clinical signs of pericardial effusion on examination, further inpatient medical evaluation was recommended. All laboratory tests were normal. After a brief hospitalization and inpatient evaluation, she was transferred to residential care. Her post-discharge treatment plan included referral to a dietitian, continued care through an individual therapist, and monthly follow-up for medical monitoring.*

## References

1. American Psychiatric Association, editor. Diagnostic and statistical manual of mental disorders. 5th ed. American Psychiatric Association; 2013. https://doi.org/10.1176/appi.books.9780890425596.
2. Udo T, Grilo CM. Prevalence and correlates of DSM-5–defined eating disorders in a nationally representative sample of U.S. Adults Biol Psychiatry. 2018;84:345–54.
3. Hornberger LL, Lane MA, et al. Identification and Management of Eating Disorders in children and adolescents. Pediatrics. 2021;147(1):e2020040279.
4. Suokas JT, Suvisaari JM, Gissler M, Löfman R, Linna MS, Raevuori A, Haukka J. Mortality in eating disorders: a follow-up study of adult eating disorder patients treated in tertiary care, 1995-2010. Psychiatry Res. 2013;210:1101–6.
5. Keshaviah A, Edkins K, Hastings ER, Krishna M, Franko DL, Herzog DB, Thomas JJ, Murray HB, Eddy KT. Re-examining premature mortality in anorexia nervosa: a meta-analysis redux. Compr Psychiatry. 2014;55:1773–84.
6. Swanson SA, Crow SJ, Le Grange D, Swendsen J, Merikangas KR. Prevalence and correlates of eating disorders in adolescents: results from the national comorbidity survey replication adolescent supplement. Arch Gen Psychiatry. 2011;68:714–23.
7. Steinhausen HC. Outcome of eating disorders. Child Adolesc Psychiatr Clin N Am. 2009;18:225–42.
8. Derenne J. Eating disorders in transitional age youth. Child Adolesc Psychiatr Clin N Am. 2019;28:567–72.
9. Fairburn CG, Cooper Z. Eating disorders, DSM-5 and clinical reality. Br J Psychiatry. 2011;198:8–10.
10. Chao AM, Nicole Cifra R, Heather Dlugosz M, et al. Eating disorders: a guide to medical care. 2021.
11. White JV, Guenter P, Jensen G, Malone A, Schofield M. Academy malnutrition work group, et al. consensus statement: academy of nutrition and dietetics and American Society for Parenteral and Enteral Nutrition: characteristics recommended for the identification and documentation of adult malnutrition (undernutrition). JPEN J Parenter Enteral Nutr. 2012;36(3):275–83.
12. Texas Children's Hospital, editor. Texas children's hospital pediatric nutrition reference guide. 12th ed. Houston, TX: Texas Children's Hospital; 2019.
13. Golden NH, Katzman DK, Sawyer SM, Ornstein RM, Rome ES, Garber AK, Kohn M, Kreipe RE. Position Paper of the Society for Adolescent Health and Medicine: medical management of restrictive eating disorders in adolescents and young adults. J Adolesc Health. 2015;56(1):121–5. https://doi.org/10.1016/j.jadohealth.2014.10.259. PMID: 25530605.
14. Müller MJ, Bosy-Westphal A. Adaptive thermogenesis with weight loss in humans. Obesity. 2013;21:218–28.
15. Sachs KV, Harnke B, Mehler PS, Krantz MJ. Cardiovascular complications of anorexia nervosa: a systematic review. Int J Eat Disord. 2016;49:238–48.
16. Resources—Academy for Eating Disorders. https://www.aedweb.org/resources/about-eating-disorders/treatment-options. Accessed 18 Apr 2022.
17. Hay P. Current approach to eating disorders: a clinical update. Intern Med J. 2020;50:24–9.
18. CIGNA standards and guidelines/medical necessity criteria for treatment of mental health disorders. 2020.
19. Intergovernmental Panel on Climate Change. Summary for policymakers. In: Climate change 2013—the physical science basis. 1st ed. Cambridge University Press; 2014. p. 1–30. https://www.cambridge.org/core/product/identifier/CBO9781107415324A009/type/book_part.
20. Leitner M, Burstein B, Agostino H. Prophylactic phosphate supplementation for the inpatient treatment of restrictive eating disorders. J Adolesc Health. 2016;58:616–20.
21. Katzman DK, Garber AK, Kohn M, Golden NH. Refeeding hypophosphatemia in hospitalized adolescents with anorexia nervosa: a position statement of the society for adolescent health and medicine. J Adolesc Health. 2014;55:455–7.

22. Eating disorders and weight management. Society of Clinical Psychology. https://div12.org/diagnosis/eating-disorders-and-weight-management/. Accessed 18 Apr 2022.
23. Yager J, Devlin M, Halmi K, Herzog D, Mitchell III J, Powers P, Zerbe K. Guideline watch (august 2012): practice Guideline for the treatment of patients with eating disorders, 3rd edition. J Lifelong Learn Psychiatry 2014:12.
24. Yager J, Devlin MJ, Halmi KA, Herzog DB, Mitchell JE, Powers P, Zerbe KJ. Practice guideline for the treatment of patients with eating disorders third edition. Am J Psychiatry. 2006;163:1–128.
25. Marcus M, Wildes J. Evidence-based psychological treatments for eating disorders. In: Gabbard's treatments of psychiatric disorders. 5th ed. American Psychiatric Publishing; 2014. https://doi.org/10.1176/appi.books.9781585625048.gg30.
26. Wilson GT, Shafran R. Eating disorders guidelines from NICE. Lancet (London, England). 2005;365:79–81.
27. NICE Guideline. Eating disorders: recognition and treatment. 2017.
28. Lock J, Le Grange D. Treatment manual for anorexia nervosa: a family-based approach. 2nd ed. New York: Guilford Press; 2015.
29. Chen EY, Weissman JA, Zeffiro TA, Yiu A, Eneva KT, Arlt JM, Swantek MJ. Family-based therapy for young adults with anorexia nervosa restores weight. Int J Eat Disord. 2016;49:701–7.
30. Chen EY, Le Grange D, Doyle AC, Zaitsoff S, Doyle P, Roehrig JP, Washington B. A case series of family-based therapy for weight restoration in young adults with anorexia nervosa. J Contemp Psychother. 2010;40:219–24.
31. Dimitropoulos G, Landers AL, Freeman V, Novick J, Ma BA, Garber A, Daniel GL. Open trial of family-based treatment of anorexia nervosa for transition age youth. J Can Acad Child Adolesc Psychiatry. 2018;27(1):50–61.
32. Dray J, Wade TD. Is the transtheoretical model and motivational interviewing approach applicable to the treatment of eating disorders? A review. Clin Psychol Rev. 2012;32:558–65.
33. Macdonald P, Hibbs R, Corfield F, Treasure J. The use of motivational interviewing in eating disorders: a systematic review. Psychiatry Res. 2012;200:1–11.
34. Weiss CV, Mills JS, Westra HA, Carter JC. A preliminary study of motivational interviewing as a prelude to intensive treatment for an eating disorder. J Eat Disord. 2013;1(1):34.
35. Crow SJ. Pharmacologic treatment of eating disorders. Psychiatr Clin North Am. 2019;42:253–62.
36. Couturier J, Isserlin L, Spettigue W, Norris M. Psychotropic medication for children and adolescents with eating disorders. Child Adolesc Psychiatr Clin N Am. 2019;28:583–92.
37. Davis H, Attia E. Pharmacotherapy of eating disorders. Curr Opin Psychiatry. 2017;30:452–7.
38. Starr TB, Kreipe RE. Anorexia nervosa and bulimia nervosa: brains, bones and breeding. Curr Psychiatry Rep. 2014;16(5):441.
39. Misra M, Klibanski A. Anorexia nervosa and bone. J Endocrinol. 2014;221:R163–76.
40. Innovation Accelerator Program M, for Medicare C, Services M. Overview of substance use disorder (SUD) care clinical guidelines: a resource for states developing SUD delivery system reforms. 2017.

# Part VI

# Case-Based Examples of Management of the Young Adult with a Chronic Childhood Condition

# Attention-Deficit/Hyperactivity Disorder (ADHD)

23

Elissa M. Monteiro, Kashia A. Rosenau, Alice A. Kuo, David S. Stein, Elizabeth B. Harstad, and William J. Barbaresi

## Case Presentation 1

Ascher is a 24-year-old man who presents to you with a broken arm due to a car accident. He has a history of abnormally high-speed car, bike, and recreational accidents which have resulted in several broken bones. In the second grade, his teachers alerted his parents of the difficulty he was experiencing with schoolwork. His teacher reported he was frequently sent out of class for getting out of his seat at inappropriate times and for distracting his classmates. Following this discussion, Ascher's parents approached his pediatrician who referred the family to a neuropsychologist. Soon after, Ascher was formally diagnosed with attention-deficit hyperactivity disorder (ADHD) combined type [1]. At that time, the results of the neuropsychological testing revealed that Ascher had an average IQ. Throughout late elementary, middle, and high school, Ascher tried several stimulant medications with suboptimal improvement in his ADHD symptoms. Eventually, he responded well to dexmethylphenidate XR daily on weekdays and dexmethylphenidate after school as needed to complete his homework. This second dose was key given his mother's report of significant challenges during homework time. Between the ages of 10 and 20, Ascher required emergency room care on 4 occasions due to lacerations (twice) and fractures of his arm and leg. In high school, he began to engage with peers who used alcohol and marijuana; at this time, he began to use marijuana on a daily basis and has continued to smoke marijuana regularly since. Ascher received special education services through late elementary, middle, and high school, primarily due to difficulty in reading and writing skills, as well as organizing and completing his work on time. His teachers recommended he go to vocational school, but ultimately, he chose to attend a community college. The summer after his high school graduation, he discontinued treatment with stimulant medication. Unfortunately, Ascher failed to graduate from community college due to his absence from class and a pattern of missed deadlines for assignments that resulted in him failing three of

E. M. Monteiro (✉)
School of Education, University of California Riverside, Riverside, CA, USA
e-mail: emont062@ucr.edu

K. A. Rosenau
David Geffen School of Medicine, University of California Los Angeles, Los Angeles, CA, USA
e-mail: k.rose@ucla.edu; krosenau@mednet.ucla.edu

A. A. Kuo
Division of Medicine-Pediatrics and Preventive Medicine, University of California, Los Angeles, CA, USA
e-mail: akuo@mednet.ucla.edu

D. S. Stein · E. B. Harstad · W. J. Barbaresi
Division of Developmental Medicine, Department of Medicine, Boston Children's Hospital, Harvard Medical School, Boston, MA, USA


A. A. Kuo et al. (eds.), *Care of Adults with Chronic Childhood Conditions*,
https://doi.org/10.1007/978-3-031-54281-7_23

his five classes. He is currently working a management job in the food industry. He regularly drinks alcohol and reports the use of illegal drugs but denies symptoms of dependence. At his follow-up visit from injuries related to a recent car accident, Ascher informs you that he was diagnosed with ADHD as a child and, because he is experiencing significant problems with distractibility, disorganization, and explosive anger in the workplace, he would like to resume treatment.

## Case Discussion 1

The case of Ascher highlights many of the common challenges seen among adult males with ADHD. Adults with ADHD typically have increased rates of medical problems, specifically in physical health, mental health, and substance abuse. Adults with ADHD exhibit poor habits related to smoking and limited exercise [2, 3] and tend to engage in more risky behaviors. Healthcare costs throughout childhood are double for subjects with ADHD compared to their non-ADHD peers in a 9-year study of median annual healthcare costs [4, 5]. Ascher does not currently exhibit substantial physical health challenges. However, his ongoing challenges with organization, keeping a job, and intermittent substance abuse may predict poorer habits and resultant physical health problems as he ages. In addition, ADHD is associated with impairments in driving, which appears to be related to increased distractibility, risk-taking, and impulsive behaviors while driving for those with ADHD relative to controls, who also engage in more defensive driving practices [6, 7]. Ascher was involved in a recent accident and subsequent emergency room visit as an adult, suggesting that his driving impairment has persisted from high school to adulthood.

Ascher uses alcohol, marijuana, and illicit drugs consistent with the increased rates of substance abuse in adults with ADHD. Individuals seeking substance abuse treatment have far higher rates of ADHD [8], and adults with a history of childhood ADHD exhibit higher rates of substance dependence in adulthood, including new onset dependence [9]. Thus, Ascher's high rates of substance use may be an indicator of risk for further substance use problems, including dependence, in adulthood. However, the fact that Ascher is seeking treatment may be a positive prognostic indicator to mitigate the risk of substance use disorder. Male adolescents with ADHD who were treated with stimulant medication showed reduced rates of substance use disorders relative to those who were untreated [10], and recent studies suggest that adults with ADHD who are medically treated also have reduced risk for substance abuse [11].

Ascher chose a common route for secondary and postsecondary education by attending a public high school and then enrolled in community college. However, Ascher did not graduate from community college, a common outcome among persons with ADHD. Individuals with ADHD typically struggle in school, with higher rates of learning disabilities [12, 13], enrollment in special education, absenteeism, and dropout, coupled with lower academic achievement scores and rates of high school graduation [14]. While we do not have specific information about Ascher's academic achievement, his failure to complete community college in the context of high average cognition suggests he experiences academic challenges. Notably, treatment with stimulant medication in childhood and adolescence moderates negative school outcomes. While we do not have specific data on vocational outcomes, several studies have demonstrated the efficacy of medication treatment in treating core symptoms of ADHD in adults [15, 16]. Further, the childhood and adolescent data and Ascher's history and trajectory (i.e., that he graduated high school while being treated and did not complete community college without treatment) suggest that resumption of medical treatment may be beneficial for him. Stimulant treatment has also been shown to improve driving in adults with ADHD [17].

## Case Presentation 2

Mia Garcia is a 23-year-old woman who presents with concerns related to her ability to remain focused on her coursework. She is currently enrolled in college to become a nurse and has been experiencing significant difficulty with time management, organization, and task completion. As a young child, Mia experienced some difficulties related to reading in elementary school, and she recalls her teachers working with her one-on-one during recess to get her basic sight words memorized and forcing her to read aloud. She reports having to spend much more time to complete tasks compared to her peers throughout elementary, middle, and high school. On average, she received Bs and Cs in her classes, often due to incomplete or incorrect assignments. Despite these challenges, Mia enjoyed her science courses and tended to receive As in those classes. Her teacher exclaimed that her interest in science seemed to improve her motivation in class. While she still tended to get out of her seat and often needed more frequent breaks than peers, she remained interested in the topic during science classes. Given the large amount of effort Mia put into school in order to keep up with her peers, she took a break from academics after graduating high school. Mia's mental health fluctuated during these few years. Two years after graduating from high school, she was given a formal diagnosis of depression by a clinical psychologist. During this time, she also struggled with regulating her alcohol consumption which started to separate her from her friends. She worked as an administrative assistant in a medical office near her home. After 5 years in this role, she decided to go to college to be a nurse. Once again, finally, she felt excited about science again and looked forward to having a regular schedule and a purpose. However, after her first month of classes, Mia quickly began to feel overwhelmed by her course load. She was enrolled in the minimum credits for her program and taking general education courses to prepare her for the nursing track and she noticed she was struggling much more than her peers to manage deadlines from multiple courses, organize her materials, and follow the pace of her lecture. She also noticed she felt restless during her lectures, she tended to fidget with materials in her backpack, and this seemed to distract students seated around her. Finally, after receiving a failing grade on a test that she studied for only the night before, Mia was referred by a professor to her university's student disability services department. It was at this time that she was first formally assessed using neuropsychological instruments which revealed she met the criteria for ADHD. She felt relieved, she had finally received an explanation for the problems she always knew she struggled with but did not know how to explain.

## Case Discussion 2

The case of Mia illustrates many of the stories of females with ADHD. ADHD is often under-identified in females given that the female ADHD phenotype tends to present differently than males [18]. Specifically, females tend to present with ADHD inattentive subtype and, therefore, tend not to be referred by teachers due to behavioral challenges in school [19]. As a result, females with ADHD tend to be diagnosed later in life [19]. Females with ADHD often experience learning challenges throughout their academic career and into college [18]. Importantly, like males, females with ADHD present with attentional difficulties, executive function deficits like disorganization, time management, impulsivity, and reward processing challenges [20].

Mia also exhibited struggles with mental health issues, including depression diagnosed in early adulthood. Adults with persistent ADHD, as seems to be the case for Mia, are much more likely to experience co-occurring psychiatric disorders, at a rate of 81 versus 35% of non-ADHD controls in one large cohort study [21, 22]. The risk of death from suicide in those with ADHD versus controls is also substantially elevated [22], and Mia's struggles with depression likely place her at higher risk for suicidality.

In the social domain, Mia is exhibiting many of the typical challenges for adults with ADHD. Individuals with ADHD are noted to have more difficulties with personal relationships [23]. While not the case for Mia, some adults with ADHD become parents at an early age [24]. This might predict financial challenges given that many adults with ADHD struggle to hold a job consistently due to apparent difficulties with executive function, particularly organization. Unfortunately, adults with ADHD are more likely to struggle to meet job requirements, to be perceived negatively by employers and to be fired from jobs [25].

Mia suffers from persistent ADHD, as will be discussed further, and characteristics of treatment for adults with ADHD differ from that of childhood ADHD, often taking the form of cognitive behavioral therapy and skill-based coaching.

Treatment approaches for childhood ADHD are well established. The American Academy of Pediatrics [26] has issued a guideline for the diagnosis and treatment of ADHD in children and adolescents. In preschool-age children, behavior therapy focused on parent training is the first-line intervention, and this can be followed by combined treatment with stimulant medication if behavioral treatment is insufficient. In school-aged children, the guidelines recommend combined treatment that includes medication, behavioral therapies, and school-based accommodations. When combined, these treatments are the most effective in addressing core symptoms; associated social, emotional, and academic issues; and allow for maintenance on lower doses of stimulant medication. These treatment recommendations are based on the Multimodal Treatment of ADHD Study [27–30] which represents the largest and most rigorous comparative trial of ADHD treatments in children and adolescents.

For adults with ADHD, medication treatment is effective in symptom management and is well tolerated [31]. Medication is the primary mode of intervention and leads to improved functioning, though long-term functional outcomes have not been sufficiently studied to date. In addition to medical intervention; however, there is evidence that psychotherapy and specifically targeted cognitive behavioral therapy (CBT) have a role in the treatment of adults with ADHD [32]. CBT may address skill deficits such as issues with executive function—likely at least in part due to improved understanding and enhanced self-awareness—and may also help to manage comorbid psychiatric conditions that have a major impact on functioning. For Mia, who struggles with executive function and has a history of depression, CBT would be an effective adjunct to psychotropic medication. It is also important to note that skill deficits and their impact on employment may be somewhat moderated by working with a rehabilitation agency. State rehabilitation agencies work with adults who have any impairing condition, including ADHD, and who would benefit from vocational assessments, job training, or job placement assistance.

Mia would likely benefit from accommodations provided by her professors and advocacy skills taught by her university's student disability resource center.

## Definition

ADHD is a neurobehavioral condition characterized by significant inattention and/or hyperactivity/impulsivity across at least two different settings, such as home and work. Symptoms must be present from early childhood, by age 12 years according to the Diagnostic and Statistical Manual of Mental Disorders (DSM)-5 [1], although it is possible for symptoms to only become apparent with increasing attentional and organizational demands of late childhood or even adulthood. Individuals can be diagnosed with ADHD of the predominantly inattentive presentation, ADHD of the predominantly hyperactive/impulsive presentation, or ADHD of the combined presentation. For adults, five out of nine of the inattentive and/or five out of nine of the hyperactive/impulsive symptoms are the minimum criteria necessary to fulfill diagnostic criteria, whereas for children the threshold is higher, with six symptoms of either required (see Box 23.1) [1]. Some research suggests that only four symptoms either inattention or hyperactive/impulsivity should be sufficient to meet diagnostic criteria for adults and that requiring five symptoms may be too restrictive [22].

**Box 23.1 DSM-5 Diagnostic Criteria for ADHD [1]**

**Inattention**

- Fails to give close attention to detail or makes careless mistakes in schoolwork, at work, or with other activities
- Has trouble holding attention on tasks or play activities
- Does not seem to listen when spoken to directly
- Does not follow through on instructions and fails to finish schoolwork, chores, or duties in the workplace (e.g., loses focus, side-tracked)
- Has trouble organizing tasks and activities
- Avoids, dislikes, or is reluctant to do tasks that require mental effort over a long period of time (such as schoolwork or homework)
- Loses things necessary for tasks and activities (e.g., school materials, pencils, books, tools, wallets, keys, paperwork, eyeglasses, and mobile telephones)
- Often easily distracted
- Often forgetful in daily activities

**Hyperactivity and Impulsivity**

- Fidgets with or taps hands or feet or squirms in seat
- Leaves seat in situations when the remaining seat is expected
- Runs about or climbs in situations where it is not appropriate (adolescents or adults may be limited to feeling restless)
- Unable to play or take part in leisure activities quietly
- Is often "on the go," acting as if "driven by a motor"
- Often talks excessively
- Blurts out an answer before a question has been completed
- Has trouble in waiting for his/her turn
- Often interrupts or intrudes on others (e.g., butts into conversations or games)

The predominant features of ADHD may differ in children versus adults, with adults showing more inattention and relatively less hyperactivity. Common manifestations of ADHD in adulthood include difficulties with organizing activities, prioritizing tasks, and meeting deadlines, as well as quitting jobs without any alternatives, reckless driving, and terminating valued relationships [16, 33]. Many adults with ADHD experience mood lability, irritability, and low frustration tolerance, which can result in the inability to manage uncomfortable emotions and the tendency to become overwhelmed and sometimes explode [34, 35].

## Epidemiology

The prevalence of ADHD among US adults ages 18–44 years is reported to be 4.4% [36]. However, this prevalence estimate may vary depending on which methods (such as simple reporting of symptoms versus use of structured diagnostic interview) are used to assess for an ADHD diagnosis in adults [37]. Furthermore, given that the prevalence rates of children have risen dramatically in the last decade [38] more work must be done to investigate current prevalence rates of ADHD among the US adult population. There is evidence to suggest ADHD is underdiagnosed in lower-income or minority racial/ethnic groups due to limited access to diagnostic services and lower quality of treatment [38, 39]. Increased availability of specialists in underserved areas and culturally competent approaches to assessing ADHD in African Americans may help to decrease this disparity [39, 40]. Paradoxically, cultural, racial, and language bias may also lead to the overidentification of ethnic minority children as having conduct-related problems related to ADHD [41]. While ADHD remains to be more common in males than females, pediatric studies report that males are two to three times more likely to have ADHD [42, 43]. However, strong arguments contend that the difference in prevalence rates between males and females could be due to differential rates of referral. Identification in young girls tends to come later due to the difference in phenotype between men and women; men tend to present with the combined subtype, and women tend to present with the inattentive subtype [18, 44, 45].

## Factors to Consider in Making a Diagnosis in Adults

The Diagnostic and Statistical Manual of Mental Disorders (DSM-5) criteria for ADHD were developed to diagnose ADHD in children, and thus, it may be difficult to directly apply these criteria to adults. According to the DSM-5, signs and symptoms of ADHD must be present prior to age 12 years [1]—although this criterion can pose a challenge when adults seek treatment for ADHD, since there are conflicting findings on the accuracy of adult recall of childhood ADHD symptoms [46, 47]. However, studies have demonstrated that adults can accurately report their childhood ADHD symptoms when they were asked about specific symptoms as part of a structured diagnostic interview [37]. If possible, a review of childhood medical records or school report cards/progress notes could help to determine if childhood symptoms were present.

Another challenge with determining a diagnosis of ADHD during adulthood is that symptoms must cause impairment in two or more settings [1]. While a childhood diagnosis relies on the use of rating scales completed by teachers and parents, it may not be possible to obtain ADHD rating scales from informants such as employers and spouses in adulthood, given concerns about patient confidentiality. Self-report of impairment may not be accurate since respondents often rate themselves overly positively [48]. The use of a brief, structured, diagnostic interview of ADHD symptoms, and related impairments may more accurately identify adult ADHD [37]. The Mini International Neuropsychiatric Interview (M.I.N.I. ADHD) [49] is an example of a structured diagnostic interview that can be administered by clinicians to help determine whether or not an adult presenting with ADHD concerns meets diagnostic criteria for ADHD. There is also emerging work to support the effectiveness of digital toolkits to support healthcare providers' practice in the diagnosis, treatment, and management of adult ADHD [50].

It is always important to assess for other medical conditions that can cause inattention and/or hyperactivity/impulsivity, such as depression, anxiety, mood disorders, substance use, thyroid disease, or sleep disorders. These conditions must be considered as they may cause ADHD-like symptoms and/or they may co-occur with ADHD.

Additionally, the potential for malingering for an adult presenting with new onset ADHD symptoms should be considered, as an ADHD diagnosis could be sought for secondary gain (such as to obtain stimulant medications, which have a high rate of abuse and diversion). However, it is important to emphasize that there is no evidence that adults with ADHD themselves abuse stimulant medications; rather, they have increased rates of substance use disorders involving alcohol, marijuana, and, less commonly, other drugs of abuse [3, 8]. While brain imaging and electroencephalographic studies are used in research settings to better understand brain function in ADHD, they are not currently recommended for clinical diagnosis or management, in the absence of other neurological concerns.

## Risk Factors

The etiology of ADHD is not fully understood, although genetics and environmental factors likely both play a role in the development of ADHD. ADHD is a polygenic condition with an important number of genes involved, as confirmed by a genome-wide association study on ADHD reporting 12 significant loci associated with ADHD [51]. Many of the associated genes are involved in processes of neurotransmission, neuritogenesis, synaptogenesis, or receptor location in the synapses [52]. Of particular interest to current work in this area are two genes: a neurotrophin called "brain-derived neurotrophic factor: (BDNF) and a molecule involved in dopaminergic signaling (DAT) [53].

Familial and twin studies show that the risk of ADHD in parents and siblings of children with ADHD is increased two to eight [54, 55], and heritability has been estimated at 76% [56]. A number of genes involved in dopamine and serotonin pathways may underlie the symptoms of ADHD [56]. Additionally, one case–control study showed that children with ADHD had a higher rate of copy number variants than controls (15.6 vs. 7.5%), thus supporting the genetic contribution to ADHD.

While genetics clearly play a role in the development of ADHD, findings from studies evaluating the association between environmental factors and ADHD are less definitive. In utero environmental exposures including prenatal exposure to tobacco, alcohol, or illicit substances may increase risk for ADHD [57]. Elevated blood lead levels are associated with an increased risk for ADHD [58].

The incidence of ADHD is also associated with several environmental factors during different stages of prenatal central nervous system development [53]. Premature birth is a salient risk factor; it has been reported that ADHD occurs 2.6 to 4 times more frequently in babies born with low weight [53, 59, 60]. One US population-based cross-sectional study found that children with higher levels of urinary metabolites of organophosphate pesticides were more likely to meet diagnostic criteria for ADHD [61]. Another research group confirmed this association and, by introducing pesticide to mice during development, revealed a mechanism that suggests developmental pyrethroid exposure is a risk factor for ADHD [62].

## Pathophysiology

A recent study that compared the cortical thickness and surface area of children, adolescents, and adults diagnosed with ADHD and their same-age neurotypical counterparts revealed structural differences in the cortical surface area of children with ADHD, compared to neurotypical children, but not in adolescents or adults with ADHD [63]. Brain imaging studies indicate that there is dysfunction of the fronto-subcortical and parietal circuits in adults with ADHD, with the most prominent abnormalities in the prefrontal cortex and its projections to subcortical structures [64, 65]. Pediatric studies have shown reduced global activation and reduced local activation in the area of the basal ganglia and the anterior frontal lobe [66]. Neuroimaging studies also show that ADHD is associated with a delay in cortical maturation [67]. Animal studies suggest that an imbalance between the norepinephrine and dopamine systems in the prefrontal cortex (decrease in dopaminergic activity and increase in norepinephrine activity) contributes to the development of ADHD [68]. In a small human study, patients with ADHD were reported to have an increase in dopamine transporter density compared to controls, meaning that the dopamine was cleared from the synapse too quickly and there was relatively less available dopamine [69]. However, a recent meta-analysis of structural and functional neuroimaging studies found that there is no significant convergent across structural and functional regional alterations in individuals with ADHD. It is possible this lack of convergence can be attributable to clinical heterogeneity, experimental and analytical flexibility, and positive publication bias. Alternatively, the lack of convergence in functional and neuroimaging studies of the ADHD brain could point toward a more distributed, network-based pathology lacking a consistent expression at any particular location [70].

## Associated Conditions

ADHD in adults is associated with a high rate of comorbid conditions. ADHD is associated with higher rates of obesity, which in turn can cause various medical problems, such as hypertension and hyperlipidemia, although ADHD itself is not reported to be directly linked to these conditions or to higher rates of cancer [71]. Some of the most commonly reported comorbid conditions for adults with ADHD are substance use disorders, antisocial personality disorders, mood disorders, anxiety, and depression [43, 72]. With increasing age, psychiatric comorbidities may become more evident and problematic. Therefore, it is imperative to routinely screen for, and treat if present, any comorbid conditions for adults with ADHD.

Adults with ADHD may experience a range of adverse psychosocial outcomes, and ADHD should be seen as a significant chronic health condition that confers an increased risk for early death related to suicide. One longitudinal, population-based study confirmed that childhood ADHD is associated with a significantly increased risk for early death from suicide, with the highest risk for those with comorbid substance use disorders or other comorbid psychiatric disorders [8, 43, 72, 73]. Other problems associated with adult ADHD include reduced educational achievement, unemployment, increased risk of traffic and other accidents, and criminality [2, 22, 74].

## Special Issues in Transition to Adulthood

Given the adverse impact of both core ADHD symptoms and commonly occurring comorbidities, youth with ADHD must be followed closely during their transition to adulthood.

## Treatment, Monitoring, and Side Effects

Treatment of both ADHD symptoms and comorbidities should be optimized. Medication treatment for ADHD usually involves stimulant medications, such as methylphenidate or amphetamine preparations, both of whose suspected mechanism of action is to increase the amount of available dopamine [75]. While stimulant medications have a higher likelihood of reducing ADHD symptoms of inattention, impulsivity, and hyperactivity compared to other medications [26], atomoxetine has US Food and Drug Administration (FDA) approval for the treatment of ADHD in adults, and alpha-agonists and antidepressants also have some evidence suggesting they may reduce ADHD symptoms in adults [75]. Table 23.1 provides a list of commonly prescribed medications to treat adult ADHD. When medication is used to treat ADHD, it is started at a relatively low dose and the dose is titrated upward until ADHD symptoms are appropriately controlled, side effects become intolerable, or the maximum dosage of medication is reached. In children and adolescents, the use of standardized ADHD rating scales at baseline and after dose changes (which usually occur 1 week to 1 month apart) can help to determine if the core symptoms of ADHD have diminished with medication treatment. For the reasons noted earlier in this chapter, it can be more difficult to obtain valid information about ADHD symptoms in adults. There are self-report questionnaires available, primarily based on the DSM-IV TR diagnostic criteria for ADHD (1). However, the symptoms of ADHD in DSM-IV TR, versus the recently published DSM-5 criteria, differ primarily in the number of symptoms required for a diagnosis [1], so DSM-IV TR-based questionnaires are still clinically useful and newer versions will undoubtedly become available. Examples include the Adult ADHD Self-Report Scale-V1.1 (ASRS-V1.1) [76] and the Conners' Adult ADHD Rating Scales [77]. Perhaps more importantly, assessment of treatment response should include a review of aspects of function that are impacted by the patient's ADHD symptoms, such as task completion at work, interactions with peers and significant others, and driving. Specific targets of treatment will vary, and the assessment of treatment should be guided by an understanding of the areas of function that were determined to be most significantly impacted by ADHD symptoms at baseline, prior to the initiation of treatment.

Common side effects of stimulant medications include diminished appetite, delayed sleep onset, headaches, and irritability. Rare, but more serious side effects, include psychosis (more common in those with underlying mood disorder already associated with psychosis) and priapism. Monitoring of heart rate and blood pressure is warranted at clinical visits (initially monthly while making dosage changes and then every

**Table 23.1** Commonly prescribed medications to treat adult ADHD

| Class | Trade name | Generic name | Side effects | Dosing considerations |
|---|---|---|---|---|
| **Stimulants** | | | | |
| Methylphenidate | Ritalin<br>Ritalin LA<br>Ritalin SR | Methylphenidate | **Common**: Diminished appetite, delayed sleep onset, headaches, and irritability<br>**Rare**: Psychosis, priapism | Initial dose: 20 mg/day<br>Adjust in weekly 20 mg increments |
| | Metadate CD | Methylphenidate | | Initial dose: 20 mg/day<br>Adjust in weekly 10–20 mg increments |
| | Focalin<br>Focalin XR | Dexmethylphenidate | | Dexmethylphenidate:<br>Initial dose: 5 mg/day<br>Adjust in weekly 2.5 mg increments<br>Dexmethylphenidate extended release:<br>Initial dose: 5 mg/day<br>Adjust in weekly 5 mg increments |
| | Concerta | Methylphenidate | | Initial dose: 18–36 mg/day<br>Adjust in weekly 18 mg increments |
| Amphetamine | Adderall<br>Adderall XR | Mixed amphetamine salts | | Mixed amphetamine salts:<br>Initial dose: 5 mg/day or BID<br>Adjust in weekly 2.5 mg increments<br>Mixed amphetamine salts, extended release:<br>Initial dose: 10 mg/day<br>Adjust in 5–10 mg weekly increments |
| | Vyvanse | Lisdexamfetamine | | Initial dose: 30 mg/day<br>Adjust in 20 mg weekly increments |
| **Nonstimulants** | | | | |
| Selective norepinephrine reuptake inhibitor | Strattera | Atomoxetine | Gastrointestinal distress, headache, sedation, suicidal ideation, transient growth effects, elevated blood pressure, or heart rate<br>**Rare**: Hepatotoxicity, priapism | Initial dose: 40 mg/day, increase to 80 mg/day after 3 days<br>Increase after 2–4 weeks if optimal response not achieved |
| Alpha agonists | Kapvay | Clonidine | Gastrointestinal distress, headache, decreased blood pressure or heart rate, sedation | Initial dose: 0.1 mg/day<br>Adjust in 0.1 mg increments weekly |
| | Intuniv | Guanfacine | | Initial dose: 1 mg/day<br>Adjust in increments of no more than 1 mg weekly |

3–4 months) because stimulant medications are associated with a slight increase in systolic and diastolic blood pressure (3–5 mmHg) and heart rate (5 beats per minute) [78]. Recent data on cardiovascular risks of stimulant medications suggest no increased risk of a serious cardiac event from stimulant medications for those with an otherwise healthy heart [79, 80]. Consultation with a cardiologist should be considered for patients with underlying cardiac defects, arrhythmias, or cardiac complaints while on stimulant medications. Stimulant medications are considered pregnancy class C; thus, prescribing during pregnancy should be done after careful risk/benefit consideration for each patient. While primary care providers may manage many patients with ADHD, consultation with a neurologist or psychiatrist should be considered for complicated cases, such as in patients with severe comorbid mental health disorders or substance abuse. Whether used as an adjunct to medication treatment or alone, there is accumulating research suggesting that participation in cognitive behavioral therapy can help reduce ADHD symptoms for adults [32, 81]. Therefore, both medication and psychotherapy should be considered as potential treatment options for adults with ADHD.

### Workplace Accommodations

In addition to medication and therapy, workplace accommodations may benefit adults with ADHD. ADHD is associated with higher levels of unemployment compared to control groups [25]. In one study involving a workplace simulation laboratory, adults with ADHD reported internal restlessness, intolerance of boredom, and difficulty maintaining vigilance, which are likely to adversely impact workplace performance [82]. Adults with ADHD may benefit from accommodations in the workplace, such as frequent breaks.

## Conclusion

### Additional Considerations

Screening for substance use disorders, anxiety, and depression should be part of routine clinical care for adolescents and adults with ADHD, given the high risk for these comorbidities to occur and the benefits that early detection and intervention can provide (Appendix). Anticipatory guidance around safe stimulant prescribing practices is also recommended, given the high rate of misuse and diversion of stimulant medications [83]. Counseling should include directions to keep stimulant medication in a secure location and information about the risks of stimulant abuse and diversion. Caregivers should provide oversight at the time that the adolescent or young adult assumes responsibility for medication administration. Given the symptoms that characterize ADHD, individuals with ADHD tend to struggle with medication adherence [84] Using a weekly pillbox and use of daily timers set by phones or watches can allow the individual with ADHD autonomy over self-administration and also enable a visual check-in from a caregiver or significant other to ensure that the medication is taken each day.

Given the chronic nature of ADHD and its association with adverse employment, relationships, and overall health outcomes, regular clinic visits with an adult provider are necessary to monitor treatment, assess for comorbidities, and ensure optimal outcomes.

## Appendix

| Attention-deficit/hyperactivity disorder (ADHD) condition fact sheet | |
|---|---|
| Definition | Attention-deficit/hyperactivity disorder (ADHD) is a chronic neurodevelopmental disorder that often affects individuals throughout the lifespan. ADHD is characterized by impairing symptoms of inattention and/or hyperactivity/impulsivity across at least two different settings, such as home and work<br>• Associated deficits in executive function (organization, planning) are common |
| Epidemiology | • The prevalence of ADHD among US adults ages 18–44 years is reported to be 4.4%<br>• ADHD is more common in males than females, with pediatric studies reporting that males are two to three times more likely to have ADHD, while the male-to-female ratio is lower among affected adults<br>• Rates of diagnosed ADHD are lower among minority populations, potentially due to under-identification<br>• ADHD is significantly more common among first-degree relatives of affected individuals, reflecting the high heritability of ADHD |
| Special considerations | Individuals with ADHD have high rates of comorbid mental health and other chronic conditions including |
| | • Depression/mood disorders<br>• Suicidality<br>• Anxiety disorders<br>• Substance use disorders<br>• Learning disorders<br>• Antisocial personality disorder<br>• Obesity |
| | Individuals often have impairment in multiple domains including<br>• Employment and occupational functioning<br>• Relationships<br>• Driving |

## References


1. American Psychiatric Association, American Psychiatric Association. Diagnostic and statistical manual of mental disorders: DSM-5. 5th ed. Washington, DC: American Psychiatric Association; 2013. p. 947.
2. Björk A, Rönngren Y, Selander J, Vinberg S, Hellzen O, Olofsson N. Health, lifestyle habits, and physical fitness among adults with ADHD compared with a random sample of a Swedish general population. Soc Health Vulnerability. 2018;9(1):1553916.
3. Spera V, Pallucchini A, Maiello M, Carli M, Maremmani AGI, Perugi G, et al. Substance use disorder in adult-attention deficit hyperactive disorder patients: patterns of use and related clinical features. IJERPH. 2020;17(10):3509.
4. Matza LS, Paramore C, Prasad M. Cost Eff Resour Alloc. 2005;3(1):5.
5. Leibson CL. Use and costs of medical care for children and adolescents with and without attention-deficit/hyperactivity disorder. JAMA. 2001;285(1):60.
6. Bron TI, Bijlenga D, Breuk M, Michielsen M, Beekman ATF, Kooij JJS. Risk factors for adverse driving outcomes in Dutch adults with ADHD and controls. Accid Anal Prev. 2018;111:338–44.
7. Groom MJ, van Loon E, Daley D, Chapman P, Hollis C. Driving behaviour in adults with attention deficit/hyperactivity disorder. BMC Psychiatry. 2015;15(1):175.
8. Magon R, Müller U. ADHD with comorbid substance use disorder: review of treatment. Adv Psychiatry Treat. 2012;18(6):436–46.
9. Molina BSG, Pelham WE. Attention-deficit/hyperactivity disorder and risk of substance use disorder: developmental considerations, potential pathways, and opportunities for research. Annu Rev Clin Psychol. 2014;10(1):607–39.
10. Katusic SK, Barbaresi WJ, Colligan RC, Weaver AL, Leibson CL, Jacobsen SJ. Psychostimulant treatment and risk for substance abuse among Young adults with a history of attention-deficit/hyperactivity disorder: a population-based, birth cohort study. J Child Adolesc Psychopharmacol. 2005;15(5):764–76.
11. Young S, Woodhouse E. Assessment and treatment of substance use in adults with ADHD: a psychological approach. J Neural Transm. 2021;128(7):1099–108.
12. Pfeifer MA, Reiter EM, Cordero JJ, Stanton JD. Inside and out: factors that support and hinder the self-advocacy of undergraduates with ADHD and/or specific learning disabilities in STEM. LSE. 2021;20(2):ar17.
13. Willcutt EG, McGrath LM, Pennington BF, Keenan JM, DeFries JC, Olson RK, et al. Understanding

comorbidity between specific learning disabilities. New Dir Child Adolesc Dev. 2019;2019(165):91–109.
14. Barry TD, Lyman RD, Klinger LG. Academic underachievement and attention-deficit/hyperactivity disorder: the negative impact of symptom severity on school performance. J Sch Psychol. 2002;40:259–83.
15. Perugi G, Pallucchini A, Rizzato S, Pinzone V, De Rossi P. Current and emerging pharmacotherapy for the treatment of adult attention deficit hyperactivity disorder (ADHD). Expert Opin Pharmacother. 2019;20(12):1457–70.
16. Geffen J, Forster K. Treatment of adult ADHD: a clinical perspective. Ther Adv Psychopharmacol. 2018;8(1):25–32.
17. Aduen PA, Cox DJ, Fabiano GA, Garner AA, Kofler MJ. Expert recommendations for improving driving safety for teens and adult drivers with ADHD. ADHD Rep. 2019;27(4):8–14.
18. Groenewald C, Emond A, Sayal K. Recognition and referral of girls with attention deficit hyperactivity disorder: case vignette study. Child Care Health Dev. 2009;35(6):767–72.
19. Young S, Adamo N, Ásgeirsdóttir BB, Branney P, Beckett M, Colley W, et al. Females with ADHD: an expert consensus statement taking a lifespan approach providing guidance for the identification and treatment of attention-deficit/hyperactivity disorder in girls and women. BMC Psychiatry. 2020;20(1):404.
20. Holthe MEG, Langvik E. The strives, struggles, and successes of women diagnosed with ADHD as adults. SAGE Open. 2017;7(1):215824401770179.
21. D'Agati E, Curatolo P, Mazzone L. Comorbidity between ADHD and anxiety disorders across the lifespan. Int J Psychiatry Clin Pract. 2019;23(4):238–44.
22. Barbaresi WJ, Colligan RC, Weaver AL, Voigt RG, Killian JM, Katusic SK. Mortality, ADHD, and psychosocial adversity in adults with childhood ADHD: a prospective study. Pediatrics. 2013;131(4):637–44.
23. Sodano SM, Tamulonis JP, Fabiano GA, Caserta AM, Hulme KF, Hulme KL, et al. Interpersonal problems of young adults with and without attention-deficit/hyperactivity disorder. J Atten Disord. 2021;25(4):562–71.
24. Barkley RA, Murphy KR, Fischer M. ADHD in adults: what the science says. New York: Guilford Press; 2008. p. 500.
25. Adamou M, Arif M, Asherson P, Aw TC, Bolea B, Coghill D, et al. Occupational issues of adults with ADHD. BMC Psychiatry. 2013;13(1):59.
26. Wolraich ML, Hagan JF, Allan C, Chan E, Davison D, Earls M, et al. Clinical practice guideline for the diagnosis, evaluation, and treatment of attention-deficit/hyperactivity disorder in children and adolescents. Pediatrics. 2019;144(4):25.
27. Jensen PS, Hinshaw SP, Swanson JM, Greenhill LL, Conners CK, Arnold LE, et al. Findings from the NIMH multimodal treatment study of ADHD (MTA): implications and applications for primary care providers. J Dev Behav Pediatr. 2001;22(1):60–73.
28. A 14-month randomized clinical trial of treatment strategies for attention-deficit/hyperactivity disorder. Arch Gen Psychiatry. 1999;56:14.
29. MTA Cooperative Group. National Institute of Mental Health multimodal treatment study of ADHD follow-up: 24-month outcomes of treatment strategies for attention-deficit/hyperactivity disorder. Pediatrics. 2004;113(4):754–61.
30. MTA Cooperative Group. National Institute of Mental Health multimodal treatment study of ADHD follow-up: changes in effectiveness and growth after the end of treatment. Pediatrics. 2004;113(4):762–9.
31. Montano B. Diagnosis and treatment of ADHD in adults in. Prim Care. 2004;4
32. Young Z, Moghaddam N, Tickle A. The efficacy of cognitive behavioral therapy for adults with ADHD: a systematic review and meta-analysis of randomized controlled trials. J Atten Disord. 2020;24(6):875–88.
33. Huang H, Huang H, Spottswood M, Ghaemi N. Approach to evaluating and managing adult attention-deficit/hyperactivity disorder in primary care. Harv Rev Psychiatry. 2020;28(2):100–6.
34. Christiansen H, Hirsch O, Albrecht B, Chavanon ML. Attention-deficit/hyperactivity disorder (ADHD) and emotion regulation over the life span. Curr Psychiatry Rep. 2019;21(3):17.
35. Shushakova A, Ohrmann P, Pedersen A. Exploring deficient emotion regulation in adult ADHD: electrophysiological evidence. Eur Arch Psychiatry Clin Neurosci. 2018;268(4):359–71.
36. Kessler RC, Adler L, Barkley R, Biederman J, Conners CK, Demler O, et al. The prevalence and correlates of adult ADHD in the United States: results from the National Comorbidity Survey Replication. AJP. 2006;163(4):716–23.
37. Barbaresi WJ, Weaver AL, Voigt RG, Killian JM, Katusic SK. Comparing methods to determine persistence of childhood ADHD into adulthood: a prospective, population-based study. J Atten Disord. 2018;22(6):571–80.
38. Danielson ML, Bitsko RH, Ghandour RM, Holbrook JR, Kogan MD, Blumberg SJ. Prevalence of parent-reported ADHD diagnosis and associated treatment among U.S. children and adolescents, 2016. J Clin Child Adolesc Psychol. 2018;47(2):199–212.
39. Ramsay JR. Health care systems issues and disparities in ADHD Care for African American Adults. J Clin Psychiatry. 2014;75(12):e32–2.
40. Rostain AL, Ramsay JR, Waite R. Culturally competent strategies for assessing and treating ADHD in African American adults: (commentary). J Clin Psychiatry. 2015;76(05):592–6.
41. Slobodin O, Masalha R. Challenges in ADHD care for ethnic minority children: a review of the current literature. Transcult Psychiatry. 2020;57(3):468–83.
42. Visser SN, Danielson ML, Bitsko RH, Holbrook JR, Kogan MD, Ghandour RM, et al. Trends in the parent-report of health care provider-diagnosed and medicated attention-deficit/hyperactivity disorder:

United States, 2003–2011. J Am Acad Child Adolesc Psychiatry. 2014;53(1):34–46.e2.
43. Policy approaches and practices for the inclusion of students with attention-deficit hyperactivity disorder (ADHD). (OECD Education Working Papers; vol. 238). Report No.: 238; 2020. https://www.oecd-ilibrary.org/education/policy-approaches-and-practices-for-the-inclusion-of-students-with-attention-deficit-hyperactivity-disorder-adhd_49af95e0-en.
44. Quinn PO, Madhoo M. A review of attention-deficit/hyperactivity disorder in women and girls: uncovering this hidden diagnosis. Prim Care Companion CNS Disord. 2014;16(3):PCC.13r01596.
45. London AS, Landes SD. Cohort change in the prevalence of ADHD among U.S. adults: evidence of a gender-specific historical period effect. J Atten Disord. 2021;25(6):771–82.
46. Barkley RA, Fischer M, Smallish L, Fletcher K. The persistence of attention-deficit/hyperactivity disorder into young adulthood as a function of reporting source and definition of disorder. J Abnorm Psychol. 2002;111(2):279–89.
47. Dias G, Mattos P, Coutinho G, Segenreich D, Saboya E, Ayrão V. Agreement rates between parent and self-report on past ADHD symptoms in an adult clinical sample. J Atten Disord. 2008;12(1):70–5.
48. Faraone SV, Antshel KM. Diagnosing and treating attention-deficit/hyperactivity disorder in adults. World Psychiatry. 2008;7(3):131–6.
49. Sheehan DV. The mini-international neuropsychiatric interview (M.I.N.I.): the development and validation of a structured diagnostic psychiatric interview for DSM-IV and ICD-10. J Clin Psychiatry. 1998;59(Suppl 20):22–33;quiz 34–57.
50. Loskutova NY, Lutgen CB, Callen EF, Filippi MK, Robertson EA. Evaluating a web-based adult ADHD toolkit for primary care clinicians. J Am Board Fam Med. 2021;34(4):741–52.
51. ADHD Working Group of the Psychiatric Genomics Consortium (PGC), Early Lifecourse & Genetic Epidemiology (EAGLE) Consortium, 23andMe Research Team, Demontis D, Walters RK, Martin J, et al. Discovery of the first genome-wide significant risk loci for attention deficit/hyperactivity disorder. Nat Genet. 2019;51(1):63–75.
52. Martinez-Morga M, Quesada-Rico MP, Bueno C, Martinez S. [Neurobiological bases of autistic spectrum disorder and attention deficit hyperactivity disorder: neural differentiation and synaptogenesis]. Rev Neurol. 2018;66(S01):S97–102.
53. Núñez-Jaramillo L, Herrera-Solís A, Herrera-Morales WV. ADHD: reviewing the causes and evaluating solutions. JPM. 2021;11(3):166.
54. On behalf of the International Multicentre persistent ADHD CollaboraTion (IMpACT), Franke B, Faraone SV, Asherson P, Buitelaar J, Bau CHD, et al. The genetics of attention deficit/hyperactivity disorder in adults, a review. Mol Psychiatry. 2012;17(10):960–87.
55. Smith AK, Mick E, Faraone SV. Advances in genetic studies of attention-deficit/hyperactivity disorder. Curr Psychiatry Rep. 2009;11(2):143–8.
56. Faraone SV, Mick E. Molecular genetics of attention deficit hyperactivity disorder. Psychiatr Clin N Am. 2010;33(1):159–80.
57. Carlsson T, Molander F, Taylor MJ, Jonsson U, Bölte S. Early environmental risk factors for neurodevelopmental disorders—a systematic review of twin and sibling studies. Dev Psychopathol. 2021;33(4):1448–95.
58. Kim JH, Kim JY, Lee J, Jeong GH, Lee E, Lee S, et al. Environmental risk factors, protective factors, and peripheral biomarkers for ADHD: an umbrella review. Lancet Psychiatry. 2020;7(11):955–70.
59. Aylward GP. Neurodevelopmental outcomes of infants born prematurely. J Dev Behav Pediatr. 2005;26(6):427–40.
60. Momany AM, Kamradt JM, Nikolas MA. A meta-analysis of the association between birth weight and attention deficit hyperactivity disorder. J Abnorm Child Psychol. 2018;46(7):1409–26.
61. Bouchard MF, Bellinger DC, Wright RO, Weisskopf MG. Attention-deficit/hyperactivity disorder and urinary metabolites of organophosphate pesticides. Pediatrics. 2010;125(6):e1270–7.
62. Richardson JR, Taylor MM, Shalat SL, Guillot TS, Caudle WM, Hossain MM, et al. Developmental pesticide exposure reproduces features of attention deficit hyperactivity disorder. FASEB J. 2015;29(5):1960–72.
63. Hoogman M, Muetzel R, Guimaraes JP, Shumskaya E, Mennes M, Zwiers MP, et al. Brain imaging of the cortex in ADHD: a coordinated analysis of large-scale clinical and population-based samples. AJP. 2019;176(7):531–42.
64. Cortese S, Kelly C, Chabernaud C, Proal E, Di Martino A, Milham MP, et al. Toward systems neuroscience of ADHD: a meta-analysis of 55 fMRI studies. AJP. 2012;169(10):1038–55.
65. Kasparek T, Theiner P, Filova A. Neurobiology of ADHD from childhood to adulthood: findings of imaging methods. J Atten Disord. 2015;19(11):931–43.
66. Rubia K, Smith AB, Brammer MJ, Toone B, Taylor E. Abnormal brain activation during inhibition and error detection in medication-naive adolescents with ADHD. AJP. 2005;162(6):1067–75.
67. Shaw P, Eckstrand K, Sharp W, Blumenthal J, Lerch JP, Greenstein D, et al. Attention-deficit/hyperactivity disorder is characterized by a delay in cortical maturation. Proc Natl Acad Sci USA. 2007;104(49):19649–54.
68. Russell VA, Sagvolden T, Johansen EB. Animal models of attention-deficit hyperactivity disorder. Behav Brain Funct. 2005;1(1):9.
69. Dougherty DD, Bonab AA, Spencer TJ, Rauch SL, Madras BK, Fischman AJ. Dopamine transporter density in patients with attention deficit hyperactivity disorder. Lancet. 1999;354(9196):2132–3.
70. Samea F, Soluki S, Nejati V, Zarei M, Cortese S, Eickhoff SB, et al. Brain alterations in children/

adolescents with ADHD revisited: a neuroimaging meta-analysis of 96 structural and functional studies. Neurosci Biobehav Rev. 2019;100:1–8.
71. Aguirre Castaneda RL, Kumar S, Voigt RG, Leibson CL, Barbaresi WJ, Weaver AL, et al. Childhood attention-deficit/hyperactivity disorder, sex, and obesity. Mayo Clin Proc. 2016;91(3):352–61.
72. Tsai FJ, Tseng WL, Yang LK, Gau SSF. Psychiatric comorbid patterns in adults with attention-deficit hyperactivity disorder: treatment effect and subtypes. PLoS ONE. 2019;14(2):e0211873.
73. Sun S, Kuja-Halkola R, Faraone SV, D'Onofrio BM, Dalsgaard S, Chang Z, et al. Association of Psychiatric Comorbidity with the risk of premature death among children and adults with attention-deficit/hyperactivity disorder. JAMA Psychiatry. 2019;76(11):1141.
74. Arnold LE, Hodgkins P, Kahle J, Madhoo M, Kewley G. Long-term outcomes of ADHD: academic achievement and performance. J Atten Disord. 2020;24(1):73–85.
75. Wilens TE, Morrison NR, Prince J. An update on the pharmacotherapy of attention-deficit/hyperactivity disorder in adults. 2012:34.
76. Hines JL, King TS, Curry WJ. The adult ADHD self-report scale for screening for adult attention deficit-hyperactivity disorder (ADHD). J Am Board Fam Med. 2012;25(6):847–53.
77. Conners CK, Erhardt D, Epstein JN, Parker JDA, Sitarenios G, Sparrow E. Self-ratings of ADHD symptoms in adults I: factor structure and normative data. J Atten Disord. 1999;3(3):141–51.
78. Wilens TE, Hammerness PG, Biederman J, Kwon A, Spencer TJ, Clark S, et al. Blood pressure changes associated with medication treatment of adults with attention-deficit/hyperactivity disorder. J Clin Psychiatry. 2005;66(02):253–9.
79. Habel LA, Cooper WO, Sox CM, Chan KA, Fireman BH, Arbogast PG, et al. ADHD medications and risk of serious cardiovascular events in young and middle-aged adults. JAMA. 2011;306(24):2673.
80. Schelleman H, Bilker WB, Kimmel SE, Daniel GW, Newcomb C, Guevara JP, et al. Methylphenidate and risk of serious cardiovascular events in adults. AJP. 2012;169(2):178–85.
81. Fullen T, Jones SL, Emerson LM, Adamou M. Psychological treatments in adult ADHD: a systematic review. J Psychopathol Behav Assess. 2020;42(3):500–18.
82. Fried R, Surman C, Hammerness P, Petty C, Faraone S, Hyder L, et al. A controlled study of a simulated workplace laboratory for adults with attention deficit hyperactivity disorder. Psychiatry Res. 2012;200(2–3):949–56.
83. Harstad E, Levy S, et al. Attention-deficit/hyperactivity disorder and substance abuse. Pediatrics. 2014;134(1):e293–301.
84. Adler LD, Nierenberg AA. Review of medication adherence in children and adults with ADHD. Postgrad Med. 2010;122(1):184–91.

## Suggested Reading

Barkley RA, Murphy KR, Fischer M. ADHD in adults: what the science says. New York, NY: The Guilford Press; 2008.
Barkley RA. Taking charge of adult ADHD. New York, NY: The Guilford Press; 2010.

## Patient/Caregiver Resources

Barkley RA. Taking charge of adult ADHD. New York, NY: The Guilford Press; 2010.
Children and adults with attention deficit disorder. www.chadd.org.

# Autism

# 24

Heather Saha, Christina Nicolaidis, Alice A. Kuo, and Christopher D. Hanks

*We use identity-first language (e.g. "autistic person"), a neurodiversity paradigm, and other strengths-based concepts and terms in an effort to promote anti-ableist practices in medicine* [1].

## Case Presentation

Allen is a 21-year-old autistic male with mild intellectual disability who presents to establish care. He is accompanied by his mother who says he refused to return to his previous internal medicine physician because the physician "did not know what to do with him." One year ago, his pediatrician had suggested that they find an adult doctor, but they have had difficulty finding the right physician. Allen graduated from high school and spent some time in a vocational training program. After completing that, he struggled to find work and spent about 1 year at home with no regular daily activities. He recently obtained some support through his local Board of Developmental Disabilities, and he is now working part-time at a local grocery store bagging groceries and retrieving shopping carts with a job coach for support. They feel he is capable of more than this but have not been able to find the right fit for him.

Allen appears well-groomed. He answers questions with short responses and at times takes longer than expected to answer. He is unable to answer some of the questions about his medical history. His mother at times needs to reword the questions asked so that he can understand them. His mother reports he had attention-deficient/hyperactivity disorder (ADHD) and was on a stimulant through high school, but he has not taken it for several years. He is also on an atypical antipsychotic, which was started 8 years ago due to explosive behavioral outbursts. He has not had any outbursts for years, and they are not sure if he should continue this medication or not. They

H. Saha (✉) · C. D. Hanks
Department of Internal Medicine, The Center for Autism Services and Transition, The Ohio State University Wexner Medical Center, Hilliard, OH, USA
e-mail: heather.saha@osumc.edu; christopher.hanks@osumc.edu

C. Nicolaidis
School of Social Work, Portland State University, Portland, OR, USA

Division of General Internal Medicine, Oregon Health and Science University, Portland, OR, USA
e-mail: nicol22@pdx.edu

A. A. Kuo
Division of Medicine-Pediatrics and Preventive Medicine, University of California, Los Angeles, CA, USA
e-mail: akuo@mednet.ucla.edu


A. A. Kuo et al. (eds.), *Care of Adults with Chronic Childhood Conditions*,
https://doi.org/10.1007/978-3-031-54281-7_24

also wonder if restarting his stimulant would help him focus at work. He exhibits some intermittent rocking in his chair and several episodes of hand-flapping that become more prominent as the visit progresses. Exam is only remarkable for being overweight. He declined the genital exam.

Allen reports that when he is not at work he spends most of his day playing video games or watching videos online. His mother expresses concern about his weight, which has been steadily increasing since he graduated from high school. Additionally, he resists brushing his teeth and bathing himself because he does not like how the toothpaste and soap feel. She also notes that he is struggling to develop relationships with friends and has seemed more withdrawn recently. When asked about these things, he is reluctant to discuss them.

## Case Discussion

This case illustrates some of the challenges that autistic individuals face when they reach adulthood. Many autistic people struggle to maintain close relationships with others once they leave the structured environment of high school. Autistic youth can be "disconnected" in the years after aging out of school, meaning that they are not in any employment or postsecondary education setting. Additionally, parents of autistic young adults may struggle to find the balance of allowing autonomy and independence while ensuring safety and support for their children.

In Allen's case, he is hesitant to express himself and communicate with his physician. This can occur due to several causes, including anxiety, challenges with communicating feelings and needs, expressive communication challenges, or sensory processing difficulties. His physician should explore how he best communicates and seek accommodations to help him remain engaged in the encounter. The provider should try to use precise, literal language to help improve the effectiveness of his or her communication. Encouraging Allen to come prepared with questions that are preplanned or written down may be beneficial. Additionally, Allen is demonstrating challenges that could benefit from services such as occupational therapy (OT) to improve his self-care skills and address possible sensory processing challenges associated with bathing and brushing his teeth. If addressing these types of challenges is a priority for Allen, then services may potentially help improve his level of independence, as well as functional and meaningful participation in other activities of interest.

Since Allen is autistic and has an intellectual disability, it is standard of care to refer him for genetic testing because some gene mutations that have been linked to autism can also be associated with cancers or other medical conditions, leading to a need to adjust the cancer-screening timeline or monitor for other health complications.

Allen's mother coached and supported him through this encounter, which allowed Allen to stay more involved in the discussion. However, many parents or caregivers struggle to find the right balance in supporting independence while also ensuring essential information is conveyed. Providers may need to coach parents to allow the individual to interact with the provider at their highest potential. Parents and caregivers can perform important roles in helping patients learn their medical needs and learn to self-advocate. Depending on patient preference, effort should be made to allow the patient some time with the physician without a parent or caregiver present to allow the development of comfort with the medical provider and allow discussion of topics that may be difficult to discuss with others present.

This case raises several important medical and social issues. Obesity is common in all adults, but particularly for autistic adults on psychotropic medications. His "disconnectedness" over the past several years may be contributing to this, as he has limited opportunity to get out of the home, be active, interact with others, and develop friendships. Assisting Allen and his parents in identifying opportunities for work that fit his strengths, interests, and needs will be important for him to maintain a healthy lifestyle. Making recommendations to Allen or his parents to connect with the Department of Vocational Rehabilitation, a local Family Resource Center, or the public Department of Developmental

Services in the area is a good place to help them get started.

Finally, many autistic people are on psychiatric medications for mood disorders such as anxiety and/or depression, ADHD, or other mental health issues. Commonly used medications include selective serotonin reuptake inhibitors (SSRIs), antipsychotics, and stimulants, as well as antiepileptic medications. Many of these medications have significant adverse effects and need monitoring with laboratories or other clinical assessments. Additionally, polypharmacy concerns are common in patients on multiple psychotropic medications. In this case, the provider should consider a trial discontinuation of the atypical antipsychotic, as the risks associated with antipsychotics may outweigh the benefit in this patient who has not had an aggressive outburst in many years. In many cases, primary care providers initially may not feel comfortable managing these medications, and gaining these skills would be helpful to more comprehensively serve these patients in the primary care setting. However, if a primary care provider does not feel comfortable or does not want to gain these skills, then patients should be referred to a psychiatrist or neurologist who has experience managing these medications.

## Medical Model Versus Social Model of Disability

Of relevance to this case study and discussion is the concept of the medical model versus the social model of disability. For several decades, approaches and interventions for autistic individuals have largely focused on the individual, their perceived impairment(s), and remediation of skills so that individuals can progress along the typical developmental pathway of their peers. This medical model has defined how we see and describe autistic individuals, the interventions that have been developed over the past several decades, and the treatments to which we often refer individuals and families. While it is known that autistic individuals may experience significant challenges in areas such as social and communication skills and sensory processing, we should also have an understanding of autism through the lens of the social model. The social model views disability as a result of societal and environmental barriers. As medical providers, we should consider the individual within their context and the social and environmental factors that may be influencing our interactions with individuals or making a visit to the clinic challenging. Examples of this include our own personal biases and assumptions and environmental factors, such as lights or sounds in the waiting room, and patients' lifetime experiences of trauma and discrimination. Many of the tips provided in this chapter focus on low-cost accommodations that could be implemented in practice. These accommodations can help create a more supportive environment and increase the chances of a successful check-up or office visit for these patients and, quite frankly, all patients.

While it is important to understand the individual challenges experienced by autistic people and the impact of social and environmental factors, it is also important to acknowledge the individual strengths of our patients. Examples of strengths commonly found in autistic individuals include detailed thinking, good long-term memory, the ability to hyperfocus, creativity, and the ability to analyze information [2, 3]. However, it is imperative not to expect that an individual autistic person will have any particular set of stereotypically positive or negative characteristics. Moreover, autistic people may experience autistic traits as either advantageous or disadvantageous (or both) depending on the social context, the ability to control the behaviors, and the extent to which the traits are expressed [3]. Identifying and focusing on the strengths of all your patients can assist individuals in seeing their own strengths. While this can positively affect the attitudes and beliefs of the individuals and parents, it can also help providers identify and make proper referrals to services and community programs and can assist individuals and families to realize the different opportunities one could pursue in adulthood with the proper supports in place.

The following sections provide information on the phenomenology and epidemiology of autism, co-occurring conditions, and special issues arising during the transition to adulthood that may be important for primary care providers to be aware of. We also provide brief descriptions of potential supports for autistic people and practical tips for facilitating health care.

## Background

### Definition

Autism is a complex, lifelong neurodevelopmental condition that is marked by differences in social communication and interaction, and repetitive or restrictive patterns of behavior, interests, or activities [4]. Signs can be present in early childhood or may not become obvious until later childhood or adulthood, when demands increase [4]. Autistic individuals may also experience a lack of coordination, motor planning, and atypical sensory processing, such as oversensitivity to auditory, tactile, and visual input [5, 6]. Intellectual disability may or may not be present [7] and may be particularly difficult to assess, especially in autistic people who are nonspeaking or have significant communication challenges. Autistic traits and non-autistic people's responses to such traits often result in decreased social participation, especially in autistic people who have had negative experiences in social situations. Relationships with other autistic people or with non-autistic people may vary greatly depending on their attitudes, expectations, and behaviors, environmental factors, and other personal and contextual factors. Autistic characteristics and their outward manifestation may change over time with development and life stages [4, 8, 9]. Autistic adolescents and adults also often learn to mask many of their autistic traits, which may have some short-term benefits, but may also increase the risk of mental health problems [10].

### Prevalence

The prevalence of autism diagnosis has increased from 6.7 per 1000 (1 in 150) to 23 per 1000 (1 in 44) children from 2002 to 2018 [7]. The reasons for the increasing prevalence of autism remain unclear; however, it is suspected that it is related to factors such as increased awareness and identification practices [11, 12]. In addition, it has been found that prevalence does not change with age [13]. While autism is reported to occur in all racial/ethnic and socioeconomic groups, prevalence estimates vary between these groups, as gender [14, 15], ethnic, and racial disparities continue to exist in the identification of autism, suggesting autism may be underrecognized in some groups [16, 17].

### Genetic Factors

Genetic factors have long been thought to influence autism and are one of the most extensively studied factors in epidemiologic research. Studies have found a 40–90% heritability rate [18, 19] and associations with a variety of genetic syndromes. Associated syndromes are more common in patients with global developmental delay or intellectual disability. These include fragile X syndrome, 15q11-13 duplications, tuberous sclerosis complex, Angelman syndrome, Rett syndrome, Cohen syndrome, Down syndrome, Noonan syndrome, and PTEN-associated macrocephaly syndromes [20]. However, most autistic people do not have monogenic genetic findings. Rather, genetic differences associated with autism are believed to arise from a wide variety of genetic variants and de novo mutations [21, 22]. Hundreds of mutated genes have been found to be associated with autism although many of these associations have not been confirmed [23]. Recent findings suggest that autism is associated with inherited genetic factors, estimated at 80% heritability [24]. Studies suggest these multifactorial genetic situations include gene–gene interaction [25], gene–environment interaction [26], epigenetic programming early in life [27–30], and windows of vulnerability that may influence autism [31] during fetal development and in early childhood. Some studies suggest there are associations between autism and prenatal exposures and perinatal factors [32–37]. However, these studies have significant limitations, and more recent studies suggest prenatal environmental factors have minimal contribution to the development of autism [24].

## Associated Conditions

Autism has been commonly researched within the disciplines of psychiatry and neurology. However, evidence has shown that autistic individuals experience high rates of co-occurring mental and physical conditions, shifting the focus from solely neurodevelopmental and behavioral to a more complex process. Research indicates that some medical conditions are more prevalent in autistic individuals compared to the non-autistic population, including gastrointestinal problems, severe headaches and migraines, sleep disorders, and epilepsy [38]. Autistic adults are also at heightened risk for chronic health conditions, such as diabetes, coronary heart disease, cancer [39], and mental health conditions [38, 40, 41], possibly due to lack of access to high-quality health care, the trauma experienced by living in an ableist world, and other social determinants of health. These co-occurring conditions have been found to negatively impact autistic individuals' behaviors, communication, cognition, and sensory processing.

## Genetic Testing and Cancer Implications

It is known that autism is highly heritable, and hundreds of genes have now been implicated. Recent estimates attribute 10–30% of cases of autism to rare variants, either de novo or inherited [42]. As the genetic background of autism is increasingly understood, an overlap with genetic predisposition for different cancers has been recognized. Involvement of the PI3K–Akt–mTOR signaling pathway (PTEN, FMR1, NF1, TSC1, TSC2) was one of the first identified; however, further identification of many more genes has shown that the majority of this overlap is due to mutations in genes involved in chromatin remodeling and genome maintenance, transcription factors, and signal transduction pathways causing nuclear changes [43]. While there are epidemiological data suggesting higher rates of cancer in autistic children, adolescents, and young adults, the incidence of cancer in adults still appears to be most highly correlated with age [43]. Genetic testing for autistic individuals can allow for more specific individualized counseling on heritability and can more appropriately target those individuals who are at increased risk for co-occurring conditions such as cancer or other conditions (e.g., increased risk of psychosis associated with 22q11 deletion) and adjust their screening, diagnostic evaluation, and therapeutic recommendations [44]. In the United States, current guidelines advise chromosomal microarray and Fragile X testing be offered to patients on the autism spectrum, and there is growing support for whole exome sequencing as well [42, 45].

We recognize that the ethics of genetic testing for autism have lagged behind the technology and that autistic self-advocates and allies are very concerned with the potential eugenics approach to prenatal counseling (i.e., genetic testing to terminate a pregnancy if the fetus may be identified as potentially autistic). We raise attention to this controversy in order to help providers be more mindful in their discussions of prenatal testing with patients and their families.

**Box 24.1 Genetics and Cancer-Screening**

- The American Academy of Neurology and the Child Neurology Society recommend referring autistic individuals for high-resolution chromosome studies (karyotype) and DNA analysis for Fragile X, particularly if
  - Intellectual disability is present (or cannot be excluded).
  - There is a family history of Fragile X or undiagnosed intellectual disability.
  - Dysmorphic features are present.

Note, however, that there is little likelihood of positive karyotype or Fragile X testing in the presence of autism without intellectual disability

- Genetic counseling for autistic individuals (and their families) should always accompany genetic evaluation.
- Routinely include age-appropriate cancer-screening procedures during health maintenance visits.

## Seizure Disorder

Autistic individuals are reported to experience higher rates of epilepsy than the general population, with a prevalence rate of 12.5% in children, which increases to 26% by adolescence [46, 47]. Seizures are associated with increased age, lower intellectual functioning, and decreased adaptive behavior. Epilepsy can be easily misdiagnosed in individuals with intellectual disabilities as a result of misinterpretation of behavioral, physiological, and psychological events [48]. Being undiagnosed or misdiagnosed can potentially have fatal implications. Therefore, further evaluation, such as electroencephalogram (EEG) and/or referral to a specialist should be considered when patients present with changes in behavior that could be related to seizures [49].

## Gastrointestinal Disorders and Nutritional Concerns

Autistic individuals experience higher rates of gastrointestinal problems, including diarrhea, constipation, vomiting, bloating, and abdominal pain. This has been attributed to the interplay between the gut microbiome and the central nervous system and possible differences in GI physiology in autistic individuals as compared to non-autistic people [50]. It is quite common for autistic people to have marked food selectivity. In many but not all cases, food selectivity may be related to sensory aversions to certain tastes, smells, textures, or combinations, sensory-seeking behaviors, and/or the desire for consistency [50]. Evaluation and management of gastrointestinal problems in autistic individuals are not yet fully understood [51]; however, it is recommended that autistic individuals should receive the same thoroughness and standard of care as non-autistic patients. Additionally, nutritional assessments and counseling should consider patients' sensory issues. No evidence currently favors any one diet compared to another in this patient population. If an overly selective diet is causing significant nutritional concerns, providers should work with autistic patients to gradually increase the variety of foods, while respecting the patient's preferences and need for consistency. Gastrointestinal workup should be considered with change in behavior.

## Sleep Disturbances

Sleep disturbances are commonly reported in autistic individuals across the lifespan at higher rates than either their non-autistic peers or those with other neurodevelopmental conditions [52–55]. Sleep disturbances can negatively impact daily functioning and quality of life [56, 57]. Sleep onset insomnia and sleep maintenance insomnia are especially common in autistic individuals [58]. They may also be a result of obstructive sleep apnea and gastrointestinal reflux and have been associated with emotional and behavioral problems and psychiatric conditions [59]. Melatonin, clonidine, and other behavioral interventions (i.e., improving sleep hygiene, mindfulness, cognitive behavioral therapy) have been found to be effective in improving sleep [52, 60]. However, providers recommending sleep hygiene should take care not to imply that an autistic patient's sleep difficulties are being primarily driven by poor habits related to autism.

## Mental Health Conditions

Autistic individuals are reported to experience high rates of mental health conditions [38, 40, 41], with anxiety, depression, and PTSD being the most commonly reported co-occurring conditions. In addition, reports suggest around 30% of autistic individuals meet the criteria for ADHD

[61]. While anxiety is reported to occur in autistic children, studies have indicated that anxiety often increases in adolescence and adulthood. Assessment and diagnosis of anxiety, depression, or other mental health issues can be challenging as individuals may have communication challenges including difficulties communicating feelings and symptoms or completing standardized screening instruments. The reasons for increased rates of co-occurring mental health problems are not fully understood, but there is reason to believe that lifetime trauma, social exclusion, ableism, and lack of adequate supports may contribute. Multiple studies also suggest that "masking" or "camouflaging" autistic traits (and the therapies that attempt to "cure" autistic people or teach them to mask their autistic traits) may be associated with worse mental health outcomes in adulthood [10, 62, 63].

Autistic burnout is a widely discussed phenomenon in autistic spaces that has only recently started to be explored in the research or clinical literature [64, 65]. It is characterized by long-term (>3 months) exhaustion, loss of skills, and reduced tolerance to stimuli. It often occurs at times of major life transitions and may be particularly common and severe during the transition to adulthood (especially as young adults move away from home, enter postsecondary education, or obtain new jobs). Autistic people themselves describe it as resulting from chronic life stress and a protracted mismatch between expectations and abilities without adequate support. Autistic burnout may have a profound impact on people's lives, including their mental and physical health, capacity for independent living, social interactions, employment, quality of life, and risk of suicide. While studies have not investigated potential treatments, autistic people report that acceptance, social support, time off school or work, reduced expectations, and being allowed to unmask were important to their ability to recover from burnout [64]. It is critical for providers to recognize autistic burnout, as it may drastically affect other recommendations.

Suicidal ideation and behaviors are also unfortunately very common (often reported by a majority of participants in autistic samples), and suicide is the leading cause of premature mortality in autistic adults [66, 67]. The odds of dying by suicide is seven to nine times higher in autistic populations than in general populations and may be up to 13 times higher in autistic females. While, as in general populations, depression may play a role in suicidal thoughts or behaviors, there may be additional pathways to suicide that may not be responsive to traditional treatments for depression [68]. As such, it is important for providers to consider issues such as autistic burnout and availability of support when trying to address suicidal ideation or prevent suicide attempts.

## Sexuality

Sexuality is an important and positive part of adulthood for a majority of adults, including autistic adults [69]. While the reported rates of sexual behaviors with a partner are somewhat lower in autistic adults compared to the non-autistic population, particularly when there is coexisting intellectual disability or lower overall functioning, many autistic people engage in partnered sexual behavior and the rate of solitary sexual behaviors is similar to the rate in the general population [70]. Many autistic adults report not receiving adequate or developmentally appropriate sexual education in adolescence. Conservative estimates suggest that autistic individuals are two to three times more likely to experience sexual victimization and abuse than non-autistic peers [70]. Autistic traits combined with insufficient sexual education can impact sexual experiences. Some autistic individuals experience challenges with social inference skills, and this may impact their experience with intimate relationships, courting behavior, or initiating sexual encounters [71]. All of these factors may create barriers to autistic individuals' expression of their sexuality, but if properly understood may allow these individuals to experience meaningful expression of their sexuality. For example, the recognition that an autistic person's sensory sensitivities and sensory-seeking may affect their sexual experiences in both positive and negative ways can potentially lead to strategies to enhance or enable engagement in sexual activity [69]. Healthcare providers should engage in open conversations about sexual expression and behaviors with autistic patients as they would with non-autistic patients with a goal of supporting positive sexual experience and prevention and treatment of sex-related health conditions.

## Gender Identity

There is growing evidence for a higher proportion of diverse gender identities in the autistic population compared to those who are not autistic. Multiple studies have noted an overlap between traits associated with autism and gender non-conformity [70, 72]. Evidence also suggests higher rates of gender dysphoria in autistic individuals compared to non-autistic peers, particularly females [70, 72], with one hypothesis suggesting that gender expression may be affected by sensory differences or a modified experience of gender identity due to neurodivergence. More research is needed to better understand the gender-related experience of autistic individuals, but all these factors highlight the importance of discussing gender identity with all patients regardless of their ability and method of communication.

## Special Issues That Arise in the Transition to Adulthood

It is estimated that approximately 500,000 autistic individuals will transition into young adulthood each year in the United States. Autistic youth are especially vulnerable during the transition to adulthood due to the inherent characteristics of autism, such as differences in communication and social interaction, [4], co-occurring physical and mental health problems [38], and societal biases and discrimination [73]. These challenges often result in complex service needs that cut across sectors and require high levels of care coordination, further complicating this transitional period [74–77].

Based on Part B of the Individuals with Disabilities Education Act (IDEA), children and youth are eligible to receive special education-related services from 3 to 22 years of age [78]. IDEA ensures that while children are in school and of eligible age, they are entitled to a free and appropriate public education (FAPE) with services that will help them access the curriculum in the least restricted environment (LRE) and prepare them for adulthood within the areas of education, employment, and independent living [78]. However, on reaching their 22nd birthday, individuals essentially experience a "services cliff" where they go from receiving several hours of services to no services, despite the need for continued supports and services to assist them during and after the transition to community-based settings.

Although this is a time of much-needed support, the gap between service needs and receipt increases as many autistic individuals exit the special education system and attempt to access adult systems of care. Evidence has shown less optimal outcomes for autistic young adults with high rates of disconnectedness upon leaving high school [79, 80]. It is reported that one-third of young adults are disconnected after high school (never had a job or continued education after high school) and approximately 26% receive no services that would help them become employed, continue their education, or live more independently [80]. In addition, only 36% ever attend postsecondary education and 58% work for pay outside of the home between high school and their early 20s [80].

The recent COVID-19 pandemic has highlighted the fragility of the many of these supports. Disruption in services impacted the health of autistic individuals and their caregivers, particularly those with more challenges. It also decreased opportunities for independence and vocational training [81, 82]. Loss of employment during the pandemic resulted in worsening mental health for autistic young adults [83].

Evidence suggests that some autistic individuals need support or accommodations in areas such as self-care and daily living skills into adulthood [84–86]. In addition, during adolescence and adulthood, when social expectation demands often increase, challenges in social communication may become increasingly problematic [87]. Autistic traits persist into adulthood [88] and many may benefit from continued support throughout life, whether in educational, vocational, or other settings [86, 89, 90]. Educating and assisting autistic individuals and their families to connect to services within their community—such as university disability service centers, the Department of Vocational Rehabilitation, the Department of Developmental Services, and community centers—may help reduce disconnectedness and improve outcomes for autistic adults.

## Approaches to Success

Autistic traits can vary widely. Families may pursue approaches including behavioral, psychological, or educational. Interventions are generally targeted at improving social communication and interaction, increasing and maintaining adaptive behaviors and functional skills, and increasing meaningful participation. Below are common interventions provided to autistic individuals.

## Applied Behavioral Analysis

Applied behavioral analysis (ABA) is an intervention for young autistic children that uses principles of learning theory to try to bring about meaningful and positive change in behavior. The goal of ABA is to increase and maintain functional and adaptive behaviors, decrease maladaptive behaviors, teach new skills, and generalize skills to other environments. Functional behavioral assessments include identifying antecedents, behaviors, and consequences of behavior and developing individualized plans that will increase the frequency of a targeted behavior and adaptive behavior. It is important to note that although ABA is commonly used in autistic children, autistic rights advocates have raised significant concerns about ABA, including it being de-humanizing; having the misguided and unachievable goal of "curing" autism, leading to masking, trauma, and mental health issues; encouraging compliance and thus putting autistic people at increased risk for abuse; and not adequately taking into account the social and environmental contexts that influence autistic behaviors [91, 92]. Furthermore, little to no evidence supports this intervention for autistic adults.

## Psychotherapy

Psychotherapy (talk therapy) has been shown to be effective in autistic patients with a variety of mental health conditions. Cognitive behavioral therapy is the best studied form of psychotherapy in this population, but early evidence suggests other forms of psychotherapy may also be effective [93–95]. There is often a lack of mental health providers trained to serve autistic adults [96, 97]. Successful psychotherapy is dependent on both the ability of the autistic individual to participate meaningfully and the skill and experience of the therapist in working with autistic patients [98]. Thus, efforts should be made to identify mental health providers with experience treating autistic patients, if possible.

## Speech and Language Therapy

Speech and language therapy aims to improve social communication and interaction, self-advocacy, and other language impairments in autistic patients. Language delay is common in autistic people and can range from learning to speak altogether to errors in syntax (how words are arranged to form phrases and sentences), semantics (rules related to the meaning and content of words), pragmatics (social aspects of language), narrative speech (ability to retell a story with sequencing and details), or reciprocal speech (ability to participate in turn-taking). A common mistake with autistic children is to terminate speech therapy once the child has achieved any language (i.e., generating words); however, the quality of language must be considered in order to communicate effectively with peers. Echolalia and scripted speech (i.e., repetition of phrases heard elsewhere, most commonly television or movies) may be less effective means of communication.

Stuttering may occur in autistic individuals, particularly those with significant anxiety. Speech therapy should be offered to teach these patients to slow down their speech, feel less tense, and speak more freely in public spaces.

Intervention includes a variety of modalities to help support and improve social interaction and verbal and nonverbal communication, including activity schedules/visual supports and/or augmentative and alternative communication (AAC). AAC includes supplementing or replacing natural speech with aided or unaided symbols. Examples of these devices include but are not limited to Picture Exchange Communication System (PECS), speech-generative devices, and manual signs or gestures. These approaches have been proven to be effective in improving communication skills, social skills and interactions, and self-advocacy and self-determination in autistic individuals [99]. Although many will have had some speech therapy during childhood, communication needs and life experiences are different as individuals reach adulthood. Often, it is assumed that autistic people who were not able to learn to use AAC when they were first exposed to it at an early age cannot benefit from such technologies. They are thus deprived of opportunities to try again as they mature and develop. Small studies suggest it is reasonable to revisit this in adulthood for individuals who may benefit from improving their communication options [100].

## Occupational Therapy

The focus of occupational therapy (OT) is to assist individuals to achieve their highest degree of independence. OT aims to improve performance and participation in daily occupations, such as self-care routines, leisure activities, and school- or work-related tasks. Evidence suggests that OT can help autistic individuals improve independence at home, with driving and community mobility, and in vocational settings [101, 102]. Additionally, OT can use sensory integration (SI) therapy for individuals experiencing sensory integration difficulties that may impact their ability to adapt and interact with their environment. Sensory integration therapy is commonly used in autistic children and has been shown to be effective [103]. There is limited evidence for its use in adults, but it could be considered to assist individuals struggling with sensory-related issues that limit their social or vocational opportunities.

## Practical Tips to Facilitate Health Care

Challenges with communication, social interactions, and sensory processing experienced by autistic individuals can make it more difficult for medical providers to identify health complications in these patients. Autistic adults report greater unmet healthcare needs, lower use of preventive services, and greater use of the emergency department than non-autistic adults [104], placing them at risk for less optimal health outcomes. Evidence suggests that poor provider and patient-level interactions contribute to negative healthcare experiences [105]. Studies have identified many modifiable barriers to health care for autistic adults [106, 107].

However, recent evidence suggests that if health care is delivered in an accessible way, autistic individuals can have improved continuity of care, are more likely to receive health screenings, vaccinations, and other preventive services, and report higher satisfaction with care [108–111].

Inpatient care can be particularly challenging for some autistic individuals as they are sometimes dependent on a routine that is disrupted or struggle with the complex sensory environment of the hospital setting. This can lead to challenges which may lead to difficulty completing necessary care [112]. Processes and tools, such as autism-specific care plans, which can be easily implemented, have been shown to be beneficial, improving the patient experience and provider comfort in caring for these patients [113, 114].

The following sections provide practical tips from the Academic Autistic Spectrum Partnership in Research and Education (AASPIRE) Healthcare Toolkit, an online set of tools and resources for healthcare providers, autistic adults, and their supporters. The complete Toolkit is available at: www.autismandhealth.org . The centerpiece of the Toolkit, the Autism Healthcare Accommodations Tool, allows patients (or their supporters) to create a personalized accommodations report for their providers. Preliminary research suggests that the use of the Toolkit may increase satisfaction with patient-provider communication, increase patient self-efficacy, and reduce barriers to care [115].

## Communication and Interaction

Autistic individuals are reported to have various strengths and challenges in verbal and nonverbal communication, receptive and expressive skills, and ability to process the information. Some evidence suggests that they prefer non-telephonic communication. Options for communication have improved with the advent of email, texting, and telehealth [116]. In addition, autistic individuals commonly use language literally and prefer information to be provided in a way that is precise, concrete, and specific (Box 24.2). Understanding a patient's communication needs is very important to providing quality care.

**Box 24.2**
Tips on communication and interaction

- Do not assume that a patient cannot understand healthcare information or communicate when he/she does not speak fluently. In addition, do not assume that a patient who speaks fluently does not have significant communication challenges.
- Obtain individualized information on communication needs and preferences.
- Be precise, concrete, and specific.
- Do not assume a patient is distracted or inattentive because he/she is fidgeting, making repetitive movements, or avoiding eye contact.
- Give adequate time for individuals to process the information they need to see, hear, or feel before they respond.

## Sensory Challenges

Autistic individuals can have varying approaches to sensory processing. Individuals may be hyperresponsive or hyporesponsive to sounds, lights, smells, touch, or taste. As a result, some environments can be overstimulating for some individuals. Environments that are not sensitive to their sensory need can have a negative impact on their healthcare experience and social interactions. In addition, individuals may have difficulties with body awareness, making it difficult for them to discriminate between different tactile inputs and location of symptoms. Therefore, understanding these sensory challenges and creating a sensory-friendly environment can create more positive experiences for the autistic patient (Box 24.3).

**Box 24.3**
Tips on sensory challenges

- Use natural light or make the lighting dim.
- See the patient in a quiet room.
- Avoid unnecessarily touching the patient and warn him/her if you will use touch for a physical examination.
- Suggest that the patient bring manipulatives or other physical supports to help reduce or increase sensory stimuli.

## Planning and Organizing

Some autistic people experience difficulties with executive functioning within the areas of planning, organizing, and sequencing information. Autistic people also commonly have difficulties adapting to new environments and situations, creating a need for routine and consistency. See Box 24.4 for tips on the types of supports that can assist individuals in making decisions, following through with information, and decreasing the stress of attending a healthcare appointment.

**Box 24.4**
Tips on planning and organizing

- Identify patient needs and necessary accommodations prior to the visit by having patients complete a pre-visit assessment or complete a Personalized Accommodations Report by going to www.autismhealth.org/AHAT.
- Let the patient and/or his/her supporter know what will occur at the appointment.
- Provide visual supports to help the patient through the healthcare routine.
- Write up step-by-step instructions.
- Have staff assist the patient in scheduling follow-up visits, referrals, or tests.
- Contact and follow-up with the patient and/or supporter after the visit.

## Exams and Procedures

Tolerating examinations, tests, and procedures may be challenging for autistic people due to the reasons mentioned previously. See Box 24.5 for tips to help autistic people better tolerate these medical procedures.

**Box 24.5**
Tips on exams and procedures

- Explain to the patient what is going to be done before doing it.
- Slowly expose individuals to different equipment and perform a "trial run" if possible.
- Give patients extra time to process information he/she sees, hears, or feels before they respond.
- Have staff assist the patient in scheduling follow-up visits, referrals, or tests.
- Use a numbing spray, cream, or provide the patient with antianxiety medication, if necessary, before a blood draw.

Trypanophobia, or an intense fear of needles, occurs in 10% of the general population and is likely higher in prevalence for those with sensory issues and/or generalized anxiety. Programs such as the Needle Anxiety Program at UCLA can offer a variety of approaches including a numbing spray or cream, distracting device (i.e., Buzzy Bee), and antianxiety medication prior to the office visit or during the visit (via inhalation, e.g., inhaled midazolam) to decrease the anxiety for any procedure involving needles, such as immunizations or phlebotomy. Using restraints for these procedures (i.e., a number of people to hold the patient down) should be discouraged, particularly as patients get older/bigger, as this approach leads to safety concerns for both patients and providers and is undignified for the patient. Patients with trypanophobia should not be on "alternative lab schedules" or not receive recommended immunizations, as this results in substandard care.

## Conclusion

Understanding the challenges that autistic individuals experience and how social and environmental factors affect them can allow for better provider–patient interactions and successful check-ups and can assist providers in making proper referrals to services and community resources (Appendix). Utilizing the tips discussed earlier and creating a supportive environment can help improve your practice and delivery of care to autistic adults and their families.

## Appendix

| Autism fact sheet | | |
|---|---|---|
| Definition | **Autism is a lifelong neurodevelopmental condition characterized by**<br>• Differences in social communication and interaction<br>• Repetitive or restrictive patterns of behavior, interests, or activities<br>• Additional traits include lack of coordination, motor planning, and differences in sensory processing<br>• Individuals may or may not have co-occurring intellectual disability | |
| Epidemiology | • In the United States, 23 per 1000 (1 in 44) children aged 8 years have autism<br>• Autism is four times more common in males (1 in 42) than in females<br>• Prevalence of autism in white non-Hispanic children is 26.5 per 1000, 28.5 per 1000 black non-Hispanic children, and 19.4 per 1000 in Hispanic children<br>• Identical twins have an increased likelihood of autism and will occur 36–95% of the time and 0–31% of the time in nonidentical twins<br>• Parents with 1 autistic child have a 2–18% chance of having a second autistic child | |
| Special considerations | **Autistic people have high rates of co-occurring physical and mental health conditions, including** [38–41] | |
| | • Eczema<br>• Allergies<br>• Asthma<br>• Ear and respiratory infections<br>• Gastrointestinal problems | • Severe headaches and migraines<br>• Sleep disorders<br>• Epilepsy<br>• ADHD<br>• Anxiety and depression |
| | **Individuals are at heightened risk for chronic conditions, including**<br>• Diabetes<br>• Coronary heart disease<br>• Cancer | |
| Recommended screening | **All autistic individuals should have genetic screening, particularly**<br>• Females<br>• Coexisting intellectual disability<br>• Known autistic sibling or other first-degree family member | |

## References


1. Bottema-Beutel K, Kapp SK, Lester JN, Sasson NJ, Hand BN. Avoiding ablest language: suggestions for autism researchers. Autism Adulthood. 2021;3(1):18–29.
2. Robertson SM. Neurodiversity, quality of life, and autistic adults: shifting research and professional focuses onto real-life challenges. Disabil Stud Q. 2009;30(1). http://dsq-sds.org/article/view/1069. Accessed 12 Aug 2016.
3. Russell G, Kapp SK, Elliott D, Elphick C, Gwernan-Jones R, Owens C. Mapping the autistic advantage from the accounts of adults diagnosed with autism: a qualitative study. Autism Adulthood. 2019;1(2):124–33.
4. American Psychiatric Association. Diagnostic and statistical manual of mental disorders. 5th ed. Arlington: American Psychiatric Association; 2013.
5. Kern JK, Trivedi MH, Garver CR, Grannemann BD, Andrews AA, Savla JS, et al. The pattern of sensory processing abnormalities in autism. Autism. 2006;10(5):480–94.
6. Fournier KA, Hass CJ, Naik SK, Lodha N, Cauraugh JH. Motor coordination in autism spectrum disorders: a synthesis and meta-analysis. J Autism Dev Disord. 2010;40(10):1227–40.
7. Maenner MJ, Shaw KA, Bakian AV, et al. Prevalence and characteristics of Autism Spectrum disorder among children aged 8 years—Autism and developmental disabilities monitoring network, 11 sites, United States 2018. MMWR Surveill Summ. 2021;70(SS-11):1–16.
8. Sukhodolsky DG, Scahill L, Gadow KD, Arnold LE, Aman MG, McDougle CJ, et al. Parent-rated anxiety symptoms in children with pervasive developmental disorders: frequency and association with core autism symptoms and cognitive functioning. J Abnorm Child Psychol. 2008;36(1):117–28.
9. Cheely CA, Carpenter LA, Letourneau EJ, Nicholas JS, Charles J, King LB. The prevalence of youth with autism spectrum disorders in the criminal justice system. J Autism Dev Disord. 2012;42(9):1856–62.
10. Pearson A, Rose K. A conceptual analysis of autistic masking: understanding the narrative of stigma and the illusion of choice. Autism Adulthood. 2021;3(1):52–60.
11. Blumberg SJ, Bramlett MD, Kogan MD, Schieve LA, Jones JR, Lu MC. Changes in prevalence of parent-reported autism spectrum disorder in school-aged U.S. Children: 2007 to 2011–2012. Natl Health Stat Rep. 2013;65:1–11.
12. Schieve LA, Rice C, Devine O, Maenner MJ, Lee L-C, Fitzgerald R, et al. Have secular changes in perinatal risk factors contributed to the recent autism prevalence increase? Development and application of a mathematical assessment model. Ann Epidemiol. 2011;21(12):930–45.
13. Brugha TS, McManus S, Bankart J, Scott F, Purdon S, Smith J, et al. Epidemiology of autism spectrum disorders in adults in the community in England. Arch Gen Psychiatry. 2011;68(5):459–65.
14. Giarelli E, Wiggins LD, Rice CE, Levy SE, Kirby RS, Pinto-Martin J, et al. Sex differences in the evaluation and diagnosis of autism spectrum disorders among children. Disabil Health J. 2010;3(2):107–16.
15. Loomes R, Hull L, Polmear Lock Mandy W. What is the male-to-female ratio in Autism Spectrum disorder? A systematic review and meta-analysis. J Am Acad Child Adolesc Psychiatry. 2017;56(6):466–74.
16. Mandell DS, Wiggins LD, Carpenter LA, Daniels J, DiGuiseppi C, Durkin MS, et al. Racial/ethnic disparities in the identification of children with autism spectrum disorders. Am J Public Health. 2009;99(3):493–8.
17. Jo H, Schieve LA, Rice CE, Yeargin-Allsopp M, Tian LH, Blumberg SJ, et al. Age at autism spectrum disorder (ASD) diagnosis by race, ethnicity, and primary household language among children with special health care needs, United States, 2009–2010. Matern Child Health J. 2015;19(8):1687–97.
18. Folstein SE, Rosen-Sheidley B. Genetics of autism: complex aetiology for a heterogeneous disorder. Nat Rev Genet. 2001;2(12):943–55.
19. Bailey A, Lecouteur A, Gottesman I, Bolton P, Simonoff E, Yuzda E, et al. Autism as a strongly genetic disorder—evidence from a British twin study. Psychol Med. 1995;25(1):63–77.
20. Richards C, Jones C, Groves L, Moss J, Oliver C. Prevalence of autism spectrum disorder phenomenology in genetic disorders: a systematic review and meta-analysis. Lancet Psychiatry. 2015;2(10):909–1618.
21. O'Roak BJ, Vives L, Fu W, Egertson JD, Stanaway IB, Phelps IG, et al. Multiplex targeted sequencing identifies recurrently mutated genes in autism spectrum disorders. Science. 2012;338(6114):1619–22.
22. O'Roak BJ, State MW. Autism genetics: strategies, challenges, and opportunities. Autism Res. 2008;1(1):4–17.
23. De Rubeis S, He X, Goldberg AP, Poultney CS, Samocha K, Cicek AE, et al. Synaptic, transcriptional and chromatin genes disrupted in autism. Nature. 2014;515(7526):209–15.
24. Bai D, et al. Association of Genetic and Environmental Factors with autism in a 5-counry cohort. JAMA Psychiatry. 2019;76(10):1035.
25. Hallmayer J, Cleveland S, Torres A, Phillips J, Cohen B, Torigoe T, et al. Genetic heritability and shared environmental factors among twin pairs with autism. Arch Gen Psychiatry. 2011;68(11):1095–102.
26. Grafodatskaya D, Chung B, Szatmari P, Weksberg R. Autism spectrum disorders and epigenetics. J Am Acad Child Adolesc Psychiatry. 2010;49(8):794–809.
27. Taylor SE, Way BM, Welch WT, Hilmert CJ, Lehman BJ, Eisenberger NI. Early family environment, current adversity, the serotonin transporter promoter polymorphism, and depressive symptomatology. Biol Psychiatry. 2006;60(7):671–6.

28. Wadhwa PD, Buss C, Entringer S, Swanson JM, editors. Developmental origins of health and disease: brief history of the approach and current focus on epigenetic mechanisms. Seminars in reproductive medicine. NIH Public Access; 2009.
29. Kuzawa CW, Thayer ZM. Timescales of human adaptation: the role of epigenetic processes. Epigenomics. 2011;3(2):221–34.
30. Borghol N, Suderman M, McArdle W, Racine A, Hallett M, Pembrey M, et al. Associations with early-life socio-economic position in adult DNA methylation. Int J Epidemiol. 2012;41(1):62–74.
31. Dietert RR, Dietert JM. Potential for early-life immune insult including developmental immunotoxicity in autism and autism spectrum disorders: focus on critical windows of immune vulnerability. J Toxicol Environ Health B Crit Rev. 2008;11(8):660–80.
32. Gardener H, Spiegelman D, Buka SL. Prenatal risk factors for autism: comprehensive meta-analysis. Br J Psychiatry. 2009;195(1):7–14.
33. Suren P, Roth C, Bresnahan M, Haugen M, Hornig M, Hirtz D, et al. Association between maternal use of folic acid supplements and risk of autism spectrum disorders in children. JAMA J Am Med Assoc. 2013;309(6):570–7.
34. Rogers EJ. Has enhanced folate status during pregnancy altered natural selection and possibly autism prevalence? A closer look at a possible link. Med Hypotheses. 2008;71(3):406–10.
35. Lyall K, Schmidt RJ, Hertz-Picciotto I. Maternal lifestyle and environmental risk factors for autism spectrum disorders. Int J Epidemiol. 2014;43(2):443–64.
36. Leeming R, Lucock M. Autism: is there a folate connection? J Inherit Metab Dis. 2009;32(3):400–2.
37. Gardener H, Spiegelman D, Buka SL. Perinatal and neonatal risk factors for autism: a comprehensive meta-analysis. Pediatrics. 2011;128(2):344–55.
38. Kohane IS, McMurry A, Weber G, MacFadden D, Rappaport L, Kunkel L, et al. The co-morbidity burden of children and young adults with autism spectrum disorders. PLoS One. 2012;7(4):e33224.
39. Tyler CV, Schramm SC, Karafa M, Tang AS, Jain AK. Chronic disease risks in young adults with autism spectrum disorder: forewarned is forearmed. Am J Intellect. 2011;116(5):371–80.
40. Levy SE, Giarelli E, Lee LC, Schieve LA, Kirby RS, Cunniff C, et al. Autism spectrum disorder and co-occurring developmental, psychiatric, and medical conditions among children in multiple populations of the United States. J Dev Behav Pediatr. 2010;31(4):267–75.
41. Joshi G, Petty C, Wozniak J, Henin A, Fried R, Galdo M, et al. The heavy burden of psychiatric comorbidity in youth with autism spectrum disorders: a large comparative study of a psychiatrically referred population. J Autism Dev Disord. 2010;40(11):1361–70.
42. Vorstman JA, Parr J, Moreno-De-Luca D, Anney R, Nurnberger J, Hallmayer J. Autism genetics: opportunities and challenges for clinical translation. Nat Rev Genetics. 2017;18(6):362–76.
43. Crawley JN, Heyer WD, LaSalle JM. Autism and cancer share risk genes, pathways, and drug targets. Trends Genet. 2016;32(3):139–46.
44. Tharpar A, Rutter M. Genetic advances in autism. J Autism Dev Disord. 2021;51(12):4321–32.
45. Srivastava S, et al. Meta-analysis and multidisciplinary consensus statement: exome sequencing is a first-tier clinical diagnosis test for individuals with neurodevelopmental disorders. Genet Med. 2019;21(11):2413–21.
46. Woolfenden S, Sarkozy V, Ridley G, Coory M, Williams K. A systematic review of two outcomes in autism spectrum disorder—epilepsy and mortality. Dev Med Child Neurol. 2012;54(4):306–12.
47. Viscidi EW, Triche EW, Pescosolido MF, McLean RL, Joseph RM, Spence SJ, et al. Clinical characteristics of children with autism spectrum disorder and co-occurring epilepsy. PLoS One. 2013;8(7):e67797.
48. Chapman M, Iddon P, Atkinson K, Brodie C, Mitchell D, Parvin G, et al. The misdiagnosis of epilepsy in people with intellectual disabilities: a systematic review. Seizure. 2011;20(2):101–6.
49. Stokes T, Shaw E, Juarez-Garcia A, Camosso-Stefinovic J, Baker R. Clinical guidelines and evidence review for the epilepsies: diagnosis and management in adults and children in primary and secondary care. London: Royal College of General Practitioners; 2004. p. 397.
50. Risori MV, Quagliariello A, Reddel S, et al. Autism, Gastrointestinal symptoms and modulation of gut microbiota by nutritional interventions. Nutrients. 2019;11(11):2812.
51. Buie T, Campbell DB, Fuchs GJ III, Furuta GT, Levy J, Vandewater J, et al. Evaluation, diagnosis, and treatment of gastrointestinal disorders in individuals with ASDS: a consensus report. Pediatrics. 2010;125(Suppl 1):S1–18.
52. Malow BA. Sleep disorders, epilepsy, and autism. Ment Retard Dev Disabil Res Rev. 2004;10(2):122–5.
53. Øyane NM, Bjorvatn B. Sleep disturbances in adolescents and young adults with autism and Asperger syndrome. Autism. 2005;9(1):83–94.
54. Polimeni MA, Richdale AL, Francis AJ. A survey of sleep problems in autism, Asperger's disorder and typically developing children. J Intellect Disabil Res. 2005;49(Pt 4):260–8.
55. Matson JL, Ancona MN, Wilkins J. Sleep disturbances in adults with autism spectrum disorders and severe intellectual impairments. J Ment Health Res Intellect Disabil. 2008;1(3):129–39.
56. Patzold LM, Richdale AL, Tonge BJ. An investigation into sleep characteristics of children with autism and Asperger's disorder. J Paediatr Child Health. 1998;34(6):528–33.
57. Schreck KA, Mulick JA, Smith AF. Sleep problems as possible predictors of intensified symptoms of autism. Res Dev Disabil. 2004;25(1):57–66.

58. Singh K, Zimmerman AW. Sleep in autism spectrum disorder and attention deficit hyperactivity disorder. Semin Pediatr Neurol. 2015;22(2): 113–25.
59. Sivertsen B, Posserud MB, Gillberg C, Lundervold AJ, Hysing M. Sleep problems in children with autism spectrum problems: a longitudinal population-based study. Autism. 2012;16(2):139–50.
60. Meltzer LJ, Mindell JA. Nonpharmacologic treatments for pediatric sleeplessness. Pediatr Clin N Am. 2004;51(1):135–51.
61. Leyfer OT, Folstein SE, Bacalman S, Davis NO, Dinh E, Morgan J, et al. Comorbid psychiatric disorders in children with autism: interview development and rates of disorders. J Autism Dev Disord. 2006;36(7):849–61.
62. Miller D, Rees J, Pearson A. "Masking is life": experiences of masking in autistic and nonautistic adults. Autism Adulthood. 2021;3(4):330–8.
63. Bradley L, Shaw R, Baron-Cohen S, Cassidy S. Autistic adults' experiences of camouflaging and its perceived impact on mental health. Autism Adulthood. 2021;3(4):320–9.
64. Raymaker DM, Teo AR, Steckler NA, et al. "Having all of your internal resources exhausted beyond measure and being left with no clean-up crew": defining autistic burnout. Autism Adulthood. 2020;2(2):132–43.
65. Mantzalas J, Richdale AL, Adikari A, Lowe J, Dissanayake C. What is autistic burnout? A thematic analysis of posts on two online platforms. Autism Adulthood. 2022;4(1):52–65.
66. Hirvikoski T, Mittendorfer-Rutz E, Boman M, Larsson H, Lichtenstein P, Bolte S. Premature mortality in autism spectrum disorder. Br J Psychiatry. 2016;208(3):232–8.
67. Hedley D, Uljarevic M. Systematic review of suicide in autism spectrum disorder: current trends and implications. Curr Dev Disord Rep. 2018;5(1):65–76.
68. Pelton MK, Crawford H, Robertson AE, Rodgers J, Baron-Cohen S, Cassidy S. Understanding suicide risk in autistic adults: comparing the interpersonal theory of suicide in autistic and non-autistic samples. J Autism Dev Disord. 2020;50(10):3620–37.
69. Gray S, Kirby A, Holmes L. Autistic narratives of sensory features, sexuality, and relationships. Autism Adulthood. 2021;3(3):238–46.
70. Pecora LA, Hooley M, Sperry L, Mesibov BG, Stokes MA. Sexuality and gender issues in individuals with autism spectrum disorder. Child Adolesc Psychiatr Clin N Am. 2020;29(3):543–56.
71. Sedgewick F, Crane L, Hill V, Pellicano E. Friends and lovers: the relationships of autistic and neurotypical women. Autism adulthood. 2019;1(2): 112–23.
72. George R, Stokes M. Gender identity and sexual orientation in autism spectrum disorder. Autism. 2018;22(8):970–82.
73. Billawala A, Wolbring G. Analyzing the discourse surrounding autism in the New York times using an ableism lens. Disabil Stud Q. 2014;34(1). https://doi.org/10.18061/dsq.v34i1.3348. Accessed 12 Aug 2016.
74. Brookman-Frazee LI, Taylor R, Garland AF. Characterizing community-based mental health services for children with autism spectrum disorders and disruptive behavior problems. J Autism Dev Disord. 2010;40(10):1188–201.
75. Garland AF, Hough RL, Landsverk JA, Brown SA. Multi-sector complexity of systems of care for youth with mental health needs. Child Serv Soc Policy Res Pract. 2001;4(3):123–40.
76. Burns BJ, Costello EJ, Angold A, Tweed D, Stangl D, Farmer E, et al. Children's mental health service use across service sectors. Health Aff. 1995;14(3):147–59.
77. Farmer TW, Farmer EM. Developmental science, systems of care, and prevention of emotional and behavioral problems in youth. Am J Orthopsychiatry. 2001;71(2):171–81.
78. Committee on Health E, Labor, and Pensions. Senate report 108–185—individuals with disabilities education act. Washington, DC: U.S. Government Publishing Office; 2003.
79. Wei X, Wagner M, Hudson L, Jennifer WY, Shattuck P. Transition to adulthood employment, education, and disengagement in individuals with autism spectrum disorders. Emerg Adulthood. 2014;3:2167696814534417.
80. Roux AM, Shattuck PT, Rast JE, Rava JA, Anderson KA. National autism indicators report: transition into young adulthood. Philadelphia, PA: Life Course Outcomes Research Program, A.J. Drexel Autism Institute, Drexel University; 2015.
81. Bhat A. Analysis of the SPARK study COVID-19 parent survey: early impact of the pandemic on access to services, child/parent mental health, and benefits of online services. Autism Res. 2021;14(11):2454–70.
82. Baweja R, Brown S, Edwards E, Murray M. COVID-19 pandemic and impact on patients with autism spectrum disorder. J Autism Dev Disord. 2021;10:1–10.
83. Taylor J, et al. Job loss predicts worsening depressive symptoms for young adults with autism: a COVID-19 natural experiment. Autism Res. 2022;15(1):93–102.
84. Matthews NL, Smith CJ, Pollard E, Ober-Reynolds S, Kirwan J, Malligo A. Adaptive functioning in autism spectrum disorder during the transition to adulthood. J Autism Dev Disord. 2015;45(8):2349–60.
85. Smith LE, Maenner MJ, Seltzer MM. Developmental trajectories in adolescents and adults with autism: the case of daily living skills. J Am Acad Child Adolesc Psychiatry. 2012;51(6):622–31.
86. Bal VH, Kim SH, Cheong D, Lord C. Daily living skills in individuals with autism spectrum disorder from 2 to 21 years of age. Autism. 2015;19(7):774–84.

87. Mitchel K, Regehr K, Reaume J, Feldman M. Group social skills training for adolescents with Asperger syndrome or high functioning autism. J Dev Disabil. 2010.
88. Seltzer MM, Shattuck P, Abbeduto L, Greenberg JS. Trajectory of development in adolescents and adults with autism. Ment Retard Dev Disabil Res Rev. 2004;10(4):234–47.
89. Taylor JL, Seltzer MM. Changes in the autism behavioral phenotype during the transition to adulthood. J Autism Dev Disord. 2010;40(12):1431–46.
90. Accardo A, Kuder SJ, Woodruff J. Accommodations and support services preferred by college students with autism spectrum disorder. Autism. 2019;23(3):574–83.
91. Jones J, Lerman DC, Lechago S. Assessing stimulus control and promoting generalization via video modeling when teaching social responses to children with autism. J Appl Behav Anal. 2014;47(1):37–50.
92. Winkenfeld DA, McCarthy AM. Ethical concerns with applied behavior analysis for autism spectrum "disorder". Kennedy Inst Ethics J. 2020;30(1):31–69.
93. White SW, Schry AR, Miyazaki Y, Ollendick TH, Scahill L. Effects of verbal ability and severity of autism on anxiety in adolescents with asd: one-year follow-up after cognitive behavioral therapy. J Clin Child Adolesc Psychol. 2015;44(5):839–45.
94. Spain D, Sin J, Chalder T, Murphy D, Happe F. Cognitive behaviour therapy for adults with autism spectrum disorders and psychiatric co-morbidity: a review. Res Autism Spectr Dis. 2015;9:151–62.
95. Spain D, et al. Cognitive behavioural therapy for adults with autism spectrum disorder and psychiatric comorbidity: a review. Res Autism Spectr Disord. 2015;9:151–62.
96. Maddox BB, Brabbe S, Beidas RS, et al. "I wouldn't know where to start": perspectives from clinicians, agency leaders, and autistic adults on improving community mental health services for autistic adults. Autism. 2020;24(4):919–30.
97. Maddox BB, Gaus VL. Community mental health services for autistic adults: good news and bad news. Autism in Adulthood. 2019;1(1):15–9.
98. Anderberg E, et al. Sticking with it: psychotherapy outcomes for adults with autism spectrum disorder in a university counselling center setting. Autism Res. 2017;10(12):2048–55.
99. Ganz J, Earles-Vollrath T, Heath A, Parker R, Rispoli M, Duran J. A meta-analysis of single case research studies on aided augmentative and alternative communication systems with individuals with autism spectrum disorders. J Autism Dev Disord. 2012;42(1):60–74.
100. Holyfield C, Drager K, Kremkow J, Light J. Systematic review of AAC intervention research for adolescents and adults with autism spectrum disorder. Augment Altern Commun. 2017;33(4):201–12.
101. Deka D, Feeley C, Lubin A. Travel patterns, needs, and barriers of adults with autism spectrum disorder. Transp Res Rec. 2016;2542:9–16.
102. Marcotte J, et al. Supporting independence at home of people with autism spectrum disorder: literature review. Can J Occup Ther. 2020;87(2):100–16.
103. Schoen S, et al. A systematic review of ayres sensory integration for children with autism. Autism Res. 2019;12(1):6–19.
104. Nicolaidis C, Raymaker D, McDonald K, Dern S, Boisclair WC, Ashkenazy E, et al. Comparison of healthcare experiences in autistic and non-autistic adults: a cross-sectional online survey facilitated by an academic-community partnership. J Gen Intern Med. 2013;28(6):761–9.
105. Nicolaidis C, Raymaker DM, Ashkenazy E, et al. "Respect the way I need to communicate with you": healthcare experiences of adults on the autism spectrum. Autism. 2015;19(7):824–31.
106. Raymaker DM, McDonald KE, Ashkenazy E, et al. Barriers to healthcare: instrument development and comparison between autistic adults and adults with and without other disabilities. Autism. 2017;21(8):972–84.
107. Mason D, Ingham B, Urbanowicz A, et al. A systematic review of what barriers and facilitators prevent and enable physical healthcare services access for autistic adults. J Autism Dev Disord. 2019:1–14.
108. Hand B, et al. Specialized primary care medical home: a positive impact on continuity of care among autistic adults. Autism. 2021;25(1):258–65.
109. Hand B, et al. Effects of a specialized primary care facility on preventative services use among autistic adults: a retrospective claims study. J Gen Intern Med. 2021;36(6):1682–8.
110. Hand B, et al. Patient and caregiver experience at a specialized primary care center for autistic adults. J Comp Eff Res. 2020;9(16):1131–40.
111. Hart L, et al. Implementation and evolution of a primary care-based program for adolescents and young adults on the autism spectrum. J Autism Dev Disord. 2021:1–10.
112. Salvatore G, Simmons C, Tremoulet P. Physician perspectives on severe behaviour and restraint use in a hospital setting for patients with autism spectrum disorder. J Autism Dev Disord. 2022;52(10):4412–25.
113. Broder-Fingert S, et al. A pilot study of autism specific care plans during hospital admission. Pediatrics. 2016;137(Suppl 2):2196–204.
114. Carter J, et al. Brief report: meeting the needs of medically hospitalized adults with autism: a provider and patient toolkit. J Autism Dev Disord. 2017;47:1510–29.
115. Nicolaidis C, Raymaker D, McDonald K, et al. The development and evaluation of an online healthcare toolkit for autistic adults and their primary care providers. J Gen Intern Med. 2016;31(10):1180–9.
116. Howard P, Sedgewick F. 'Anything but the phone!': communication mode preferences in the autism community. Autism. 2021;28(8):2265–78.

# Cerebral Palsy

# 25

Thomas W. Davis, Jonathan Tolentino, Stephanie M. J. Lee, Catherine Zaw, and Gregg Talente

## Case Presentation

Ann is a 20-year-old woman with cerebral palsy (CP) presenting to your office to establish care. She is accompanied by her mother at this visit. Ann was last seen by her primary care pediatrician 2 years ago before moving away to college. She has recently left school and moved back home after a 2-week hospitalization for pneumonia which forced her to withdraw from school. The hospital physician instructed her to find a primary care physician for follow-up.

Ann appears as a well-groomed young woman sitting in one of the wheelchairs from your office. She expresses that her main goal for the visit is to get well enough to return to school for the next semester. Since her hospitalization, she has had increased difficulty with ambulation and routine daily activities requiring more assistance from her parents than normal. She has also lost 12 pounds.

Ann's medical history is significant for premature birth at 32 weeks gestation. She was diagnosed with cerebral palsy in infancy. Her cognitive development was normal. Speech early on was impacted by mild dysarthria which improved with speech therapy as a child. She had significant gross and fine motor delay and spasticity predominantly in her left arm and leg. She has had difficulty with swallowing and with weight gain and maintenance throughout her life and has a gastrostomy tube in place, though she has not used this in the last few years. In addition to her recent hospitalization, she has been hospitalized a few other times for pneumonia as a child. Her only current medication is ibuprofen which she uses as needed but somewhat frequently for hip and back pain.

On review of systems, Ann reports fatigue, back and left hip pain, the weight loss previously mentioned, and some recent difficulty swallowing some foods since her discharge. She also reports issues with constipation. She states that previously she could ambulate independently using a cane for balance but that since her hospitalization she has needed additional assistance and because of this has limited her activities considerably compared to when she was in school. She states that the nurses had her use the office

T. W. Davis
Departments of Internal Medicine and Pediatrics, Geisinger Commonwealth School of Medicine, Danville, PA, USA
e-mail: twdavis@geisinger.edu

J. Tolentino · S. M. J. Lee · C. Zaw
Departments of Internal Medicine and Pediatrics, University of Miami/Jackson Health Systems, Miami, FL, USA
e-mail: jxt1084@med.miami.edu; stephanie.lee@jhsmiami.org; catherine.zaw@jhsmiami.org

G. Talente (✉)
Departments of Internal Medicine and Pediatrics, University of South Carolina School of Medicine, Columbia, SC, USA
e-mail: gregg.talente@uscmed.sc.edu


A. A. Kuo et al. (eds.), *Care of Adults with Chronic Childhood Conditions*,
https://doi.org/10.1007/978-3-031-54281-7_25

wheelchair to make it easier for her to get back to the exam room.

On exam, her vital signs are normal. Her body mass index (BMI) is 18 kg/m$^2$. She is a thin but well-appearing young woman. She has some difficulty transferring to the exam table. Her musculoskeletal exam is significant for mild scoliosis and hypertonicity, particularly in the left arm and leg, with a mild reduction of extension of the left knee. She has tenderness over the lumbar region of the back and the left hip on palpation and reports pain on movement of the left hip on exam.

## Case Discussion

This case illustrates many of the problems adults with cerebral palsy face and highlights the most important aspect of managing adults with cerebral palsy. What is most important is exactly what Ann states as her goals: wellness, functioning, and participation in normal aspects of adult life. In Ann's case, this includes attaining higher education and maintaining her social connections with friends. The case fails though to fully capture what it means to be an adult with cerebral palsy because cerebral palsy is a variable condition, and each person's experience, problems, and needs are unique despite many commonalities.

The primary symptoms of cerebral palsy are spasticity, joint contractures, motor control difficulties, and musculoskeletal deformities. These lead to issues with mobility, fine motor dexterity, and, in some, communication and learning. These issues can in turn lead to decreased overall health, less independence, and less participation in normal aspects of adult life, all of which are illustrated in Ann's case.

While the underlying insult in cerebral palsy is not progressive, individuals can have deterioration in the severity of their symptoms that can cause ongoing loss of function as they age. Contractures can worsen over time and strength can deteriorate. Inactivity is the most common risk factor for this, so it is not surprising that Ann's hospitalization has led to decreased functioning. In caring for cerebral palsy patients, constant surveillance and early intervention to preserve strength and function are important. Collaboration with a physical and occupational therapist to develop a plan to assist Ann to regain the mobility she had prior to hospitalization would be the recommended approach.

Pain control is another important component of managing adults with cerebral palsy. Many have chronic pain which can result from the inherent spasticity of the condition or several other sources. It can also have a significant impact on function. It is clear from the history that Ann is dealing with pain even though this is not her main complaint. Assessment of the severity and its impact on her function would be a critical component of her care. Simple interventions such as anti-inflammatory medications and physical therapy are effective, but in some patients, more aggressive interventions are needed. If her pain is related to uncontrolled spasticity and proves difficult to control, assistance from a physiatrist and consideration of interventions like botulinum A toxin injection or intrathecal baclofen is necessary.

Cerebral palsy is associated with several other conditions, some of which are demonstrated in this case. Ann reports difficulties with swallowing and weight loss, with her low BMI suggesting that her nutritional status may be less than ideal, as well as issues with constipation. An important aspect of managing patients with cerebral palsy is to have familiarity with the many issues they may face, to do a thorough review of systems, and manage these issues as they are discovered. In Ann's case, it might be beneficial to consider consultation with a nutritionist supplementing her diet, possibly by use of her gastrostomy tube. A bowel regimen consisting of increased fiber in the diet, increased hydration, and the initiation of an osmotic laxative might help with her constipation.

Patients with cerebral palsy present a unique challenge to hospital-based providers. Ann's pneumonia was likely more serious because of her cerebral palsy, and because of her prolonged hospitalization, she has had a decrease in her motor function that has forced her to leave school. Among individuals with cerebral palsy, infection is the most common reason for admission followed by uncontrolled epilepsy and gastrointestinal issues. While the management of her pneumonia may not differ from that of other patients in terms of antibiotic choice, for example, Ann has needs and issues that are unique from other hospitalized patients. Managing her associated comorbidities, maintaining strength and motor function as well as nutritional needs, and addressing psychosocial issues can all impact outcomes for patients with cerebral palsy who are hospitalized.

The key to managing Ann as a patient begins with listening to her stated goals. Cerebral palsy is a chronic condition that cannot be cured. What is important is helping Ann to live with cerebral palsy the way she wants. Ann's stated main goal is to help her regain enough strength and mobility to restart school. This may be done with simple exercises guided by a physical therapist, or it may require finding new solutions to increase her mobility and ability to participate at school. In addition, to best help her with her goals, a thorough evaluation with specific attention to possible problems related to her cerebral palsy should be undertaken. Finally, routine preventive health should be provided. At this time, Ann requires only sexually transmitted infection (STI) screening, but as she ages additional preventive measures should not be neglected, though they frequently are in adults with cerebral palsy. She should also receive counseling on reproductive health issues as part of her initial evaluation.

## Definition

Cerebral palsy is defined as a group of permanent disorders affecting the development of movement and posture causing activity limitations and attributed to nonprogressive injury of the developing fetal or infant brain [1]. This encompasses a broad spectrum of conditions with diverse symptoms and presentations. Individuals with cerebral palsy are often further classified by the location of the brain lesion, the types of motor symptoms displayed, and the severity of the symptoms.

Classification by brain lesion requires magnetic resonance imaging (MRI) and typically divides cases into cortical, pyramidal tract, extrapyramidal tract, and cerebellar groupings. Symptom classification usually divides patients based on the primary motor symptom: spasticity, dyskinesia, athetoid, or ataxic cerebral palsy. Another classification is by the affected extremities, dividing cerebral palsy into diplegic, hemiplegic, and quadriplegic groups [1]. Scales exist that are commonly used to classify cerebral palsy based on the severity of motor dysfunction. The Gross Motor Function Classification System (GMFCS) and the Minimal Ability Classification System (MACS) are two that are commonly used in the literature on cerebral palsy [2, 3].

While classification has its importance for research and transfer of knowledge, no system of classification can truly represent the needs of an individual patient and, practically, classification is less important than assessing an individual's functional needs, risks, and treatment goals. This focus on function is what led the International Classification of Functioning Disability and Health (ICF) sponsored by the World Health Organization (WHO) to promote a shift in how we discuss disability. Traditionally, we think of conditions using a linear model, where disease leads to a damaged organ or organ system which in turn leads to disability. The WHO recommends instead an integrative model focusing on the condition and the contextual factors both impacting and impacted by the condition, promoting a focus on functional activity in the framework of the patient's condition [4]. Practically, the use of a classification system like the GMFCS (described in detail later in the section on Ambulatory Presentation) can be a useful tool to assist in communication between providers sharing the care of a young adult with cerebral palsy and in communication with the patient and family about prognosis.

## Prevalence

Cerebral palsy occurs in 2–3 of 1000 children born [1]. The prevalence of cerebral palsy has been mostly stable over time. Risk factors for cerebral palsy include prematurity and low birth weight. Most infants born with cerebral palsy will live into adulthood. Studies suggest that 98% of children with cerebral palsy not classified as severe reach age 20 years and up to 85% of children with severe cerebral palsy reach age 20 years. It is estimated that there are about half a million adults with cerebral palsy living in the United States.

Life expectancy of adults with cerebral palsy is less than that of the general population though a significant percentage of patients reach age 50 years and older [1]. In patients with higher function, mortality is similar to that of the general population; however, those who have lost the ability to ambulate by age 60 years are more likely to have poorer survival. Mortality in patients in the third and fourth decade of life is usually due to respiratory complications, while mortality in the fourth and fifth decade of life is usually due to cardiovascular or oncologic diseases [5–8]. Intellectual disability was found to be the greatest single predictor of mortality, while severe motor impairment increased the risk for early mortality [9].

## Pathophysiology

Cerebral palsy is most commonly caused by interference in brain development in utero, though it has been attributed to injury occurring perinatally. Hypoxic injury or neonatal asphyxia was traditionally thought to be the cause of the injury, though currently asphyxia is believed to impact only 10–20% of cases of cerebral palsy. Other causes of developmental injury leading to cerebral palsy include genetic causes, infection, and thromboembolic causes [1].

## Ambulatory Presentation

Patients with cerebral palsy will often present with abnormalities in motor function secondary to abnormal tone, weakness, difficulty with mobility and balance, and poor control of motor movement, with accompanying abnormalities in sensation, cognition, communication, and behavior [10]. While cerebral palsy is often considered a nonprogressive disorder, the motor abilities of adults with cerebral palsy often decline over time, affecting gross and fine motor function and ambulation [11].

Several non-neuromuscular comorbidities are associated with cerebral palsy that should be co-managed among the primary care provider, neurologist, physiatrist, and other subspecialists (see Table 25.1). Most commonly seen disorders include musculoskeletal disorders, epilepsy, intellectual disability, speech disorders, obesity,

**Table 25.1** Common comorbidities associated with adults with cerebral palsy [1, 10, 11, 14]

| | |
|---|---|
| **HEENT** | **Gastrointestinal** |
| Saliva control | Gastroesophageal reflux disease (GERD) |
| Visual problems | Delayed gastric emptying |
| Strabismus | Constipation |
| Visual field defects | Bowel dysfunction |
| Myopia | Problems with feeding, swallowing |
| Hypermetropia | Bower motility |
| Severe visual and hearing impairment | Poor nutrition and growth |
| Speech disorders | **Urological** |
| Poor dental health | Bladder dysfunction |
| **Neurological** | **Psychological** |
| Epilepsy (severe CP) | Chronic pain |
| Partial epilepsy (unilateral spastic CP) | Chronic fatigue |
| Sensorineural hearing loss | **Bone health** |
| **Infectious disease** | Hip dislocation |
| High rates of infection | Scoliosis |
| Cellulitis and decubitus ulcers | Cervical instability and spinal arthritis |
| Urinary tract infection (UTI) | Osteopenia and osteoporosis |

*HEENT* head, ears, eyes, nose, and throat; *CP* cerebral palsy

dysphagia, bladder and gastrointestinal problems, and dental problems [5, 12, 13]. Patients with more severe functional impairment and higher GMFCS scores have increasing problems with advancing age, including disorders associated with decreased movement such as osteopenia [5].

## Hospital Presentation

Patients with cerebral palsy will present to the hospital for a variety of reasons. (see Table 25.2) With age, there are shifts in reasons for admission among cerebral palsy patients. In youth, epilepsy, pneumonia, and orthopedic conditions represent many inpatient admissions. While epilepsy and respiratory conditions are also the most significant reasons for admissions among young adults with cerebral palsy, other issues start to develop around this time as well, such as lower gastrointestinal (GI) problems, nutritional issues (malnutrition and dehydration), and especially mental health concerns.

Adult CP patients predominantly seek hospital admission due to emergency rather than planned care, and length of stay for adult patients tends to be longer than that of children [15]. As is the case among the general population, many of the reasons for inpatient admissions are highly preventable and are inversely correlated with appropriate access to primary care. The priority is the prevention of hospitalizations through understanding and anticipation of complications of cerebral palsy.

**Table 25.2** Common causes of hospital admission for adults with cerebral palsy [15]

| | |
|---|---|
| **Neurological** | **Renal** |
| Epilepsy | Dehydration and metabolic disturbance |
| Convulsions | Chronic kidney disease |
| Shunt dysfunction | Urinary tract infection (UTI) |
| Dystonia | **Infectious disease** |
| Baclofen pump placement or dysfunction | Sepsis |
| **Orthopedic** | Bacteremia |
| Fracture or other injury | Cellulitis and decubitus ulcers |
| Scheduled procedures | **Other** |
| **Pulmonary** | Drug complications or side effects |
| Pneumonia | Mental health |
| Pneumonitis | |
| **Gastrointestinal** | |
| Malnutrition | |
| Constipation | |
| Feeding tube malfunction | |
| Ileus | |

## Quality of Life

Multiple studies have shown that the reported health and quality of life of patients with cerebral palsy is lower compared to the general population populations, particularly in the domains of motor and social functioning, but better compared to other diseases such as multiple sclerosis [16–19]. Adults with CP report a deterioration of gross motor function and quality of life as they age, with the greatest decline occurring by the mid-40s rather than during the young adult transition period [16, 18, 20, 21]. Physical function has a greater effect on reported quality of life in adolescent CP patients, while psychological and emotional aspects play a greater role in older patients [19, 22]. Other factors that influence quality of life include sports participation, chronic pain, chronic fatigue, deterioration of function, living alone, unemployment, and low sense of coherence [23, 24]. Many cerebral palsy patients separate physical health from overall health, and one study reported that the subjective well-being and general satisfaction of life in a cross section of adults with CP was not decreased [25].

## Transition Issues

Most patients presenting to the general internist for continuity of care usually have come from a pediatric institution that provides care involving a multidisciplinary team, including physical therapists, occupational therapists, orthopedic surgeons, physiatrists, and neurologists to provide coordinated care [1, 10, 26–29]. In addition, many adult practitioners are unfamiliar with the unique needs of CP patients and struggle in dealing with the needs of cognitively limited patients with impaired communication skills, factors which can contribute to access issues for these emerging adults [26, 30, 31]. There is considerable heterogeneity among the CP population, ranging from autonomous patients with normal intelligence to those with severe cognitive deficits requiring coordinated specialty and supportive care [32]. New clinical and transition programs are being designed at some pediatric and adult centers targeting the adult cerebral palsy patients, but long-term outcomes for these programs remain limited. Regardless, most care for adults with CP will take place in traditional adult primary care practices [33–36].

CP patients find it difficult to transition because of attachment to child-centered providers, youth and parental reluctance to transition to adult care, and unease and limited training among adult providers in the management of cerebral palsy [37]. The lack of cooperation or communication between providers, the feeling of abandonment among patients, and the lack of knowledge or support through the transition period further complicate the process [38, 39]. The transition process also presents a new focus in shift of care from the normalization of function, which is a primary focus of therapy treatments in childhood, to the accommodation of function, which is increasingly becoming the focus of therapy across the lifespan [40]. Compared to their peers, patients with CP lag behind in several milestones in achieving independence in transition, such as housing, employment, and relationships [41]. In addition, many patients will remain dependent on parents for both emotional and financial support, causing stress for both patients and parents [42, 43].

## Ambulatory Management of CP Patients

### Neuromuscular Function Issues

Primary care providers will comanage with physical therapists, occupational therapists, physiatrists, and possibly neurologists and orthopedic surgeons on many of the neuromuscular issues associated with the adults with cerebral palsy. The GMFCS is commonly used to describe function in cerebral palsy patients (see Box 25.1) [2].

**Box 25.1 Expanded and Revised Gross Motor Function Classification System for Children 12–18 Years [2]**

**GMFCS Level I**: Youth walk at home, school, outdoors, and in the community. Youth are able to climb curbs and stairs without physical assistance or a railing. They perform gross motor skills such as running and jumping, but speed, balance, and coordination are limited.

**GMFCS Level II**: Youth walk in most settings but environmental factors and personal choice influence mobility choices. At school or work, they may require a hand-held mobility device for safety and climb stairs holding onto a railing. Outdoors and in the community, youth may use wheeled mobility when traveling long distances.

**GMFCS Level III**: Youth are capable of walking using a hand-held mobility device. Youth may climb stairs holding onto a railing with supervision or assistance. At school, they may self-propel a manual wheelchair or use powered mobility. Outdoors and in the community youth are transported in wheelchair or use powered mobility.

**GMFCS Level IV**: Youth use wheeled mobility in most settings. Physical assistance of 1–2 people is required for transfers. Indoors, youth may walk short distances with physical assistance and use wheeled mobility or a body support walker when positioned. They may operate a powered chair, otherwise are transported in a manual wheelchair.

**GMFCS Level V**: Youth are transported in a manual wheelchair in all settings. Youth are limited in their ability to maintain antigravity head and trunk postures and control leg and arm movements. Self-mobility is severely limited, even with the use of assistive technology.

*GMFCS:* Gross Motor Function Classification System.

Based on available data among patients with cerebral palsy, an estimated 21–43% are hemiplegic, 29–35% are diplegic, and 12–22% are quadriplegic; approximately one-fifth of adult patients had dyskinesia [3, 44, 45]. Between 28 and 77% of adults with CP report the use of a wheelchair, with up to 40% of wheelchair users being ambulatory previously [3, 10, 11, 45, 46]. Some CP adults stop ambulating by choice as they age due to fatigue and pain, leading to inactivity, deconditioning, and contractures. The decline in function is less common between childhood and early adulthood, but up to one-fourth may show a decline in gross neuromuscular function later into adult life, with declines occurring between the second and fourth decades [10, 18, 21, 47, 48]. The decline may be a function of changes in muscle flexibility, increased spasticity, falls, fractures, pain, and fatigue [11]. It is more common in those with more severe neuromuscular disease [49].

The management of neuromuscular problems in patients with cerebral palsy requires the coordination between physical therapy, occupational therapy, and physiatry [27–29]. The primary medical therapies include muscle relaxants and anti-dystonic drugs (Tables 25.3 and 25.4) [1]. Baclofen is most often used and has been very effective; however, sudden withdrawal can lead to rebound spasticity, seizures, and hallucinations [50]. Second-line agents, such as tizanidine and dantrolene, are effective in reducing spasticity, but their use is limited by their side effect profile. Physiatry will typically be able to assist with the use of other interventions, such as the use of botulinum toxin (Botox) injections. Botox has shown some efficacy in the pediatric population, and initial studies using Botox in the adult CP population have demonstrated improvement in function [50, 51]. Botox effects usually peak within 4–6 weeks of delivery but wane after 12 weeks; patients will need repeated planned injections every 12 weeks [50]. Physical therapy will be able to assist in interventions for mobility, improvements in biomechanics, assistive technology, and movement dysfunction [29].

More invasive therapies include selective dorsal rhizotomy, which severs problematic nerve roots and intrathecal baclofen pump placement.

**Table 25.3** Medical management of patients with dystonia [52]

| Medication | Target population | Typical dose |
|---|---|---|
| Carbidopa-levodopa | Early-onset dystonia | Begin 1 mg/kg/day divided BID to TID. Increase by 1 mg/kg/week, up to 5 mg/kg/day for at least 4 weeks. |
| Benzodiazepines | Early-onset dystonia<br>Late-onset dystonia | Clonazepam: 0.5–10 mg QD<br>Diazepam: 2–100 mg QD<br>Lorazepam 0.5–8 mg QD |
| Baclofen | Craniofacial dystonia<br>Early-onset dystonia | Begin 2.5–5 mg QHS<br>Increase by 2.5 or 5 mg QD to a total daily dose of 80 mg |
| Trihexyphenidyl | Early-onset dystonia<br>Late-onset dystonia | Adults typically tolerate 8–12 mg QD |
| Tetrabenazine | Tardive dystonia | 12.5 mg–200 mg QD |

Adapted with permission from Bragg et al. [52]

**Table 25.4** Medical management of patients with spasticity [50]

| Medication | Indication | Typical dose | Side effects |
|---|---|---|---|
| Baclofen | Preferred oral antispasticity drug | Starting dose 5 mg three times daily; titration 5–10 mg weekly; maximum dose 90–120 mg/day divided into three doses; lower doses in renal failure; and taper by up to 15 mg/week | Weakness, drowsiness, dizziness, sexual dysfunction, and urinary incontinence. Sudden withdrawal may cause rebound spasticity, seizures, and hallucinations. Should be used with caution during pregnancy |
| Tizanidine | Second-line treatment if baclofen is not tolerated or ineffective | Starting dose 2 mg at bedtime; titration, increased by 2 mg weekly; maximum dose 36 mg/day divided into three or four doses; taper by 4 mg/week | Dry mouth, gastrointestinal disturbance, hypotension, and acute hepatitis. Monitor liver enzyme levels |
| Dantrolene | Second-line treatment if baclofen is not tolerated or ineffective | Starting dose 25 mg/day; titration, increase in steps of 25 mg/week; maximum dose 100 mg three or four times daily, taper by 25 mg/week | Hepatotoxicity, weakness, dizziness, and diarrhea. Monitor liver enzyme levels |
| Gabapentin | Spasticity associated with pain | 300 mg once daily on day 1, then 300 mg twice daily on day 2, then 300 mg three times daily on day 3, and then increased according to response in steps of 300 mg every 2 or 3 days, up to a maximum of 3600 mg daily | Weight gain, gastrointestinal disturbance, confusion, depression, hostility, and sleep disturbances. Need electrocardiography to monitor for QT interval prolongation |

Reprinted with permission from Nair and Mardsen [50]

Selective dorsal rhizotomies are usually performed in ambulatory patients and improve body function and spasticity but have not been demonstrated to influence long-term activity and participation [1, 53]. Intrathecal baclofen has been shown to be effective in reducing short-term spasticity, but its effect on gross motor function, improvement in comfort, ease of care, and quality of life is not as well-established [54, 55].

## Orthopedic Issues: Fractures, Joint Deformities, and Surgical Interventions

A number of orthopedic issues affect patients with cerebral palsy, many of which are the result of long-standing contractures [48]. Hip displacement is fairly common, affecting up to one-third of patients with cerebral palsy, especially the nonambulatory patients [1, 56]. Hip dislocation most commonly occurs in patients with quadriplegia and can be painful and affect function [48]. Neuromuscular scoliosis affects between 15 and 80% of patients with CP, particularly the nonambulatory and less functional patients [48, 56, 57]. Other orthopedic issues can be seen as well (see Table 25.5).

Collaborative care among primary care, orthopedic surgery, physical therapy, and physiatry is necessary to assure management with the focus on improvement in function. Scoliosis should be monitored into adulthood as curve angles may continue to progress even after skeletal maturity is achieved and the need for future corrective surgery may need to be entertained to avoid complications such as restrictive lung pathologies [56, 57]. Providers need to be aware that cerebral palsy patients can develop common orthopedic conditions like spinal stenosis and osteoarthritis later in life [58, 59].

**Table 25.5** Secondary orthopedic conditions [45]

| |
|---|
| Patella Alta |
| Hip displacement |
| Spondylosis |
| Cervical stenosis |
| Scoliosis |
| Foot deformities |

## Osteopenia

Poor bone health (osteopenia and osteoporosis) and the risk for fracture associated with low bone mineral density are common in cerebral palsy. Low bone mineral density is often found much earlier in cerebral palsy patients than among the general population [60, 61]. Physicians caring for adults with cerebral palsy need to be aware of this and consider early screening and intervention. Risk factors for developing low bone mineral density in patients with cerebral palsy include poor nutrition, worse severity of neurologic symptoms, nonambulatory status, poor vitamin D and calcium intake, and periods of immobility [62]. Unfortunately, there is not enough data available to develop a standard recommendation for evaluation with dual-energy X-ray absorptiometry in the cerebral palsy population.

Treatment of low bone mineral density in cerebral palsy should involve nutritional interventions, vitamin D and calcium supplementation, and increased physical activity. Studies in cerebral palsy patients suggest a benefit from the use of bisphosphonates, however the specific CP patients to target as well as the ideal timing for initiation of this intervention remains unclear [63–67].

### Pain

Pain is a common and important problem in adults with cerebral palsy. Multiple studies suggest that up to two-thirds of patients with cerebral palsy suffer from pain in one or more sites for longer than 3 months duration [68]. Thus, many adult cerebral palsy patients meet the criteria for suffering from chronic pain. The incidence of chronic pain in cerebral palsy increases with increasing age [69]. Back pain is the most common site of pain with hip and leg pain being the next most common [70].

Evaluation and management of pain in cerebral palsy are best undertaken with a detailed history and examination to determine the cause of the pain. If feasible, specific interventions for the underlying cause, such as repair of dental issues and treatment of gastroesophageal reflux, should be undertaken. Otherwise, management of pain in cerebral palsy should be done according to the principles used to treat all chronic pain.

Management of pain with medication in patients with cerebral palsy is best done by treating the underlying cause such as spasticity and dystonia, as described earlier. Nonsteroidal anti-inflammatory medications are also useful. The use of narcotic pain medications as with any instance of chronic noncancer pain should be used judiciously and as a last resort.

## Gastrointestinal Issues

There are four common gastrointestinal issues associated with cerebral palsy. Their impact can range from mild to severe. They can be a source of pain, have an impact on function and participation, and impact risk for morbidity and mortality. Thus, screening for and management of gastrointestinal issues in adult cerebral palsy patients is an important aspect of care.

Dysphagia and difficulty swallowing are common [71]. These issues are frequently diagnosed in childhood and often infancy. Speech therapy is the most common intervention. Placement of a gastrostomy tube is done when swallowing issues present too great a risk for aspiration or inhibit adequate nutrition. Progression of dysphagia in adulthood is typically caused by acute illness or poor nutritional status.

Gastroesophageal reflux is very common in cerebral palsy. It can present at any age as simple heartburn, respiratory symptoms, or as anemia alone [72]. Because reflux is related to the central developmental brain injury and resulting motor dysfunction, it can be refractory to medical therapy. Despite this, the initial intervention is acid blockade with histamine-2 (H2) receptor antagonists or proton pump inhibitors. In severe, refractory cases fundoplication should be considered, especially if comorbid complications such as recurrent aspiration pneumonitis or pneumonia develop [71].

Constipation is another frequent GI issue seen in cerebral palsy. It results from delayed colonic transit and incoordination of the anal sphincter and pelvic floor musculature [73, 74]. It is often exacerbated by immobility and dietary factors. Treatment of constipation should include dietary fiber, hydration, and, when needed, the use of osmotic laxatives or stimulants [75].

Poor nutrition is also common in cerebral palsy patients. Typically, it is due to other gastrointestinal issues, particularly dysphagia. Studies suggest that many patients have a poor diet without adequate nutrients [76]. Assessment of nutritional status, tracking of weight with attention to periods of weight loss, and collaboration with a nutritionist are recommended in managing adults with cerebral palsy [71].

### Urinary Dysfunction and Urinary Tract Infections

Urinary dysfunction including incontinence is common in cerebral palsy patients [77, 78]. Conservative nonsurgical management of urinary dysfunction is successful in 75–91% of CP patients; such management includes toileting education, medications such as oxybutynin, padding, perineal hygiene, and, when needed, clean intermittent catheterization for bladder management [79, 80]. Urinary tract infections are most often seen with poor perineal hygiene and the use of an external urinary collection device or an indwelling Foley catheter [81]. Outpatient management of urinary tract infections, which should be considered complex urinary tract infections in the CP patient population, should be based upon established guidelines for urinary tract infections in the general population and local antibiotic resistance patterns [82].

## Vision, Hearing, and Communication

Addressing communication, vision, and hearing deficits should be a priority in managing adults with cerebral palsy. Commonly diagnosed visual, hearing, and communication comorbidities among individuals with cerebral palsy were previously described (see Table 25.1). Vision and hearing problems may develop later on in adulthood, whereas communication issues are more likely to be noted early in childhood [11, 83].

Regardless, all three areas should be screened for by adult providers in routine health assessments.

Dysarthria is the most common cause of communication limitations in cerebral palsy patients [84]. Dysarthria is caused by interference with the muscle function related to speech production [11]. Speech therapy is the first intervention for dysarthria. Studies have suggested that intrathecal baclofen can improve dysarthria. Assistive technology should be considered in more severe cases. Receptive communication issues can also occur in cerebral palsy patients with comorbid intellectual disability.

### Health Maintenance and Other Primary Care Concerns

All established age-appropriate preventive health screening, vaccination, and counseling recommendations for adults are applicable and should be completed for adults with cerebral palsy. Unique challenges in the delivery of these services exist among individuals with CP. For example, the delivery of preventive and therapeutic dental health frequently requires sedation. Positioning for routine examination can also be a barrier. Regardless, it is critical for adult primary care providers to complete recommended interventions in this population as well as be attentive to some unique concerns.

Numerous studies have shown an increased incidence of cardiovascular disease markers and cardiovascular disease outcomes early in adults with cerebral palsy [85–89]. Cerebral palsy patients may have a degree of muscle atrophy and decreased bone density, and despite a normal BMI, have excess body fat. Metabolic syndrome and cardiovascular risk factors may present early [86, 88]. Increased morbidity and mortality due to cardiovascular diseases are seen at a younger-than-expected age among adults with cerebral palsy [6, 85, 87]. Attention to weight management, lifestyle changes, and early screening are recommended, though no clear guidelines exist.

Recent studies have also identified evidence of polypharmacy among adults with cerebral palsy [90]. This has been associated with increased mortality, chronic kidney disease, and liver disease [91]. Given the numerous problems and comorbidities associated with cerebral palsy and the systemic challenges in accessing care in the adult healthcare system for this patient population, there is a real danger of excessive medication use. Providers should be vigilant in performing medication reconciliation and in stopping unnecessary medications.

## Psychosocial Issues/Mental Health

For young adults with CP, psychosocial well-being improves as patients age. Although psychosocial well-being is not strongly associated with overall functional status, participation by cerebral palsy patients of normal intelligence in daily activities and in social roles (i.e., leisure activities, community living, and employment) is more restricted, especially in those with lower motor function, advanced age, and lower education level [17, 92, 93]. Nearly two-thirds reportedly have difficulty with mobility, recreation, and housing, and nearly half have difficulties with personal care and employment [94]. Loneliness in patients with cerebral palsy was noted to be higher than in the general population [95]. Patients with CP are more likely to participate in leisure activities if mobility is good and if the environment facilitates leisure (such as adaptive transport, accompanying services, and computer aids) [96].

Educational attainment is possible for many patients with cerebral palsy, with a good proportion completing high school and college if appropriate support systems and accommodations are in place [45]. Completion of community college or supplemental job training does improve the chances for employment opportunities. For patients with developmental disabilities who are unable to continue onto higher education, special education high schools end at age 21 years and can provide a useful bridge to additional adult educational enrichment programs in the community [10].

Employment rates remain low, with reported rates between 10 and 48% [10, 44, 45, 96]. Patients with higher IQ, higher education, better mobility, supportive family, improved physical health, decreased pain, completion of regular high school, improved speech ability, and normal hearing and vision are more likely to have regular employment [10].

For living arrangements, approximately 60–80% of young adult CP patients live with their parents, while approximately 60% of older CP patients in the age range of 30–40 years live independently [45]. Among older CP adults, approximately 20–28% are either married or live with a partner. However, at least 60% report difficulties with mobility, recreation, and housing, and about one-fourth report issues with personal care and employment [94]. Patients with more severe forms of spastic cerebral palsy and with developmental disabilities can often reside in group homes and assisted living arrangements [10, 45].

An increased incidence of mental health comorbidities is noted in adults with cerebral palsy [85, 97]. Among other conditions, both anxiety and depression are noted to be prevalent [98]. Providers should screen adults with cerebral palsy routinely for mental health concerns consistent with recommendations among the general population.

### Reproductive Health and Sexuality

As with all patients, reproductive health and sexuality are important aspects of ambulatory care for patients with cerebral palsy. Just as in other adults, the needs regarding reproductive health vary between individuals based on gender and sexual orientation, personal views and experiences, and culture. The extent of their disease symptoms and the patient's level of function may impact each individual's needs in this area [99, 100]. It is a mistake to ignore this area in caring for these patients. Regardless of the extent of their symptoms and functional limitations, cerebral palsy patients actively participate in healthy relationships and actively engage in sex. Between 52 and 76% of young adults have been in a relationship, with one-quarter report being in a current relationship [101–103]. A little over half of young adults with CP report being sexually active, but compared to nondisabled peers, rates of experiences are lower [102–104]. Generalists should provide appropriate preventive care for CP adults, including education regarding sexuality, treatment, and evaluation of sexual difficulties and prevention of sexually transmitted infections.

## Hospital Management of CP Patients

### General Hospital Management Considerations

Given the complexity of the CP patients, the care of adults with cerebral palsy in the hospital setting presents many challenges. Providers should recognize the importance of considering the patient as a whole and not limit focus to the admitting diagnosis. While the pathogenesis for many of the reasons patients with CP end up in the hospital does not differ from the same issues in a patient without CP, the extent of the patient's CP-related symptoms and comorbidities increases the risk for complications, prolonged hospitalization, and long-term effects on function and general wellness after discharge. Compared to non-CP patients, there is a higher proportion of patients admitted for pneumonia, epilepsy, and other respiratory conditions in CP patients [105]. The patient's socioeconomic status and social support system can have a significant impact on outcomes. Unfortunately, very little published data exist to guide hospital-based providers in the complex needs of patients with cerebral palsy when they are admitted to the hospital.

Independence and self-management vary with disease severity in CP patients. Therefore, involving family and caregivers early and throughout the hospitalization is of utmost importance, not only for the patient's well-being and continuity of care but also to establish good rapport among the caregivers involved in the care of the patient with CP [106]. When possible, collaboration with the patient's primary care provider and where appropriate specialty providers is also beneficial. Unfortunately, many young adult CP patients admitted to the adult hospital are still cared for by pediatric providers, which can present a barrier to collaboration, a barrier that will have to be overcome either by system design within the healthcare organization or by a concerted effort of the inpatient team [106].

As with other complex patients, discharge planning and application of the standards for high-quality hospital-to-ambulatory transition management is critical. CP patients are at high risk for loss of function after hospitalization, so attention to rehabilitation needs should be prioritized. Again, good communication with the patient, their family, and the ambulatory providers is critical to avoiding errors and complications.

## Neurological Issues

The most common neurologic reason for admission among patients with cerebral palsy is breakthrough seizures, with varying degrees of severity [105]. A significant number of adults with CP have hydrocephalus, and many require prior surgical intervention with VP shunt placements, which can easily have complications leading to admission. Shunt malfunctions can cause an array of complications: shunt infection, overdrainage (slit-ventricle syndrome), underdrainage, subdural hematoma, multiloculated hydrocephalus, material degradation, seizures, and abdominal complications. Additionally, many patients with cerebral palsy and more severe spasticity are admitted for placement of a baclofen pump or for issues arising from required maintenance or dysfunction of a baclofen pump. Cerebrospinal fluid (CSF) leaks, headaches, mechanical problems with pump or catheter, infections, wound dehiscence, and seroma are all possible complications requiring inpatient care. The most frequent problems with pumps requiring an unplanned secondary surgery are end-of-battery life, pump/catheter problems, and CSF leak.

## Orthopedic Issues

As in childhood, a number of admissions in adults with CP are for planned orthopedic interventions intended to help manage spasticity and its complications in order to improve or maintain function. There is a higher-than-normal risk for complications after such scheduled procedures [107]. Admission for fractures, hip dislocation, and other acquired orthopedic issues increases in adult cerebral palsy patients [105].

## Pulmonary Issues

Respiratory infections, specifically pneumonia, are among the most common reasons for admission in adults with cerebral palsy [15, 105]. While underlying lung disease is not a feature of CP, more impacted adults with CP may suffer from restrictive lung disease due to scoliosis and contracture. The neuromuscular issues related to CP can impact the management of secretions, risk for aspiration, and recovery from even common respiratory pathogens. Attention to respiratory therapy needs is important in all hospitalized adults with CP but even more critical in those admitted for primary pulmonary disease.

## Gastrointestinal Issues

In adults with cerebral palsy receiving nutrition through a gastrostomy tube, tube-related issues are a common cause for admission [15]. Peristomal wound infections, clogged feeding tubes, and leaking tubes are common, and while at times, these issues can be managed in the outpatient setting, access to intervention often leads to admission to ensure continued hydration and metabolic needs are met. Such complications, while not completely avoidable, can be minimized through regular skin and stomal care, avoiding excessive traction on the G-tube, and avoiding thick enteral feeds, bulking agents, and medications that need to be delivered through the G-tube.

Constipation is common in CP. Admission for ileus, impaction, and failure of outpatient bowel regimens is sometimes required. In patients admitted for other issues, the hospital course can be extended by iatrogenic worsening of bowel issues. Therefore, in all admitted patients, discussions should be made with caretakers and nursing staff to understand and continue, if possible, home bowel regimens while the patient remains hospitalized. Further, avoidance of unnecessary interventions that might worsen bowel function is recommended.

### Renal Issues

Due to chronic issues with poor nutrition, dysphagia, and dependence on enteral feeding regimens, common presenting problems in adults with cerebral palsy being admitted to the hospital are dehydration and other metabolic abnormalities. This is often seen in the setting of other acute issues such as infection and gastrostomy tube dysfunction but can occur in isolation. Acute kidney injury due to dehydration or intrarenal causes such as medication side effects or infection is also common. Due to the high incidence of urinary dysfunction in these patients, urinary tract infections are also common. While many can be treated in the outpatient setting, pyelonephritis and sepsis often lead to admission.

## Infectious Disease Considerations

Infections of the respiratory and genitourinary systems account for a large proportion of admissions among adults with cerebral palsy. Skin infections are also common. Many adults with cerebral palsy will present with sepsis or bacteremia as a complication of their underlying infection. In treating sepsis, bacteremia, or other infections that require hospitalization in adults with cerebral palsy, nosocomial infections should be considered. Further, due to possible frequent prior treatment with antibiotics in all settings, providers should be vigilant for resistant pathogens.

Cerebral palsy patients who are quadriplegic and have significant limitations in mobility are at risk for complications associated with skin breakdown. While the literature in the ambulatory nonhospitalized cerebral palsy patients is limited, we know that patients with CP admitted to the hospital are at risk for skin-related complications [108]. Most commonly, postsurgical infections after spinal fusion are due to gram-negative bacilli [109]. About 21% of paraplegic and 23% of quadriplegic patients have pressure ulcers, commonly affecting the sacrum, ischium, and heel [109, 110]. Management of pressure ulcers requires appropriate staging using the European Pressure Ulcer Advisory Panel (EPUAP) guidelines [111]. Nonsurgical management by general internists should be done in consultation with a wound care provider and often includes hydrocolloid and hydrogel dressings for stage I and stage II ulcers. Complex stage II ulcers and higher should be managed with a wound care provider, and recalcitrant ulcers typically will require co-management with a plastic surgeon [110, 112]. Suspicion for an infected ulcer should include workup for potential osteomyelitis, including obtaining serum inflammatory markers and blood cultures and appropriate imaging such as MRI (care should be taken for those who have prior surgical hardware placed for comorbid conditions such as scoliosis).

## Conclusion

**Overview and Recommendations for Practice**

1. The goal of therapy for adults with CP should be to maximize function even if accomplished through the use of assistive technology so that these individuals can achieve their life goals.
2. Providers should familiarize themselves with the treatments for the neuromuscular complications of CP, be comfortable medically managing dystonia and spasticity with oral medications, and identify referral sources for more invasive treatments if required.
3. Ambulatory management of adults with CP should include surveillance for the common

complications associated with cerebral palsy as listed in Table 25.1.

4. Adults with CP should receive all the normal counseling and preventive health measures appropriate for their age.
5. In the hospital setting providers treating adults with cerebral palsy need to be attentive to not only the presenting problem but also the risk for complications in hospitalized adults with cerebral palsy and the potential impact of prolonged hospitalization on function after discharge.
6. Good communication with caregivers and ambulatory providers along with best practices for transition on discharge is essential to hospital care in these patients.
7. Important partners in managing adults with CP should include a physical therapist, a physiatrist, an orthopedist, and other specialists as needed based on the individual's unique problems.

## References


1. Colver A, Fairhurst C, Pharoah PO. Cerebral palsy. Lancet. 2014;383(9924):1240–9.
2. Palisano R, Rosenbaum P, Walter S, Russell D, Wood E, Galuppi B. Development and reliability of a system to classify gross motor function in children with cerebral palsy. Dev Med Child Neurol. 1997;39(4):214–23.
3. Stevenson CJ, Pharoah PO, Stevenson R. Cerebral palsy—the transition from youth to adulthood. Dev Med Child Neurol. 1997;39(5):336–42.
4. World Health Organization. International classification of functioning, disability, and health. Geneva, Switzerland: World Health Organization; 2001.
5. Turk MA. Health, mortality, and wellness issues in adults with cerebral palsy. Dev Med Child Neurol. 2009;51(Suppl 4):24–9.
6. Strauss D, Cable W, Shavelle R. Causes of excess mortality in cerebral palsy. Dev Med Child Neurol. 1999;41(9):580–5.
7. Strauss D, Ojdana K, Shavelle R, Rosenbloom L. Decline in function and life expectancy of older persons with cerebral palsy. NeuroRehabilitation. 2004;19(1):69–78.
8. Blair E, Langdon K, McIntyre S, Lawrence D, Watson L. Survival and mortality in cerebral palsy: observations to the sixth decade from a data linkage study of a total population register and National Death Index. BMC Neurol. 2019;19(1):111.
9. Blair E, Watson L, Badawi N, Stanley FJ. Life expectancy among people with cerebral palsy in Western Australia. Dev Med Child Neurol. 2001;43(8):508–15.
10. Glew GM, Bennett FC. Cerebral palsy grown up. J Dev Behav Pediatr. 2011;32(6):469–75.
11. Haak P, Lenski M, Cooley Hidecker MJ, Li M, Paneth N. Cerebral palsy and aging. Dev Med Child Neurol. 2009;51(Suppl 4):16–23.
12. Mezaal MA, Nouri KA, Abdool S, Al Safar K, Nadeem ASM. Cerebral palsy in adults consequences of non progressive pathology. Open Neurol J. 2009;3:24–6.
13. Henderson CM, Rosaco M, Robinson LM, Meccarello J, Janicki MP, Turk MA, et al. Functional impairment severity is associated with health status among older persons with intellectual disability and cerebral palsy. J Intellect Disabil Res. 2009;53(11):887–97.
14. Liptak GS. Health and well being of adults with cerebral palsy. Curr Opin Neurol. 2008;21(2):136–42.
15. Morgan P, Enticott J, Nikam R, Tracy J. Profile of hospital admissions for adults with cerebral palsy: a retrospective study. Dev Med Child Neurol. 2020;62(8):939–45.
16. Young NL, Rochon TG, McCormick A, Law M, Wedge JH, Fehlings D. The health and quality of life outcomes among youth and young adults with cerebral palsy. Arch Phys Med Rehabil. 2010;91(1):143–8.
17. Tan SS, van Meeteren J, Ketelaar M, Schuengel C, Reinders-Messelink HA, Raat H, et al. Long-term trajectories of health-related quality of life in individuals with cerebral palsy: a multicenter longitudinal study. Arch Phys Med Rehabil. 2014;95(11):2029–39.
18. Morgan PE, Soh SE, McGinley JL. Health-related quality of life of ambulant adults with cerebral palsy and its association with falls and mobility decline: a preliminary cross sectional study. Health Qual Life Outcomes. 2014;12:132.
19. Jovanović M, Lakićević M, Stevanović D, Milić-Rasić V, Slavnić S. Community-based study of health-related quality of life in spinal cord injury, muscular dystrophy, multiple sclerosis, and cerebral palsy. Disabil Rehabil. 2012;34(15):1284–90.
20. Usuba K, et al. Changes in gross motor function and health-related quality of life in adults with cerebral palsy: an 8-year follow-up study. Arch Phys Med Rehabil. 2014;95(11):2071–7. e1.
21. Morgan P, McGinley J. Gait function and decline in adults with cerebral palsy: a systematic review. Disabil Rehabil. 2014;36(1):1–9.
22. Tarsuslu T, Livanelioglu A. Relationship between quality of life and functional status of young adults and adults with cerebral palsy. Disabil Rehabil. 2010;32(20):1658–65.
23. Groff DG, Lundberg NR, Zabriskie RB. Influence of adapted sport on quality of life: perceptions

of athletes with cerebral palsy. Disabil Rehabil. 2009;31(4):318–26.
24. Roebroeck ME, Jahnsen R, Carona C, Kent RM, Chamberlain MA. Adult outcomes and lifespan issues for people with childhood-onset physical disability. Dev Med Child Neurol. 2009;51(8):670–8.
25. Hergenroder H, Blank R. Subjective Well-being and satisfaction with life in adults with spastic cerebral palsy: a pilot study of a randomized sample. Dev Med Child Neurol. 2009;51(5):389–96.
26. Young NL. The transition to adulthood for children with cerebral palsy: what do we know about their health care needs? J Pediatr Orthop. 2007;27(4):476–9.
27. Cassidy C, Campbell N, Madady M, Payne M. Bridging the gap: the role of physiatrists in caring for adults with cerebral palsy. Disabil Rehabil. 2016;38(5):493–8.
28. Kibele A. Occupational therapy's role in improving the quality of life for persons with cerebral palsy. Am J Occup Ther. 1989;43(6):371–7.
29. Orlin MN, Cicirello NA, O'Donnell AE, Doty AK. The continuum of care for individuals with lifelong disabilities: role of the physical therapist. Phys Ther. 2014;94(7):1043–53.
30. Schor NF. Life at the interface: adults with "pediatric" disorders of the nervous system. Ann Neurol. 2013;74(2):158–63.
31. Young NL, Barden WS, Mills WA, Burke TA, Law M, Boydell K. Transition to adult-oriented health care: perspectives of youth and adults with complex physical disabilities. Phys Occup Ther Pediatr. 2009;29(4):345–61.
32. Merrick H, McConachie H, LeCouteur A, Mann K, Parr JR, Pearce MS, et al. Characteristics of young people with long term conditions close to transfer to adult health services. BMC Health Serv Res. 2015;15:435.
33. Linroth R. Meeting the needs of young people and adults with childhood-onset conditions: Gillette lifetime specialty healthcare. Dev Med Child Neurol. 2009;51(Suppl 4):174–7.
34. Tsybina I, Kingsnorth S, Maxwell J, Bayley M, Lindsay S, McKeever P, et al. Longitudinal evaluation of transition services ("LETS study"): protocol for outcome evaluation. BMC Pediatr. 2012;12:51.
35. Watson R, Parr JR, Joyce C, May C, LeCouteur AS. Models of transitional care for young people with complex health needs: a scoping review. Child Care Health Dev. 2011;37(6):780–91.
36. Colver AF, Merrick H, Deverill M, LeCouteur A, Parr J, Pearce MS, et al. Study protocol: longitudinal study of the transition of young people with complex health needs from child to adult health services. BMC Public Health. 2013;13:675.
37. Binks JA, Barden WS, Burke TA, Young NL. What do we really know about the transition to adult-centered health care? A focus on cerebral palsy and spina bifida. Arch Phys Med Rehabil. 2007;88(8):1064–73.
38. Larivière-Bastien D, Bell E, Majnemer A, Shevell M, Racine E. Perspectives of young adults with cerebral palsy on transitioning from pediatric to adult healthcare systems. Semin Pediatr Neurol. 2013;20(2):154–9.
39. Blackman JA, Conaway MR. Adolescents with cerebral palsy: transitioning to adult health care services. Clin Pediatr (Phila). 2014;53(4):356–63.
40. Moll LR, Cott CA. The paradox of normalization through rehabilitation: growing up and growing older with cerebral palsy. Disabil Rehabil. 2013;35(15):1276–83.
41. Donkervoort M, Wiegerink DJHG, van Meeteren J, Stam HJ, Roebroeck ME, Transition Research Group South West Netherlands. Transition to adulthood: validation of the Rotterdam transition profile for young adults with cerebral palsy and normal intelligence. Dev Med Child Neurol. 2009;51(1):53–62.
42. Björquist E, Nordmark E, Hallstrom I. Parents' experiences of health and needs when supporting their adolescents with cerebral palsy during transition to adulthood. Phys Occup Ther Pediatr. 2016;36(2):204–16.
43. Maggs J, Palisano R, Chiarello L, Orlin M, Chang H-J, Polansky M. Comparing the priorities of parents and young people with cerebral palsy. Disabil Rehabil. 2011;33(17–18):1650–8.
44. Andersson C, Mattsson E. Adults with cerebral palsy: a survey describing problems, needs, and resources, with special emphasis on locomotion. Dev Med Child Neurol. 2001;43(2):76–82.
45. Frisch D, Msall ME. Health, functioning, and participation of adolescents and adults with cerebral palsy: a review of outcomes research. Dev Disabil Res Rev. 2013;18(1):84–94.
46. Bottos M, Feliciangeli A, Sciuto L, Gericke C, Vianello A. Functional status of adults with cerebral palsy and implications for treatment of children. Dev Med Child Neurol. 2001;43(8):516–28.
47. Jonsson U, Eek MN, Suunerhagen KS, Himmelmann K. Changes in walking ability, intellectual disability, and epilepsy in adults with cerebral palsy over 50 years: a population-based follow-up study. Dev Med Child Neurol. 2021;63(7):839–45.
48. Tosi LL, Maher N, Moore DW, Goldstein M, Aisen ML. Adults with cerebral palsy: a workshop to define the challenges of treating and preventing secondary musculoskeletal and neuromuscular complications in this rapidly growing population. Dev Med Child Neurol. 2009;51(Suppl 4):2–11.
49. Chui HC, Ada L, Chen C. Changes in walking performance between childhood and adulthood in cerebral palsy: a systematic review. Dev Neurorehabil. 2020;23(6):343–8.
50. Nair KP, Marsden J. The management of spasticity in adults. BMJ. 2014;349:g4737.

51. Charles PD, Gill CE, Taylor HM, Putman MS, Blair CR, Roberts AG, et al. Spasticity treatment facilitates direct care delivery for adults with profound intellectual disability. Mov Disord. 2010;25(4):466–73.
52. Bragg DC, Sharma N. Update on treatments for dystonia. Curr Neurol Neurosci Rep. 2014;14(6):454.
53. Grunt S, Becher JG, Vermeulen RJ. Long-term outcome and adverse effects of selective dorsal rhizotomy in children with cerebral palsy: a systematic review. Dev Med Child Neurol. 2011;53(6):490–8.
54. Hasnat MJ, Rice JE. Intrathecal baclofen for treating spasticity in children with cerebral palsy. Cochrane Database Syst Rev. 2015;11:CD004552.
55. Bonouvrié LA, Becher JG, Vles JS, Vermeulen RJ, Buizer AI, IDYS Study Group. The effect of intrathecal baclofen in dyskinetic cerebral palsy: the IDYS trial. Ann Neurol. 2019;86(1):79–90.
56. Burns F, Stewart R, Reddihough D, Scheinberg A, Ooi K, Graham HK. The cerebral palsy transition clinic: administrative chore, clinical responsibility, or opportunity for audit and clinical research? J Child Orthop. 2014;8(3):203–13.
57. Hägglund G, Pettersson K, Czuba T, Persson-Bunke M, Rodby-Bousquet E. Incidence of scoliosis in cerebral palsy. Acta Orthop. 2018;89(4):443–7.
58. Hung CW, Matsumoto H, Ball JR, Plachta S, Dutkowsky JP, Kim H, et al. Symptomatic cervical spinal stenosis in spastic cerebral palsy. Dev Med Child Neurol. 2020;62(10):1147–53.
59. French ZP, Torres RV, Whitney DG. Elevated prevalence of osteoarthritis among adults with cerebral palsy. Rehabil Med. 2019;51(8):575–81.
60. Jaffe JS, Timell AM. Prevalence of low bone density in institutionalized men with developmental disabilities. J Clin Densitom. 2003;6(2):143–7.
61. Smeltzer SC, Zimmerman VL. Usefulness of the SCORE index as a predictor of osteoporosis in women with disabilities. Orthop Nurs. 2005;24(1):33–9.
62. Sheridan KJ. Osteoporosis in adults with cerebral palsy. Dev Med Child Neurol. 2009;51(Suppl 4):38–51.
63. Henderson RC, Lark RK, Kecskemethy HH, Miller F, Harcke HT, Bachrach SJ. Bisphosphonates to treat osteopenia in children with quadriplegic cerebral palsy: a randomized, placebo-controlled clinical trial. J Pediatr. 2002;141(5):644–51.
64. Allington N, Vivegnis D, Gerard P. Cyclic administration of pamidronate to treat osteoporosis in children with cerebral palsy or a neuromuscular disorder: a clinical study. Acta Orthop Belg. 2005;71(1):91–7.
65. Batch JA, Couper JJ, Cowell CT, Zacharin M. Use of bisphosphonate therapy for osteoporosis in childhood and adolescence. J Paediatr Child Health. 2003;39(2):88–92.
66. Grissom LE, Kecskemethy HH, Bachrach SJ, McKay C, Harcke HT. Bone densitometry in pediatric patients treated with pamidronate. Pediatr Radiol. 2005;35(5):511–7.
67. Plotkin H, Coughliin S, Kreikemeier R, Heldt K, Bruzoni M, Lerner G. Low doses of pamidronate to treat osteopenia in children with severe cerebral palsy: a pilot study. Dev Med Child Neurol. 2006;48(9):709–12.
68. Vogtle LK. Pain in adults with cerebral palsy: impact and solutions. Dev Med Child Neurol. 2009;51(Suppl 4):113–21.
69. Schwartz L, Engel JM, Jensen MP. Pain in persons with cerebral palsy. Arch Phys Med Rehabil. 1999;80(10):1243–6.
70. Engel JM, Jensen MP, Hoffman AJ, Kartin D. Pain in persons with cerebral palsy: extension and cross validation. Arch Phys Med Rehabil. 2003;84(8):1125–8.
71. Pohl JF, Cantrell A. Gastrointestinal and nutritional issues in cerebral palsy. Pract Gastroenterol. 2006;30(6):14–22.
72. Sood MR, Rudolph CD. Gastroesophageal reflux in adolescents. Adolesc Med Clin. 2004;15(1):17–36, vii–viii.
73. Park ES, Park CI, Cho S-R, Na S-I, Cho YS. Colonic transit time and constipation in children with spastic cerebral palsy. Arch Phys Med Rehabil. 2004;85(3):453–6.
74. Agnarsson U, Warde C, Clayden GS, Evans S. Anorectal function of children with neurological problems. II: cerebral palsy. Dev Med Child Neurol. 1993;35(10):903–8.
75. Green LGG, Hurwitz E. Primary care of children with cerebral palsy. Clin Fam Pract. 2003;5:467.
76. Brown MC, Marciniak CH, Garrett AM, Gaebler-Spira DJ. Diet quality in adults with cerebral palsy: a modifiable risk factor for cardiovascular disease prevention. Dev Med Child Neurol. 2021;63(10):1221–8.
77. Yildiz N, Akkoç Y, Ersöz M, Gündüz B, Erhan B, Yesil H, et al. Cross-sectional study of urinary problems in adults with cerebral palsy: awareness and impact on the quality of life. Neurol Sci. 2017;38(7):1193–203.
78. Cotter KJ, Levy ME, Goldfarb RA, Liberman D, Katorski J, Myers JB, et al. Urodynamic findings in adults with moderate to severe cerebral palsy. Urology. 2016;95:216–21.
79. Murphy KP, Boutin SA, Ide KR. Cerebral palsy, neurogenic bladder, and outcomes of lifetime care. Dev Med Child Neurol. 2012;54(10):945–50.
80. Goldfarb RA, Pisansky A, Fleck J, Hoversten P, Cotter KJ, Katorski J, et al. Neurogenic lower urinary tract dysfunction in adults with cerebral palsy: outcomes following a conservative management approach. J Urol. 2016;195(4Pt1):1009–13.
81. Murphy KP, Molnar GE, Lankasky K. Medical and functional status of adults with cerebral palsy. Dev Med Child Neurol. 1995;37(12):1075–84.
82. Grigoryan L, Trautner BW, Gupta K. Diagnosis and management of urinary tract infections in the outpatient setting: a review. JAMA. 2014;312(16):1677–84.

83. Heydarian S, Abbasadabi MM, Khabazkhoob M, Hoseini-Yazdi H, Gharib M. Vision abnormalities in children and young adults with cerebral palsy: a systematic review. Semin Opthalmol. 2022;37(4):471–9.
84. Schölderle T, Staiger A, Lampe R, Strecker K, Ziegler W. Dysarthria in adults with cerebral palsy: clinical presentation and impacts on communication. J Speech Lang Hear Res. 2016;59(2):216–28.
85. Peterson MD, Lin P, Kamdar N, Hurvitz EA, Mahmoudi E. Psychological, cardiometabolic, and musculoskeletal morbidity and multimorbidity among adults with cerebral palsy and spina bifida: a retrospective cross-sectional study. Am J Phys Med Rehabil. 2021;100(10):940–5.
86. Hammam N, Becher H, Andersen J, Manns PJ, Whittaker JL, Pritchard L. Early indictors of cardiovascular disease are evident in children and adolescents with cerebral palsy. Disabil Health J. 2021;14(4):101–12.
87. Peterson MD, Lin P, Kamdar N, Mahmoudi E, Schmidt MM, Haapala JH, et al. Cardiometabolic morbidity in adults with cerebral palsy and spina bifida. Am J Med. 2020;133(12):e695–705.
88. Heyn PC. Prevalence of metabolic syndrome and cardiovascular disease risk factors in adults with cerebral palsy. Dev Med Child Neurol. 2019;61(4):477–83.
89. Wu CW. Risk of stroke among patients with cerebral palsy: a population based study. Dev Med Child Neurol. 2017;59(1):52–6.
90. Whitney DG. Polypharmacy among privately insured adults with cerebral palsy: a retrospective study. J Manag Care Spec Pharm. 2020;26(9):1153–61.
91. Whitney DG. Polypharmacy is a risk factor for mortality, severe chronic kidney disease, and liver disease among privately insured adults with cerebral palsy. J Manag Care Spec Pharm. 2021;27(1):51–63.
92. Livingston MH, Rosenbaum PL, Russell DJ, Palisano RJ. Quality of life among adolescents with cerebral palsy: what does the literature tell us? Dev Med Child Neurol. 2007;49(3):225–31.
93. Donkervoort M, et al. Determinants of functioning of adolescents and young adults with cerebral palsy. Disabil Rehabil. 2007;29(6):453–63.
94. Van der Slot WM, Nieuwenhuijsen C, van den Berg-Emons RJG, Wensink-Boonstra AE, Stam HJ, Roebroeck ME, et al. Participation and health-related quality of life in adults with spastic bilateral cerebral palsy and the role of self-efficacy. J Rehabil Med. 2010;42(6):528–35.
95. Balandin S, Berg N, Waller A. Assessing the loneliness of older people with cerebral palsy. Disabil Rehabil. 2006;28(8):469–79.
96. Boucher N, Dumas F, Maltais DB, Richards CL. The influence of selected personal and environmental factors on leisure activities in adults with cerebral palsy. Disabil Rehabil. 2010;32(16):1328–38.
97. Peterson MD, Lin P, Kamdar N, Mahmoudi E, Marsack-Topolewski CN, Haapala H, et al. Psychological morbidity among adults with cerebral palsy and spina bifida. Psychol Med. 2021;51(4):694–701.
98. Smith KJ, Peterson MD, O'Connell NE, Victor C, Liverani S, Anokye N, et al. Risk of depression and anxiety in adults with cerebral palsy. JAMA Neurol. 2019;76(3):294–300.
99. Gray SH, Wylie M, Christensen S, Khan A, Williams D, Glader L. Puberty and menarche in young females with cerebral palsy and intellectually disability: a quantitative study of caregivers' experiences. Dev Med Child Neurol. 2021;63(2):190–5.
100. Hayward K, Chen AY, Forbes E, Byrne R, Greenberg MB, Fowler EG. Reproductive healthcare experiences of women with cerebral palsy. Diabil Health J. 2017;10(3):413–8.
101. Wiegerink DJ, Stam HJ, Ketelaar M, Coehn-Kettenis PT, Roebroeck ME. Personal and environmental factors contributing to participation in romantic relationships and sexual activity of young adults with cerebral palsy. Disabil Rehabil. 2012;34(17):1481–7.
102. Wiegerink DJ, Stam HJ, Gorter JW, Cohen-Kettenis PT, Roebroeck ME, Transition Research Group Southwest Netherlands. Development of romantic relationships and sexual activity in young adults with cerebral palsy: a longitudinal study. Arch Phys Med Rehabil. 2010;91(9):1423–8.
103. Wiegerink DJ, Roebroeck ME, van der Slot WM, Stam HJ, Cohen-Kettenis PT, Transition Research Group South West Netherlands. Importance of peers and dating in the development of romantic relationships and sexual activity of young adults with cerebral palsy. Dev Med Child Neurol. 2010;52(6):576–82.
104. Wiegerink D, Roebroeck M, Bender J, Stam H, Cohen-Kettenis, Transition Research Group South West Netherlands. Sexuality of Young adults with cerebral palsy: experienced limitations and needs. Sex Disabil. 2011;29(2):119–28.
105. Chiang K-L, Huang C-Y, Fan H-C, Kuo F-C. Prolonged length of stay for acute hospital admissions as the increasing of age: a nationwide population study for Taiwan's patients with cerebral palsy. Pediatr Neonatol. 2019;60(1):74–82.
106. Hemsley B, Balandin S, Togher L. 'We need to be the centrepiece': adults with cerebral palsy and complex communication needs discuss the roles and needs of family carers in hospital. Disabil Rehabil. 2008;30(23):1759–71.
107. DiFazio R, Vessey JA, Miller P, Van Nostrand K, Snyder B. Postoperative complications after hip surgery in patients with cerebral palsy: a retrospective matched cohort study. J Pediatr Orthop. 2016;36(1):56–62.
108. Ailey SH, Johnson TJ, Fogg L, Friese TR. Factors related to complications among adult patients with intellectual disabilities hospitalized at an academic medical center. Intellect Dev Disabil. 2015;53(2):114–9.

109. Chidambaran V, Gentry C, Ajuba-Iwuji C, Sponsellar PD, Ain M, Lin E, et al. A retrospective identification of gastroesophageal reflux disease as a new risk factor for surgical site infection in cerebral palsy patients after spine surgery. Anesth Analg. 2013;117(1):162–8.
110. Giuglea C, Marinescu S, Florescu IP, Jecan. Pressure sores—a constant problem for plegic patients and a permanent challenge for plastic surgery. J Med Life. 2010;3(2):149–53.
111. National Pressure Ulcer Advisory Panel, European Pressure Ulcer Advisory Panel, and Pan Pacific Pressure Injury Alliance. Prevention and treatment of pressure ulcers: quick reference guide. In: Haesler E, editor. Osborne Park, Australia: Cambridge Media; 2014.
112. Bass MJ, Phillips LG. Pressure sores. Curr Probl Surg. 2007;44(2):101–43.

## Resources for Family with Cerebral Palsy

Centers for Independent Living. http://www.ilru.org/projects/cil-net/cil-center-and-association-directory.

The CP Group. A group for adults with cerebral palsy. http://thecpgroup.org/.

United Cerebral Palsy. www.ucp.org.

## Suggested Reading

Colver A, Fairhurst C, Pharoah PO. Cerebral palsy. Lancet. 2014;383(9924):1240–9.
Glew GM, Bennett FC. Cerebral palsy grown up. J Dev Behav Pediatr. 2011;32(6):469–75.

# Childhood and Adolescent Cancer Survivors

# 26

Yannis K. Valtis, Linda S. Overholser, and Larissa Nekhlyudov

## Case Presentation

A 26-year-old woman presents for evaluation to establish care with a new gynecologist and for an annual well-woman exam. She reports that she was previously diagnosed with Hodgkin lymphoma (HL). She is unsure of all the details of her history but recalls where she received part of her treatment; some of her prior clinical visit notes are available through the electronic medical record. At 14 years of age, she presented with fatigue and difficulty keeping up with her peers on her school track team. On evaluation, she was found to have enlarged lymph nodes of the right supraclavicular fossa. A biopsy revealed nodular sclerosing HL. Imaging studies found bulky mediastinal and supraclavicular lymphadenopathy. Records indicate that she was treated with doxorubicin, bleomycin, vinblastine, and dacarbazine (ABVD) chemotherapy over the course of 5 months in 2010, which consisted of doxorubicin (total dose 200 mg/m$^2$), bleomycin (80 IU/m$^2$), vinblastine (32 mg/m$^2$), and dacarbazine (3000 mg/m$^2$) as well as mantle chest radiation at a dose of 21 Gy. On follow-up evaluation 12 months later, she was found to have a relapse. She received an autologous stem cell transplant and received a myeloablative conditioning regimen with carmustine, etoposide, cytarabine, and melphalan. Since that time, she has been disease-free.

At the time of the visit, she had no specific medical concerns. She reports having regular menstrual cycles at the time she was diagnosed and then stopped having menses during treatment. Since treatment, she has had irregular menses, currently managed on oral contraceptives. She also has intermittent headaches for which she takes an occasional ibuprofen. She has received appropriate post-transplant immunizations, including *Haemophilus influenzae b*, hepatitis A and B, DTaP, influenza, meningococcal, pneumococcal, and inactivated polio vaccines.

During her treatment, her mother drove her to the Boston area from Maine, where she lived at the time. She was often away from her friends and school. She has two sisters, who are 4 and 6 years older. They lived at home with their father during her treatment. After treatment was completed, she returned to school and was able to resume her studies with no difficulties but struggled in social situations. While her sisters and

Y. K. Valtis
Department of Medicine, Memorial Sloan Kettering Cancer Center, New York, NY, USA
e-mail: kalogii@mskcc.org

L. S. Overholser (✉)
Division of General Internal Medicine, University of Colorado Anschutz Medical Campus, Aurora, CO, USA
e-mail: linda.overholser@cuanschutz.edu

L. Nekhlyudov
Department of Medicine, Brigham and Women's Hospital, Boston, MA, USA
e-mail: lnekhlyudov@partners.org


A. A. Kuo et al. (eds.), *Care of Adults with Chronic Childhood Conditions*,
https://doi.org/10.1007/978-3-031-54281-7_26

friends understood her illness, she felt that they were somewhat distant. She became very self-conscious about her appearance and the changes her body had been through. She avoided social situations and developed anxiety about dating. She began using alcohol around age 17 to help her cope. At this time, psychological counseling was suggested and was thought to have been helpful. She began focusing on artwork, finding this to be a great way for her to express herself and her emotions.

She has not been followed in oncology for about 10 years as she has found it to be quite difficult to travel to Boston to continue to receive follow-up care there. She is currently working as a receptionist in a gym in Maine after having completed 2 years in a community college and then transferring to a university to complete her bachelor's degree. She is single and still experiences binge drinking behavior mostly on weekends. She does not smoke but does vape tobacco products. She also uses marijuana recreationally but does not use any other drugs. She is planning to move to New York City, where one of her sisters has moved, to pursue art or fashion design. She plans to find a job there after she relocates and to live temporarily with her sister.

At her mother's request, she presents for this initial gynecological evaluation just to "make sure all is okay" before she relocates. She is not sure what she is going to do about her health insurance once she moves; her current insurance plan is a high-deductible health plan. She is unsure if she will remain on her parents' health insurance plan once she moves.

Review of systems reveals no additional concerns. There is no family history of malignancy, though the family history is notable for diabetes mellitus and hypertension on her maternal side.

On physical examination, she is a well-appearing woman in no acute distress. Her height is 5 ft 3 in., and her body mass index (BMI) is 27 kg/m$^2$. Examination of her head, eyes, ears, nose, and throat is normal. Her neck is supple with no palpable thyromegaly, thyroid masses, nor lymphadenopathy. Heart rhythm is regular, with no murmurs, and carotid arteries are without bruits. Her lungs are clear to auscultation. Her abdomen is soft and nondistended with no palpable masses nor hepatosplenomegaly. Extremities are without edema, and she has normal distal pulses. Neurological examination is unremarkable with a normal sensory and motor exam. She completed a screening psychosocial instrument that suggests depression and anxiety. Her breast examination is unremarkable though her breast tissue is dense. Gynecological examination is unremarkable and a Papanicolaou test to screen for cervical cancer is performed without complication.

Laboratory evaluation reveals normal blood count, serum creatinine, and electrolytes, with a borderline elevation of serum glucose and total cholesterol level. Her thyroid-stimulating hormone (TSH) level is slightly elevated.

## Case Discussion

This patient is a long-term survivor of childhood/adolescent cancer, treated with multiagent chemotherapy, chest radiation, and an autologous stem cell transplant. She has presented to a gynecologist for her well woman examination and does not have a regular primary care provider for other medical issues. This evaluation should allow for an initial discussion of survivorship care planning (including a possible consultation with a specialized clinic) and the importance of long-term follow-up and health promotion as well as the importance of establishing care with an adult primary care provider, setting the stage for risk-based care. Because treatment information is available for review, some recommendations can already be made.

In this chapter, a few of the more prevalent conditions that may be identified and are relevant to the presented case are discussed. This chapter is not meant to be inclusive of all potential chronic medical conditions among adult survivors of childhood cancer. Further, the field of cancer survivorship continues to evolve as new data emerges. We provide resources that clinicians will be able to use for future reference as survivorship research advances. A most valuable resource is the North American based Children's Oncology Group

*Long-term Follow-up Guidelines for Survivors of Childhood, Adolescent, and Young Adult Cancers* (COG LTFU Guidelines), found online at www.survivorshipguidelines.org [1]. This set of recommendations reviews potential late effects as organized by treatment exposure, such as chemotherapy and radiation. Similar clinical guidance recommendations have been developed in many other countries. In 2010, the International Late Effects of Childhood Cancer Guideline Harmonization Group was developed in order to help align clinical guidance for surveillance of late and long-term effects across national and international groups [2]. The use of these guidelines is further described in the following sections.

## Risk of and Surveillance for Recurrence of Primary Cancer

The patient is close to 12 years post-diagnosis and 11 years from completion of therapy. Her risk of recurrence of HL at this time is low. Though there are no current specific recommendations for surveillance of HL and her current risk for recurrence is low, she is advised to continue to be vigilant and report any new or unusual symptoms to a healthcare provider.

## Management and Surveillance for Late Effects of Therapy

Some of the more prominent late effects of her chemotherapy will first be considered. Her regimen included doxorubicin, which is an anthracycline chemotherapeutic agent and as such is associated with cardiomyopathy. This is an example of a *late effect*, a medical condition that develops some time after the original exposure. Based on current COG LTFU guidelines, given the age of the patient and dose of her exposure (200 mg/m$^2$) in combination with mantle chest radiation, echocardiograms every 2 years would be recommended. A stress test may also be obtained if she endorses new cardiovascular symptoms such as shortness of breath or chest pain with exertion. Physical examination should include listening for carotid bruits and carotid ultrasound 10 years after treatment completion could be considered because of her exposure to radiation therapy with potential exposure to the neck area. Close monitoring is also recommended during pregnancy, as will be discussed later in this chapter. Her regimen also included vinblastine, a vinca plant alkaloid, which may be associated with peripheral motor or sensory neuropathy, though not likely to develop at this time as this is more typically a *long-term effect*, a medical condition that arises at the time of treatment exposure and persists over time. Bleomycin is an anti-tumor antibiotic that can cause acute pulmonary toxicity but can also lead to pulmonary late effects, including pulmonary fibrosis.

As she has received mantle radiation and does not have documented pulmonary function tests (PFTs) on record, baseline PFTs should be obtained. Otherwise, she should be assessed regularly for any new pulmonary symptoms. Dacarbazine (less likely), melphalan, and carmustine are alkylating agents, which can lead to several important late effects, including ovarian function suppression. In this patient who was already menstruating at the time of treatment, secondary amenorrhea could occur. Though menstrual cycles resumed after treatment, an important late effect would be an increased risk for premature ovarian failure and reduced window for fertility. The development of premature ovarian failure would increase this patient's risks for important metabolic and/or physical side effects such as osteoporosis, dyslipidemia, cardiovascular disease, and sexual dysfunction. As she is of childbearing age and fertility may partially recover over time, it is imperative to understand this patient's preferences for childbearing. To address these risks proactively, ongoing monitoring and referral to reproductive endocrinology is recommended. Alkylating agents can also increase the risk for secondary acute myeloid leukemia and myelodysplasia, typically for up to 10 years after exposure. During that time, patients should undergo periodic evaluation to assess for fatigue as well as easy bruising or bleeding, with a complete blood count if clinically indicated. Given that she is beyond the 10-year high-risk period, no routine testing would be recommended. High doses of cytarabine could lead to neurocognitive deficits; a referral for neuropsychological evaluation could be considered if concerns are expressed.

Radiation therapy is associated with a number of potential late effects including subsequent malignancies in the area of radiation involving the skin, subcutaneous tissue, and organs. As such, she is at risk for skin cancer as well as precancerous skin lesions and should be monitored for this as well as advised to take precautions such as using sunscreen diligently. Despite her young age, she is at significantly elevated risk for breast cancer and should begin high-risk screening for breast cancer, which includes mammography and breast MRI as she is already past due the currently recommended timeline to begin that screening (age 25 or 8 years after exposure to radiation therapy, whichever occurs last). Additionally, she is at increased risk for thyroid diseases, including hypothyroidism, thyroid nodules and thyroid cancer. She should have a neck examination as part of her yearly physical and if any thyroid abnormalities are noted, she should be referred for an ultrasound. A consultation with an endocrinologist could be considered. She is also at increased risk for lung cancer and screening may be considered (especially given her smoking history). The patient should also be counseled to have routine influenza and COVID-19 vaccinations.

## Psychosocial Concerns

The patient has endorsed a number of concerns with family and social functioning since her diagnosis and treatment. She has been to therapy in the past and is currently still having depressive symptoms and anxiety. These are common in young adult survivors of cancer and should be recognized and closely monitored. She may benefit from referral to a mental health provider to help with strategies for self-management and coping, and medication management if deemed appropriate. Since she is moving to a new city, she might be at risk for worsening of functioning in the absence of a support network other than her sister. She may benefit from connecting with others who have experienced cancer at an early age, perhaps at a local cancer center or through online resources.

## Health Promotion

This case illustrates important opportunities for health promotion and counseling regarding health behaviors. Her cardiovascular risk factors, including use of tobacco products, should be rigorously managed. Though she is not currently in a relationship, she is unsure of her fertility status, and she should not consider herself infertile based on her irregular menstrual cycles alone. Though the individual in this case presentation is taking oral contraceptives, if she were not then she should have counseling and take precautions to avoid pregnancy if she is sexually active with a male partner until her fertility status is confirmed in order to avoid unintended pregnancy.

She has developed some concerning health behaviors as a way to cope with her stress and would benefit from regular assessment and counseling regarding these health behaviors. Priority should be given to vaping cessation, and referral to a tobacco cessation specialist may be helpful. Smoking is a known risk factor for comorbid medical conditions that cause the highest rates of morbidity and mortality in the childhood cancer survivor population: cardiovascular disease, pulmonary disease, and second primary cancers. She should be counseled about the health effects of alcohol and the risks of binge drinking; referral to alcohol use support groups can be considered. Finally, she should be encouraged to engage in regular physical activity and exercise as well as adhere to a healthy diet and to maintain a healthy weight. Having a regular source of primary care can be especially important in this aspect of her follow-up care. Guidelines for physical activity and nutrition in cancer survivors are available and have been recently updated [3], but evidence shows that childhood cancer survivors are not faring any better than the general population at following these guidelines [4].

Under the Affordable Care Act, she can remain on her parents' insurance until the age of 26 years in the United States. She should be sure to get appropriate information from her parents or from another trusted resource in the practice or in the community such as a social worker or a patient navigator once she gets established with her new provider.

## Overview

### Definition and Epidemiology of Childhood Cancers

Childhood and adolescent cancer is defined as any malignancy diagnosed before the age of 20 and treated with cancer therapy [5]. The number of survivors of pediatric cancers in the United States (USA) and worldwide has grown significantly over the past half-century, largely due to the development of increasingly effective treatment modalities and protocols. Surveillance, epidemiology, and end results (SEER) data show that patients diagnosed before age 20 now have a 5-year (5-year) survival rate of more than 85% in contrast to only 50% just 35 years ago [6]. Acute lymphoblastic leukemia (ALL), the most common childhood malignancy, has seen a staggering improvement in 5-year survival rates from only 11.1% in the 1960s to 91.1% in the 2000s [7]. This improved survival has translated into more than 380,000 childhood and adolescent cancer survivors living in the USA as of January 1, 2010 [8]. With the improved survival in this population as well as the increasing complexity of treatment regimens has come a growing recognition of treatment-related late effects. These late effects confer an increased rate of mortality as well as morbidity in the form of chronic health conditions [9].

The National Academy of Medicine (formerly the Institute of Medicine (IOM)) considers childhood cancer according to 12 different categories. They are, leukemias, central nervous system tumors, lymphomas, carcinomas/malignant epithelial neoplasms, germ cell/gonadal neoplasms, soft tissue sarcomas, malignant bone tumors, sympathetic nervous system tumors, renal tumors, retinoblastoma, hepatic tumors, and, last, other unspecified cancers. The characteristics of each of these cancer types are described further in the IOM report "Childhood Cancer Survivorship: Improving Care and Quality of Life" [10]. Cancer therapy may include chemotherapy, radiation therapy, surgery, and bone marrow transplant. Immunotherapies and cell-based therapies, like chimeric antigen receptor T-cell (CAR-T), are increasingly used for certain pediatric malignancies. The spectrum of cancer therapy also includes blood products, supportive medication for side effects, as well as anti-infective and marrow-stimulating medications. While cancer therapies halt the progression of cancer, among those who survive cancer, chronic medical conditions arise due to late and long-term effects of such therapies. Additionally, cancer survivors are at risk for relapse of the original malignancy as well as development of second primary neoplasms related to their treatment or to their underlying genetic risk.

### Pathophysiology of Chronic Conditions Among Cancer Survivors

In considering the varied therapies that a cancer patient might receive, the associated late and long-term effects that an individual patient may experience are largely related to a "field" effect. This means that any tissue (such as skin, subcutaneous tissue, and underlying organs), whether normal or cancerous, exposed to therapy is at highest risk for late effects. Host factors such as the age of exposure, gender, pubertal status, family history of illness, or current health behaviors may affect the presentation and/or severity of a late effect. Cytotoxic chemotherapy is intended to kill cancer cells; its systemic administration often leads to effects on normal cells as well. Some classic examples include cardiomyocyte damage due to anthracyclines such as doxorubicin, peripheral neuropathy from platinum-based therapies, and gastroenteritis at the time of chemotherapy administration [11–16]. Radiotherapy is generally directed to cancerous tissue; still, even with advances in radiotherapy modeling, surrounding normal tissue often receives high doses of radiation through scatter, leading to inflammation, fibrosis, and/or tissue destruction [9]. Hormonal therapies are used frequently with hormone-sensitive cancers such as breast cancer. This treatment modality is much less commonly used in pediatric cancers, noting that when they are, hormone therapies can lead to disruptions of the endocrine system [4]. Surgical resection of cancer can lead to localized and surrounding anatomical disruption of normal structure and scarring. For example, in a patient with resection of brain cancer, there can be significant residual neurological complications. For a patient with significant lymphatic and bone resection for a pelvic sarcoma can be associated with lymphedema and musculoskeletal pain, loss of motion, or other abnormalities [4]. Targeted therapies, like immunotherapies, were largely created to minimize systemic effects; still, some of the targeted pathways are nonspecific. For example, therapy targeting vascular endothelial growth factor (VEGF) receptors on cancer cells can have the additional effect of inducing thrombosis in normal vessels [17]. Late and long-term effects of these newer regimens are still unknown. Many of these cumulative late and long-term effects associated with cancer treatment have been likened to a process of accelerated aging; proposed mechanisms include cellular senescence, telomere shortening, hematopoietic stem cell stresses, damage to DNA, and epigenetic modifications as a result of treatment [18].

## Common Chronic Adult Conditions in This Population

Over the past three decades, several cohort studies, such as the Childhood Cancer Survivor Study (CCSS) [19], the St. Jude's Lifetime cohort study [20], and the British Columbia cohort [21], as well as many European cohorts [22], have provided instrumental information about the effects of cancer treatment on the development of chronic conditions among adult survivors of childhood cancer. This forms the basis for much of what we have learned about long-term survivorship in this population.

Childhood cancer survivors are at risk for premature morbidity as adults compared to sibling controls without a history of cancer [23, 24]. The rate of increase in the prevalence of adverse health status, activity limitations, and functional impairment appears to be accelerated over time compared to sibling controls as well [25]. It has been estimated that by 45 years of age, 95% of childhood cancer survivors have at least one chronic health condition, and 80% have a condition described as serious or life-threatening [26]. While the risk of primary cancer recurrence decreases as children and adolescents age, their risk for other medical morbidities outpaces their peers without a history of cancer. Examples of such conditions include important endocrine, cardiac, pulmonary, and neurocognitive conditions discussed in this section [27–31]. In addition to medical morbidity, individuals with a history of childhood cancer are considered to have higher risks of premature death, with the most likely causes being from secondary cancers as well as cardiac and pulmonary conditions [32–35]. Studies in this population indicate that survivors are 3.3 times more likely than their siblings without cancer to have any chronic condition and 8.2 times more likely to have a severe condition. Initial long-term follow-up studies suggest that this disparity in health risks persists as individuals age [36] and have also prompted changes to treatment regimens in an effort to reduce this significant late morbidity. Recent observational studies from the CCSS suggest that the cumulative incidence of health outcomes rated as severe, disabling, life-threatening, or fatal has improved over time for those individuals treated from 1990 to 1999 compared to those treated between 1970 and 1979 [37] though still remains higher than sibling controls. Likewise, the gap in life expectancy for childhood cancer survivors has improved over time for individuals treated during the same three decades from 1970 to 1999, particularly for those individuals treated only with chemotherapy and with no exposure to radiation therapy [38].

## Endocrine Concerns

Endocrinopathies occurring as late and long-term effects of childhood cancer are prevalent and varied. Effects on various hormonally active organs can be related to direct effects, for example direct tumor invasion or surgery, radiation directly to the affected organ systems (i.e., pituitary or thyroid gland), or chemotherapeutic agents. Thyroid hormone derangements, growth hormone (GH) deficiency, and risks for premature menopause are examples. A discussion of the endocrine late effects as it relates to fertility and reproduction follows in the "Special Issues in Adolescent and Young Adult Transition" section appearing later in this chapter. Bone health of cancer survivors is discussed in the "Orthopedic Issues" section. Long-term follow-up studies in this population to date indicate that radiation therapy exposure, including total body irradiation in preparation for bone marrow transplant, and alkylating agents appear to confer the highest risk for various endocrinopathies [39, 40].

In regard to disorders of the hypothalamic-pituitary axis (HPA), growth hormone (GH) deficiency, precocious puberty, and central hypothyroidism are the most prevalent. Cranial radiation therapy is considered to be the primary risk factor. Total dose of cranial radiation therapy and increasing time after exposure appear to be the most important pieces of information to consider when evaluating risk [41, 42]. Doses greater than 18 Gy confer risk for GH deficiency and central precocious puberty through dysregulation of luteinizing hormone (LH) and follicle-stimulating hormone (FSH) [43], while doses greater than 30 Gy also put the thyroid-stimulating hormone (TSH) and adrenocorticotropic hormone (ACTH) pathways at risk. GH deficiency is known to be associated with visceral adiposity, dyslipidemia, and reduced bone density and is important to recognize as a potential contributing risk factor for morbidity in adults [44]. The preponderance of evidence suggests that growth hormone replacement therapy is efficacious in cancer survivors with established growth hormone deficiency [45], but some observational studies have shown a small risk of solid neoplasms in survivors treated with GH [46]. Consultation with an endocrinologist would be prudent if such therapy is being considered.

Disorders of the thyroid gland are common in adults with a history of pediatric cancer. Radiation appears to be the major culprit, whether it is cranial irradiation resulting in central hypothyroidism or primary hypothyroidism related to direct effects on the thyroid gland. Tyrosine kinase inhibitor therapy, increasingly utilized for treatment of certain pediatric cancers, has also been associated with hypothyroidism [47]. As a late or long-term effect, primary hypothyroidism occurs more frequently than central hypothyroidism. The risk for hypothyroidism approaches 50% at 20 years of follow-up in individuals who were treated for Hodgkin lymphoma, where radiation to the neck and chest area are common modalities for treatment [48]. Risk does not appear to plateau over time. In addition to functional thyroid disorders, both thyroid nodules and thyroid cancer are seen more commonly in individuals with a history of treatment for childhood cancer. When completing an evaluation for thyroid disease in an adult with a history of radiation exposure to the head/neck area, thyroid function tests—including a free T4 level if central hypothyroidism is being considered—in addition to a careful neck exam yearly is recommended according to the Children's Oncology Group Long-Term Follow-Up (COG LTFU) Guidelines. While thyroid ultrasound should be considered in the workup of thyroid nodules, a prospective observational study of survivors of Hodgkin lymphoma suggested no benefit to routine ultrasound screening for thyroid cancer [49]. However, if the thyroid examination is limited (for example in an obese patient), an ultrasound may be considered.

The endocrine risks described previously may overlap with other late effects that serve as risk factors for the development of cardiovascular disease—a major cause of morbidity and mortality in the general adult population. For reasons that have not yet been fully elucidated, among individuals treated for cancer as children, the risk of being overweight or obese over time is most strongly correlated with treatment for ALL or brain tumors. Individuals with a history of childhood cancer were about twice as likely as their siblings without cancer to develop diabetes mellitus, even after adjustment for body mass index [50]. In a large study of 1713 adult survivors of childhood cancers, 48% were found to be obese; in 42% of those patients, the obesity was deemed attributable to cancer treatment [26]. Notably, survivors also developed diabetes at significantly younger ages than their sibling counterparts. In multivariate analysis, important risk factors included abdominal radiation therapy, total body radiation, treatment under the age of 5 years, physical inactivity, and BMI above 25 kg/m$^2$ [51]. A later study indicated that overall childhood cancer survivors were not more likely to be obese but were more likely over time to be taking medications for hypertension, dyslipidemia, or diabetes [52]. The prevalence of metabolic syndrome in small studies of adult survivors of childhood cancer ranges from 12.6 to 33% with 17–25 years of follow-up [53–55]. The COG LTFU Guidelines recommend that all patients treated with abdominal or total body irradiation undergo screening for diabetes (through fasting blood sugar or hemoglobin A1c) and hyperlipidemia (through lipid panel) every 2 years [56].

## Cardiovascular Concerns

Many long-term follow-up studies have now described the ongoing risks of cardiovascular disease related to childhood cancer treatment [57]. The risk of cardiovascular morbidity and mortality is significant.

A well-recognized late effect includes the development of cardiomyopathy related to anthracyclines. Anthracycline-associated cardiomyopathy as a late effect in childhood cancer survivors appears to be dose-related, and knowing the cumulative dose impacts the surveillance strategy. Concomitant therapy with chest irradiation can further increase the risk for cardiomyopathy as well as the risk of myocardial infarction, valvular heart disease, and pericardial disease [58]. A threshold for anthracycline exposure of 250 mg/m$^2$ increases risk for congestive heart failure, pericardial disease, and valvular heart disease [59]. Radiation exposure above 1500 cGy increases risk for each of the aforementioned cardiovascular outcomes. Risk factors for toxicity include younger age at exposure, higher cumulative doses of chemotherapy, and increasing time since exposure, which means that symptoms may develop years, sometimes decades, later [60]. Importantly, early identification and prompt treatment of cancer therapy-related heart failure can lead to substantial improvement or even normalization of ejection fraction [61]. Coronary artery disease is another serious complication. Survivors of childhood cancer have a greater than tenfold risk of ischemic heart disease compared to their siblings [9]. Atherosclerotic disease is not limited to diseases affecting the heart, and stroke could also be a consequence associated with childhood cancer treatment, with cranial and mantle radiation therapy being significant risk factors. The Childhood Cancer Survivor Study included 13,060 cancer survivors and 4023 siblings to establish risk factors for cardiovascular disease and led to the creation of a risk-prediction tool that incorporates age, prior chemo- and radiotherapy, and metabolic syndrome to assess the risk of individual cancer survivors [62]. This tool can be used to devise appropriate monitoring plans with echocardiograms and other modalities based on the risk of each patient. In general, patients who received high doses of anthracyclines (equivalent to 250 mg/m$^2$ of doxorubicin or more), those who received high doses of radiation (>30 Gy in an area affecting the heart), or those who received both anthracyclines and radiation should have an echocardiogram every 2 years and referral to a cardiologist should also be considered.

Childhood cancer survivors are also at risk for hypertension and hyperlipidemia, both of which can exacerbate coronary disease and cardiomyopathies. Survivors are 2.6 times more likely than the general population to develop hypertension, although no clear associations have been drawn between specific cancer therapies and hypertension development [63]. Survivors of stem cell transplantation are at high risk for hypercholesterolemia and hypertriglyceridemia with acute GVHD thought to be an independent risk factor [64]. Additionally, survivors of testicular cancer treated with chemotherapy and radiotherapy are at risk for lipid disorders and cardiovascular disease [65]. In consideration of the high prevalence of cardiovascular disease in the general population and evidence for further increases in risk among the childhood cancer survivors, a screening strategy for high blood pressure, diabetes, and lipid abnormalities in the childhood cancer survivor that is more aggressive compared to an individual of the same age without a history of cancer is indicated and could potentially lead to a reduction in the cardiovascular mortality currently seen.

Of note, pregnancy can exacerbate an underlying subclinical heart failure. It is recommended that women who have had abnormalities identified previously be closely monitored during pregnancy, and an echocardiogram during the third trimester and possibly postpartum may be considered. These women should be managed accordingly by a high-risk obstetric or maternal-fetal medicine specialist. Women with no prior abnormalities identified may have repeat testing done during a pregnancy at the discretion of the medical provider.

## Pulmonary Disease

Though onset of disease and symptoms can be subtle, late effects related to pulmonary disease are a major source of morbidity, with a prevalence rivaling that of long-term cardiovascular disease after 25 years of follow-up. A longitudinal cohort study of 121 childhood cancer survivors from the CCSS that controlled for smoking status, presence of heart failure, and exercise demonstrated that cancer survivors had a higher risk of developing impairments in diffusing capacity and restrictive lung defects compared to age-matched peers without a history of cancer [66]. Notably in this study, a reduced diffusion capacity was associated with more symptoms. Pulmonary conditions are also associated with an increased risk of death, and individuals with a history of childhood cancer are 8.8 times more likely to die from pulmonary disease than their peers of similar age after 30 years of follow-up [67]. Pulmonary issues are typically associated with radiation, with select chemotherapeutic agents (bleomycin, busulfan, and nitrosureas [carmustine, lomustine]), with a history of lung or chest surgery, or due to a combination of these exposures.

Radiation can lead to direct cell damage, pulmonary vasculature damage and leakage, interstitial inflammation, and progress to fibrosis with development of restrictive lung disease over time. Radiation exposure to the chest wall or thoracic spine could also potentially affect chest wall development, contributing to pulmonary symptoms. These changes may not only impact an individual's quality of life and physical functioning but might also limit the ability to utilize procedures that involve radiation from a diagnostic testing perspective (i.e., use of computed tomography [CT] scanning to follow lung nodules) or from a therapeutic perspective (such as the use of radiation therapy for breast cancer in later years). It is important to have a sense of the cumulative dose of radiation received and the volume of lung tissue exposed. Significant pulmonary toxicity typically occurs when over 10% of the lung tissue is exposed [68]. Contemporary strategies that can minimize the risk of radiation-induced tissue damage include intensity-modulated radiation therapy (IMRT) and stereotactic body radiation therapy (SBRT). Younger age at the time of radiation exposure to the lungs appears to be associated with a higher risk for late pulmonary effects [69].

Of the chemotherapy agents that lead to pulmonary toxicity, bleomycin has been well described. Bleomycin therapy can lead to acute pneumonitis, bronchiolitis obliterans and early- or late-onset fibrosis. Damage secondary to bleomycin is believed to occur via injury to the pulmonary vasculature and production of free radicals in the lungs. Pulmonary complications may occur in response to the use of high-dose oxygen in lungs that have been exposed to bleomycin, such as that used during prolonged surgical procedures or with activities that require high doses of oxygen exposure such as scuba diving. While patients with bleomycin exposure have been previously thought to have high perioperative complication risks, modern cohorts have not confirmed this [70]. The pulmonary toxicity that occurs with bleomycin exposure is dose dependent and thus it is helpful to know the cumulative dose of bleomycin used. Small studies have reported that nitrosureas have been associated with the development of late-onset pulmonary fibrosis, and this toxicity also appears to be dose dependent [71, 72]. More recent studies indicate that it is the combination of these chemotherapeutic agents with radiation or radiation alone, rather than chemotherapeutic agents alone, that seem to confer the highest risk of late-onset or long-term pulmonary toxicity [66, 73, 74].

Pulmonary function testing, with evaluation of diffusion capacity (diffusion capacity of the lungs for carbon monoxide [DLCO]) and spirometry, is a useful modality to screen for lung dysfunction in general in pediatric cancer survivors [75]. Such testing is not recommended on a routine basis (in the COG LFTU Guidelines) but rather at baseline, generally upon entry into long-term follow-up and as needed if symptoms arise. These recommendations have been found to have high yield for surveillance [76]. For the primary care provider (PCP), it is recommended to assess smoking status in all cancer survivors and to reinforce the importance of smoking cessation among individuals at risk for pulmonary complications based on the aforementioned exposures. Additionally, PCPs should recommend yearly influenza vaccination and pneumococcal vaccination to childhood cancer survivors who have a history of pulmonary toxic cancer treatments.

Low-dose computed tomography (CT) screening for lung cancer is recommended for individuals at elevated risk for lung cancer in the general population [77, 78]. Childhood cancer survivors who have received chest or mantle radiation therapy and especially those who report a smoking history may be at especially high risk for lung cancer, though the guidance regarding lung cancer screening in this population is less clear. Participation in lung cancer screening and follow-up as currently recommended does require CT imaging, which creates further exposure to potentially toxic radiation; this may be a limiting factor in individuals who have already received significant doses of chest or mantle radiation as children or adolescents. A cost-effectiveness analysis of low-dose CT lung cancer screening in survivors of Hodgkin lymphoma published in 2014 did conclude that annual screening was cost-effective and resulted in a significant life expectancy benefit for survivors who received chest radiation and were smokers but not necessarily for those who were non-smokers [79]. The COG LTFU Guidelines recommend discussing the risks and benefits of lung cancer screening with childhood cancer survivors who received radiation therapy to the chest, axilla, or total body irradiation (TBI). Referral to a lung cancer screening clinic if available may be appropriate.

## Immunologic Considerations

Most modalities of cancer treatment (cytotoxic chemotherapy, radiation or surgical removal of immune organs, stem cell transplantation, and immunotherapies) impair the immune system, and the timeline of immune reconstitution is dependent on the patient and the specific treatments used. In general, the risk for infections is highest during and immediately after treatment and decreases with time. In general, though survivors of hematological cancers, such as lymphoma and leukemia, who have completed treatment more than 2 years prior, may have prolonged immune dysfunction, they are not considered to be immunocompromised. There is some evidence that patients treated with standard chemotherapy for ALL and solid tumors might lose protective humoral immunity against vaccine-preventable diseases [80]. Revaccination of cancer survivors treated with standard chemotherapy is currently not routine practice in the United States. However, the European Conference on Infections in Leukemia recently recommended routine booster vaccination for ALL survivors [81], while a recent review from the Children's Oncology Group suggested that shared decision-making should be undertaken with cancer survivors to discuss empiric revaccination or titer measurement [82].

The long-term immune impairment caused by allogeneic stem cell transplant is well documented; the timing of immune recovery is dependent on the indication for transplant, the type of conditioning, stem cell source, and the presence of and treatment for graft-versus-host disease (GVHD). T cells might require up to 2 years to return to their pre-transplant functional level, while B cells might need up to 5 years [83]. Both acute and chronic GVHD, as well as their treatments, can prolong immune dysfunction and place patients at risk for infections. Generally, recipients of both autologous (patient receives their own hematopoietic stem cells after intensive chemotherapy) and allogeneic (patient receives donor hematopoietic stem cells from another person) stem cell transplants lose immunity to many vaccine-preventable diseases, and routine revaccination is recommended for several diseases by the Infectious Disease Society of America [84]. Of note, several live vaccines are contraindicated in stem cell transplant patients with chronic GVHD. Additionally, anti-microbial prophylaxis with antibiotic agents, usually stopped after cellular engraftment, may be continued for longer periods for patients with chronic GVHD or splenectomy (including high-dose abdominal radiation causing functional splenic dysfunction) [85].

Newer immune-based therapies for childhood cancers, including immune checkpoint inhibitors, bispecific T-cell engagers, and chimeric antigen receptor T cells (CAR-T), modulate the immune system in various ways; their effect on long-term immunity and the optimal management of patients that have received them is an area of active research. There are currently no consensus recommendations for vaccinations after CAR-T therapy, although some investigators have suggested possible vaccination schedules [86]. Of note, many patients who received B-cell-directed CAR-T therapy are found to have prolonged B-cell aplasia and thus require immunoglobulin replacement therapy.

## Orthopedic Issues

Cancer survivors are at risk for impaired bone health, which can lead to orthopedic issues such as fractures and osteonecrosis (avascular necrosis), often necessitating surgery and significantly burdening their quality of life.

One of the main manifestations of impaired bone health in this population is decreased bone mineral density (BMD). Children with ALL often have low BMD at presentation and exhibit further decreases in BMD during treatment, although several investigators have suggested that the BMD often improves in the following years. Among survivors of other cancers, estimates for prevalence of low BMD range between 41% (for Hodgkin Lymphoma) and 65% (for osteosarcoma) [87]. These effects are a result of a multitude of bone health risk factors that cancer patients are subject to immobilization as a result of surgery or pain, hormonal deprivation secondary to endocrine insults, chemotherapeutic agents (especially corticosteroids) with direct and indirect bone toxicities, radiotherapy, and suboptimal nutritional status during treatment, all of which conspire to cause bone damage in cancer survivors [88].

Another orthopedic injury of significance to ALL survivors is osteonecrosis (ON), thought to be a result of steroid and asparaginase exposure during treatment [89]. ON can affect any joint and ultimately results in mechanical collapse of the joint and necessitates surgical replacement. Recent research suggests that patients who receive treatment during adolescence and young adulthood are particularly vulnerable to osteonecrosis [90]. Beyond age, other risk factors include sex, steroid and asparaginase exposure, genetic polymorphisms, and the presence of the metabolic syndrome (hypertension, hyperlipidemia, obesity) [91].

Given the frequency and severity of orthopedic issues in childhood cancer survivors, the COG LTFU guidelines recommend a dual energy X-ray absorptiometry (DEXA) scan 2 years after completion of cancer therapy for those who are at high risk of low BMD [92]. When a DEXA study is ordered for young adult males and females with a history of childhood, adolescent, or young adult cancer, caution is needed in interpreting results, as normative Z-scores may need to be used in lieu of T-scores. Optimizing bone health through ensuring adequate intake of Vitamin D and calcium is also recommended, while directed pharmacologic therapies like bisphosphonates are used by some centers for those with confirmed low BMD [93]. Lastly, ALL survivors should be carefully counseled regarding the risk of ON, and any new joint complaints should lead to prompt evaluation with MRI and orthopedic surgery referral if ON is identified.

## Neurocognitive Issues

The prevalence of neurocognitive problems is increased overall compared to non-cancer sibling controls in both younger and older childhood cancer survivors. Mechanisms of damage to cortical brain tissue can result from direct invasion of central nervous system tumors or from cancer treatment and include glial cell damage, demyelination, scarring from surgical resection or disruption of the cerebral vasculature. Younger children are at greater risk for long-term neurocognitive deficits [94, 95]. Neurocognitive deficits related to cancer treatment can have long-lasting consequences; they can affect schooling, employment opportunities, and social interactions. Well-described risk factors that impact neurologic functioning include cranial radiation therapy, intrathecal chemotherapy, and high-dose steroids. The types of childhood cancer most commonly associated with long-term neurologic deficits, other than primary childhood brain tumors, include Hodgkin lymphoma and ALL, most likely due to the use of radiation and/or intrathecal chemotherapy in treatment. Deficits may occur in specific domains of cognitive functioning such as processing speed, memory, or attention as examples, and neuropsychological testing can be useful in identifying and following specific areas of concern. In ALL alone, specific deficits described include impaired attention, decreased executive functioning, visual-spatial deficits, and impaired mathematic abilities, with those treated before the age of 5 years being most sensitive to late and long-term effects [96, 97]. Behavior could be affected as well; self-reported behavioral problems increase with each passing year after treatment. Primary care and other health care providers should be prepared to help patients and their caregivers seek resources if needed at school, work, or other community settings. The COG LTFU Guidelines Task Force on Neurocognitive/Behavioral Complications after Childhood Cancer has developed specific guidance to help those caring for childhood cancer survivors [98].

## Second Primary Neoplasms

The late effect with the highest rate of mortality in childhood cancer survivors is the finding of second primary neoplasms (SPNs). For example, individuals diagnosed with Hodgkin lymphoma as a child or adolescent have a 14-fold increased risk of developing a SPN compared to the general population. Additionally, long-term follow-up studies of childhood cancer survivor cohorts are beginning to make available the identification of specific risk profiles that influence the risk of developing a SPN [99].

This increased risk of developing a SPN can be attributed to the late effects of primary cancer treatment but also to possible inherited cancer predisposition syndromes, such as Li–Fraumeni syndrome, as well as the development of behavioral risk factors. With regard to treatment-related SPNs, both chemotherapy and radiation therapy can be associated with increased risks of SPNs. Alkylating agents can be associated with secondary blood cancers up to 10 years following administration and a complete blood count is used to help identify these cancers. Radiation-induced cancers tend to have a slower course with the risk increasing many years after therapy and not appearing to plateau [100]. Importantly, secondary malignancies tend to occur in the field of radiation. Classic examples include the development of breast cancer following chest or mantle radiation, increased risk for colon cancer following abdominal/pelvic radiation, meningiomas following cranial radiation, sarcomas following radiation to the extremities or soft tissues, and skin cancer in any involved field.

For those cancers that have screening guidelines available (breast, colorectal, and now lung cancer), a history of radiation exposure can significantly alter both the age at and frequency with which screening and testing should occur; such guidance is again provided in the COG LTFU guidelines. For less common cancers for which no screening recommendations for the general population exist, additional evaluation or screening may be advised based on the treatment history as well as a potentially lower threshold to pursue testing based on new symptoms; examples include increased risks of skin cancer (melanoma and non-melanoma skin cancers), thyroid cancers, soft tissue sarcomas, or brain meningiomas in patients who received radiation therapy to respective affected body parts. In individuals for whom radiation has been a significant part of past therapy or past cumulative doses are unknown, consultation with a radiation oncologist can be valuable to help assess potential risks and guide recommended surveillance.

### Breast Cancer

The risk for breast cancer starts to increase within about 8 years after radiation exposure, and the risk does not appear to plateau over time [101]. Radiation appears to be the biggest treatment-related risk factor, though there is some emerging evidence that high-dose anthracycline chemotherapy (>250 mg/m$^2$) may also substantially increase risk [102]. In a recent study of female childhood cancer survivors, by the age of 50 the risk of breast cancer was 30%, with an even higher incidence among survivors of Hodgkin lymphoma [103]. This is similar to the risk of breast cancer in women with a BRCA1/2 mutation. This study also demonstrated that the risk was elevated even for smaller doses of radiation delivered as whole lung radiation compared to higher doses of mantle radiation. If a female has received alkylating agents with resulting ovarian function suppression, the risk may be decreased though to what degree is not known, and high-risk screening is still recommended. The COG LTFU guidelines recommend that females who received at least 10 Gy of radiation therapy to the chest (including total body irradiation [TBI]) have clinical breast exams yearly starting at puberty and then every 6 months, in addition to yearly mammogram starting at the age of 25 or 8 years after exposure, whichever occurs later. As an adjunct to mammogram screening, breast magnetic resonance imaging (MRI) should also be done annually; these can be staggered at 6-month intervals. If breast tissue was exposed to radiation therapy during treatment to the upper abdomen, then a similar approach could be considered [104]. If a breast MRI is not feasible or acceptable, then a breast ultrasound could be considered. It is estimated that up to one-half of breast-cancer-related deaths in this population could be avoided using this screening strategy [105].

### Colorectal Cancer

Childhood cancer survivors are at a significantly increased risk of developing colorectal cancer compared to their peers [106, 107]. After a mean follow-up of almost 30 years in one cohort study, individuals treated for Hodgkin lymphoma developed colorectal cancer beginning as early as 12 years after treatment exposure, and by the age of 50, the cumulative incidence approaches that of individuals with a strong family history of colorectal cancer. The COG LTFU guidelines recommend colorectal cancer screening for childhood cancer survivors who received abdominal, spinal, or pelvic radiation or TBI starting at 5 years after treatment exposure or at the age of 30, whichever occurs later [28]. A recent modeling study supports this more aggressive screening approach, describing that a higher percentage of deaths from colorectal cancer in this population could be avoided using this strategy compared to the screening strategy currently recommended by the US Preventive Services Task Force (USPSTF) for those at average risk [108].

### Lung Cancer

Among second primary cancers in a 40-year observational study of Hodgkin lymphoma survivors, lung cancer ranked highly among the excess cancers [100]. In another study of Hodgkin lymphoma survivors, the cumulative incidence of lung cancer by the age of 50 was double that of non-smokers in the general population. The COG LTFU guidelines recommend shared decision-making around screening for lung cancer using spiral CT scanning for childhood cancer survivors who are at highest risk. Smoking likely increases the risk and could serve as a prompt for conversations around lung cancer screening in cancer survivors.

### Thyroid Cancer

The risk for thyroid cancer appears to develop as a late effect and is associated with a radiation dose between 10 and 30 Gy. The COG LTFU guidelines recommend a yearly neck exam and a referral for ultrasound if nodules are palpated or if the clinical examination is insufficient, for example in an obese patient. Normal thyroid function tests do not exclude the presence of thyroid cancer. If any abnormalities are noted, consultation with an endocrinologist is recommended where available.

## Genetic Considerations

With any of the aforementioned late and long-term effects, obtaining a multigenerational family history is important. Based on observational studies, having been diagnosed with and treated for childhood cancer does not in itself appear to confer an increased risk of congenital abnormalities or cancer in offspring outside of a hereditary cancer syndrome [109, 110]. Childhood cancer can, however, be an important clue to inherited cancer syndromes, such as the Li–Fraumeni syndrome. Individuals with suggestive family histories for hereditary cancer syndromes should be considered for genetic risk assessment, counseling and testing if deemed appropriate, and those that are found to carry typical hereditary mutations may require careful and aggressive surveillance for the development of secondary cancers as adults [111]. Family history can also further clarify potential future risks for important health conditions such as cardiovascular disease or predisposition to psychiatric illness. This is a rapidly evolving field and the understanding of multigenic risk scores for several types of cancer is likely to change in the next 5 years.

## Special Issues in Adolescent and Young Adult Transition

### Fertility

Any young adult who was treated for cancer as a child should have a thorough assessment of fertility status, reproductive history, and especially future plans for childbearing, as young adulthood represents a phase of life that is especially pertinent to these topics, and cancer treatment can significantly impact reproductive health. In both women and men, consideration should be given to both reproductive hormone functioning and direct treatment effects to reproductive organs (i.e., ovaries, testes) as well as the stage of pubertal development at the time of exposure. Cranial irradiation can lead to derangements of the reproductive gonadotropins luteinizing hormone (LH) and follicle-stimulating hormone (FSH), but generally this is seen at higher doses [112].

Premature ovarian insufficiency (POI) is defined by the International Late Effects of Childhood Cancer Guideline Harmonization Group (IGHG) as a clinical condition in any adult female at age <40 years characterized by absence of menstrual cycles for >4 months and two elevated FSH levels in the menopausal range [113]. POI is seen at a significantly increased rate in females with a history of childhood cancer compared with their female siblings and may reduce the span of time that a woman has to consider bearing children [114, 115]. Use of certain chemotherapy agents and radiation exposure to the ovaries appear to be risk factors [115].

Chemotherapeutic agents most commonly described to have an adverse effect on ovarian function include alkylating agents (cyclophosphamide, ifosfamide, procarbazine, busulfan, melphalan, thiotepa) and nitrosoureas (carmustine, lomustine) [116, 117]. The cyclophosphamide equivalent dosage (CED) score can assist in quantifying the exposure to alkylating agents and the potential risk for infertility [118, 119]. Ovarian radiation exposure as low as 10 Gy, but especially greater than 20 Gy, has been associated with acute ovarian failure, which may become permanent [120, 121]. For those women who received a combination of pelvic irradiation and alkylating agents, the cumulative incidence of developing POI may approach 30%. In women, the resumption of menstrual cycles after chemotherapy does not necessarily signify a return to normal fertility, nor does the absence of menstrual cycles guarantee infertility. Impaired spermatogenesis in males is more likely to occur with CED doses above 4000 mg/m$^2$ [118].

For both men and women who are sexually active and are uncertain of their fertility status, it is important to reinforce that infertility should not be assumed based on prior cancer treatment and to use recommended methods of contraception if pregnancy is not desired. Evaluation in men includes a semen analysis, which is the most direct way to evaluate fertility status, though methods are available to accomplish an evaluation if a male survivor is unable to ejaculate. Semen analysis should be done at least 12 months after completion of cancer treatment; sperm count and quality may improve over time depending upon treatment-related factors as well as gonadal age and developmental stage at exposure [122]. In women, testing can include traditional measures of fertility, LH and FSH levels, as well as more advanced testing such as anti-Müllerian hormone (AMH) levels (which can be tested while a patient is on oral contraceptives) and antral follicle counts [123]. When testing is done, women should have discontinued hormones or hormonal contraceptive therapy, and testing should be completed if possible on day three of the menstrual cycle [113]. Much of this should be done with the assistance of a reproductive medicine specialist. In the absence of a genetic or hereditary basis for the original cancer, it is also important to know that cancer treatment is not associated with an increased risk of birth defects [124, 125]. In women, direct radiation to the pelvic field involving the uterus, cervix, or birth canal could result in scarring, which can pose an increased risk for pregnancy complications.

## Access to Care

The adolescent and young adult age is one of transition-transition from childhood to adulthood, from school to work, from dependent to independent. This transition can include changes in financial security, location, and support structure. With the previously described late effects noted, this flux can lead to inconsistent access to health care in a population at high risk of chronic disease.

Many survivors of childhood cancer are not fully aware of their therapies and the risk of sequelae [126, 127]. Also, this is a mobile patient population at risk for inconsistent follow-up. In one study from CCSS data, during a 2-year study period, only 31% of childhood and adolescent cancer survivors had received any survivor-focused care, and 11% had received no medical care at all [128]. Importantly, many patients undergo a transition in health insurance status during young adulthood, as they move to attend college, pursue jobs, or leave their parents' insurance. Lapses in adequate insurance coverage place young adults at particular risk for missing necessary cancer surveillance and preventative care previously discussed. Hence, specific discussions about insurance transitioning should be held with patients who complete cancer treatment and their parents, and involvement of social work or financial services might be helpful.

The IOM recommended the use of survivorship care plans (SCP) to facilitate the transfer of information to all providers [129] though these have been challenging to implement universally. The SCP includes the cancer diagnosis, a summary of the treatment received, any complications related to therapy, and potential long-term and late effects of which to be aware [130]. A survivorship visit allows for review of treatment as well as development of a care plan for follow-up. The education, both in person and on paper through the SCP, may help patients understand their cancer history and treatment and allows for outlining a plan for follow-up. Patients can share these treatment summaries and SCP documents with any provider as they navigate the medical system. Dedicated survivorship clinics exist in many major cancer centers and can be very helpful in facilitating transition to adult providers and outlining important screening recommendations for the PCP.

PCPs may need guidance on gathering treatment information and formulation of a plan for monitoring long-term survivors of childhood cancer. Such guidance may be derived by a "survivorship care planning visit," which may be offered by oncologists, a local cancer center, or specialized pediatric oncology long-term follow-up program. Novel models of survivorship care planning are emerging and may be available in primary care settings (see Box 26.1).

**Box 26.1 Elements of Survivorship Care Planning**

- Surveillance for recurrence
- Monitoring for and managing psychosocial and medical late effects
- Providing screening recommendations for second cancers
- Providing health education to survivors regarding their diagnoses, treatment exposures, and potential late and long-term effects
- Providing referrals to specialists and resources as indicated
- Familial genetic risk assessment (as appropriate)
- Guidance about diet, exercise, and health promotion activities
- Providing resources to assist with financial and insurance issues
- Empowering survivors to advocate for their own healthcare needs

## Psychosocial Considerations

Research suggests that depression, anxiety, fear or cancer recurrence, and post-traumatic stress disorder (PTSD) are seen in survivors at disproportionately high numbers [131]. Newer studies indicate that this increased risk is found in certain subsets of patients. The patterns of psychological morbidity can change over time [132]. A 2013 longitudinal study of childhood cancer survivors in the CCSS between 1994 and 2010 demonstrated that individuals may exhibit persistently high, decreasing, increasing, or persistently low levels of distress over time. In those with depression, a cluster of poor physical health, cancer-related pain, and emotional concerns can place these patients at higher risk for suicidal ideation [133]. Anxiety is shown to be associated with survivors who are female, unmarried, unemployed have low household income, lower educational attainment, a chronic health condition, or lack health insurance [134]. The prevalence of anxiety and PTSD appears to be related to family functioning. Literature shows that in one sample of adolescent survivors with PTSD, 75% came from families with poor family functioning [135, 136].

Sexual dysfunction may be a significant problem for young adult cancer survivors, as studies suggest that up to two-thirds of cancer survivors struggle with sexual health issues [137]. Etiologies might include anatomic and endocrine changes related to cancer therapy, as well as the psychological impact of cancer treatment and cancer-related anxiety. Additionally, a cancer diagnosis occurring during adolescence or young adulthood may impact an individual's sexual identity development and peer social and dating relationships [138, 139]. This may be a topic that young adults do not feel comfortable discussing with their care providers or close family members. Creating a supportive environment in the clinic can provide encouragement and empowerment to young adults deciding how much to share with their providers.

While there is certainly distress seen in survivorship, there are studies showing positive outcomes of the cancer experience such as resiliency, post-traumatic growth, and benefit finding [140–142]. Optimism, a leukemia diagnosis (compared to central nervous system or solid tumors), and a belief that the illness still affected their lives were associated with a tendency toward benefit finding. Many survivors speak toward positive changes in self, relationships, and life goals as a result of the traumatic experience of cancer and cancer therapy.

It is also important to remember that significant illness in childhood can affect the achievement of developmental milestones. As such, the childhood cancer survivor can be found to have less satisfaction in social functioning and emotional health [143]. This can play a role in future academic achievement, vocational success, and personal relationships.

To optimally address the psychosocial concerns of cancer survivors, centers and providers should undertake a multi-disciplinary approach. Psychoeducation, the process of providing developmentally appropriate education on what to expect to the cancer survivor, has been shown to be effective in breast cancer survivors [144]. Psychotherapy, usually in the form of cognitive behavioral therapy, has been used extensively to treat mood disorders common among survivors, such as depression and anxiety, but also to address specific fears or concerns, such as the fear of cancer recurrence. Medication treatment might be appropriate for some cancer survivors with anxiety and depression. Lastly, the psychosocial stressors on the parents and the entire family unit of the cancer survivor must be acknowledged, and family-based interventions can be considered in the appropriate setting.

## Equity Considerations

While all survivors of childhood cancer face barriers in accessing optimal survivorship care as discussed above, certain groups are particularly vulnerable due to structural inequities. In 2021, the Agency for Healthcare Research and Quality (AHRQ) produced a comprehensive technical brief outlining disparities and barriers to pediatric survivorship care and discussing mitigation strategies [145]. They identified inequities in access to and quality of care along the following dimensions: sex, race, ethnicity, insurance status, rural residence, income, education, and employment. In the primary literature, several studies have demonstrated that patients of color and those with public or no insurance are particularly vulnerable to lapses in survivorship care [146, 147].

Several strategies have been proposed to address these inequities, and these include technology-based interventions, patient education, survivorship clinics, and location-based strategies (such as co-locating an oncologist and primary care physician) [148]. The optimal mix of strategies will depend on the patient population and health system specifics at hand. Overall, any survivorship systems need to be designed with the awareness of structural racism and other inequities that characterize the American and other healthcare systems and place particular patient groups at significant risk for poor outcomes.

## Conclusion

There are a host of considerations when taking care of the adult survivor of childhood cancer, particularly during the transitional period of adolescence and young adulthood. With knowledge of the medical, psychological, and social complications of cancer therapy, as well as access to supportive resources, providers can be instrumental in helping childhood cancer survivors navigate the seas of young adulthood and optimize their future health and well-being (Appendix).

## Appendix

| Childhood cancer survivor fact sheet | |
|---|---|
| Definitions | A childhood cancer survivor is defined as a someone diagnosed and treated for cancer before the age of 20 years<br>Survivors are at risk for cancer therapy-related chronic medical conditions (long-term and late effects):<br>• Long-term effects are adverse effects as a result of therapy that develop during treatment and persist for several years<br>• Late effects are adverse effects related to cancer therapy that may only develop many years later |
| Epidemiology | • If diagnosed with cancer before age 20 years, now have a 5-year survival of more than 85% [2]<br>• Improved survival has translated into more than 380,000 childhood and adolescent cancer survivors living in the USA [3]<br>• During a 2-year study period, only 31% of CCS had received any survivor-focused care, and 11% had received no medical care at all [59] |
| Common chronic conditions (pathophysiology) | Survivors are at risk for complications related to underlying organ damage from cancer therapy; these therapies include chemotherapy, radiation therapy, surgery, bone marrow transplant, targeted therapies, and transfusions<br>Survivors are particularly at increased risk for the following conditions:<br>• Diabetes/insulin resistance<br>• Radiation-induced endocrinopathies (e.g., growth hormone, thyroid)<br>• Cardiovascular disease including cardiomyopathy and atherosclerotic disease<br>• Restrictive and/or obstructing pulmonary disease<br>• Neurocognitive issues including memory, concentration<br>• Secondary malignancies, particularly in the radiation field<br>• Hypogonadism and reduced fertility |
| Challenges in transition | • Population is mobile and may have inconsistent follow-up<br>• Changing insurance status can make care for chronic conditions difficult<br>• Psychological needs that may require specialized counseling |
| Resources | Provider resources<br>• COG guidelines: http://www.survivorshipguidelines.org/<br>• ASCO practice guidelines: https://www.asco.org/news-initiatives/current-initiatives/cancer-care-initiatives/survivorship-compendium<br>• National Cancer Institute: http://www.cancer.gov/cancertopics/aya/survivorship<br>• SurvivorLink CME modules: http://www.cancersurvivorlink.org/CME/Index.aspx?v=HCP<br>Patient resources:<br>• Cancer.Net: http://www.cancer.net/survivorship<br>• Stupid cancer: http://stupidcancer.org/<br>• Planet cancer: http://myplanet.planetcancer.org/<br>• Cancer and careers: http://www.cancerandcareers.org/en<br>• Fertility resources: http://www.myoncofertility.org/<br>• First descents: https://firstdescents.org/ |

## References


1. Children's Oncology Group. Long-term follow-up guidelines for survivors of childhood, adolescent, and young adult cancers. 2016. http://www.survivorshipguidelines.org/
2. Kremer LCM, Mulder RL, Oeffinger KC, Bhatia S, Landier W, Levitt G, et al. A worldwide collaboration to harmonize guidelines for the long-term follow-up of childhood and young adult cancer survivors: a report from the international late effects of Childhood Cancer Guideline Harmonization Group: guidelines for childhood cancer survivors. Pediatr Blood Cancer. 2013;60(4):543–9.
3. Rock CL, Thomson CA, Sullivan KR, Howe CL, Kushi LH, Caan BJ, et al. American Cancer Society nutrition and physical activity guideline for cancer survivors. CA Cancer J Clin. 2022;72(3):230–62.
4. Berdan CA, Tangney CC, Scala C, Stolley M. Childhood cancer survivors and adherence to the American Cancer Society guidelines on

nutrition and physical activity. J Cancer Surviv. 2014;8(4):671–9.
5. Cleeland CS, Allen JD, Roberts SA, Brell JM, Giralt SA, Khakoo AY, et al. Reducing the toxicity of cancer therapy: recognizing needs, taking action. Nat Rev Clin Oncol. 2012;9(8):471–8.
6. Howlader N, Noone AM, Krapcho M, Miller D, Brest A, Yu M, Ruhl J, Tatalovich Z, Mariotto A, Lewis DR, Chen HS, Feuer EJ, Cronin KA, editors. SEER cancer statistics review, 1975–2018. National Cancer Institute. https://seer.cancer.gov/csr/1975_2018/index.html\.
7. Pui CH, Evans WE. A 50-year journey to cure childhood acute lymphoblastic leukemia. Semin Hematol. 2013;50(3):185–96.
8. Ward E, DeSantis C, Robbins A, Kohler B, Jemal A. Childhood and adolescent cancer statistics, 2014: cancer in children and adolescents. CA A Cancer J Clin. 2014;64(2):83–103.
9. Oeffinger KC, Mertens AC, Sklar CA, Kawashima T, Hudson MM, Meadows AT, et al. Chronic health conditions in adult survivors of childhood cancer. N Engl J Med. 2006;355(15):1572–82.
10. Hewitt M, Weiner SL, Simone JV, National Cancer Policy Board, Institute of Medicine, National Research Council, editors. Childhood cancer survivorship: improving care and quality of life. Washington, DC: National Academies Press; 2003.
11. Albini A, Pennesi G, Donatelli F, Cammarota R, De Flora S, Noonan DM. Cardiotoxicity of anticancer drugs: the need for cardio-oncology and cardio-oncological prevention. J Natl Cancer Inst. 2010;102(1):14–25.
12. Curigliano G, Mayer EL, Burstein HJ, Winer EP, Goldhirsch A. Cardiac toxicity from systemic cancer therapy: a comprehensive review. Prog Cardiovasc Dis. 2010;53(2):94–104.
13. Sonis ST. Regimen-related gastrointestinal toxicities in cancer patients. Curr Opin Support Palliat Care. 2010;4(1):26–30.
14. Sul JK, Deangelis LM. Neurologic complications of cancer chemotherapy. Semin Oncol. 2006;33(3):324–32.
15. Mohty B, El-Cheikh J, Yakoub-Agha I, Moreau P, Harousseau JL, Mohty M. Peripheral neuropathy and new treatments for multiple myeloma: background and practical recommendations. Haematologica. 2010;95(2):311–9.
16. Hagiwara H, Sunada Y. Mechanism of taxane neurotoxicity. Breast Cancer (Tokyo, Japan). 2004;11(1):82–5.
17. Force T, Kerkela R. Cardiotoxicity of the new cancer therapeutics—mechanisms of, and approaches to, the problem. Drug Discov Today. 2008;13(17–18):778–84.
18. Wang S, Prizment A, Thyagarajan B, Blaes A. Cancer treatment-induced accelerated aging in cancer survivors: biology and assessment. Cancers. 2021;13(3):427.
19. Robison LL, Mertens AC, Boice JD, Breslow NE, Donaldson SS, Green DM, et al. Study design and cohort characteristics of the childhood cancer survivor study: a multi-institutional collaborative project. Med Pediatr Oncol. 2002;38(4):229–39.
20. Hudson MM, Ness KK, Nolan VG, Armstrong GT, Green DM, Morris EB, et al. Prospective medical assessment of adults surviving childhood cancer: study design, cohort characteristics, and feasibility of the St. Jude lifetime cohort study. Pediatr Blood Cancer. 2011;56(5):825–36.
21. McBride ML, Rogers PC, Sheps SB, Glickman V, Broemeling AM, Goddard K, et al. Childhood, adolescent, and young adult cancer survivors research program of British Columbia: objectives, study design, and cohort characteristics. Pediatr Blood Cancer. 2010;55(2):324–30.
22. Winther JF, Kenborg L, Byrne J, Hjorth L, Kaatsch P, Kremer LCM, et al. Childhood cancer survivor cohorts in Europe. Acta Oncol. 2015;54(5):655–68.
23. Hudson MM, Mertens AC, Yasui Y, Hobbie W, Chen H, Gurney JG, et al. Health status of adult long-term survivors of childhood cancer: a report from the childhood cancer survivor study. JAMA. 2003;290(12):1583–92.
24. Suh E, Stratton KL, Leisenring WM, Nathan PC, Ford JS, Freyer DR, et al. Late mortality and chronic health conditions in long-term survivors of early-adolescent and young adult cancers: a retrospective cohort analysis from the childhood cancer survivor study. Lancet Oncol. 2020;21(3):421–35.
25. Hudson MM, Oeffinger KC, Jones K, Brinkman TM, Krull KR, Mulrooney DA, et al. Age-dependent changes in health status in the childhood cancer survivor cohort. JCO. 2015;33(5):479–91.
26. Hudson MM, Ness KK, Gurney JG, Mulrooney DA, Chemaitilly W, Krull KR, et al. Clinical ascertainment of health outcomes among adults treated for childhood cancer. JAMA. 2013;309(22):2371–81.
27. Diller L, Chow EJ, Gurney JG, Hudson MM, Kadin-Lottick NS, Kawashima TI, et al. Chronic disease in the childhood cancer survivor study cohort: a review of published findings. J Clin Oncol. 2009;27(14):2339–55.
28. Hudson MM, Mulrooney DA, Bowers DC, Sklar CA, Green DM, Donaldson SS, et al. High-risk populations identified in childhood cancer survivor study investigations: implications for risk-based surveillance. J Clin Oncol. 2009;27(14):2405–14.
29. Lipshultz SE, Adams MJ, Colan SD, Constine LS, Herman EH, Hsu DT, et al. Long-term cardiovascular toxicity in children, adolescents, and young adults who receive cancer therapy: pathophysiology, course, monitoring, management, prevention, and research directions: a scientific statement from the American Heart Association. Circulation. 2013;128(17):1927–95.
30. Robison LL, Hudson MM. Survivors of childhood and adolescent cancer: life-long risks and responsibilities. Nat Rev Cancer. 2014;14(1):61–70.

31. Oeffinger KC, Mertens AC, Sklar CA, Yasui Y, Fears T, Stovall M, et al. Obesity in adult survivors of childhood acute lymphoblastic leukemia: a report from the childhood cancer survivor study. J Clin Oncol. 2003;21(7):1359–65.
32. Yeh JM, Nekhlyudov L, Goldie SJ, Mertens AC, Diller L. A model-based estimate of cumulative excess mortality in survivors of childhood cancer. Ann Intern Med. 2010;152(7):409–17.
33. Armstrong GT, Liu Q, Yasui Y, Neglia JP, Leisenring W, Robison LL, et al. Late mortality among 5-year survivors of childhood cancer: a summary from the childhood cancer survivor study. J Clin Oncol. 2009;27(14):2328–38.
34. Mertens AC, Liu Q, Neglia JP, Wasilewski K, Leisenring W, Armstrong GT, et al. Cause-specific late mortality among 5-year survivors of childhood cancer: the childhood cancer survivor study. J Natl Cancer Inst. 2008;100(19):1368–79.
35. Mertens AC, Yasui Y, Neglia JP, Potter JD, Nesbit ME, Ruccione K, et al. Late mortality experience in five-year survivors of childhood and adolescent cancer: the childhood cancer survivor study. J Clin Oncol. 2001;19(13):3163–72.
36. Armstrong GT, Kawashima T, Leisenring W, Stratton K, Stovall M, Hudson MM, et al. Aging and risk of severe, disabling, life-threatening, and fatal events in the childhood cancer survivor study. J Clin Oncol. 2014;32(12):1218–27.
37. Gibson TM, Mostoufi-Moab S, Stratton KL, Leisenring WM, Barnea D, Chow EJ, et al. Temporal patterns in the risk of chronic health conditions in survivors of childhood cancer diagnosed 1970–99: a report from the childhood cancer survivor study cohort. Lancet Oncol. 2018;19(12):1590–601.
38. Yeh JM, Ward ZJ, Chaudhry A, Liu Q, Yasui Y, Armstrong GT, et al. Life expectancy of adult survivors of childhood cancer over 3 decades. JAMA Oncol. 2020;6(3):350–7.
39. Chemaitilly W, Sklar CA. Endocrine complications in long-term survivors of childhood cancers. Endocr Relat Cancer. 2010;17(3):R141–59.
40. Gurney JG, Kadan-Lottick NS, Packer RJ, Neglia JP, Sklar CA, Punyko JA, et al. Endocrine and cardiovascular late effects among adult survivors of childhood brain tumors. Cancer. 2003;97(3):663–73.
41. Mulder RL, Kremer LCM, et al. Prevalence and risk factors of radiation-induced growth hormone deficiency in childhood cancer survivors: a systematic review. Cancer Treat Rev. 2009;35(7):616–32.
42. Tonorezos ES, Hudson MM, Edgar AB, Kremer LC, Sklar CA, Wallace WHB, et al. Screening and management of adverse endocrine outcomes in adult survivors of childhood and adolescent cancer. Lancet Diabetes Endocrinol. 2015;3(7):545–55.
43. Darzy KH. Radiation-induced hypopituitarism after cancer therapy: who, how and when to test. Nat Clin Pract Endocrinol Metab. 2009;5(2):88–99.
44. Link K, Moëll C, Garwicz S, Cavallin-Ståhl E, Björk J, Thilén U, et al. Growth hormone deficiency predicts cardiovascular risk in young adults treated for acute lymphoblastic leukemia in childhood. J Clin Endocrinol Metab. 2004;89(10):5003–12.
45. Tamhane S, Sfeir JG, Kittah NEN, Jasim S, Chemaitilly W, Cohen LE, et al. GH therapy in childhood cancer survivors: a systematic review and meta-analysis. J Clin Endocrinol Metab. 2018;103(8):2794–801.
46. Ergun-Longmire B, Mertens AC, Mitby P, Qin J, Heller G, Shi W, et al. Growth hormone treatment and risk of second neoplasms in the childhood cancer survivor. J Clin Endocrinol Metab. 2006;91(9):3494–8.
47. Torino F, Corsello SM, Longo R, Barnabei A, Gasparini G. Hypothyroidism related to tyrosine kinase inhibitors: an emerging toxic effect of targeted therapy. Nat Rev Clin Oncol. 2009;6(4):219–28.
48. Sklar C, Whitton J, Mertens A, Stovall M, Green D, Marina N, et al. Abnormalities of the thyroid in survivors of Hodgkin's disease: data from the childhood cancer survivor study. J Clin Endocrinol Metab. 2000;85(9):3227–32.
49. Metzger ML, Howard SC, Hudson MM, Gow KW, Li C-S, Krasin MJ, et al. Natural history of thyroid nodules in survivors of pediatric Hodgkin lymphoma. Pediatr Blood Cancer. 2006;46(3):314–9.
50. Meacham LR, Sklar CA, Li S, Liu Q, Gimpel N, Yasui Y, et al. Diabetes mellitus in long-term survivors of childhood cancer. Increased risk associated with radiation therapy: a report for the childhood cancer survivor study. Arch Intern Med. 2009;169(15):1381–8.
51. Armstrong GT, Oeffinger KC, Chen Y, Kawashima T, Yasui Y, Leisenring W, et al. Modifiable risk factors and major cardiac events among adult survivors of childhood cancer. J Clin Oncol. 2013;31(29):3673–80.
52. Meacham LR, Chow EJ, Ness KK, Kamdar KY, Chen Y, Yasui Y, et al. Cardiovascular risk factors in adult survivors of pediatric cancer–a report from the childhood cancer survivor study. Cancer Epidemiol Biomarkers Prev. 2010;19(1):170–81.
53. Gurney JG, Ness KK, Sibley SD, O'Leary M, Dengel DR, Lee JM, et al. Metabolic syndrome and growth hormone deficiency in adult survivors of childhood acute lymphoblastic leukemia. Cancer. 2006;107(6):1303–12.
54. Hoffman KE, Derdak J, Bernstein D, Reynolds JC, Avila NA, Gerber L, et al. Metabolic syndrome traits in long-term survivors of pediatric sarcoma. Pediatr Blood Cancer. 2008;50(2):341–6.
55. van Waas M, Neggers SJCMM, Pieters R, van den Heuvel-Eibrink MM. Components of the metabolic syndrome in 500 adult long-term survivors of childhood cancer. Ann Oncol. 2010;21(5):1121–6.
56. Children's Oncology Group. Long-term follow-up guidelines for survivors of childhood, adolescent, and young adult cancers. http://www.survivorship-guidelines.org/.

57. de Ville de Goyet M, Moniotte S, Brichard B. Cardiotoxicity of childhood cancer treatment: update and current knowledge on long-term follow-up. Pediatr Hematol Oncol 2012;29(5):395–414.
58. van der Pal HJH, van Dalen EC, Kremer LCM, Bakker PJM, van Leeuwen FE. Risk of morbidity and mortality from cardiovascular disease following radiotherapy for childhood cancer: a systematic review. Cancer Treat Rev. 2005;31(3):173–85.
59. Mulrooney DA, Yeazel MW, Kawashima T, Mertens AC, Mitby P, Stovall M, et al. Cardiac outcomes in a cohort of adult survivors of childhood and adolescent cancer: retrospective analysis of the childhood cancer survivor study cohort. BMJ. 2009;339:b4606.
60. Lipshultz SE, Alvarez JA, Scully RE. Anthracycline associated cardiotoxicity in survivors of childhood cancer. Heart. 2008;94(4):525–33.
61. Cardinale D, Colombo A, Lamantia G, Colombo N, Civelli M, De Giacomi G, et al. Anthracycline-induced cardiomyopathy. J Am Coll Cardiol. 2010;55(3):213–20.
62. Chow EJ, Chen Y, Hudson MM, Feijen EAM, Kremer LC, Border WL, et al. Prediction of ischemic heart disease and stroke in survivors of childhood cancer. J Clin Oncol. 2018;36(1):44–52.
63. Gibson TM, Li Z, Green DM, Armstrong GT, Mulrooney DA, Srivastava D, et al. Blood pressure status in adult survivors of childhood cancer: a report from the St. Jude lifetime cohort study. Cancer Epidemiol Biomarkers Prev. 2017;26(12):1705–13.
64. Blaser BW, Kim HT, Alyea EP, Ho VT, Cutler C, Armand P, et al. Hyperlipidemia and statin use after allogeneic hematopoietic stem cell transplantation. Biol Blood Marrow Transplant. 2012;18(4):575–83.
65. Haugnes HS, Wethal T, Aass N, Dahl O, Klepp O, Langberg CW, et al. Cardiovascular risk factors and morbidity in long-term survivors of testicular cancer: a 20-year follow-up study. JCO. 2010;28(30):4649–57.
66. Armenian SH, Landier W, Francisco L, Herrera C, Mills G, Siyahian A, Supab N, Wilson K, Wolfson JA, Horak D, Bhatia S. Long-term pulmonary function in survivors of childhood cancer. J Clin Oncol. 2015;33(14):1592–600.
67. Armstrong GT, Liu Q, Yasui Y, Neglia JP, Leisenring W, Robison LL, Mertens AC. Late mortality among 5-year survivors of childhood cancer: a summary from the childhood cancer survivor study. J Clin Oncol. 2009;27(14):2328–38.
68. Visscher H, Otth M, Feijen EAML, Nathan PC, Kuehni CE. Cardiovascular and pulmonary challenges after treatment of childhood cancer. Pediatr Clin N Am. 2020;67(6):1155–70.
69. Khan F, Williams AM, Weiner DJ, Constine LS. Impact of respiratory developmental stage on sensitivity to late effects of radiation in pediatric cancer survivors. Adv Radiat Oncol. 2020;5(3):426–33.
70. Calaway AC, Foster RS, Adra N, Masterson TA, Albany C, Hanna NH, Einhorn LH, Cary C. Risk of bleomycin-related pulmonary toxicities and operative morbidity after postchemotherapy retroperitoneal lymph node dissection in patients with good-risk germ cell tumors. J Clin Oncol. 2018;36(29):2950–4.
71. O'Driscoll BR, Hasleton PS, Taylor PM, Poulter LW, Gattameneni HR, Woodcock AA. Active lung fibrosis up to 17 years after chemotherapy with carmustine (BCNU) in childhood. N Engl J Med. 1990;323(6):378–82.
72. Lohani S, O'Driscoll BR, Woodcock AA. 25-year study of lung fibrosis following carmustine therapy for brain tumor in childhood. Chest. 2004;126:1007.
73. Mulder RL, Thonissen NM, van der Pal HJ, et al. Pulmonary function impairment measured by pulmonary function tests in long-term survivors of childhood cancer. Thorax. 2011;66:1065–71.
74. Dietz AC, Chen Y, Yasui Y, Ness KK, Hagood JS, Chow EJ, Stovall M, Neglia JP, Oeffinger KC, Mertens AC, Robison LL, Armstrong GT, Mulrooney DA. Risk and impact of pulmonary complications in survivors of childhood cancer: a report from the childhood cancer survivor study. Cancer. 2016;122(23):3687–96.
75. Landier W, Bhatia S, Eshelman DA, Forte KJ, Sweeney T, Hester AL, et al. Development of risk-based guidelines for pediatric cancer survivors: the children's oncology group long-term follow-up guidelines from the children's oncology group late effects committee and nursing discipline. J Clin Oncol. 2004;22(24):4979–90.
76. Landier W, Armenian SH, Lee J, Thomas O, Wong FL, Francisco L, et al. Yield of screening for long-term complications using the children's oncology group long-term follow-up guidelines. J Clin Oncol. 2012;30(35):4401–8.
77. US Preventive Services Task Force, Krist AH, Davidson KW, Mangione CM, Barry MJ, Cabana M, et al. Screening for lung cancer: US Preventive Services Task Force recommendation statement. JAMA. 2021;325(10):962–70.
78. Lorigan P, Radford J, Howell A, Thatcher N. Lung cancer after treatment for Hodgkin's lymphoma: a systematic review. Lancet Oncol. 2005;6(10):773–9.
79. Wattson DA, Hunink MGM, DiPiro PJ, Das P, Hodgson DC, Mauch PM, et al. Low-dose chest computed tomography for lung cancer screening among Hodgkin lymphoma survivors: a cost-effectiveness analysis. Int J Radiat Oncol Biol Phys. 2014;90(2):344–53.
80. Zignol M, Peracchi M, Tridello G, Pillon M, Fregonese F, D'Elia R, et al. Assessment of humoral immunity to poliomyelitis, tetanus, hepatitis B, measles, rubella, and mumps in children after chemotherapy. Cancer. 2004;101(3):635–41.
81. Mikulska M, Cesaro S, de Lavallade H, Di Blasi R, Einarsdottir S, Gallo G, et al. Vaccination of patients with haematological malignancies who did not have transplantations: guidelines from the 2017 European conference on infections in Leukaemia (ECIL 7). Lancet Infect Dis. 2019;19(6):e188–99.

82. Guilcher GMT, Rivard L, Huang JT, Wright NAM, Anderson L, Eissa H, et al. Immune function in childhood cancer survivors: a Children's oncology group review. Lancet Child Adolesc Health. 2021;5(4):284–94.
83. Ogonek J, Kralj Juric M, Ghimire S, Varanasi PR, Holler E, Greinix H, et al. Immune reconstitution after allogeneic hematopoietic stem cell transplantation. Front Immunol. 2016;7:507.
84. Rubin LG, Levin MJ, Ljungman P, Davies EG, Avery R, Tomblyn M, et al. 2013 IDSA clinical practice guideline for vaccination of the immunocompromised host. Clin Infect Dis. 2014;58(3):309–18.
85. Tomblyn M, Chiller T, Einsele H, Gress R, Sepkowitz K, Storek J, et al. Guidelines for preventing infectious complications among hematopoietic cell transplantation recipients: a global perspective. Biol Blood Marrow Transplant. 2009;15(10):1143–238.
86. Los-Arcos I, Iacoboni G, Aguilar-Guisado M, Alsina-Manrique L, Díaz de Heredia C, Fortuny-Guasch C, et al. Recommendations for screening, monitoring, prevention, and prophylaxis of infections in adult and pediatric patients receiving CAR T-cell therapy: a position paper. Infection. 2021;49(2):215–31.
87. Wilson CL, Ness KK. Bone mineral density deficits and fractures in survivors of childhood cancer. Curr Osteoporos Rep. 2013;11(4):329–37.
88. Marcucci G, Beltrami G, Tamburini A, Body JJ, Confavreux CB, Hadji P, et al. Bone health in childhood cancer: review of the literature and recommendations for the management of bone health in childhood cancer survivors. Ann Oncol. 2019;30(6):908–20.
89. Kunstreich M, Kummer S, Laws HJ, Borkhardt A, Kuhlen M. Osteonecrosis in children with acute lymphoblastic leukemia. Haematologica. 2016;101(11):1295–305.
90. Valtis YK, Stevenson KE, Place AE, Silverman LB, Vrooman LM, Gotti G, et al. Orthopedic toxicities among adolescents and young adults treated in DFCI ALL consortium trials. Blood Adv. 2022;6(1):72–81.
91. Valtis YK, Place AE, Silverman LB, Vrooman LM, DeAngelo DJ, Luskin MR. Orthopaedic adverse events among adolescents and adults treated with asparaginase for acute lymphoblastic leukaemia. Br J Haematol. 2022;198(3):421–30.
92. Children's Oncology Group. Long term follow up guideline for survivors of childhood, adolescent, and young adult cancers, version 5.0: bone health. Monrovia, CA: Children's Oncology Group; 2018. www.survivorshipguidelines.org.
93. Lim SW, Ahn JH, Choi A, Cho WH, Lee JA, Kim DH, et al. Efficacy of pamidronate in pediatric osteosarcoma patients with low bone mineral density. Ann Pediatr Endocrinol Metab. 2016;21(1):21–5.
94. Prasad PK, Hardy KK, Zhang N, Edelstein K, Srivastava D, Zeltzer L, et al. Psychosocial and neurocognitive outcomes in adult survivors of adolescent and early young adult cancer: a report from the childhood cancer survivor study. J Clin Oncol. 2015;33(23):2545–52.
95. Kadan-Lottick NS, Zeltzer LK, Liu Q, et al. Neurocognitive functioning in adult survivors of childhood non-central nervous system cancers. J Natl Cancer Inst. 2010;102:881–93.
96. Edelstein K, D'Agostino N, Bernstein LJ, Nathan PC, Greenberg ML, Hodgson DC, et al. Long-term neurocognitive outcomes in young adult survivors of childhood acute lymphoblastic leukemia. J Pediatr Hematol Oncol. 2011;33(6):450–8.
97. Krull KR, Brinkman TM, Li C, Armstrong GT, Ness KK, Srivastava DK, et al. Neurocognitive outcomes decades after treatment for childhood acute lymphoblastic leukemia: a report from the St Jude lifetime cohort study. J Clin Oncol. 2013;31(35):4407–15.
98. Nathan PC. Guidelines for identification of, advocacy for, and intervention in neurocognitive problems in survivors of childhood cancer: a report from the Children's Oncology Group. Arch Pediatr Adolesc Med. 2007;161(8):798.
99. Holmquist et al. Risk of solid subsequent malignant neoplasms after childhood Hodgkin lymphoma—identification of high-risk populations to guide surveillance: a report from the Late Effects Study Group. Cancer; 2019.
100. Schaapveld M, Aleman BMP, van Eggermond AM, Janus CPM, Krol ADG, van der Maazen RWM, et al. Second cancer risk up to 40 years after treatment for Hodgkin's lymphoma. N Engl J Med. 2015;373(26):2499–511.
101. Bhatia S, Yasui Y, Robison LL, Birch JM, Bogue MK, Diller L, et al. High risk of subsequent neoplasms continues with extended follow-up of childhood Hodgkin's disease: report from the late effects study group. J Clin Oncol. 2003;21(23):4386–94.
102. Ehrhardt MJ, Howell CR, Hale K, Baassiri MJ, Rodriguez C, Wilson CL, et al. Subsequent breast cancer in female childhood cancer survivors in the St Jude lifetime cohort study (SJLIFE). J Clin Oncol. 2019;37(19):1647–56.
103. Moskowitz CS, Chou JF, Wolden SL, Bernstein JL, Malhotra J, Novetsky Friedman D, et al. Breast cancer after chest radiation therapy for childhood cancer. J Clin Oncol. 2014;32(21):2217–23.
104. Mulder RL, Hudson MM, Bhatia S, Landier W, Levitt G, Constine LS, et al. Updated breast cancer surveillance recommendations for female survivors of childhood, adolescent, and young adult cancer from the international guideline harmonization group. J Clin Oncol. 2020;38(35):4194–207.
105. Yeh JM, Lowry KP, Schechter CB, Diller LR, Alagoz O, Armstrong GT, et al. Clinical benefits, harms, and cost-effectiveness of breast cancer screening for survivors of childhood cancer treated with chest radiation: a comparative modeling study. Ann Intern Med. 2020;173(5):331–41.
106. Henderson TO, Oeffinger KC, Whitton J, Leisenring W, Neglia J, Meadows A, et al. Secondary gastrointestinal cancer in childhood cancer survivors: a

cohort study. Ann Intern Med. 2012;156(11):757–66, W-260.
107. Holmqvist AS, Chen Y, Berano Teh J, Sun C, Birch JM, van den Bos C, et al. Risk of solid subsequent malignant neoplasms after childhood Hodgkin lymphoma-identification of high-risk populations to guide surveillance: a report from the late effects study group. Cancer. 2019;125(8):1373–83.
108. Gini A, Meester RGS, Keshavarz H, Oeffinger KC, Ahmed S, Hodgson DC, et al. Cost-effectiveness of colonoscopy-based colorectal cancer screening in childhood cancer survivors. J Natl Cancer Inst. 2019;111(11):1161–9.
109. Hawkins MM. Is there evidence of a therapy-related increase in germ cell mutation among childhood cancer survivors? J Natl Cancer Inst. 1991;83(22):1643–50.
110. Madanat-Harjuoja LM, Malila N, Lahteenmaki P, Pukkala E, Mulvihill JJ, Boice JD Jr, et al. Risk of cancer among children of cancer patients—a nationwide study in Finland. Int J Cancer. 2010;126(5):1196–205.
111. McBride KA, Ballinger ML, Killick E, Kirk J, Tattersall MH, Eeles RA, et al. Li–Fraumeni syndrome: cancer risk assessment and clinical management. Nat Rev Clin Oncol. 2014;11(5):260–71.
112. Green DM, Kawashima T, Stovall M, Leisenring W, Sklar CA, Mertens AC, et al. Fertility of female survivors of childhood cancer: a report from the childhood cancer survivor study. J Clin Oncol. 2009;27(16):2677–85.
113. van Dorp W, Mulder RL, Kremer LCM, et al. Recommendations for premature ovarian insufficiency surveillance for female survivors of childhood, adolescent, and young adult cancer: a report from the international late effects of childhood cancer guideline harmonization Group in Collaboration with the PanCareSurFup consortium. J Clin Oncol. 2016;34(28):3440–50.
114. Sklar CA, Mertens AC, Mitby P, Whitton J, Stovall M, Kasper C, et al. Premature menopause in survivors of childhood cancer: a report from the childhood cancer survivor study. J Natl Cancer Inst. 2006;98(13):890–6.
115. Green DM, Sklar CA, Boice JD, Mulvihill JJ, Whitton JA, Stovall M, et al. Ovarian failure and reproductive outcomes after childhood cancer treatment: results from the childhood cancer survivor study. J Clin Oncol. 2009;27(14):2374–81.
116. Bath LE, Wallace WHB, Critchley HOD. Late effects of the treatment of childhood cancer on the female reproductive system and the potential for fertility preservation. BJOG Int J Obstetr Gynaecol. 2002;109(2):107–14.
117. Sklar C. Maintenance of ovarian function and risk of premature menopause related to cancer treatment. JNCI Monogr. 2005;2005(34):25–7.
118. Green DM, Liu W, Kutteh WH, Ke RW, Shelton KC, Sklar CA, et al. Cumulative alkylating agent exposure and semen parameters in adult survivors of childhood cancer: a report from the St Jude lifetime cohort study. Lancet Oncol. 2014;15(11):1215–23.
119. Green DM, Nolan VG, Goodman PJ, Whitton JA, Srivastava D, Leisenring WM, et al. The cyclophosphamide equivalent dose as an approach for quantifying alkylating agent exposure: a report from the childhood cancer survivor study. Pediatr Blood Cancer. 2014;61(1):53–67.
120. Thomson AB, Critchley HOD, Kelnar CJH, Wallace WHB. Late reproductive sequelae following treatment of childhood cancer and options for fertility preservation. Best Pract Res Clin Endocrinol Metab. 2002;16(2):311–34.
121. Chemaitilly W, Mertens AC, Mitby P, Whitton J, Stovall M, Yasui Y, et al. Acute ovarian failure in the childhood cancer survivor study. J Clin Endocrinol Metab. 2006;91(5):1723–8.
122. Skinner R, Mulder RL, Kremer LC, et al. Recommendations for gonadotoxicity surveillance in male childhood, adolescent, and young adult cancer survivors: a report from the international late effects of childhood cancer guideline harmonization group in collaboration with the PanCareSurFup consortium. Lancet Oncol. 2017;18(2):e75–90.
123. Metzger ML, Meacham LR, Patterson B, Casillas JS, Constine LS, Hijiya N, et al. Female reproductive health after childhood, adolescent, and young adult cancers: guidelines for the assessment and management of female reproductive complications. J Clin Oncol. 2013;31(9):1239–47.
124. Sankila R, Olsen JH, Anderson H, Garwicz S, Glattre E, Hertz H, et al. Risk of cancer among offspring of childhood-cancer survivors. Association of the Nordic Cancer Registries and the Nordic Society of Paediatric Haematology and Oncology. N Engl J Med. 1998;338(19):1339–44.
125. Signorello LB, Mulvihill JJ, Green DM, Munro HM, Stovall M, Weathers RE, et al. Congenital anomalies in the children of cancer survivors: a report from the childhood cancer survivor study. J Clin Oncol. 2012;30(3):239–45.
126. Kadan-Lottick NS, Robison LL, Gurney JG, Neglia JP, Yasui Y, Hayashi R, et al. Childhood cancer survivors' knowledge about their past diagnosis and treatment: childhood cancer survivor study. JAMA. 2002;287(14):1832–9.
127. Oeffinger KC, Wallace WH. Barriers to follow-up care of survivors in the United States and the United Kingdom. Pediatr Blood Cancer. 2006;46(2):135–42.
128. Nathan PC, Greenberg ML, Ness KK, Hudson MM, Mertens AC, Mahoney MC, et al. Medical care in long-term survivors of childhood cancer: a report from the childhood cancer survivor study. J Clin Oncol. 2008;26(27):4401–9.
129. Hewitt M, Greenfield S, Stovall E, editors. From cancer patient to cancer survivor: lost in transition. Washington, DC: Institute of Medicine and National Research Council; 2005.
130. ASCO Survivorship guidelines. http://www.instituteforquality.org/practice-guidelines.

131. Hobbie WL, Stuber M, Meeske K, Wissler K, Rourke MT, Ruccione K, et al. Symptoms of posttraumatic stress in young adult survivors of childhood cancer. J Clin Oncol. 2000;18(24):4060–6.
132. Brinkman TM, Zhu L, Zeltzer LK, Recklitis CJ, Kimberg C, Zhang N, et al. Longitudinal patterns of psychological distress in adult survivors of childhood cancer. Br J Cancer. 2013;109(5):1373–81.
133. Recklitis CJ, Diller LR, Li X, Najita J, Robison LL, Zeltzer L. Suicide ideation in adult survivors of childhood cancer: a report from the childhood cancer survivor study. J Clin Oncol. 2010;28(4):655–61.
134. Langeveld NE, Grootenhuis MA, Voûte PA, de Haan RJ. Posttraumatic stress symptoms in adult survivors of childhood cancer. Pediatr Blood Cancer. 2004;42(7):604–10.
135. Ozono S, Saeki T, Mantani T, Ogata A, Okamura H, Nakagawa S-i, et al. Psychological distress related to patterns of family functioning among Japanese childhood cancer survivors and their parents. Psycho-Oncology. 2010;19(5):545–52.
136. Alderfer MA, Navsaria N, Kazak AE. Family functioning and posttraumatic stress disorder in adolescent survivors of childhood cancer. J Fam Psychol. 2009;23(5):717–25.
137. Livestrong. "I learned to live with it" is not good enough: challenges reported by post-treatment cancer survivors in the LIVESTRONG surveys. A LIVESTRONG report. 2010. http://www.livestrong.org/pdfs/3-0/LSSurvivorSurveyReport_final. Accessed 23 July 2014.
138. Evan EE, Kaufman M, Cook AB, Zeltzer LK. Sexual health and self-esteem in adolescents and young adults with cancer. Cancer. 2006;107(7):1672–9.
139. Aubin S, Perez S. The Clinician's toolbox: assessing the sexual impacts of cancer on adolescents and young adults with cancer (AYAC). Sex Med. 2015;3(3):198–212.
140. Barakat LP, Alderfer MA, Kazak AE. Posttraumatic growth in adolescent survivors of cancer and their mothers and fathers. J Pediatr Psychol. 2006;31(4):413–9.
141. Zebrack BJ, Stuber ML, Meeske KA, Phipps S, Krull KR, Liu Q, et al. Perceived positive impact of cancer among long-term survivors of childhood cancer: a report from the childhood cancer survivor study. Psycho-Oncology. 2012;21(6):630–9.
142. Michel G, Taylor N, Absolom K, Eiser C. Benefit finding in survivors of childhood cancer and their parents: further empirical support for the benefit finding scale for children. Child Care Health Dev. 2010;36(1):123–9.
143. Zeltzer LK, Lu Q, Leisenring W, Tsao JCI, Recklitis C, Armstrong G, et al. Psychosocial outcomes and health-related quality of life in adult childhood cancer survivors: a report from the childhood cancer survivor study. Cancer Epidemiol Biomarkers Prev. 2008;17(2):435–46.
144. Rowland JH, Meyerowitz BE, Crespi CM, Leedham B, Desmond K, Belin TR, et al. Addressing intimacy and partner communication after breast cancer: a randomized controlled group intervention. Breast Cancer Res Treat. 2009;118(1):99–111.
145. Mobley EM, Moke DJ, Milam J, Ochoa CY, Stal J, Osazuwa N, et al. Disparities and barriers to pediatric cancer survivorship care. Rockville, MD: Agency for Healthcare Research and Quality (US); 2021. (AHRQ Comparative Effectiveness Technical Briefs). http://www.ncbi.nlm.nih.gov/books/NBK568475/.
146. Milam JE, Meeske K, Slaughter RI, Sherman-Bien S, Ritt-Olson A, Kuperberg A, et al. Cancer-related follow-up care among Hispanic and non-Hispanic childhood cancer survivors: the project forward study. Cancer. 2015;121(4):605–13.
147. Barakat LP, Schwartz LA, Szabo MM, Hussey HM, Bunin GR. Factors that contribute to post-treatment follow-up care for survivors of childhood cancer. J Cancer Surviv. 2012;6(2):155–62.
148. Mobley EM, Moke DJ, Milam J, Ochoa CY, Stal J, Osazuwa N, et al. Interventions to address disparities and barriers to pediatric cancer survivorship care: a scoping review. J Cancer Surviv. 2022;16(3):667–76.

# Congenital Heart Disease

# 27

Joseph Truglio, Kali Hopkins, and Barry Love

## Case Presentations

R.A. is a 20-year-old cisgender female with repaired Tetralogy of Fallot (ToF) presenting to an adult medical practice for follow-up. She was diagnosed prenatally with ToF and had a surgical correction at 2 years of age. A workup for syndromes associated with ToF was unrevealing. After her repair, she demonstrated age-appropriate growth but mild developmental delay and was followed regularly by her pediatrician and pediatric cardiologist. She received speech therapy, physical therapy, and occupational therapy in grade school. She started college 2 years ago. She is now sexually active with 1 cisgender male partner. She is using condoms for sexually transmitted infection protection and is interested in discussing additional contraception options. She has not seen a doctor since the year before starting college. On review of symptoms, she reports intermittent dizziness when exercising. During high school, she ran regularly, but she now becomes short of breath and dizzy after approximately 5 min of jogging. She denies any syncopal episodes. She last saw her pediatric cardiologist 5 years ago.

E.W. is a 52-year-old man with a history of atrioventricular (AV) canal and Down syndrome presenting to an adult medical practice for preoperative assessment for dental rehabilitation under general anesthesia. He had an AV canal repair as an infant and was followed by his pediatric cardiology team well into adulthood. He lived with his mother until his 30 s. He has since lived in a group home. Eight years ago, he was diagnosed with type 2 diabetes mellitus and hypertension. He takes metformin and empagliflozin for his diabetes. His most recent hemoglobin A1c was 9%, but he has been unable to reliably take insulin. His hypertension is well controlled on lisinopril and chlorthalidone. He has moderate developmental delay and is accompanied by an aid from the group home where he has lived for the past 15 years.

## Case Discussions

Over the past four decades, there has been an epidemiological shift wherein the majority of patients with congenital heart disease (CHD) are now adults. More recently, there has been a significant increase in the number of adults over 40 years of age with CHD. Successes in repairing

J. Truglio (✉)
Departments of Internal Medicine, Pediatrics and Medical Education, Icahn School of Medicine at Mount Sinai, New York, NY, USA
e-mail: joseph.truglio@mssm.edu

K. Hopkins · B. Love
Department of Pediatrics, Icahn School of Medicine at Mount Sinai, New York, NY, USA
e-mail: Kali.Hopkins@mountsinai.org; barry.love@mssm.edu


A. A. Kuo et al. (eds.), *Care of Adults with Chronic Childhood Conditions*,
https://doi.org/10.1007/978-3-031-54281-7_27

and managing even highly complex CHD have thus created a large, ever-growing, and heterogeneous population of adults with congenital heart disease (ACHD).

The above cases illustrate the wide variety of common themes presented to PCPs of ACHD. R.A. is a young woman in college, transitioning from pediatric to adult care. She had a complex heart lesion repaired as a child. Despite successful surgical repair and a lack of associated syndromes, R.A. experienced developmental delay. A 2014 prospective, longitudinal study found that 75% of children with congenital heart disease had developmental delay, despite only 19% of patients in this study having a genetic syndrome [1]. After a period of very close follow-up, R.A. had a significant lapse in care, and she now presents with dizziness, concerning for potential complications of her cardiac repair. A recent study of adults with complex congenital heart disease found that 63% had a lapse in care while transitioning from pediatric to adult care. The median lapse was 10 years in duration. Unfortunately, those patients with a lapse in care were more than three times more likely to require urgent cardiac intervention [2]. R.A. is also in need of sexual and reproductive health counseling as well as guidance regarding appropriate physical activity. Finally, although R.A. underwent genetic testing as a child, it would be reasonable to offer genetic counseling and possible re-testing, as new tests have become available and new syndromes have been recognized in the past 20 years.

E.W. also has a history of CHD requiring repair as a child. Unlike R.A., he has diagnosed a syndrome—Down syndrome—associated with his CHD. E.W.'s Down syndrome has manifested as moderate developmental delay resulting in him living in a group home. It has been estimated that as many as 25% of patients with congenital heart disease have an associated genetic syndrome with comorbid conditions [3, 4]. For E.W., his care should be provided in the context of his chronological and developmental age. At 52 years of age, E.W. has developed comorbid cardiovascular conditions including diabetes mellitus and hypertension. A 2015 American Heart Association (AHA) Scientific Paper is dedicated to the unique needs of the growing population of ACHD over the age of 40 [5]. As seen in E.W., many patients over 40 years of age with CHD are at increased risk for acquired cardiovascular disease in addition to the late complications of their underlying CHD. The screening and management of acquired cardiovascular disease and cardiovascular risk factors in ADCH should consider the patient's underlying CHD lesion and should be done in partnership with an ACHD specialist. E.W. has a repaired AV canal. His diabetes and hypertension do not require any special management from a cardiac perspective. E.W. presents in need of perioperative management for non-cardiac surgery. Performing a preoperative assessment for this patient will require consideration of his CHD, his most recently acquired conditions, and his overall developmental status. A thorough history and physical exam should focus on any changes in his cardiac status with special attention paid to his risk for hemodynamic compromise and infective endocarditis risk related to the surgery. A baseline electrocardiogram (EKG) is indicated, given the risk of arrhythmias associated with the underlying lesion. If no murmur is noted on physical exam, an AV canal repaired more than 6 months prior with no evidence of subsequent complication is a low-risk lesion that does not require any particular perioperative management and should not require endocarditis prophylaxis. Additionally, beyond E.W.'s cardiac condition, his underlying genetic syndrome and any associated conditions should be addressed. Commonly associated conditions related to Down syndrome that may require special attention perioperatively include atlantoaxial instability, potential endocrine disorders such as diabetes and hypothyroidism, and any immune dysfunction.

## Definition and Pathophysiology

Congenital heart disease refers to a wide range of structural defects of the heart and major blood vessels that are present at birth. The pathophysiology of CHD is incredibly complex, with numerous genetic mutations, chromosomal abnormalities, epigenetic insults, and environmental exposures implicated in abnormal cardiogenesis [4]. An identifiable genetic or environmental cause is found in approximately 20–30% of cases of congenital heart disease. As many as 18–25% of congenital heart defects are associated with a congenital syndrome or chromosomal abnormality, most commonly Down syndrome and 22q11.2 deletion, and less commonly Williams syndrome, Noonan syndrome, and Turner syndrome [3, 4].

## Epidemiology

The prevalence of CHD at birth ranges from 6 to 13 per 1000 live births [6–8]. While there are no national adult congenital heart disease registries, current estimates are that there are well over 1,250,000 adults in the United States with CHD. More than 50% of these patients had a moderate-to-severe complexity heart lesion at birth. Survival rates into adulthood for children with CHD vary, from 98% for mild and 96% for moderate to 56% for severe complexity lesions [9]. Due to such high survival rates and improved care for adults with CHD, the ACHD population is currently growing at a rate of approximately 5% annually, with the vast majority of ACHD (90% of those with mild, 75% with moderate, and 40% with complex lesions) living past 60 years of age [5, 10].

## Common Adult Conditions in This Population

Multiple guidelines exist for the management of ACHD. The most recent guidelines are the 2018 American College of Cardiology/American Heart Association (ACC/AHA) Guidelines for Adults with Congenital Heart Disease and the 2020 European Society of Cardiology (ESC) Guidelines for the Management of Adults Congenital Heart Disease [11, 12]. While primarily written for specialists, these resources provide guidance for all clinicians who care for ACHD. Both sets of guidelines have detailed recommendations for specific conditions common to ACHD. They also provide distinct yet overlapping classification systems for the complexity of individual CHD lesions, with attention paid to both the anatomy and physiology at play. Such frameworks can help guide PCPs in their co-management and help identify patients who require varying levels of specialty and subspecialty expertise.

Adult conditions associated with CHD depend upon the presence of an associated congenital syndrome or chromosomal abnormality, the complexity of the underlying CHD lesion, and the age of the patient. Associated syndromes will often require the PCP to coordinate with several subspecialists as well as ancillary services such as physical and occupational therapy. Complications directly related to CHD should be managed in conjunction with an ACHD specialist. These include heart failure, arrhythmia (often atrial tachycardias), vascular complications (pulmonary hypertension, aortic root dilation, aneurysm formation, venous insufficiency), and risk for sudden cardiac death. Such complications can occur at any age. As ACHD age, they may also develop risk factors for acquired heart disease, most notably hypertension, diabetes, and hyperlipidemia. The diagnosis and management of these risk factors may vary from that in the general population depending on the underlying CHD and any associated syndromes. PCPs should be comfortable managing such risk factors in most ACHD and should be able to recognize when co-management with an ACHD specialist is indicated. Subsequent acquired heart disease, including coronary artery disease and ischemic heart failure, should be co-managed with a cardiologist experienced in ACHD.

Finally, several themes commonly arise when caring for ACHD regardless of the patient's age or physical condition. These include counseling around physical activity and employment, sexual and reproductive health, genetic counseling, and antibiotic prophylaxis for infective endocarditis.

## Screening, Diagnosis, and Management of Cardiovascular Risk Factors

Adults with CHD may be at higher risk for the development of ventricular dysfunction, arrhythmias, and heart failure. The management of acquired heart disease in ACHD should be managed in conjunction with an ACHD specialist. However, PCPs should be comfortable identifying and managing cardiovascular risk factors in ACHD, including hypertension, diabetes, hyperlipidemia as well as providing smoking cessation resources when needed. National and international guidelines for these risk factors can usually be applied to ACHD, but there are several notable exceptions.

### Hypertension

There may be an increased prevalence of hypertension in the ACHD population [13]. The approach to screening, diagnosis, and management of hypertension in adults with CHD is similar to that within the general population with a few exceptions (see Table 27.1). Coarctation of the aorta (CoA) places patients at higher risk for developing hypertension, even after the lesion is repaired [14]. Close monitoring for hypertension, including ambulatory blood pressure monitoring when available, is reasonable for patients with repaired CoA. For patients who have a persistent gradient across the coarctation site on echocardiogram after repair, an ACHD cardiologist should be consulted to evaluate for possible stenting of this lesion. The choice of antihypertensive agent for patients with CoA depends on the presence of associated syndromes and the presence and location of any aortic aneurysm. For patients with Marfan's syndrome or an aortic aneurysm, an angiotensin-converting enzyme (ACE) inhibitor or angiotensin receptor blocker (ARB) should be considered as a first-line agent. If the aneurysm involves the renal arteries, however, ACE inhibitors (ACEIs) and ARBs should be used with caution and renal function closely monitored. Patients with unrepaired cyanotic heart disease or those with persistent cyanosis are at high risk for developing nephropathy from glomerular sclerosis [15, 16]. ACEIs and diuretics should therefore be avoided if possible to prevent further decline in renal function. Finally, Eisenmenger physiology—when pulmonary pressures rise above those of systemic pressures—is typically seen in long-standing, unrepaired complex CHD. Management of systemic hypertension in these patients must be done in conjunction with an ACHD specialist, and the use of vasodilating agents should be avoided to prevent exacerbation of right-to-left shunting.

### Diabetes Mellitus

The incidence of diabetes in the overall ACHD population seems to be similar to that of the general population [17]. However, certain syndromes that are also associated with congenital heart disease, such as Down syndrome and Williams syndrome, may place patients at increased risk for type 1 or type 2 diabetes mellitus. A comprehensive review of such syndromes is beyond the scope of this chapter. Clinicians caring for such patients should familiarize themselves with any syndrome-specific screening guidelines. Regardless of any increased incidence of diabetes, adults with CHD are likely at higher risk for complications from diabetes. The American Heart Association therefore recommends considering screening for diabetes in all adults with congenital heart disease who are over 40 years of age with body mass index ≥25 kg/m$^2$, regardless of additional risk factors, with repeat screening every 3 years [5]. The management of diabetes in ACHD is similar to that in the general population. However, in patients with diabetic nephropathy who also have cyanotic lesions, ACEIs and ARBs should generally be avoided. As is the case for all patients with diabetes, statin therapy should be initiated in ACHD who have diabetes unless contraindicated.

**Table 27.1** Lesion-specific recommendations for management of cardiovascular risk factors in ACHD

| Lesion/condition | CV risk factor | Physiology | Management |
|---|---|---|---|
| Unrepaired cyanotic heart disease or persistent cyanosis | Hypertension | Nephropathy from glomerular sclerosis | Avoid nonsteroidal anti-inflammatory drugs<br>Avoid ACEIs, ARBs, and diuretic use if possible |
| | Diabetes | Risk for decline in renal function with ACEI and ARBs | Avoid ACEIs and ARBs for renal protection |
| Coarctation of the aorta | Hypertension | Increased incidence of hypertension even with repair | Cardiology evaluation for persistent gradient requiring stenting<br>Consider ACEIs or ARBs in setting of aneurysm or Marfan's syndrome, but use caution if renal arteries are involved |
| | Hyperlipidemia | Increased risk for coronary artery atherosclerosis | Consider earlier initiation of statin therapy and an LDL goal of 70 mg/dL or less |
| Eisenmenger physiology | Hypertension | Elevated pulmonary pressures with shunting | Avoid vasodilating agents to limit right-to-left shunting |
| Bioprosthetic valves in aortic position | Hyperlipidemia | Increased risk for coronary artery atherosclerosis | Consider earlier initiation of statin therapy and an LDL goal of 70 mg/dL or less |
| Transposition of the great vessels | Hyperlipidemia | Sympathetic nerve injury during arterial switch operation | Consider earlier initiation of statin therapy and an LDL goal of 70 mg/dL or less |

*ACE* angiotensin-converting enzyme; *ACEI* angiotensin-converting enzyme inhibitor; *ARB* angiotensin receptor blocker; *LDL* low-density lipoprotein

## Hyperlipidemia

With the exception of specific lesions that increase a patient's risk for coronary artery disease, the role of statin therapy is the same in ACHD as in the general population. Patients with surgically repaired d-transposition of the great vessels are at increased coronary artery disease risk, likely due to injury of the sympathetic nerves that supply the coronary arteries during the arterial switch operation [18–20]. Patients with coarctation of the aorta and potentially patients with bioprosthetic valves in the aortic position are also at increased risk [21, 22]. It is reasonable therefore to have a lower threshold to initiate statin therapy in these patients and to aim for a target LDL of 70 mg/dL or less.

## Perioperative Management for Non-cardiac Surgeries in Adults with Congenital Heart Disease

Perioperative management of patients involves providing an assessment of the patient's risk of a perioperative cardiac event, optimizing the patient to reduce this and other risks, and providing recommendations for the management of any chronic illnesses around the time of surgery. The vast majority of ACHD may safely undergo non-cardiac surgeries with appropriate perioperative management. However, traditional cardiac risk calculators [23, 24] may not adequately assess the perioperative risk for ACHD. Further, most current recommendations regarding perioperative care of adults with complex congenital heart disease are based on expert opinion or small case series. An effective approach to ACHD perioperative care includes the traditional Revised Cardiac Risk Index used for adults without CHD *plus* an assessment of the patients' congenital heart disease, as described by the 2018 ACC/AHA and/or the 2020 ESC guidelines, and any associated conditions [11, 12].

In general, cardiac surgeries are not "cures" for congenital heart disease. The hemodynamics and electrophysiology may remain dynamic and change over time. It is reasonable even in the absence of symptoms for some workup to be done for nearly all adults with CHD undergoing non-cardiac surgery. Previous guidelines advised complete blood count, chest X-ray, EKG, and echocardiogram pre-operatively [25]. For adults with simple, uncomplicated, repaired lesions such as ventricular septal defects, atrial septal defects, and patent ductus arteriosus who have a normal physical exam and no new symptoms, it is reasonable to limit testing to the above, especially for simple surgery. Conversely, all patients with moderate-to-high-risk lesions (see Table 27.2) should undergo a risk assessment by an ACHD expert regardless of the stability of

**Table 27.2** Select moderate, high, and highest risk conditions for perioperative adverse events associated with non-cardiac surgery

| Highest risk | High risk | Moderate risk |
|---|---|---|
| Fontan procedure | Pulmonary hypertension | Prosthetic valve or conduit |
| Severe pulmonary arterial hypertension | Severe systemic ventricular dysfunction (LVEF <35%) | Intra-cardiac shunt |
| Cyanotic congenital heart disease | NYHA class III or IV heart failure | Moderate left-sided heart obstruction |
| Complex CHD with residual heart failure | Severe left-sided obstructive lesions | Moderate systemic ventricular dysfunction |
| Valvular heart disease with need for anticoagulation | | |
| CHD complicated by malignant arrhythmia | | |

**Note that this list is not comprehensive and that both underlying anatomy and current physiology of a patient's CHD should be considered when assessing risk**

*LVEF* left ventricular ejection fraction; *NYHA* New York Heart Association; *CHD* congenital heart disease

their symptoms. The 2018 ACC/AHA Guidelines highlight additional factors that are associated with increased risk of morbidity and mortality when ACHD undergo non-cardiac surgery, with emphases added to consider the anatomy and current physiology as well as overall patient characteristics when assessing risk. These include cyanosis, congestive heart failure, poor general health, younger age, pulmonary hypertension, surgeries involving the respiratory and nervous system, complex congenital heart disease, and urgent or emergent surgeries. Guidelines recommend managing patients with these conditions or any patient with higher risk lesions at an ACHD center [11, 12, 25, 26].

## Physical Activity and Employment

PCPs play a critical role in empowering ACHD to live full and meaningful lives. This includes encouraging all patients to engage in safe physical activity and developmentally appropriate, meaningful employment. Patients with CHD often have their physical activity limited to decrease the risk of sudden cardiac death. ACHD is also far less likely to be employed as compared with otherwise healthy, age-matched adults [27]. This is at times due to patient, caregiver, and clinician fear of adverse events due to physical exertion. Unfortunately, few data are available regarding routine physical activity or employment restrictions for ACHD. Historically, restrictive guidelines for exclusion from sport for patients with cardiac conditions including ACHD were considered to be the "gold standard" [28]. Prevention of sudden cardiac death was deemed to be highest priority goal at the expense of healthy sports participation for a large number of patients that are probably at lower risk [29–31].

It must be noted, however, that any individual patient's risk must be assessed with consideration of his or her underlying lesion, surgical repairs, complications, acquired conditions, and associated syndromes. While exercise testing can potentially be helpful in risk-stratifying patients, Holter monitoring or long-term event monitoring is also reasonable tests when arrhythmias are suspected [32].

A more recent 2015 AHA/ACC Scientific Statement is much more liberal and incorporates a "shared decision making" model rather than a paternalistic, widely prohibitive approach to athletics [33]. This paradigm is more useful when promoting activity in ACHD of all ages, be it "sports or activities of daily living" or meaningful employment. Subsequent publications confirm the importance of individualizing the risk assessment, considering the anatomic and physiologic state of the patient's CHD lesion and the dynamic and static aspects of the activity [34, 35].

## Sexual and Reproductive Health

Sexual and reproductive health are arguably the most neglected health domains for adults with CHD. Congenital malformations are the most common causes of maternal cardiac morbidity and mortality in the United States [36]. Despite this risk, women with CHD are often not counseled on pregnancy-related risk or appropriate contraception. Data show that one in five sexually active women with CHD use a contraindicated birth control option, 28% do not use any contraception, and nearly half have not received counseling on pregnancy-related risk [37]. Given the genetic risk for CHD in the offspring of ACHD and the impact of functional limitations on sexual activity, sexual and reproductive health should be addressed in all ACHD, regardless of their sexual orientation or gender identity, age, or perceived physical abilities. The role of the PCP is to advocate for appropriate counseling on sexual and reproductive health and identify when patients need to be referred to subspecialists. The most common issues include contraceptive counseling, pregnancy and delivery, genetic counseling, functional limitations that impact sexual activity, and management of perimenopausal symptoms. The 2022 Supreme Court decision in Dobbs v. Jackson highlights the need for PCPs to advocate for the sexual and reproductive health of patients with congenital heart disease. This includes being aware of evolving state and federal laws as well as local and regional resources for patients and families.

## Contraceptive Counseling

The vast majority of women with CHD can have their contraception managed by their PCP. This is especially important as young adults transition from pediatric-oriented to adult-oriented care. The Adult Congenital Heart Association advocates that "no matter how complex a woman's heart there is a safe and effective birth control option for her" [38]. The World Health Organization Medical Eligibility Criteria for Contraceptive Use provides guidance for the safety of contraceptive options for a wide variety of underlying medical conditions [39]. The major concern in adults with CHD is the risk of thromboembolism. Estrogen-containing birth control increases the risk of thromboembolism and is therefore not recommended for adults with cyanotic lesions, pulmonary arterial hypertension, prior Fontan procedure, or atrial fibrillation. The risk of thromboembolism in these conditions must be individualized for each patient and weighed against their family planning goals and risks of pregnancy in conjunction with an ACHD specialist and gynecologist.

Progesterone-only forms of contraception are often the preferred alternative. However, the risk of fluid overload should be discussed in patients with heart failure, and lifestyle factors must be considered given the need for strict adherence. Intrauterine devices (IUDs) are also a popular choice and are widely available in a variety of hormone and non-hormone-containing versions. There are concerns regarding infections with IUD use, particularly in ACHD who may be at increased risk of infective endocarditis (IE). However, studies have shown only a modest 1.4 times increase in risk of IE in women with ACHD using IUDs [25].

Table 27.3 outlines common high-risk conditions for venous thromboembolism (VTE) with the use of estrogen, as well as possible alternative contraception options [39, 40].

## Management of Perimenopausal Symptoms

The use of hormone replacement therapy (HRT) in the general population for management of perimenopausal symptoms remains controversial but is generally accepted for patients with low estimated atherosclerotic cardiovascular disease risk profiles for short periods of time (typically less than 5 years) [41]. For women with ACHD, the risk of venous thromboembolism due to their CHD must be considered prior to any HRT. For women with lesions considered high-risk for VTE (see Table 27.3), estrogen-containing HRT should be avoided. Alternative treatments include vaginal estrogen creams and non-hormonal lubricants for vaginal dryness and high-dose vitamin E and selective serotonin reuptake inhibitors for vasomotor symptoms.

**Table 27.3** Common high-risk lesions for thrombosis with the use estrogen-containing birth control or estrogen hormone replacement

| High-risk lesions | Alternative contraceptive options |
|---|---|
| Atrial fibrillation/flutter not on anticoagulation | Non-estrogen intrauterine devices |
| Bjork–Shiley or Starr–Edwards valve | Progesterone-only pill ("mini pill") |
| Dilated left atrium >4 cm | Depot medroxyprogesterone acetate |
| Cyanotic heart disease | Etonogestrel implant |
| Pulmonary arteriovenous malformation | Barrier methods |
| Prior thrombotic event | |
| Left ventricular dysfunction with ejection fraction <30% | |
| Kawasaki disease with coronary involvement | |
| Complicated valvular heart disease (pulmonary hypertension, risk of atrial fibrillation, history of infective endocarditis) | |

For women with lower risk lesions in whom HRT is an option, the lowest dose of estrogen for the shortest period of time is recommended [42]. In general, transdermal estrogen preparations deliver lower, more consistent doses of estrogen than oral preparations.

## Sexual Dysfunction

Sexual dysfunction and anxiety around sexual activity may impact adults of all ages with CHD, regardless of the severity of the underlying lesion. In a study of ACHD patients ranging in age from 18 to 57 years, 20% of individuals surveyed responded "yes" when asked the following: "being insecure about having sex," "being afraid of having sex," or "worrying about your sex life" [43]. Ninety-four percent of these patients had mild cardiovascular disease and were New York Heart Association (NYHA) functional class I or II. The American Heart Association recommends that "sexual activity is reasonable for most CHD patients who do not have decompensated or advanced heart failure, severe and/or significantly symptomatic valvular disease, or uncontrolled arrhythmias" [44]. Unfortunately, these guidelines are based predominantly on expert opinion and little data exist to help guide clinicians on counseling ACHD around sexual activity and sexual dysfunction. A reasonable approach considers the patient's chronological age and developmental stage, the severity of his or her underlying CHD lesion, and any subsequent physical and mental conditions (please refer to Chap. 7 on "Sexual and Reproductive Health" of this textbook for a more detailed discussion of sexual and reproductive health considerations for adults with intellectual and developmental disabilities).

Types of sexual dysfunction may vary based on patient age, the severity of the underlying cardiac lesion and any medical and surgical treatments. A study of women aged 18–75 found cardiac symptoms with sexual activity occurred in 6–26% of cisgender women, with presence and severity of symptoms related to the severity of the underlying lesion [45]. Similar studies in cisgender men reveal erectile dysfunction (ED) in 10–42% of patients [46, 47]. However, the likelihood of ED is unrelated to the severity of the underlying condition and similar to rates in the general population. PCPs for ACHD should not assume the presence or absence of sexual activity or sexual dysfunction. Rather, assessment of sexual and reproductive health must be included as part of the routine care of any adult patient.

## Gender-Affirming Therapy

PCPs can play a critical role ensuring access to appropriate medications for ACHD requiring gender-affirming therapies. The vast majority of ACHD can safely take gender-affirming medications. Depending on the medical class used, safety issues to consider include thromboembolism, QTc prolongation, and electrolyte disturbances (Table 27.4). PCPs should work alongside patients and, when needed, their ACHD specialists to weigh the risks and benefits of each of

**Table 27.4** Gender-affirming hormone therapies for ACHD

| Therapy | Goal | Risk | Suggested approach |
|---|---|---|---|
| Estrogen | Feminization | Thromboembolism | Follow similar approach to hormonal birth control decisions<br>May consider holding 2-weeks pre-operatively, but often safe to continue perioperatively |
| Spironolactone | Feminization | Hyperkalemia | Monitor electrolytes, especially if concomitant renal dysfunction or ACEI/ARB use |
| Gonadotropin-releasing hormone (GnRH) analogues | Delay puberty | Potential prolongation of QTc interval | Periodic EKG monitoring is reasonable and can consider avoiding if evidence of QTc prolongation |

*ACEI* angiotensin-converting-enzyme inhibitors; *ARB* angiotensin receptor blocker

these medications as they relate to the patient's individual CHD and gender expression goals.

Perioperative management of gender-affirming surgery in patients with ACHD should generally be approached using the same framework as all non-cardiac surgeries as previously described. Of particular importance is discussing with the patient the risks and benefits of continuing estrogen therapy perioperatively. Such decisions should be made jointly with the patient and in consultation with their ACHD specialist based on individual thromboembolic risk.

## Genetic Screening

An identifiable genetic or environmental cause is found in approximately 20–30% of cases of CHD, with chromosomal abnormalities identified in approximately 10% of infants with CHD [3, 4, 48]. Common associated syndromes include DiGeorge syndrome, Down syndrome, Holt-Oram syndrome, Klinefelter syndrome, Noonan Syndrome, Turner syndrome, and Williams syndrome [11]. For patients with CHD, defining a genetic cause may help identify other organ systems at risk for complications, may provide prognostic information, and may help clarify the risk of CHD in their offspring and other family members [49, 50]. Guidelines suggest genetic evaluation of patients with CHD, especially complex CHD, and genetic risk factors [51, 52]. Guidelines for older ACHD reinforce the importance of such screening and highlight the need to consider re-evaluating patients periodically as new genetic tests become available and new syndromes are recognized [5]. In general, guidelines call for a thorough history and physical exam to identify any non-cardiac manifestations of possible syndromes and a detailed, three-generation family history with attention to CHD and other birth defects, consanguinity, and spontaneous abortions. PCPs should work closely with ACHD cardiologists and, when available, cardiovascular geneticists to ensure that ACHD with genetic risks is offered genetic counseling and genetic testing and that the results of such testing are integrated into their overall care.

## Infective Endocarditis Prophylaxis

The use of antibiotics for the prevention of infective endocarditis (IE) must balance the risk reduction of IE from antibiotics against the risk of adverse reactions to antibiotics and the development of antibiotic-resistant organisms. ACHD may be at higher risk for developing IE and at higher risk for adverse outcomes from IE. In the general population, the incidence of IE after dental procedures is less than 1 per 100,000. For patients with predisposing conditions, the incidence is 9 per 100,000. In this population, pre-procedural antibiotics reduce this risk to ~2/100,000 [53]. CHD is present in 11–13% of cases of IE [54]. However, studies of adults with certain congenital heart lesions have found the incidence of IE to be 35 times higher than that of the general population [55]. It is therefore critical to recognize the conditions and lesions that place a patient at increased risk for IE. Table 27.5 presents the cardiac conditions that are associated with the highest risk of IE or adverse events from IE [25, 56]. Prior IE and a history of heart transplant can be obtained by a thorough medical history. Residual defects near patches or prosthetic devices tend to have high velocity jets, resulting in easily audible murmurs. Prosthetic valves and prosthetic materials used in valve repairs also produce characteristic murmurs. Therefore, a patient's likelihood of having a high-risk condition for IE and need for additional workup can easily be assessed by the PCP through a careful history and physical exam.

An appreciation of high-risk conditions and lesions will help guide the PCP in prescribing appropriate prophylactic antibiotics, expediting treatment of possible sources of IE and raising the index of suspicion for patients presenting with clinical features of IE.

The appropriate prophylactic antibiotics for infective endocarditis are based primarily on the patient's allergies. Table 27.5 also shows the recommended regimens for antibiotic prophylaxis for dental procedures in adults. The 2007 American Heart Association guidelines advise the use of these antibiotics in patients at high risk for IE prior to dental procedures [56]. Their use prior

**Table 27.5** Recommendations for primary and secondary prevention of infective endocarditis

| High-risk lesions for which IE prophylaxis with dental procedures is reasonable | Regiments for antibiotic prophylaxis for dental procedures in adults[a] | Procedures where antibiotic prophylaxis is indicated |
|---|---|---|
| Prosthetic cardiac valve or prosthetic material used for cardiac valve repair, including trans-catheter valve replacements | 1. Amoxicillin 2 g orally<br>2. Ampicillin 2 g IM/IV, cefazolin 1 g IM/IV, or ceftriaxone 1 g IM/IV if unable to take PO<br>3. Cephalexin 2 g or clindamycin 600 mg or azithromycin/clarithromycin 500 mg if allergic to PCN or ampicillin<br>4. Cefazolin, ceftriaxone, or clindamycin if allergic to PCN or ampicillin AND unable to take PO | Dental procedures (manipulation of gingiva or apical region of teeth, or mucosal perforation)) [22, 50]<br>Procedures involving infected skin/soft tissues (may need to modify antibiotic based on known/suspected pathogen)<br>Consider for incisions or biopsies through respiratory tissue (may need to modify antibiotic based on known/suspected pathogen)<br>Consider during complicated vaginal deliveries for patient with unrepaired cyanotic lesions or prosthetic valves [22] |
| Previous infective endocarditis | | |
| Congenital heart disease:<br>• Unrepaired cyanotic CHD, including palliative shunts and conduits<br>• Completely repaired congenital heart defect with prosthetic material or device, whether placed by surgery or by catheter intervention, during the first 6 months after the procedure<br>• Repaired CHD with residual defects at the site or adjacent to the site of a prosthetic device (which inhibit endothelialization) | | |
| Cardiac transplant recipients who develop cardiac valvulopathy | | |

*IE* infective endocarditis; *CHD* congenital heart disease; *PCN* penicillin

[a] All antibiotics to be given as a single dose 30–60 min prior to procedure. If missed, can be dosed up to 2 h post-procedure

to genitourinary procedures is no longer recommended. However, the 2008 American College of Cardiology/American Heart Association Guidelines for the Management of Adults with Congenital Heart Disease recommend considering IE prophylaxis with antibiotics in patients with prosthetic valves or unrepaired cyanotic CHD undergoing complex vaginal deliveries, despite lack of evidence of efficacy [25].

## Mental Health, Neurodevelopmental, and Cognitive Issues

The prevalence of mood and anxiety disorders among ACHD is higher than the general population, and there remains a large gap in appropriate treatment [57, 58]. Untreated anxiety and depression can have a significant impact on quality of life and has been shown to increase healthcare utilization in inpatient, outpatient, and emergency settings as well as increased comorbidities and mortality among ACHD [59, 60]. Studies also show that mood disorders increase rates of nonadherence, which can have a detrimental impact on the health of patients with ACHD [59]. Screening for mental health disorders, including substance use disorders, in those with ACHD should be a priority for PCPs, keeping in mind that these patients face significant challenges, including early mortality concerns, adjustment to new therapies such as implanted cardiac devices or upcoming surgeries, physical limitations, and challenges regarding the transition from pediatric to adult care. The risk of mood and anxiety disorders is amplified by a patient's perceived health status, not necessarily the clinician's assessment of their health status, thus making it imperative to screen all patients with ACHD [57]. Neurodevelopmental disorders, due to underlying genetic syndromes or related to complex surgical repairs, are at times undiagnosed in childhood and should therefore be considered by adult clinicians. Additionally, the risk of dementia, including early-onset dementia, is significantly higher in ACHD compared to the general population [61]. PCPs should feel empowered to treat or to refer for psychotherapy or pharmacotherapy in patients diagnosed with mental health disorders.

## Inpatient Considerations

As the population of ACHD increases, so too do the number of inpatient admissions of ACHD [62, 63]. The increase is in large part due to the increased age and complexity of this patient population as well as an increase in comorbidities, such as hypertension and diabetes. However, the number of admissions in patients with simple lesions is also on the rise [62]. A significant number of patients are present in emergency settings, particularly after a period of inconsistent cardiac care. This often occurs during the transition from pediatric to adult care [62]. This transition period is also a time of decentralization of care from large centers, where the majority of pediatric cardiac and surgical care occurs, to the spectrum of small to large centers where ACHD receive their care [63, 64]. Although the AHA/ACC Guideline for Management of Adults with Congenital Heart Disease recommends care at centers experienced in congenital heart disease for those with complex disease, many patients present in emergency settings or seek care locally [11, 65].

The majority of admissions among ACHD are for cardiovascular reasons, including arrhythmia, congestive heart failure, valve disease, and cerebrovascular accidents [62, 65]. Other important causes include pulmonary hypertension, pregnancy, and respiratory disorders [62, 63]. Compared to adults without CHD admitted for heart failure, those with CHD experience longer lengths of stay, increased invasive procedures, and increased risk of in-hospital mortality [65]. Clinicians should be cognizant of these increased risks despite the younger age of the population and consider early utilization of resources in physical therapy, occupational therapy, and nutrition while the patient is hospitalized.

ACHD is at increased risk for arrhythmia compared to the general population, particularly certain sub-groups, such as patients with single ventricle physiology. Monitoring telemetry is therefore important while in the hospital when electrolyte derangements and fluid shifts commonly occur. Maintaining appropriate serum electrolyte levels can also help reduce the risk of arrhythmia.

Additional considerations during patient care of ACHD include careful attention to prevention of venous thromboembolism, particularly among those at increased risk of stroke due to atrial-level shunting or right-to-left shunting of blood. For patients with baseline cyanosis, meticulous de-airing of intravenous lines should be performed to prevent cerebral air emboli.

Inpatient hospitalizations can provide a unique opportunity for educating patients about their heart disease and the importance of routine cardiac care. Providers should screen for mental health disorders and medication nonadherence that may contribute to hospital re-admission. Finally, many ACHD have post-traumatic stress disorder related to medical therapies in childhood [61]. Hospitalization may be triggering for these individuals and extra support from social work, chaplaincy, or family should be considered throughout their admission.

## Conclusion

The primary care of ACHD requires a patient-centered approach that considers the presence of any associated syndrome or chromosomal abnormality, the complexity of the underlying CHD lesion, and the chronological and developmental age of the patient (see Appendix). The role of the PCP in caring for ACHD is to partner with and advocate for the patient in understanding his or her heart and the individualized care required.

## Appendix

<table>
<tr><th colspan="3">Adult Congenital Heart Disease (ACHD) fact sheet</th></tr>
<tr><td>Definition</td><td colspan="2">Congenital heart disease (CHD) refers to a wide range of structural defects of the heart and major blood vessels that are present at birth</td></tr>
<tr><td>Epidemiology</td><td colspan="2">• The prevalence of congenital heart disease at birth ranges from 6 to 13 per 1000 live births<br>• There are more than 1.2 million adults with congenital heart disease (ACHD) in the United States<br>– 50% of ACHD had a moderate-to-severe complexity heart lesion at birth.<br>– The total ACHD population is growing at a rate of approximately 5% per year</td></tr>
<tr><td rowspan="6">Special considerations</td><td colspan="2">ACHD are at risk for complications from their underlying CHD and often require special management for acquired CV risks</td></tr>
<tr><td>Common complications of CHD:<br>• Heart failure<br>• Arrhythmia<br>• Vascular complications<br>• Sudden death</td><td>Cardiovascular risk factors requiring special management:<br>• Diabetes<br>• Hyperlipidemia<br>• Hypertension</td></tr>
<tr><td colspan="2">Perioperative management of ACHD should include traditional revised cardiac risk index (RCRI) assessments and consideration of the patient's CHD (anatomy AND physiology) and any associated syndromes<br>• Consideration should be given to managing patients with high-risk lesions in a center specialized in perioperative care for patients with ACHD</td></tr>
<tr><td colspan="2">Sexual and reproductive health:<br>• Thrombotic risk should be assessed when considering estrogen-containing medications for contraception, the management of perimenopausal symptoms, or in gender-affirming care<br>• ACHD should be assessed for sexual dysfunction in the context of their overall development, the severity of their underlying cardiac lesion, and any ongoing cardiovascular therapies</td></tr>
<tr><td colspan="2">Genetic screening:<br>• An identifiable genetic or environmental cause is found in approximately 20–30% of cases of congenital heart disease<br>• All ACHD with genetic risks should be offered genetic counseling and genetic testing</td></tr>
<tr><td colspan="2">Prevention of infective endocarditis (IE):<br>• High-risk lesions for IE particularly to ACHD include unrepaired cyanotic CHD, repaired lesions within the first 6 months post-procedure, and repaired lesions with residual defects at or adjacent to the site of a prosthetic device</td></tr>
</table>

## References


1. Mussatto KA, Hoffmann RG, Hoffman GM, Tweddell JS, Bear L, Cao Y, Brosig C. Risk and prevalence of developmental delay in young children with congenital heart disease. Pediatrics. 2014;133(3):e570–7.
2. Yeung E, Kay J, Roosevelt GE, Brandon M, Yetman AT. Lapse of care as a predictor for morbidity in adults with congenital heart disease. Int J Cardiol. 2008;125(1):62–5.
3. Beauchesne LM, Warnes CA, Connolly HM, Ammash NM, Grogan M, Jalal SM, Michels VV. Prevalence and clinical manifestations of 22q11.2 microdeletion in adults with selected conotruncal anomalies. J Am Coll Cardiol. 2005;45:595–8.
4. Cowan JR, Stephanie MW. Genetics and genetic testing in congenital heart disease. Clin Perinatol. 2015;42:373–99.
5. Bhatt AB, Foster E, Kuehl K, Alpert J, Brabeck S, Crumb S, et al. On behalf of the American Heart Association Council on Clinical Cardiology. Congenital heart disease in the older adult: a scientific statement from the American Heart Association. Circulation. 2015;131:131.
6. Tanner K, Sabrine N, Wren C. Cardiovascular malformations among preterm infants. Pediatrics. 2005;116(6):e833–8.
7. Wren C, Irving CA, Griffiths JA, O'Sullivan JJ, Chaudhari MP, Haynes SR, et al. Mortality in infants with cardiovascular malformations. Eur J Pediatr. 2012;17(2):281.
8. Khoshnood B, Lelong N, Houyel, Thieulin AC, Jouannic JM, Magnier S, et al. Prevalence, timing of diagnosis and mortality of newborns with congenital heart defects: a population-based study. Heart. 2012;98(22):1667–73.
9. Warnes CA, Liberthson R, Danielson GK, Dore A, Harris L, Hoffman JI, et al. Task force 1: the changing profile of congenital heart disease in adult life. J Am Coll Cardiol. 2001;37:1170–5.
10. van der Bom T, Mulder BJ, Meijboom FJ, van Dijk AP, Pieper PG, Vliegen HW, Konings TC, Zwinderman AH, Bouma BJ. Contemporary survival of adults with congenital heart disease. Heart. 2015;101:19891995.
11. Stout KK, Daniels CJ, Aboulhosn J, Bozkurt B, Broberg CS, Colman JM, et al. 2018 AHA/ACC guideline for the management of adults with congenital heart disease: executive summary. J Am Coll Cardiol. 2019;73:1494–563.
12. Baumgartner H, De Backer J, Babu-Narayan SV, et al. 2020 ESC guidelines for the management of adult congenital heart disease. Eur Heart J. 2021;42(6):563–645.
13. Billett J, Cowie MR, Gatzoulis MA, Vonder Muhll IF, Majeed A. Comorbidity, healthcare utilization and process of care measures in patients with congenital heart disease in the UK: cross-sectional, population-based study with case–control analysis. Heart. 2008;94:1194–9.
14. Kenny D, Hijazi ZM. Coarctation of the aorta: from fetal life to adulthood. Cardiol J. 2011;18:487–95.
15. Flanagan MF, Hourihan M, Keane JF. Incidence of renal dysfunction in adults with cyanotic congenital heart disease. Am J Cardiol. 1991;68:403–6.
16. Perloff JK, Latta H, Barsotti P. Pathogenesis of the glomerular abnormality in cyanotic congenital heart disease. Am J Cardiol. 2000;86:1198–204.
17. Moons P, Van Deyk K, Dedroog D, Troost E, Budts W. Prevalence of cardiovascular risk factors in adults with congenital heart disease. Eur J Cardiovasc Prev Rehabil. 2006;13:612–6.
18. Gagliardi MG, Adorisio R, Crea F, Versacci P, Di Donato R, Sanders SP. Abnormal vasomotor function of the epicardial coronary arteries in children five to eight years after arterial switch operation: an angiographic and intracoronary Doppler flow wire study. J Am Coll Cardiol. 2005;46:1565–72.
19. Kondo C, Nakazawa M, Momma K, Kusakabe K. Sympathetic denervation and reinnervation after arterial switch operation for complete transposition. Circulation. 1998;97:2414–9.
20. Pasquali SK, Marino BS, Powell DJ, McBride MG, Paridon SM, Meyers KE, et al. Following the arterial switch operation, obese children have risk factors for early cardiovascular disease. Congenit Heart Dis. 2010;5:16–24.
21. Gilmanov D, Bevilacqua S, Mazzone A, Glauber M. Do statins slow the process of calcification of aortic tissue valves? Interact Cardiovasc Thorac Surg. 2010;11:297–301.
22. Paraskevas KI, Mikhailidis DP. Statins may not prevent structural valve degeneration of aortic bioprosthetic valves, but should probably be prescribed to patients undergoing heart valve surgery nonetheless. Interact Cardiovasc Thorac Surg. 2010;11:302.
23. Goldman L, Caldera DL, Nussbaum SR, Southwick FS, Krogstad D, Murray B, et al. Multifactorial index of cardiac risk in noncardiac surgical procedures. N Engl J Med. 1977;297(16):845–50.
24. Lee TH, Marcantonio ER, Mangione CM, Thomas EJ, Polanczyk CA, Cook EF, et al. Derivation and prospective validation of a simple index for prediction of cardiac risk of major noncardiac surgery. Circulation. 1999;100(10):1043–9.
25. Warnes CA, Williams RG, Bashore TM, Child JS, Connolly HM, Dearani JA, et al. ACC/AHA 2008 guidelines for the management of adults with congenital heart disease: a report of the American College of Cardiology/American Heart Association task force on practice guidelines (writing committee to develop guidelines for the management of adults with congenital heart disease). Circulation. 2008;118:e714–833.
26. Ammash NM, Connolly HM, Abel MD, Warnes CA. Noncardiac surgery in Eisenmenger syndrome. J Am Coll Cardiol. 1999;33:222–7.

27. Simko LC, McGinnis KA, Schembri J. Educational needs of adults with congenital heart disease. J Cardiovasc Nurs. 2006;21:85–94.
28. Graham TP Jr, Driscoll DJ, Gersony WM, Newburger JW, Rocchini A, Towbin JA. Task force 2: congenital heart disease. J Am Coll Cardiol. 2005;45:1326–33.
29. Driscoll DJ, Edwards WD. Sudden unexpected death in children and adolescents. J Am Coll Cardiol. 1985;5:118B–21B.
30. Garson AJ, McNamara DG. Sudden death in a pediatric cardiology population, 1958 to 1983: relation to prior arrhythmias. J Am Coll Cardiol. 1985;5:134B–7B.
31. Maron BJ. Sudden death in young athletes. N Engl J Med. 2003;349:1064–75.
32. Inuzuka R, Diller GP, Borgia F, Benson L, Tay EL, Alonso-Gonzalez R, et al. Comprehensive use of cardiopulmonary exercise testing identifies adults with congenital heart disease at increased mortality risk in the medium term. Circulation. 2012;125:250–9.
33. Van Hare GF, Ackerman MJ, Evangelista JK, et al. AHA/ACC scientific statement. Eligibility and disqualification recommendations for competitive athletes with cardiovascular abnormalities: task force 4: congenital heart disease. J Am Coll Cardiol. 2015;21:2372–84.
34. Van Hare GF, Ackerman MJ, Evangelista JAK, et al. Eligibility and disqualification recommendations for competitive athletes with cardiovascular abnormalities: task force 4: congenital heart disease: a scientific statement from the American Heart Association and American College of Cardiology. Circulation. 2015;132(22):e281–91.
35. Levine BD, Baggish AL, Kovacs RJ, et al. Eligibility and disqualification recommendations for competitive athletes with cardiovascular abnormalities: task force 1: classification of sports: dynamic, static, and impact: a scientific statement from the American Heart Association and American College of Cardiology. Circulation. 2015;132(22):e262–6.
36. Siu SC, Sermer M, Colman JM, Alvarez AN, Mercier LA, Morton BC, et al. Prospective multicenter study of pregnancy outcomes in women with heart disease. Circulation. 2001;104:515–21.
37. Vigl M, Kaemmerer M, Seifert-Klauss V, Niggemeyer E, Nagdyman N, Trigas V, et al. Contraception in women with congenital heart disease. Am J Cardiol. 2010;106(9):1317–21.
38. The Adult Congenital Heart Association. ACHA Q and A: birth control for women with congenital heart disease. 2008.
39. Berry-Bibee E, Curtis K, Dragoman M, Gaffield ML, Jatlaoui T, Kim C, et al. Medical eligibility criteria for contraceptive use. 5th ed. Geneva: The World Health Organization; 2015.
40. Silversides CK, Sermer M, Siu S. Choosing the best contraceptive method for the adult with congenital heart disease. Curr Cardiol Rep. 2009;11:298–305.
41. Santen RJ, Allred DC, Ardoin SP, Archer DF, Boyd N, Braunstein GD, et al. Endocrine Society. Postmenopausal hormone therapy: an Endocrine Society scientific statement. J Clin Endocrinol Metab. 2010;95(suppl 1):s1–66.
42. Canobbio MM, Perloff JK, Rapkin AJ. Gynecological health of females with congenital heart disease. Int J Cardiol. 2005;98:379–87.
43. Moons P, Van Deyk K, Marquet K, De Bleser L, Budts W, De Geest S. Sexual functioning and congenital heart disease: something to worry about? Int J Cardiol. 2007;121:30–5.
44. Levine GN, Steinke EE, Bakaeen FG, Bozkurt B, Cheitlin MD, Conti JB, et al. Sexual activity and cardiovascular disease: a scientific statement from the American Heart Association. Circulation. 2012;125:1058–72.
45. Vigl M, Kaemmerer M, Niggemeyer E, Nagdyman N, Seifert-Klauss V, Trigas V, et al. Sexuality and reproductive health in women with congenital heart disease. Am J Cardiol. 2010;105:538–41.
46. Cook SC, Arnott LM, Nicholson LM, Cook LR, Sparks EA, Daniels CJ. Erectile dysfunction in men with congenital heart disease. Am J Cardiol. 2008;102:1728–30.
47. Vigl M, Hager A, Bauer U, Niggemeyer E, Wittstock B, Köhn FM, et al. Sexuality and subjective wellbeing in male patients with congenital heart disease. Heart. 2009;95:1179–83.
48. Hartman RJ, Rasmussen SA, Botto LD, et al. The contribution of chromosomal abnormalities to congenital heart defects: a population-based study. Pediatr Cardiol. 2011;32:1147–57.
49. Burchill L, Greenway S, Silversides CK, Mital S. Genetic counseling in the adult with congenital heart disease: what is the role? Curr Cardiol Rep. 2011;13:347–55.
50. Cowan J, Morales A, Dagua J, Hershberger RE. Genetic testing and genetic counseling in cardiovascular genetic medicine: overview and preliminary recommendations. Congest Heart Fail. 2008;14:97–105.
51. Pierpont ME, Basson CT, Benson DW Jr, Gelb BD, Giglia TM, Goldmuntz E, et al. Genetic basis for congenital heart defects: current knowledge: a scientific statement from the American Heart Association congenital cardiac defects committee, council on cardiovascular disease in the young. Circulation. 2007;115:3015–38.
52. Silversides CK, Marelli A, Beauchesne L, Dore A, Kiess M, Salehian O, et al. Canadian cardiovascular society 2009 consensus conference on the management of adults with congenital heart disease: executive summary. Can J Cardiol. 2010;26:143–50.
53. Duval X, Alla F, Hoen B, Danielou F, Larrieu S, Delahaye F, et al. Estimated risk of endocarditis in adults with predisposing cardiac conditions undergo-

ing dental procedures with or without antibiotic prophylaxis. Clin Infect Dis. 2006;42:e102.
54. van der Meer JT, Thompson J, Valkenburg HA, Michel MF. Epidemiology of bacterial endocarditis in The Netherlands, I. Patient characteristics. Arch Intern Med. 1992;152:1863–8.
55. Hayes CJ, Gersony WM, Driscoll DJ, Keane JF, Kidd L, O'Fallon WM, et al. Second natural history study of congenital heart defects. Results of treatment of patients with pulmonary valvar stenosis. Circulation. 1993;87(suppl 2):I28–37.
56. Wilson W, Taubert KA, Gewitz M, Lockhart PB, Baddour LM, Levison M, et al. Prevention of infective endocarditis: guidelines from the American Heart Association: a guideline from the American Heart Association Rheumatic Fever, Endocarditis, and Kawasaki Disease Committee, Council on Cardiovascular Disease in the Young, and the Council on Clinical Cardiology, Council on Cardiovascular Surgery and Anesthesia, and the Quality of Care and Outcomes Research Interdisciplinary Working Group. Circulation. 2007;116:1736–54.
57. Kovacs AH, Saidi AS, Kuhl EA, Sears SF, Silversides C, Harrison JL, et al. Depression and anxiety in adult congenital heart disease: predictors and prevalence. Int J Cardiol. 2009;137:158–64.
58. Westhoff-Bleck M, Briest J, Fraccarollo D, Hilfiker-Kleiner D, Winter L, Maske U, et al. Mental disorders in adults with congenital heart disease: unmet needs and impact on quality of life. J Affect Disord. 2016;204:180–6.
59. Benderly M, Kalter-Leibovici O, Weitzman D, Blieden L, Buber J, Dadashey A, et al. Depression and anxiety are associated with high health care utilization and mortality among adults with congenital heart disease. Int J Cardiol. 2019;276:81–6.
60. Desai R, Patel K, Dave H, Shah K, DeWitt N, Fong HK, et al. Nationwide frequency, sequential trends, and impact of co-morbid mental health disorders on hospitalizations, outcomes, and healthcare resource utilization in adult congenital heart disease. Am J Cardiol. 2020;125:1256–62.
61. Jacobsen RM. Outcomes in adult congenital heart disease: neurocognitive issues and transition of care. Pediatr Clin N Am. 2020;67:963–71.
62. Agarwal S, Sud K, Menon V. Nationwide trends in adult congenital heart disease across 2003–2012. J Am Heart Assoc. 2016;5:e002330.
63. Opotowsky AR, Siddiqi OK, Webb GD. Trends in hospitalizations for adults with congenital heart disease in the U.S. J Am Coll Cardiol. 2009;54:460–7.
64. Gurvitz MZ, Inkelas M, Lee M, Stout K, Escarce J, Chang R. Changes in hospitalization patterns among patients with congenital heart disease during the transition from adolescence to adulthood. J Am Coll Cardiol. 2007;49:875–82.
65. Nitloudi D, Dimopoulos K, Tzifa A, Karvounis H, Giannakoulas G. Hospitalizations in adult patients with congenital heart disease: an emerging challenge. Heart Fail Rev. 2021;26:347–53.

## Resources

### General Resources

Congenital Heart Disease Clinic Directory. Includes a listing of centers designated as an Adult Congenital Heart Disease Clinic. https://www.cardiosmart.org/Heart-Conditions/Congenital-Heart-Defects/CHD.

The International Society for Adults with Congenital Heart Disease. http://isachd.org.

### Clinical Guidelines and Scientific Statements

### General Guidelines

2018 AHA/ACC guideline for the management of adults with congenital heart disease. https://doi.org/10.1161/CIR.0000000000000603.

2020 ESC guidelines for the management of adult congenital heart disease. https://www.escardio.org/Guidelines/Clinical-Practice-Guidelines/Grown-Up-Congenital-Heart-Disease-Management-of.

AHA Scientific Statement. Congenital heart disease in the older adult. http://circ.ahajournals.org/content/early/2015/04/20/CIR.0000000000000204.full.pdf.

AHA/ACC guideline for the management of patients with valvular heart disease. https://doi.org/10.1161/CIR.0000000000000923.

American Heart Association. Guidelines for the prevention of infective endocarditis. https://www.heart.org/en/health-topics/infective-endocarditis.

British Society for Antimicrobial Chemotherapy. Guidelines for the prevention of infective endocarditis. http://jac.oxfordjournals.org/content/57/6/1035.full.pdf.

Report of the National Heart, Lung, and Blood Institute Working Group on Research in Adult Congenital Heart Disease. https://pubmed.ncbi.nlm.nih.gov/16487831/.

### Physical Activity

AHA Scientific Statement. Promotion of physical activity for children and young adults with congenital heart disease. http://circ.ahajournals.org/content/127/21/2147.full.pdf.

### Reproductive Health

AHA Scientific Statement. Sexual activity and cardiac health. https://doi.org/10.1161/CIR.0b013e3182447787.

World Health Organization. Medical eligibility criteria for contraceptive use. https://www.who.int/publications/i/item/9789241549158.

## Genetic Resources

Information on labs for gene testing. www.genetest.org.
National Institutes of Health Genetics Home Reference. Congenital heart disease. https://medlineplus.gov/genetics/condition/critical-congenital-heart-disease/.
Online mendelian inheritance in man. http://www.omim.org.

## Patient Resources

Adult Congenital Heart Association. "For the patient". https://doi.org/10.1161/CIR.0000000000000603.
Adult Congenital Heart Association. Free printable handouts of specific conditions: https://www.achaheart.org/your-heart/resources/download-materials/.
Adult Congenital Heart Association. Q and A—birth control for women with congenital heart disease. https://www.uclahealth.org/sites/default/files/documents/birthcontrolforchd.pdf.
American Heart Association. Conditions: congenital defects, adults and children. https://www.heart.org/en/health-topics/congenital-heart-defects.
Insurance and the Affordable Care Act. https://www.healthcare.gov/glossary/affordable-care-act/

# Cystic Fibrosis

# 28

Christine M. Bojanowski, Ross C. Klingsberg, and Michael Landry

## Case Presentation

Dillon T., a 19-year-old young man, presents for his initial visit to establish care with an adult primary care physician. Although he plans to attend a Cystic Fibrosis Foundation-accredited care center, he recognizes that he needs a physician closer to home as he lives 3 h away from the nearest cystic fibrosis (CF) center. Dillon was diagnosed with CF shortly after birth secondary to meconium ileus. His sweat chloride test result was 105 mmol/L, and his genotype is homozygous Phe508del. Up until this visit, Dillon was treated by a pediatric pulmonologist for his health care. His parents are divorced, and Dillon has been cared for by his mother. He has completed high school and will be starting college in the fall close to home but will be living on campus. He is 1 year delayed in his education secondary to multiple hospitalizations that necessitated his starting kindergarten a year later. At that time, he required a percutaneous endoscopic gastrostomy (PEG) tube for supplemental feeding as he was severely underweight. The PEG tube has since been removed, and his weight has improved on oral pancreatic enzyme supplementation.

His past medical history is also significant for complications related to CF, namely pneumothorax at age 17 years. This required chest tube placement but was resolved without further intervention. When he goes to the beach with family and friends, he is self-conscious about the surgical scars on his chest and abdomen.

Dillon is prescribed daily airway clearance therapy consisting of the following inhaled medications via a nebulizer: a short-acting bronchodilator, hypertonic saline (7%), dornase alpha, and an antipseudomonal antibiotic. He also has a pneumatic oscillating vest (a.k.a. "The Vest"), which he uses for chest physiotherapy. He has a daily cough, worse in the morning upon awakening, which produces yellow/green sputum. He admits to intermittent noncompliance with performing his airway clearance therapy twice daily as prescribed. He says that he

C. M. Bojanowski
Department of Medicine, Tulane University School of Medicine, New Orleans, LA, USA
e-mail: cbojanowski@tulane.edu

R. C. Klingsberg (✉)
Department of Medicine, Tulane University School of Medicine, New Orleans, LA, USA

Department of Internal Medicine, Southeast Louisiana Veterans Healthcare System and Tulane University School of Medicine, New Orleans, LA, USA
e-mail: rklingsb@tulane.edu

M. Landry
Department of Internal Medicine, Southeast Louisiana Veterans Healthcare System and Tulane University School of Medicine, New Orleans, LA, USA
e-mail: mlandry@tulane.edu


A. A. Kuo et al. (eds.), *Care of Adults with Chronic Childhood Conditions*,
https://doi.org/10.1007/978-3-031-54281-7_28

has better adherence on school days. He frequently oversleeps and skips treatments when his routine is unstructured on holidays, during the summer, and on the weekends. He is admitted for intravenous (IV) antibiotics once or twice per year for exacerbations of his CF-related bronchiectasis. Sputum cultures have shown methicillin-resistant *Staphylococcus aureus* (MRSA) and *Pseudomonas aeruginosa,* and screening for nontuberculous mycobacterial respiratory infections has been negative. He takes azithromycin, 500 mg, three times per week year-round.

He takes pancreatic enzyme replacement therapy with meals to treat exocrine pancreatic insufficiency. Dillon almost never forgets this medication because without pancreatic enzymes he suffers severe gastrointestinal discomfort and produces oily foul-smelling stools. He has occasionally required osmotic laxatives for constipation. Dillon was also found to have glucose intolerance on an oral glucose tolerance test (OGTT) performed last year. He does not take insulin. He has a congenital bilateral absence of the vas deferens (CBAVD). He has had unprotected sex on multiple occasions because he has been told that male CF patients are infertile. He has tried smoking tobacco and vaping e-cigarettes on a few occasions with his friends but noticed that he suffered dyspneic episodes afterward. He reports occasional alcohol intake but denies binge drinking.

He recently started taking triple protein modulator therapy (elexacaftor–tezacaftor–ivacaftor). He has since noted an increase in his weight and improved cough, energy, and exercise tolerance. While he is happy with this new medication, these improvements have made him anxious about his future. He is noting increased insomnia and is scoring higher in the clinic on anxiety and depression screens.

He emphasizes his hope that he will be able to establish an adult-oriented practice, as his pediatric provider has told him he now needs to start seeing an adult provider. He admits that he was quite apprehensive about making this appointment and has canceled several prior appointments due to anxiety over this transition.

## Case Discussion

Dillon has a classic presentation of cystic fibrosis (CF, "Appendix") [1]. He also has the most common genetic cause of CF, two copies of F508del (a.k.a. Phe508del), a deletion of the amino acid phenylalanine at position 508 of the cystic fibrosis transmembrane conductance regulator (CFTR) protein. More than 2100 variations in the CFTR gene have been discovered. Of those, approximately 400 CFTR variants have been identified as pathogenic, meaning that if an individual has one of these mutations on each chromosome inherited from his or her parents, he or she will have CF disease and symptoms (https://cftr2.org).

The remaining mutations vary across a spectrum of CF and CFTR-related disease presentations and symptom manifestations. They may cause CF with a full spectrum of symptoms, CF with variable symptoms, milder forms of CF, or have no effect or association with CF [2]. The clinical spectrum for symptom manifestation in CF ranges from asymptomatic individuals to chronic rhinosinusitis to male infertility to the symptoms classically associated with CF.

The diagnosis of CF is often made soon after birth when there is no meconium passed. As Dillon's case illustrates, abdominal distention, feeding intolerance, and vomiting appear, suggesting a meconium ileus. This is a common initial presentation for patients with CF and occurs in approximately 20% of newborns that are eventually diagnosed with CF by the sweat chloride test, which is considered the gold standard for diagnosis [3].

Pancreatic dysfunction causes both endocrine and exocrine symptom manifestations in CF patients. Dillon has been diagnosed with CF-related diabetes (CFRD). It is important for primary care physicians to recognize CFRD as the most common comorbidity in people with CF, occurring in ~20% of adolescents and 40–50% of adults. Appropriate screening and workup for symptoms related to diabetes presentation should be considered in CF patients [4].

While CFRD shares features of type 1 and type 2 diabetes mellitus, CFRD is a distinct clinical entity. It is primarily caused by insulin insufficiency, although fluctuating levels of insulin resistance related to acute and chronic illness also play a role. Interestingly, there are no documented cases of death from atherosclerotic vascular disease in patients with CFRD despite the fact that some patients with CFRD now live into their sixth and seventh decades [5].

The diagnosis of CFRD is made by performing an oral glucose tolerance test (OGTT): measurement of fasting glucose followed by a 75-gram glucose challenge and a 2-h post-challenge plasma glucose measurement. A plasma glucose ≥200 mg/dL is diagnostic of CF-related diabetes. Dillon's glucose tolerance test result was a glucose level of 285 mg/dL. The hemoglobin A1c (HgA1c) test is not sufficiently sensitive for diagnosis of CFRD and thus should not be used as a screening test. A HgA1C level <6.5% does not rule out CFRD because this value is often spuriously low in CF patients. However, a HgA1C ≥6.5% does confirm the diagnosis of CFRD. Furthermore, a fasting plasma glucose ≥126 mg/dL will also confirm the diagnosis [5].

Dillon's history is also notable for the presence of a pneumothorax. This complication, along with hemoptysis, is more common among individuals with CF as compared to the general population, and specific guidelines exist for management. It is critical to note that pleurodesis, a therapy used to treat recurrent pneumothorax, may be deferred after a single pneumothorax in CF. Pleurodesis may have a negative effect on future candidacy for lung transplantation, which may be critical for extending Dillon's life expectancy [6].

Dillon is infertile, as are most men with CF. Naturally, men with CF are subject to the same sexually transmitted infections as men without CF, and safe sex practices are to be encouraged. If parenthood is desired, genetic counseling is advised, and spermatozoa can be surgically harvested by a urologist. Many men with CF elect to have sperm donated instead. Finally, it must be remembered and incorporated into counseling that women with CF remain fertile and may become pregnant without fertility treatment.

## Definition, Epidemiology, and Natural History of Cystic Fibrosis

The association between abnormal sweat chloride, salt loss, and illness in children was made in the nineteenth century as shown by the adage, "Woe to the child who tastes salty from a kiss on the brow, for he is cursed and soon must die." In 1938, Dorothy Anderson made the first association between pancreatic disease, lung disease, and intestinal disease. Dr. Anderson called the disease, "cystic fibrosis of the pancreas." She was the first to utilize pancreatic enzyme replacement therapy (PERT) to treat affected children [7].

In 1952, Paul di Sant'Agnese discovered abnormalities in sweat electrolytes that are associated with CF. A sweat test was subsequently developed and improved over the next decade. This test remains in widespread use for establishing the diagnosis of cystic fibrosis. In 1989, Francis Collins, Lap-Chee Tsui, and John R. Riordan discovered the first gene mutation for CF, F508del (see case discussion). The nomenclature for this mutation has evolved from "delta F508" to "F508del" to "Phe508del," with the latter being the most current and accurate terminology.

For a child to be born with CF, one gene with CFTR abnormalities must be inherited from each parent (CF gene homozygous). People carrying one gene for CF are clinically unaffected but carry the risk of passing on this gene to subsequent offspring (CF gene heterozygous). One out of 25–30 Caucasians is a carrier for a CF-causing gene mutation. CF is the most common lethal genetic mutation in persons of non-Latinx European descent [8].

It is important to recognize though that abnormalities in the CFTR gene can be found in all races and ethnic backgrounds. This recognition is of critical importance as non-White infants with CF carry mutations that are less likely to be identified on prenatal newborn screens, and thus, diagnoses are more likely to be missed at birth among these populations. Therefore, these individuals are diagnosed later in life as compared to their White counterparts. Furthermore, people with CF who identify as Black, Latinx, or Asian are over two times more likely to have failure to thrive and have nearly a twofold higher risk of death before the age of 18 years. Access to lung transplantation is also worse in these populations.

The cystic fibrosis transmembrane conductance regulator (CFTR) is in an epithelial cell surface chloride channel. Changes in CFTR function have the greatest deleterious effects on the respiratory tract and the pancreas in most patients. Cystic fibrosis causes bronchiectasis, and CF has become a paradigm for this condition. Bronchiectasis causes airflow obstruction and a chronic productive cough. Most patients who die from complications of CF do so because of respiratory failure.

The life expectancy for patients living with CF has increased dramatically secondary to therapeutic advances in nutrition, pancreatic enzyme replacement therapy, inhaled airway clearance therapy (mucolytics), anti-inflammatory medications, and aggressive use of antibiotic therapy. In 1970, the median predicted survival was 16 years. Today, the median predicted survival is 50 years of age. Many of the CFTR variants can now be targeted by highly effective modulator therapy (HEMT). There are currently four different CFTR protein modulator therapies available. These drugs, which are primarily given in combination, work by helping the CFTR protein form the correct three-dimensional shape so that it can successfully traffic to the cell surface ("correctors") or by binding to the defective protein at the cell surface and improving the activity of the chloride channel ("potentiators"). These treatments, which were introduced into the market within the past 10 years and are prescribed only through specialists, have been shown to improve lung function (using forced expiratory volume in 1 s [$FEV_1$] as a surrogate), decrease pulmonary exacerbations, decrease sweat chloride levels, and improve weight and quality of life. An increase in survival has led to many patients needing to transition their care from pediatric providers to adult physicians including primary care and specialists [9].

Currently, there are approximately 31,000 patients within the United States and 70,000 worldwide living with CF. Most of the patients in the United States participate in the CF Foundation's Data Registry [1]. Patient information is collected by CF care centers that are accredited by the CF Foundation (CFF). There are more than 130 CF care centers that form a nationwide network. These centers are held accountable for informing best practices and infection-control guidelines (https://www.cff.org/medical-professionals/clinical-care-guidelines).

## Care of Cystic Fibrosis and Associated Medical Conditions

### Overview

The routine care of CF is best provided by one of the nationwide CFF-accredited care centers. Many of the medications require experience with prescribing, prior authorization from third-party payers, and specialty pharmacy dispensing. The time and costs involved in the provision of these services would be prohibitive to a clinic that sees an occasional CF patient. The current guidelines for CF-specific care include quarterly clinic visits with the submission of sputum samples for analysis via specialized CF culture and pulmonary function testing. All accredited CF care centers have multidisciplinary care teams that include physicians, nurses, social workers, dietitians, respiratory therapists, and clinical coordinators. Another key service delivered by accredited CF centers is the collection of data that is included in the CF Foundation Registry. This is a valuable resource for tracking the CF population as a whole, leading to improved clinical care delivery and population health management. Lastly, CF centers are at the center of clinical trials and play a critical role in ground-breaking drug development. A list of current clinical trials in CF can be found online at https://apps.cff.org/trials/finder.

The development of the care center network by the CFF occurred in the early 1960s. These centers were established to ensure the rapid adoption of new CF therapies and developments by providers to maximize care for CF patients. In addition to providing care, these centers serve as a focus for CF clinical trials, where new CF therapeutics are first introduced. It is in the best interest of patients with CF to be seen regularly at CFF-accredited care centers [10].

Primary care physicians (PCPs) play an important role in the lives of patients with CF. Even medium-to-large CF care centers do not have daily clinics. As mentioned, some patients live far from CF care centers. Since many of the CF care needs are chronic and recurring, a primary care clinic visit may be able to address problems early and prevent hospitalization (Table 28.1) [11]. Some examples would be helping with adherence issues, treating minor gastrointestinal disturbances such as constipation, and initiating oral antibiotics for mild exacerbations.

## Respiratory System

In CF, the respiratory tract secretions lining the airways are thicker than normal. In fact, the alternate name for CF, "mucoviscidosis," is more descriptive of the underlying pathophysiology of this disease. Most current therapies are aimed at mobilizing the thick airway secretions and decreasing the overgrowth of characteristic bacteria. A typical CF airway clearance regimen starts with a bronchodilator. All patients with bronchiectasis have airflow obstruction, and the current thinking is that subsequent therapies are most effective if they are preceded by a bronchodilator such as albuterol.

Following administration of a bronchodilator, 4 mL of 7% hypertonic saline is inhaled by nebulization. This agent is inexpensive and is an effective way of drawing water from the lung interstitium into the surface layer of the airway. This will decrease the viscosity and allow easier expectoration of secretions by the patient. Current guidelines recommend hypertonic saline twice daily. Some patients find this therapy highly effective and utilize it more frequently. Nebulized hypertonic saline twice daily has been shown to decrease the frequency of exacerbations and improve pulmonary function in terms of forced vital capacity (FVC) and forced expiratory volume in 1 s ($FEV_1$) [12]. Unfortunately, a small number of patients do not tolerate 7% hypertonic saline because of bronchospasm or cough. In these patients, 3% hypertonic saline or isotonic 0.9% saline can be utilized. Inhaled mannitol, a mucoactive hyperosmotic agent, has also been approved by the U.S. Food and Drug Administration (FDA) as an add-on therapy in CF and is another alternative means to hydrate the airways.

**Table 28.1** Fundamentals of chronic cystic fibrosis therapy

| Airway clearance | Antimicrobials | Nutrition | CFTR modulation |
|---|---|---|---|
| Physical vibration<br>• Manual percussion<br>• Oscillating vest<br>• Flutter valve<br>• Vigorous exercise | • Nebulized tobramycin (alternate months)<br>• Aztreonam lysine<br>• Colistimethate | • High-caloric/high-salt diet<br>• Fat-soluble vitamin supplementation (A, D, E, and K) | Genotype-specific oral medications<br>• Ivacaftor<br>• Lumacaftor/ivacaftor<br>• Tezacaftor/ivacaftor<br>• Elexacaftor/tezacaftor/ivacaftor |
| Surface hydration<br>• Inhaled hypertonic saline<br>• Mannitol inhalation powder | • Oral azithromycin (anti-inflammatory) | | |
| Mucolysis<br>• Dornase alfa | • Aggressive antibiotic therapy for exacerbations | | |

Modified with permission from Boyle [11]
Not all patients will perform all therapies listed. Treatments are individualized

Most patients with CF take a mucolytic agent: dornase alfa. This nebulized enzymatic solution cleaves the long nucleic acid chains that accumulate in the mucosal layer from lysed neutrophils found in purulent sputum. It is taken once or twice daily. Combining nebulized medications is not advisable because it dilutes the concentration of the solutions and decreases effectiveness. Unlike hypertonic saline, dornase alpha is not associated with bronchospasm.

All patients with CF should participate in some form of vigorous exercise. This not only helps mobilize respiratory secretions but also helps to strengthen the overall musculature, leading to increased efficiency of the cough. Patients with CF experience all the benefits of exercise that non-CF patients experience, and this should be encouraged at all clinical encounters.

Many patients with CF, however, do not exercise regularly. Alternative airway clearance therapies are frequently used. These include active cycle breathing techniques; high-frequency pneumatic chest wall oscillation devices (such as "The Vest"); Acapella (flutter) valves, which create a vibrating column of air upon forceful exhalation; and manual chest physical therapy. All of these modalities seek to apply vibrating energy to the airways to help mobilize secretions for expectoration. Evidence is limited in supporting one modality above another; thus, what works best for an individual patient is what should be encouraged regularly [13].

Following the airway clearance techniques, patients with pseudomonas colonization often take a nebulized antipseudomonal antibiotic. Currently, there are commercially available nebulized forms of tobramycin and aztreonam in widespread use among CF patients. Specialized pharmacies may create nebulized forms of colistin and amikacin, although these are less commonly used. Nebulized antibiotics are taken after hypertonic saline and dornase alfa.

Since bronchiectasis is an obstructive disease, many patients with CF also take asthma medications such as long-acting beta-agonists and inhaled corticosteroids. Making a distinction between the obstruction of asthma and the obstruction of bronchiectasis may be difficult and may only be a matter of semantics, as the treatments for airflow obstruction are the same in both conditions [14]. Patients are encouraged to take their inhaled medications in the following order: bronchodilator, hypertonic saline, dornase alfa, inhaled antibiotics, and long-acting beta-agonists/inhaled corticosteroids (if prescribed).

## Gastrointestinal System

The gastrointestinal system can be severely affected despite the use of pancreatic enzyme replacement therapy (PERT). Patients may suffer from mild to severe functional bowel disorders and from mild to severe liver cirrhosis.

Adult patients with CF have frequent episodes of diarrhea alternating with constipation and/or the distal intestinal obstruction syndrome (DIOS). Constipation refers to the inability to evacuate the colon, whereas DIOS refers to the inability to evacuate the distal small intestine. Both constipation and DIOS may require hospitalization for IV fluids, nasogastric suctioning, anti-emetics, pain control, and aggressive use of osmotic cathartic agents such as polyethylene glycol to help relieve bowel obstruction.

When CF patients present with acute abdominal pain, physicians must consider a broad differential diagnosis, which includes complications such as intussusception. PERT is not without risk. Fibrosing colonopathy and colonic strictures are associated with the prolonged use of high doses of lipase supplementation. Patients present with signs and symptoms of DIOS as described above and may require operative intervention. To avoid complications such as this, the CFF recommends that PERT doses not exceed 2500 lipase units/kg/meal. As with the general population, gallbladder disease and acute appendicitis are common causes of acute abdominal symptoms that should be considered.

The complications from cirrhosis are like the complications from other causes of chronic liver disease and include the complications of portal hypertension: esophageal varices, splenomegaly, thrombocytopenia, and gastrointestinal bleeding.

It is now widely recognized that there is a significantly increased incidence of gastrointestinal malignancies in the CF population, particularly in patients with CF-related diabetes mellitus and in those who have received transplantations. Based on available data from the CFF Patient Registry, the median age of colorectal cancer in people with CF is up to 20–30 years younger as compared to the general public. At this time, the recommendation of the CFF is to initiate colonoscopy screening at age 40 with rescreening every 5 years. Screening should be initiated earlier in patients who have received lung transplantations and should be considered earlier in patients with CF-related diabetes. Many CF centers are now affiliated with gastroenterologists with specialized training and experience with CF to assist in managing CF-related gastrointestinal symptoms.

## Endocrine System

The incidence of CF-related diabetes (CFRD) increases with age, as was previously reviewed in the case discussion. CFRD should not be confused with type 1 diabetes mellitus. Unlike type 1 diabetics, most CF patients with diabetes can still produce insulin at a basal rate. Consequently, CF patients rarely experience diabetic ketoacidosis (DKA). If a CF patient presents with DKA, one should suspect coexisting type 1 diabetes mellitus.

CFRD is also different from type 2 diabetes mellitus. Patients with CF often suffer from protein–calorie malnutrition, and thus, insulin resistance is not observed as it is in type 2 diabetes mellitus. Therefore, patients with CFRD should not be restricted calorically as one would in the treatment of type 2 diabetes mellitus. In fact, a cornerstone of CF care is encouraging and promoting a high-calorie/high-protein diet. Most CF patients benefit from some form of caloric and nutritional medical food supplementation. Additionally, their diets should be supplemented with the fat-soluble vitamins (A, D, E, and K) due to malabsorption of these vitamins secondary to pancreatic insufficiency.

The treatment of CF-related diabetes starts with moderate aerobic exercise, maintaining a normal diet and monitoring blood glucose levels. Pharmacologic treatment consists of insulin therapy. Oral hypoglycemic agents should not be used in CF-related diabetes, as they are not as effective as insulin in improving nutritional and metabolic outcomes [4].

People with CF are also at increased risk for reduced bone mineral density, with some studies suggesting 50–75% of adults with CF have low bone density and increased rates of fractures. Several factors likely contribute to this risk, including malabsorption of vitamin D, physical inactivity, poor nutritional status, and glucocorticoid therapy [15]. Optimizing nutritional status is the priority for these patients. Several studies have looked at bisphosphonates in CF, and while this intervention has been shown to increase bone density, bisphosphonates have not been shown to reduce fracture risk in people with CF. PCPs can play a vital role in disease prevention by assisting patients in the prevention and treatment of these comorbidities.

## Acute Care

Unfortunately, since CF is a relatively rare disease, CF care centers often have ambulatory sessions only a few days per week and do not always have availability on the days when patients need to seek acute care. Patients with CF are subject to many of the same acute medical issues as people without CF. They need many of the same medical services that do not require specialized CF knowledge or treatment including preventive health care. Some examples include routine immunizations, testing for influenza or coronavirus disease 2019 (COVID-19), routine gynecologic care, and symptomatic treatment for acute medical issues. Ideally, a primary care physician would have an open-communication access to a CF care center particularly when antibiotics are being considered. It is also optimal for patients to be established with providers in the local healthcare system before needing acute interventions, as CF patients often have complicated medical histories and physical exam findings.

## Transplant Evaluation

When people with CF no longer experience clinical improvement with IV antibiotics or experience exacerbations at greater frequency and/or of greater severity, suffer complications of CF such as recurrent pneumothoraces or episodes of massive hemoptysis, become oxygen-dependent, or have $FEV_1$ measurements less than 30–35% of predicted, lung transplantation should be considered. Transplant criteria include an adequate social support system to ensure follow-up after hospital discharge and adherence to a complex treatment regimen. Certain infections, notably *Mycobacterium abscessus* and *Burkholderia cenocepacia*, are widely considered contraindications to lung transplantation, as patients tend to have much worse outcomes if these infections are present before transplantation. When patients undergo lung transplantation, they typically transfer care from CF specialists at CF centers to specialists at the lung transplant centers. These patients will still benefit from locally established primary, preventive, and acute care management, as the distance from their transplant center may be similarly far to that from the CF center.

## Primary and Preventive Care

Persons living with CF are subject to the same non-CF issues as the general population. Having a non-CF specialist general physician can be an asset to the patient and a rewarding collaboration for the physician. Patients who are located greater distances from CF centers often have the greatest need to find local primary care providers and non-CF specialists. Important primary and preventive care considerations among this patient population would be immunizations (including but not limited to pneumococcal, influenza, and COVID-19 as per evolving CDC recommendations), mammograms by the age of 40 per the American Cancer Society recommendations, colonoscopy screenings by the age of 40, and dual-energy X-ray absorptiometry tests (DEXA) to assess bone density every 1–5 years depending on the results as discussed above. Particularly for patients with CFRD, it is important to screen for complications such as retinopathy and renal disease and for common comorbidities such as hypertension.

## Medical and Mental Health Assessment

Living with CF creates tremendous physical, psychological, and financial burdens for patients and their families. Patients with CF are aware of their limited life expectancy. The treatments are expensive and time-consuming. Patients are afflicted with a chronic cough that may be disruptive to close personal contacts and in group settings such as classrooms. Exacerbations of bronchiectasis are unpredictable and may disrupt planned activities and employment. Extended hospital stays and frequent clinic visits can become part of a hopeless cycle for some. Disease progression often leads to decreased exercise tolerance and inability to complete activities of daily living.

Given the tremendous psychosocial burden this creates patients with CF are prone to anxiety, depression, and other psychological disorders such as sleep disturbance, substance abuse, and suicide. These issues fluctuate as patients transit from childhood into adolescence and adulthood. Dramatic differences exist between pediatric and adult healthcare systems including physical location, structure, patient responsibilities, and caregiver's mindsets. Physicians should be sure to screen for mental health issues in addition to treating the acute and chronic conditions associated with CF [16].

## Substance Abuse

The psychological burden of the disease is great, and persons with CF are susceptible to forming destructive dependencies on alcohol, sedatives, and analgesic drugs. The same defense and denial mechanisms may occur in the non-CF population. Thus, detecting illicit substance abuse and dependency requires a high level of suspicion. Irregular behaviors, difficulty answering and returning phone calls, noncompliance with medication regimens, complaints of sleep disturbances, or missed appointments may provide early clues to substance abuse issues. Avoidance of tobacco use and other inhalants such as marijuana and e-cigarettes is critical given the impact on the pulmonary system in these patients.

## Medication Management

CF centers are best suited to help patients manage the specialty medications and interventions used for CF. These include dornase alfa, nebulized antibiotics, pneumatic compression devices, and CFTR modulator. These new medications may only be prescribed by CF specialists and require prior authorization from third-party payers. However, the regimen does not change frequently, and primary physicians are well-suited to reinforce adherence to high-calorie/high-protein diet exercise and airway clearance therapy. Primary care providers can play a critical role in reinforcing the need for medication compliance.

## Reproductive Health

In general, men with cystic fibrosis are infertile, with rates estimated at 95% [17]. The abnormal CFTR gene causes the absence of the vas deferens during development. Women, on the other hand, remain fertile and must be counseled on appropriate prophylaxis if pregnancy is not desired. Men who desire children may have sperm harvested by a specialty urologist. Many patients seek assisted reproduction and utilize sperm donation. Adolescents and young adults need counseling on safe sex practices; this may need to be especially reinforced among male CF patients who may consider condom use less important given their low fertility rates. Pregnant female CF patients are considered high-risk and often require care by a high-risk obstetrician [18]. For women, routine gynecologic care is recommended. It has been suggested that there is an increased risk for women with CF to have cervical dysplasia. As with colorectal cancer, this risk is increased in those who have received transplantations [19, 20].

## Palliative Care

End-of-life care is individualized. Some patients are not eligible or choose not to undergo lung transplant evaluation. End-of-life considerations are best managed by the physician with the greatest rapport with the patient and family. This may be the CF multidisciplinary team, though the primary care provider may also be suited for engaging in this discussion. When CF progresses to respiratory failure and mechanical ventilation, the prognosis is uniformly poor. People with CF rarely recover from respiratory failure requiring mechanical ventilation. Thus, advance planning may prevent days on mechanical ventilation that create anxiety and discomfort for the patient and the family.

## Inpatient Issues: Coordinating Care with Cystic Fibrosis Specialists

Although most routine care can be handled by local physicians, there will be times when clinical conditions arise that necessitate specialty care by physicians trained in CF. Pulmonary complications of CF including bronchiectasis, hemoptysis, and pneumothoraces are life-threatening emergencies that require prompt attention by specialists. Hemoptysis and pneumothorax occur with greater frequency in the patients with CF as compared to the general population.

### Bronchiectasis

People with CF are prone to frequent exacerbations of bronchiectasis, and these episodes are best treated in care centers with experience treating CF. Exacerbations may occur several times per year in the most severely affected patients. Conversely, some people with CF rarely experience exacerbations. The frequency of exacerbations increases as the disease progresses. Based upon clinical trials and collective experience of experienced CF care physicians, exacerbations are best treated as aggressively as possible as soon as they are recognized. This usually includes either oral antibiotics for mild exacerbations or IV antibiotics for moderate to severe exacerbations. The choice of antibiotic should be based on the CF respiratory cultures and on the previous antibiotic history of the patient.

When a person with CF presents with acute symptoms of increased productive cough, fatigue, lassitude, and weight loss, physicians not familiar with CF may erroneously attribute symptoms to "bronchitis." Indeed, the chest radiograph may be unchanged, but the loss of lung function that occurs during CF exacerbations may not be recovered unless aggressive treatment regimens are initiated early in the exacerbation.

The determination of when to treat for an exacerbation of CF is a clinical judgment. When symptoms are mild, oral antibiotics may be used at the highest dose tolerable by the patient. A typical regimen for a mild exacerbation in a patient with *Pseudomonas aeruginosa* and *methicillin-resistant Staphylococcus aureus (MRSA)* includes ciprofloxacin 750 mg two times daily and trimethoprim/sulfamethoxazole (double strength) two times daily. Typically, treatment durations last from 10 to 21 days.

Many people with CF experience exacerbations and more rapid declines in lung function because of lapses in their CF airway clearance regimen. Experienced CF providers will observe this phenomenon frequently. Patients drift away from their daily routine of airway clearance and their lung function declines precipitously. Consequently, reinstitution of airway clearance is a priority during exacerbations. Unfortunately, not all decreases in lung function are reversible, and so, a lifelong program of adherence to airway clearance therapy must be continually reinforced.

## Hemoptysis

For some patients, scant hemoptysis may occur daily and thus not require acute evaluation. However, when hemoptysis is noted for the first time or increases in severity, it may be associated with an exacerbation of bronchiectasis. Hemoptysis is characterized as either mild/moderate or severe/massive. This distinction can be based on the volume of blood expectorated. As a general rule, any hemoptysis greater than a cup (approximately 8 oz or 240 mL) constitutes "massive" hemoptysis. Massive hemoptysis should be managed in an acute hospital setting with access to interventional radiology.

There are no clear guidelines for the management of hemoptysis. However, expert opinion is that hypertonic saline and dornase alfa should be discontinued in the setting of massive hemoptysis. Bronchoscopy adds little to the acute evaluation and should not be performed routinely. Bronchial arterial imaging in the form of a bronchial arterial computed tomography (CT) angiogram is often requested as it may help the radiologist locate the bleeding vessel. This test requires special coordination with the radiologist as the timing of contrast administration is different from the timing of contrast administration for a pulmonary artery imaging study.

When hemoptysis continues or escalates despite antibiotic treatment and cessation of hypertonic saline and dornase alfa, inhaled or oral tranexamic acid can be considered, but bronchial artery embolization may be required. The most serious complication of this procedure is inadvertent embolization of an anatomical variant spinal-penetrating arterial branch of the bronchial artery. When this variant is present, embolization can lead to irreversible lower extremity paralysis. The bronchial arterial imaging study can aid in identifying this variant.

## Pneumothorax

Pneumothoraces are encountered less frequently than hemoptysis. Small pneumothoraces in clinically stable patients may be observed for resolution, but large pneumothoraces require tube thoracostomy for evacuation. Positive pressure ventilation should be avoided during episodes of pneumothorax. Recurrent pneumothoraces are sometimes referred to as pleurodesis. However, in patients with advanced lung disease ($FEV_1$ < 40% of predicted) and a large pneumothorax, pleurodesis should be deferred until an evaluation for lung transplantation has been performed. Pleurodesis can make removal of the diseased lung prohibitive during the lung transplant procedure.

## Transition Care Management for People with Cystic Fibrosis

The transition from pediatric to adult medical care can be a stressful time for people with CF and their families. Adult healthcare systems have significant differences in patient care delivery compared with pediatric systems of care, with one of the most significant differences being in care management responsibility. Pediatric systems of care often focus primarily on the parents for healthcare education and care management. Adult healthcare system providers often assume, sometimes incorrectly, that the adult patient can manage their own healthcare independently. The transition process will vary from person to person. Some people with CF are ready to assume personal responsibility for their care and well-being when they reach the age 18 or 19 years, while others are not. Caregivers should keep in mind that maintaining and refilling a long list of medications, keeping follow-up appointments every 3 months, and addressing payment are extremely time-consuming tasks for parents and patients. Some individuals rise to the challenge of independence earlier, while others need more help. Many adolescents and young adults have adapted to the "sick role," as their care may have led to extended hospital stays where extra attention and special gifts/care are bestowed upon them. It can be extremely challenging at times for adolescents to transition from this system where they may be coddled, to their own detriment, to a system that they may perceive as uncaring and indifferent.

Pediatricians often arbitrarily develop their own criteria for transitioning their patients to adult care. Some employ a specific age cutoff, others delay until the conclusion of the first year of college, a number transition the adolescent/young adult when the patient presents to an emergency room with an acute illness, and some transition after the patient becomes sexually active or pregnant. Once a pediatrician transitions a patient, they will usually never see them again. The transition can be emotionally traumatic for some patients as they may have come to trust and rely on a specific physician for nearly 20 years and often through very serious illnesses. This transition can also be difficult for pediatric care providers as they may have developed special bonds with patients and their families over many years. They may have seen these patients through life-challenging events and share concerns that adult healthcare providers may not exhibit the same depth of understanding regarding their patient's issues as they do. Optimal transitions should be planned and occur during times of well-being in the chronic disease process if possible and should be viewed as a well-coordinated process rather than as an event. The stress of transition during a sudden acute medical issue can lead to unnecessary stress for the patient and their family [21].

A particular time of concern is the first year of college for those people with CF who attend. During the first year of immersion in campus life, people with CF often decrease their adherence to therapy. A therapeutic alliance with providers and patience on the part of providers and caregivers is critical in helping the young adult navigate this difficult life change. Treatment adherence usually improves after the first year of college, once daily routines are established.

To better plan for transition, the pediatric team and parents may begin teaching the responsibility for obtaining medications, adherence, and follow-up to the patient as the patient approaches their teenage years. As a patient approaches the transition to adult medicine, the adult and pediatric teams should meet and discuss the needs of each patient. There should be a clear plan prior to the last pediatric visit that delineates the adult physician who will assume care for the person with CF. When the transition occurs smoothly, some of the lapses in treatment can be averted.

Many physicians involved in the care of patients diagnosed with a chronic disease of childhood advocate that transition should begin at diagnosis. Understandably, physical transition will be deferred until the clinically appropriate time. However, early discussions about the process of transitioning to an adult healthcare system help to assure successful experiences and outcomes. In some centers, adult healthcare providers will meet with parents and pediatric patients during their initial pediatric visits to initiate the concept that a transition plan will need to be enacted at the appropriate time. Care of adolescents and adult CF patients requires a CF-trained specialist. However, the best patient-centered outcomes include the care and input from a multidisciplinary team that will include non-CF-trained physicians in addition to CF care centers.

## Conclusion

The progress made to prolong and improve the lives of people with CF is one of the greatest success stories of modern medicine. With a current life expectancy of around 50 years and with time-consuming and costly therapies that fall far short of a cure, there remains much work to be done for this vulnerable and dependent population. Thus, there is an important role for primary care physicians who are part of a care team and can recognize acute situations that require more urgent specialist involvement. PCPs play vital roles in the lives of people with CF and support both patients and families while increasing patient independence both medically and socially. Caring for patients with CF can be among the most rewarding of doctor–patient relationships.

## Appendix

| Cystic fibrosis (CF) fact sheet | |
|---|---|
| Definition and symptoms | **Cystic fibrosis (CF) is an inherited lifelong condition characterized by**<br>• Inherited abnormalities in the cystic fibrosis transmembrane conductance regulator (CFTR), an epithelial cell membrane protein and chloride channel<br>• Abnormal CFTR protein disrupts chloride transport and water movement across secretory epithelial membranes<br>• Thick (viscous) mucus buildup in the lungs, pancreas, and other organs<br>• Bronchiectasis (persistent lung infections and progressive obstructive airway disease)<br>• Persistent coughing, at times with phlegm<br>• Hemoptysis and pneumothorax<br>• Exocrine pancreatic enzyme insufficiency with poor growth or weight gain in spite of good appetite<br>• Frequent greasy, bulky stools, or difficulty with bowel movements<br>• Male (not female) infertility |
| Prevalence | In the United States<br>• About 31,000 people are living with cystic fibrosis (70,000 worldwide)<br>• Approximately 1000 new cases of CF are diagnosed each year<br>• More than 75% of people with CF are diagnosed by age 2 years<br>• Over half of the CF population is aged 18 years or older<br>• Predicted median survival: 50 years |
| Genetics and epidemiology | Epidemiology<br>• CF is the most common disorder of autosomal recessive inheritance in Caucasians<br>• In general, it occurs in 1/3000 Caucasian, 1/6000 Hispanic, 1/10,000 African-American, and 1/90,000 Asian American births<br>Genetics:<br>• More than 2100 mutations in the CFTR gene have been identified<br>• The most common CF-causing mutation is Phe508del<br>• The most common CF-causing genes are screened for at birth<br>• People with only one copy of the defective CF gene are called carriers, but they do not have the disease. Each time two CF carriers have a child; the chances are as follows:<br>– 25% (1 in 4) of the offspring will have CF<br>– 50% (1 in 2) of the offspring will be a carrier but will not have CF<br>– 25% (1 in 4) of the offspring will not be a carrier and will not have CF |

| Cystic fibrosis (CF) fact sheet | |
|---|---|
| Characteristics of adults with CF 18 years and older | • 8.4% masters/doctoral-level degree<br>• 30.7% college graduate<br>• 29.3% some college<br>• 24.1% high school diploma<br>• 44.9% married/co-habitating<br>• 40.0% full-time employment<br>• 99.1% have medical insurance<br>• Phe508del homozygotes—44.5% of CF population<br>• Phe508del heterozygotes—41.2% of CF population |
| Associated conditions | Individuals with CF have high rates of comorbid physical and mental health conditions, including<br>• Bronchiectasis<br>• Airway colonization and chronic infections with *Pseudomonas aeruginosa*, *Staphylococcus aureus*, and *Burkholderia* spp.<br>• Allergic bronchopulmonary aspergillosis<br>• Nontuberculous mycobacterial infection<br>• Exocrine pancreatic insufficiency<br>• CF-related diabetes<br>• Fat-soluble vitamin (A, D, E, and K) deficiency<br>• Osteopenia/osteoporosis<br>• Male infertility<br>• Hepatobiliary disease (cirrhosis, gallstones, biliary disease)<br>• Pancreatitis<br>• Intestinal obstruction, intussusception<br>• Chronic pain<br>• Depression, anxiety, substance abuse, and suicide |
| Challenges in transition | • Learning to manage time, finances, housing, employment, education, medication, and frequent physician visits<br>• Challenges impacting the transition to adulthood include<br>– Parental educational and financial status<br>– Proximity to specialized CF care centers<br>– Financial burden of medications and inability to work due to illness<br>– Unpredictable nature of exacerbations requiring intensification of care and usually IV antibiotics and disruption of usual activities<br>– Reluctance on the part of patient and parents/caregivers and pediatric providers to initiate transition<br>– Difficulty identifying adult generalist willing to accept patient into practice |

Adapted from Cystic Fibrosis Patient Registry Annual Data Report 2020 [1]

## References


1. Cystic Fibrosis Foundation. Cystic Fibrosis Patient Registry Annual Data Report. 2020. https://www.cff.org/medical-professionals/patient-registry
2. United States Cystic Fibrosis Foundation, Johns Hopkins University, the hospital for sick children. Clinical and functional translation of CFTR. 2011. www.cftr2.org.
3. Farrell PM, Rosenstein BJ, White TB, Accurso FJ, Castellani C, Cutting GR, et al. Guidelines for diagnosis of cystic fibrosis in newborns through older adults: cystic fibrosis foundation consensus report. J Pediatr. 2008;153(2):S4–14.
4. Moran A, Dunitz J, Nathan B, Saeed A, Lolme B, Thomas W. Cystic fibrosis-related diabetes: current trends in prevalence, incidence, and mortality. Diabetes Care. 2009;32(9):1626–31.
5. Moran A, Brunzell C, Cohen RC, Katz M, Marshall BC, Onady G, et al. Clinical care guidelines for cystic fibrosis-related diabetes. Diabetes Care. 2010;33(12):2697–708.
6. Flume PA, Mogayzel PJ, Robinson KA, Rosenblatt RL, Quittell L, Marshall BC. Cystic fibrosis pulmonary guidelines. Pulmonary complications: hemoptysis and pneumothorax. Am J Respir Crit Care Med. 2010;182(3):298–306.
7. Anderson DH. Cystic fibrosis of the pancreas and its relation to celiac disease: a clinical and pathologic study. Am J Dis Child. 1938;56(2):344–99.
8. Tobias E, Connor M, Ferguson-Smith M. Ch 15. Strong family history—typical Mendelian disease. In: Tobias ES, editor. Essential medical genetics, 6E. Hoboken, NJ: Wiley; 2011. p. 312.
9. MacKenzie T, Gifford AH, Sabadosa KA, Quinton HB, Knapp EA, Goss CH, Marshall BC. Longevity of patients with cystic fibrosis in 2000 to 2010

and beyond: survival analysis of the cystic fibrosis foundation patient registry. Ann Intern Med. 2014;161(4):233–41.
10. Beall RJ. The cystic fibrosis foundation. In: Yankaskas JR, Knowles MR, editors. Cystic fibrosis in adults. Riverwoods, IL: Walters Kluwer Publishers; 1999. p. 477–84.
11. Boyle MP. Adult cystic fibrosis. JAMA. 2007;298(15):1787–93.
12. Donaldson SH, Bennett WD, Zeman KL, Knowles MR, Tarran R, Boucher RC. Mucus clearance and lung function in cystic fibrosis with hypertonic saline. N Engl J Med. 2006;354(3):241–50.
13. Chaudary N, Balasa G. Airway clearance therapy in cystic fibrosis patients insights from a clinician providing cystic fibrosis care. Int J Gen Med. 2021;14:2513–21.
14. Flume PA, Robinson KA, O'Sullivan BP, Finder JD, Vender RL, Willey-Courand DB, et al. Cystic fibrosis pulmonary guidelines: airway clearance therapies. Respir Care. 2009;54(4):522–37.
15. Aris RM, Merkel PA, Bachrach LK, Borowitz DS, Boyle MP, Elkin SL, et al. Guide to bone health and disease in cystic fibrosis. J Clin Endocrinol Metab. 2005;90(3):1888–96.
16. Quittner AL, Abbott J, Georgiopoulos AM, Goldbeck L, Smith B, Hempstead SE, et al. International committee on mental health in cystic fibrosis: Cystic Fibrosis Foundation and European Cystic Fibrosis Society consensus statements for screening and treating depression and anxiety. Thorax. 2016;71(1):26–34.
17. Popli K, Stewart J. Infertility and its management in men with cystic fibrosis: review of literature and clinical practices in the UK. Hum Fertil (Camb). 2007;10(4):217–21.
18. Yankaskas JR, Marshall BC, Sufian B, Simon RH, Rodman D. Cystic fibrosis adult care. Chest. 2004;125(1 Suppl):1S–39S.
19. Rousset-Jablonski C, Reynaud Q, Nove-Josserand R, Ray-Coquard I, Mekki Y, Golfier F, Durieu I. High proportion of abnormal pap smear tests and cervical dysplasia in women with cystic fibrosis. Eur J Obstet Gynecol Reprod Biol. 2018;221:40–5.
20. Thornton C, somayaji R, Chu A, Parkins M. Human papillomavirus (HPV) and cervical dysplasia in adult female cystic fibrosis (CF) lung transplant recipients. Thora. 2022;77(6):625–7. https://doi.org/10.1136/thoraxjnl-2021-218461.
21. Okumur MJ, Kleinhenz ME. Cystic fibrosis transitions of care: lessons learned and future directions for cystic fibrosis. Clin Chest Med. 2016;37(1):119–26.

# 29 Transitioning Adolescents and Young Adults with Type 1 Diabetes to Adulthood

Rachel D'Amico and Elizabeth O. Buschur

## Case Presentation

Mark is a 22-year-old young man with type 1 diabetes mellitus diagnosed at age 15. He is being seen at the Diabetes Transition Clinic for the first time after last being seen about 5 months ago in the pediatric endocrinology clinic. He presents with his mother. Mark states he has not been checking blood sugars for several months. He takes basal insulin (glargine) every day and denies missing any doses. He is also prescribed short-acting insulin for meals and correction but has not taken this in several months. When asked why, he says he does not care. He denies difficulty affording insulin or supplies. On review of prior records, his hemoglobin A1c has been between 11% to greater than 14% since 1–2 years after diagnosis. He complains of blurry vision, polyuria, polydipsia, fatigue, and depression. He is not interested in seeing a counselor regarding his depression. Mark appears to be a thin young man, well-groomed, and quiet. He wears a hat covering his eyes somewhat. His exam is unremarkable, including his thyroid and foot exam. Hemoglobin A1c is >14%. He works the night shift at a warehouse. His mother with whom he lives works during the day. Mark sleeps during the day. His eating schedule is somewhat erratic—usually two meals per day with the largest before going to work in the evening. He denies smoking and illicit drug use. He occasionally drinks beer but denies any binge drinking behavior. His mother's main concern which she asks about is how long do complications of diabetes take to occur. She would like her son to change his behavior but is not sure how to help him, and admits that she does not see him awake much due to their differing work schedules. Mark states that he isn't worried about the complications of diabetes as he believes they are unavoidable even if he controls his diabetes.

## Case Discussion

This case illustrates the importance of necessary adherence to glucose checks, insulin injection administration, and careful dietary assessment which people with diabetes live with on a daily basis, and challenges that are specific to young adults. During the pediatric time period, glucose checks, insulin dosing, and meal planning are often team-based with the individual child, his family, and his teacher and/or school nurse play-

R. D'Amico
Division of General Internal Medicine, Department of Internal Medicine, The Ohio State University, Columbus, OH, USA
e-mail: rachel.d'amico@osumc.edu

E. O. Buschur (✉)
Division of Endocrinology, Metabolism, and Diabetes, Department of Internal Medicine, The Ohio State University, Columbus, OH, USA
e-mail: elizabeth.buschur@osumc.edu


A. A. Kuo et al. (eds.), *Care of Adults with Chronic Childhood Conditions*,
https://doi.org/10.1007/978-3-031-54281-7_29

ing collaborative roles. During adolescence, teens with diabetes often seek independence and at times will rebel against self-care behaviors. Furthermore, many adolescents and young adults with diabetes have coexisting depression, anxiety, and other mental health disorders that need treatment. During the teenage years, diabetes self-care behaviors should become incorporated into the young adult's normal routine.

## Definition and Pathophysiology of Disease

Type 1 diabetes is one of the most common chronic conditions affecting children. The American Diabetes Association/Worldwide Health Organization (ADA/WHO) criteria for the diagnosis of diabetes include fasting blood glucose ≥126 mg/dL at least twice, HbA1c ≥ 6.5%, or any random glucose ≥200 mg/dL. Type 1 diabetes results from the autoimmune destruction of the pancreatic beta cells resulting in complete insulin deficiency. It is most commonly present in childhood, although some people are diagnosed as adults. Type 1 diabetes occurs in genetically susceptible individuals who often have a family history of autoimmune disease and is thought to be triggered by environmental agents. The autoimmune process is thought to occur over months to years before clinical symptoms (polyuria, polydipsia, polyphagia, weight loss) occur and hyperglycemia is diagnosed.

## Epidemiology

The incidence of type 1 diabetes is increasing worldwide, with the US estimated incidence rate increasing by 1.4% annually [1]. In a Swedish registry of 1666 adults, blood samples were obtained from 1630 (97.8%). Those subjects with diabetes, positive autoantibodies (glutamic decarboxylase (GAD) antibody and/or islet cell antibody (ICA)), and/or c-peptide levels less than 0.25 nmol/L (0.7%) were classified as having type 1 diabetes [2]. In this large Swedish population, the incidence of type 1 diabetes in 0–19-year-olds was 37.8 per 100,000 and year (36.1–39.6, 95% confidence interval (CI)) and in 20–100-year-olds was 27.1 (25.6–27.4) per 100,000 and year [2]. There was a bimodal distribution with equal peaks in 0–9-year-olds and 50–80-year-olds. In contrast, the incidence of type 2 diabetes among adults in this population was higher at 378 (375–380) per 100,000 and year. There were 101 adults that had one or more autoantibodies positive; GAD antibody was the most common in 90%, ICA in 71%, and both GAD and ICA in 61% [2]. There were no significant gender differences in type 1 diabetes in any age group, except for some trends in pediatric subgroups.

A second study examined the time trends and prevalence of type 1 diabetes in Europe [3]. Incidence rates of newly diagnosed type 1 diabetes for 0–14-year-old children were reported from 22 European countries during the period of 1989–2013. There was a pooled increased incidence of 3.4% annually, with the maximum increase (6.6% per year) noted in a Polish center. Rates of increase were similar between genders from the ages of 0–9, but increased rates of incidence were noted in boys from 10 to 14 years compared to girls.

The United States has the highest number of new diagnoses of type 1 diabetes annually in the world [4], with an estimated 27,000 new cases annually in children and 37,000 new cases in adults [5]. Several studies have examined the prevalence and trends of diabetes in the United States [6]. Data from the National Survey of Children's Health in 2006 found an estimated prevalence of diabetes (both types 1 and 2 diabetes) among children in the United States to be 3.2 per 1000 (95% CI 2.6–3.7), for a total of an estimated 229,240 children [7]. There were differences among race and obesity status: non-Latinx White children had a higher prevalence of diabetes (3.8 per 1000 children) compared with other racial and ethnic categories (2.2 per 1000 children) [7]. Between 2001 and 2015, the annual incidence of type 1 diabetes in children increased by 1.9% per annum [5]. In The SEARCH for Diabetes in Youth Study, non-Latinx White youth had the highest prevalence in the younger group (1.06 cases per 1000 youth). Among younger children, type 1 diabetes accounted for the majority of cases (more than 80%), and among the older group, there were higher estimates of type 2 diabetes ranging from 6 to 76% [8].

The reason why type 1 diabetes prevalence is increasing over time is unknown but is thought to be related to environmental triggers for beta cell dysfunction in genetically vulnerable individuals. This is supported by findings that populations with similar genetic risks for type 1 diabetes have different disease incidence when separated by socioeconomic borders [9]. Proposed environmental triggers include maternal viral infections during pregnancy, older maternal age, viral infections in childhood, and adverse childhood experiences [10]. Vitamin D intake and a diet higher in omega-3 fatty acids have been associated with lower type 1 diabetes incidence [10].

## Considerations in Hospitalization

Admission for diabetic complications in patients with type 1 diabetes is most frequently due to diabetic ketoacidosis (DKA), which is diagnosed by blood glucose >200 mg/dL, venous pH < 7.30, bicarbonate <15 mmol/L, and positive urine and serum ketones [11]. DKA is responsible for an estimated 500,000 hospital days per year and accounts for half of all deaths in patients with diabetes younger than 24 years old [12]. Hospitalization is unfortunately common in the transitional age population; adolescence (defined as 13–25 years old) is associated with increased DKA risk, as is lower socioeconomic status, female sex, and mental illness [13]. Modifiable risk factors for DKA, like substance use and infrequent healthcare encounters [14], are more common in the adolescent and young adult population. The most severe complication from DKA is cerebral edema, which is more common in patients under 20 years old [15].

Acute management of DKA centers around fluid resuscitation, electrolyte normalization, and initiation of IV insulin infusion. Insulin should be continuously infused until acidosis has resolved; if blood glucose normalizes prior to acidosis resolution, concurrent dextrose infusions should be used to prevent hypoglycemia. Hypoglycemia during inpatient admission is associated with increased hospital duration and mortality [16]. After acidosis and hyperglycemia have resolved, the patient should be transitioned to a home-going subcutaneous insulin regimen. Prevention of further episodes of DKA is critical, as the history of a previous episode of DKA is a risk factor for future occurrences [13]. Arranging regular follow-ups with primary care and their endocrinologist prior to discharge is key for continued management. Diabetes education that includes information on sick day management, as well as emergency hotlines where patients can call for medical advice when blood glucose or ketones are high, have shown to decrease further episodes of DKA [13].

## Common Adult Conditions in the Type 1 Diabetes Population

### Mood Disorders

Psychosocial challenges commonly occur during periods of transition for young adults; however, they are more pronounced for patients with diabetes due to their associated disease-related emotional distress. At diagnosis, many patients with diabetes report feeling scared, angry, alone, and depressed when thinking about having diabetes [17]. Most patients worry about the future and the possibility of developing serious complications related to their diabetes, and some develop a significant fear of hypoglycemia and its adverse effects. Many feel discouraged and overwhelmed by their diabetes regimen; there is "burnout" from the constant effort to manage diabetes, and guilt and anxiety regarding poor adherence. Patients with diabetes also report concern about reactions and uncomfortable interactions around family friends, or coworkers who do not have diabetes [18]. About one in three adolescents [19] and half of adults with type 1 diabetes [20] express diabetes distress, which is related to poorer glycemic control and decreased self-efficacy [19]. Diabetes distress and depression both are associated with a higher incidence of cardiovascular disease risk factors, such as elevated body mass index (BMI) and high cholesterol [21]. As a result, the American Diabetes Association's "Standards of Medical Care in Diabetes—2021" position statement recommends routine screening for psychosocial problems including diabetes-related distress, depression, anxiety, and eating disorders so they can be addressed [22].

Depression has been clearly identified as a common comorbid condition in patients with diabetes. Almost one in three adolescents with type 1 diabetes report a history of anxiety or depression, and 14% were symptomatic in the last year [23]. Recent studies demonstrate that about 10% of adult patients with type 1 diabetes have comorbid depression [24] while over 20% of older adolescent females with type 2 diabetes exhibit significant depressive symptoms [25]. Depression in patients with type 1 diabetes has been found to be associated with non-White races and longer disease duration [26]. Depression has not only been identified as a risk factor for decreased adherence [27] and poor glycemic control [28] but also for increased morbidity and mortality in patients with diabetes [24]. Adolescents and young adults who screened positive for mental illness had twice the odds of poor glycemic control [29]. Given the high prevalence of depression in the diabetic population and the serious implications it has for morbidity and mortality, it is very important for the provider to identify and treat mood disorders. Not only has depression treatment been shown to improve symptoms and improve glycemic control [30], but it has also had a significant economic benefit from the health plan perspective [31].

Anxiety is the most frequently diagnosed psychiatric disorder in the general adolescent population [32] and poses unique challenges to patients with diabetes. Studies demonstrate that 21–32% of youth with type 1 diabetes have symptoms of anxiety [33, 34]. Similar to depression, symptoms of anxiety have been associated with decreased blood glucose monitoring and poorer glycemic control among adolescents with type 1 diabetes [34]. However, somatic symptoms of anxiety such as increased heart rate and perspiration, dizziness, lightheadedness, and abdominal discomfort [35] are very similar to those associated with hypoglycemia and may make it difficult for patients with diabetes to appropriately understand their glycemic levels [36].

## Overweight and Obesity

Stereotypically, adolescents with type 1 diabetes are lean in contrast to those with type 2 diabetes who are often obese. However, with the global increases in overweight and obesity, more than 36% of children under 18 years of age with type 1 diabetes are overweight or obese (BMI $\geq$ 85th percentile) [37]. Young adults with type 1 diabetes have been found to be overweight at higher rates than the general population and have on average higher body fat mass [38]. Children of Latinx race and female gender are at the highest risk of obesity [37]. Other risk factors for higher BMI changes during childhood which may lead to overweight and obesity include intensification of insulin regimen (a higher number of injections per day or insulin pump therapy) and higher total daily insulin dose, lower BMI at diabetes onset, pubertal diabetes, and long diabetes duration [39]. While the reasons for obesity development are complex, multiple barriers to healthy weight maintenance affect individuals with type 1 diabetes. For example, individuals with type 1 diabetes are less likely to be physically active than nondiabetic peers [40], diabetes management with dietary changes can be potentially dangerous, and insulin therapy can cause weight gain as a side effect.

Children and adolescents with type 1 diabetes should be counseled on the independent risks of overweight and obesity on cardio-metabolic complications. Minorities and young girls with type 1 diabetes, especially those diagnosed between ages 10 and 15 years of age, have been shown to be at highest risk of overweight and obesity and may benefit from targeted counseling and lifestyle modification for weight maintenance during the course of diabetes treatment, with frequent titration of insulin with dietary and weight changes.

## Disordered Eating

Eating disorders are a well-known problem for patients with diabetes. According to the DSM-V, an eating disorder is characterized by a persistent disturbance of eating that impairs health or psychosocial functioning. Disturbed eating behavior is common in late adolescent and young adult women in the general population [41]; however, adolescents with type 1 diabetes are about 2.5 times more likely to develop an eating disorder [42]. Subclinical eating disorder symptoms have been noted in over 39% of women with type 1 diabetes [43]. These rates are likely under-reported, as most studies use non-diabetic-specific questionnaires that don't include questions about diabetic-specific concerns, like insulin omission [44]. This causes catabolism of lipids and induced glycosuria which causes the excretion of calories in the urine and is a behavior unique to patients with diabetes given the role insulin therapy plays in the disease. It has been recognized by the DSM-V as either an inappropriate compensatory feature of bulimia nervosa or as a purging disorder [45]. Also termed "diabulimia," insulin restriction is one of the most common weight control methods for patients with diabetes, and has been reported in up to 60% of patients with diabetes treated with insulin [46].

Many factors specific to diabetes have been shown to predispose patients to developing eating disorders. The age of onset of diabetes in adolescence [47] as well as the cycle of weight loss at disease onset and subsequent weight gain with the initiation of insulin therapy [48] correlate with the risk of subsequent development of an eating disorder. Many patients with diabetes and eating disorders identified a feeling of a lack of control related to their diabetes, which they attempted to regain with disordered eating and insulin use [49]. Diabetes management requires significant focus on when and what to eat, and the dietary restraint demanded is thought to contribute by leading to craving and then binging on "forbidden foods" without appropriate insulin coverage [50]. Similarly, episodes of hypoglycemia may trigger disordered eating because the associated intense hunger can lead to binging and subsequent guilt about over-eating [51]. These circumstances make individuals who develop eating disorders very likely to relapse if they recover; one study found a probability of recurrence was 53% within 6 years after remission [52].

Eating disorders are especially serious for patients with diabetes because they are associated with increased morbidity and mortality. Multiple studies have shown worse metabolic control with higher hemoglobin A1c in patients with diabetes who have an eating disorder compared to those who do not [45, 53]. Purposeful insulin omission has severe consequences, including higher rates of retinopathy and nephropathy, as well as almost threefold increased mortality [49].

To avoid the severe consequences of an eating disorder, it is important for healthcare providers to prevent and identify eating disorders. They should be sensitive to a preoccupation with body weight, discuss dissatisfaction with body image [54], and minimize risk factors that have been shown to lead to an eating disorder by promoting flexibility with treatment and a nondepriving diet[50]. It is notable that BMI is not correlated with the risk of developing an eating disorder, and thus should not be used to determine who to screen [54]. A high index of suspicion is required to identify an eating disorder in patients with diabetes as they frequently conceal and deny that they have a problem and do not often use unhealthy weight control behaviors like vomiting, laxatives, or skipping meals as their peers without diabetes do, but rather often omit insulin. The following clinical signs should alert physicians of a possible eating disorder: poor glycemic control, recurrent episodes of DKA, recurrent hypoglycemic episodes, frequently missed medical appointments, refusal to be weighed, and preoccupation with appearance [45]. Multiple screening tools that are specific to diabetic patients have been developed that can help with detection and diagnosis [44, 55].

## Thyroid Disease

Autoimmune thyroid disease is the most common coexisting autoimmune condition among people with type 1 diabetes [56]. Autoimmune thyroiditis manifesting as hypothyroidism (Hashimoto's thyroiditis) is more common than autoimmune hyperthyroidism (Graves' disease). An estimated 21% of children with type 1 diabetes have positive thyroid antibodies (antithyroid peroxidase or antithyroglobulin antibodies) [57], while an estimated 9% of patients with type 1 diabetes develop autoimmune primary hypothyroidism [58]. Autoimmune thyroid disease is more common among women than men with type 1 diabetes [56] as well as more common with increasing age. Autoimmune thyroid disease and type 1 diabetes have been shown to share many predisposing genetic mutations [59]. Coexisting thyroid disease can complicate the management of diabetes during the transition of care, as uncontrolled thyroid disease can worsen hypoglycemia (for hyperthyroidism), weight changes, depression, anxiety, insomnia, fatigue, and other problems that may be common among adolescents and young adults with diabetes. A study of children with type 1 diabetes and coexisting autoimmune thyroid disease showed they are at higher risk for both hypoglycemia and diabetic ketoacidosis, as opposed to type 1 diabetes alone [60]. The American Diabetes Association recommends regular screening of children, adolescents, and young adults with type 1 diabetes for the development of thyroid disease at the time of diabetes diagnosis and every 1–2 years after, or sooner if they develop symptoms of hypothyroidism [61]. In addition to thyroid disease, other autoimmune diseases may also accompany type 1 diabetes including celiac disease, and much less commonly adrenal insufficiency (Addison's disease), pernicious anemia, among others.

## Celiac Disease

Similar to autoimmune thyroid disease, celiac disease is an additional autoimmune disease that is common among people with type 1 diabetes. Celiac disease is more common among patients with type 1 diabetes (estimates between 3.5 and 5.6% of patients with type 1 diabetes) than those without type 1 diabetes [62, 63]. An estimated 7–10% of patients with type 1 diabetes have positive antiendomysial antibodies or tissue transglutaminase antibodies [64]. Risk factors for the development of celiac disease include female gender, younger age at diagnosis of diabetes[62], and presence of autoimmune thyroid disease [64]. A concomitant diagnosis of celiac disease increases a patient's risk of developing diabetic microvascular complications, like retinopathy and nephropathy [65], as well as hyperlipidemia [66]. Many patients with type 1 diabetes and celiac disease will present without symptoms or with vague symptoms including recurrent hypoglycemia, unpredictable glycemic patterns, growth failure, and low bone density or fractures [67]. As most cases of celiac disease will be diagnosed within 5 years of diabetes diagnosis [68], the American Diabetes Association recommends screening children with type 1 diabetes for celiac on diagnosis, within 2 years and again within 5 years of diabetes diagnosis, as well as if any new symptoms arise [22].

## Complications of Diabetes

One of the most compelling reasons for strict diabetes management is that multiple longitudinal randomized trials have shown that poor glycemic control is associated with long-term vascular complications of diabetes, including nephropathy, retinopathy, neuropathy, and cardiovascular disease [69, 70]. Typically, vascular complications of diabetes do not clinically manifest until adulthood, but their pathogenesis begins much earlier at disease onset. For example, studies have shown increased arterial stiffness in adolescents with poorly controlled diabetes [71]. Furthermore, microvascular complications of diabetes have been diagnosed at times in emerging adulthood. There has been no significant difference in terms of screening for complications of diabetes between pediatric and adult medical care, but one study of 108 subjects with type 1 diabetes showed that background retinopathy increased from 5% to 29% from age 18 to 24 years [72]. Table 29.1 shows recommended screening tests and their timing for patients with type 1 diabetes.

**Table 29.1** Screening for complications and coexisting conditions of diabetes

| Condition | Test | Frequency |
|---|---|---|
| Blood glucose control | Hemoglobin A1c | At least two times a year in patients who meet treatment goals (and have stable glycemic control)<br>Quarterly in patients whose therapy has changed or who are not meeting glycemic goals |
| Retinopathy | Dilated eye exam by a trained eye services professional | Patients *with* evidence of retinopathy should be screened annually<br>Patients *without* evidence of retinopathy should be screened every 2 years |
| Nephropathy | Urine spot microalbumin/creatinine ratio | Annually |
| Autonomic neuropathy | Ask about symptoms of sexual dysfunction and gastroparesis | Annually |
| Peripheral neuropathy | Physical exam focused on ankle reflexes, dorsalis pedis pulses, vibratory sensation, and 5.07 monofilament touch sensation | Patients at *very high risk* should be seen every 3 months by a wound care nurse<br>Patients at *increased risk* and *average risk* should be screened annually |
| Hypertension | Blood pressure measurement by a trained professional | Every visit |
| Hyperlipidemia | Lipids | At the time of diabetes diagnosis or at initial medical evaluation. If LDL is <100 mg/dL, recheck lipids every 5 years. If lipids are abnormal, check annually. If HbA1c is >9%, check more often (i.e., every 2 years) |
| Electrolyte and chemistry abnormalities | Serum creatinine and potassium | At least annually |
| Depression and diabetes-related distress | Patient Health Questionnaire (PHQ-2) and either the Diabetes Distress Scale (DDS) or Problem Areas in Diabetes (PAID)-1 scale | Screen at each visit (quarterly) |
| Celiac disease | Anti-tissue transglutaminase antibody | Regular screening of children at diagnosis and also every 2–3 years or if clinically suspected. Screening in adults with signs or symptoms of celiac disease, unexplained hypoglycemia, glycemic patterns, or low bone density |
| Thyroid disease | TSH | Every 1–2 years or sooner if symptoms of hypothyroidism |
| Obesity | BMI | Quarterly |
| Periodontal disease | Routine dental exam | Every 6 months |
| Unplanned pregnancy | Counsel on reproductive and sexual health | Every visit (quarterly) |
| Immunizations | Hepatitis B vaccine | 3-dose series ages 19–59. Age 60 and older depending on risk |
| | Pneumococcal polysaccharide (PPSV23) vaccine | Once between age 19 and 64 years<br>Booster after age 65 (at least 5 years after previous dose) |
| | Influenza vaccine | Annually |

*LDL* low-density lipoproteins, *TSH* thyroid-stimulating hormone, *BMI* body mass index

Diabetic nephropathy rates have decreased over the past several decades with improvements in hemoglobin A1c [73]. Men, older patients, and patients with cumulative poor glycemic control are all at higher risk for the development of microalbuminuria and chronic kidney disease (CKD) [74]. While improved glycemic control can decrease rates of developing CKD, renal involvement is very common even for those with well-controlled disease. Rates of microalbuminuria within 50 years of type 1 diabetes diagnosis have been shown to be around 88% [75]. Tobacco use significantly increases the risk of progression of microalbuminuria to nephropathy [76]. Hypertension also is an independent risk for nephropathy [77].

Around 6–16% of children with type 1 diabetes are diagnosed with hypertension [78], which is a risk factor for the development of albuminuria [79]. Therefore, blood pressure measurement and screening for hypertension should be done at each visit for diabetes care. In children and adolescents with diabetes, prehypertension is defined as systolic or diastolic blood pressure between the 90th and 95th percentiles or blood pressure ≥120/80, whichever is higher, at three different time points. Hypertension is defined as systolic or diastolic blood pressure ≥95th percentile for age, gender, and height (or ≥130/80, whichever is higher) at three different time points. Lifestyle changes (diet and exercise) should be recommended for teens with blood pressure readings in the prehypertension range. Medical treatment is indicated for adolescents and young adults with blood pressure in the hypertensive range or for those with blood pressure in the prehypertensive range despite lifestyle changes for 3–6 months. An Angiontensin-converting enzyme (ACE) inhibitor is the recommended first-line pharmacologic treatment if needed as this class of drugs has been shown to protect against the development of progressive nephropathy in patients with diabetes [80], and appears to provide endothelial protection for teenagers with diabetes [81]. If an ACE inhibitor is prescribed to female patients of childbearing age, it is recommended to counsel on the teratogenic potential of this class of medications [80]. The goal blood pressure on treatment is <90th percentile for age or <120/80. Strict blood pressure management is critical to decrease the risk of cardiovascular disease, as patients with type 1 diabetes are at threefold higher risk of cardiovascular disease and have higher mortality associated with cardiac events [82].

Symptomatic neuropathy is uncommon in teens with type 1 diabetes, although there are patients who are genetically predisposed to neuropathy development [83]; however, subclinical neurologic impairment has been identified in many youth with type 1 diabetes [84], particularly those with chronic hyperglycemia and recurrent DKA [85]. Both peripheral and autonomic nervous systems may be affected by the classic symmetric distal sensory loss in peripheral neuropathy versus abnormal heart rate variability, postural blood pressure abnormalities, and impairment of pupillary dilation. Cardiac autonomic dysfunction may be associated with pubertal development and more often occurs in those patients with poor glycemic control [86], and is associated with a higher rate of cardiovascular mortality [87]. Screening for peripheral neuropathy should be done annually with monofilament and vibratory sensation testing. As in older adults with diabetes, better glycemic control can lead to improvements in nerve function in teens and young adults with diabetes, and the protective effect of good glycemic control can last for over 10 years [88].

Cardiovascular disease and dyslipidemia are common in adults with type 1 diabetes. Adults with type 1 diabetes are about twice as likely to have cardiovascular disease and mortality secondary to cardiac disease compared to matched controls without diabetes [89]. Age at diagnosis of type 1 diabetes has a significant impact on risk, as those diagnosed with diabetes before age 10 had about a 30x increased risk of coronary artery disease compared to the general population [90]. Although very few teens have had cardiovascular disease events, strict glycemic control can provide protection against cardiac disease for up to 30 years [91]. Changes in lipids and cardiac function have also been noted to begin to occur in childhood, including reductions in left ventricular size and stroke volume [92], atherosclerotic changes [93], and increases in vascular stiffness [94]. The American Diabetes Association recommends screening children and adolescents with type 1 diabetes with a lipid panel (ideally fasting) when initial glycemic control has been achieved and age is >2 years. If LDL is less than 100 mg/dL, a lipid screen should be repeated at 9–11 years of age and then repeated every 3 years if within goal. If lipids are abnormal, annual lipids are recommended, and if hemoglobin A1c is elevated greater than 9%, screening should occur more often (i.e., every 2 years). Exercise has been shown to reduce cardiometabolic risk and should be advised to all children and young adults with diabetes [95]. Diet, exercise, and better glycemic control are recommended if hyperlipidemia is diagnosed. HMG-CoA reductase inhibitors (statins) are recommended in patients older than 10 years if lifestyle changes and improvements in hemoglobin A1c do not achieve target lipid goals (LDL < 160 mg/dL or < 130 mg/dL with one or more cardiovascular risk factors) [22]. If a statin is prescribed to a female of reproductive age, it is recommended to counsel her on discontinuation prior to conception as there have been poor fetal outcomes related to the statins [96].

1. Special issues that arise in those with diabetes who transition to adulthood
   (a) Alcohol, tobacco, and illicit drug use

   The prevalence of tobacco, alcohol, and illicit drug use in young adults with diabetes approximates that of the general population [97]. In general, substance abuse has negative effects on adolescent health, but it can affect patients with type 1 diabetes to a more significant degree by increasing their risk for acute and chronic complications of diabetes [98]. It is critical that adolescent and young adult patients with diabetes are counseled on both the short- and long-term consequences of substance use and involved in developing risk reduction strategies if necessary.

   Cigarette smoking is associated with worsened glycemic control[99], increased development and progression of retinopathy [100], neuropathy [101], microalbuminuria, and impairment of renal function [102]. It is also a well-known risk factor for cardiovascular disease [103]. Because diabetes itself is a cardiovascular risk factor, cigarette smoking significantly heightens the risk of premature death due to stroke and coronary artery disease [102]. Active smoking increases the risk of both cardiovascular disease and mortality by around 50% in people with diabetes [104]. Prevention and cessation of cigarette smoking is an important goal for physicians caring for patients with diabetes. Standard of care cessation aids, like varenicline, can be used safely and effectively in patients with diabetes [105].

   It is well known that alcohol is a risk factor for hypoglycemia in patients with type 1 diabetes, likely due to the inhibition of gluconeogenesis in the liver [106]. This can be especially dangerous as moderate alcohol intake has been shown to cause decreased awareness of hypoglycemia in patients with type 1 diabetes despite exaggerated physiological changes [107]. Alcohol use also increases the risk of developing neuropathy [108]. Physicians should routinely educate diabetic patients about the risk of nocturnal hypoglycemia with alcohol and counsel them on risk reduction techniques of eating with alcohol, snacking before bed, and considering reducing insulin dosage[109].

   Around 24% of adults with type 1 diabetes endorse substance use in the last year, with around 3% showing signs of substance dependency [110]. Substance abuse has been shown to be a significant contributing factor to noncompliance in patients with diabetes [111]. Cocaine has been found to be a risk factor for diabetic ketoacidosis, either due to its association with insulin therapy omission or its effects on counterregulatory hormones [112]. Marijuana use has also been associated with double the risk of diabetic ketoacidosis [113].

(b) Sexual health, contraception, and preconception planning

The number of women with preexisting diabetes who become pregnant and deliver babies is increasing [114]. Unfortunately, unplanned pregnancy is common for women with diabetes. More than one-half of women with diabetes have experienced unplanned pregnancies [115]. Contraceptive use is lower in women with diabetes than in women without diabetes [115]. Only half of young adults with diabetes who reported being sexually active had ever used birth control to prevent pregnancy [116].

It is critical to include reproductive and sexual health care in transition planning to prevent unplanned pregnancy and to optimize the health outcomes of women with diabetes and their infants. Multiple studies have demonstrated high rates of spontaneous abortions and major congenital malformations in infants of mothers with type 1 diabetes who have poor glycemic control during pregnancy [117]. Women with type 1 diabetes are at 2.5× increased risk of pregnancy complications with an increased risk of maternal and infant mortality [118]. However, tight glycemic control preconception and during pregnancy can significantly decrease these risks [119], and the use of continuous glucose monitoring to improve awareness of hyperglycemia has been shown to improve neonatal outcomes [120]. Many medications common to diabetic regimens, like statins and ACE inhibitors, are teratogenic and need to be titrated off prior to conception to decrease the risk of congenital defects [121].

To minimize the risk of devastating malformations, the American Diabetes Association recommends that all women of childbearing potential receive preconception counseling [122]. However, most women do not. Less than half of teenagers with diabetes had discussed birth control with a healthcare professional and 31% reported that they would not feel comfortable bringing the subject up [123]. In women up to age 45, only 26% reported receiving contraceptive advice specific to diabetes [124], and more than 75% of young adults were not aware of the maternal and fetal risks in women with diabetes and the need for good glycemic control [125].

In a survey of primary care physicians who care for adolescents with chronic health conditions, all agreed that reproductive and sexual health is one of the most important issues, but many did not feel prepared to discuss it with their patients [126]. Over half of endocrinology providers stated that they were very uncomfortable discussing contraception, and only 28% brought up reproductive health proactively [127]. To help clarify the goals of preconception care, the American Diabetes Association has outlined two key objectives: (1) Educate patients on the risk of malformations associated with unplanned pregnancies and poor glycemic control. (2) Provide effective contraception to all women with diabetes who are at childbearing age (unless the patient has good metabolic control and is trying to conceive). Contraceptive choice should focus on which is the most effective method for the patient as there are no specific contraindications to any contraceptive methods in patients with diabetes. Women who received reproductive health education in adolescence are more likely to utilize contraception and preconception planning in adulthood [128]. The Centers for Disease Control has also developed recommendations for preconception care that can help in the development of a reproductive health plan [129].

(c) Americans with Disabilities Act and school/work accommodations

The Americans with Disabilities Act [130] protects teens and young adults with diabetes against workplace discrimination. An employer cannot fail to hire or fail to promote a young adult due to diabetes, nor can they terminate an individual because of diabetes, and must not discriminate with regard to employer-paid health insurance. An employer should provide reasonable accommodations if requested by the employee. Similarly, in educational settings, teens and young adults with diabetes may request reasonable accommodations for learning if needed. Directing undergraduate students to register with their Disabilities Services Office is the first step in requesting accommodations. At many universities, the Disabilities Services Office will provide an accommodation letter that the student can provide to each of their teachers at the beginning of the semester. Providers should assist adolescents with diabetes and their families in anticipating what accommodations they may need, such as having glucose testing supplies and insulin always available, the ability to reschedule testing based on diabetic complications (acute hypo- or hyperglycemia), and access to appropriate storage conditions for insulin. Both the American Diabetes Association's Going Away to College [131] and the College Diabetes Network website [132] have resources about standardized testing and asking for possible testing accommodations.

(d) Financial issues

Financial concerns may pose a significant barrier to successful transition from pediatric to adult medical care for patients with diabetes, as the mean annual cost of type 1 diabetes is around $17,000 and is continuing to rise due to increasing costs of insulin [133]. Patients with diabetes may have difficulty affording supplies, including glucometer test strips, insulin, and associated supplies, or continuous glucose monitoring supplies. Government programs and medication assistance programs may be able to help. Patients can be recommended to check if they are eligible for the hospital's financial assistance program, the Bureau for Children with Medical Handicaps for their state, and prescription assistance programs. The College Diabetes Network website has several resources on obtaining and affording diabetes supplies and health insurance [134].

(e) Changing living situations

As patients with diabetes move away from home it is very important that they inform the people they will be living with about their diabetes. If they are going to college, this would include their roommate and residence hall advisor. It is helpful to provide some basic information to these people on what diabetes is to clear up misconceptions. It may be useful to demonstrate how supplies including glucagon work. Most importantly, the roommate should be made aware of the dangers of hypoglycemia, how to recognize it, and what to do if the patient becomes confused or unarousable. This would entail calling 911 and administer glucose gel or glucagon either via injection or intranasal [135]. Because patients may find starting a conversation about their diabetes challenging, the College Diabetes Network has developed tools and tips on how to talk with friends and roommates about diabetes [132]. The Juvenile Diabetes Research Foundation (JDRF) has also developed a letter that can be used to facilitate this discussion [136]. Similarly, the College Diabetes Network has resources for preparing to talk to one's roommate about having diabetes [136].

(f) Family-oriented care to self-care behaviors and adherence

Fundamental differences between pediatric "family oriented" care and adult care are well recognized. In pediatric setting, care is provided in a family-focused model that tries to accommodate the child and family's needs with significant support. Parents are highly involved because children do not have the cognitive skills to independently manage their diabetes. In the adult model, patients are treated as autonomous individuals, provided with information and recommendations, and expected to independently make decisions about their disease management. Visits tend to be shorter, less holistic, and more focused on medical problems. The contrast between these two models can be upsetting for young adults with diabetes as they transition to adult models of care [98]. Furthermore, patients struggle with self-care and adherence as they attempt to manage their diabetes in a model that demands independence during transition. Over the 2-year period following the transition to adult care, research demonstrates a significant deterioration in treatment adherence as well as glycemic control in young adults with type 1 diabetes [137].

2. Approaching transfer of care in patients with diabetes

(a) Barriers to transfer

The American Diabetes Association released a policy on transfer of adolescents with diabetes to adult care in 2011, recommending that pediatric providers start preparing adolescents 1 year prior to planned transfer, provide a written patient summary to the adult endocrinologist, and adult endocrinologists have a protocol in place to identify adults lost to follow-up and provide linkage to resources [98]. Despite these recommendations, many adolescents with type 1 diabetes struggle with transitioning their care to adult endocrinology for a variety of reasons. Fragmented care is associated with a higher risk of DKA and mortality [138], and even when transfer of care is achieved it is marked by worsening glycemic control compared to those who remain in pediatric care [139]. For these reasons, it is critical the transfer of care to adult care is studied more and solutions to barriers are identified.

Some of the struggles with the transfer of care center around lack of standardization of transition timeline and process among pediatric endocrinologists. There is no agreed-upon age for transfer of care; it is often around ages 18–21, a time when some patients are in college. This can complicate the transfer of care as there are many other changes at this time, patients may not live in the same city as their providers, and schoolwork can often take priority over appointments with new providers [140]. Transfer of control of disease management from parents to adolescents can also cause significant discomfort and stress, leading to young adults feeling uncomfortable taking the lead in their care [141]. Because of this, while adult providers may assume young adults are knowledgeable about their disease, they oftentimes need re-education about diabetes management [142].

Insufficient communication between providers and training on transition of care also contributes to complicating transfer. Almost half of pediatric endocrinologists noted a lack of training on transition of care; those who had received training were more likely to provide medical records to adult providers and less likely to have patients return after transfer [143]. Around 40% of pediatric endocrinologists also expressed concern about a lack of adult endocrinologist experience in the care of young adults and type 1 diabetes [143]. In a survey of adult endocrinologists, only 36% reported often or always receiving medical records from pediatric endocrinologists and 11% reported receiving patient summaries, although over 70% felt this was crucial to care continuity [144]. Fewer than half of adult endocrinologists reported being familiar with the American Diabetes Association's transition of care policy [145].

(b) Models of transition

Due to the concern that transfer of care to adult medicine is a vulnerable time for young adults with diabetes, multiple models have been utilized to improve care. It is recommended that the transition of care starts around ages 12–14, to allow ample time to explore potential barriers and establish self-reliance in disease control before transferring to an adult provider [146]. While there is not one established model to seamlessly transition care, a few have shown promising evidence for bridging the gap between pediatric and adult care, and planned transition overall shows a decrease in hospitalizations for DKA [147].

Increased involvement from providers during the transfer of care is crucial to ensuring a successful handoff. Combined visits (sometimes also called "transition clinic visits") with pediatric and adult endocrinologists can help improve clinic attendance and glycemic control [148]. This typically takes place in the pediatric office, and usually consists of one to two visits; it allows the patient to meet the adult endocrinologist in a familiar setting and feel there is a collaborative relationship with their pediatric endocrinologists, something patients and their families often say is important to them in choosing an adult provider [149]. Transition coordinators, frequently nurses or diabetes educators, can be helpful with scheduling appointments, individualized problem-solving, and follow-up for missed appointments. Studies that utilized both a transition clinic and transition coordinator showed the most significant improvements in self-reliance and disease control [147]. Transition coordinators are critical in reaching patients who are lost to follow-up, as most transition of care efforts take place in the clinical setting; in one study, a transition coordinator decreased loss to follow-up from 47.1% to 11.9% in patients with diabetes transferring to adult care [150].

Support from peers can also improve the transition to adult care. Many patients with diabetes acknowledge that when parents and caregivers become less central to their diabetes care, working with others who have been through a similar experience is an important method of problem-solving and coping [151]. Young adults with diabetes who participated in a peer support group had improvement in glycemic control and diabetes self-care [152]. Casual evening groups with medical providers and educational events have been shown to improve clinic attendance in adolescent patients [153].

Technology can be utilized to improve transition. Telemedicine visits, particularly school-based telemedicine, have been shown to improve glycemic control and glucose monitoring [154]. While mobile health applications have been utilized successfully with adolescents with other chronic conditions [155, 156], so far this benefit has not been shown to extend to adolescents with diabetes. One study showed a slight improvement in the frequency of blood glucose monitoring but no change in overall glycemic control among teens using an app that highlighted trends in glucose values and cited possible causes and fixes of out-of-range values [157]. Another study showed that the intervention group using a mobile app had worsened glycemic control compared to the control group [158].

## Chronic Condition Fact Sheet

### Type 1 Diabetes

#### What Is Type 1 Diabetes?

Type 1 diabetes is an autoimmune condition that affects the body's ability to break down food (sugar) into energy. In people without diabetes, the pancreas makes insulin which helps turn food into energy. In people with type 1 diabetes, the pancreas does not work properly, and insulin is not made at all (or in very small amounts). The body cannot survive without insulin.

#### How Is Type 1 Diabetes Treated?

People with type 1 diabetes need to inject insulin or use an insulin pump. They also need to check their blood sugar multiple times per day to see how much insulin to give.

#### What Is a Low Blood Sugar and How Is It Treated?

A low blood sugar means there is not enough glucose (sugar) in the blood. Low blood sugar levels occur with too much insulin, too little food, or an imbalance of food, insulin, and also sometimes with exercise, stress, and illness. Symptoms of low blood sugars include being shaky, dizzy, tired, sweaty, confused, irritable, pale, blurry vision, and hungry. Low blood sugar is treated with quick-acting carbohydrates such as juice, regular soda, or glucose tablets.

#### What Is a High Blood Sugar and How Is It Treated?

A high blood sugar means there is too much glucose (sugar) in the blood and too little insulin. Too high blood sugars can result from not taking insulin or taking too little insulin as well as stress and sickness. Symptoms include fatigue, increased thirst, dry skin, urinating frequently, blurry vision, and headache. Treatment of a high blood sugar includes insulin, increasing fluids, and monitoring blood sugars.

#### What Are the Risks of Not Controlling Blood Sugars?

Over time, high blood sugars can damage the body's eyes, heart, kidneys, and nerves.

#### What Are the Common Issues Emerging Adults with Diabetes Face?

Depression and anxiety are more common in teens and young adults with diabetes. Eating disorders are also more common in people with diabetes compared to those without diabetes. Other autoimmune problems occasionally occur including thyroid problems or celiac disease.

#### Can Women with Diabetes Have Children?

Women with diabetes can have healthy, normal pregnancies. It is recommended to have very tight blood sugar control before and during pregnancy (hemoglobin A1c goal before pregnancy $<7\%$ and during pregnancy $<6\%$). For this reason, it is recommended for women with diabetes to plan and prepare for pregnancy.

## Appendix

| Type 1 diabetes condition fact sheet | |
|---|---|
| Definition | Type 1 diabetes is an autoimmune condition that affects the pancreas' ability to make insulin needed to break down food (sugar) into energy needed for survival. It is defined by any of the following criteria:<br>• Fasting plasma glucose ≥126 mg/dL (7.0 mmol/L). Fasting is defined as no caloric intake for at least 8 h<br>• 2-h plasma glucose ≥200 mg/dL (11.1 mmol/L) during an oral glucose tolerance test<br>• A1C ≥ 6.5% (48 mmol/mol)<br>• In a patient with classic symptoms of hyperglycemia or hyperglycemic crisis, a random plasma glucose ≥200 mg/dL (11.1 mmol/L) |
| Epidemiology | • Prevalence of diabetes (both types 1 and 2 diabetes) among children in the United States is 3.2 per 1000<br>• Non-Hispanic white children have a higher prevalence of diabetes (3.8 per 1000 children) compared with other racial and ethnic categories (2.2 per 1000 children) |
| Special considerations | • *Depression and anxiety* are more common and more pronounced in patients with diabetes due to the associated disease-related emotional distress<br>• *Disordered eating* is 2.4 times more common in adolescent women with diabetes than those without, and the prevalence of insulin omission for weight loss affects up to 40% of young adult females with type 1 diabetes<br>• *Reproductive health* is critical to discuss to prevent unplanned pregnancy and to optimize the health outcomes of diabetic women and their infants. More than one-half of women with diabetes have experienced unplanned pregnancies and more than 75% were not aware of the maternal and fetal risks and the need for good glycemic control<br>• *Long-term vascular complications* are associated with poor glycemic control and should be routinely screened for to identify any nephropathy, retinopathy, neuropathy, and cardiovascular disease<br>• *Obesity* in patients with diabetes disproportionally affects minorities and young girls, especially those diagnosed between ages 10 and 15 years of age<br>• *Associated autoimmune diseases* that should be routinely screened for include thyroid disease and celiac disease<br>• *Alcohol, tobacco, and illicit drug use* can increase the risk for complications in patients with type 1 diabetes; physicians should routinely educate patients about the risk of cigarettes and nocturnal hypoglycemia with alcohol |
| Recommended screening | See Table 29.1 |

## References


1. Mayer-Davis EJ, Lawrence JM, Dabelea D, et al. Incidence trends of type 1 and type 2 diabetes among youths, 2002–2012. N Engl J Med. 2017;376(15):1419–29.
2. Thunander M, Petersson C, Jonzon K, et al. Incidence of type 1 and type 2 diabetes in adults and children in Kronoberg, Sweden. Diabetes Res Clin Pract. 2008;82(2):247–55.
3. Patterson CC, Harjutsalo V, Rosenbauer J, et al. Trends and cyclical variation in the incidence of childhood type 1 diabetes in 26 European centres in the 25 year period 1989-2013: a multicentre prospective registration study. Diabetologia. 2019;62(3):408–17.
4. Patterson C, Guariguata L, Dahlquist G, Soltész G, Ogle G, Silink M. Diabetes in the young—a global view and worldwide estimates of numbers of children with type 1 diabetes. Diabetes Res Clin Pract. 2014;103(2):161–75.
5. Rogers MAM, Kim C, Banerjee T, Lee JM. Fluctuations in the incidence of type 1 diabetes in the United States from 2001 to 2015: a longitudinal study. BMC Med. 2017;15(1):199.
6. Menke A, Casagrande S, Geiss L, Cowie CC. Prevalence of and trends in diabetes among adults in the United States, 1988-2012. JAMA. 2015;314(10):1021–9.
7. Lee JM, Herman WH, McPheeters ML, Gurney JG. An epidemiologic profile of children with diabetes in the U.S. Diabetes Care. 2006;29(2):420–1.
8. SEARCH for Diabetes in Youth Study Group, Liese AD, D'Agostino RB, et al. The burden of diabetes

mellitus among US youth: prevalence estimates from the SEARCH for diabetes in youth study. Pediatrics. 2006;118(4):1510–8. https://doi.org/10.1542/peds.2006-0690.
9. Kondrashova A, Reunanen A, Romanov A, et al. A six-fold gradient in the incidence of type 1 diabetes at the eastern border of Finland. Ann Med. 2005;37(1):67–72.
10. Rewers M, Ludvigsson J. Environmental risk factors for type 1 diabetes. Lancet. 2016;387(10035):2340–8.
11. Raghupathy P. Diabetic ketoacidosis in children and adolescents. Indian J Endocrinol Metab. 2015;19(Suppl 1):S55–7.
12. Kitabchi AE, Umpierrez GE, Miles JM, Fisher JN. Hyperglycemic crises in adult patients with diabetes. Diabetes Care. 2009;32(7):1335–43.
13. Ehrmann D, Kulzer B, Roos T, Haak T, Al-Khatib M, Hermanns N. Risk factors and prevention strategies for diabetic ketoacidosis in people with established type 1 diabetes. Lancet Diabetes Endocrinol. 2020;8(5):436–46.
14. Holt RIG, DeVries JH, Hess-Fischl A, et al. The management of type 1 diabetes in adults. A consensus report by the American Diabetes Association (ADA) and the European Association for the Study of Diabetes (EASD). Diabetologia. 2021.
15. Wolfsdorf J, Glaser N, Sperling MA, American Diabetes Association. Diabetic ketoacidosis in infants, children, and adolescents: a consensus statement from the American Diabetes Association. Diabetes Care. 2006;29(5):1150–9.
16. Umpierrez G, Korytkowski M. Diabetic emergencies—ketoacidosis, hyperglycaemic hyperosmolar state and hypoglycaemia. Nat Rev Endocrinol. 2016;12(4):222–32.
17. DeCosta P, Grabowski D, Skinner TC. The psychosocial experience and needs of children newly diagnosed with type 1 diabetes from their own perspective: a systematic and narrative review. Diabet Med J Br Diabet Assoc. 2020;37(10):1640–52.
18. Polonsky WH, Anderson BJ, Lohrer PA, et al. Assessment of diabetes-related distress. Diabetes Care. 1995;18(6):754–60.
19. Hagger V, Hendrieckx C, Sturt J, Skinner TC, Speight J. Diabetes distress among adolescents with type 1 diabetes: a systematic review. Curr Diab Rep. 2016;16(1):9.
20. Fisher L, Hessler D, Polonsky W, Strycker L, Masharani U, Peters A. Diabetes distress in adults with type 1 diabetes: prevalence, incidence and change over time. J Diabetes Complicat. 2016;30(6):1123–8.
21. McCarthy MM, Whittemore R, Gholson G, Grey M. Diabetes distress, depressive symptoms, and cardiovascular health in adults with type 1 diabetes. Nurs Res. 2019;68(6):445–52.
22. American Diabetes Association. 13. Children and adolescents: standards of medical Care in Diabetes—2021. Diabetes Care. 2021;44(Supplement 1):S180–99.
23. Nguyen LA, Pouwer F, Winterdijk P, et al. Prevalence and course of mood and anxiety disorders, and correlates of symptom severity in adolescents with type 1 diabetes: results from diabetes LEAP. Pediatr Diabetes. 2021;22(4):638–48.
24. Trief PM, Xing D, Foster NC, et al. Depression in adults in the T1D exchange clinic registry. Diabetes Care. 2014;37(6):1563–72.
25. Anderson BJ, Edelstein S, Abramson NW, et al. Depressive symptoms and quality of life in adolescents with type 2 diabetes: baseline data from the TODAY study. Diabetes Care. 2011;34(10):2205–7.
26. Knight A, Weiss P, Morales K, et al. Identifying differences in risk factors for depression and anxiety in pediatric chronic disease: a matched cross-sectional study of youth with lupus/mixed connective tissue disease and their peers with diabetes. J Pediatr. 2015;167(6):1397–1403.e1.
27. Gonzalez JS, Safren SA, Cagliero E, et al. Depression, self-care, and medication adherence in type 2 diabetes: relationships across the full range of symptom severity. Diabetes Care. 2007;30(9):2222–7.
28. Lustman PJ, Anderson RJ, Freedland KE, de Groot M, Carney RM, Clouse RE. Depression and poor glycemic control: a meta-analytic review of the literature. Diabetes Care. 2000;23(7):934–42.
29. Bernstein CM, Stockwell MS, Gallagher MP, Rosenthal SL, Soren K. Mental health issues in adolescents and Young adults with type 1 diabetes: prevalence and impact on glycemic control. Clin Pediatr (Phila). 2013;52(1):10–5.
30. Uchendu C, Blake H. Effectiveness of cognitive-behavioural therapy on glycaemic control and psychological outcomes in adults with diabetes mellitus: a systematic review and meta-analysis of randomized controlled trials. Diabet Med J Br Diabet Assoc. 2017;34(3):328–39.
31. Simon GE, Katon WJ, Lin EHB, et al. Cost-effectiveness of systematic depression treatment among people with diabetes mellitus. Arch Gen Psychiatry. 2007;64(1):65–72.
32. Dierker LC, Albano AM, Clarke GN, et al. Screening for anxiety and depression in early adolescence. J Am Acad Child Adolesc Psychiatry. 2001;40(8):929–36.
33. Rechenberg K, Whittemore R, Grey M. Anxiety in youth with type 1 diabetes. J Pediatr Nurs. 2017;32:64–71.
34. Buchberger B, Huppertz H, Krabbe L, Lux B, Mattivi JT, Siafarikas A. Symptoms of depression and anxiety in youth with type 1 diabetes: a systematic review and meta-analysis. Psychoneuroendocrinology. 2016;70:70–84.
35. Ginsburg GS, Riddle MA, Davies M. Somatic symptoms in children and adolescents with anxiety disorders. J Am Acad Child Adolesc Psychiatry. 2006;45(10):1179–87.
36. Herzer M, Hood KK. Anxiety symptoms in adolescents with type 1 diabetes: association with blood

glucose monitoring and glycemic control. J Pediatr Psychol. 2010;35(4):415–25.
37. Minges KE, Whittemore R, Weinzimer SA, Irwin ML, Redeker NS, Grey M. Correlates of overweight and obesity in 5529 adolescents with type 1 diabetes: the T1D exchange clinic registry. Diabetes Res Clin Pract. 2017;126:68–78.
38. Szadkowska A, Madej A, Ziółkowska K, et al. Gender and age—dependent effect of type 1 diabetes on obesity and altered body composition in young adults. Ann Agric Environ Med AAEM. 2015;22(1):124–8.
39. Fröhlich-Reiterer EE, Rosenbauer J, Bechtold-Dalla Pozza S, et al. Predictors of increasing BMI during the course of diabetes in children and adolescents with type 1 diabetes: data from the German/Austrian DPV multicentre survey. Arch Dis Child. 2014;99(8):738–43. https://doi.org/10.1136/archdischild-2013-304237.
40. Colberg SR, Laan R, Dassau E, Kerr D. Physical activity and type 1 diabetes: time for a rewire? J Diabetes Sci Technol. 2015;9(3):609–18.
41. Fairburn CG, Beglin SJ. Studies of the epidemiology of bulimia nervosa. Am J Psychiatry. 1990;147(4):401–8.
42. Toni G, Berioli M, Cerquiglini L, et al. Eating disorders and disordered eating symptoms in adolescents with type 1 diabetes. Nutrients. 2017;9(8):906.
43. Young V, Eiser C, Johnson B, et al. Eating problems in adolescents with type 1 diabetes: a systematic review with meta-analysis. Diabet Med J Br Diabet Assoc. 2013;30(2):189–98.
44. Markowitz JT, Butler DA, Volkening LK, Antisdel JE, Anderson BJ, Laffel LMB. Brief screening tool for disordered eating in diabetes: internal consistency and external validity in a contemporary sample of pediatric patients with type 1 diabetes. Diabetes Care. 2010;33(3):495–500.
45. Pinhas-Hamiel O, Hamiel U, Levy-Shraga Y. Eating disorders in adolescents with type 1 diabetes: challenges in diagnosis and treatment. World J Diabetes. 2015;6(3):517–26.
46. Deiana V, Diana E, Pinna F, et al. Clinical features in insulin-treated diabetes with comorbid diabulimia, disordered eating behaviors and eating disorders. Eur Psychiatry. 2016;33(S1):S81–1.
47. Takii M, Uchigata Y, Kishimoto J, et al. The relationship between the age of onset of type 1 diabetes and the subsequent development of a severe eating disorder by female patients. Pediatr Diabetes. 2011;12(4 Pt 2):396–401.
48. Jones JM, Lawson ML, Daneman D, Olmsted MP, Rodin G. Eating disorders in adolescent females with and without type 1 diabetes: cross sectional study. BMJ. 2000;320(7249):1563–6.
49. Coleman SE, Caswell N. Diabetes and eating disorders: an exploration of 'Diabulimia'. BMC Psychol. 2020;8(1):101.
50. Rodin G, Olmsted MP, Rydall AC, et al. Eating disorders in young women with type 1 diabetes mellitus. J Psychosom Res. 2002;53(4):943–9.
51. Verrotti A, Catino M, De Luca FA, Morgese G, Chiarelli F. Eating disorders in adolescents with type 1 diabetes mellitus. Acta Diabetol. 1999;36(1–2):21–5.
52. Colton PA, Olmsted MP, Daneman D, et al. Eating disorders in girls and women with type 1 diabetes: a longitudinal study of prevalence, onset, remission, and recurrence. Diabetes Care. 2015;38(7):1212–7.
53. Cecilia-Costa R, Volkening LK, Laffel LM. Factors associated with disordered eating behaviours in adolescents with type 1 diabetes. Diabet Med. 2019;36(8):1020–7.
54. Rohde P, Stice E, Marti CN. Development and predictive effects of eating disorder risk factors during adolescence: implications for prevention efforts. Int J Eat Disord. 2015;48(2):187–98.
55. Zuijdwijk CS, Pardy SA, Dowden JJ, Dominic AM, Bridger T, Newhook LA. The mSCOFF for screening disordered eating in pediatric type 1 diabetes. Diabetes Care. 2014;37(2):e26–7.
56. Wägner AM, Santana A, Herńndez M, et al. Predictors of associated autoimmune diseases in families with type 1 diabetes: results from the type 1 diabetes genetics consortium. Diabetes Metab Res Rev. 2011;27(5):493–8.
57. Riquetto ADC, de Noronha RM, Matsuo EM, et al. Thyroid function and autoimmunity in children and adolescents with type 1 diabetes mellitus. Diabetes Res Clin Pract. 2015;110(1):e9–e11.
58. Nederstigt C, Uitbeijerse BS, Janssen LGM, Corssmit EPM, de Koning EJP, Dekkers OM. Associated autoimmune disease in type 1 diabetes patients: a systematic review and meta-analysis. Eur J Endocrinol. 2019;180(2):135–44.
59. Li L, Liu S, Yu J. Autoimmune thyroid disease and type 1 diabetes mellitus: same pathogenesis; new perspective? Ther Adv Endocrinol Metab. 2020;11:204201882095832.
60. Ogarek N, Mrówka A, Jarosz-Chobot P. Thyroid diseases—ally or enemy of type 1 diabetes in children and adolescents? Pediatr Endocrinol Diabetes Metab. 2021:42740.
61. American Diabetes Association. 4. Comprehensive medical evaluation and assessment of comorbidities: standards of medical care in diabetes—2021. Diabetes Care. 2021;44(Supplement 1):S40–52.
62. Craig ME, Prinz N, Boyle CT, et al. Prevalence of celiac disease in 52,721 youth with type 1 diabetes: international comparison across three continents. Diabetes Care. 2017;40(8):1034–40.
63. Puñales M, Bastos MD, Ramos ARL, et al. Prevalence of celiac disease in a large cohort of young patients with type 1 diabetes. Pediatr Diabetes. 2019;20(4):414–20.
64. Warncke K, Fröhlich-Reiterer EE, Thon A, et al. Polyendocrinopathy in children, adolescents, and young adults with type 1 diabetes: a multicenter

analysis of 28,671 patients from the German/Austrian DPV-Wiss database. Diabetes Care. 2010;33(9):2010–2.

65. Rohrer TR, Wolf J, Liptay S, et al. Microvascular complications in childhood-onset type 1 diabetes and celiac disease: a multicenter longitudinal analysis of 56,514 patients from the German-Austrian DPV database. Diabetes Care. 2015;38(5):801–7.
66. Warncke K, Liptay S, Fröhlich-Reiterer E, et al. Vascular risk factors in children, adolescents, and young adults with type 1 diabetes complicated by celiac disease: results from the DPV initiative. Pediatr Diabetes. 2016;17(3):191–8.
67. Verkasalo M, Kuitunen P, Leisti S, Perheentupa J. Growth failure from symptomless celiac disease. A study of 14 patients. Helv Paediatr Acta. 1978;33(6):489–95.
68. Pham-Short A, Donaghue KC, Ambler G, Phelan H, Twigg S, Craig ME. Screening for celiac disease in type 1 diabetes: a systematic review. Pediatrics. 2015;136(1):e170–6.
69. Diabetes Control and Complications Trial Research Group, Nathan DM, Genuth S, et al. The effect of intensive treatment of diabetes on the development and progression of long-term complications in insulin-dependent diabetes mellitus. N Engl J Med. 1993;329(14):977–86.
70. Pambianco G, Costacou T, Ellis D, Becker DJ, Klein R, Orchard TJ. The 30-year natural history of type 1 diabetes complications: the Pittsburgh epidemiology of diabetes complications study experience. Diabetes. 2006;55(5):1463–9.
71. Urbina EM, Isom S, Bell RA, et al. Burden of cardiovascular risk factors over time and arterial stiffness in youth with type 1 diabetes mellitus: the SEARCH for diabetes in youth study. J Am Heart Assoc. 2019;8(13):e010150.
72. Sparud-Lundin C, Ohrn I, Danielson E, Forsander G. Glycaemic control and diabetes care utilization in young adults with type 1 diabetes. Diabet Med J Br Diabet Assoc. 2008;25(8):968–73.
73. Nordwall M, Bojestig M, Arnqvist HJ, Ludvigsson J. Declining incidence of severe retinopathy and persisting decrease of nephropathy in an unselected population of type 1 diabetes-the Linköping diabetes complications study. Diabetologia. 2004;47(7):1266–72.
74. Perkins BA, Bebu I, de Boer IH, et al. Risk factors for kidney disease in type 1 diabetes. Diabetes Care. 2019;42(5):883–90.
75. Costacou T, Orchard TJ. Cumulative kidney complication risk by 50 years of type 1 diabetes: the effects of sex, age, and calendar year at onset. Diabetes Care. 2018;41(3):426–33.
76. Papadopoulou-Marketou N, Paschou SA, Marketos N, Adamidi S, Adamidis S, Kanaka-Gantenbein C. Diabetic nephropathy in type 1 diabetes. Minerva Med. 2018;109(3):218–28.
77. Amin R, Widmer B, Prevost AT, et al. Risk of microalbuminuria and progression to macroalbuminuria in a cohort with childhood onset type 1 diabetes: prospective observational study. BMJ. 2008;336(7646):697–701.
78. Downie ML, Ulrich EH, Noone DG. An update on hypertension in children with type 1 diabetes. Can J Diabetes. 2018;42(2):199–204.
79. Guntsche Z, Saraví FD, Reynals EA, Rauek B, Rauek M, Guntsche EM. Parental hypertension and 24 h-blood pressure in children prior to diabetic nephropathy. Pediatr Nephrol Berl Ger. 2002;17(3):157–64.
80. Standards of medical care in diabetes—2015: summary of revisions. Diabetes Care. 2015;38 Suppl:S4.
81. Chiesa ST, Marcovecchio ML, Benitez-Aguirre P, et al. Vascular effects of ACE (angiotensin-converting enzyme) inhibitors and statins in adolescents with type 1 diabetes. Hypertens Dallas Tex 1979. 2020;76(6):1734–43.
82. Lee SI, Patel M, Jones CM, Narendran P. Cardiovascular disease and type 1 diabetes: prevalence, prediction and management in an ageing population. Ther Adv Chronic Dis. 2015;6(6):347–74.
83. Kallinikou D, Soldatou A, Tsentidis C, et al. Diabetic neuropathy in children and adolescents with type 1 diabetes mellitus: diagnosis, pathogenesis, and associated genetic markers. Diabetes Metab Res Rev. 2019;35(7):e3178.
84. Jaiswal M, Lauer A, Martin CL, et al. Peripheral neuropathy in adolescents and young adults with type 1 and type 2 diabetes from the SEARCH for diabetes in youth follow-up cohort: a pilot study. Diabetes Care. 2013;36(12):3903–8.
85. Cameron FJ, Northam EA, Ryan CM. The effect of type 1 diabetes on the developing brain. Lancet Child Adolesc Health. 2019;3(6):427–36.
86. Pop-Busui R, Low PA, Waberski BH, et al. Effects of prior intensive insulin therapy on cardiac autonomic nervous system function in type 1 diabetes mellitus: the diabetes control and complications trial/epidemiology of diabetes interventions and complications study (DCCT/EDIC). Circulation. 2009;119(22):2886–93.
87. Dimitropoulos G, Tahrani AA, Stevens MJ. Cardiac autonomic neuropathy in patients with diabetes mellitus. World J Diabetes. 2014;5(1):17–39.
88. Albers JW, Herman WH, Pop-Busui R, et al. Effect of prior intensive insulin treatment during the diabetes control and complications trial (DCCT) on peripheral neuropathy in type 1 diabetes during the epidemiology of diabetes interventions and complications (EDIC) study. Diabetes Care. 2010;33(5):1090–6.
89. Htay T, Soe K, Lopez-Perez A, Doan AH, Romagosa MA, Aung K. Mortality and cardiovascular disease in type 1 and type 2 diabetes. Curr Cardiol Rep. 2019;21(6):45.
90. Rawshani A, Sattar N, Franzén S, et al. Excess mortality and cardiovascular disease in young adults with type 1 diabetes in relation to age at onset: a nationwide, register-based cohort study. Lancet Lond Engl. 2018;392(10146):477–86.

91. Diabetes Control and Complications Trial (DCCT)/ Epidemiology of Diabetes Interventions and Complications (EDIC) Study Research Group. Intensive diabetes treatment and cardiovascular outcomes in type 1 diabetes: the DCCT/ EDIC study 30-year follow-up. Diabetes Care. 2016;39(5):686–93.
92. Gøtzsche O, Darwish A, Gøtzsche L, Hansen LP, Sørensen KE. Incipient cardiomyopathy in young insulin-dependent diabetic patients: a seven-year prospective Doppler echocardiographic study. Diabet Med J Br Diabet Assoc. 1996;13(9):834–40.
93. Järvisalo MJ, Putto-Laurila A, Jartti L, et al. Carotid artery intima-media thickness in children with type 1 diabetes. Diabetes. 2002;51(2):493–8.
94. Maahs DM, Dabelea D, D'Agostino RB, et al. Glucose control predicts 2-year change in lipid profile in youth with type 1 diabetes. J Pediatr. 2013;162(1):101–107.e1.
95. Absil H, Baudet L, Robert A, Lysy PA. Benefits of physical activity in children and adolescents with type 1 diabetes: a systematic review. Diabetes Res Clin Pract. 2019;156:107810.
96. Petersen EE, Mitchell AA, Carey JC, et al. Maternal exposure to statins and risk for birth defects: a case-series approach. Am J Med Genet A. 2008;146A(20):2701–5.
97. Potter K, Virtanen H, Luca P, et al. Knowledge and practice of harm-reduction behaviours for alcohol and other illicit substance use in adolescents with type 1 diabetes. Paediatr Child Health. 2019;24(1):e51–6.
98. Peters A, Laffel L, American Diabetes Association Transitions Working Group. Diabetes care for emerging adults: recommendations for transition from pediatric to adult diabetes care systems: a position statement of the American Diabetes Association, with representation by the American College of Osteopathic Family Physicians, the American Academy of Pediatrics, the American Association of Clinical Endocrinologists, the American Osteopathic Association, the Centers for Disease Control and Prevention, Children with Diabetes, The Endocrine Society, the International Society for Pediatric and Adolescent Diabetes, Juvenile Diabetes Research Foundation International, the National Diabetes Education Program, and the Pediatric Endocrine Society (formerly Lawson Wilkins Pediatric Endocrine Society). Diabetes Care. 2011;34(11):2477–85.
99. Lycett D, Nichols L, Ryan R, et al. The association between smoking cessation and glycaemic control in patients with type 2 diabetes: a THIN database cohort study. Lancet Diabetes Endocrinol. 2015;3(6):423–30.
100. Tyrberg M, Nyström L, Arnqvist HJ, et al. Overweight, hyperglycemia and tobacco use are modifiable risk factors for onset of retinopathy 9 and 17years after the diagnosis of diabetes—a retrospective observational nation-wide cohort study. Diabetes Res Clin Pract. 2017;133:21–9.
101. Braffett BH, Gubitosi-Klug RA, Albers JW, et al. Risk factors for diabetic peripheral neuropathy and cardiovascular autonomic neuropathy in the diabetes control and complications trial/epidemiology of diabetes interventions and complications (DCCT/ EDIC) study. Diabetes. 2020;69(5):1000–10.
102. Haire-Joshu D, Glasgow RE, Tibbs TL. Smoking and diabetes. Diabetes Care. 1999;22(11):1887–98.
103. Valerio G, Mozzillo E, Zito E, et al. Alcohol consumption or cigarette smoking and cardiovascular disease risk in youth with type 1 diabetes. Acta Diabetol. 2019;56(12):1315–21.
104. Pan A, Wang Y, Talaei M, Hu FB. Relation of smoking with total mortality and cardiovascular events among patients with diabetes mellitus: a meta-analysis and systematic review. Circulation. 2015;132(19):1795–804.
105. Tonstad S, Lawrence D. Varenicline in smokers with diabetes: a pooled analysis of 15 randomized, placebo-controlled studies of varenicline. J Diabetes Investig. 2017;8(1):93–100.
106. White ND. Alcohol use in Young adults with type 1 diabetes mellitus. Am J Lifestyle Med. 2017;11(6):433–5.
107. Kerr D, Macdonald IA, Heller SR, Tattersall RB. Alcohol causes hypoglycaemic unawareness in healthy volunteers and patients with type 1 (insulin-dependent) diabetes. Diabetologia. 1990;33(4):216–21.
108. Alessi SM, Foster NC, Rash CJ, et al. Alcohol use and clinical outcomes in adults in the type 1 diabetes exchange. Can J Diabetes. 2020;44(6):501–6.
109. Tetzschner R, Nørgaard K, Ranjan A. Effects of alcohol on plasma glucose and prevention of alcohol-induced hypoglycemia in type 1 diabetes-a systematic review with GRADE. Diabetes Metab Res Rev. 2018;34(3).
110. Petry NM, Foster NC, Cengiz E, Tamborlane WV, Wagner J, Polsky S. Substance use in adults with type 1 diabetes in the T1D exchange. Diabetes Educ. 2018;44(6):510–8.
111. Umpierrez GE, Kelly JP, Navarrete JE, Casals MM, Kitabchi AE. Hyperglycemic crises in urban blacks. Arch Intern Med. 1997;157(6):669–75.
112. Warner EA, Greene GS, Buchsbaum MS, Cooper DS, Robinson BE. Diabetic ketoacidosis associated with cocaine use. Arch Intern Med. 1998;158(16):1799–802.
113. Kinney GL, Akturk HK, Taylor DD, Foster NC, Shah VN. Cannabis use is associated with increased risk for diabetic ketoacidosis in adults with type 1 diabetes: findings from the T1D exchange clinic registry. Diabetes Care. 2020;43(1):247–9.
114. Lawrence JM, Contreras R, Chen W, Sacks DA. Trends in the prevalence of preexisting diabetes and gestational diabetes mellitus among a racially/ ethnically diverse population of pregnant women, 1999-2005. Diabetes Care. 2008;31(5):899–904.
115. Vahratian A, Barber JS, Lawrence JM, Kim C. Family-planning practices among women with

diabetes and overweight and obese women in the 2002 National Survey for Family Growth. Diabetes Care. 2009;32(6):1026–31.
116. Giraudo F, Lalanne I, Valdés I, Gajardo A, Charron-Prochownik D, Codner E. Risky sexual behaviors in adolescents and young adult women with type 1 diabetes: an overlooked problem. Pediatr Diabetes. 2021.
117. Kitzmiller JL, Buchanan TA, Kjos S, Combs CA, Ratner RE. Pre-conception care of diabetes, congenital malformations, and spontaneous abortions. Diabetes Care. 1996;19(5):514–41.
118. McCance DR, Casey C. Type 1 diabetes in pregnancy. Endocrinol Metab Clin N Am. 2019;48(3):495–509.
119. Feldman AZ, Brown FM. Management of Type 1 diabetes in pregnancy. Curr Diab Rep. 2016;16(8):76.
120. Feig DS, Donovan LE, Corcoy R, et al. Continuous glucose monitoring in pregnant women with type 1 diabetes (CONCEPTT): a multicentre international randomised controlled trial. Lancet Lond Engl. 2017;390(10110):2347–59.
121. Mukherjee MS, Coppenrath VA, Dallinga BA. Pharmacologic management of types 1 and 2 diabetes mellitus and their complications in women of childbearing age. Pharmacotherapy. 2015;35(2):158–74.
122. Preconception care of women with diabetes. Diabetes Care. 2004;27(Supplement 1):S76-S78.
123. Schwarz EB, Sobota M, Charron-Prochownik D. Perceived access to contraception among adolescents with diabetes: barriers to preventing pregnancy complications. Diabetes Educ. 2010;36(3):489–94.
124. Osman A, Hoffman A, Moore S, van der Spuy Z. Reproductive knowledge and use of contraception among women with diabetes. South Afr Med J Suid-Afr Tydskr Vir Geneeskd. 2015;105(9):760–4.
125. Charron-Prochownik D, Sereika SM, Wang SL, et al. Reproductive health and preconception counseling awareness in adolescents with diabetes: what they don't know can hurt them. Diabetes Educ. 2006;32(2):235–42.
126. Scal P. Transition for youth with chronic conditions: primary care physicians' approaches. Pediatrics. 2002;110(6 Pt 2):1315–21.
127. Kohn JR, Hilliard ME, Lyons SK, Fox KA, Kushner JA. Identifying and addressing gaps in reproductive health education for adolescent girls with type 1 diabetes. PLoS One. 2018;13(11):e0206102.
128. Sereika SM, Becker D, Schmitt P, et al. Operationalizing and examining family planning vigilance in adult women with type 1 diabetes. Diabetes Care. 2016;39(12):2197–203.
129. Johnson K, Posner SF, Biermann J, et al. Recommendations to improve preconception health and health care—United States. A report of the CDC/ATSDR Preconception Care Work Group and the Select Panel on Preconception Care. MMWR Recomm Rep Morb Mortal Wkly Rep Recomm Rep. 2006;55(RR-6):1–23.
130. Americans with Disabilities Act. https://www.dol.gov/general/topic/disability/ada. Accessed 1 Dec 2015
131. Gordon K, Rapp JA, Dimmick BL, Jackson C. Going to college with diabetes: a self advocacy guide for students. http://main.diabetes.org/dorg/PDFs/Advocacy/Discrimination/going-to-college-with-diabetes.pdf. Accessed 1 Dec 2015.
132. On Your Own But Not Alone. College Diabetes Network.
133. Crossen S, Xing G, Hoch JS. Changing costs of type 1 diabetes care among US children and adolescents. Pediatr Diabetes. 2020;21(4):644–8.
134. Insurance. https://collegediabetesnetwork.org/insurance. Accessed 31 Aug 2021.
135. Mellinger DC. Preparing students with diabetes for life at college. Diabetes Care. 2003;26(9):2675–8.
136. Juvenile Diabetes Research Foundation. Letter to My Roommate. https://hscweb3.hsc.usf.edu/wp-content/uploads/2012/02/Dear_Roommate.pdf. Accessed 30 Nov 2015.
137. Rausch JR, Hood KK, Delamater A, et al. Changes in treatment adherence and glycemic control during the transition to adolescence in type 1 diabetes. Diabetes Care. 2012;35(6):1219–24.
138. Mays JA, Jackson KL, Derby TA, et al. An evaluation of recurrent diabetic ketoacidosis, fragmentation of care, and mortality across Chicago, Illinois. Diabetes Care. 2016;39(10):1671–6.
139. Lotstein DS, Seid M, Klingensmith G, et al. Transition from pediatric to adult care for youth diagnosed with type 1 diabetes in adolescence. Pediatrics. 2013;131(4):e1062–70.
140. Ness MM, Saylor J, Selekman J. Barriers and facilitators influencing parental transition of college-bound youth with type 1 diabetes mellitus: an integrative review. Curr Diab Rep. 2019;19(8):57.
141. Ersig AL, Tsalikian E, Coffey J, Williams JK. Stressors in teens with type 1 diabetes and their parents: immediate and long-term implications for transition to self-management. J Pediatr Nurs. 2016;31(4):390–6.
142. Baretić M, Matovinović Osvatić M, Pavić E, et al. Type 1 diabetes from adolescence to adulthood: is there a permanent need for nutrition education and re-education? Minerva Endocrinol. 2018;43(1):27–33.
143. Agarwal S, Garvey KC, Raymond JK, Schutta MH. Perspectives on care for young adults with type 1 diabetes transitioning from pediatric to adult health systems: a national survey of pediatric endocrinologists. Pediatr Diabetes. 2017;18(7):524–31.
144. Garvey KC, Telo GH, Needleman JS, Forbes P, Finkelstein JA, Laffel LM. Health care transition in Young adults with type 1 diabetes: perspectives of adult endocrinologists in the U.S. Diabetes Care. 2016;39(2):190–7.
145. Michaud S, Dasgupta K, Bell L, et al. Adult care providers' perspectives on the transition to adult care for emerging adults with type 1 diabetes: a cross-

sectional survey. Diabet Med J Br Diabet Assoc. 2018;35(7):846–54.
146. Six Core Elements of Health Care Transition. https://www.gottransition.org/six-core-elements/. Accessed 25 July 2021.
147. Schultz AT, Smaldone A. Components of interventions that improve transitions to adult care for adolescents with type 1 diabetes. J Adolesc Health Off Publ Soc Adolesc Med. 2017;60(2):133–46.
148. Levy-Shraga Y, Elisha N, Ben-Ami M, et al. Glycemic control and clinic attendance of emerging adults with type 1 diabetes at a transition care clinic. Acta Diabetol. 2016;53(1):27–33.
149. van Staa AL, Jedeloo S, van Meeteren J, Latour JM. Crossing the transition chasm: experiences and recommendations for improving transitional care of young adults, parents and providers. Child Care Health Dev. 2011;37(6):821–32.
150. Butalia S, Crawford SG, McGuire KA, Dyjur DK, Mercer JR, Pacaud D. Improved transition to adult care in youth with type 1 diabetes: a pragmatic clinical trial. Diabetologia. 2021;64(4):758–66.
151. Tong A, Wong G, Hodson E, Walker RG, Tjaden L, Craig JC. Adolescent views on transition in diabetes and nephrology. Eur J Pediatr. 2013;172(3):293–304.
152. Markowitz JT, Laffel LMB. Transitions in care: support group for young adults with type 1 diabetes: support group for young adults with type 1 diabetes. Diabet Med. 2012;29(4):522–5.
153. Van Walleghem N, Macdonald CA, Dean HJ. Evaluation of a systems navigator model for transition from pediatric to adult care for young adults with type 1 diabetes. Diabetes Care. 2008;31(8):1529–30.
154. Guljas R, Ahmed A, Chang K, Whitlock A. Impact of telemedicine in managing type 1 diabetes among school-age children and adolescents: an integrative review. J Pediatr Nurs. 2014;29(3):198–204.
155. Farooqui N, Phillips G, Barrett C, Stukus D. Acceptability of an interactive asthma management mobile health application for children and adolescents. Ann Allergy Asthma Immunol. 2015;114(6):527–9.
156. Le Marne FA, Butler S, Beavis E, Gill D, Bye AME. EpApp: development and evaluation of a smartphone/tablet app for adolescents with epilepsy. J Clin Neurosci. 2018;50:214–20.
157. Goyal S, Nunn CA, Rotondi M, et al. A Mobile app for the self-Management of Type 1 diabetes among adolescents: a randomized controlled trial. JMIR Mhealth Uhealth. 2017;5(6):e82.
158. Castensøe-Seidenfaden P, Husted GR, Jensen AK, et al. Testing a smartphone app (young with diabetes) to improve self-management of diabetes over 12 months: randomized controlled trial. JMIR Mhealth Uhealth. 2018;6(6):e141.

## Suggested Reading

American Association of Clinical Endocrinologists. Find an endocrinologist.
American College of Physicians. Pediatric to adult care transitions initiative. https://www.acponline.org/clinical-information/high-value-care/resources-for-clinicians/pediatric-to-adult-care-transitions-initiative.
American Diabetes Association. Standards of medical care in diabetes—2015 and diabetes care for emerging adults: recommendations for transition from pediatric to adult diabetes care systems.
Endocrine society managing the transition of care for patients with type 1 diabetes (including A recommended approach to planning for pediatric practices and a recommended approach to the adolescent transitioning to adult practice). https://www.endocrine.org/education-and-practice-management/quality-improvement-resources/clinical-practice-resources/transition-of-care.
Got transition six core elements (elements of health care transition for clinicians) https://www.gottransition.org/six-core-elements/.
Hormone Health Network. Find an endocrinologist.
Juvenile Diabetes Research Foundation.
National Diabetes Education Program. Transition resources pediatric to adult health care.

## Patient/Caregiver Resources

American Association of Clinical Endocrinologists.
American Diabetes Association's. Going to college with diabetes: a self advocacy guide for students.
Americans with Disabilities Act. http://www.dol.gov/dol/topic/disability/ada.htm.
College Diabetes Network. Preparing for college, life on campus, between visits and other resources. http://www.collegediabetesnetwork.org.
Endocrine Society Transitions of Care for Diabetes Resources. https://www.endocrine.org/improving-practice/transitions.
Hormone Health Network. Find an endocrinologist.
Juvenile Diabetes Research Foundation. https://www.jdrf.org/wp-content/docs/JDRF_School_Advisory_Toolkit.pdf including "Letter to My Roommate" (https://hscweb3.hsc.usf.edu/wp-content/uploads/2012/02/Dear_Roommate.pdf) and Type 1 Diabetes Teen Toolkit. https://www.jdrf.org/wp-content/uploads/2013/10/JDRFTEENTOOLKIT.pdf.
National Diabetes Education Program. http://ndep.nih.gov/transitions/resourceslist.aspx.

# Down Syndrome

# 30

Kristin M. Jensen, Peter D. Bulova, and Stephanie Santoro

## Case Presentations

These three patients were each referred to the adult Down syndrome center for evaluation of a decline in skills and possible Alzheimer's type dementia.

Bobby is a 24-year-old male with Down syndrome with a history of depression. He is followed by a therapist and was doing well until 6 months ago. He often prefers to be alone, and they wondered if this could be a sign of depression. However, his parents have noticed significant changes in his behavior, function, and perseveration/hallucination about imaginary characters that he has not had before. They are concerned that his movements are significantly delayed; it can take him 2 h to eat a meal because of the slowness with moving food to his mouth. They mentioned that before this started, Bobby had a hard time with his sister's move to college out-of-state.

Susan is a 33-year-old female with Down syndrome with a history of hypothyroidism and a repaired ventricular septal defect. She recently moved from her family home to a group home, as the health of her parents was failing. She has shown little interest in leaving the house and has had a decline in productivity at her work in a clothing shop. She has had an increase in self-talking and compulsive behaviors, making piles of her belongings and refusing to throw out old magazines or papers. She is less social and spends more time in her room.

Jonathan is a 52-year-old male with Down syndrome with a history of congenital heart disease, difficulty swallowing, and several previous bouts of aspirations pneumonia. He is currently living in a group home. He has shown a gradual decline in skills over the past 6 months, with new issues of balance disturbance and recent urinary incontinence. He demonstrates persistent forgetfulness, often having trouble remembering previous skills such as how to set the table or brush his teeth. He was found to have a new tonic–clonic seizure 5 months ago and is now on levetiracetam. He has had no further seizure episodes events.

K. M. Jensen
Departments of Pediatrics and Internal Medicine, University of Colorado School of Medicine, Aurora, CO, USA
e-mail: kristin.jensen@cuanschutz.edu

P. D. Bulova
Department of Internal Medicine, General Internal Medicine, UPMC Montefiore Hospital, University of Pittsburgh Medical Center, Pittsburgh, PA, USA
e-mail: bulovapd@upmc.edu

S. Santoro (✉)
Department of Pediatrics, Massachusetts General Hospital, Boston, MA, USA
e-mail: ssantoro3@mgh.harvard.edu


A. A. Kuo et al. (eds.), *Care of Adults with Chronic Childhood Conditions*,
https://doi.org/10.1007/978-3-031-54281-7_30

## Case Discussion

### Decline in Skills in Down Syndrome

While the case of Jonathan describes a common presentation of Alzheimer's dementia in an adult with Down syndrome, Susan's case is a "masquerader" of dementia—in this case, depression. Bobby's case refers to developmental regression (discussed below).

A great deal of attention is paid to the development of dementia in adults with Down syndrome. This is due to the fact that the pathogenesis of Alzheimer's dementia is linked to excess amyloid protein, the gene for which is found on Chromosome 21 [1]. Despite the fact that autopsy specimens of adults with Down syndrome over age 35 years show neurofibrillary plaques and tangles, Alzheimer's dementia is a clinical diagnosis and does not develop universally in this population [2]. Current estimates of the prevalence of Alzheimer's dementia among individuals with Down syndrome are 10% in those ages 40–49 years, 20% in those ages 50–60 years, and 40% in those over 60 years of age. There are very few cases of true Alzheimer's dementia before age 40 years [3].

Because Alzheimer's dementia is a clinical diagnosis, most of the data used relies on the first-hand descriptions of caregivers, who tend to focus on patient behaviors that impact the caregivers. This can lead to an overestimation of the diagnosis when compared to results from direct assessment. Additionally, clinicians are predisposed to over-diagnose dementia, as the clinical diagnosis of dementia is difficult to make, and the inevitability of dementia is presumed in adults with Down syndrome [4]. Traditional tools such as the mini-mental status exam are unreliable and unusable in nearly half of adults with Down syndrome [4]. The current health guidelines for adults with Down syndrome suggest screening with the EDSD-NTG or other instruments, such as the ABDQ [5, 6]. A dementia assessment must include both a medical and psychiatric evaluation, as multiple conditions can mimic the decline in skills of Alzheimer's. One must assess emotional and motivational changes in addition to memory changes.

There are distinguishing differences between the presentations of Alzheimer's dementia in those with Down syndrome compared to those without Down syndrome. The incidence of adult-onset seizure development is much higher in those with dementia and Down syndrome [7]. They often develop incontinence, sleep disturbance, apathy, gait changes, and personality changes [4]. At this time, the treatments available for adults with Down syndrome and dementia are mainly supportive. There are several Cochrane database reviews of different medications for the treatment of dementia in adults with Down syndrome, none of which support their use [8–12]. The largest trial of pharmaceutical intervention used memantine, which showed no benefit and actually showed a trend toward worse behaviors in the treatment group [13]. Aducanumab is an antibody against amyloid that was approved in 2021. Most organizations do not support its use in adults with Down syndrome due to side effects such as brain swelling and microhemorrhages, limited efficacy in adults without Down syndrome, and no testing in adults with Down syndrome [14]. Current recommendations focus on interventions to minimize caregiver burden, including respite care and creating an environment for the patient to maintain function.

The differential diagnosis of a decline in skills is complex and requires a comprehensive approach to care, as there are several masqueraders of dementia. The most common are psychiatric issues, including depression, anxiety, obsessive–compulsive disorder, adjustment disorder, attention-deficit disorder and psychosis [15]. There have been many patients referred for an evaluation of dementia who were later diagnosed with depression [16]. The differentiation between true Alzheimer's dementia and other causes is difficult as there are several overlapping causes of behavioral changes, such as urinary changes, mood changes, irritability, and decline in skills [17]. There is a description in the literature of "pseudo-dementia" in persons with Down syndrome, which resolves after starting an antidepressant [18]. The most common endocrine cause for a decline in skills is hypothyroidism, which is described later in this chapter [15]. Therefore, the traditional workup of reversible causes of dementia in those without Down syndrome includes a thyroid-stimulating hormone (TSH). Additionally, a serum vitamin B12 level is also recommended. The other issues particular to Down syndrome and decline in skills include sensory impairment, urinary tract infections, menopause, seizure disorder, and obstructive sleep apnea [15]. Additionally, in adolescents and young adults with Down syndrome, a decline in skills can be one feature of a regression entity characterized by mood changes as well as repetitive behaviors and may co-occur with psychosis, aggression, or catatonia, with changes in motor activity, speech, and oral intake over months to years, some of which were present in Bobby's case [19]. This will be discussed in greater detail in the "Additional Neurologic and Behavioral Issues" section of this chapter.

In summary, the differential diagnosis for a decline in skills in an adult with Down syndrome is broad and includes dementia, depression, hypothyroidism, sleep apnea, hearing loss, vision loss, seizure disorder, infection, menopause, and developmental regression [20, 21].

## Background: Definition and Epidemiology

Occurring in 1 in 700 to 1 in 1000 live births, Down syndrome is the most common identifiable genetic cause of intellectual disability [22–24]. Due to dramatic improvements in clinical care during early childhood, nearly 90% of persons with Down syndrome now survive to 20 years of age with a median life expectancy approaching 50–60 years of age [25–34]. This is a dramatic improvement compared to their life expectancy of less than 10 years of age in the 1970s [25–33]. The World Health Organization currently estimates 250,000 persons with Down syndrome live in the United States [23]. Down syndrome is caused by extra material on chromosome 21, with 93–95% of karyotypes displaying trisomy 21, 3–4% displaying translocation involving chromosome 21, and 1–3% displaying mosaic trisomy 21 [35–37]. In addition to the risk of comorbidities discussed in this chapter, persons with Down syndrome are universally affected by moderate to severe intellectual disability, which may be less severe in persons with mosaic trisomy 21 [37]. With appropriate medical, social, and educational support, persons with Down syndrome can live long, fulfilling lives.

## Special Issues in the Care of the Adult with Down Syndrome

### Additional Neurologic and Behavioral Issues

While dementia is the most common neurologic condition in adults with Down syndrome (as discussed in the case), there are several other issues that adult providers should consider. Seizures are much more common than in the general population, with a bimodal distribution—usually occurring in childhood or after the third decade of life. Up to 84% of adults with dementia develop seizures [38]. This is particularly important, as untreated seizures in the setting of dementia have been shown to hasten decline [39]. While there is an association between Down syndrome and Moyamoya disease as a cause of cerebrovascular events, this is still a rare finding [40]. Adults are at higher risk for strokes than the general population, and these can be ischemic, hemorrhagic, or cardio-embolic in etiology [41]. Adults are also found to have micro- and macro-hemorrhages in association with amyloid deposition [42]. Adult guidelines for Down syndrome agree with the American Heart Association/American Stroke Association guidelines for the primary prevention of stroke for the general population [5].

Concurrent mental health conditions are common in persons with Down syndrome, particularly depression, anxiety, obsessive-compulsive tendencies, and behavioral issues [43, 44]. Mental illness can present with a decline in skills or urinary incontinence, which can be mislabeled as Alzheimer's dementia [44]. Depression can be triggered by a stressful life event, such as separation from a parent or a death in the family. As depression is often responsive to medical therapy in those with Down syndrome, differentiating it from dementia is vital [45]. Recent epidemiological data indicate that adolescents and young adults with Down syndrome have similar rates of anxiety (18%) and depression (15%) with lower rates of bipolar (4%) and impulse control (20%) disorders when compared to persons with other forms of intellectual disability in this age group [46]. Hyperactivity and impulsive behaviors have been observed in children with Down syndrome as young as 3 years of age [47]. These can be treated with both behavioral modifications and traditional attention-deficit/hyperactivity disorder medications. In particular, persons with Down syndrome tend to thrive in systems incorporating routine and a stable environment, which is theorized to increase feelings of competence, reduce anxiety, and free up cognitive capacity [48]. There is evidence to suggest an increased prevalence of psychosis (35%) in adolescents and young adults with Down syndrome compared to peers with other etiologies of intellectual disability [46]. This finding needs to be interpreted with caution, however, as it is quite common for persons with Down syndrome to engage in self-talk as a mechanism to guide problem-solving or revisit previous conversations and activities, which can be unrelated to behavioral problems [46].

Individuals with Down syndrome have an increased risk of concurrent autistic spectrum disorder compared to the general population, with estimated prevalence rates of 5–39% [43, 49, 50]. However, many individuals with Down syndrome display symptoms of autism spectrum disorder without a true diagnosis, especially in those with more severe expressive language difficulties. Concurrent Down syndrome and autism spectrum disorder can be extremely difficult to treat, often requiring specialists who work with adolescents and adults with special needs [43]. Medical therapies, behavioral management, maintenance of a stable environment, communication supports, and reduction of stressors are all accepted forms of therapy [43, 50].

Persons with Down syndrome are also at risk for a rare developmental regression during young adulthood involving rapid, atypical loss of previously acquired skills in activities of daily living, cognition, and socialization with an increase in maladaptive behaviors [51–53]. Clinical experience suggests this regression may develop in response to transitions, hormonal/menstrual changes, or significant life events (as described in Bobby's case), with early data suggesting a link between this condition and the pathogenesis of dementia later in life [51, 53]. Given the rarity of this phenomenon, little evidence exists to recommend standard treatment modalities [51]. Evaluation of developmental regression in persons with Down syndrome should include all causes of loss of skills as discussed above.

## Cardiology

Congenital heart disease is present in 40–60% of persons with Down syndrome [54–59]. The most common forms of congenital heart disease within Down syndrome are atrioventricular septal defects, atrial septal defects, and ventricular septal defects, followed by patent ductus arteriosus, coarctation of the aorta, tetralogy of Fallot, and other forms of congenital heart disease [58, 60, 61]. Previously, congenital heart disease was responsible for high mortality rates during early childhood in Down syndrome. Now, these lesions are routinely surgically corrected with similar 5-year survival rates to non-Down syndrome children with congenital heart disease [61, 62]. Older adult patients with Down syndrome and congenital heart disease were born in an era during which surgical repair for congenital heart disease was not universal [63]. Consequently, primary care providers may encounter patients with Eisenmenger syndrome due to their nowunrepairable defects [64]. Recently, published data analyzing 10 years of a nationally representative sample of U.S. hospital admissions indicate increased inpatient mortality for adults with Down syndrome and congenital heart disease compared to adults with congenital heart disease without Down syndrome [65]. It is unclear whether this mortality difference results from differing approaches to the current care of adults with Down syndrome versus long-term sequelae of differences in the care of their congenital heart disease during early childhood versus from differences in the prevalence of specific types of congenital heart disease or from other causes. There is conflicting research if the prevalence of types of congenital heart disease is changing toward more simple defects over time [66]. All persons with congenital heart disease should be followed by a cardiologist trained in the care of adults with congenital heart disease. Subsequent follow-up will be dictated by the nature of their lesion, repair status, and associated complications [55].

In addition to congenital heart disease, adults with Down syndrome are at risk for developing acquired valve disease, most commonly mitral valve prolapse followed by aortic regurgitation and tricuspid valve prolapse [58, 67–69]. In many cases, murmurs may not be detectable. Current evidence supports obtaining an echocardiogram for those who did not have one in childhood and for patients presenting with a new murmur or any clinical signs of heart failure [58]. Likewise, electrocardiograms should be obtained for any concerns of arrhythmia [70].

Down syndrome was previously believed to be protective against the development of atherosclerosis and subsequently ischemic heart disease or cerebrovascular accidents [71]. However, autopsy studies from the 1980s demonstrate similar levels of atherosclerosis in persons with Down syndrome compared to non-Down syndrome institutionalized peers [72]. More recent studies confirm increased adverse lipid profiles among individuals with Down syndrome as compared to their siblings [73]. Although the incidence of ischemic heart disease is lower in adults with Down syndrome compared to the general population, longitudinal population studies in Denmark, Sweden, and Australia report a higher prevalence than previously documented at 6.9% of the overall Down syndrome population and 13.2% of those >50 years of age [29, 41, 74]. Despite the above discussion on cardiac risk factors in Down syndrome, adults with Down syndrome tend to have decreased risks for hypertension, with blood pressure measurements averaging approximately 10 points lower than their age-matched peers [75, 76]. Health-care guidelines for adults with Down syndrome suggest that adults with Down syndrome should follow U.S. Preventive Services Task Force (USPSTF) guidelines for the general population regarding statin use for the primary prevention of cardiovascular disease in "Adults: preventive medication" [5].

## Pulmonology

Due to both congenital malformations (e.g., pulmonary hypoplasia, laryngomalacia, hypotonia, and pulmonary hypertension) and deficiencies in their innate and adaptive immunity, respiratory illnesses such as influenza, pneumonia, and aspiration pneumonia are common in persons with Down syndrome [77–80]. Many individuals with Down syndrome experience recurrent wheezing that is thought to be related to airway malacia, generalized hypotonia, or recurrent gastroesophageal reflux disease (GERD) given often suboptimal responsiveness to traditional asthma medications [79, 81]. Aspiration can also cause pneumonia in adults with Down syndrome with dysphagia [82]. Pneumonia is the leading cause of admission to the hospital and the second leading cause of death in adults with Down syndrome, after congenital heart disease [29, 83–85]. As the rate of death from congenital heart disease decreases in adults with Down syndrome, the proportion of deaths attributable to pneumonia increases with age [29]. Therefore, primary care physicians should be vigilant in identifying and treating respiratory illnesses in persons with Down syndrome. Adults with

Down syndrome should be immunized against influenza, pneumonia, and pertussis according to the current vaccine schedule published by the Centers for Disease Control and Prevention [86]. One study found that though people with Down syndrome mount a response to the COVID-19 vaccine, the response is less robust and does not last as long as in those without Down syndrome [87]. The study investigators suggested that boosters may be more helpful for adults with Down syndrome compared to those without Down syndrome [87].

Obstructive sleep apnea is among the more common comorbidities in persons with Down syndrome, with estimated prevalence rates at 30–50% during childhood and >90% in adults [81, 88–94]. This increased risk of obstructive sleep apnea in Down syndrome is multifactorial. Persons with Down syndrome have many physical attributes that predispose them to obstructive sleep apnea including midface and maxillary hypoplasia, relative macroglossia, hypertrophy of the tonsils and adenoids, laryngomalacia, and generalized hypotonia [77, 81, 88, 89, 93]. Persons with Down syndrome also have increased risks of developing hypothyroidism and obesity, both of which are associated with obstructive sleep apnea [81, 89]. Obstructive sleep apnea can present at any age in persons with Down syndrome, with symptoms such as snoring, fatigue, restless sleep, hyperactivity, behavioral or mood changes, decline in skills, daytime sleepiness, nocturnal gasping or choking episodes, or unusual sleep postures [81, 88, 95, 96]. Overnight pulse oximetry has poor sensitivity to diagnose obstructive sleep apnea in Down syndrome, so providers should strongly consider formal polysomnography for diagnosis [81]. The consequences of untreated obstructive sleep apnea are significant and range from behavioral disturbances, decreased executive function, and learning difficulties to neuronal changes in the brain, pulmonary hypertension, and right-sided heart failure [81, 91, 97, 98]. Treatment is important, and options range from traditional positive airway pressure modalities (continuous positive airway pressure [CPAP] or bilevel positive airway pressure [BiPAP]), weight loss, or dental appliances to surgical interventions, such as tonsillectomy and adenoidectomy, and placement of a hypoglossal nerve stimulator device [81, 99].

## Gastroenterology

The primary issues pertinent to adults with Down syndrome of the gastrointestinal tract are celiac disease, dysphagia, and gastroesophageal reflux.

Down syndrome is a known risk factor for celiac disease with approximately 11% prevalence and a sixfold increased odds of developing celiac disease compared to the general population [5, 100–102]. Celiac disease can develop over one's lifetime and should not be considered a one-time diagnosis [100, 103]. Symptoms range from none to gastrointestinal (diarrhea, constipation, abdominal pain, weight loss, bloating, and flatulence) to nongastrointestinal (growth impairment, iron-deficiency anemia, metabolic bone disease, abnormal liver function tests, infertility, and skin disorders) [100, 104, 105]. In the case of persons with intellectual disabilities such as Down syndrome, celiac disease can also present with new or challenging behavioral problems, and diagnosis can be missed due to expressive language difficulties articulating symptoms [54, 103].

Screening recommendations for celiac disease among asymptomatic individuals with Down syndrome remain somewhat controversial [100, 105]. The American Academy of Pediatrics, USPSTF, and the Global Down Syndrome Foundation Medical Care Guidelines Task Force do not recommend screening asymptomatic persons for celiac disease, citing insufficient evidence to assess the benefits and burdens of this practice [5, 54, 100, 106]. However, the National Institute for Health and Care Excellence (United Kingdom) recommends offering testing for celiac disease to asymptomatic persons with a first-degree relative with celiac disease; to those with certain high-risk conditions, including autoimmune thyroid conditions and Type 1 diabetes mellitus (both of which are often seen in persons with Down syndrome); and to consider offering testing to all persons with Down syndrome [107]. All of the above organizations recommend testing in symptomatic persons [5, 54, 100, 104, 106, 107].

Serologic testing for celiac disease includes immunoglobulin A tissue transglutaminase (TTG), endomysial antibodies, or deamidated gliadin peptide (DGP) (sensitivity and specificity for IgA TTG: 95–98%, for IgA endomysial antibodies ~100%) [100]. In patients with concurrent selective IgA deficiency, IgG TTG and DGP testing are recommended (sensitivity up to 90%) [100]. Ancillary testing of HLA-DQ2 and HLA-DQ8 can be helpful in assessing the genetic risk of developing celiac disease [104]. If both HLA-DQ2 and HLA-DQ8 are negative, the diagnosis of celiac disease is highly unlikely (negative predictive value >99%) [104]. For this reason, the American College of Gastroenterology recommends ancillary testing of HLA-DQ2 and HLA-DQ8 in persons with Down Syndrome [104]. If both are negative, providers can be reassured of low genetic risk for the development of celiac disease in that patient [104].

The only effective treatment for celiac disease is a gluten-free diet [108]. While the establishment of a gluten-restrictive diet can be difficult, it is generally well-tolerated in most adults with Down syndrome. Regardless of which screening approach a provider chooses to take, one should be vigilant for signs and symptoms of this condition as earlier diagnosis and implementation of a gluten-free diet are important to decrease morbidity [100].

Dysphagia is one of the most common conditions in adults with Down syndrome, especially in older adults. One study found dysphagia in more than 50% of those over 50 years of age, with increasing prevalence associated with advancing age [109]. In a study of directly observed eating behaviors in adults with Down syndrome, 56.5% experienced coughing while eating [110]. This is of particular importance due to the high risk of aspiration, which is among the leading causes of hospitalization and death in adults with Down syndrome [111–113]. Dysphagia can also lead to malnutrition and dehydration [114]. Clinical screening for aspiration includes questions about mealtime symptoms with differing consistencies of food [113]. Radiologic evaluation for dysphagia and aspiration can involve a video-fluoroscopic swallow study or a fiber-optic endoscopic evaluation [113]. Dysphagia needs to be managed symptomatically with potential interventions including dietary restrictions on easily aspirated foods, thickening liquids, strengthening exercises, and mealtime supervision to normalize eating rate [110]. Many persons with Down syndrome eat very quickly, thereby increasing the risk for aspiration [110].

Gastroesophageal reflux is also common with estimated prevalence ranging from 9 to 20% among adults with Down syndrome [109, 112, 115, 116]. In one French review article, approximately 25% of adults with Down syndrome were found to have *Helicobacter pylori* infection, with markedly higher rates (75%) cited among institutionalized children with Down syndrome [115]. The true prevalence of gastroesophageal reflux in persons with Down syndrome is likely underestimated, however, as it is often treated empirically. Gastroesophageal reflux disease can present with abdominal pain, chest pains, involuntary weight loss, aspirations, iron-deficiency anemia, or a variety of behavioral changes [115, 117]. Treatments can involve dietary modifications (e.g., frequent small feeds of thickened food to minimize gastric distension), pharmacological therapies (e.g., histamine-2 (H2)-blockers, proton pump inhibitors, or prokinetic agents), or surgery (e.g., fundoplication) and should address the underlying causes of gastroesophageal reflux disease and its complications in the individual patient [117].

## Endocrinology

Hypothyroidism is among the more common comorbidities in persons with Down syndrome, presenting with fatigue, weight gain, decreased interest in activities, a decline in skills, cold intolerance, constipation, dry skin, and growth impairment [20, 56, 118–121]. Prevalence estimates for hypothyroidism range from 9 to 45% of persons with Down syndrome of all ages [20, 56, 119, 120, 122, 123]. Moreover, 1–6% of children with Down syndrome are born with congenital hypothyroidism [54, 124]. An additional 25–60% of persons with Down syndrome demonstrate subclinical hypothyroidism, which can be transitory and does not definitively predict progression to clinical hypothyroidism [120, 124]. The literature favors not treating subclinical hypothyroidism, but this issue remains controversial [125]. The risks for acquired hypothyroidism correlate with age in persons with Down syndrome, with the onset of autoimmune thyroid disease starting in puberty and increasing with age [124, 126]. Thyroid antibodies (anti-thyroid peroxidase [TPO] antibody, thyroglobulin antibody) are found in approximately one-third of persons with Down syndrome [124, 126]. Prior to age 12 years, hypothyroidism in persons with Down syndrome is thought to be due to poor development or hypoplasia of the thyroid gland [118, 126]. Untreated hypothyroidism can contribute to decreased cognitive function and is thus important to identify and treat. Current consensus guidelines are to screen asymptomatic adults every 1–2 years after age 21 years for hypothyroidism with a serum thyroid-stimulating hormone (TSH) level [5].

Hyperthyroidism is slightly more common in the Down syndrome population (0.65–3%) than the general population but is still relatively uncommon [124, 127, 128]. This typically presents with heat intolerance, irritability, weight loss, tachycardia, and palpitations and appears to be the result of autoimmune thyroiditis [118, 124]. Autoimmune thyroiditis can have a fluctuating course in persons with Down syndrome between hypo- and hyperthyroidism [118]. Definitive therapy for hyperthyroidism is Iodine-131 with surgical treatment reserved for patients requiring rapid resolution of thyrotoxicosis or for those with serious side effects from anti-thyroid medications [124].

There is also an increased prevalence of diabetes mellitus (DM) among children and adults with Down syndrome compared to the general population, with a higher predominance of type 1 DM than type 2 DM [119, 129–134]. More typically, type 1 DM presents in a bimodal distribution during childhood, with peaks at less than 2 years of age and again in early adolescence [135]. Reports from Denmark demonstrate a fourfold increase in the presence of Down syndrome in persons <20 years old with type 1 DM (0.38%) compared to the prevalence of Down syndrome in the background Danish population [133]. Similarly, a Scottish study demonstrated a prevalence of type 1 DM in adults with Down syndrome ranging from 1.4 to 10.6% [131]. Within a population-based study of persons with intellectual disability of all ages in Ireland, 23% of those with type 1 DM and intellectual disabilities had Down syndrome, compared to 8% of those with type 2 DM and intellectual disabilities [134]. There is additional evidence to suggest coexisting autoimmune disease with type 1 DM in persons with Down syndrome, with one study reporting 74% with coexisting thyroid autoimmunity, 14% with celiac disease, and 8% with combined diabetes, thyroid autoimmunity, and celiac disease [135]. Consensus guidelines recommended screening for diabetes at age 21 years; every 1–3 years if the person's BMI is greater than 30; and screening all adults with Down syndrome regardless of BMI every 1–3 years after age 30 years [5].

Obesity is widespread among persons with intellectual disabilities but disproportionately affects more persons with Down syndrome compared to other causes of intellectual disability [119, 136–139]. It has been reported that 25–55% of persons with Down syndrome are overweight with roughly another one-third meeting criteria for obesity [136, 138–140]. Women with Down syndrome tend to have slightly higher rates of overweight and obesity than men [136, 141]. Additionally, overweight and obesity tend to be associated with milder forms of intellectual disability [136, 141]. Likely reasons for the high prevalence of obesity within Down syndrome include lower levels of physical activity, lower resting metabolic rate, and poor nutritional choices, especially among the more independent and ambulatory populations [140–143]. Compared to non-Down syndrome peers, persons with Down syndrome tend to have higher fat and lower lean mass in their body composition, making traditional measurements of adiposity (e.g., BMI) less helpful [139, 144, 145]. Due to differences such as limb length, those with Down syndrome have a different distribution of body mass. One can use the 2015 growth charts (recently published in *Pediatrics)* that continue to age 20 years as a good approximation for adults [146]. As with the non-Down syndrome population, overweight and obesity increases the risk of musculoskeletal complications, insulin resistance, and overall mortality in persons with Down syndrome [139, 147–149] However, overweight and obesity in persons with Down syndrome do not seem to translate into metabolic syndrome [148]. To combat overweight and obesity in Down syndrome, experts have found the greatest success using a multidisciplinary approach involving physical exercise, nutrition counseling, caloric restriction, and a comprehensive behavioral management program involving the patient's family [140, 150, 151]. While regular exercise in moderate intervals does improve muscle strength and core balance in the Down syndrome population, persons with Down syndrome appear to need longer training durations (45–60 min) to improve their overall aerobic fitness [150]. Consensus guidelines recommend monitoring for weight change, and obesity should be performed annually by calculating BMI in adults with Down syndrome. The USPSTF recommendation for behavioral weight loss interventions to prevent obesity-related morbidity and mortality in adults should be followed [5].

## Musculoskeletal

The musculoskeletal issues of primary concern in adults with Down syndrome are osteopenia-osteoporosis, osteoarthritis, hip disease, and (rarely) atlantoaxial instability. The classic skeletal association with Down syndrome is atlantoaxial instability; however, this is typically of more concern in children than adults.

The more common conditions in the spine of adults with Down syndrome are osteoarthritis, cervical spondylosis, and cervical spondylotic myelopathy [152]. The prevalence of spondylosis or osteoarthritis of the cervical spine is estimated to be 33–64% among adults with Down syndrome, often localizing to higher levels of the cervical spine compared to the general population [152–157]. The severity of this appears to increase with age [152, 155, 157]. Although not specific to adults with Down syndrome, cervical spondylotic myelopathy resulting from cervical spondylosis is thought to be the most common spinal cord disorder in typically developing adults, with the symptoms of gait impairment, sensory changes, neck pain, or stiffness suggesting high risk for disease progression [152, 158].

In comparison, atlantoaxial instability is found in only 2–20% of adults with Down syndrome [5, 152–155, 159–166]. While atlantoaxial instability may be present in a radiologic study, it does not mean that subluxation and clinical symptoms will follow. It is estimated that 2% of people with Down syndrome are at risk for spinal cord compression from atlantoaxial instability, with the presence of os odontoideum and/or ossicles serving as markers of high risk in adults and children [153, 159, 167]. Risks do not appear to be influenced by gender [160]. Current guidelines for adults with Down syndrome recommend annual screening for signs and symptoms of cervical myelopathy (e.g., altered gait, new incontinence, brisk reflexes, or clonus) rather than using cervical radiographs to screen asymptomatic individuals [5]. Even the guidelines for the care of children with Down syndrome, no longer recommend routine screening for atlantoaxial instability among asymptomatic persons [54]. Although rare, it is still prudent to evaluate for atlantoaxial instability in symptomatic adults with new neurologic symptoms, as prompt intervention is necessary. Presentations can vary, with potential symptoms including cervical pain, torticollis, hyperreflexia, ataxia, quadriparesis, syncope, vertigo, change in handedness, and/or ear pain [119, 130, 160, 168–176]. One review estimated symptom prevalence for atlantoaxial dislocation as follows: 50% presented with neck pain or restriction of neck movement, 70% with numbness and/or weakness, and 90% presented with pyramidal signs [177]. Neurosurgical evaluation is recommended prior to any athletic participation with the above symptoms of atlantoaxial dislocation. Plain cervical radiographs (including imaging of sagittal alignment and instability with flexion extension) are typically sufficient for initial evaluation, although they bear the risk of false negatives [152, 178]. Further imaging with magnetic resonance imaging (preferably) or computerized tomography (CT) may be needed for definitive diagnosis [152]. Regarding athletic participation decisions, it is felt to be more appropriate to conduct a focused history and neurological examination, evaluating for gait disturbance, neck movements, tendon reflexes, and plantar responses. Any symptoms concerning atlantoaxial instability should be referred for definitive imaging and neurosurgical consultation [179]. However, it is always important to check with the individual organizations (e.g., Special Olympics) for current pre-participation screening recommendations.

Osteopenia-osteoporosis is common, with over 50% prevalence among adults with Down syndrome [180]. Down syndrome is considered an independent risk factor for low bone mineral density (BMD), with the incidence of reported fracture as high as 55% (long bones) or 30% (vertebral bodies) in adults with Down syndrome over 50 years old [20, 181–185]. Persons with Down syndrome attain peak bone mass at younger ages and experience bone loss at earlier ages and at higher rates than the typically developing population [186, 187]. Persons with Down syndrome have multiple risk factors for lower bone integrity due to decreased muscle tone/hypermobility leading to decreased physical activity and increased risk of joint dislocation; delayed puberty; hormonal factors; thyroid abnormalities; seizure disorder; high-risk medication use; low intake of calcium; vitamin D insufficiency; and autoimmune diseases [185]. In addition, there appears to be a Down syndrome-specific mechanism for decreased BMD involving suppression of bone formation and resorption [181, 188]. All adults with Down syndrome should be regularly screened for risk factors of low BMD, including thyroid function tests every 1–2 years, while assessing high-risk medication use, ensuring adequate levels of calcium and vitamin D, and promoting increased physical activity [5, 181, 188]. Given the increased risk of osteoporotic fractures in adults with Down syndrome, bone densitometry screening should be considered in both men and women with Down syndrome prior to 45–50 years of age or with their first fracture if earlier [20, 152]. Current guidelines also recommend evaluation for secondary causes of osteoporosis in adults with Down syndrome who sustain a fracture, such as hyperthyroidism, celiac disease, vitamin D deficiency, hyperparathyroidism, and medications impacting bone health [5]. Data are not yet available to guide Down syndrome-specific evidence-based interventions for osteoporosis-osteopenia or to suggest comprehensive strategies for optimal treatment once low BMD is identified [181, 186]. However, vitamin D and calcium, both integral components of bone health, are often low enough to require supplementation among persons with Down syndrome [186]. Similarly, a study in children with Down syndrome ages 7–12 years demonstrated that weight-bearing exercise and calcium intake have a synergistic effect on femoral neck BMD, suggesting that prevention plays an important role [189].

Radiographic evidence of hip abnormalities is present in nearly 30% of adults with Down syndrome, including acetabular dysplasia and acquired hip dislocation [190, 191]. Of note, hip abnormalities in persons with Down syndrome can involve congenital or developmental dislocation, developmental or acetabular dysplasia of the hip, or even acquired subluxation or dislocation occurring well into adulthood [113, 190, 191]. The etiologies of hip abnormalities in persons with Down syndrome are hypothesized to include ligamentous laxity, decreased muscle tone, and abnormal morphology of the femur and acetabulum [191]. The presence of hip instability dramatically impacts ambulation, independence, and function in this population [113, 191, 192]. One study found that the majority of adult patients with Down syndrome and co-occurring hip disease could not ambulate in the community after the age of 30 years [190]. Current care guidelines for adults with Down syndrome do not recommend screening asymptomatic individuals for hip abnormalities [113]. However, hip disease should be considered in any symptomatic adult with Down syndrome presenting with difficulties ambulating, changed gait, pain, or changes in activity. The initial evaluation may start with radiographs but CT will be needed for evaluation and surgical planning [113].

Although not yet well understood, there is emerging literature around "Down syndrome-associated arthritis" or "Arthropathy of Down syndrome," which is felt to be similar to juvenile idiopathic arthritis [193–195]. Patients with Down syndrome-associated arthritis most frequently present with polyarticular arthritis, although it can manifest as an oligoarticular disease [193–195]. This condition typically lacks elevation of inflammatory markers, rheumatoid factor, or anti-nuclear antibody, contributing to diagnostic confusion and long delays prior to diagnosis [193, 194]. Referral to and management by rheumatology is appropriate for this condition.

Data are not yet available to guide evidence-based preventive therapeutic interventions among young adults with Down syndrome [181]. Given the increased risk of osteoporotic fractures in adults with Down syndrome, the general consensus recommends screening adults for osteoporosis starting in their 40s or with their first fracture if earlier than 40 years of age [20]. As noted previously, a study in children with Down syndrome ages 7–12 years demonstrated that weight-bearing exercise and calcium intake have a synergistic effect on femoral neck BMD [189]. This suggests that prevention plays an important role. More research is needed to determine the specific mechanism of low BMD in this population as well as their fracture risk prior to recommending pharmacologic interventions [121].

## Reproductive Health

Reproductive health for persons with Down syndrome is an area that is often poorly addressed by healthcare providers [196]. Both men and women with Down syndrome can experience delays in puberty and have decreased fertility compared to the general population [197–200].

Women with Down syndrome can have regular ovulatory menstrual cycles although there is evidence to suggest the presence of ovarian hypoplasia and gonadal dysfunction with decreased follicular growth, decreased number of oocytes, and decreased ovarian sensitivity to follicle-stimulating hormone (FSH) [200, 201]. The most common gynecologic complaints among women with Down syndrome are menstrual, such as menorrhagia, dysmenorrhea, irregular bleeding, and hygiene concerns. Women with Down syndrome may go through menopause at younger ages than women without Down syndrome and typically go through menopause at younger ages than women with other forms of intellectual disability (often between 44 and 47 years of age) [196, 202, 203] Earlier onset of menopause in women with Down syndrome appears to be associated with a two- to threefold increased risk of Alzheimer's dementia and earlier age of onset for Alzheimer's dementia [203]. Receipt of preventive reproductive healthcare in women with Down syndrome, however, is quite low compared to the typically developing population despite the fact that current guidelines recommend routine gynecologic care starting in adolescence, including discussion of contraception and sexually transmitted infections [54]. To this point, recently published studies indicate that less than half of women aged 18 years and older ever received a gynecologic examination and less than one-third of women with Down syndrome ever received a Papanicolaou test [204, 205]. Many women with Down syndrome are able to conceive and bear children [197, 198, 206]. Approximately 50% of their children will have Down syndrome, and these children are at increased risk for other congenital malformations [207]. Determination regarding whether pregnancy in a woman with Down syndrome is considered high risk will depend upon her cognitive level and co-occurring medical conditions (e.g., cardiac, thyroid, hepatic diseases, and/or seizure disorder) [208].

Men with Down syndrome are typically considered sterile with evidence of germ cell hypoplasia demonstrated by elevated luteinizing hormone (LH) and FSH hormone levels, lower testosterone levels, and smaller testicular volume [201, 209]. However, there have been case reports of children being fathered by men with complete trisomy 21 [210, 211].

Persons with intellectual disability, such as Down syndrome, are at increased risk for sexual exploitation and abuse due to factors, such as isolation, communication deficits, small peer groups, limited mutual support services, multiple living situations, and/or transient caregivers [208, 212, 213]. Similarly, persons with Down syndrome are at risk for sexually transmitted infections when consistent and correct use of barrier methods (e.g., condoms) are not used [208]. Consequently, it is important to educate persons with Down syndrome about their reproductive capacity, to assess their sexual practices and/or desires, to screen for abuse, and to address these concerns clinically [212]. Primary care providers should consider reviewing contraceptive methods to prevent sexually transmitted infections or undesired pregnancy and should routinely offer age-, gender-, and risk-factor appropriate reproductive health screenings in a disability-friendly manner [20, 212].

A review of a large cohort of individuals with DS followed at one clinic found that relative to controls, individuals with DS had lesser odds of experiencing breast (OR: 0.20 [0.11, 0.38]), and cervical (OR: 0.29 [0.21, 0.40]) cancers [214]. Although this provides reassurance, screening is infrequent with only 29–36% of women age 21 years and older receiving screens for cervical cancer and only 46–49% of women age 40 years and older receiving mammograms [204]. For women with Down syndrome, the ideal timing and duration for cervical and breast cancer screening is yet to be determined.

## Visual and Hearing Issues

The disability caused by people with Down syndrome with ophthalmologic pathology cannot be underestimated. Especially in adults who often have compromised hearing and balance issues, poor vision can manifest with an Alzheimer's-like picture of withdrawal from social situations and a decline in skills. Many patients will not complain of visual loss and will instead only exhibit behavioral changes. This issue and the high prevalence of visual abnormalities make routine screening a necessity. While there is no unanimous consensus regarding the frequency of screening, our review of the literature suggests a routine ophthalmologic exam every 2 years in adults is warranted [20].

All structures of the eye are at increased risk of abnormalities: the cornea, retina, iris, and lens as well as the eyelid. The prevalence is much higher in those with more severe cognitive limitations. The overall incidence of some vision compromise is as high as 75% in people with DS aged 30 years and older [215]. Of note, those with mosaic Down syndrome are also at a significantly increased risk for structural abnormalities [216]. The most common abnormalities in adults are cataracts, strabismus, refractive errors, and presbyopia, all of which are more common compared to the general population. In one large study, 42% of 455 adults with Down syndrome were found to have cataracts with incidences of 37.8% in the 40–49 year age range and 100% in the 70–79 year age range [215]. This is of particular significance, as many physicians are wary of recommending cataract surgery for this population. In actuality, the benefits of surgery are mixed. The surgical outcomes are generally good, but the patient's visual abilities often remain compromised due to other ocular comorbidities [217].

Caring for the ophthalmologic issues in adults with Down syndrome is often challenging. Visual impairments in those with intellectual disabilities can lead to behavioral changes such as self-injurious behavior. This may manifest as self-stimulatory behaviors such as eye poking/pressing or staring into bright lights. Finding an ophthalmic specialist experienced in caring for individuals with intellectual disabilities can be invaluable, as problems with cooperation with the exam are common, and creative solutions with more engaging visual tests may be necessary. There are several forms of testing that have proved successful in these settings [218].

According to one source, approximately 40–77% of adults with Down syndrome have disabling hearing loss [219]. The incidence of hearing loss increases sharply after age 40. It is at this point when the incidence differs dramatically from the general population [33]. Recognizing and treating sensory impairments is critical, as they can present as a decline in skills, thereby diminishing quality of life and/or being misdiagnosed as dementia. Bone conduction devices, such as bone-anchored hearing aids (BAHAs), have been found to be effective interventions in some patients with Down syndrome with high rates of daily usage and high satisfaction scores [220, 221].

## Hematology-Oncology

Persons with Down syndrome have increased risks for hematologic conditions, ranging from idiopathic macrocytosis and mild polycythemia to myelodysplastic syndrome to actual leukemias [74, 222–225]. Studies show a high frequency of leukopenia, idiopathic macrocytosis, and mild polycythemia in the Down syndrome population, often without underlying disease [222]. Elevations in the mean corpuscular volume are frequently found in infants with Down syndrome and can persist throughout their lives [226]. In one observational study, approximately two-thirds of persons with Down syndrome had an elevated mean corpuscular volume, and one-third had mild leukopenia [226]. Although myelodysplastic syndrome is often transient in individuals with Down syndrome, this can progress to leukemia and/or marrow failure in both children and adults [226, 227].

Leukemia in Down syndrome is predominantly found in the pediatric population, with >90% of cases occurring before age 20 years [149, 223]. Acute myeloid leukemia and acute lymphoblastic leukemia seem to occur with equal frequencies within the Down syndrome population [225]. Although leukemia in Down syndrome is generally associated with a poor prognosis, childhood acute megakaryoblastic leukemia is unusually sensitive to chemotherapy with excellent outcomes [223, 228, 229].

Persons with Down syndrome have a decreased but nonzero risk of developing most solid tumors compared to the general population [74, 225]. However, combined analyses of nearly 30 years of cancer registry data from Denmark and Sweden observed a modest increase in risk of liver, testicular, and male penile cancers among adults with Down syndrome compared to non-Down syndrome rates in these countries [74]. These same registries documented the presence of solid tumor neoplasms in persons with Down syndrome in numerous organ systems, including cancers of the colon, testes, breast, liver, penis, stomach, brain, endometrium, parathyroid, kidney, and small intestine [74]. There have been additional case reports of male breast cancer in adults with Down syndrome [230, 231].

Primary care providers of adults with Down syndrome should retain a high index of suspicion for underlying hematologic or solid tumor neoplasms. Solid tumor screening should be dictated by clinical symptoms, family history, and risk factors. Providers should follow complete blood counts in situations that would raise one's suspicions for hematologic processes, such as easy bruising, petechiae, fatigue, or change in feeding patterns, and refer to specialty providers as appropriate [54, 224].

## Inpatient Considerations

Reviews have shown that the most common cause of hospitalization for individuals with Down syndrome is pneumonia/aspiration syndrome (29.6%) and the most common comorbidity is GERD/dysphagia (70.3%) [112]. The presence of GERD/dysphagia or seizure disorder was shown to be significantly associated with multiple admissions and readmission within 1 month ($P < 0.05$) [112]. The mortality rate in this study was 4.9%, and the rate of intensive care unit admission was 8.6% [112]. In comparison to adults in the general population, adults with DS had a mean age at admission of 48.6 ± 8.8 years, with a median length of stay of 3 days (interquartile range 4 days) [112]. Male patients were hospitalized longer than female patients (mean 5.0 versus 2.8 days; $p < 0.05$), and patients who lived at home were admitted at earlier ages than those who presented from residential health-care facilities (mean 41.5 vs. 52.2 years; $p < 0.001$). Indeed, a scoping review of the literature found that pneumonia and respiratory infections are more prevalent and more severe in individuals with Down syndrome compared to healthy controls [85].

A retrospective chart review of a 10-year cohort found that respiratory illnesses are a common cause of health-care utilization among patients with DS, particularly early in childhood and later in life. Patients were seen predominately in outpatient settings. When an inpatient setting was needed, individuals frequently required higher levels of care [82]. A recent survey during the COVID-19 pandemic found that hospitalized COVID-19 patients <18 years with DS had a higher incidence of respiratory symptoms, fever, and several medical complications from COVID-19 than patients <18 years without DS. Older age, obesity, and epilepsy were significant risk factors for hospitalization among pediatric COVID-19 patients with DS, and age and thyroid disorder were significant risk factors for acute respiratory distress syndrome. Mortality rates were low in all pediatric COVID-19 patients (with and without DS), contrasting with previous findings in adults with DS (who exhibited higher mortality than those without DS). Children with DS are at increased risk for more severe presentations of COVID-19 [232].

A large international survey of 1046 patients with COVID and DS was compared to a British study of 100 Hospitalized patients with and without Down syndrome. In the international study, the most frequent signs and symptoms of COVID-19 were fever, cough, and shortness of breath. Pain and nausea were reported less frequently ($p < 0.01$), whereas altered consciousness/confusion were reported more frequently ($p < 0.01$). In the comparison to the British study, risk factors for hospitalization and mortality were similar to the general population (e.g., age, male gender, diabetes, obesity, and dementia) with the addition of congenital heart defects as a risk factor for hospitalization. Mortality rates increased from age 40 years compared to controls, even after adjusting for known risk factors for COVID-19 mortality [233].

Regardless of the cause of admission, there may be unique considerations for the inpatient team caring for individuals with Down syndrome who are hospitalized. First, individuals with Down syndrome often thrive with routine and develop behavioral "grooves" [234]. The fact that they are admitted to the hospital, in a new bed, with new people, and with new rules is likely to be impactful for someone with Down syndrome regardless of the reason for admission. Many individuals with Down syndrome do well with consistency, and steps to increase routine in the hospital could be beneficial, such as maintaining a consistent bedside nurse, maintaining a consistent physician, and adding consistency to their day to follow their home routine when possible. Additionally, communication is an important consideration for individuals with Down syndrome who are admitted, especially given the variable levels of communication skills among this population [235]. Some considerations might include the use of visual aids to enhance communication, including family and guardians in discussions, and/or the use of communication devices, such as augmentative and alternative communication (AAC) devices if the individual with Down syndrome uses that at home [236]. Patients with Down syndrome often have strengths in visual learning and benefit from the use of social stories. Other considerations to support individuals with Down syndrome during inpatient stays might include sitters for sundowning if diagnosed with dementia, sitters for support of behavior, and bringing familiar items from home.

In the care of hospitalized adults with Down syndrome, guidance can also be drawn from many geriatric studies and standards of care due to the many overlapping concerns and comorbidities between these populations [237]. Patient-centered care is extremely important across interdisciplinary teams for this population [238]. It is also important to screen for malnutrition, dysphagia, and dehydration on admission to optimize nutrition and possibly decrease hospital-acquired infections [239]. Additionally, the use of behavior therapy with standard of care may reduce apathy and agitation and improve activities of daily living for hospitalized adults with Down syndrome [240].

## Conclusions

While every person with Down syndrome is unique, there are several issues that are common throughout the population. It is important to have a systematic approach to both health maintenance and active medical issues, as multiple organ systems can be involved. One must take a comprehensive approach to the diagnosis of decline in skills, paying particular attention to mental health issues. While all people with Down syndrome may develop amyloid deposition in the brain, not all will develop clinical dementia. In addition, a medical workup is warranted for unexplained behavioral changes as common conditions such as hyperthyroidism, sleep apnea, and sensory changes may present this way.

<table>
<tr><th colspan="3">Down syndrome (DS) fact sheet</th></tr>
<tr><td>Definition</td><td colspan="2">Down syndrome is a genetic condition resulting from the triplication of all or a portion of chromosome 21 (trisomy 21). Down syndrome is characterized by:<br>• Intellectual disability, ranging from mild to profound<br>• Common physical findings include hypotonia, epicanthic folds, flat nasal bridge, upward-slanting palpebral fissures, high arched palate, narrow ear canals, short stature, single transverse palmar crease, and wide-spacing between the first and second toes<br>• Persons with Down syndrome have increased risks for congenital and acquired conditions involving most organ systems as described below</td></tr>
<tr><td>Epidemiology</td><td colspan="2">• In the United States, Down syndrome occurs in 1/700–1/1000 live births. Affecting approximately 250,000 persons<br>• Karyotypes for persons with Down syndrome are as follows:<br>– 93–95% of persons with Down syndrome have complete trisomy 21<br>– 3–4% have a chromosomal translocation involving chromosome 21<br>– 1–3% have mosaic trisomy 21</td></tr>
<tr><td rowspan="4">Special considerations</td><td colspan="2">In addition to intellectual and developmental disabilities, adults with Down syndrome have high rates of comorbid physical and mental health conditions, including:</td></tr>
<tr><td>• Congenital heart disease<br>• Hypothyroidism<br>• Hearing abnormalities<br>• Vision abnormalities<br>• Gastroesophageal reflux<br>• Celiac disease</td><td>• Obesity<br>• Obstructive sleep apnea<br>• Behavioral/mental health disorders<br>• Acquired cardiac valve disease<br>• Cervical spinal instability</td></tr>
<tr><td colspan="2">Adults with Down syndrome also experience accelerated aging, which can involve:</td></tr>
<tr><td>• Early dementia<br>• Osteoporosis</td><td>• Osteoarthritis<br>• Dysphagia</td></tr>
</table>

| Down syndrome (DS) fact sheet | | |
|---|---|---|
| Recommended screening | In addition to appropriate age and gender primary health screenings, we recommend the following screenings for adults with Down syndrome: | |
| | **Yearly:**<br>• Hypothyroidism<br>• Obesity | **Every 1–2 years:**<br>• Hearing<br>• Vision |
| | As directed by comorbidities, risk factors, and clinical presentation: | |
| | • Echocardiogram<br>• Sleep study<br>• Bone densitometry | • Cervical spine imaging<br>• Celiac disease screening labs |

## References


1. Zigman WB, Devenny DA, Krinsky-McHale SJ, Jenkins EC, Urv TK, Wegiel J, et al. Alzheimer's disease in adults with Down syndrome. Int Rev Res Ment Retard. 2008;36:103–45.
2. Lott IT, Head E. Alzheimer disease and Down syndrome: factors in pathogenesis. Neurobiol Aging. 2005;26(3):383–9.
3. Livingston G, Strydom A. Improving Alzheimer's disease outcomes in Down's syndrome. Lancet. 2012;379(9815):498–500.
4. Nieuwenhuis-Mark RE. Diagnosing Alzheimer's dementia in Down syndrome: problems and possible solutions. Res Dev Disabil. 2009;30(5):827–38.
5. Tsou AY, Bulova P, Capone G, Chicoine B, Gelaro B, Harville TO, et al. Medical care of adults with Down syndrome: a clinical guideline. JAMA. 2020;324(15):1543–56.
6. Prasher V, Farooq A, Holder R. The adaptive behaviour dementia questionnaire (ABDQ): screening questionnaire for dementia in Alzheimer's disease in adults with Down syndrome. Res Dev Disabil. 2004;25(4):385–97.
7. Menendez M. Down syndrome, Alzheimer's disease and seizures. Brain and Development. 2005;27(4):246–52.
8. Mohan M, Bennett C, Carpenter PK. Memantine for dementia in people with Down syndrome. Cochrane Database Syst Rev. 2009;1:CD007657.
9. Mohan M, Bennett C, Carpenter PK. Galantamine for dementia in people with Down syndrome. Cochrane Database Syst Rev. 2009;1:CD007656.
10. Mohan M, Bennett C, Carpenter PK. Rivastigmine for dementia in people with Down syndrome. Cochrane Database Syst Rev. 2009;1:CD007658.
11. Mohan M, Carpenter PK, Bennett C. Donepezil for dementia in people with Down syndrome. Cochrane Database Syst Rev. 2009;1:CD007178.
12. Livingstone N, Hanratty J, McShane R, Macdonald G. Pharmacological interventions for cognitive decline in people with Down syndrome. Cochrane Database Syst Rev. 2015;10:CD011546.
13. Hanney M, Prasher V, Williams N, Jones EL, Aarsland D, Corbett A, et al. Memantine for dementia in adults older than 40 years with Down's syndrome (MEADOWS): a randomised, double-blind, placebo-controlled trial. Lancet. 2012;379(9815):528–36.
14. Chicoine B, Head E, Hendrix J, Janicki MP, Keller SM, Radner R, et al. Aducanumab and persons with Down syndrome: what do we do now? A D U H E L M & D S. https://2e626e23-9885-43be-a9e4-d60d120ed14f.filesusr.com/ugd/8c1d0a_a8d8434e60644c869a3fb3944142b8ad.pdf.
15. Chicoine B, McGuire D, Rubin SS. Specialty clinic perspectives. In: Janicki MP, Dalton AJ, editors. Dementia, aging, and intellectual disabilities: a handbook. London, England New York, New York: Routledge; 1999.
16. Warren AC, Holroyd S, Folstein MF. Major depression in Down's syndrome. Br J Psychiatry. 1989;155:202–5.
17. Burt DB. Dementia and depression. In: Janicki MP, Dalton AJ, editors. Dementia, aging, and intellectual disabilities: a handbook. London, England New York, New York: Routledge; 1999.
18. Tsiouris JA, Patti PJ. Drug treatment of depression associated with dementia or presented as 'pseudodementia' in older adults with Down syndrome. J Appl Res Intellect. 1997;10(4):312–22.
19. Santoro SL, Cannon S, Capone G, Franklin C, Hart SJ, Hobensack V, et al. Unexplained regression in Down syndrome: 35 cases from an international Down syndrome database. Genet Med. 2020;22(4):767–76.
20. Jensen KM, Bulova PD. Managing the care of adults with Down's syndrome. BMJ. 2014;349:g5596.
21. Fortea J, Zaman SH, Hartley S, Rafii MS, Head E, Carmona-Iragui M. Alzheimer's disease associated with Down syndrome: a genetic form of dementia. The Lancet Neurology. 2021;20(11):930–42.
22. Centers for Disease Control and Prevention. Data and statistics: occurrence of Down syndrome. http://www.cdc.gov/ncbddd/birthdefects/downsyndrome/data.html.

23. World Health Organization. Genes and human disease. 2012. http://www.who.int/genomics/public/geneticdiseases/en/print.html.
24. Parker SE, Mai CT, Canfield MA, Rickard R, Wang Y, Meyer RE, et al. Updated National Birth Prevalence estimates for selected birth defects in the United States, 2004-2006. Birth Defects Res A Clin Mol Teratol. 2010;88(12):1008–16.
25. Lose EJ, Robin NH. Caring for adults with pediatric genetic diseases: a growing need. Curr Opin Pediatr. 2007;19(6):611–2.
26. Centers for Disease Control and Prevention. Racial disparities in median age at death of persons with Down syndrome—United States, 1968-1997. MMWR Morb Mortal Wkly Rep. 2001;50(22):463–5.
27. Glasson EJ, Sullivan SG, Hussain R, Petterson BA, Montgomery PD, Bittles AH. The changing survival profile of people with Down's syndrome: implications for genetic counselling. Clin Genet. 2002;62(5):390–3.
28. Presson AP, Partyka G, Jensen KM, Devine OJ, Rasmussen SA, McCabe LL, et al. Current estimate of Down syndrome population prevalence in the United States. J Pediatr. 2013;163(4):1163–8.
29. Englund A, Jonsson B, Zander CS, Gustafsson J, Anneren G. Changes in mortality and causes of death in the Swedish Down syndrome population. Am J Med Genet A. 2013;161A(4):642–9.
30. Zhu JL, Hasle H, Correa A, Schendel D, Friedman JM, Olsen J, et al. Survival among people with Down syndrome: a nationwide population-based study in Denmark. Genet Med. 2013;15(1):64–9.
31. Wu J, Morris JK. The population prevalence of Down's syndrome in England and Wales in 2011. Eur J Hum Genet. 2013;21(9):1016–9.
32. Kucik JE, Shin M, Siffel C, Marengo L, Correa A, Congenital Anomaly Multistate P, et al. Trends in survival among children with Down syndrome in 10 regions of the United States. Pediatrics. 2013;131(1):e27–36.
33. Glasson EJ, Dye DE, Bittles AH. The triple challenges associated with age-related comorbidities in Down syndrome. J Intellect Disabil Res. 2014;58(4):393–8.
34. Antonarakis SE, Skotko BG, Rafii MS, Strydom A, Pape SE, Bianchi DW, et al. Down syndrome. Nat Rev Dis Primers. 2020;6(1):1–20.
35. Mutton D, Alberman E, Hook EB. Cytogenetic and epidemiological findings in Down syndrome, England and Wales 1989 to 1993. National down Syndrome Cytogenetic Register and the Association of Clinical Cytogeneticists. J Med Genet. 1996;33(5):387–94.
36. Mulcahy MT. Down's syndrome in Western Australia: cytogenetics and incidence. Hum Genet. 1979;48(1):67–72.
37. Bittles AH, Glasson EJ. Clinical, social, and ethical implications of changing life expectancy in Down syndrome. Dev Med Child Neurol. 2004;46(4):282–6.
38. Lott IT. Neurological phenotypes for Down syndrome across the life span. Prog Brain Res. 2012;197:101–21.
39. Lott IT, Doran E, Nguyen VQ, Tournay A, Movsesyan N, Gillen DL. Down syndrome and dementia: seizures and cognitive decline. J Alzheimers Dis. 2012;29(1):177–85.
40. Hwang SW, Jea A. A review of the neurological and neurosurgical implications of Down syndrome in children. Clin Pediatr (Phila). 2013;52(9):845–56.
41. Sobey CG, Judkins CP, Sundararajan V, Phan TG, Drummond GR, Srikanth VK. Risk of major cardiovascular events in people with Down syndrome. PLoS One. 2015;10(9):e0137093.
42. Wilcock DM, Schmitt FA, Head E. Cerebrovascular contributions to aging and Alzheimer's disease in Down syndrome. Biochim Biophys Acta. 2016;1862(5):909–14.
43. Capone G, Goyal P, Ares W, Lannigan E. Neurobehavioral disorders in children, adolescents, and young adults with Down syndrome. Am J Med Genet C Semin Med Genet. 2006;1 42C(3):158–72.
44. Mantry D, Cooper SA, Smiley E, Morrison J, Allan L, Williamson A, et al. The prevalence and incidence of mental ill-health in adults with Down syndrome. J Intellect Disabil Res. 2008;52(Pt 2):141–55.
45. Walker JC, Dosen A, Buitelaar JK, Janzing JG. Depression in Down syndrome: a review of the literature. Res Dev Disabil. 2011;32(5):1432–40.
46. Dykens EM, Shah B, Davis B, Baker C, Fife T, Fitzpatrick J. Psychiatric disorders in adolescents and young adults with Down syndrome and other intellectual disabilities. J Neurodev Disord. 2015;7(1):9.
47. Capone GT, Brecher L, Bay M. Guanfacine use in children with Down syndrome and comorbid attention-deficit hyperactivity disorder (ADHD) with disruptive behaviors. J Child Neurol. 2016;31(8):957–64.
48. Glenn S, Cunningham C, Nananidou A, Prasher V, Glenholmes P. Routinised and compulsive-like behaviours in individuals with Down syndrome. J Intellect Disabil Res. 2015;59(11):1061–70.
49. Lott IT, Dierssen M. Cognitive deficits and associated neurological complications in individuals with Down's syndrome. Lancet Neurol. 2010;9(6):623–33.
50. Channell MM, Phillips BA, Loveall SJ, Conners FA, Bussanich PM, Klinger LG. Patterns of autism spectrum symptomatology in individuals with Down syndrome without comorbid autism spectrum disorder. J Neurodev Disord. 2015;7(1):5.

51. Devenny D, Matthews A. Regression: atypical loss of attained functioning in children and adolescents with Down syndrome. In: Hodapp RM, editor. International review of research in developmental disabilities. Oxford: Academic Press; 2011. p. 233–64.
52. Prasher VP. Disintegrative syndrome in young adults. Ir J Psychol Med. 2002;19(3):101.
53. Tamasaki A, Saito Y, Ueda R, Ohno K, Yokoyama K, Satake T, et al. Effects of donepezil and serotonin reuptake inhibitor on acute regression during adolescence in Down syndrome. Brain and Development. 2016;38(1):113–7.
54. Bull MJ. Health supervision for children with Down syndrome. Pediatrics. 2011;128(2):393–406.
55. Warnes CA, Liberthson R, Danielson GK, Dore A, Harris L, Hoffman JI, et al. Task force 1: the changing profile of congenital heart disease in adult life. J Am Coll Cardiol. 2001;37(5):1170–5.
56. Maatta T, Maatta J, Tervo-Maatta T, Taanila A, Kaski M, Iivanainen M. Healthcare and guidelines: a population-based survey of recorded medical problems and health surveillance for people with Down syndrome. J Intellect Develop Disabil. 2011;36(2):118–26.
57. Tan M, Xu C, Sim SK, Seow AL, Tan TH, Quek SC. Types and distribution of congenital heart defects associated with trisomy 21 in Singapore. J Paediatr Child Health. 2013;49(3):223–7.
58. Lin AE, Basson CT, Goldmuntz E, Magoulas PL, McDermott DA, McDonald-McGinn DM, et al. Adults with genetic syndromes and cardiovascular abnormalities: clinical history and management. Genet Med. 2008;10(7):469–94.
59. Lin AE, Santoro S, High FA, Goldenberg P, Gutmark-Little I. Editors. Congenital heart defects associated with aneuploidy syndromes: new insights into familiar associations. Am J Med Genet C Semin Med Genet. 2020;184(1):53–63.
60. Stoll C, Dott B, Alembik Y, Roth MP. Associated congenital anomalies among cases with Down syndrome. Eur J Med Genet. 2015;58(12):674–80.
61. Ko JM. Genetic syndromes associated with congenital heart disease. Korean Circ J. 2015;45(5):357–61.
62. Pierpont ME, Basson CT, Benson DW Jr, Gelb BD, Giglia TM, Goldmuntz E, et al. Genetic basis for congenital heart defects: current knowledge: a scientific statement from the American Heart Association Congenital cardiac defects committee, council on cardiovascular disease in the young: endorsed by the American Academy of Pediatrics. Circulation. 2007;115(23):3015–38.
63. Champagne CR, Lewis M, Gilchrist DM. Should we mend their broken hearts? The history of cardiac repairs in children with Down syndrome. Pediatrics. 2014;134(6):1048–50.
64. Diller GP, Alonso-Gonzalez R, Kempny A, Dimopoulos K, Inuzuka R, Giannakoulas G, et al. B-type natriuretic peptide concentrations in contemporary Eisenmenger syndrome patients: predictive value and response to disease targeting therapy. Heart. 2012;98(9):736–42.
65. Baraona F, Gurvitz M, Landzberg MJ, Opotowsky AR. Hospitalizations and mortality in the United States for adults with Down syndrome and congenital heart disease. Am J Cardiol. 2013;111(7):1046–51.
66. Santoro SL, Steffensen EH. Congenital heart disease in Down syndrome—a review of temporal changes. J Congenit Cardiol. 2021;5(1):1–14.
67. Geggel RL, O'Brien JE, Feingold M. Development of valve dysfunction in adolescents and young adults with Down syndrome and no known congenital heart disease. J Pediatr. 1993;122(5 Pt 1):821–3.
68. Goldhaber SZ, Brown WD, Sutton MG. High frequency of mitral valve prolapse and aortic regurgitation among asymptomatic adults with Down's syndrome. JAMA. 1987;258(13):1793–5.
69. Goldhaber SZ, Rubin IL, Brown W, Robertson N, Stubblefield F, Sloss LJ. Valvular heart disease (aortic regurgitation and mitral valve prolapse) among institutionalized adults with Down's syndrome. Am J Cardiol. 1986;57(4):278–81.
70. Majdalany DS, Burkhart HM, Connolly HM, Abel MD, Dearani JA, Warnes CA, et al. Adults with Down syndrome: safety and long-term outcome of cardiac operation. Congenit Heart Dis. 2010;5(1):38–43.
71. Murdoch JC, Rodger JC, Rao SS, Fletcher CD, Dunnigan MG. Down's syndrome: an atheroma-free model? Br Med J. 1977;2(6081):226–8.
72. Chaney RH. Neurogenic atherosclerosis in mentally retarded persons. J Ment Defic Res. 1987;31(Pt 3):235–40.
73. Adelekan T, Magge S, Shults J, Stallings V, Stettler N. Lipid profiles of children with Down syndrome compared with their siblings. Pediatrics. 2012;129(6):e1382–7.
74. Hill DA, Gridley G, Cnattingius S, Mellemkjaer L, Linet M, Adami HO, et al. Mortality and cancer incidence among individuals with Down syndrome. Arch Intern Med. 2003;163(6):705–11.
75. Rodrigues AN, Coelho LC, Goncalves WL, Gouvea SA, Vasconcellos MJ, Cunha RS, et al. Stiffness of the large arteries in individuals with and without Down syndrome. Vasc Health Risk Manag. 2011;7:375–81.
76. Roy-Vallejo E, Galván-Román JM, Moldenhauer F, Real de Asua D. Adults with Down syndrome challenge another paradigm: when aging no longer entails arterial hypertension. J Clin Hypertens. 2020;22(7):1127–33.
77. McDowell KM, Craven DI. Pulmonary complications of Down syndrome during childhood. J Pediatr. 2011;158(2):319–25.
78. Ram G, Chinen J. Infections and immunodeficiency in Down syndrome. Clin Exp Immunol. 2011;164(1):9–16.

79. Weijerman ME, Brand PL, van Furth MA, Broers CJ, Gemke RJ. Recurrent wheeze in children with Down syndrome: is it asthma? Acta Paediatr. 2011;100(11):e194–7.
80. Broers CJ, Gemke RJ, Weijerman ME, Kuik DJ, van Hoogstraten IM, van Furth AM. Frequency of lower respiratory tract infections in relation to adaptive immunity in children with Down syndrome compared to their healthy siblings. Acta Paediatr. 2012;101(8):862–7.
81. Lal C, White DR, Joseph JE, van Bakergem K, LaRosa A. Sleep-disordered breathing in Down syndrome. Chest. 2015;147(2):570–9.
82. Blake JM, Estrada Gomez D, Skotko BG, Torres A, Santoro SL. Pneumonia and respiratory infection in Down syndrome: a 10-year cohort analysis of inpatient and outpatient encounters across the lifespan. Am J Med Genet A. 2021;185:2878.
83. Tenenbaum A, Chavkin M, Wexler ID, Korem M, Merrick J. Morbidity and hospitalizations of adults with Down syndrome. Res Dev Disabil. 2012;33(2):435–41.
84. Bittles AH, Bower C, Hussain R, Glasson EJ. The four ages of Down syndrome. Eur J Pub Health. 2007;17(2):221–5.
85. Santoro SL, Chicoine B, Jasien JM, Kim JL, Stephens M, Bulova P, et al. Pneumonia and respiratory infections in Down syndrome: a scoping review of the literature. Am J Med Genet A. 2021;185(1):286–99.
86. Centers for Disease Control and Prevention. Recommended adult immunization schedule—United States, 2014. 2014. http://www.cdc.gov/vaccines/schedules/hcp/imz/adult.html.
87. Sali M, Carfi A, DiPaola A, Boza MP, Zampino G, Sanguinetti M, et. al. SARS-CoV-2 vaccine humoral response in adults with Down syndrome. Clin Microbiol Infect 2022, 28, 1155.e1.
88. Ono J, Chishaki A, Ohkusa T, Sawatari H, Nishizaka M, Ando S. Obstructive sleep apnea-related symptoms in Japanese people with Down syndrome. Nurs Health Sci. 2015;17(4):420–5.
89. Trois MS, Capone GT, Lutz JA, Melendres MC, Schwartz AR, Collop NA, et al. Obstructive sleep apnea in adults with Down syndrome. J Clin Sleep Med. 2009;5(4):317–23.
90. Shott SR. Down syndrome: common otolaryngologic manifestations. Am J Med Genet C Semin Med Genet. 2006;142C(3):131–40.
91. Marcus CL, Keens TG, Bautista DB, von Pechmann WS, Ward SL. Obstructive sleep apnea in children with Down syndrome. Pediatrics. 1991;88(1):132–9.
92. de Miguel-Diez J, Villa-Asensi JR, Alvarez-Sala JL. Prevalence of sleep-disordered breathing in children with Down syndrome: polygraphic findings in 108 children. Sleep. 2003;26(8):1006–9.
93. Pandit C, Fitzgerald DA. Respiratory problems in children with Down syndrome. J Paediatr Child Health. 2012;48(3):E147–52.
94. Rosen D. Management of obstructive sleep apnea associated with Down syndrome and other craniofacial dysmorphologies. Curr Opin Pulm Med. 2011;17(6):431–6.
95. Capone GT, Aidikoff JM, Taylor K, Rykiel N. Adolescents and young adults with Down syndrome presenting to a medical clinic with depression: co-morbid obstructive sleep apnea. Am J Med Genet A. 2013;161(9):2188–96.
96. Myers KA, Mrkobrada M, Simel DL. Does this patient have obstructive sleep apnea?: the rational clinical examination systematic review. JAMA. 2013;310(7):731–41.
97. Breslin J, Spano G, Bootzin R, Anand P, Nadel L, Edgin J. Obstructive sleep apnea syndrome and cognition in Down syndrome. Dev Med Child Neurol. 2014;56(7):657–64.
98. Halbower AC, Degaonkar M, Barker PB, Earley CJ, Marcus CL, Smith PL, et al. Childhood obstructive sleep apnea associates with neuropsychological deficits and neuronal brain injury. PLoS Med. 2006;3(8):e301.
99. Diercks GR, Wentland C, Keamy D, Kinane TB, Skotko B, de Guzman V, et al. Hypoglossal nerve stimulation in adolescents with Down syndrome and obstructive sleep apnea. JAMA Otolaryngol Head Neck Surg. 2018;144(1):37–42.
100. Kumral D, Syed S. Celiac disease screening for high-risk groups: are we doing it right? Dig Dis Sci. 2020;65:2187–95.
101. Liu E, Wolter-Warmerdam K, Marmolejo J, Daniels D, Prince G, Hickey F. Routine screening for celiac disease in children with Down syndrome improves case finding. J Pediatr Gastroenterol Nutr. 2020;71(2):252–6.
102. Marild K, Stephansson O, Grahnquist L, Cnattingius S, Soderman G, Ludvigsson JF. Down syndrome is associated with elevated risk of celiac disease: a Nationwide case-control study. J Pediatr. 2013;163(1):237–42.
103. Ostermaier KK, Weaver AL, Myers SM, Stoeckel RE, Katusic SK, Voigt RG. Incidence of celiac disease in Down syndrome: a longitudinal, population-based birth cohort study. Clin Pediatr (Phila). 2020;59(12):1086–91.
104. Rubio-Tapia A, Hill ID, Kelly CP, Calderwood AH, Murray JA. American College of Gastroenterology clinical guideline: diagnosis and management of celiac disease. Am J Gastroenterol. 2013;108(5):656–76.
105. Pavlovic M, Berenji K, Bukurov M. Screening of celiac disease in Down syndrome—old and new dilemmas. World J Clin Cases. 2017;5(7):264–9.
106. Bibbins-Domingo K, Grossman DC, Curry SJ, Barry MJ, Davidson KW, Doubeni CA, et al. Screening for celiac disease: US preventive services task force recommendation statement. JAMA. 2017;317(12):1252–7.

107. Richey R, Howdle P, Shaw E, Stokes T. Recognition and assessment of coeliac disease in children and adults: summary of NICE guidance. BMJ Br Med J. 2009;338:b1684.
108. Mooney PD, Hadjivassiliou M, Sanders DS. Coeliac disease. BMJ. 2014;348:g1561.
109. Hermans H, Evenhuis HM. Multimorbidity in older adults with intellectual disabilities. Res Dev Disabil. 2014;35(4):776–83.
110. Smith CH, Teo Y, Simpson S. An observational study of adults with Down syndrome eating independently. Dysphagia. 2014;29(1):52–60.
111. Landes SD, Stevens JD, Turk MA. Cause of death in adults with Down syndrome in the United States. Disabil Health J. 2020;13(4):100947.
112. Chenbhanich J, Wu A, Phupitakphol T, Atsawarungruangkit A, Treadwell T. Hospitalisation of adults with Down syndrome: lesson from a 10-year experience from a community hospital. J Intellect Disabil Res. 2019;63(3):266–76.
113. Capone G, Stephens M, Santoro S, Chicoine B, Bulova P, Peterson M, et al. Co-occurring medical conditions in adults with Down syndrome: a systematic review toward the development of health care guidelines. Part II. Am J Med Genet A. 2020;182(7):1832–45.
114. Lazenby T. The impact of aging on eating, drinking, and swallowing function in people with Down's syndrome. Dysphagia. 2008;23(1):88–97.
115. Ravel A, Mircher C, Rebillat A-S, Cieuta-Walti C, Megarbane A. Feeding problems and gastrointestinal diseases in Down syndrome. Arch Pediatr. 2020;27(1):53–60.
116. Böhmer C, Niezen-de Boer M, Klinkenberg-Knol E, Devillé W, Nadorp J, Meuwissen S. The prevalence of gastroesophageal reflux disease in institutionalized intellectually disabled individuals. Am J Gastroenterol. 1999;94(3):804–10.
117. Macchini F, Leva E, Torricelli M, Valadè A. Treating acid reflux disease in patients with Down syndrome: pharmacological and physiological approaches. Clin Exp Gastroenterol. 2011;4:19–22.
118. Popova G, Paterson WF, Brown A, Donaldson MD. Hashimoto's thyroiditis in Down's syndrome: clinical presentation and evolution. Horm Res. 2008;70(5):278–84.
119. Steingass KJ, Chicoine B, McGuire D, Roizen NJ. Developmental disabilities grown up: Down syndrome. J Dev Behav Pediatr. 2011;32(7):548–58.
120. Prasher V, Gomez G. Natural history of thyroid function in adults with Down syndrome—10-year follow-up study. J Intellect Disabil Res. 2007;51(Pt 4):312–7.
121. Whooten R, Schmitt J, Schwartz A. Endocrine manifestations of Down syndrome. Curr Opin Endocrinol Diabetes Obes. 2018;25(1):61–6.
122. Jensen KM, Taylor LC, Davis MM. Primary care for adults with Down syndrome: adherence to preventive healthcare recommendations. J Intellect Disabil Res. 2013;57(5):409–21.
123. Brodtmann A. Hashimoto encephalopathy and Down syndrome. Arch Neurol. 2009;66(5):663–6.
124. King K, O'Gorman C, Gallagher S. Thyroid dysfunction in children with Down syndrome: a literature review. Ir J Med Sci. 2014;183(1):1–6.
125. Amr NH. Thyroid disorders in subjects with Down syndrome: an update. Acta Bio Med Acta Biomed. 2018;89(1):132–9.
126. Ivarsson SA, Ericsson UB, Gustafsson J, Forslund M, Vegfors P, Anneren G. The impact of thyroid autoimmunity in children and adolescents with Down syndrome. Acta Paediatr. 1997;86(10):1065–7.
127. Goday-Arno A, Cerda-Esteva M, Flores-Le-Roux JA, Chillaron-Jordan JJ, Corretger JM, Cano-Perez JF. Hyperthyroidism in a population with Down syndrome (DS). Clin Endocrinol. 2009;71(1):110–4.
128. Londhey VA, Rajadhyaksh GC, Barhate KS, More AV, Dedhia CR. Hyperthyroidism in a case of Down syndrome. J Assoc Physicians India. 2010;58:568–9.
129. Roizen NJ, Patterson D. Down's syndrome. Lancet. 2003;361(9365):1281–9.
130. Smith DS. Health care management of adults with Down syndrome. Am Fam Physician. 2001;64(6):1031–8.
131. Anwar AJ, Walker JD, Frier BM. Type 1 diabetes mellitus and Down's syndrome: prevalence, management and diabetic complications. Diabet Med. 1998;15(2):160–3.
132. Schmidt F, Kapellen TM, Wiegand S, Herbst A, Wolf J, Frohlich-Reiterer EE, et al. Diabetes mellitus in children and adolescents with genetic syndromes. Exp Clin Endocrinol Diabetes. 2012;120(10):579–85.
133. Bergholdt R, Eising S, Nerup J, Pociot F. Increased prevalence of Down's syndrome in individuals with type 1 diabetes in Denmark: a nationwide population-based study. Diabetologia. 2006;49(6):1179–82.
134. Taggart L, Coates V, Truesdale-Kennedy M. Management and quality indicators of diabetes mellitus in people with intellectual disabilities. J Intellect Disabil Res. 2013;57(12):1152–63.
135. Aitken RJ, Mehers KL, Williams AJ, Brown J, Bingley PJ, Holl RW, et al. Early-onset, coexisting autoimmunity and decreased HLA-mediated susceptibility are the characteristics of diabetes in Down syndrome. Diabetes Care. 2013;36(5):1181–5.
136. Stancliffe RJ, Lakin KC, Larson S, Engler J, Bershadsky J, Taub S, et al. Overweight and obesity among adults with intellectual disabilities who use intellectual disability/developmental disability services in 20 U.S. states. Am J Intell Dev Disabil. 2011;116(6):401–18.

137. Rimmer JH, Yamaki K, Davis BM, Wang E, Vogel LC. Obesity and overweight prevalence among adolescents with disabilities. Prev Chronic Dis. 2011;8(2):A41.
138. Rimmer JH, Yamaki K, Lowry BM, Wang E, Vogel LC. Obesity and obesity-related secondary conditions in adolescents with intellectual/developmental disabilities. J Intellect Disabil Res. 2010;54(9): 787–94.
139. Real de Asua D, Parra P, Costa R, Moldenhauer F, Suarez C. Evaluation of the impact of abdominal obesity on glucose and lipid metabolism disorders in adults with Down syndrome. Res Dev Disabil. 2014;35(11):2942–9.
140. Wong C, Dwyer J, Holland M. Overcoming weight problems in adults with Down syndrome. Nutr Today. 2014;49(3):109–19.
141. de Winter CF, Bastiaanse LP, Hilgenkamp TI, Evenhuis HM, Echteld MA. Overweight and obesity in older people with intellectual disability. Res Dev Disabil. 2012;33(2):398–405.
142. Hsieh K, Rimmer JH, Heller T. Obesity and associated factors in adults with intellectual disability. J Intellect Disabil Res. 2014;58(9):851–63.
143. Allison DB, Gomez JE, Heshka S, Babbitt RL, Geliebter A, Kreibich K, et al. Decreased resting metabolic rate among persons with Down syndrome. Int J Obes Relat Metab Disord. 1995;19(12):858–61.
144. Gonzalez-Aguero A, Ara I, Moreno LA, Vicente-Rodriguez G, Casajus JA. Fat and lean masses in youths with Down syndrome: gender differences. Res Dev Disabil. 2011;32(5):1685–93.
145. Gonzalez-Aguero A, Vicente-Rodriguez G, Ara I, Moreno LA, Casajus JA. Accuracy of prediction equations to assess percentage of body fat in children and adolescents with Down syndrome compared to air displacement plethysmography. Res Dev Disabil. 2011;32(5):1764–9.
146. Zemel BS, Pipan M, Stallings VA, Hall W, Schadt K, Freedman DS, et al. Growth charts for children with Down syndrome in the United States. Pediatrics. 2015;136(5):e1204–11.
147. Pau M, Galli M, Crivellini M, Albertini G. Relationship between obesity and plantar pressure distribution in youths with Down syndrome. Am J Phys Med Rehabil. 2013;92(10): 889–97.
148. Real de Asua D, Parra P, Costa R, Moldenhauer F, Suarez C. A cross-sectional study of the phenotypes of obesity and insulin resistance in adults with Down syndrome. Diabetes Metab J. 2014;38(6): 464–71.
149. Yang Q, Rasmussen SA, Friedman JM. Mortality associated with Down's syndrome in the USA from 1983 to 1997: a population-based study. Lancet. 2002;359(9311):1019–25.
150. Li C, Chen S, Meng How Y, Zhang AL. Benefits of physical exercise intervention on fitness of individuals with Down syndrome: a systematic review of randomized-controlled trials. Int J Rehabil Res. 2013;36(3):187–95.
151. Curtin C, Bandini LG, Must A, Gleason J, Lividini K, Phillips S, et al. Parent support improves weight loss in adolescents and young adults with Down syndrome. J Pediatr. 2013;163(5):1402–8.e1.
152. Capone GT, Chicoine B, Bulova P, Stephens M, Hart S, Crissman B, et al. Co-occurring medical conditions in adults with Down syndrome: a systematic review toward the development of health care guidelines. Am J Med Genet A. 2018;176(1):116–33.
153. Burke SW, French H, Roberts J, Johnston C 2nd, Whitecloud T 3rd, Edmunds J Jr. Chronic atlanto-axial instability in Down syndrome. JBJS. 1985;67(9):1356–60.
154. Maclachlan RA, Fidler KE, Yeh H, Hodgetts PG, Pharand G, Chau M. Cervical-spine abnormalities in institutionalized adults with downs-syndrome. J Intellect Disabil Res. 1993;37:277–85.
155. Miller J, Capusten B, Lampard R. Changes at the base of skull and cervical spine in Down syndrome. Can Assoc Radiol J. 1986;37(2):85–9.
156. Van Dyke DC, Gahagan CA. Down syndrome: cervical spine abnormalities and problems. Clin Pediatr (Phila). 1988;27(9):415–8.
157. Tangerud Å, Hestnes A, Sand T, Sunndalsfoll S. Degenerative changes in the cervical spine in Down's syndrome. J Intellect Disabil Res. 1990;34(2):179–85.
158. Wang L, Hee HT, Wong HK. Cervical spondylotic myelopathy: a brief review of its pathophysiology, presentation, assessment, natural history and management. Orthop Trauma. 2011;25(3):181–9.
159. El-Khouri M, Mourao MA, Tobo A, Battistella LR, Herrero CFP, Riberto M. Prevalence of atlanto-occipital and atlantoaxial instability in adults with Down syndrome. World Neurosurg. 2014;82(1–2):215–8.
160. Pueschel SM, Scola FH. Atlantoaxial instability in individuals with Down syndrome: epidemiologic, radiographic, and clinical studies. Pediatrics. 1987;80(4):555–60.
161. Alvarez N, Rubin L. Atlantoaxial instability in adults with Down syndrome: a clinical and radiological survey. Appl Res Ment Retard. 1986;7(1):67–78.
162. Cooke LB, Lansdall-Welfare R. Atlanto-axial instability in adults with Down's syndrome: a survey of a long-stay hospital population. West Engl Med J. 1991;106(1):7–8.
163. Elliott S, Morton R, Whitelaw R. Atlantoaxial instability and abnormalities of the odontoid in Down's syndrome. Arch Dis Child. 1988;63(12):1484–9.
164. Ferguson RL, Putney ME, Allen BL Jr. Comparison of neurologic deficits with atlanto-dens intervals in patients with Down syndrome. J Spinal Disord. 1997;10(3):246–52.

165. French HG, Burke SW, Roberts JM, Johnston C 2nd, Whitecloud T, Edmunds J. Upper cervical ossicles in Down syndrome. J Pediatr Orthop. 1987;7(1):69–71.
166. Roy M, Baxter M, Roy A. Atlantoaxial instability in Down syndrome-guidelines for screening and detection. J R Soc Med. 1990;83(7):433–5.
167. Cohen WI. Current dilemmas in Down syndrome clinical care: celiac disease, thyroid disorders, and atlanto-axial instability. Am J Med Genet C Semin Med Genet. 2006;142C(3):141–8.
168. Lott IT, editor Dementia in Down syndrome. Down syndrome medical interest group national symposium, Phoenix, AZ; 2015.
169. Cohen WI. Down syndrome preventive medical check list. Down Syndrome Quarterly. 1999;4(3):1–16.
170. Vanderbilt Kennedy Center for Research on Human Development. Health care for adults with intellectual and developmental disabilities—toolkit for primary care providers: checklist—Down syndrome. 2014. http://vkc.mc.vanderbilt.edu/etoolkit/physical-health/health-watch-tables-2/down-syndrome/.
171. Van Riper M, Cohen WI. Caring for children with Down syndrome and their families. J Pediatr Health Care. 2001;15(3):123–31.
172. Roizen NJ. Medical care and monitoring for the adolescent with Down syndrome. Adolesc Med. 2002;13(2):345–58. vii
173. Pueschel SM, Anneren G, Durlach R, Flores J, Sustrova M, Verma IC. Guidelines for optimal medical care of persons with Down syndrome. International league of societies for persons with mental handicap (ILSMH). Acta Paediatr. 1995;84(7):823–7.
174. Davidson MA. Primary care for children and adolescents with Down syndrome. Pediatr Clin N Am. 2008;55(5):1099–111. xi
175. Taggard DA, Menezes AH, Ryken TC. Treatment of Down syndrome-associated craniovertebral junction abnormalities. J Neurosurg. 2000;93(2 Suppl):205–13.
176. Radcliff K, Kepler C, Reitman C, Harrop J, Vaccaro A. CT and MRI-based diagnosis of craniocervical dislocations: the role of the occipitoatlantal ligament. Clin Orthop Relat Res. 2012;470(6):1602–13.
177. Sun YY, Boniello AJ, Poorman CE, Chang AL, Wang S, Passias PG. A review of the diagnosis and treatment of atlantoaxial dislocations. Global Spine J. 2014;4:197–210.
178. Hengartner AC, Whelan R, Maj R, Wolter-Warmerdam K, Hickey F, Hankinson TC. Evaluation of 2011 AAP cervical spine screening guidelines for children with Down syndrome. Childs Nerv Syst. 2020;36(11):2609–14.
179. Tomlinson C, Campbell A, Hurley A, Fenton E, Heron N. Sport preparticipation screening for asymptomatic atlantoaxial instability in patients with Down syndrome. Clin J Sport Med. 2020;30(4):293–5.
180. Schrager S, Kloss C, Ju A. Prevalence of fractures in women with intellectual disabilities: a chart review. J Intellect Disabil Res. 2007;51(4):253–9.
181. Hawli Y, Nasrallah M, El-Hajj Fuleihan G. Endocrine and musculoskeletal abnormalities in patients with Down syndrome. Nat Rev Endocrinol. 2009;5(6):327–34.
182. Dreyfus D, Lauer E, Wilkinson J. Characteristics associated with bone mineral density screening in adults with intellectual disabilities. J Am Board Fam Med. 2014;27(1):104–14.
183. Geijer JR, Stanish HI, Draheim CC, Dengel DR. Bone mineral density in adults with Down syndrome, intellectual disability, and nondisabled adults. Am J Intellect Dev Disabil. 2014;119(2):107–14.
184. Van Allen MI, Fung J, Jurenka SB. Health care concerns and guidelines for adults with Down syndrome. Am J Med Genet. 1999;89(2):100–10.
185. McKelvey KD, Fowler TW, Akel NS, Kelsay JA, Gaddy D, Wenger GR, et al. Low bone turnover and low bone density in a cohort of adults with Down syndrome. Osteoporos Int. 2013;24(4):1333–8.
186. LaCombe JM, Roper RJ. Skeletal dynamics of Down syndrome: a developing perspective. Bone. 2020;133:115215.
187. Costa R, Gullón A, De Miguel R, de Asúa DR, Bautista A, García C, et al. Bone mineral density distribution curves in Spanish adults with Down syndrome. J Clin Densitom. 2018;21(4):493–500.
188. Srikanth R, Cassidy G, Joiner C, Teeluckdharry S. Osteoporosis in people with intellectual disabilities: a review and a brief study of risk factors for osteoporosis in a community sample of people with intellectual disabilities. J Intellect Disabil Res. 2011;55(1):53–62.
189. Reza SM, Rasool H, Mansour S, Abdollah H. Effects of calcium and training on the development of bone density in children with Down syndrome. Res Dev Disabil. 2013;34(12):4304–9.
190. Hresko MT, McCarthy JC, Goldberg MJ. Hip disease in adults with Down syndrome. J Bone Joint Surg Br. 1993;75(4):604–7.
191. Maranho D, Fuchs K, Kim Y-j, Novais EN. Hip instability in patients with Down syndrome. J Am Acad Orthop Surg. 2018;26(13):455–62.
192. Kelley SP, Wedge JH. Management of hip instability in trisomy 21. J Pediatr Orthop. 2013;33:S33–S8.
193. Nicek A, Talib N, Lovell D, Smith C, Becker ML, Jones JT. Assessment and treatment of Down syndrome-associated arthritis: a survey of pediatric rheumatologists. Pediatr Rheumatol Online J. 2020;18(1):1–7.

194. Olson JC, Bender JC, Levinson JE, Oestreich A, Lovell DJ. Arthropathy of Down syndrome. Pediatrics. 1990;86(6):931–6.
195. Juj H, Emery H. The arthropathy of Down syndrome: an underdiagnosed and under-recognized condition. J Pediatr. 2009;154(2):234–8.
196. Toler F. Females with Down syndrome: lost opportunities in primary care. J Am Assoc Nurse Pra. 2015;27(7):356–62.
197. McGuire DE, Chicoine BA. Life issues of adolescents and adults with Down syndrome. In: Cohen WI, Nadel L, Madnick ME, editors. Down syndrome: visions for the 21st century. New York, NY: Wiley-Liss, Inc; 2002. p. 221–45.
198. Edwards J. Sexuality, marriage, and parenting for persons wtih Down syndrome. In: Pueschel SM, editor. The young person with Down syndrome: transition from adolescence to Adulthoodq. Baltimore, MD: Paul H. Brookes Publishing Company; 1988. p. 187–204.
199. Pueschel SM, Orson JM, Boylan JM, Pezzullo JC. Adolescent development in males with Down syndrome. Am J Dis Child. 1985;139(3):236–8.
200. Cento RM, Proto C, Guido M, Lanzone A. Postmenarchal Down's syndrome: a theoretical model of growth hormone action on ovarian function. Gynecol Endocrinol. 2001;15(1):81–8.
201. Hsiang YH, Berkovitz GD, Bland GL, Migeon CJ, Warren AC. Gonadal function in patients with Down syndrome. Am J Med Genet. 1987;27(2):449–58.
202. Schupf N, Zigman W, Kapell D, Lee JH, Kline J, Levin B. Early menopause in women with Down's syndrome. J Intellect Disabil Res. 1997;41(Pt 3):264–7.
203. Schupf N, Lee JH, Pang D, Zigman WB, Tycko B, Krinsky-McHale S, et al. Epidemiology of estrogen and dementia in women with Down syndrome. Free Radic Biol Med. 2018;114:62–8.
204. Jensen KM, Campagna EJ, Juarez-Colunga E, Prochazka AV, Runyan DK. Low rates of preventive healthcare service utilization among adolescents and adults with Down syndrome. Am J Prev Med. 2021;60(1):1–12.
205. Smith AJB, Applebaum J, Tanner EJ, Capone G. Gynecologic Care in Women wiht Down syndrome: findings from a National Registry. Obstet Gynecol. 2020;136:518–23.
206. Angelopoulou N, Souftas V, Sakadamis A, Matziari C, Papameletiou V, Mandroukas K. Gonadal function in young women with Down syndrome. Int JGynaecol Obstet. 1999;67(1):15–21.
207. Bovicelli L, Orsini LF, Rizzo N, Montacuti V, Bacchetta M. Reproduction in Down syndrome. Obstet Gynecol. 1982;59(6 Suppl):13S–7S.
208. Van Dyke DC, McBrien D, Sherbondy A. Issues of sexuality in Down syndrome. Down Syndr Res Pract. 1995;3(10/26/21):65–9.
209. Suzuki K, Nakajima K, Kamimura S, Takasugi K, Suzuki Y, Sekine H, et al. Eight case reports on sex-hormone profiles in sexually mature male Down syndrome. Int J Urol. 2010;17(12):1008–10.
210. Pradhan M, Dalal A, Khan F, Agrawal S. Fertility in men with Down syndrome: a case report. Fertil Steril. 2006;86(6):1765 e1-3.
211. Sheridan R, Llerena J Jr, Matkins S, Debenham P, Cawood A, Bobrow M. Fertility in a male with trisomy 21. J Med Genet. 1989;26(5):294–8.
212. Scheepers M, Kerr M, O'Hara D, Cooper S-A, Davis R, Fujiura G, et al. Reducing health disparity in people with intellectual disabilities: a report from health issues special interest research Group of the International Association for the scientific study of intellectual disabilities. J Policy Pract Intellect Disabil. 2005;2(3/4):249–55.
213. Schor DP. Sex and sexual abuse in developmentally disabled adolescents. Semin Adolesc Med. 1987;3(1):1–7.
214. Chicoine B, Rivelli A, Fitzpatrick V, Chicoine L, Jia G, Rzhetsky A. Prevalence of common disease conditions in a large cohort of individuals with Down syndrome in the United States. J Patient Cent Res Rev. 2021;8(2):86–97.
215. Krinsky-McHale SJ, Jenkins EC, Zigman WB, Silverman W. Ophthalmic disorders in adults with Down syndrome. Curr Gerontol Geriatr Res. 2012;2012:974253.
216. Motley WW 3rd, Saltarelli DP. Ophthalmic manifestations of mosaic Down syndrome. J AAPOS. 2011;15(4):362–6.
217. Li EY, Chan TC, Lam NM, Jhanji V. Cataract surgery outcomes in adult patients with Down's syndrome. Br J Ophthalmol. 2014;98(9):1273–6.
218. Li J, Wong K, Park AS, Fricke TR, Jackson AJ. The challenges of providing eye care for adults with intellectual disabilities. Clin Exp Optom. 2015;98(5):420–9.
219. Keiser H, Montague J, Wold D, Maune S, Pattison D. Hearing loss of Down syndrome adults. Am J Ment Defic. 1981;85(5):467–72.
220. Grojean M, Wollet A, Knollman P. Bone conduction hearing device use for the management of hearing loss in children and young adults with Down syndrome. In: Down syndrome medical interest group national symposium; 2021.
221. Eng B, Mass J, Stephens M. Evaluation of co-morbid medical conditions in adults with Down syndrome: treatment of hearing loss—grading the evidence and identifying research gaps. In: Down syndrome medical interest group national symposium; 2021.
222. Akin K. Macrocytosis and leukopenia in Down's syndrome. JAMA. 1988;259(6):842.
223. Seewald L, Taub JW, Maloney KW, McCabe ER. Acute leukemias in children with Down syndrome. Mol Genet Metab. 2012;107(1–2): 25–30.

224. McLean S, McHale C, Enright H. Hematological abnormalities in adult patients with Down's syndrome. Ir J Med Sci. 2009;178(1):35–8.
225. Hasle H, Clemmensen IH, Mikkelsen M. Risks of leukaemia and solid tumours in individuals with Down's syndrome. Lancet. 2000;355(9199):165–9.
226. Dixon N, Kishnani PS, Zimmerman S. Clinical manifestations of hematologic and oncologic disorders in patients with Down syndrome. Am J Med Genet C. 2006;142C(3):149–57.
227. Roizen NJ, Amarose AP. Hematologic abnormalities in children with Down syndrome. Am J Med Genet. 1993;46(5):510–2.
228. Cheng YZ, Wang HF, Wang HP, Chen ZM, Jin J. Trisomy 21 in patients with acute leukemia. Am J Hematol. 2009;84(3):193–5.
229. Malinge S, Izraeli S, Crispino JD. Insights into the manifestations, outcomes, and mechanisms of leukemogenesis in Down syndrome. Blood. 2009;113(12):2619–28.
230. Devata S, Pfiefer K. Doubly unexpected: Down syndrome and male breast cancer. In: Society of general internal medicine annual meeting, June 2010, Minneapolis, MN. 2010. p. S508.
231. Bratman SV, Horst KC, Carlson RW, Kapp DS. Solid malignancies in individuals with Down syndrome: a case presentation and literature review. J Natl Compr Cancer Netw. 2014;12(11):1537–45.
232. Emes D, Hüls A, Baumer N, Dierssen M, Puri S, Russell L, et al. Covid-19 in children with Down syndrome: data from the trisomy 21 research society survey. J Clin Med. 2021;10(21):5125.
233. Hüls A, Costa AC, Dierssen M, Baksh RA, Bargagna S, Baumer NT, et al. An international survey on the impact of COVID-19 in individuals with Down syndrome. medRxiv. 2020.
234. McGuire D, Chicoine B. Mental wellness in adults with Down syndrome: a guide to emotional and behavioral strengths and challenges. 2nd ed. Woodbine House; 2021.
235. Matthews TJ, Allain DC, Matthews AL, Mitchell A, Santoro SL, Cohen L. An assessment of health, social, communication, and daily living skills of adults with Down syndrome. Am J Med Genet A. 2018;176(6):1389–97.
236. Multimodal AAC for individuals with Down syndrome. Wilkinson KM, Finestack LH, editors. Baltimore, MD: Brooke Publishing; 2020.
237. Luchi RJ, Gammack JK, Narcisse VJ III, Storey CP Jr. Standards of care in geriatric practice. Annu Rev Med. 2003;54(1):185–96.
238. Wieland D, Kramer BJ, Waite MS, Rubenstein LZ. The interdisciplinary team in geriatric care. Am Behav Sci. 1996;39(6):655–64.
239. Rypkema G, Adang E, Dicke H, Naber T, De Swart B, Disselhorst L, et al. Cost-effectiveness of an interdisciplinary intervention in geriatric inpatients to prevent malnutrition. J Nutr Health Aging. 2004;8(2):122–7.
240. Staal JA, Amanda S, Matheis R, Collier L, Calia T, Hanif H, et al. The effects of Snoezelen (multisensory behavior therapy) and psychiatric care on agitation, apathy, and activities of daily living in dementia patients on a short term geriatric psychiatric inpatient unit. Int J Psychiatry Med. 2007;37(4):357–70.

## Suggested Reading

Bull MJ. Health supervision for children with Down Syndrome. Pediatrics. 2011;128(2):393–406.

Jensen KM, Bulova PD. Managing the care of adults with Down's syndrome. BMJ. 2014;349:g5596.

Smith DS. Health care management of adults with Down syndrome. Am Fam Physician. 2001;64(6):1031–8.

Tsou AY, Bulova P, Capone G, Chicoine B, Gelaro B, Harville TO, Martin BA, McGuire DE, McKelvey KD, Peterson M, Tyler C, Wells M, Whitten MS. Medical care of adults with Down syndrome: A clinical guideline. Global Down Syndrome Foundation Medical Care guidelines for adults with Down syndrome workgroup. JAMA. 2020;324(15):1543–56.

## Patient/Caregiver Resources

Advocate Health Care Adult Down Syndrome Center. https://www.advocatehealth.com/health-services/adult-down-syndrome-center/.

Alzheimer's and Down Syndrome. http://alzheimers.gov/down_syndrome.html.

Canadian Down Syndrome Society. http://www.cdss.ca/.

Down Syndrome Clinic to You (DSC2U). http://www.DSC2U.org/.

Down Syndrome Education International. https://www.dseinternational.org/en-us/.

DS-Connect. https://dsconnect.nih.gov/.

Global Down Syndrome Foundation. https://www.globaldownsyndrome.org/.

Massachusetts General Hospital, Down Syndrome Program. https://www.massgeneral.org/children/down-syndrome/patient-handouts.

National Down Syndrome Congress. https://www.ndsc-center.org/.
National Down Syndrome Society. http://www.ndss.org/.
The ARC. http://www.thearc.org/.
University of Pittsburgh, Down Syndrome Center. https://www.upmc.com/services/adult-down-syndrome-center..

## Medical Providers

American Academy of Developmental Medicine and Dentistry. http://aadmd.org/.
Down Syndrome Australia. http://www.downsyndrome.org.au/.
Down Syndrome Medical Interest Group of the United Kingdom & Ireland. http://www.dsmig.org.uk/.
Down Syndrome Medical Interest Group—USA. http://dsmig-usa.org/.
Vanderbilt University. Health watch table—Down syndrome. http://vkc.mc.vanderbilt.edu/etoolkit/physical-health/health-watch-tables-2/down-syndrome/T21 Research Society. https://www.T21rs.org.

# 31 Human Immunodeficiency Virus

Kimberly C. Bates and Megan Brundrett

## Case Presentation

Jon is a 17-year-old male presenting to his primary care physician (PCP) for an adolescent wellness visit and sports physical. He has a history of asthma, well controlled on an inhaled corticosteroid and a pre-exercise short-acting beta agonist. He complains of a facial rash and difficulty gaining weight despite efforts of increased caloric intake and strength conditioning 4 days per week. On social screening, he does not smoke tobacco products but does smoke marijuana two to three times per week and has unprotected sexual activity. His vital signs are age-appropriate, and his weight is 4 kilograms less than his last exam 12 months prior. On physical exam, he has mild cervical lymphadenopathy that is nontender, mobile, and less than 1 cm in size. He has some flaking of his skin in a beard distribution on his face but no acne. The rest of the exam is within normal limits. Because he is sexually active, he is screened for gonorrhea and chlamydia via a urine sample. He is cleared to participate in sports, given mild cleansing instructions for his facial rash, and is asked to return in 12 months.

Laboratory results return and are positive for gonorrhea and negative for chlamydia. A confidential call to Jon is made to schedule follow-up for in-office treatment of gonorrhea. Jon returns to the office 3 weeks later because it is difficult to arrange a time outside of school when his mother is not aware. He is treated with intramuscular ceftriaxone per current guidelines. His PCP reviews his visit from the previous year and notes that he was sexually active at that time too but had deferred gonorrhea or chlamydia testing due to concerns regarding confidentiality. Today, Jon denies any penile discharge, fevers, or joint pains. Further sexual history is obtained. Jon became sexually active at age 15. He had both male and female partners in the past, but for the past 18 months has preferred male partners. He has engaged in oral, vaginal, and anal sex, all without condom usage. He has a total of six lifetime partners and three of those partners he met using an application (app) on his phone and did not know much about them, including their real names or age. With those three partners, he engaged in receptive and insertive anal sex without a condom. His parents are not aware that he is sexually active, and he has not discussed any sexual preferences with them because he is concerned about how they would feel if he told them he was gay. More laboratory studies are completed at the

K. C. Bates (✉)
Department of Medicine, Creighton University School of Medicine; Graduate Medical Education, Dignity Health St. Rose Dominican, Las Vegas, NV, USA
e-mail: kimberly.bates@dignityhealth.org

M. Brundrett
Departments of Internal Medicine and Pediatrics; Medical Director, FACES Program, Nationwide Children's Hospital, Columbus, OH, USA
e-mail: megan.brundrett@nationwidechildrens.org


A. A. Kuo et al. (eds.), *Care of Adults with Chronic Childhood Conditions*,
https://doi.org/10.1007/978-3-031-54281-7_31

**Table 31.1** Laboratory test results from Jon's visit

| Laboratory test | Result |
|---|---|
| Rapid plasma reagin (RPR) | Positive, titer 1:64 |
| Gonorrhea—pharyngeal | Negative |
| Gonorrhea—rectal | Positive |
| Chlamydia—pharyngeal | Negative |
| Chlamydia—rectal | Positive |
| HIV-1 and HIV-2 antigen/ antibody screen (fourth-generation test) | Preliminary positive |
| Reflex confirmatory testing: HIV-antibody differentiation | HIV-1 antibody positive HIV-2 antibody negative |

*HIV* human immunodeficiency virus

visit, including testing for syphilis and HIV as well as additional testing for gonorrhea and chlamydia using pharyngeal and rectal swabs. Safe sex is discussed, including condom use and risks related to using apps as a minor [2]. He is scheduled to return for a confidential visit in 2 weeks when all laboratory tests will be resulted.

Laboratory test results returned 1 week later (see Table 31.1):

Jon returns to the office for laboratory results and brings his mother with him. He asks his mother to sit in the waiting room while he is given the results. After he is given the results, he invites his mother into the exam room, and the results are disclosed by Jon and his PCP.

## Case Considerations

1. What is the prevalence of acquiring HIV during adolescence?
2. What is the importance of quickly engaging in care and starting on ART youth living with HIV?
3. What is the role of the PCP in preventing HIV in youth and young adults?

## HIV Epidemiology

Compared to older adults with HIV, YAWH ages 13–24 years are more ethnically diverse, have larger female representation, have higher rates of poverty, and consist of both perinatally infected youth and those who acquired HIV during adolescence and young adulthood via sexual activity and/or injection drug use. YAWH experience significant disparities regarding HIV diagnosis and treatment. Although the number of new HIV infections in YAWH decreased from 2014 to 2018, YAWH continue to account for the largest percentage of PWH who are undiagnosed (44.9%), and therefore are more likely to unknowingly continue to transmit the virus. In 2018, the largest number of HIV infections occurred among young men who have sex with men (MSM) of color, specifically Black/African American young men, who accounted for 47% of HIV infections in MSM aged 25–34 years and 48% of HIV infections in MSM aged 13–24 years. Although adolescents and young adults ages 13–24 years constitute a small percentage of the total population of diagnosed people living with HIV (32,219/1,042,270 [3.1%] in 2018), they accounted for 21% of new infections in 2018. The annual estimated number of HIV infections in youth ages 13–24 has steadily decreased, but this improvement has not been seen in the 25–34 age group, where numbers of new HIV infections have been stable since 2015 and the overall proportion of total HIV infections has increased (in relation to all other age groups with new HIV infections) [1]. Transgender women with HIV are overrepresented in the young adult cohort of those with HIV. A 2016 analysis of the Ryan White HIV/AIDS Program (with over 530,000 PWH aged 13 and older) showed nearly 40% of transgender women in the program were in the 13–34 age group, compared to 23% of cisgender men and cisgender women, and transgender women in the program were predominantly of racial/ethnicity minority status (over 88%) [3].

## Diagnosis of HIV and Initiation of Antiretroviral Therapy

Making a diagnosis of HIV is dependent on one being tested for HIV. Understanding the risk factors for HIV acquisition and the community prevalence of HIV infection can increase testing rates. The Centers for Disease Control and Prevention (CDC) recommends routine screening for HIV at least once in a lifetime for persons aged 13–64 years. Those with risk factors for HIV acquisition should have more frequent testing, such as annually. Risk factors include male-to-male sexual intercourse, injection drug use, exchanging sex for drugs or money, sexual partners with known HIV diagnosis, and unknown HIV status of sexual partners or sexual partners with risk factors for HIV acquisition. It is also recommended that women be screened for HIV with every pregnancy, regardless of risk factors [4].

The signs and symptoms of HIV can vary based on time since acquisition. Acute HIV infection (usually within the first 6 weeks) can present with lymphadenopathy, pharyngitis, myalgias, fever, and rash. Laboratory findings can include leukopenia, thrombocytopenia, and elevated transaminases. These are nonspecific signs and symptoms and can be attributed to different viral syndromes, such as influenza or mononucleosis, or to streptococcal pharyngitis, leading to clinicians' failure to recognize and test for HIV [5]. Patients may also have mild or no symptoms during this time. Fourth-generation HIV testing, which detects both HIV-1 and HIV-2 antibodies and p24 antigen, is recommended for screening for HIV. During acute infection, the HIV antibody is negative, but either the p24 antigen and/or HIV RNA is present, representing viremia without antibody conversion. Typically, a viral load of >20,000 copies/mL is needed for a p24 antigen response; therefore, in the first few days of infection, if there is clinical suspicion for HIV, a sample for HIV RNA quantitative testing should be obtained as well. Knowing the prevalence of HIV in the community can help increase clinician awareness and prompt HIV testing for patients with flu-like symptoms, especially in communities with a prevalence of ≥0.1% [5]. It is also helpful to screen for HIV acquisition risk factors which, if present, should decrease the threshold for testing for acute HIV in a patient with a nonspecific flu-like illness.

Recent HIV is defined as the period within 6 months of HIV acquisition. During this time, patients may present with symptoms similar to acute infection or may be asymptomatic. Screening with a fourth-generation combination immunoassay is recommended for diagnosis. If the initial test is reactive, confirmatory testing with antibody differentiation for HIV-1 or HIV-2 antibody should be completed. Both acute and recent HIV infections are associated with high levels of viremia and infectivity. Previous recommendations delayed ART based on CD4+ lymphocyte count, but delaying treatment has been shown to significantly increase morbidity and mortality [6, 7]. The current guidelines recommend starting ART as soon as possible, including same-day (rapid start) options which have been shown to be safe and effective [8]. If ART is started the same day as a positive qualitative or quantitative HIV RNA test, an additional sample of blood should be drawn for confirmatory testing with HIV antibody differentiation and HIV RNA quantitative testing. Early or rapid start ART decreases time to viral suppression and reduces the risk of HIV transmission through sexual activity [9].

Chronic HIV is infection that has lasted greater than 6 months. The presentation has a wide spectrum including recognition on asymptomatic routine testing, minor symptoms such as weight loss and lymphadenopathy or fulminant HIV with opportunistic infections such as *Pneumocystis jiroveci* pneumonia (PJP). When CD4+ lymphocytes are <200 cells/mm$^3$, the risk of opportunistic infections increases due to decreased immune defenses. Discussion of such infections are beyond the scope of this chapter but are often the presenting symptoms when HIV is diagnosed during an acute hospitalization. It is important to treat both the opportunistic infections and HIV concurrently in most cases [5, 10]. Adequate HIV treatment improves immune function and in some cases is the only treatment for opportunistic infections such as progressive multifocal leukoencephalopathy and cryptosporidiosis. The exception to this is cryptococcal meningitis and tuberculosis meningitis, in which ART can be withheld initially as the underlying infections are treated due to the risk of immune reconstitution syndrome [11, 12].

Regardless of length of time since infection, U.S. Department of Health and Human Services (HHS) guidelines recommend similar ART regimens in treatment-naïve individuals. The typical regimens include two nucleoside reverse transcriptase inhibitors (NRTIs) plus either an integrase strand transfer inhibitor (INSTI), protease inhibitor (PI) and booster, or a non-nucleoside reverse transcriptase inhibitor (NNRTI) [5]. In the 2021 U.S. Department of HHS guidelines, specific initial treatment recommendations include the combination therapy of NRTIs and an INSTI. For rapid start, ART either bictegravir/tenofovir alafenamide/emtricitabine once daily or dolutegravir plus tenofovir alafenamide (or tenofovir disoproxil)/emtricitabine once daily can be used. Neither regimen requires HIV genotypic resistance testing prior to starting therapy; however, such testing should be obtained at the start of therapy for future reference and to ensure the current treatment regimen is appropriate [5]. Other regimens are recommended as first line, as well, but certain criteria must be met prior to initiation. Dolutegravir/abacavir/lamivudine is a once daily combination regimen, but HLA-B *5701 negativity must be documented before starting the regimen due to the risk of abacavir hypersensitivity, a potentially life-threatening reaction to abacavir. Therefore, this medication cannot be used in rapid start circumstances. The two-drug combination dolutegravir/lamivudine is also recommended as a first-line option but cannot be used if initial HIV RNA viral load is >500,000 copies/mL and/or if genotypic resistance results have not returned. Neither of the latter two therapies should be used in individuals with coinfection of hepatitis B. There are many different classes and combinations of ART, and an individual may have certain circumstances that make one ART regimen more appropriate than another. For those who are not treatment naïve, different considerations including comorbidities, past ART exposure, genotypic resistance patterns, adherence, and pill burden will affect the clinical decision when choosing therapy [5].

## HIV Care Continuum and Engagement in Care

The HIV Care Continuum (HIVCC) outlines the stages from diagnosis through viral suppression (diagnosis, linkage to care within 30 days, engagement in care, continuing in care, and viral suppression). Disparities exist for YAWH throughout the care continuum, with a lower percentage of those aged 13–24 years receiving an HIV diagnosis, receiving HIV medical care, being retained in HIV medical care, and achieving viral suppression compared to other age groups [13–15]. CDC data from 2019 show race/ethnicity, injection drug use, and male-to-male sexual transmission are all associated with lower percentages of both linkage to care and viral suppression within 6 months of diagnosis. Black/African American young adults and young men who have sex with men (YMSM), particularly YMSM who use injection drugs, are less likely to have a CD4+ lymphocyte count or viral load test within 1 month of diagnosis or achieve a viral load <200 copies/mL at 6 months [16].

Progress along the HIVCC was evaluated in 1411 newly diagnosed youth (aged 12–24 years) from urban HIV care centers in the United States [15]. The group was representative of the youth HIV epidemic nationwide: predominantly racial/ethnic minorities (72% Black/African American, 18% Latinx), predominantly sexual and gender minorities, including lesbian, gay, bisexual, and transgender youth (63%) and with a majority of infections through MSM transmission (63%). In this cohort, only 75% of those diagnosed were linked to care within 6 weeks of diagnosis, and less than 34% had two HIV medical visits within 1 year. During the median follow-up of 48 months, only 12% showed evidence of viral suppression. For those who made the first appointment (linkage), 80% were engaged in care (having one additional visit within the first 16 weeks of the linkage visit), but only 45% were retained in care. Of the youth who were prescribed ART, only 35% had evidence of at least one suppressed viral load, suggesting that in this population there are additional barriers (outside of access and engagement in HIV primary care) to achieving and maintaining viral load suppression. Because of factors such as lack of knowledge of diagnosis, decreased retention in care with ART, and decreased viral suppression, youth living with HIV have increased deaths attributable to HIV compared to older aged groups [17].

Early referral to HIV care focusing on adolescents has been shown to improve linkage to care for youth newly diagnosed with HIV, but there is scant literature on successful long-term retention strategies focusing solely on this group, despite clear understanding of their challenges and overall poor outcomes in the HIV Care Continuum [18–21]. Research focusing on alternative strategies for engaging this population are ongoing, including investigating internet and mobile health (mHealth) strategies as well as peer navigation and adherence interventions, with focus on sexual, gender, racial, and ethnic minority YAWH. Adolescence is a common time of gaps in primary care so for young adults diagnosed with HIV in late adolescence, HIV primary care may constitute their first foray into adult care. Adult generalists are likely to encounter YAWH at all points in the HIVCC, including young adults who are initially diagnosed with HIV after transitioning from pediatric to adult care.

## HIV Care Transition from Pediatric and Adolescent Care Settings

The time of transition from pediatric to adult care settings can be a challenging time for any youth with a chronic illness, including young adults with HIV. The majority of young adults with HIV live in Africa, with five African countries (South Africa, Kenya, Tanzania, Uganda, and Nigeria) bearing the brunt of adolescent HIV diagnoses worldwide. Transition practices vary widely between low-income and high-income countries, with low-income countries often finding transfer of health care to adult care settings occurring more due to aging out of pediatric care settings rather than a true planned transition. Outside of the United States, healthcare transitions tend to occur at earlier ages in YAWH compared to the United States. In many African and European cohorts, the median age of transition fell between 15 and 18 years of age compared to U.S. cohorts who often do not transition from pediatric care until after 18–20 years of age [22–30]. A recent meta-analysis on transition and clinical outcomes in YAWH reviewed 24 studies assessing outcomes of healthcare transitions worldwide and noted that retention rates in the 12–24 months post transition varied from 37 to 94% [31]. YAWH between the ages of 18 and 19 in these studies were most vulnerable to CD4+ lymphocyte decline and/or loss of viral suppression/viral load stability post transition. Despite considerable variability among included studies, all seem to note that transition for most YAWH is successful in the short term, though reports of worsening adherence is seen when evaluated more than 24 months post transition [32, 33]. Mortality data in outcome studies of YAWH post transition are rarely reported, but if reported, death post transition was most strongly associated with poor adherence to therapy pretransition and to unsuppressed viral loads at the time of transition, despite the availability of potentially suppressive regimens [24, 32–36]. These deaths may reflect excess mortality arising from pretransition morbidity that was not well controlled at the time of transition (for example, low CD4+ lymphocyte counts and poor adherence to opportunistic infection prophylaxis).

## Successful Models of Transition for Youth with HIV

Several successful models of healthcare transition for youth with HIV (YWH) have been developed and implemented in the United States. The Adolescent Master Protocol (AMP) Up cohort looked at 455 youth, a cohort that was predominantly female (61%) and Black/African American (68%), with a significant minority of patients with Latinx ethnicity (29%). Self-management skills were assessed using an eight-question self-administered instrument, with a score of 7 or more strongly associated with increased retention in care post transition (adjusted odds ratio, 3.4) [37]. Key determinants of successful transition for YWH in U.S. cohorts include a connection between pediatric and adult HIV providers, interdisciplinary team coordination, availability of intervention services, and recognition and management of social determinants of health and related co-morbidities before and during the transition to adult care [28, 29, 31]. Most concerning for YAWH, most studies have not shown a correlation between successful transition and viral load suppression.

In a comparison of two clinical programs in an academic, urban HIV clinic, YAWH who were lost to follow-up tended to be older and more likely to have acquired HIV thorough MSM transmission. A high-risk cohort of YWH in this study was more likely to have had a mental health diagnosis, prior incarceration, and less formal education after high school, all of which would be expected to increase loss to follow-up [28]. Enrollment in a youth focused care model for the younger, high-risk cohort improved retention in care compared to the usual care group. Retention in care was not associated with viral suppression in either group in the adjusted analysis, highlighting the challenges among YAWH. The greatest predictor of viral suppression post transition continues to be viral suppression prior to transition to adult care. Generalists who provide primary care for YAWH who have not achieved or maintained viral suppression should be prepared to connect this high-risk group with additional services, including peer support, if possible, to address barriers to viral suppression.

## Special Populations

### Young MSM of Color

Minority populations in the United States are overrepresented in the HIV epidemic and none more so than YMSM. African American YMSM account for more than 50% of YMSM infected with HIV, and YMSM account for more than 80% of HIV infections in males between 13 and 24 years of age [38]. Young males tend to have older sexual partners, putting themselves at increased risk for coercive sexual practices [39]. In addition, studies have shown MSM of color tend to have relatively small, homogenous sexual networks, and that HIV and other sexually transmitted infections (STIs) can rapidly spread throughout these networks [40, 41]. Providers should frequently screen HIV-positive YMSM for intimate partner violence and coercive sexual activity due to the high prevalence of both in this group, similar to what is seen among cisgender women [42–46]. Discussion of current sexual practices as well as risk assessment and screening for STIs should be a part of primary care for YMSM with HIV. Pre-exposure prophylaxis (PrEP) for HIV-negative partners of YMSM with HIV may also be a powerful tool to prevent continued spread of HIV among the sexual networks of YMSM of color. Generalists caring for HIV-positive YMSM (as well as at risk HIV-negative men) should be aware of and appropriately prescribe PrEP to decrease transmission among this group of patients.

### Black/African American Young Adults with HIV

In 2019, 41% of new HIV infections and 42% of new HIV diagnoses were among Black/African American persons, reflecting the racial/ethnic disparity in those living with HIV [1]. Although cases of new diagnoses have trended downward in Black/African Americans from 2014 to 2019 (as in all other ethnic groups), HIV still disproportionally affects the Black/African American community, and rates of viral suppression are lower among Black/African American patients. Among young adults with HIV, Black/African American persons are more likely to have experienced incarceration, more likely to have unstable housing and more likely to have poor social supports and poverty, further worsening health disparities [47–51].

African American women make up 13% of the entire U.S. female population but over 50% of women with HIV. A 2005 small case–control study of HIV-infected Black women and matched controls (Black women at risk for HIV infection) in North Carolina showed HIV-infected women were more likely to exchange basic needs or drugs for sex ($p$ value = 0.01) and were more likely to have sexual partners with a prior history of incarceration ($p$ value = 0.04) [52]. This suggests that economic disadvantage and reliance on a partner for substantive needs increase the risk for HIV infection among this group. A component of patient-centered care for young women, particularly Black/African American women, with HIV should include the evaluation of the current living situation and screening for transactional sex which may increase the risk for other STIs and intimate partner violence. There have been decreases in new HIV infections among African American women in the last decade (with a 11% decrease from 2015 to 2019), but racial and ethnic disparities persist, with the incidence of HIV infection being 13 times higher in Black/African American women than in White women and four times higher than in Latinx women [53]. Black/African American youth in the United States constitute 60% of those diagnosed with perinatally acquired HIV, and although mother to child transmission of HIV continues to be low (less than 1% of all new diagnoses), 57% of new perinatal HIV infections occur within this ethnic group [53]. This suggests significant disparities in prenatal care and maternal-to-child transmission prevention activities during pregnancy for Black/African American women in the United States. Physicians and other practitioners should be aware of the poorer outcomes in Black/African Americans with HIV, likely due to the effects of institutionalized racism and trauma in African American young adults with HIV, and should proactively connect them to trauma-informed HIV case management and peer support services if they are not already connected.

## Socioeconomically Disadvantaged Youth

Despite improved access to health care through both the Ryan White Care Act, which provides HIV primary care services for HIV-infected men, women, and children, as well as the Affordable Care Act (ACA), young adults with HIV continue to face difficulty engaging in HIV care and being retained in treatment. Poverty remains an independent risk factor for HIV infection and failure to be retained in HIV care [54, 55]. Socioeconomically disadvantaged youth and young adults have unique challenges including lack of transportation, unemployment, and lack of health insurance, particularly as they age out of Medicaid in states without Medicaid expansion through the ACA. As a result, they may require additional strategies to maintain viral suppression. To better engage YAWH, HIV primary care must address social determinants such as high unemployment rates, HIV stigma and disclosure, unstable housing, poverty, and lack of social supports. Young adults living in poverty have less opportunity to learn key self-management skills that may help them cope with chronic disease. Special attention should be placed on educating young adults about their disease and the importance of self-care in preventing additional HIV-related comorbidities. The Medical Monitoring Project, which consists of a sample of PWH who are engaged in HIV care from 23 states and/or metropolitan areas, notes that 16% of young adults ages 18–29 experienced homelessness in the previous 12 months, the highest of any age range. Evidence of housing instability, such as living temporarily with friends and transactional sex for housing, was not included, likely underestimating the incidence of unstable housing in this population. Not surprisingly, PWH who experience homelessness have lower retention in care and more difficulty achieving viral suppression. Sexual and gender minority youth (SGMY), regardless of HIV status, experience homelessness at higher rates than non-SGMY [56]. Screening for unstable housing and providing resources for safe housing, including Housing Opportunities for Persons with AIDS, are crucial for YWH, especially SGMY.

## Sexual and Gender Minority Young Adults

Transgender women are disproportionally affected by the HIV epidemic. Studies of YWH typically do not include large numbers of transgender young women, but due to the high prevalence of HIV in all transgender women (estimated to be approximately 25%), researchers are increasingly focusing on the experiences of transgender female youth. Sixty-six gender diverse young adults with HIV from 14 cities in the United States were interviewed in a qualitative study looking at specific barriers in care for this population. Key themes from this work included lack of social support and negative interactions with the healthcare system, both of which may help explain why SGMY have lower rates of viral suppression [57]. Transgender adults with HIV have better rates of viral suppression and retention in care than transgender youth, although the reason for this disparity is unclear [58]. Researchers analyzing data from 11,000 transgender persons with HIV in the Ryan White HIV/AIDS Program (RWHAP) noted significant disparities in care and viral suppression in Black/African American transgender women compared to both Black/African American cisgender men and women, results suggesting the existence of barriers due to additional stigma experienced by minority transgender women. Nearly 40% of transgender women were under age 35 and were on average 10 years younger than their cisgender counterparts, reflecting a primarily young adult population [58]. Additional research on the intersectionality of age, race, ethnicity, sexual orientation, gender, and gender identity in SGMY with HIV is needed to clarify determinants of poorer outcomes in this group. Physicians and other practitioners caring for this population should recognize the need for additional care support services (such as RWHAP case management and gender-affirming health care) to continue to engage this population in care and to achieve and maintain viral suppression.

## HIV Primary Care and Comorbidities

### HIV Primary Care Screening

Young adults with HIV should have yearly preventive medicine visits to address chronic disease management and screening for common comorbidities in addition to HIV primary care. The Infectious Diseases Society of America (IDSA) and HIV Medicine Association (HIVMA) released updated guidelines in 2021 for primary care for adults with HIV [59]. Health maintenance activities that are specific to young adults with HIV infection which could be delivered in a primary care practice have been summarized below (see Table 31.2).

### Co-Morbidities in Persons with HIV

Several metabolic complications associated with ART have been documented in YAWH, including lipodystrophy, lipoatrophy, hyperlipidemia, poor bone health, micronutrient deficiencies, and insulin resistance, although these complications are typically associated with use of older ART formulations or in youth with perinatal HIV [60, 61]. Protease inhibitors increase the risk of metabolic disorders such as hyperlipidemia and hyperglycemia. Patients on protease inhibitor therapy should be screened annually for the development of diabetes, particularly in those who are also obese. The ADVANCE trial noted increases in truncal and limb fat mass and an increase in metabolic syndromes for patients on tenofovir alafenamide (TAF) and dolutegravir (DTG), both newer antiretrovirals (ARVs) [62]. Generally, lipodystrophies are significantly less common with current regimens, however, most classes of ART cause some increase in lipid levels, particularly low-density (LDL)-C and triglycerides. There are no long-term studies of outcomes of metabolic complications of ART or the metabolic consequences of HIV infection in adolescents and young adults, particularly in the era of INSTI. Regimens using INSTIs and newer NRTIs are considered to be mostly lipid neutral.

Young women with HIV (aged 18–24 years) who are in care are more likely to be obese compared to their older counterparts [13, 63]. Obesity is a risk-enhancing factor for atherosclerotic cardiovascular disease (ASCVD) as well as metabolic diseases such as prediabetes, hypertension, and hyperlipidemia. Current ASCVD-prevention guidelines now include HIV disease as a risk-enhancing factor (as a chronic inflammatory condition), and several studies have demonstrated increased risk for early ASCVD in adults with HIV, particularly cerebrovascular accidents [64–69]. American College of Cardiology/

**Table 31.2** Health maintenance screening guidelines for primary care of patients with HIV

| Screening | Interval | Additional information |
|---|---|---|
| Anal cancer screening | At least annually | Digital rectal examination for anal lesions, anal warts, and other changes. In specialized centers, may consider anal cytology for those with receptive anal intercourse if high-resolution anoscopy is available |
| Depression screening | At least annually | Depression is the most common mental health co-morbidity in PWH |
| Diabetes and prediabetes screening | Annually and 3–6 months after starting or switching ART therapy | Screening for diabetes due to metabolic dysfunction in HIV infection. Avoid hemoglobin A1c for diagnosis in patients on ART due to independent effects of ART on hemoglobin A1c levels |
| Hyperlipidemia | Based on age and ASCVD risk | Adults aged 20–40 years without any additional risk factors (diabetes, smoking, obesity, etc.) may be screened every 5 years if normal. Since HIV is considered a risk-enhancing factor for ASCVD, more frequent testing and earlier statin therapy could be considered for those at intermediate risk. Also consider repeat lipid testing with changes in ART |
| Urinalysis for proteinuria screening | At initiation into care and consider annually | Increased risk of chronic kidney disease in certain populations, including African American, PWID, use of TDF-based regimen, history of nephrotoxic drugs, etc. |
| Trichomoniasis | At initiation into care and annually thereafter if sexually active | Increased risk of STI acquisition in women with untreated trichomoniasis and high trichomoniasis reinfection rates |
| Tobacco use screening and cessation counseling | At least annually, and at each visit for active or intermittent tobacco users | Association with smoking and disease progression in HIV and HIV-associated co-morbidities |
| STI testing-syphilis, gonorrhea and chlamydia | At initiation into care and then at least annually if sexually active. Consider every 3–6 months for those with multiple partners | Increased incidence of non-HIV STI infection in youth and young adults with HIV due to continued high-risk sexual practices and low condom use |
| Hepatitis B virus (HBV) screening, including evidence of HBV post-vaccination immunity | At initiation into care | Testing for evidence of HBV infection, which will impact choice of ART and testing for immunity to HBV as result of childhood vaccination |
| Hepatitis C virus (HCV) screening | At initiation into care and annually for sexually active MSM and PWID | Rapidly increasing incidence of acute HCV in young adults aged 20–39 years and chronic HCV in adults aged 30–39 years. PWID, and MSM continue to be additional risk factors |
| Alcohol and drug screening | At least annually, and at each visit for active users | Increased incidence of alcohol and drug use as part of high-risk sexual behaviors and negative association with viral load suppression in young adults with HIV |
| Secondary HIV prevention | At each visit if possible | Prevention of HIV transmission |
| Medication adherence | At each visit if possible | Maintenance of viral suppression |
| Intimate partner violence screening (regardless of gender identity or sexual orientation) | At least annually and more often if needed | Patients with HIV are at higher risk of intimate partner violence than general population |

(continued)

**Table 31.2** (continued)

| Screening | Interval | Additional information |
|---|---|---|
| Immunizations | Per advisory committee on immunization practices (ACIP) guidelines and previous vaccine history | In adolescents and young adults newly diagnosed with HIV, typical childhood vaccinations may require boosters due to new immunosuppression. Review timing of HIV infection and pneumococcal and meningococcal vaccines. HPV vaccination should be done if not previously completed. Hepatitis A and B vaccination should be completed if nonimmune |

Adapted with permission from [59]
*PWH* people living with HIV, *ART* antiretroviral therapy, *HIV* human immunodeficiency virus, *ASCVD* atherosclerotic cardiovascular disease, *TDF* tenofovir disoproxil fumarate, *PWID* people who inject drugs, *STI* sexually transmitted infection, *HPV* human papilloma virus

American Heart Association (ACC/AHA) guidelines for ASCVD risk assessment recommend aggressive lifestyle optimization for adults under age forty with risk factors and considering ASCVD risk estimation, although ASCVD risk scoring may not accurately reflect risk in persons with HIV. Coronary artery calcium (CAC) scoring via computed tomography to determine subclinical coronary atherosclerosis could also be considered for those with intermediate or borderline ASCVD risk scoring with multiple risk-enhancing factors (including HIV) per ACC/AHA guidelines [64, 70]. Clinicians caring for young adults with HIV and elevated cholesterol levels who have additional risk factors such as obesity, diabetes, hypertension, family history of ASCVD, or other risk factors (particularly with an elevated CAC score) may consider early initiation of statin therapy (with special attention to drug–drug interactions with many ART formulations and statins) for those under the age of 40, in part due to accelerations in atherosclerosis driven by longstanding chronic inflammation. Observational data from the CARDIA cohort (a U.S. cohort of healthy young adults) show that early adult risk factor levels (such as hyperlipidemia, hypertension, and smoking) predict later development of heart disease [71]. Given the higher rates of ASCVD risk factors such as hyperlipidemia and smoking in young adults living with HIV, this population may be at even greater risk of early CAD. Clinicians should discuss options to statins in women with HIV of childbearing age, including contraception if considering statin use, due to teratogenic effects of this drug class.

Effects of ART on long-term bone development and bone mineral density (BMD) in YWH are unknown, but among adults with HIV, early data suggested decreases in BMD due to ART have been associated with increased risk of fractures in Caucasian and Black/African American patients [72]. Decreases in bone density with tenofovir disoproxil appear to be reversible, with bone density returning to normal after cessation in those on tenofovir disoproxil-based therapy for PrEP [73–75]. Low CD4+ counts reflecting severe immunodeficiency have been shown to adversely affect bone health in adults with HIV [76–79]. There are no evidence-based recommendations on the use of dual-energy X-ray absorptiometry (DEXA) scanning for osteopenia and osteoporosis screening in young adults with HIV, but osteoporosis prevention activities such as weight-bearing exercise, treatment of vitamin D deficiency, and adequate dietary sources of calcium and protein to support bone health are reasonable recommendations [80].

Studies have shown that PWH have a higher prevalence of smoking compared to age-matched persons without HIV [81–84]. Young adults with HIV are also more likely to use tobacco compared to age-matched peers [85]. HIV infection is associated with airflow obstruction on spirometry and may accelerate or exacerbate tobacco-related lung disease such as chronic obstructive pulmonary disease (COPD) and emphysema [86, 87]. YAWH, particularly those with perinatally acquired HIV, are at further risk of chronic lung disease in adulthood due to longstanding chronic inflammation as well as opportunistic infections of the lungs such as *Pneumocystis jirovecii* pneumonia during childhood. These effects may be demonstrated by restrictive or fibrotic changes in the lung as well as exercise intolerance. Tobacco use may exacerbate these changes and at an earlier age than expected [87–89]. Tobacco cessation is crucial for PWH who smoke and should be addressed at every visit.

## Cancer Screening

PWH are at risk for AIDS-related and non-AIDS-related cancers [90, 91]. AIDS-related cancers include cervical cancer, Kaposi sarcoma, and non-Hodgkin lymphoma. In addition, PWH are at higher risk of cancers caused by human papilloma virus (HPV), including cervical cancer, anogenital cancer, and oropharyngeal cancer, and this risk is present for both men and women, regardless of the type of sexual activity [92, 93]. PWH have a higher prevalence of both cancer risk factors and oncogenic HPV infection of the oral and genital track compared to the general U.S. population, which may have an additive effect when combined with immunosuppression from HIV [94–97]. Due to the elevated risk of invasive cervical cancer in women with HIV, cervical cancer screening recommendations are slightly different compared to women without HIV (see Table 31.3) [10, 98, 99]. Guidelines for the management of abnormal cervical cytology in women with HIV aged 21–29 years recommend colposcopy for atypical squamous cells of undetermined significance (ASC-US) with positive HPV reflex testing or greater cytology. If HPV reflex testing cannot be performed on the obtained specimen, cytology should be repeated in 6–12 months, with referral for colposcopy if ASC-US or greater. For women with HIV aged 30 years or older, guidelines are similar with the exception that even with normal cytology, all women with high-risk HPV positive results should be referred for colposcopy [10].

People with HIV have a 30-fold increase in lifetime risk for anal cancer and a four-fold increase in 5-year mortality from invasive anal cancer compared to HIV-unaffected individuals. This disparity continues to exist even when controlling for history of receptive anal intercourse [93, 100]. PWH have a higher incidence of all HPV-related cancers (cervical, vulvar, anal, and oropharyngeal) compared to the general population, and CD4 count is inversely associated with the development of HPV-related cancers [10]. Other than cervical cancer, there are no current guidelines for screening for other HPV-related

**Table 31.3** Recommendations for cervical cancer screening in women with HIV compared to women without HIV

| | Ages 21–29 years[a] | | Age 30 years or greater[b] | |
|---|---|---|---|---|
| | HIV (+) | HIV (−) | HIV (+) | HIV (−) |
| Initiation of screening | Age 21 | Age 21 | At time of HIV diagnosis | At initial evaluation if not previously screened |
| Type of screening | Pap test (cytology) only | Pap test (cytology) only | Pap test (cytology) only<br>Pap (cytology) + HPV co-testing | Pap (cytology) + HPV co-testing OR hrHPV testing alone OR cytology alone |
| Screening interval | Every 12 months for 3 years and, if negative, every 3 years[c] | Every 3 years | Cytology: Every 12 months for 3 years and, if negative, every 3 years<br>Co-testing (cytology + HPV testing) every 3 years | Cytology every 3 years<br>hrHPV testing alone every 5 years<br>Co-testing (cytology +HPV testing) every 5 years |

Adapted with permission from [95]

[a]Recommendations for the initiation of cervical cancer screening for young adults with HIV at 21 years instead of the initiation of sexual activity have changed due to low incidence of invasive cervical cancer under age 25 years [97]

[b]For women without HIV, screening should continue until age 65 years. No evidence-based recommendations exist for screening cessation in women with HIV

[c]Until age 29 years. Aged 30 years and over, women should preferably receive co-testing if available

*HIV* human immunodeficiency virus, *Pap* papanicolaou, *HPV* human papilloma virus, *hrHPV* high-risk HPV standalone testing

cancers for people with HIV. HIVMA/IDSA Clinical Practice Guideline for the Primary Care Management of Persons with HIV recommends anal Pap testing for those with genital warts or a history of receptive anal intercourse if access to specialized follow up is available [59]. With the recently completed Anal Cancer HSIL Outcome Research (ANCHOR) study, stopped early in late 2021 due to the success of treatment of anal HSIL (high-grade squamous intraepithelial lesions) in preventing progression to anal cancer, screening and treatment guidelines for anal dysplasia in PWH are likely forthcoming in the upcoming years [101]. While awaiting official recommendations, the PCP should at a minimum discuss anal cancer screening with YAWH and identify a high-quality referral center, performing high volumes of high-resolution anoscopy (HRA) screening should the patient wish to pursue screening. In addition, the visual screening of oropharyngeal and anal areas for abnormalities should be done no less than annually, and clinicians should have a low threshold for specialist referral and biopsy for suspicious lesions.

There are no guidelines for screening for the other two AIDS-defining malignancies (Kaposi sarcoma and non-Hodgkin [B-cell] lymphoma) or other non-AIDS defining malignancies specific to PWH. It should be noted that PWH have a higher overall incidence of malignancy compared to their age-matched peers. PWH also have a higher incidence of liver and lung cancer, and unlike the AIDS-defining cancers, incidence has not decreased in the ART era [102–105]. Similar to the general population, incidence for both cancers increases with age, but PWH may present at an earlier age than expected compared to the general population. At this time, routine non-HPV cancer screening should be based on screening recommendations for the general population.

## Sexual and Reproductive Health

YWH commonly acquire other STIs, noted either at the time of initial diagnosis or during routine follow-up visits. Analyses of perinatally infected patients in the Pediatric HIV/AIDS Cohort Study (PHACS) registry showed that 62% of sexually active HIV-positive youth reported unprotected sexual activity [106]. A single-center, retrospective analysis of urban YWH (primarily through perinatal acquisition) also documented a high prevalence of unprotected sexual activity as measured by STI acquisition. In this cohort, 76% of youth reported using barrier contraceptive methods "intermittently," yet during the 3-year period studied, 67% contracted an STI. Risk factors for STI acquisition in this cohort included lack of HIV virological control and number of sexual partners. Notably, sexual preference was not seen to be an indicator of STI risk in this cohort, with those with same-sex or opposite-sex partners having similar risks for STI acquisition [107]. Some studies have shown that YWH use barrier protection less often than youth without HIV, particularly those with higher numbers of sexual partners [108]. The percentage of sexually active U.S. youth who report using a condom during their last sexual intercourse has consistently been less than 70% over the last two decades and has continued to decline since 2003 [109, 110]. Condom usage for SGMY is consistently lower than that among heterosexual youth as well [109]. For the adult provider, it is important to recognize that STI risk-reduction education has not resulted in increased condom use and decreased STI acquisition for the current generation of adolescents and young adults. Changes in state laws limiting sexual and reproductive health education (for example, the percentage of schools that required HIV prevention education decreased from 2000 to 2016) and lack of condom availability programs in schools (with only 7% of high schools offering condom availability programs [CAPs] in 2014) may have contributed to the low uptake of STI prevention activities among youth [111]. Adolescents and young adults with HIV are no more likely to utilize STI risk-reduction strategies and should therefore be counseled on secondary risk reduction for HIV transmission and STIs at every visit. Clinicians should screen for *Neisseria gonorrhoeae* and *Chlamydia trachomatis* (rectal, pharyngeal, and urethral based on method of intercourse), and syphilis in sexually active young men and women with HIV at least annually and more often in those with multiple sexual partners and other risk factors such as lack of condom usage, transactional sex, and anal intercourse. All PWH should receive one time hepatitis C screening, with annual screening in young MSM and people who inject drugs (PWID) [112–114].

Sexual dysfunction is not an uncommon comorbidity in persons with HIV. Men with HIV may have sexual dysfunction, stemming from medical (such as testosterone deficiency), psychological (such as internalized HIV stigma), medication-related (such as ART side effects), or HIV-related or HIV-exacerbated comorbidities (hyperlipidemia, vascular disease, etc.). Hypogonadism, one of the endocrine comorbidities in HIV, has symptoms such as erectile dysfunction, muscle mass loss, and fatigue. In transgender men and women and MSM, sexual dysfunction can also be related to their sexual minority status. Transgender men and women should be referred to specialists in transgender sexual health, as issues around body image and gender identity can further complicate any sexual issues resulting from their HIV status.

## Partner Disclosure

Disclosure may increase opportunities for social support and improve overall quality of life in PWH but may also result in stigma, discrimination, and rejection, particularly among racial, ethnic, sexual, and gender minorities. YAWH may face stigma related to HIV disclosure, presenting a barrier to partner disclosure and potentially increasing HIV transmission to sexual partners. YAWH receiving care in the Adolescent Trials Networks for HIV clinics (ATN) were unlikely to disclose their HIV status to casual sexual partners, regardless of viral suppression status, although many more were likely to have disclosed to past and/or current steady sexual partners, similar to behavior in adults with HIV [115–120]. Although HIV disclosure in adults has been associated with greater engagement in care and improved adherence, this may not be the same in YAWH [117, 121, 122]. YWH may experience negative repercussions (family rejection, bullying and violence, and loss of housing) from broader disclosure that make them less likely to disclose to sexual partners. Qualitative studies of youth and HIV disclosure often describe instances of rejection, isolation, fear, internalized stigma, and other negative experiences [116, 117, 120]. Generalists caring for YAWH should also be aware of the laws in their state regarding HIV disclosure. As of 2021, 12 states in the United States still have laws that require persons with HIV who are aware of their status to disclose to any sexual partner, with maximum sentence lengths of over one year for most states who require disclosure [123]. Additional 20 states have included HIV into their communicable disease laws. Notably, state laws may not incorporate or reflect the current HIV prevention landscape of the Undetectable = Untransmittable (U=U) campaign and PrEP usage. YWH may be unaware of these laws, placing them at potential legal risk.

## Medical Concerns in Pregnant Women with HIV

Literature on peripartum complications in pregnant women with HIV is mixed, with some early studies showing an increased risk for preterm labor and low birth weight deliveries and more recent cohorts showing no difference between women with and without HIV when controlled for conditions such as pre-existing co-morbidities and age [124]. Notably, women with HIV who conceive and deliver are more likely to be Black/African American, to have come from low socioeconomic status, and to smoke, all characteristics associated with preterm delivery in women without HIV [125, 126]. Pregnant women with perinatally acquired HIV are more likely to have existing co-morbidities compared to women who acquire HIV through sexual activity, although several studies have not shown any difference in maternal or infant outcomes comparing these two groups [127–129].

## Reproductive Health in Young Women and Transgender Males with HIV

HIV does not appear to affect fertility for young women with HIV, and pregnancies are common in this group. As in all women of reproductive age, the PCP should counsel young women with HIV on options for contraception if desired. Because ARVs have multiple drug–drug interactions, previously there were concerns regarding both the effectiveness of hormonal contraception as well as a possible association with injectable hormonal contraception and HIV transmission among women receiving ARVs [130]. The U.S. Guidelines for the Medical Eligibility for Contraception recently reaffirmed that women with HIV can use any form of hormonal contraception (both progesterone-only and combination estrogen–progesterone regimens) without restriction [131]. Women who are interested in pregnancy prevention should be started on hormonal contraception (oral, injectable, or preferably, long-acting reversible contraception [LARC]) immediately to prevent unwanted pregnancy.

Transgender males represent a small population of those living with HIV, and most studies do not have enough representation to report outcomes specifically for this population. However, sexual health recommendations for transgender males with HIV do not differ from those without HIV. Particularly, transgender males should be offered gender-affirming therapy, including options for reducing or eliminating menstrual cycles, if desired.

## Maternal to Child Transmission Prevention

Mother-to-child transmission of HIV is less than 1% if women are taking ART during the pregnancy, achieve viral suppression near delivery, and their infants receive appropriate antiviral prophylaxis [132]. Prevention of transmission begins with identifying women who have been infected with HIV and by testing all women when they enter prenatal care. If testing is initially negative, third-trimester HIV testing should also be obtained if the mother has risk factors for HIV acquisition or lives in an area with incidence ≥0.1%. This will identify any women who were infected later in pregnancy and allow time to start ART before delivery [132].

All women who have a new diagnosis of HIV during pregnancy should be connected to HIV care and started on ART as soon as possible, even before genotypic-resistance testing results have returned, as the risk of transmission of HIV is inversely associated with length of maternal viral suppression. In women with HIV (WWH), preconception counseling should be focused on maintaining viral suppression and continuing ART before and throughout pregnancy. Most common ART regimens are considered safe during pregnancy and without known teratogenic effects. Because of this, most women should continue their prepregnancy ART during pregnancy [132].

In treatment-naïve women or women newly diagnosed with HIV during pregnancy, a regimen of either tenofovir/emtricitabine or abacavir/lamivudine, plus either an INSTI or PI is acceptable. Special considerations include women with hepatitis B virus coinfection who should be on tenofovir/emtricitabine and those considering usage of abacavir for whom HLA- B*5701 testing should be completed prior to starting therapy. Women who do not achieve viral suppression within 4 weeks of delivery and have a viral load of >1000 copies/mL should be given intrapartum zidovudine and undergo cesarean section delivery at 38 weeks to reduce the risk of intrapartum HIV transmission [132].

Infants at very low risk of perinatal transmission (those whose mother is on ART during pregnancy and has achieved and maintained viral suppression without concerns for adherence) are started on zidovudine twice daily for 4 weeks. All other infants should be started on triple therapy with zidovudine, lamivudine, and nevirapine as presumptive HIV therapy [132]. These medications should be managed by a pediatric infectious disease specialist, and serial testing of HIV DNA or RNA should be completed. It is particularly important to avoid testing for HIV antibodies in an infant of a WWH as maternal antibodies cross the placenta and will be positive, causing unnecessary alarm.

## HIV Prevention Strategies and Pre-Exposure Prophylaxis

With declining perinatal transmission, most HIV acquisition in youth occurs during sexual activity and, to a lesser extent, through injection drug use. HIV prevention strategies should be reviewed with all individuals at increased risk for HIV. Prevention strategies include use of barrier protection (condoms) during sexual activity, being regularly tested for HIV, being tested and treated for other STIs, and using clean needles/not sharing needles during injection drug use. Importantly, viral suppression is another important aspect of HIV prevention. Known worldwide as the U=U campaign, an individual can prevent sexual transmission of HIV to others by taking ART and achieving and maintaining viral suppression for 6 months. In serodiscordant relationships, the partner with HIV should be counseled to achieve viral suppression prior to having unprotected sex.

An additional effective option for HIV prevention is the use of PrEP for those at increased risk for HIV acquisition. PrEP is 99% effective at preventing sexual transmission of HIV and 74% effective at preventing HIV transmission through injection drug use. Prior to starting PrEP, one must have a negative HIV test, and if there is any concern or signs/symptoms of acute infection, an HIV RNA quantitative should be completed. There are two options for oral PrEP: tenofovir disoproxil fumarate (TDF)/emtricitabine and tenofovir alafenamide (TAF)/emtricitabine. Both are FDA approved as a once daily combination medication for adolescents and adults weighing ≥35 kilograms or 77 pounds.

TDF/emtricitabine is approved for use in cisgender and transgender men and women and those using injection drugs. It is currently the only oral PrEP formulation approved in women and for receptive vaginal intercourse. It has been well studied and shown to be safe and effective [133, 134]. Because of the risk of nephrotoxicity, TDF/emtricitabine should be used in those with creatine clearance CrCl >60 mL/min/1.73 m$^2$. In PrEP studies in adults, there have been some mild elevations in creatinine which resolved with discontinuation of therapy but no reports of renal failure [135, 136]. TDF/emtricitabine has been associated with reversible BMD loss, but at this time there are no recommendations to screen with DEXA while on this medication. Common side effects of TDF/emtricitabine are headache, abdominal pain, and weight loss [137].

TAF/emtricitabine is approved to prevent the sexual transmission of HIV in only cisgender men and transgender women and is not approved for receptive vaginal intercourse or injection drug use. The medication is associated with less risk for nephrotoxic effects and bone loss due to lower levels of tenofovir in the plasma. The most common side effect of TAF/emtricitabine is diarrhea.

Cabotegravir, an INSTI, was recently approved for PrEP in cisgender and transgender men and women older than 12 years of age and 35 kg. This medication is injected bimonthly after an initial introductory period of two injections 1 month apart. This medication does not rely on daily medication and therefore has the opportunity to enhance adherence for those that struggle with daily medications [138].

Effectiveness of these medications is directly related to medication adherence, which can be challenging in the adolescent and young adult population. Barriers to PrEP in youth contribute to a lower uptake compared with adults. Youth less than 18 years old face minor consent issues depending on local or state statutes and likely are still on caregiver insurance plans, making confidentiality pertaining to medication access difficult. Other barriers include lack of support, transportation issues, and lack of access outside of school hours. In the Adolescent Trials Network for HIV Interventions (ATN) demonstration project, adherence to PrEP declined when office visits were spaced to every 12 weeks. Close follow-up should be considered when prescribing adolescents PrEP, with a review of barriers and assessment of adherence being performed at each visit [139].

## Stigma, Mental Health and Substance Abuse

### HIV-Related Stigma

Stigma related to diagnosis with HIV is significantly associated with poor adherence to ART, lack of viral suppression, and to mental health disorders [116, 140–142]. Due to this association, HIV-related stigma research has been set as a priority at the National Institutes of Health, including the development of a national indicator to measure HIV-related stigma [143]. Youth and young adults with HIV experience more stigma compared to their older counterparts as measured by the Berger HIV stigma scale [144]. Young adults aged 18–29 years continue to have the highest median HIV stigma scores (42.9 in 2019 compared to 38.3 for all ages) [13]. Addressing HIV stigma through education, avoidance of stigmatizing language, and peer and professional mental health support focusing on dealing with internalized stigma are key components to improving the lives of young adults with HIV.

### Mental Health and Substance Abuse

Prevalence of depression and anxiety is increasing among U.S. adolescents, most notably since the beginning of the COVID-19 pandemic. Parents and caregivers report that among youth aged 12–17 years, 6% have been diagnosed with depression, over 10% with anxiety, and 58% of those diagnosed with a mental/behavioral health condition have received counseling or other treatment [145, 146]. One in three high school students self-reported persistent feelings of sadness or hopelessness, and over one in six have considered attempting suicide, with persistent sadness and hopelessness and suicidal ideation increasing over the period from 2009 to 2019, regardless of race and ethnicity [145, 147, 148]. Sexual minority youth were twice as likely to have reported persistent feelings of sadness or hopelessness during the previous year compared to heterosexual students (66.3% vs. 32.2%) and were over three times as likely to have seriously considered a suicide attempt (46.8% vs. 14.5%) [149]. These findings are likely to be even more significant among YWH [150]. Cohorts of youth and young adults with HIV transitioning to adult care have demonstrated high rates of psychiatric comorbidities ranging from 15% to 60% [29, 151–154]. Despite similar rates of psychiatric disorders, youth with perinatally acquired HIV (pHIV) were twice as likely to attempt suicide compared to HIV-exposed but uninfected peers, regardless of sexual orientation or demographics, with most attempts occurring between 14 and 18 years of age [155, 156]. This suggests that living with HIV conferred a greater risk of suicidical ideation. Mental health conditions persist at the age of transition as well. In a group of youth with pHIV at the time of care transition, 21% of the transitioned cohort were subsequently diagnosed with anxiety or depression in adult care [24]. Patient cohorts studied in two U.S. urban HIV youth transition clinics noted that 30% of the total study population had pre-existing psychiatric comorbidities, even though only one arm of one clinical program focused on accepting youth with prior mental health disorders [29]. A study of psychiatric disorders and ART adherence in adolescents and young adults with pHIV assessed participants for symptoms of common mental health disorders and found that of 179 participants, 53% met criteria for a psychiatric disorder, with generalized anxiety being the most common [153]. Close to 20% of a transition-age cohort of youth adults with pHIV had evidence of significant depressive symptoms, designated as a Center for Epidemiological Studies-Depression Scale (CES-D-10) score $\geq$ 10 [37]. Additionally, mental health disorders and symptomology have also been correlated with substance use disorder (SUD) and lack of viral suppression in YWH [157]. Youth and young adults with HIV can reasonably be considered at high risk for mental health co-morbidities and should be screened at least annually for depression and anxiety. Clinicians caring for this group should have a low threshold for mental health referral. In addition, medication side effects and interactions, particularly with antipsychotics and ART, must be evaluated prior to initiation of therapy. Consultation with a psychiatrist with experience caring for persons with HIV may be warranted.

SUD includes tobacco, alcohol, marijuana, opiates, and illicit drugs such as heroin or cocaine. Cohort studies in the United States show high levels of SUD in YAWH, with tobacco, marijuana, and alcohol predominantly used [158]. When compared to their White counterparts, youth of color are equally likely to engage in weekly substance use but more likely to experience substance-related problems due to other structural problems such as poverty, exposure to violence, and institutionalized racism, limiting access to diagnosis and treatment [158]. These issues are only magnified in youth of color with HIV. The use of illicit drugs (cocaine, inhalants, heroin, methamphetamines hallucinogens, or ecstasy) have steadily decreased over the previous 10 years in White and Latinx youth, but rates in Black/African American youth have not changed [159]. A sample of 823 YWH (median age 21 years) recruited from adolescent HIV clinics in ATN were assessed using the ASSIST (Alcohol, Smoking and Substance Abuse Screening Test) tool for substance use, with 20–25% reporting weekly alcohol use, monthly marijuana use, and/or any other drug use (cocaine, inhalants, sedatives, hallucinogens, opioids, or methamphetamine) within the previous 3 months [160]. Over half of the group met criteria for moderate or high-risk marijuana use, and greater than 25% met criteria for moderate or high-risk alcohol use. Substance use was strongly associated with STIs in this cohort of YWH, suggesting a correlation with SUD and high-risk behaviors among this group. Prevalence of substance use in newly diagnosed YAWH also appears to be high, with 52% reporting any substance use (excluding tobacco and including street hormones) within the previous 6 months [15]. Any substance use in this study was associated with a decreased likelihood of viral suppression (HR 0.68) in YAWH linked to HIV care.

Injection drug use continues to be low among all youth but is associated with increased risk of HIV and hepatitis C virus (HCV) infection. Youth and young adults aged 13–34 years made up 47% of new HIV diagnoses among people who inject drugs PWID in 2018, and 5% of all new HIV diagnoses were in youth who reported injection drug use (IDU) [1, 13, 53]. An increasing percentage of those new infections are in White, nonurban communities, many without ready access to harm-reduction strategies such as syringe services programs and medication-assisted treatment [161]. IDU has been linked to the skyrocketing rates of HCV infection in young adults, with 67% of those with newly diagnosed hepatitis C reporting IDU. HIV/HCV coinfection is common, with 21% of people with HIV having HIV/HCV coinfection [113].

In 2019, about 7% of high school students reported misusing prescription opiates, with Black/African American and Latinx students reporting misuse more than White students, reversing a trend of White youth being more likely to report substance abuse compared to youth of color [159]. Youth with sexual contacts of the same sex were over twice as likely to misuse prescription opiates compared to those who reported sexual contacts of the same sex (20.3% vs. 8.3%). Given the percentage of YWH who identify as YMSM, specific screening for prescription opiate misuse is likely warranted. Multiple screening and assessment tools that combine tobacco, alcohol, and drug use are readily available (the National Institute for Drug Abuse has a repository of evidence-based tools), and generalists should choose and utilize at least one comprehensive tool no less than annually for young adults with HIV who have transitioned to adult care. Given the frequency of substance use in this population, greater than annual screening, with assessment and referral for medication-assisted treatment, when necessary, should be considered.

## Conclusion

Many youth and young adults are living with HIV, and life expectancy continues to approach that of persons without HIV. Youth and YAWH manage a lifelong chronic medical condition with many associated comorbidities. As such, they require clinicians skilled in chronic disease management and preventive health care in order to lead long, healthy lives. Skilled PCPs are essential in the care of all patients with chronic disease but perhaps more so in a population for which quality of life and survival are directly dependent on strict medication adherence. As more data on the natural history of adolescents and young adults with HIV become available, physicians will need to remain up to date on recommendations for disease screening, chronic disease management, and prevention of associated comorbidities for those living with HIV (Appendix). As these patients transition to adult services, special attention should be given to the challenges unique to young adults living with HIV, including HIV stigma and mental health concerns, secondary HIV prevention, sexual and reproductive health concerns, and comorbidities due to long-term immunodeficiency and medication adherence.

## Appendix

| Human immunodeficiency virus (HIV) condition fact sheet | |
|---|---|
| Definition | Human immunodeficiency virus (HIV) is a retrovirus that infects CD4+ lymphocytes resulting in immunodeficiency and chronic inflammation<br>Chronic immunodeficiency from HIV infection is manageable with lifelong antiretroviral therapy (ART) |
| Epidemiology | ART has resulted in extended life expectancy for youth and young adults with perinatal HIV infection<br>In the United States, approximately 1 in 5 new HIV infections annually are in persons aged 13–24 years, and sexual and ethnic minorities are significantly over-represented in this population<br>Youth and young adults with HIV are more likely than their adult peers to experience adverse social determinants of health such as homelessness and poverty |
| Special considerations | Adolescents and young adults with HIV face unique challenges |
| | HIV disease progression due to age-related disparities throughout the HIV care continuum (diagnosis, linkage, engagement and retention, and viral suppression)<br>Mental health and substance use disorders<br>Increased HIV stigma and fear of disclosure to peers/family<br>Comorbidities including HPV-related malignancies, cardiometabolic disease, and AIDS-defining malignancies<br>Sexual and reproductive health issues including increased prevalence of sexually transmitted infections and preconception counseling for young women with HIV and transgender sexual health |
| Recommended screening | Age-appropriate screening, including screening for intimate partner violence, housing instability, substance use disorder and mental health disorders, particularly in sexual and gender minorities<br>Additional recommend screening to include:<br>Increased frequency of STI screening and testing<br>Increased frequency of hepatitis C screening<br>Enhanced cervical cancer screening (and potentially anal cancer screening)<br>Age-appropriate vaccinations<br>Human papilloma virus (HPV), meningococcal, pneumococcal, and hepatitis A virus vaccination if not already completed<br>Potential boosters of childhood vaccinations depending on level of immunodeficiency |
| Prevention | Preexposure prophylaxis is approved for use in adolescents and young adults, and those at increased risk for HIV acquisition should be offered this as prevention |

## References


1. CDC. HIV Surveillance Report, 2019. In: Diagnoses of HIV Infection in the United States and Dependent Areas, 2019, vol. 32; 2021. https://www.cdc.gov/hiv/library/reports/hiv-surveillance.html.
2. Saberi P, Neilands TB, Lally MA, Hosek SG, Hightow-Weidman L. The association between use of online social networks to find sex partners and sexually transmitted infection diagnosis among Young men who have sex with men and transgender women living with HIV. J Int Assoc Provid AIDS Care. 2019;18:2325958219867324.
3. Mandsager P, Marier A, Cohen S, Fanning M, Hauck H, Cheever LW. Reducing HIV-related Health disparities in the Health Resources and Services Administration's Ryan white HIV/AIDS program. Am J Public Health. 2018;108:S246–50. https://pubmed.ncbi.nlm.nih.gov/30383416
4. CDC. Getting Tested|Testing|HIV Basics|HIV/AIDS|CDC. 2022. https://www.cdc.gov/hiv/basics/hiv-testing/getting-tested.html.
5. Panel on Antiretroviral Guidelines for Adults and Adolescents. Guidelines for the Use of Antiretroviral Agents in Adults and Adolescents Living with HIV. 2022. https://clinicalinfo.hiv.gov/en/guidelines/hiv-clinical-guidelines-adult-and-adolescent-arv/early-acute-and-recent-hiv-infection.
6. Group TA 12136 S, Danel C, Moh R, Gabillard D, Badje A, Le Carrou J, et al. A trial of early Antiretrovirals and isoniazid preventive therapy in Africa. N Engl J Med. 2015;373:808–22.
7. Group ISS, Lundgren JD, Babiker AG, Gordin F, Emery S, Grund B, et al. Initiation of Antiretroviral Therapy in Early Asymptomatic HIV Infection. N Engl J Med. 2015;373:795–807.
8. Martin TCS, Abrams M, Anderson C, Little SJ. Rapid antiretroviral therapy among individuals with acute and early HIV. Clin Infect Dis. 2021;73:130–3.
9. Cohen MS, Chen YQ, McCauley M, Gamble T, Hosseinipour MC, Kumarasamy N, et al. Antiretroviral therapy for the prevention of HIV-1transmission. N Engl J Med. 2016;375:830–9.
10. Panel on Opportunistic Infections in Adults and Adolescents with HIV. Guidelines for the Prevention and Treatment of Opportunistic Infections in Adults and Adolescents with HIV: Recommendations from the Centers for Disease Control and Prevention, the National Institutes of Health, and the HIV Medicine Association of the Infectious Diseases Society of America. 2022. https://clinicalinfo.hiv.gov/en/guidelines/adult-and-adolescent-opportunistic-infection/whats-new-guidelines.
11. Boulware DR, Meya DB, Muzoora C, Rolfes MA, Huppler Hullsiek K, Musubire A, et al. Timing of antiretroviral therapy after diagnosis of cryptococcal meningitis. N Engl J Med. 2014;370:2487–98.
12. Török ME, Yen NT, Chau TT, Mai NT, Phu NH, Mai PP, et al. Timing of initiation of antiretroviral therapy in human immunodeficiency virus (HIV)--associated tuberculous meningitis. Clin Infect Dis. 2011;52:1374–83.
13. CDC. Behavioral and clinical characteristics of persons with diagnosed HIV infection--medical monitoring project, United States, 2019 cycle. 2022. https://www.cdc.gov/hiv/library/reports/hiv-surveillance-special-reports/no-28/index.html.
14. Li Z, Purcell DW, Sansom SL, Hayes D, Hall HI. Vital signs: HIV transmission along the continuum of care — United States, 2016. MMWR. 2019;68:267–72.
15. Kapogiannis BG, Koenig LJ, Xu J, Mayer KH, Loeb J, Greenberg L, et al. The HIV continuum of care for adolescents and young adults attending 13 Urban US HIV care centers of the NICHD-ATN-CDC-HRSA SMILE Collaborative J Acquir Immune Defic Syndr 2020;84:92–100. https://www.ncbi.nlm.nih.gov/pmc/articles/PMC7147723/.
16. U.S. Health and Human Services America's HIV Epidemic Analysis Dashboard (AHEAD). 2019. https://ahead.hiv.gov/.
17. Bosh KA, Johnson AS, Hernandez AL, Prejean J, Taylor J, Wingard R, et al. Vital signs: deaths among persons with diagnosed HIV infection, United States, 2010-2018. MMWR. 2020;69:1717–24.
18. Philbin MM, Tanner AE, DuVal A, Ellen JM, Xu J, Kapogiannis B, et al. HIV testing, care referral, and linkage to care intervals affect time to engagement in Care for Newly Diagnosed HIV-infected adolescents in 15 adolescent medicine clinics in the United States. JAIDS. 2016;72:222–9.
19. Miller RL, Chiaramonte D, Strzyzykowski T, Sharma D, Anderson-Carpenter K, Fortenberry JD. Improving timely linkage to care among newly diagnosed HIV-infected youth: results of SMILE. J Urban Health. 2019;96:845–55.
20. Philbin MM, Tanner AE, DuVal A, Ellen JM, Xu J, Kapogiannis B, et al. Factors affecting linkage to care and engagement in care for newly diagnosed HIV-positive adolescents within fifteen adolescent medicine clinics in the United States. AIDS Behav. 2014;18:1501–10.
21. Philbin MM, Tanner AE, DuVal A, Ellen JM, Kapogiannis B, Fortenberry JD. Understanding care linkage and engagement across 15 adolescent clinics: provider perspectives and implications for newly HIV-infected youth. AIDS Educ Prev. 2017;29:93–104.
22. Badejo OA, Menson WNA, Sam-Agudu NA, Pharr J, Erekaha S, Bruno T, et al. Pediatric to adult healthcare transitioning for adolescents living with HIV in Nigeria: a national survey. PLoS One. 2018;13:e0198802.
23. Collins IJ, Foster C, Tostevin A, Tookey P, Riordan A, Dunn D, et al. Clinical status of adolescents with perinatal HIV at transfer to adult care in the UK/Ireland. Clin Infect Dis. 2017;64:1105–12. https://pubmed.ncbi.nlm.nih.gov/28329212

24. Foster C, Ayers S, Mcdonald S, Frize G, Chhabra S, Pasvol TJ, et al. Clinical outcomes post transition to adult services in young adults with perinatally acquired HIV infection: mortality, retention in care and viral suppression. AIDS. 2020;34:261–6.
25. Continisio GI, Lo Vecchio A, Basile FW, Russo C, Cotugno MR, Palmiero G, et al. The transition of care from pediatric to adult health-care services of vertically HIV-infected adolescents: a pilot study. Front Pediatr. 2020;8:322.
26. Zanoni BC, Archary M, Subramony T, Sibaya T, Psaros C, Haberer JE. 'It was not okay because you leave your friends behind': a prospective analysis of transition to adult care for adolescents living with perinatally-acquired HIV in South Africa. Vulnerable Child Youth Stud. 2021;16:206–20. https://doi.org/10.1080/17450128.2021.1876965.
27. Halyard AS, Doraivelu K, Camacho-González AF, Del Río C, Hussen SA. Examining healthcare transition experiences among youth living with HIV in Atlanta, Georgia, USA: A longitudinal qualitative study. J Int AIDS Soc. 2021;24:e25676.
28. Griffith D, Snyder J, Dell S, Nolan K, Keruly J, Agwu A. Impact of a youth-focused care model on retention and virologic suppression among young adults with HIV cared for in an adult HIV clinic. JAIDS. 2019;80:e41–7.
29. Griffith D, Jin L, Childs J, Posada R, Jao J, Agwu A. Outcomes of a comprehensive retention strategy for youth with HIV after transfer to adult Care in the United States. Pediatr Infect Dis. 2019;38:722–6.
30. Neilan AM, Lu F, Gebo KA, Diaz-Reyes R, Huang M, Parker RA, et al. Higher acuity resource utilization with older age and poorer HIV control in adolescents and Young adults in the HIV research network. JAIDS. 2020;83:424–33.
31. Ritchwood TD, Malo V, Jones C, Metzger IW, Atujuna M, Marcus R, et al. Healthcare retention and clinical outcomes among adolescents living with HIV after transition from pediatric to adult care: a systematic review. BMC Public Health. 2020;20:1195.
32. Davies MA, Tsondai P, Tiffin N, Eley B, Rabie H, Euvrard J, et al. Where do HIV-infected adolescents go after transfer?—tracking transition/transfer of HIV-infected adolescents using linkage of cohort data to a health information system platform. J Int AIDS Soc. 2017;20:21668.
33. Weijsenfeld AM, Smit C, Cohen S, Wit FWNM, Mutschelknauss M, van der Knaap LC, et al. Virological and social outcomes of HIV-infected adolescents and Young adults in The Netherlands before and after transition to adult care. Clin Infect Dis. 2016;63:1105–12.
34. Xia Q, Abraham B, Shah D, Ramaswamy C, Braunstein SL, Torian LV. Transition from paediatric to adult care among persons with perinatal HIV infection in new York City, 2006-2015. AIDS. 2018;32:1821–8.
35. Asad H, Collins IJ, Goodall RL, Crichton S, Hill T, Doerholt K, et al. Mortality and AIDS-defining events among young people following transition from paediatric to adult HIV care in the UK. HIV Med. 2021;22:631–40.
36. Fish R, Judd A, Jungmann E, O'Leary C, Foster C, (HYPNet) HYPN. Mortality in perinatally HIV-infected young people in England following transition to adult care: an HIV Young persons network (HYPNet) audit. HIV Med. 2014;15:239–44.
37. Tassiopoulos K, Huo Y, Patel K, Kacanek D, Allison S, Siminski S, et al. Healthcare transition outcomes among Young adults with perinatally acquired human immunodeficiency virus infection in the United States. Clin Infect Dis. 2020;71:133–41.
38. CDC. HIV in the United States by age-HIV in youth. 2022. https://www.cdc.gov/hiv/group/age/index.html.
39. Imahashi M, Fujimoto K, Kuhns LM, Amith M, Schneider JA. Network overlap and knowledge of a partner's HIV status among young men who have sex with men. AIDS Care. 2019;31:1533–9.
40. Tieu HV, Liu TY, Hussen S, Connor M, Wang L, Buchbinder S, et al. Sexual networks and HIV risk among Black men who have sex with men in 6 U.S. Cities. 2015;10:e0134085.
41. Hernández-Romieu AC, Sullivan PS, Rothenberg R, Grey J, Luisi N, Kelley CF, et al. Heterogeneity of HIV prevalence among the sexual networks of Black and white men who have sex with men in Atlanta: illuminating a mechanism for increased HIV risk for Young Black men who have sex with men. Sex Transm Dis. 2015;42:505–12.
42. Finneran C, Stephenson R. Intimate partner violence, minority stress, and sexual risk-taking among U.S. men who have sex with men. J Homosex. 2014;61:288–306.
43. Kubicek K, McNeeley M, Collins S. Young men who have sex with men's experiences with intimate partner violence. J Adolsec Res. 2016;31:143–75.
44. Stephenson R, Finneran C. Minority stress and intimate partner violence among gay and bisexual men in Atlanta. Am J Mens Health. 2017;11:952–61.
45. Stults CB, Javdani S, Greenbaum CA, Kapadia F, Halkitis PN. Intimate partner violence and substance use risk among young men who have sex with men: the P18 cohort study. Drug Alcohol Depend. 2015;154:54–62.
46. Freedner N, Freed LH, Yang YW, Austin SB. Dating violence among gay, lesbian, and bisexual adolescents: results from a community survey. J Adolsec Health. 2002;31:469–74.
47. Sullivan PS, Knox J, Jones J, Taussig J, Valentine Graves M, Millett G, et al. Understanding disparities in viral suppression among Black MSM living with HIV in Atlanta Georgia. J Int AIDS Soc. 2021;24:e25689.
48. Millett GA, Peterson JL, Flores SA, Hart TA, Jeffries WL, Wilson PA, et al. Comparisons of disparities and risks of HIV infection in black and other men

who have sex with men in Canada, UK, and USA: a meta-analysis. Lancet. 2012;380:341–8.
49. Dawit R, Trepka MJ, Duncan DT, Li T, Pires SF, Brock P, et al. Neighborhood factors associated with racial/ethnic disparities in achieving sustained HIV viral suppression among Miami-Dade County Ryan white program clients. AIDS Patient Care STDs. 2021;35:401–10.
50. Sheehan DM, Dawit R, Gbadamosi SO, Fennie KP, Li T, Gebrezgi M, et al. Sustained HIV viral suppression among men who have sex with men in the Miami-Dade County Ryan white program: the effect of demographic, psychosocial, provider and neighborhood factors. BMC Public Health. 2020;20:326–020–8442–1.
51. Xia Q, Robbins RS, Lazar R, Torian LV, Braunstein SL. Racial and socioeconomic disparities in viral suppression among persons living with HIV in new York City. Ann Epidemiol. 2017;27:335–41.
52. CDC. HIV transmission among black women--North Carolina, 2004. MMWR Morb Mortal Wkly Rep. 2005;54:89–94.
53. CDC. Estimated HIV incidence and prevalence in the United States, 2014–2018. HIV Surveillance Supplemental Report 2020. 2020; 25(1). http://www.cdc.gov/hiv/library/reports/hiv-surveillance.html.
54. CDC. Social determinants of health among adults with diagnosed HIV infection, 2018. HIV Surveillance Supplemental Report 2020. 2020; 25(3). http://www.cdc.gov/hiv/library/reports/hiv-surveillance.html.
55. CDC. Social determinants of health among adults with diagnosed HIV infection, 2019. HIV Surveillance Supplemental Report 2022; 2022. 27(2). http://www.cdc.gov/hiv/library/reports/hiv-surveillance.html.
56. Morton MH, Samuels GM, Dworsky A, Patel S. Missed opportunities: LGBTQ youth homelessness in America. Chapin Hall at the University of Chicago; 2018. p. 1–16. http://eric.ed.gov/ERICWebPortal/detail?accno=ED603005.
57. Harper GW, Jadwin-Cakmak L, Popoff E, Campbell BA, Granderson R, Wesp LM, et al. Transgender and other gender-diverse Youth's progression through the HIV continuum of care: socioecological system barriers. AIDS Patient Care STDs. 2019;33:32–43.
58. Klein PW, Psihopaidas D, Xavier J, Cohen SM. HIV-related outcome disparities between transgender women living with HIV and cisgender people living with HIV served by the Health Resources and Services Administration's Ryan white HIV/AIDS program: a retrospective study. PLoS Med. 2020;17:e1003125.
59. Thompson MA, Horberg MA, Agwu AL, Colasanti JA, Jain MK, Short WR, et al. Primary care guidance for persons with human immunodeficiency virus: 2020 update by the HIV medicine Association of the Infectious Diseases Society of America. Clin Infect Dis. 2021;73:e3572–605.
60. Barlow-Mosha L, Eckard AR, McComsey GA, Musoke PM. Metabolic complications and treatment of perinatally HIV-infected children and adolescents. J Int AIDS Soc. 2013;16:18600.
61. Lagathu C, Béréziat V, Gorwood J, Fellahi S, Bastard JP, Vigouroux C, et al. Metabolic complications affecting adipose tissue, lipid and glucose metabolism associated with HIV antiretroviral treatment. Expert Opin Drug Saf. 2019;18:829–40.
62. Venter WDF, Sokhela S, Simmons B, Moorhouse M, Fairlie L, Mashabane N, et al. Dolutegravir with emtricitabine and tenofovir alafenamide or tenofovir disoproxil fumarate versus efavirenz, emtricitabine, and tenofovir disoproxil fumarate for initial treatment of HIV-1 infection (ADVANCE): week 96 results from a randomised, phase 3, non-inferiority trial. Lancet HIV. 2020;7:e666–76.
63. Murthy VL, Abbasi SA, Siddique J, Colangelo LA, Reis J, Venkatesh BA, et al. Transitions in metabolic risk and long-term cardiovascular Health: coronary artery risk development in Young adults (CARDIA) study. J Am Heart Assoc. 2016;5:e003934. https://doi.org/10.1161/JAHA.116.003934.
64. Virani Salim S, Morris Pamela B, Anandita A, Ballantyne Christie M, Birtcher Kim K, Kris-Etherton Penny M, et al. 2021 ACC expert consensus decision pathway on the management of ASCVD risk reduction in patients with persistent hypertriglyceridemia: a report of the american college of cardiology solution set oversight committee. J Am Coll Cardiol. 2021;78:960–93.
65. Grundy SM, Stone NJ, Bailey AL, Beam C, Birtcher KK, Blumenthal RS, et al. 2018 AHA/ACC/AACVPR/AAPA/ABC/ACPM/ADA/AGS/APhA/ASPC/NLA/PCNA guideline on the Management of Blood Cholesterol: a report of the American College of Cardiology/American Heart Association task force on clinical practice guidelines. Circulation. 2019;139(25):e1082–143.
66. So-Armah K, Benjamin LA, Bloomfield GS, Feinstein MJ, Hsue P, Njuguna B, et al. HIV and cardiovascular disease. Lancet HIV. 2020;7:e279–93.
67. So-Armah K, Freiberg MS. HIV and cardiovascular disease: update on clinical events, special populations, and novel biomarkers. Curr HIV/AIDS Rep. 2018;15:233–44.
68. Alonso A, Barnes AE, Guest JL, Shah A, Shao IY, Marconi V. HIV infection and incidence of cardiovascular diseases: an analysis of a large healthcare database. J Am Heart Assoc. 2019;8:e012241.
69. Stone L, Looby SE, Zanni MV. Cardiovascular disease risk among women living with HIV in North America and Europe. Curr Opin HIV/AIDS. 2017;12:585–93.
70. Lloyd-Jones DM, Braun LT, Ndumele CE, Smith SC Jr, Sperling LS, Virani SS, et al. Use of risk assessment tools to guide decision-making in the primary prevention of atherosclerotic cardiovascular disease: a special report from the American Heart

Association and American College of Cardiology. JACC. 2019;73:3153–67.

71. Loria CM, Liu K, Lewis CE, Hulley SB, Sidney S, Schreiner PJ, et al. Early adult risk factor levels and subsequent coronary artery calcification: the CARDIA study. JACC. 2007;49:2013–20.
72. Triant VA, Brown TT, Lee H, Grinspoon SK. Fracture prevalence among human immunodeficiency virus (HIV)-infected versus non-HIV-infected patients in a large U.S. healthcare system. J Clin Endocrinol Metab. 2008;93:3499–504.
73. Glidden DV, Mulligan K, McMahan V, Anderson PL, Guanira J, Chariyalertsak S, et al. Brief report: recovery of bone mineral density after discontinuation of Tenofovir-based HIV pre-exposure prophylaxis. JAIDS. 2017;76:177–82.
74. Havens PL, Perumean-Chaney SE, Patki A, Cofield SS, Wilson CM, Liu N, et al. Changes in bone mass after discontinuation of Preexposure prophylaxis with Tenofovir Disoproxil fumarate/Emtricitabine in Young men who have sex with men: extension phase results of adolescent trials network protocols 110 and 113. Clin Infect Dis. 2020;70:687–91.
75. Mirembe BG, Kelly CW, Mgodi N, Greenspan S, Dai JY, Mayo A, et al. Bone mineral density changes among Young, healthy African women receiving Oral Tenofovir for HIV Preexposure prophylaxis. JAIDS. 2016;71:287–94.
76. Kwak MK, Lee EJ, Park JW, Park SY, Kim B, Kim TH, et al. CD4 T cell count is inversely associated with lumbar spine bone mass in HIV-infected men under the age of 50 years. Osteoporos Int. 2019;30:1501–10.
77. Kim-Chang J, Wilson L, Chan C, Fischer B, Venturi G, Goodenow MM, et al. Tenofovir has minimal effect on biomarkers of bone Health in youth with HIV receiving initial antiretroviral therapy. AIDS Res Hum Retrovir. 2019;35:746–54.
78. Yong MK, Elliott JH, Woolley IJ, Hoy JF. Low CD4 count is associated with an increased risk of fragility fracture in HIV-infected patients. JAIDS. 2011;57:205–10.
79. Grijsen ML, Vrouenraets SM, Steingrover R, Lips P, Reiss P, Wit FW, et al. High prevalence of reduced bone mineral density in primary HIV-1-infected men. AIDS. 2010;24:2233–8.
80. Starup-Linde J, Rosendahl SB, Storgaard M, Langdahl B. Management of Osteoporosis in patients living with HIV—A systematic review and meta-analysis. JAIDS. 2020;83:1–8.
81. Lifson AR, Lando HA. Smoking and HIV: prevalence, health risks, and cessation strategies. Curr HIV/AIDS Rep. 2012;9:223–30.
82. Mdodo R, Frazier EL, Dube SR, Mattson CL, Sutton MY, Brooks JT, et al. Cigarette smoking prevalence among adults with HIV compared with the general adult population in the United States: cross-sectional surveys. Ann Intern Med. 2015;162:335–44.
83. Johnston PI, Wright SW, Orr M, Pearce FA, Stevens JW, Hubbard RB, et al. Worldwide relative smoking prevalence among people living with and without HIV. AIDS. 2021;35:957–70.
84. Lam JO, Levine-Hall T, Hood N, Alexeeff SE, Horberg MA, Young-Wolff KC, et al. Smoking and cessation treatment among persons with and without Hiv in a U.S. integrated health system. Drug Alcohol Depend. 2020;213:108128.
85. Gamarel KE, Westfall AO, Lally MA, Hosek S, Wilson CM. Tobacco use and sustained viral suppression in youth living with HIV. AIDS Behav. 2018;22:2018.
86. Verboeket SO, Wit FW, Kirk GD, Drummond MB, van Steenwijk RP, van Zoest RA, et al. Reduced forced vital capacity among human immunodeficiency virus-infected middle-aged individuals. J Infect Dis. 2019;219:1274–84.
87. Singhvi D, Bon J, Morris A. Obstructive lung disease in HIV-phenotypes and pathogenesis. Curr HIV/AIDS Rep. 2019;16:359–69.
88. Ronit A, Benfield T, Mocroft A, Gerstoft J, Nordestgaard BG, Vestbo J, et al. Diagnostic performance of clinical characteristics to detect airflow limitation in people living with HIV and in uninfected controls. HIV Med. 2018;19:751–5.
89. Qin S, Vodovotz L, Zamora R, Fitzpatrick M, Kessinger C, Kingsley L, et al. Association between inflammatory pathways and phenotypes of pulmonary dysfunction using cluster analysis in persons living with HIV and HIV-uninfected individuals. JAIDS. 2020;83:189–96.
90. Horner M-J, Shiels MS, Pfeiffer RM, Engels EA. Deaths attributable to cancer in the US human immunodeficiency virus population during 2001–2015. Clin Infect Dis. 2020;72:e224–31.
91. Reid E, Suneja G, Ambinder RF, Ard K, Baiocchi R, Carchman E, et al. Cancer in people with HIV, version 1.2022, NCCN clinical practice guidelines in oncology. Pennsylvania, PA: NCCN; 2022. https://www.nccn.org/professionals/physician_gls/pdf/hiv.pdf.
92. Darwich L, Videla S, Cañadas MP, Piñol M, García-Cuyàs F, Vela S, et al. Distribution of human papillomavirus genotypes in anal cytological and histological specimens from HIV-infected men who have sex with men and men who have sex with women. Dis Colon Rectum. 2013;56:1043–52.
93. Palefsky JM, Lensing SY, Belzer M, Lee J, Gaur AH, Mayer K, et al. High prevalence of anal high-grade squamous intraepithelial lesions, and prevention through human papillomavirus vaccination, in Young men who have sex with men living with human immunodeficiency virus. Clin Infect Dis. 2021;73:1388–96.
94. Perkins RB, Guido RL, Saraiya M, Sawaya GF, Wentzensen N, Schiffman M, et al. Summary of current guidelines for cervical cancer screening and Management of Abnormal Test Results: 2016-2020. J Women's Health. 2021;30:5–13.
95. Perkins RB, Guido RS, Castle PE, Chelmow D, Einstein MH, Garcia F, et al. 2019 ASCCP risk-based

management consensus guidelines for abnormal cervical cancer screening tests and cancer precursors. J Lower Genit Tract Dis. 2020;24:102–31.
96. Fontham ETH, Wolf AMD, Church TR, Etzioni R, Flowers CR, Herzig A, et al. Cervical cancer screening for individuals at average risk: 2020 guideline update from the American Cancer Society. CA Cancer J Clin. 2020;70:321–46.
97. Rositch AF, Levinson K, Suneja G, Monterosso A, Schymura MJ, McNeel TS, et al. Epidemiology of cervical adenocarcinoma and squamous cell carcinoma among women living with HIV compared to the general population in the United States. Clin Infect Dis. 2021;74:814–20.
98. NIH. Guidelines for the Prevention and Treatment of Opportunistic Infections in HIV-Exposed and HIV-Infected Children. 2013. 2022. https://clinicalinfo.hiv.gov/en/guidelines/pediatric-opportunistic-infection/human-papillomavirus.
99. Stier EA, Engels E, Horner M-J, Robinson WT, Qiao B, Hayes J, et al. Cervical cancer incidence stratified by age in women with HIV compared with the general population in the United States, 2002-2016. AIDS. 2021;35:1851–6.
100. Colón-López V, Shiels MS, Machin M, Ortiz AP, Strickler H, Castle PE, et al. Anal cancer risk among people with HIV infection in the United States. J Clin Oncol. 2018;36:68–75.
101. Palefsky JM, Lee JY, Jay N, Goldstone SE, Darragh TM, Dunlevy HA, ANCHOR investigators group, et al. Treatment of anal high-grade squamous intraepithelial lesions to prevent anal cancer. N Engl J Med. 2022;386:2273–82.
102. Sun J, Althoff KN, Jing Y, Horberg MA, Buchacz K, Gill MJ, et al. Trends in hepatocellular carcinoma incidence and risk among persons with HIV in the US and Canada, 1996-2015. JAMA Netw Open. 2021;4:e2037512.
103. Silverberg MJ, Lau B, Achenbach CJ, Jing Y, Althoff KN, D'Souza G, et al. Cumulative incidence of cancer among persons with HIV in North America: a cohort study. Ann Intern Med. 2015;163:507–18.
104. Winstone TA, Man SFP, Hull M, Montaner JS, Sin DD. Epidemic of lung cancer in patients with HIV infection. Chest. 2013;143:305–14.
105. Haddad DN, Sandler KL, Henderson LM, Rivera MP, Aldrich MC. Disparities in lung cancer screening: a review. Ann Am Thorac Soc. 2020;17:399–405.
106. Tassiopoulos K, Moscicki AB, Mellins C, Kacanek D, Malee K, Allison S, et al. Sexual risk behavior among youth with perinatal HIV infection in the United States: predictors and implications for intervention development. Clin Infect Dis. 2013;56:283–90.
107. Brownstein PS, Gillespie SE, Leong T, Chahroudi A, Chakraborty R, Camacho-Gonzalez AF. The association of uncontrolled HIV infection and other sexually transmitted infections in metropolitan Atlanta youth. United States. Pediatr Infect Dis J. 2015;34:e119–24.
108. Hein K, Dell R, Futterman D, Rotheram-Borus MJ, Shaffer N. Comparison of HIV+ and HIV−adolescents: risk factors and psychosocial determinants. Pediatrics. 1995;95:96–104.
109. Szucs LE, Lowry R, Fasula AM, Pampati S, Copen CE, Hussaini KS, et al. Condom and contraceptive use among sexually active high school students—youth risk behavior survey, United States, 2019. MMWR. 2020;69:11–8.
110. CDC. Trends in the prevalence of sexual behaviors and HIV Testing National YRBS: 1991—2019. 2020. https://www.cdc.gov/healthyyouth/data/yrbs/factsheets/2019_sexual_trend_yrbs.htm.
111. CDC. School Health policies and practices study (SHPPS). CDC; 2016. https://www.cdc.gov/healthyyouth/data/shpps/pdf/shpps-results_2016.pdf.
112. Ghany MG, Morgan TR. Hepatitis C Guidance 2019 Update: American Association for the Study of Liver Diseases–Infectious Diseases Society of America Recommendations for Testing, Managing, and Treating Hepatitis C Virus Infection. Hepatology. 2020;71:686–721.
113. CDC. People coinfected with HIV and viral hepatitis. 2021. https://www.cdc.gov/hepatitis/populations/hiv.htm.
114. Schillie S, Wester C, Osborne M, Wesolowski L, Ryerson AB. CDC recommendations for hepatitis C screening among adults—United States, 2020. MMWR. 2020;69:1–17.
115. van den Berg JJ, Gamarel KE, Westfall AO, Fortenberry JD, Hosek SG, Wilson CM, et al. Transmission risk among youth living with HIV. J Adolsec Health. 2020;67:61–8.
116. Dunn Navarra AM, Whittemore R, Bakken S, Rosenberg MJ, Gormley M, Bethea J, et al. Adherence self-management and the influence of contextual factors among emerging adults with human immunodeficiency virus. Nurs Res. 2020;69:197–209.
117. Fields EL, Bogart LM, Thurston IB, Hu CH, Skeer MR, Safren SA, et al. Qualitative comparison of barriers to antiretroviral medication adherence among perinatally and behaviorally HIV-infected youth. Qual Health Res. 2017;27:1177–89.
118. Halperin J, Pathmanathan I, Richey LE. Disclosure of HIV status to social networks is strongly associated with increased retention among an urban cohort in New Orleans. AIDS Patient Care STDs. 2013;27:375–7.
119. WHO. HIV status disclosure to sexual partners: Rates, barriers and outcomes for women. 2004. https://apps.who.int/iris/handle/10665/42717.
120. Gabbidon K, Chenneville T, Peless T, Sheared-Evans S. Self-disclosure of HIV status among youth living with HIV: a global systematic review. AIDS Behav. 2020;24:114–41.
121. Elopre L, Hook EW, Westfall AO, Zinski A, Mugavero MJ, Turan J, et al. The role of early HIV

status disclosure in retention in HIV care. AIDS Patient Care STDs. 2015;29:646–50.

122. Modi RA, McGwin GL, Willig JH, Westfall AO, Griffin RL, Amico R, et al. Factors associated with HIV disclosure status among iENGAGE cohort of new to HIV care patients. AIDS Patient Care STDs. 2020;34:213–27.
123. CDC. HIV and STD Criminalization Laws. 2021. https://www.cdc.gov/hiv/policies/law/states/exposure.html.
124. Thompson KD, Meyers DJ, Lee Y, Cu-Uvin S, Wilson IB. HIV-positive and HIV-negative women with Medicaid have similar rates of stillbirth and preterm birth. Womens Health Rep. 2022;3:1–9.
125. Cohn ER, Korte JE, Lazenby GB. Absence of antenatal care and antiretroviral therapy associated with preterm delivery in women with HIV: an 11-year retrospective cohort in South Carolina. J Health Care Poor Underserved. 2021;32:1461–74.
126. Berhie S, Yee L, Jao J. The reproductive years of women with perinatally acquired HIV: from gynecologic care to obstetric outcomes. Infect Dis Clin N Am. 2019;33:817–33.
127. Venkatesh KK, Morrison L, Tuomala RE, Stek A, Read JS, Shapiro DE, et al. Profile of chronic comorbid conditions and obstetrical complications among pregnant women with human immunodeficiency virus and receiving antiretroviral therapy in the United States. Clin Infect Dis. 2021;73:969–78.
128. O'Brien BE, Williams PL, Huo Y, Kacanek D, Chadwick EG, Powis KM, et al. Repeat pregnancies among US women living with HIV in the SMARTT study: temporal changes in HIV disease status and predictors of preterm birth. JAIDS. 2020;85:346–54.
129. Venkatesh KK, Edmonds A, Westreich D, Dionne-Odom J, Weiss DJ, Sheth AN, et al. Associations between HIV, antiretroviral therapy and preterm birth in the US Women's interagency HIV study, 1995-2018: a prospective cohort. HIV Med. 2022;23:406–16.
130. Krishna GR, Haddad LB. Interactions between hormonal contraception and anti-retroviral therapy: an updated review. Curr Obstet Gynecol Rep. 2020;9:98–104.
131. Tepper NK, Curtis KM, Cox S, Whiteman MK, Update to U.S. Medical Eligibility Criteria for Contraceptive Use. Updated recommendations for the use of contraception among women at high risk for HIV infection. MMWR. 2016;2020(69):405–10.
132. US Department of Health and Human Services. Panel on Treatment of HIV During Pregnancy and Prevention of Perinatal Transmission Recommendations for the Use of Antiretroviral Drugs During Pregnancy and Interventions to Reduce Perinatal HIV Transmission in the United States. 2021. https://clinicalinfo.hiv.gov/en/guidelines/perinatal/whats-new-guidelines.
133. Baeten JM, Donnell D, Ndase P, Mugo NR, Campbell JD, Wangisi J, et al. Antiretroviral prophylaxis for HIV prevention in heterosexual men and women. New Engl J Med. 2012;367:399–410.
134. Rodger AJ, Cambiano V, Bruun T, Vernazza P, Collins S, Degen O, et al. Risk of HIV transmission through condomless sex in serodifferent gay couples with the HIV-positive PARTNER taking suppressive antiretroviral therapy (PARTNER): final results of a multicentre, prospective, observational study. Lancet. 2019;393:2428–38.
135. Mugwanya K, Baeten J, Celum C, Donnell D, Nickolas T, Mugo N, et al. Low risk of proximal tubular dysfunction associated with Emtricitabine-Tenofovir Disoproxil fumarate Preexposure prophylaxis in men and women. J Infect Dis. 2016;214:1050–7.
136. Mugwanya KK, Wyatt C, Celum C, Donnell D, Mugo NR, Tappero J, et al. Changes in glomerular kidney function among HIV-1-uninfected men and women receiving emtricitabine-tenofovir disoproxil fumarate preexposure prophylaxis: a randomized clinical trial. JAMA Intern Med. 2015;175:246–54.
137. CDC. Preexposure prophylaxis for the prevention of HIV infection in the United States---2021 Update: a clinical practice guideline. 2021. https://www.cdc.gov/hiv/pdf/risk/prep/cdc-hiv-prep-guidelines-2021.pdf.
138. U.S. Food and Drug Administration. FDA News Release: FDA approves first injectable treatment for HIV pre-exposure prevention. 2021. https://www.fda.gov/news-events/press-announcements/fda-approves-first-injectable-treatment-hiv-pre-exposure-prevention.
139. Hosek SG, Landovitz RJ, Kapogiannis B, Siberry GK, Rudy B, Rutledge B, et al. Safety and feasibility of antiretroviral Preexposure prophylaxis for adolescent men who have sex with men aged 15 to 17 years in the United States. JAMA Pediatr. 2017;171:1063–71.
140. Christopoulos KA, Neilands TB, Dilworth S, Lisha N, Sauceda J, Mugavero MJ, et al. Internalized HIV stigma predicts subsequent viremia in US HIV patients through depressive symptoms and ART adherence. AIDS. 2020;34:1665–71.
141. Earnshaw VA, Eaton LA, Collier ZK, Watson RJ, Maksut JL, Rucinski KB, et al. HIV stigma, depressive symptoms, and substance use. AIDS Patient Care STDs. 2020;34:275–80.
142. Rao D, Andrasik MP, Lipira L. HIV stigma among Black women in the United States: intersectionality, support, Resilience. Am J Public Health. 2018;108:446–8.
143. Greenwood GL, Wilson A, Bansal GP, Barnhart C, Barr E, Berzon R, et al. HIV-related stigma research as a priority at the National Institutes of Health. AIDS Behav. 2021;26:5–26.
144. Berger BE, Ferrans CE, Lashley FR. Measuring stigma in people with HIV: psychometric assessment of the HIV stigma scale. Res Nurs Health. 2001;24:518–29.

145. Data Resource Center for Child and Adolescent Health. Child and Adolescent Health Measurement Initiative. 2019–2020 National Survey of Children's Health (NSCH) data query. 2022. www.childhealthdata.org.
146. Bitsko RH, Claussen AH, Lichstein J, Black LI, Jones SE, Danielson ML, et al. Mental Health surveillance among children—United States, 2013-2019. MMWR. 2022;71:1–42.
147. Ivey-Stephenson AZ, Demissie Z, Crosby AE, Stone DM, Gaylor E, Wilkins N, et al. Suicidal ideation and behaviors among high school students—youth risk behavior survey, United States 2019. MMWR. 2020;69:47–55.
148. Johns MM, Lowry R, Andrzejewski J, Barrios LC, Demissie Z, McManus T, et al. Transgender identity and experiences of violence victimization, substance use, suicide risk, and sexual risk behaviors among high school students—19 states and large Urban School districts, 2017. MMWR. 2019;68:67–71.
149. Kann L, Olsen EO, McManus T, Kinchen S, Chyen D, Harris WA, et al. Sexual identity, sex of sexual contacts, and Health-risk behaviors among students in grades 9–12—youth risk behavior surveillance, selected sites, United States, 2001–2009. MMWR. 2011;60:1–133.
150. Pei J-H, Pei Y, Ma T, Du Y, Wang X-L, Zhong J, et al. Prevalence of suicidal ideation, suicide attempt, and suicide plan among HIV/AIDS: a systematic review and meta-analysis. J Affect Disord. 2021;292(295–304):1005085.
151. Ayano G, Demelash S, Abraha M, Tsegay L. The prevalence of depression among adolescent with HIV/AIDS: a systematic review and meta-analysis. AIDS Res Therapy. 2021;18:23–021–00351–1.
152. Benton TD, Kee Ng WY, Leung D, Canetti A, Karnik N. Depression among youth living with HIV/AIDS. Child Adolesc Psychiatr Clin N Am. 2019;28:447–59.
153. Bucek A, Leu C-S, Benson S, Warne P, Abrams EJ, Elkington KS, et al. Psychiatric disorders, antiretroviral medication adherence and viremia in a cohort of perinatally HIV-infected adolescents and Young adults. Pediatr Infect Dis J. 2018;37:673–7.
154. Tsegay L, Ayano G. The prevalence of suicidal ideation and attempt among Young people with HIV/AIDS: a systematic review and meta-analysis. Psychiatry Q. 2020;91:1291–304.
155. Kreniske P, Mellins CA, Dolezal C, Korich R, Leu CS, Wiznia A, et al. Sounding the alarm: perinatally HIV-infected youth more likely to attempt suicide than their uninfected cohort peers. J Adolsec Heath. 2019;65:702–5.
156. Kreniske P, Mellins CA, Dolezal C, Morrison C, Shea E, Fisher PW, et al. Predictors of attempted suicide among youth living with perinatal HIV infection and perinatal HIV-exposed uninfected counterparts. JAIDS. 2021;88:348–55.
157. Amico KR, Crawford J, Ubong I, Lindsey JC, Gaur AH, Horvath K, et al. Correlates of high HIV viral load and antiretroviral therapy adherence among Viremic youth in the United States enrolled in an adherence improvement intervention. AIDS Patient Care STDs. 2021;35:145–57.
158. Gamarel KE, Brown LA, Kahler CW, Fernandez MI, Bruce D, Nichols S. Prevalence and correlates of substance use among youth living with HIV in clinical settings. Drug Alcohol Depend. 2016;169:11–8.
159. Jones CM, Clayton HB, Deputy NP, Roehler DR, Ko JY, Esser MB, et al. Prescription opioid misuse and use of alcohol and other substances among high school students—youth risk behavior survey, United States, 2019. MMWR. 2020;69:38–46.
160. Gamarel KE, Nichols S, Kahler CW, Westfall AO, Lally MA, Wilson CM. A cross-sectional study examining associations between substance use frequency, problematic use, and sexually transmitted infections among youth living with HIV. Sex Transm Infect. 2018;94:304–8.
161. Lancaster KE, Cooper HLF, Browning CR, Malvestutto CD, Bridges JFP, Young AM. Syringe service program utilization, barriers, and preferences for Design in Rural Appalachia: differences between men and women who inject drugs. Subst Use Misuse. 2020;55:2268–77.

# 32 Inflammatory Bowel Disease

Christina Awad, Elana Maser, and Anish Patel

## Case Presentation

Michelle is an 18-year-old woman with Crohn's disease who presents for an initial evaluation at an adult internal medicine office accompanied by her parents. She was diagnosed at the age of 12 years. She had severe disease, requiring two small bowel resections by ages 14 and 15 due to recurrent Crohn's strictures. Since her last surgery, she has been on biological therapy and is planning to leave college out of state in 6 months. Her parents wanted to establish care before her departure, as was recommended by their pediatrician.

Michelle is a well-groomed, well-mannered patient. She is slightly timid and quiet. Her parents speak most of the time. She only speaks when spoken to directly, with frequent interjections by her parents. She reports good compliance with her medication, but her mother notes the "missed timing" of doses on regular occasions. She appears healthy, is an appropriate weight, and has almost reached the height of her parents. There are no abnormalities other than well-healed abdominal surgical scars on the physical exam.

Michelle's parents have voiced three concerns. They are uneasy about leaving their lifelong and beloved pediatrician. They have concerns about their daughter's compliance with medications, and they are worried about their daughter having reduced access to the appropriate care while in college.

## Case Discussion

Transition is a complicated and often fearful time for families, especially for patients with severe Crohn's disease [1]. Pediatric gastroenterologists often develop strong bonds with their patients and families. However, limited time is spent preparing for the transition to adult providers [2, 3]. Difficulties arise in the transition to adult care as adult providers are faced with patients who have limited knowledge of their complicated medical, surgical, and drug history.

This case is a common scenario in the adult medicine realm. Michelle has severe Crohn's disease requiring multiple surgeries at an early age and requires biologic drugs to maintain remission. Her parents are apprehensive about letting her go alone to an out-of-state college where access to specialists or generalists who understand Crohn's disease may be scarce and access to biological drugs may be difficult.

C. Awad (✉) · A. Patel
Department of Gastroenterology, Brooke Army Medical Center, San Antonio, TX, USA
e-mail: anish.a.patel.mil@health.mil

E. Maser
Division of Gastroenterology, Icahn School of Medicine at Mount Sinai, New York, NY, USA
e-mail: elana.maser@mountsinai.org


A. A. Kuo et al. (eds.), *Care of Adults with Chronic Childhood Conditions*,
https://doi.org/10.1007/978-3-031-54281-7_32

For Michelle, developing a good rapport with and trust in her adult gastroenterologist is critical to a successful transition and ongoing care. Discussions need to focus on adherence to medication and risks to her health and quality of life if regimens are not maintained. As new generations of adolescents are more involved with technology, discussions about maintaining communication, whether via email or patient portals, could help alleviate tension among the parents and patients. To alleviate fears about Michelle's relocation out of state, identifying a local physician for emergency purposes would be helpful. She should contact her insurance provider to find a local infusion center that can administer biologics unless she could make arrangements to return for infusions. Switching biologics (often from infusion to self-injection) should be avoided if Michelle is in remission. Switching biologics puts patients at risk of a flare, which would be undesirable during this stressful period [4].

## Overview

### Epidemiology

Crohn's disease (CD) and ulcerative colitis (UC) affect over five million people worldwide, with over 1.7 million in the United States and about three million in Europe [5]. Higher rates occur in industrialized countries [6, 7]. The lifetime risk of developing inflammatory bowel disease (IBD), including CD and UC, is approximately 1%.

Over one-quarter of all patients will first be diagnosed in childhood or adolescence. While the incidence in adults seems to be stabilizing, the incidence rates in pediatrics are currently rising [8]. The annual incidence has doubled over 11 years from 1.1/100,000 to 2.4/100,000 in the pediatric population [9]. Following childhood, the diagnosis of IBD can occur at any age, but there are two peaks of higher incidence around age 20 and 50 years [7, 10].

There are no significant gender differences found in the prevalence of UC, but there is a slightly higher incidence of CD among women than men [11, 12].

IBD is thought to be a disease that primarily affects Ashkenazi Jews. However, Sephardic Jews are also involved, albeit with a lower incidence [13]. IBD is not a disease reserved only for those of Jewish descent. While these populations have the highest incidence, IBD can occur in any race [13].

### Pathophysiology

IBD includes Crohn's disease (CD) and ulcerative colitis (UC). IBD is characterized by chronic, relapsing inflammation within the gastrointestinal tract. To develop the disease, one must have a genetic predisposition and be exposed to an environmental trigger. There have been over 100 genes identified in the pathogenesis of IBD, and numerous environmental factors, including smoking, the use of oral contraceptives, and exposure to antibiotics, have been suggested, though none have been implicated [14, 15].

Current literature suggests that the inflammation results from inappropriate and ongoing activation of the innate immune system of the gut mucosa, driven by the commensal luminal flora in a genetically susceptible host [16, 17]. Once the inflammation has been initiated, it has difficulty resolving without the help of medication. It is unclear which commensal flora is responsible; however, a more limited variation in gut bacteria is typically seen in an IBD host [18]. Current understanding is that both CD and UC have a similar pathogenesis, but clinically, they have varying characteristics. The characteristic features are summarized in Table 32.1.

**Table 32.1** Comparison of Crohn's disease and ulcerative colitis

| Feature | Crohn's disease | Ulcerative colitis |
|---|---|---|
| Site of origin | Terminal ileum (can occur anywhere in gastrointestinal tract) | Colon |
| Pattern of progression | "Skip" lesions/irregular | Contiguous |
| Histopathology | Transmural disease<br>Deep ulcers, granulomas, "cobblestoning" | Submucosa/mucosa |
| Complications | Fistulas, abscesses, obstruction | Bleeding, toxic megacolon |
| Radiographic findings | String sign | Lead pipe colon |
| Clinical features | Crampy abdominal pain | Bloody diarrhea |

## Clinical Definition, Presentation, and Natural History of IBD

### Ulcerative Colitis

UC is a chronic inflammatory disease affecting the mucosal layer of the colon and rectum. The condition is relapsing and remitting. When the condition is active, also called "flaring," patients typically suffer from acute and frequent bouts of bloody diarrhea. Flares are intermittent, unpredictable, and vary in severity. Most commonly, UC is painless unless the disease is severe. Endoscopically, inflammation is continuous from the anal verge extending proximally. One-third of patients have mild disease requiring minimal medication, one-third of patients require chronic maintenance medication, and 20–30% will need colectomy [19]. Patients with UC develop colorectal cancer at twice the population risk. Therefore, guidelines suggest screening patients with annual colonoscopies, as is further discussed later in this chapter [20]. Patients with proctitis do not have an increased risk of colon cancer and should not be screened more frequently than the general population. This disease can affect the quality of life but not the duration of life. An average life span should be expected [5].

### Crohn's Disease

CD is also a chronic inflammatory condition with periods of wellness interspersed with flares. In contrast to UC, CD affects all layers of the bowel and can occur in any part of the gastrointestinal tract from mouth to anus. The most common presentation is terminal ileitis. A child may present with weight loss or poor growth and have no other symptoms. Pain is more commonly seen in patients with CD than in those with UC. Symptoms can range from mild abdominal cramping to severe diarrhea or symptoms of intestinal obstruction. Perianal disease is common and can manifest as abnormal anal skin tags, deep anal fissures, and fistulae. Endoscopically, inflammation can occur in patches with normal mucosa interspersed with inflamed mucosa. There is no single test to diagnose Crohn's disease; however, rarely are granulomas seen on histopathology. When these are seen, Crohn's can be differentiated from ulcerative colitis.

Disease course can range from mild, intermittent flares to more severe cases that are difficult to control. Up to 70% of patients with CD will require at least one surgery [21]. Risk of colon cancer is also increased in patients with CD, and like patients with UC, patients with colonic Crohn's should have annual colonoscopies, again as will be further discussed later in this chapter [22]. Patients with CD are also at higher risk for nutritional deficiencies. They should be monitored for deficiencies in folate, zinc, and vitamins B12 and D. In severe cases, total parenteral nutrition (TPN) may be required. Like UC, quality of life may be affected; however, most patients with Crohn's disease have an average life span.

## Risk Factors

The etiology of the development of mucosal inflammation is multifactorial. Current theories focus on genetic factors, immunoregulatory defects, microbial exposure, and environmental triggers [23].

## Microbial Exposure

The epithelial layer of intestinal mucosa plays an essential role in maintaining functional equilibrium within the lumen from the spectrum of microbial species and their byproducts. Barrier defects within the mucosa increase microbial and antigen presentation, leading to perturbations in the immune response, contributing to the development of IBD. Growing evidence suggests a significant dysbiosis or imbalance among protective and harmful microbiota species within the intestinal lumen [24]. IBD patients have demonstrated a lack of diversity among species, but no specific species have been implicated as a causative agent in IBD [25]. Identifying the key factors and species that shape microbiota–host interactions in the structure and function of the immune response will be essential to further understanding the pathogenesis of IBD.

## Immunoregulatory Defects

The loss of barrier function can lead to microbial and antigen penetration into the intestinal mucosa, causing immune activation. The innate and acquired immune systems are activated with antigen presentation, but differences have been demonstrated within the IBD sub-types. Crohn's disease results in T-helper-1 (Th1) and T-helper-17 (Th17) immune responses with subsequent production of proinflammatory cytokines (i.e., interleukin [IL]-12, IL-18, interferon [IFN]-γ) [26]. The cascade of proinflammatory mediators with CD leads to the activation of proteases and metalloproteinases, causing tissue destruction and sustained chronic inflammation. The mediator response with UC was previously theorized as a T-helper-2 (Th2) response but is still under investigation [26].

## Genetics

Epidemiological and clinical data from Europe and North America have provided strong evidence that CD and UC are related to polygenic disorders, and genetic factors play a role in susceptibility to IBD [27, 28]. Up to 14% of patients with IBD will report a family history of either CD or UC [29]. The relative risk of developing IBD for a first-degree relative is up to 8% for CD and 5% for UC, but the risk is increased to 30% for offspring of parents affected with IBD [30, 31]. Familial studies have demonstrated a significant genetic link with IBD; however, it appears that IBD is not inherited in a simple Mendelian fashion. Instead, it has a complex genetic basis with multiple contributing genes [32].

Genetic linkage studies have demonstrated numerous IBD loci overlapping between UC and CD, with one of the earliest and clearest linkages on chromosome 16 for the nucleotide-binding oligomerization domain 2 (NOD2), also known as caspase activation and recruitment domain 15 (CARD15) [33, 34]. NOD2/CARD15 defects have been associated with up to 25% of CD cases [35]. Homozygosity is associated with a > 20-fold increased risk of developing CD, with heterozygosity conferring a < fourfold disease risk [35, 36]. Despite having significant advances in identifying genetic risk factors, genetics may account for <25% of the pathogenesis of IBD, further suggesting the vital role played by environmental factors [29].

## Environmental

### Hygiene

Like other autoimmune diseases such as rheumatoid arthritis, IBD confers an inverse relationship with sanitation. In other words, poor sanitation appears to protect against IBD [23]. The "hygiene hypothesis" was first proposed by authors in a 1989 study citing the rising incidence of autoimmune diseases, such as IBD, in developing countries [37]. Factors including the number of siblings, larger family size, living on a farm, and pet exposures in childhood have been implicated with a reported decreased risk of developing IBD. Still, such studies were limited in size and subject to significant bias [38, 39]. Less robust associations have been made between the mode of childbirth (potential increased risk with Caesarean delivery) and the role of breastfeeding (decreased risk) in the development of IBD [40, 41].

## Smoking

One of the most substantial environmental risk factors is smoking tobacco. Patients with CD who smoke have a more aggressive disease course. They typically require more immunosuppression and earlier surgery and have a higher risk of recurrence of disease after ileocecal resection [42]. A 2006 meta-analysis demonstrated an almost two-fold risk of developing Crohn's disease associated with smoking; conversely, a strong inverse association between active smoking and UC was seen [43]. Current smoking appears to reduce the risk of developing UC. In a cohort of female nurses, there was an increased risk of developing UC within 5 years of smoking cessation. This risk remained elevated for up to 20 years [44]. Passive smoking had similar effects [45]. While it appears that smoking can reduce inflammation in patients with UC, it is not a recommended habit due to the other well-described health concerns.

## Medications

Antibiotics have been implicated as a potential risk factor for IBD due to the alteration of the gut flora. A 2014 study reported an almost two-fold risk for developing CD from prior antibiotic exposure, though the same risk did not apply to UC [46]. The association of IBD with antibiotics has also shown to be stronger with exposure in the first year of life compared with later use [47]. However, conflicting evidence from Asia has demonstrated a protective association of antibiotic exposure with IBD development [48].

Nonsteroidal anti-inflammatory drugs (NSAIDs) can potentially increase IBD risk, but the absolute risk is negligible [49, 50]. The association was strongest with higher doses and a longer duration of therapy. The conferred risk was similar for both CD and UC [51, 52]. Concerning exacerbations, there is no consistent association between acetaminophen, nonsteroidal anti-inflammatory drug (NSAID), or cyclooxygenase-2 (COX-2) inhibitor use and the risk of CD and UC exacerbations [53]. Avoidance of NSAIDs is recommended; however, occasional use likely presents an acceptable risk.

Prior case reports have suggested an association between IBD and isotretinoin, used to treat acne vulgaris [54, 55]. However, in a recent meta-analysis, pooled results from the United States claims database found no increased risk of developing IBD in patients exposed to isotretinoin compared to patients unexposed [56]. Therefore, clinicians should not necessarily avoid prescribing retinoic acid when other drugs fail.

Current oral contraceptive use poses a minor increased risk of developing Crohn's disease, which is even lower for past users [57, 58]. The same risk was not seen with UC. Lower-estrogen formulations of contraception may be safer. Because the overall risk is so low, avoidance of oral contraceptive use cannot be recommended.

## Stress

Most patients note that their disease often flares during stressful events. Large observational studies support an association between significant life stressors, anxiety, depression, and IBD development risk [59–62]. Psychological distress/factors can be implicated in the nonadherence to medications in patients with IBD [63]. The reduction of stress may lead to better symptom control and improved quality of life. Due to the unpredictable nature of the disease, anxiety is a significant concern, especially for adolescents; working with a psychologist is often helpful. Newer cognitive-behavioral techniques and mindfulness training are currently being investigated in patients with IBD [64].

## Obesity

The association between IBD and obesity remains unclear [65, 66]. Obesity is a proinflammatory state; thus, if patients work on losing weight, then there will be an assumed reduction in proinflammatory cytokines. It has been reported that obese patients have a more rapid clearance of biological agents and a suboptimal response to medical therapy [67]. IBD patients who achieve a healthy body weight through exercise and physical activity can improve their response to biological treatment and attenuation of inflammation through the anti-inflammatory state of exercise.

In CD patients, the accumulation of intra-abdominal fat may play a role in mucosal inflammation and disease progression [68]. Obese patients have been shown to have higher rates of hospitalizations and are more likely to require IBD-related surgery [69, 70]. A 2013 prospective study demonstrated that intense physical activity had a > 40% risk reduction in the development of CD, but there was no significant association with UC [71].

## Sleep

Sleep quality and duration can have an impact on IBD. Sleep deprivation has been associated with an increased risk of UC while poor sleep quality has been associated with a higher risk of relapse [72, 73].

# Clinical Considerations in Individuals with IBD

The role of the PCP in the co-management of IBD with the subspecialist is essential in optimizing the clinical care of the IBD patient.

## Sexual and Reproductive Health

Ideally, discussions about the impact IBD might have on intimacy, reproduction, and pregnancy would have already been initiated by the patient's pediatric or adolescent provider. However, this is not always the case. Conversations with an adult provider about intimacy and sexuality may be welcome [74]. In fact, this may be a helpful way for the young adult to separate from their parents and develop an independent relationship with the adult provider.

One-third of CD patients say IBD has a significant impact on their sexual life. Impaired body image has been reported in 35% of women and 13% of men [75]. There may be disfiguration of the recto-vaginal area, abdominal scars, or the presence of an ostomy. About 58% of patients report decreased libido caused by diarrhea, fever, or abdominal pain [76]. Patients need a safe place to discuss these issues. They want to know how and when to disclose their chronic condition to their partners. Unfortunately, one study reported that 40% of IBD patients feel the disease prevents an intimate relationship altogether [77]. While it may not be practical for the adult physician to provide extensive counseling, acknowledging that these are essential quality-of-life issues which can help patients feel comfortable with their new adult doctor.

Fecundity, the probability of becoming pregnant per month by unprotected intercourse, is average in female IBD patients. The exceptions are female patients who have active disease or who have undergone pelvic surgery, most commonly the creation of an ileal pouch after total colectomy [78]. There is a decrease in fertility by as much as 14–36% due to voluntary childlessness among both male and female patients with IBD. They may be afraid of passing on the disease to their offspring, be concerned about medication teratogenicity, or be worried about the difficulty of raising a child when they have active and unpredictable disease [79, 80]. By establishing a positive relationship with young adult patients, adult physicians can educate patients and help them overcome these barriers.

Pregnancy outcomes have been well studied in IBD patients. A majority of the literature demonstrates a slightly higher risk of IBD-related pregnancy complications that include preterm birth and low birth weight. Still, there is not a significantly increased risk of congenital abnormalities [81–83]. Patients should understand that these risks are caused by active inflammation, not their medications. Most drugs, including thiopurines and biologics, are safe for use during pregnancy, with one exception being methotrexate. Patients should be encouraged to continue to take their medications throughout their pregnancy to allow for the best outcome. Pregnancy has not shown a higher likelihood to induce flares, but active disease at conception has been associated with higher rates of illness worsening throughout pregnancy [84, 85].

In patients taking newer molecular therapies such as tofacitinib, smaller studies have shown pregnancy outcomes similar to those observed in the general population; however, pregnancy should be avoided until more definitive data become available [86]. Similarly, pregnancy should be avoided in patients with ozanimod, given the limited clinical experience [87].

The role of the PCP is to acknowledge the need to discuss the impact of IBD on intimacy, sexuality, and fertility with both male and female patients. It is essential to maintain good communication with the patient's gastroenterologist to convey and reinforce consistent messaging. Conflicting messages can be harmful to patients and may cause unnecessary anxiety. The strong bond between the PCP and patient allows for open discussion of these delicate yet essential topics.

## Preventive Care

Preventive care has traditionally been in the domain of the PCP. With the increased use of immunomodulators, biologics, and oral molecular therapies, providing proper preventative measures can be daunting. Important preventive health considerations for individuals with IBD include cancer screening and prevention, osteoporosis screening and prevention, and immunizations.

## Cancer Screening and Prevention

In patients with IBD, the risk of colon cancer is much higher than in the general population. It is well described that dysplasia and adenocarcinoma of the colon and rectum (CRC) are associated with longstanding colitis, a feared complication of the disease. Colorectal cancer is observed in 5.5–13.5% of all patients with ulcerative colitis and 0.4–0.8% of patients with Crohn's disease [88].

General population screening without risk factors is recommended to begin at the age of 45 years. For patients with IBD, it is recommended that patients with >8 years of extensive colitis (> 1/3 of the colon) have a surveillance colonoscopy every 1–3 years [89]. For patients with concomitant primary sclerosing cholangitis, surveillance colonoscopy should begin immediately and yearly after that. Patients with isolated ulcerative proctitis (colitis involving the rectum only) do not have an increased risk of colon cancer beyond the general population. Therefore, increased screening is not required.

Women with IBD, especially those requiring immunomodulators and biologics, have a higher prevalence of abnormal Pap smears [90, 91]. The American College of Obstetrics and Gynecology (ACOG) recommends screening women starting at 21 years of age with Pap smears and then every 3 years [92]. However, due to the increased risk in women on immunosuppressive therapy, expert recommendations are for yearly screening by cytology (if cytology alone) or every 3 years (if HPV negative) [89].

IBD patients, especially those on immunomodulators, biologics, or oral molecular therapies, have an increased risk of skin cancers compared to the general population. Thiopurine use is associated with an increased risk of non-melanoma skin cancers, particularly basal cell carcinoma and squamous cell carcinoma, with an incidence rate of 1.1 cases per 1000 person-years [93]. Concerning melanoma, patients exposed to tumor necrosis factor-alpha (TNF-α) antagonists had a twofold higher risk than unexposed patients, with an incidence rate of about 0.5 cases per 1000 person-years [94]. Experts recommend yearly visual skin exams by a dermatologist in combination with appropriate sun exposure precautions for patients on systemic immunosuppression [89].

## Osteoporosis Screening and Prevention

IBD, along with increased use of corticosteroids, puts this population at risk for osteoporosis. Nutritional assessments, such as vitamin D testing, are recommended to be performed at least annually, with appropriate repletion for those with a deficiency. Bone density assessment is in line with the U.S. Preventative Services Task Force recommendations, but with additional considerations: 1. Steroid use >3 months; 2. Inactive disease but past chronic steroid use of at least 1 year within the past 2 years; 3. Inactive disease but a maternal history of osteoporosis; 4. Inactive disease but malnourished or very thin; 5. Inactive disease but amenorrheic [95, 96]. Consideration should be made to screen patients earlier than normal if such risk factors exist.

## Immunizations

As the use rates for immunosuppressive drugs in IBD increase, optimal preventable measures such as vaccinations can help limit the risk of infectious complications. Patients often turn to their PCP, who has been responsible for administering vaccines throughout their lives. Therefore, the role of the PCP in managing vaccine administration is pivotal.

Adult patients are often unaware of the recommended adult immunization schedule, and this may be especially concerning for those who are immunosuppressed and may require additional vaccinations. Patients with inflammatory bowel disease have a higher risk of pneumonia [97]. Therefore, if the pneumococcal 13-valent (PCV13) and 23-valent vaccines (PPSV23) were not administered during childhood, adults should be provided pneumococcal 15-valent (PCV15) followed by a dose of PPSV23 ≥ 1 year later OR pneumococcal 20-valent (PCV 20). Unfortunately, current vaccination rates in IBD populations are sub-optimal, with <90% of patients receiving yearly influenza vaccinations and < 50% receiving pneumococcal vaccinations [98, 99]. To help improve these rates, patients should be advised to bring updated vaccination records to their adult providers.

There are special considerations for vaccinating patients who are on immunosuppressive therapy. Administering a live vaccine to an immunosuppressed patient can be life-threatening [100]. All live vaccines available in the United States are listed in Table 32.2. Ideally, live vaccines should be administered more than 4 weeks before initiating immunosuppression. However, there are some exceptions. For IBD patients on low levels of immunosuppression, defined as methotrexate <0.4 mg/kg per week, azathioprine <3 mg/kg per day, and 6-mercaptopurine <1.5 mg/kg per day, live vaccines such as the varicella vaccination can be considered. For highly immunosuppressed patients, defined as

**Table 32.2** Live and inactivated adult vaccines in the United States

| Live | Inactivated |
|---|---|
| Live attenuated influenza vaccine (LAIV) | Inactivated influenza vaccine (IIV4) |
| Varicella (chicken pox) | Tetanus/diphtheria/ pertussis (Tdap) |
| Zoster (shingles) | Pneumococcal (PCV15, PCV20, PPSV23) |
| Measles, mumps, and rubella (MMR) | Meningococcal (MenACWY, MenB) |
| Yellow fever | Hepatitis A and B |
| | Human papilloma virus |
| | Zoster vaccine, recombinant |

individuals with a primary immunodeficiency disorder, cancer chemotherapy, within 2 months of solid organ transplant, human immunodeficiency virus (HIV) infection with a CD4 T-cell count <200/mm$^3$, systemic corticosteroid >20 mg/d use for more than 14 days, anti-TNF agent use or rituximab use, and live vaccines should be avoided altogether [101]. Unlike live vaccines, inactivated vaccines can be administered at any point while on immunosuppression. To allow adequate time for developing protective antibodies, inactivated vaccines should be administered at least 2 weeks before initiation of immunosuppression. Therefore, it is good practice to vaccinate patients with IBD when they are well, even if they are not taking immunosuppressive regimens. This will allow for the immediate initiation of treatment should a flare occur. A complete and up-to-date vaccine dosing schedule can be found through the Centers for Disease Control and Prevention [102].

Because vaccine administration recommendations for immunosuppressed patients are rapidly evolving, including those for SARS-CoV-2, having both the PCP and the gastroenterologist participate in the co-management of patients in this area of care might significantly improve vaccination rates.

## Diet

It would be beneficial if following a specific diet could cure or improve symptoms in patients with IBD. However, because strictly controlling diet is complicated, prospective studies are limited. It is known, though, that food plays an important role. Strict enteral nutrition has shown benefits in the induction and maintenance of remission in IBD, particularly in children [103].

Patients frequently scour the internet for special diets, hoping to manage their disease without medication. Popular diets include the specific carbohydrate diet (SCD), the low-fermentable oligosaccharides, disaccharides, and monosaccharides (FODMAP) diet, the gluten-free diet, and the Mediterranean diet [104]. The DINE-CD study demonstrated improvement in symptoms in both the Mediterranean and SCD diets; however, there was a lack of superiority of the SCD relative to the MD to achieve remission at 12 weeks [105]. For some, these diets work tremendously well. For the majority, they do not. Currently, no diet can be prescribed for everyone. The most crucial point to emphasize is following a balanced healthy diet.

Avoiding dairy is also a popular fad diet, but this puts patients at an even higher risk for osteoporosis, and there is no current evidence to support this practice. A vegan diet increases the risk of vitamin D and vitamin B12 deficiencies.

There is scientific evidence that particular dietary factors may influence the risk of developing IBD. Dietary fiber intake has been associated with a lower risk of developing CD, but not UC [106]. The consumption of more significant amounts of red meat and fats, particularly polyunsaturated fatty acids (PUFAs) and omega-6 (n-6) fatty acids, increases the risk of developing IBD as opposed to a diet high in fiber, fruits, and vegetables [107]. Ingested iron, particularly iron sulfate, has been directly linked with intestinal inflammation; however, the effects of iron from red meat are unknown [108]. Dietary calcium and vitamin D are essential for IBD patients, not only for bone health but also because vitamin D is involved in anti-inflammatory pathways [109].

Specific dietary recommendations include reducing red meat and saturated fats and increasing dietary fiber, such as oatmeal. For patients with known stenosis or those in the first 6 weeks after a partial bowel resection, a low-residue diet is recommended to avoid the risk of possible obstruction. Following a low-residue diet means avoiding peanuts, popcorn, raw vegetables, skins of vegetables, and high-fiber foods.

At this time, no diet can cure or reduce the existing inflammation. The role of the PCP is to recommend eating a healthy balanced diet, replenish possible nutrient deficiencies, and encourage avoidance of extreme, possibly stressful diets. If the patient is at risk of poor nutrient intake, then a multivitamin can be supplemented.

## Drug Monitoring/Side Effect Management

Over the last decade, many therapeutic options have become available for the treatment of IBD. These drugs include mesalamine, immunomodulators, biological agents, and oral molecular agents, with multiple different mechanisms of action. Many of the medications will be under the management of a gastroenterologist, but the PCP can still play a key role when drug side effects arise or in routine lab monitoring.

One of the first-line class choices for IBD treatment is the mesalamine-based (5-ASA) drugs. Mesalamine has an advantage in UC, but there is limited data to support its use in CD [110, 111]. There are minimal side effects associated with the newer generation 5-ASA drugs. However, headaches, hair loss, and rarely pancreatitis have been reported. Because there is a small but real risk of developing interstitial nephritis, the routine assessment of renal function every 6–12 months and a yearly urinalysis are recommended [112].

Corticosteroids are often needed to provide immediate relief for patients with ulcerative colitis. They are used in UC when mesalamine does not control the inflammation and in CD when the symptoms are severe or a biologic is not readily available. Steroid use is typically recommended for shorter durations due to the significant side effect profile. Along with the known side effects of corticosteroids, patients with CD can develop fistulae or opportunistic infections. Management of side effects requires the use of steroid-sparing drugs.

Immunomodulators are steroid-sparing drugs that work by inhibiting the proliferation and activation of lymphocytes. Common medications in this class include azathioprine (AZA), 6-mercaptopurine (6-MP), and methotrexate (MTX). AZA and 6-MP are also called thiopurines and follow weight-based dosing. Gastroenterologists can optimize the dose by using biomarkers such as thiopurine methyltransferase (TPMT) activity and drug metabolites such as 6-thioguanine (6-TG) and 6-methylmeracaptopruine (6-MMP). Side effects include agranulocytosis and hepatotoxicity [113]. Other complications include autoimmune hepatitis, fatigue, and pancreatitis. Severe effects such as myelosuppression and pancreatitis can be managed with discontinuation of therapy and supportive care. To minimize complications, routine lab monitoring with complete blood count (CBC) with differential and hepatic function should be performed every 3 months. A reduction in the white blood cell (WBC) count is desired, but if it falls to $<4.0 \times 10^3$ cells/μL, the drug should be held and restarted at a lower dose once the WBC count returns to normal. Methotrexate is an alternative to thiopurines and is used more commonly in Crohn's disease in combination therapy. Significant complications include hepatotoxicity, myelosuppression, and pneumonitis, which occur in <10% of patients [114]. This agent should always be taken with folic acid to avoid anemia. Chest radiograph and baseline liver function tests, followed by an assessment of CBC with differential and hepatic function every 3 months, are recommended. Consideration for liver biopsy is suggested for patients with liver enzymes that remain persistently elevated for more than 12 months [115].

The use of biologic drugs such as anti-TNFα has had a significant impact on IBD treatment. The medications included in this class are infliximab, adalimumab, golimumab, and certolizumab. Numerous clinical trials have demonstrated efficacy in moderate-to-severe CD and UC [116–118]. These drugs are well tolerated and have minimal side effects. Side effects include infusion or injection site reactions, opportunistic infections, autoimmune hepatitis, and psoriasis. Rarely there are neurological side effects, including unmasking of underlying multiple sclerosis. The most feared side effect is hepatosplenic T-cell lymphoma. This rarely occurs, seen in approximately 4–5/10,000 patients. The demographic most often affected is men under the age of 35 years [119]. A thorough exam for lymphadenopathy and splenomegaly is required at every visit. Before drug initiation, latent tuberculosis infection and hepatitis B virus infection should be ruled out to prevent dissemination. The PCP can assist with routine lab testing, which should be drawn every 3–6 months.

Ustekinumab is a human monoclonal antibody that binds to and interferes with the proinflammatory cytokines IL-12 and IL-23. Several trials have demonstrated efficacy in CD and UC [120, 121]. Its side effect profile includes hypersensitivity reactions, the risk for infections or reactivation of latent infections, increased risk of malignancy, particularly nonmelanoma skin cancer, and noninfectious pneumonia such as interstitial pneumonia, eosinophilic pneumonia, and cryptogenic organizing pneumonia. Cases of posterior reversible encephalopathy syndrome have been reported [122].

Vedolizumab is another human monoclonal antibody, an $\alpha_4\beta_7$ integrin inhibitor used in moderate-to-severe CD and UC [123, 124]. More common side effects include arthralgia, nasopharyngitis, and headaches, but no reported cases of progressive multifocal leukoencephalopathy (PML) have been associated with vedolizumab use [125].

Janus kinase inhibitors (JAKi), including tofacitinib and upadacitinib, are the first class of oral molecular therapies available for IBD. JAKi are FDA approved for the management of moderate–severe ulcerative colitis [126, 127]. The most commonly reported adverse events include headaches, nasopharyngitis, respiratory infections, herpes zoster, and higher rates of nonmelanoma skin cancer [128]. The FDA placed a black box warning on the drug class due to higher venous thromboembolism (VTE) and all-cause mortality, including sudden cardiovascular death [128, 129]. This class of therapy should be chosen for the right patient population under the guidance of both the gastroenterologist and PCP to weigh the risks and benefits.

Ozanimod is another oral molecular therapy in the class of sphingosine I-phosphate receptor modulators (S1P). The role of S1P modulators is to prevent immune cells, such as lymphocytes, from moving out of the lymph nodes into the colon [130]. Ozanimod has been FDA approved to manage moderate-to-severe UC [131]. Some more common side effects include upper respiratory infections, elevated transaminases, headache, and arthralgias. Ozanimod is contraindicated in patients with significant cardiac comorbidities, including arrhythmias and myocardial infarction, within 6 months of starting therapy. Close monitoring by both the gastroenterologist and PCP is recommended for such patients.

## Extraintestinal Manifestations

An extraintestinal manifestation (EIM) is a disease that occurs outside the bowel and is associated with IBD. At least 25% of patients with IBD are affected [132]. While there are numerous EIMs, the most common include arthropathy, cutaneous lesions, and ocular inflammation (see Table 32.3). Unfortunately, the underlying pathogenesis of EIM development in IBD is not well

**Table 32.3** Common extra-intestinal manifestations (EIM) and relationship to IBD activity

| EIM | Paralleling disease activity | Independent of disease activity | Either parallel or independent of activity |
|---|---|---|---|
| Axial arthropathy | | X | |
| Peripheral arthropathy | **X**<br>**(type I)** | **X**<br>**(type II)** | |
| Erythema nodosum | X | | |
| Pyoderma gangrenosum | | | X |
| Oral aphthous ulcers | X | | |
| Episcleritis | X | | |
| Uveitis | | | X |
| Primary sclerosing cholangitis | | | X |

understood. EIMs can either parallel or be independent of disease activity. They can be the first presenting feature of IBD, and finding one of these conditions should trigger a referral to a gastroenterologist. Pediatric patients have been shown to have a higher prevalence of EIMs in comparison to adult patients [133]. Furthermore, because patients with IBD are often unaware of EIM, they may first seek care from their PCP. It is critical that the PCP coordinate appropriate evaluation with the gastroenterologist when this occurs.

## Arthropathy

Joint pain or inflammation is the most common EIM in IBD, occurring in up to 40% of IBD patients [134]. Peripheral arthralgia can occur in up to 10% of UC patients and 20% of CD patients. It is characterized as seronegative and classified into two distinct categories. Type I (pauciarticular) involves <5 large joints and is dependent on disease activity. Type II (polyarticular) affects >5 large joints, and its severity is independent of disease activity. Knees tend to be the most affected joints, but differentiation of Type I versus Type II is seldom clinically relevant. Treating the underlying bowel inflammation can help control joint symptoms, but further evaluation by rheumatology is recommended in refractory cases. The use of NSAIDs is discouraged due to the potential for worsening underlying IBD [49].

## Skin/Mucosal Lesions

Cutaneous disorders associated with IBD can occur in up to 15% of patients [135]. Erythema nodosum (EN) is characterized as raised, tender, red/violet subcutaneous nodules measuring up to 5 centimeters in diameter. They are typically located on the anterior surface of the lower extremities (Fig. 32.1) [136]. EN usually resolves when the bowel inflammation is treated. On the other hand, pyoderma gangrenosum (PG) has an unpredictable course and does not parallel disease activity. It is characterized initially by an erythematous pustule/nodule, followed by rapid local spread and development into a burrowing ulcer with irregular violaceous edges (Fig. 32.2) [137]. The same drugs used to treat IBD treat PG. However, refractory cases have benefited from intralesional steroids and cyclosporine [138]. PG typically involves expert consultation with a dermatologist.

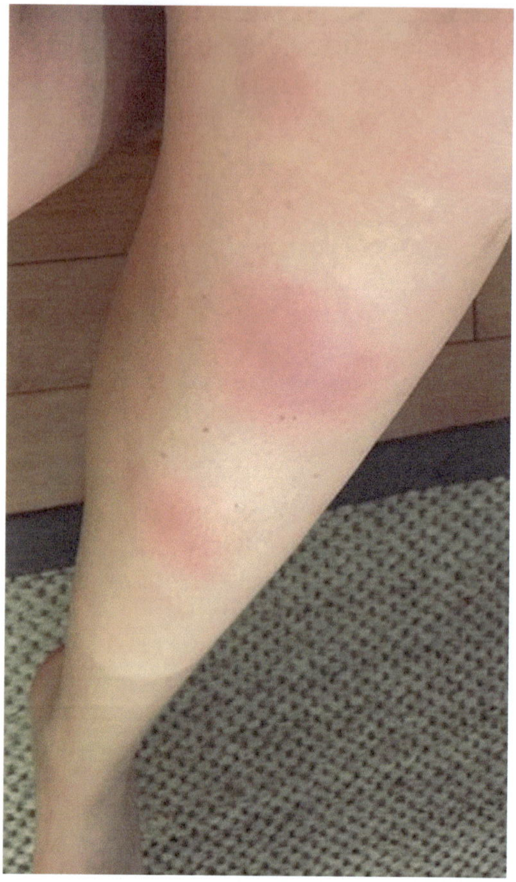

**Fig. 32.1** Erythema nodosum of the anterior left leg in a patient with ulcerative colitis. *(Courtesy of Dr. Elana Maser)*

Aphthous ulcers in the oral cavity typically occur in conjunction with IBD activity and are localized to the buccal mucosa, with occasional appearances on the tongue. Treatment typically involves therapy of underlying IBD in combination with antiseptic mouthwashes and topical steroid dental paste.

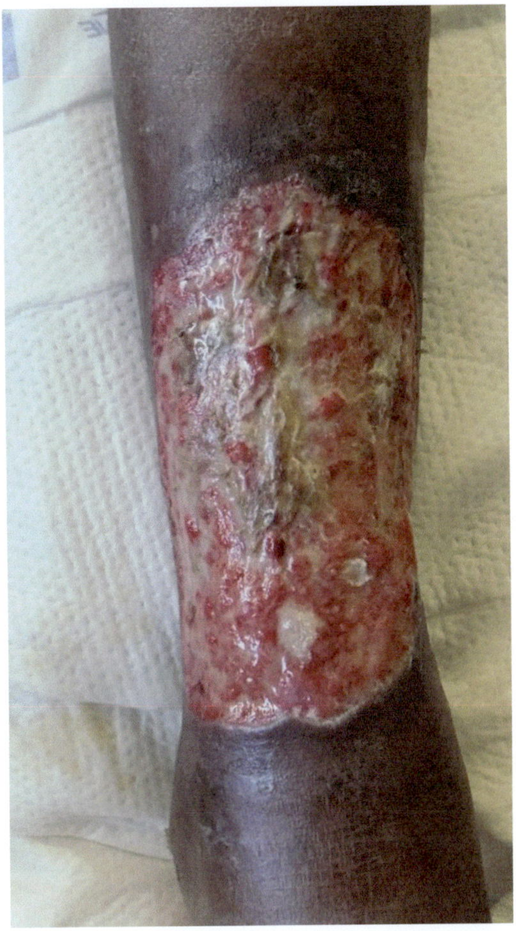

**Fig. 32.2** Pyoderma gangrenosum of the anterior left leg in a patient with ulcerative colitis. Note the "violaceous" hue along the borders. *(Courtesy of Dr. David Faleck and Dr. Serre-yu Wong)*

## Ophthalmologic Manifestations

Up to 5% of IBD patients will present with ocular manifestations [139]. Episcleritis is characterized as painless hyperemia of the conjunctiva and often parallels IBD activity. Treatment of the underlying bowel inflammation and topical steroids are used to relieve symptoms. Alternatively, the temporal correlation of uveitis with IBD is unpredictable. Uveitis may present as ocular pain, blurred vision, or photophobia. Uveitis can lead to blindness. Thus, all patients with IBD who present with any visual symptoms should be immediately referred to an ophthalmologist in addition to having an annual ophthalmological evaluation.

## Nonalcoholic Fatty Liver Disease (NAFLD)

NAFLD is one of the most common liver disorders in the United States, resulting from excess fat accumulation in the liver, which can progress to nonalcoholic steatohepatitis (NASH) [140]. IBD patients seem to have a higher susceptibility to NAFLD, and its prevalence reaches almost 40%; however, such patients lack traditional metabolic NAFLD risk factors [141, 142]. Risk factors that increase the risk for NAFLD in patients with IBD include small bowel surgery, disease activity and duration, need for parenteral nutrition, and high doses of corticosteroids [143]. The role of IBD management has an unknown effect on the development or complication risk of NAFLD. The PCP is pivotal in helping to address known metabolic risk factors, including obesity, and coordinating care with the gastroenterologist.

## Special Issues in the Transition to Adult Care

With the rising incidence of pediatric IBD, many young patients are transitioning to adult care. Adult providers need to be ready to manage young adults who may lack the readiness to cope independently with their illness. With evidence from chronic disease models, poorer outcomes have been demonstrated in young adults transitioning to adult healthcare, partly due to the expectation of increased autonomy [144, 145].

Based on a survey of adult gastroenterologists, one of the significant perceived barriers to transitioning to adult health-care settings for IBD patients was the lack of prior specific adolescent training among providers [146]. Gastroenterology fellowship programs provide minimal, if any, training in the care of adolescents. The care of young adults with other chronic conditions, such as rheumatologic and cardiac diseases, presents similar concerns [147, 148]. Adult providers will need to be aware of their patients' developing independence, differences in the communication style of adolescents and young adults, greater body image concerns among younger patients, challenges for their patients in navigating intimate relationships, and worries regarding missed school or work [149]. Lastly, coordinating insurance coverage as adolescents' transition off their parents' insurance plans is essential because treating IBD often requires expensive biologic drugs.

Some adolescents arrive at the adult gastroenterologist ready to take control of their healthcare, while others continue to communicate through their parents. Every adolescent grows at their own pace. The first step is for the provider to assess the patient's current level of independence and build from there. Part of fostering independence includes helping adolescents understand how to manage IBD. Having IBD often involves frequent lab testing, imaging, and annual screening colonoscopies, procedures that may not have needed to be initiated by their pediatric gastroenterologist.

Fostering independence also includes encouraging adolescents to communicate directly with their physicians rather than through their parents. Having this direct connection will help establish trust. As adolescents often prefer to correspond via email and text, the use of patient portals that allow for electronic communication may be helpful. There are many emerging applications (a.k.a. "apps") for disease education and monitoring.

Once communication and trust have been established, there can be an opening to discuss the impact of IBD on body image and sexuality. IBD diagnosis is often made in adolescence when body image is forming. Up to two-thirds of adult IBD patients report impaired body image, and one-third blame IBD for negatively affecting their sexual desire and satisfaction [75, 77]. The presence of disfiguring abdominal scars or the presence of an ostomy may lead patients to withdraw from active sexual relationships and have difficulty initiating new ones, especially during the sensitive adolescent period. Patients may want advice on disclosing that they have a chronic illness to their partners. Unfortunately, adequate counseling on sexual health IBD remains low, especially for women [150]. Not all PCPs or gastroenterologists feel comfortable or lack adequate time to provide comprehensive counseling to patients. However, they can explain that these critical issues are considered when making medical decisions. For example, if a colectomy is required, then it is helpful to discuss with patients that an ostomy can be well hidden under clothing and that bathing suits are designed to hide ostomies. Primary care doctors can help advocate for their patients if these sensitive topics are more easily discussed with them. Whether or not the adolescent seems well adjusted, referral to a psychologist should be offered to all patients to support them while navigating this sensitive time.

Missed school or work can be difficult for young adults as they attempt to establish themselves in their careers. The indirect costs of missed work and unemployment attributable to IBD are estimated at $3.6 billion per year [151]. Physicians can help minimize the disruption to the lives of their patients by being sensitive to the possible need to delay surgery or start a new medication when conflicts with work, school, weddings, or travel may exist. College students can be advised that they may be eligible for exam extensions or taking a leave from school if necessary. Many pharmaceutical companies offer scholarships to help support patients with IBD. There are also camps for children with Crohn's (Camp Oasis), where an adolescent can provide counsel to younger children navigating their disease and allow them to meet others with similar issues.

As they emerge into young adulthood, individuals eventually age off their parent's health insurance. A 2014 survey demonstrated that only up to 24% of young adults received counseling concerning obtaining insurance coverage [152]. Interruption in the administration of biological agents can prevent their usefulness in the future. Therefore, notifying patients to be proactive to assure they do not experience gaps in their health insurance coverage can be life changing. If possible, then access to a social worker would be helpful.

## Conclusion

Acknowledging important issues for adolescents and young adults with IBD when they arrive in an adult practice will establish trust and ultimately lead to better patient outcomes and satisfaction. It is essential to maintain careful coordination of care between the PCP and subspecialist to assure the delivery of comprehensive care to patients with IBD.

## References


1. Escher J. Transition from pediatrics to adult health care in inflammatory bowel disease. Dig Dis. 2009;27:382–6.
2. Dabadie A, Troadec F, Heresbach D, Siproudhis L, Pagenault M, Bretagne JF. Transition of patients with inflammatory bowel disease from pediatric to adult care. Gastroenterol Clin Biol. 2008;3 2(5 Pt 1):451–9.
3. El-Matary W. Transition of children with inflammatory bowel disease: big task, little evidence. World J Gastroenterol. 2009;15(30):3744.
4. Van Assche G, Vermeire S, Ballet V, Gabriels F, Noman M, D'Haens G, et al. Switch to adalimumab in patients with Crohn's disease controlled by maintenance infliximab: prospective randomised SWITCH trial. Gut. 2012;61(2):229–34.
5. Burisch J, Jess T, Martinato M, Lakatos PL, EpiCom E. The burden of inflammatory bowel disease in Europe. J Crohns Colitis. 2013;7(4):322–37.
6. Bernstein C, Wajda A, Svenson L, MacKenzie A, Koehoorn M, Jackson M. The epidemiology of inflammatory bowel disease in Canada: a population-based study. Am J Gastroenterol. 2006;101:1559–68.
7. Burisch J, Pedersen N, Cukovic-Cavka S, Brinar M, Kaimakliotis I, Duricova D, et al. East-west gradient in the incidence of inflammatory bowel disease in Europe: the ECCO-EpiCom inception cohort. Gut. 2014;63(4):588–97.
8. Sawczenko A, Sandhu BK, Logan RFA, Jenkins H, Taylor CJ, Mian S, et al. Prospective survey of childhood inflammatory bowel disease in the British Isles. Lancet. 2001;357(9262):1093–4.
9. Malaty HM, Fan X, Opekun AR, Thibodeaux C, Ferry GD. Rising incidence of inflammatory bowel disease among children: a 12-year study. J Pediatr Gastroenterol Nutr. 2010;50(1):27–31.
10. Loftus CG, Loftus EV Jr, Harmsen WS, Zinsmeister AR, Tremaine WJ, Melton LJ 3rd, et al. Update on the incidence and prevalence of Crohn's disease and ulcerative colitis in Olmsted County, Minnesota, 1940-2000. Inflamm Bowel Dis. 2007;13(3):254–61.
11. Romberg-Camps MJL, Hesselink-van de Kruijs MAM, Schouten LJ, Dagnelie PC, Limonard CB, Kester ADM, et al. Inflammatory bowel disease in South Limburg (The Netherlands) 1991-2002: incidence, diagnostic delay, and seasonal variations in onset of symptoms. J Crohns Colitis. 2009;3:115–24.
12. Trallori G, Palli D, Saieva C, Bardazzi G, Bonanomi A, D'Albasio G. A population-based study of inflammatory bowel disease in Florence over 15 years (1978-92). Scand J Gastroenterol. 1996;31:892–9.
13. Robison W, Bentlif P, JR K. Observations on 261 consecutive patients with inflammatory bowel disease seen in the Southwest United States. Dig Dis Sci. 1980;25:198–204.
14. Anderson CA, Boucher G, Lees CW, Franke A, D'Amato M, Taylor KD, et al. Meta-analysis identifies 29 additional ulcerative colitis risk loci, increasing the number of confirmed associations to 47. Nat Genet. 2011;43(3):246–52.
15. Franke A, McGovern DP, Barrett JC, Wang K, Radford-Smith GL, Ahmad T, et al. Genome-wide meta-analysis increases to 71 the number of confirmed Crohn's disease susceptibility loci. Nat Genet. 2010;42(12):1118–25.
16. Bellaguarda E, Chang EB. IBD and the gut microbiota--from bench to personalized medicine. Curr Gastroenterol Rep. 2015;17(4):15.
17. Hart AL, Ng SC, Mann E, Al-Hassi HO, Bernardo D, Knight SC. Homing of immune cells: role in homeostasis and intestinal inflammation. Inflamm Bowel Dis. 2010;16(11):1969–77.
18. Hold GL, Smith M, Grange C, Watt ER, El-Omar EM, Mukhopadhya I. Role of the gut microbiota in inflammatory bowel disease pathogenesis: what have we learnt in the past 10 years? World J Gastroenterol. 2014;20(5):1192–210.
19. Monstad I, Hovde O, Solberg IC, Moum A, B. Clinical course and prognosis in ulcerative colitis: results from population-based and observational studies. Ann Gastroenterol. 2014;27(2):95–104.
20. Kornbluth A, Sachar DB. Practice parameters Committee of the American College of G. Ulcerative colitis practice guidelines in adults: American College of Gastroenterology, practice parameters committee. Am J Gastroenterol. 2010;105(3):501–23.
21. Louis E, Collard A, Oger AF, Degroote E, El Yafi AN, FA, Belaiche J. Behaviour of Crohn's disease according to the Vienna classification: changing pattern over the course of the disease. Gut. 2001;49(6):777–82.
22. Maser EA, Sachar DB, Kruse D, Harpaz N, Ullman T, Bauer JJ. High rates of metachronous colon cancer or dysplasia after segmental resection or subtotal colectomy in Crohn's colitis. Inflamm Bowel Dis. 2013;19(9):1827–32.

23. Hanauer S. Epidemiology, pathogenesis, and treatment of IBD. Inflamm Bowel Dis. 2006;12(1):S3–9.
24. Frank DN, St Amand AL, Feldman RA, Boedeker EC, Harpaz N, Pace NR. Molecular-phylogenetic characterization of microbial community imbalances in human inflammatory bowel diseases. Proc Natl Acad Sci USA. 2007;104(34):13780–5.
25. Manichanh C, Rigottier-Gois L, Bonnaud E, Gloux K, Pelletier E, Frangeul L, et al. Reduced diversity of faecal microbiota in Crohn's disease revealed by a metagenomic approach. Gut. 2006;55(2):205–11.
26. Papadakis KA, Targan SR. Role of cytokines in the pathogenesis of inflammatory bowel disease. Annu Rev Med. 2000;51:289–98.
27. Satsangi J, Jewell D, Bell J. The genetics of inflammatory bowel disease. Gut. 1997;40(5):572–4.
28. Satsangi J, Morecroft J, Shah N, Nimmo E. Genetics of inflammatory bowel disease: scientific and clinical implications. Best Pract Res Clin Gastroenterol. 2003;17(1):3–18.
29. Khor B, Gardet A, Xavier RJ. Genetics and pathogenesis of inflammatory bowel disease. Nature. 2011;474(7351):307–17.
30. Halme L, Paavola-Sakki P, Turunen U, Lappalainen M, Farkkila M, Kontula K. Family and twin studies in inflammatory bowel disease. World J Gastroenterol. 2006;12(23):3668–72.
31. Yang H, McElree C, Roth M, Shanahan F, Targan S, Rotter J. Familial empirical risks for inflammatory bowel disease: differences between Jews and non-Jews. Gut. 1993;34(4):517–24.
32. Bouma G, Strober W. The immunological and genetic basis of inflammatory bowel disease. Nat Rev Immunol. 2003;3(7):521–33.
33. Hugot J, Laurent-Puig P, Gower-Rousseau C, Olson J, Lee J, Beaugerie L, et al. Mapping a susceptibility locus for Crohn's disease on chromosome 16. Nature. 1996;379(6568):821–3.
34. Jostins L, Ripke S, Weersma RK, Duerr RH, McGovern DP, Hui KY, et al. Host-microbe interactions have shaped the genetic architecture of inflammatory bowel disease. Nature. 2012;491(7422):119–24.
35. Hugot J, Chamaillard M, Zouali H, Lesage S, Cezard J, Belaiche J, et al. Association of NOD2 leucine-rich repeat variants with susceptibility to Crohn's disease. Nature. 2001;411(6837):599–603.
36. Ogura Y, Bonen D, Inohara N, Nicolae D, Chen F, Ramos R, et al. A frameshift mutation in NOD2 associated with susceptibility to Crohn's disease. Nature. 2001;411(6837):603–6.
37. Strachan D. Hay fever, hygiene, and household size. BMJ. 1989;299(6710):1259–60.
38. Radon K, Windstetter D, Poluda AL, Mueller B, von Mutius E, Koletzko S, et al. Contact with farm animals in early life and juvenile inflammatory bowel disease: a case-control study. Pediatrics. 2007;120(2):354–61.
39. Van Kruiningen H, Joosens M, Vermeire S, Joosens S, Debeugny S, Gower-Rousseau C, et al. Environmental factors in familial Crohn's disease in Belgium. Inflamm Bowel Dis. 2005;11(4):360–5.
40. Bager P, Simonsen J, Nielsen NM, Frisch M. Cesarean section and offspring's risk of inflammatory bowel disease: a national cohort study. Inflamm Bowel Dis. 2012;18(5):857–62.
41. Barclay A, Russell R, Wilson M, Gilmour W, Satsangi J, Wilson D. Systematic review: the role of breastfeeding in the development of pediatric inflammatory bowel disease. J Pediatr. 2009;155(3):421–6.
42. Cosnes J, Carbonnel F, Beaugerie L, Le Quintrec Y, Gendre J. Effects of cigarette smoking on the long-term course of Crohn's disease. Gastroenterology. 1996;110(2):424–31.
43. Mahid S, Minor K, Soto R, Hornung C, Galandiuk S. Smoking and inflammatory bowel disease: a meta-analysis. Mayo Clin Proc. 2006;81(11):1462–71.
44. Higuchi LM, Khalili H, Chan AT, Richter JM, Bousvaros A, Fuchs CS. A prospective study of cigarette smoking and the risk of inflammatory bowel disease in women. Am J Gastroenterol. 2012;107(9):1399–406.
45. Mahid SS, Minor KS, Stromberg AJ, Galandiuk S. Active and passive smoking in childhood is related to the development of inflammatory bowel disease. Inflamm Bowel Dis. 2007;13(4):431–8.
46. Ungaro R, Bernstein CN, Gearry R, Hviid A, Kolho KL, Kronman MP, et al. Antibiotics associated with increased risk of new-onset Crohn's disease but not ulcerative colitis: a meta-analysis. Am J Gastroenterol. 2014;109(11):1728–38.
47. Kronman MP, Zaoutis TE, Haynes K, Feng R, Coffin SE. Antibiotic exposure and IBD development among children: a population-based cohort study. Pediatrics. 2012;130(4):e794–803.
48. Gevers D, Kugathasan S, Denson LA, Vazquez-Baeza Y, Van Treuren W, Ren B, et al. The treatment-naive microbiome in new-onset Crohn's disease. Cell Host Microbe. 2014;15(3):382–92.
49. Felder J, Korelitz B, Rajapakse R, Schwarz S, Horatagis A, Gleim G. Effects of nonsteroidal antiinflammatory drugs on inflammatory bowel disease: a case-control study. Am J Gastroenterol. 2000;95(8):1949.
50. Kaufmann H, Taubin H. Nonsteroidal anti-inflammatory drugs activate quiescent inflammatory bowel disease. Ann Intern Med. 1987;107(4):513.
51. Ananthakrishnan A, Higuchi L, Huang E, Khalili H, Richter J, Fuchs C, et al. Aspirin, nonsteroidal anti-inflammatory drug use, and risk for Crohn disease and ulcerative colitis a cohort study. Ann Intern Med. 2012;156(5):350–9.
52. Tanner A, Raghunath A. Colonic inflammation and nonsteroidal anti-inflammatory drug administration: an assessment of the frequency of the problem. Digestion. 1988;41(2):116–20.
53. Moninuola OO, Milligan WLP, Khalili H. Systematic review with meta-analysis: association between acetaminophen and nonsteroidal anti-inflammatory drugs (NSAIDs) and risk of Crohn's disease and

ulcerative colitis exacerbation. Aliment Pharmacol Ther. 2018;47(11):1428–39.
54. Bankar R, Dafe C, Kohnke A, Babu P. Ulcerative colitis probably associated with isotretinoin. Indian J Gastroenterol. 2006;25(3):171–2.
55. Bernstein CN, Nugent Z, Longobardi T, Blanchard JF. Isotretinoin is not associated with inflammatory bowel disease: a population-based case-control study. Am J Gastroenterol. 2009;104(11):2774–8.
56. Lee SYJM, Nguyen ET, Bechtold ML, Nguyen DL. Does exposure to isotretinoin increase the risk for the development of inflammatory bowel disease? A meta-analysis. Eur J Gastroenterol Hepatol. 2016;28(2):210–6.
57. Khalili H, Higuchi LM, Ananthakrishnan AN, Manson JE, Feskanich D, Richter JM, et al. Hormone therapy increases risk of ulcerative colitis but not Crohn's disease. Gastroenterology. 2012;143(5):1199–206.
58. Khalili H, Higuchi LM, Ananthakrishnan AN, Richter JM, Feskanich D, Fuchs CS, et al. Oral contraceptives, reproductive factors and risk of inflammatory bowel disease. Gut. 2013;62(8):1153–9.
59. Ananthakrishnan AN, Khalili H, Pan A, Higuchi LM, de Silva P, Richter JM, et al. Association between depressive symptoms and incidence of Crohn's disease and ulcerative colitis: results from the Nurses' health study. Clin Gastroenterol Hepatol. 2013;11(1):57–62.
60. Bitton A, Dobkin PL, Edwardes MD, Sewitch MJ, Meddings JB, Rawal S, et al. Predicting relapse in Crohn's disease: a biopsychosocial model. Gut. 2008;57(10):1386–92.
61. Goodhand JR, Wahed M, Mawdsley JE, Farmer AD, Aziz Q, Rampton DS. Mood disorders in inflammatory bowel disease: relation to diagnosis, disease activity, perceived stress, and other factors. Inflamm Bowel Dis. 2012;18(12):2301–9.
62. Triantafillidis JK, Merikas E, Gikas A. Psychological factors and stress in inflammatory bowel disease. Expert Rev Gastroenterol Hepatol. 2013;7(3):225–38.
63. Dasharathy SS, Long MD, Lackner JM, Ben-Ami Shor D, Yang L, Bar N, Ha C, et al. Psychological factors associated with adherence to oral treatment in ulcerative colitis. Inflamm Bowel Dis. 2022;29(1):97–102. https://doi.org/10.1093/ibd/izac041.
64. Szigethy E. Hypnotherapy for inflammatory bowel disease across the lifespan. Am J Clin Hypn. 2015;58(1):81–99.
65. Chan SS, Luben R, Olsen A, Tjonneland A, Kaaks R, Teucher B, et al. Body mass index and the risk for Crohn's disease and ulcerative colitis: data from a European prospective cohort study (the IBD in EPIC study). Am J Gastroenterol. 2013;108(4):575–82.
66. Mendall MA, Gunasekera AV, John BJ, Kumar D. Is obesity a risk factor for Crohn's disease? Dig Dis Sci. 2011;56(3):837–44.
67. Flynn MG, McFarlin BK, Markofski M. The anti-inflammatory actions of exercise training. Am J Lifestyle Med. 2007;1(3):220–35.
68. Desreumaux P, Ernst O, Geboes K, Gambiez L, Berrebi D, Muller-Alouf H, et al. Inflammatory alterations in mesenteric adipose tissue in Crohn's disease. Gastroenterology. 1999;117(1):73–81.
69. Blain A, Cattan S, Beaugerie L, Carbonnel F, Gendre JP, Cosnes J. Crohn's disease clinical course and severity in obese patients. Clin Nutr. 2002;21(1):51–7.
70. Long MD, Crandall WV, Leibowitz IH, Duffy L, del Rosario F, Kim SC, et al. Prevalence and epidemiology of overweight and obesity in children with inflammatory bowel disease. Inflamm Bowel Dis. 2011;17(10):2162–8.
71. Khalili H, Ananthakrishnan AN, Konijeti GG, Liao X, Higuchi LM, Fuchs CS, et al. Physical activity and risk of inflammatory bowel disease: prospective study from the Nurses' health study cohorts. BMJ. 2013;347:f6633.
72. Ali T, Madhoun MF, Orr WC, Rubin DT. Assessment of the relationship between quality of sleep and disease activity in inflammatory bowel disease patients. Inflamm Bowel Dis. 2013;19(11):2440–3.
73. Ananthakrishnan AN, Khalili H, Konijeti GG, Higuchi LM, de Silva P, Fuchs CS, et al. Sleep duration affects risk for ulcerative colitis: a prospective cohort study. Clin Gastroenterol Hepatol. 2014;12(11):1879–86.
74. Drossman D, Leserman J, Li Z, Mitchell C, Zagami E, Patrick D. The rating form of IBD patient concerns: a new measure of health status. Psychosom Med. 1991;53(6):701–12.
75. Marin L, Manosa M, Garcia-Planella E, Gordillo J, Zabana Y, Cabre E, et al. Sexual function and patients' perceptions in inflammatory bowel disease: a case-control survey. J Gastroenterol. 2013;48(6):713–20.
76. Timmer A, Bauer A, Dignass A, Rogler G. Sexual function in persons with inflammatory bowel disease: a survey with matched controls. Clin Gastroenterol Hepatol. 2007;5(1):87–94.
77. Muller KR, Prosser R, Bampton P, Mountifield R, Andrews JM. Female gender and surgery impair relationships, body image, and sexuality in inflammatory bowel disease: patient perceptions. Inflamm Bowel Dis. 2010;16(4):657–63.
78. Johnson P, Richard C, Ravid A, Spencer L, Pinto E, Hanna M, et al. Female infertility after ileal pouch-anal anastomosis for ulcerative colitis. Dis Colon Rectum. 2004;47(7):1119–26.
79. Mountifield R, Bampton P, Prosser R, Muller K, Andrews JM. Fear and fertility in inflammatory bowel disease: a mismatch of perception and reality affects family planning decisions. Inflamm Bowel Dis. 2009;15(5):720–5.
80. Tavernier N, Fumery M, Peyrin-Biroulet L, Colombel JF, Gower-Rousseau C. Systematic review: fertility in non-surgically treated inflammatory bowel disease. Aliment Pharmacol Ther. 2013;38(8):847–53.

81. Fonager K, Sorensen H, Olsen J, Dahlerup J, Rasmussen S. Pregnancy outcome for women with Crohn's disease: a follow-up study based on linkage between national registries. Am J Gastroenterol. 1998;9 3(12):2426–30.
82. Mahadevan U, Sandborn WJ, Li DK, Hakimian S, Kane S, Corley DA. Pregnancy outcomes in women with inflammatory bowel disease: a large community-based study from northern California. Gastroenterology. 2007;133(4):1106–12.
83. Norgard B, Fonager K, Sorensen H, Olsen J. Birth outcomes of women with ulcerative colitis: a nationwide Danish cohort study. Am J Gastroenterol. 2000;95(11):3165–70.
84. Katz J. Pregnancy and inflammatory bowel disease. Curr Opin Gastroenterol. 2004;20(4):328–32.
85. Ujihara M, Ando T, Ishiguro K, Maeda O, Watanabe O, Hibi S, et al. Appropriate pharmaceutical management is crucial for pregnant women complicated by ulcerative colitis. Gastroenterology. 2012;142(5):S251–2.
86. Clowse MEFS, Isaacs JD, et al. Pregnancy outcomes in the tofacitinib safety databases for rheumatoid arthritis and psoriasis. Drug Saf. 2016;39(8):755–62.
87. Dubinsky MC, Mahadevan U, Charles L, Afsari S, Henry A, Comi G, et al. Pregnancy outcomes in the ozanimod clinical development program in relapsing multiple sclerosis, ulcerative colitis, and Crohn's disease. J Crohn's Colitis. 2021;15:S088–9.
88. Pohl CHA, Kruis W. Chronic inflammatory bowel disease and cancer. Hepato-Gastroenterology. 2000;47(31):57–70.
89. Syal G, Serrano M, Jain A, Cohen BL, Rieder F, Stone C, et al. Health maintenance consensus for adults with inflammatory bowel disease. Inflamm Bowel Dis. 2021;27(10):1552–63.
90. Bhatia J, Bratcher J, Korelitz B, Vakher K, Mannor S, Shevchuk M, et al. Abnormalities of uterine cervix in women with inflammatory bowel disease. World Gastroenterol. 2006;12(38):6167–71.
91. Kane S, Khatibi B, Reddy D. Higher incidence of abnormal pap smears in women with inflammatory bowel disease. Am J Gastroenterol. 2008;103(3):631–6.
92. Committee on Practice Bulletins—Gynecologists. ACOG Practice bulletin no. 131: screening for cervical cancer. Obstet Gynecol. 2012;120:1222–38.
93. Peyrin-Biroulet L, Khosrotehrani K, Carrat F, Bouvier AM, Chevaux JB, Simon T, et al. Increased risk for nonmelanoma skin cancers in patients who receive thiopurines for inflammatory bowel disease. Gastroenterology. 2011;141(5):1621–8. e1–5
94. Nyboe Andersen N, Pasternak B, Basit S, Andersson M, Svanstrom H, Caspersen S, et al. Association between tumor necrosis factor-alpha antagonists and risk of cancer in patients with inflammatory bowel disease. JAMA. 2014;311(23):2406–13.
95. Force USPST. Screening for osteoporosis: U.S. preventative services task force recommendation statement. Ann Intern Med. 2011;154(5):356–64.
96. Moscandrew M, Mahadevan U, Kane S. General health maintenance in IBD. Inflamm Bowel Dis. 2009;15(9):1399–409.
97. Long MD, Martin C, Sandler RS, Kappelman MD. Increased risk of pneumonia among patients with inflammatory bowel disease. Am J Gastroenterol. 2013;108(2):240–8.
98. Melmed GY, Ippoliti AF, Papadakis KA, Tran TT, Birt JL, Lee SK, et al. Patients with inflammatory bowel disease are at risk for vaccine-preventable illnesses. Am J Gastroenterol. 2006;101(8):1834–40.
99. Wasan SK, Calderwood AH, Long MD, Kappelman MD, Sandler RS, Farraye FA. Immunization rates and vaccine beliefs among patients with inflammatory bowel disease: an opportunity for improvement. Inflamm Bowel Dis. 2014;20(2):246–50.
100. Dezfoli S, Melmed GY. Vaccination issues in patients with inflammatory bowel disease receiving immunosuppression. Gastroenterol Hepatol (NY). 2012;8(8):504–12.
101. Rubin LG, Levin MJ, Ljungman P, Davies EG, Avery R, Tomblyn M, et al. 2013 IDSA clinical practice guideline for vaccination of the immunocompromised host. Clin Infect Dis. 2014;58(3):309–18.
102. Centers for Disease Control and Prevention: Vaccines and Immunizations. http://www.cdc.gov/vaccines/default.htm.
103. Sandhu BK, Fell JM, Beattie RM, Mitton SG, Wilson DC, Jenkins H, et al. Guidelines for the management of inflammatory bowel disease in children in the United Kingdom. J Pediatr Gastroenterol Nutr. 2010;50(Suppl 1):S1–13.
104. Borrelli O, Cordischi L, Cirulli M, Paganelli M, Labalestra V, Uccini S, et al. Polymeric diet alone versus corticosteroids in the treatment of active pediatric Crohn's disease: a randomized controlled open-label trial. Clin Gastroenterol Hepatol. 2006;4(6):744–53.
105. Lewis JD, Sandler RS, Brotherton C, Brensinger C, Li H, Kappelman MD, et. al.; DINE-CD Study Group. A randomized trial comparing the specific carbohydrate diet to a Mediterranean diet in adults with Crohn's disease. Gastroenterology. 2021;161(3):837–52.
106. Ananthakrishnan AN, Khalili H, Konijeti GG, Higuchi LM, de Silva P, Korzenik JR, et al. A prospective study of long-term intake of dietary fiber and risk of Crohn's disease and ulcerative colitis. Gastroenterology. 2013;145(5):970–7.
107. Hou JK, Abraham B, El-Serag H. Dietary intake and risk of developing inflammatory bowel disease: a systematic review of the literature. Am J Gastroenterol. 2011;106(4):563–73.
108. Weiss G. Iron in the inflammed gut: another proinflammatory hit? Gut. 2011;60(3):287–8.
109. Cantorna M, Zhu Y, Froicu M, Wittke A. Vitamin D status, 1,25-dihyroxyvitamin D3, and the immune system. Am J Clin Nutr. 2004;80(6):1717S–20S.
110. Ford AC, Kane SV, Khan KJ, Achkar JP, Talley NJ, Marshall JK, et al. Efficacy of 5-aminosalicylates

in Crohn's disease: systematic review and meta-analysis. Am J Gastroenterol. 2011;106(4):617–29.

111. Gordon GL, Zakko S, Murthy U, Sedghi S, Pruitt R, Barrett AC, et al. Once-daily mesalamine formulation for maintenance of remission in ulcerative colitis: a randomized, placebo-controlled clinical trial. J Clin Gastroenterol. 2016;50(4):318–25.
112. World M, Stevens P, Ashton M, Rainford D. Mesalazine-associated interstitial nephritis. Nephrol Dial Transplant. 1996;11:614–21.
113. Connell W, Kamm M, Ritchie J, Lennard-Jones J. Bone marrow toxicity caused by azathioprine in inflammatory bowel disease: 27 years of experience. Gut. 1993;34:1081–5.
114. Moshkowitz M, Oren R, Tishler M, Konikoff F, Graff E, Brill S, et al. The absorption of low-dose methotrexate in patients with inflammatory bowel disease. Aliment Pharmacol Ther. 1997;11:569–73.
115. Singh JA, Furst DE, Bharat A, Curtis JR, Kavanaugh AF, Kremer JM, et al. 2012 update of the 2008 American College of Rheumatology recommendations for the use of disease-modifying antirheumatic drugs and biologic agents in the treatment of rheumatoid arthritis. Arthritis Care Res (Hoboken). 2012;64(5):625–39.
116. Hanauer SB, Feagan BG, Lichtenstein GR, Mayer LF, Schreiber S, Colombel JF, et al. Maintenance infliximab for Crohn's disease: the ACCENT I randomised trial. Lancet. 2002;359(9317):1541–9.
117. Rutgeerts P, Sandborn WJ, Feagan BG, Reinisch W, Olson A, Johanns J, et al. Infliximab for induction and maintenance therapy for ulcerative colitis. N Engl J Med. 2005;353(23):2462–72.
118. Sands BE, Anderson FH, Bernstein CN, Chey WY, Feagan BG, Fedorak RN, et al. Infliximab maintenance therapy for fistulizing Crohn's disease. N Engl J Med. 2004;350(9):876–85.
119. Kotlyar DS, Osterman MT, Diamond RH, Porter D, Blonski WC, Wasik M, et al. A systematic review of factors that contribute to hepatosplenic T-cell lymphoma in patients with inflammatory bowel disease. Clin Gastroenterol Hepatol. 2011;9(1):36–41.e1.
120. Feagan BG, Sandborn WJ, Gasink C, Jacobstein D, Lang Y, Friedman JR, et al. Ustekinumab as induction and maintenance therapy for Crohn's disease. N Engl J Med. 2016;375(20):1946–60.
121. Sands BE, Sandborn WJ, Panaccione R, O'Brien CD, Zhang H, et al. Ustekinumab as induction and maintenance therapy for ulcerative colitis. N Engl J Med. 2019;381(13):1201–14.
122. Galvan-Banqueri M, Gil RM, Santos Ramos B, Bautista Paloma FJ. Biological treatments for moderate-to-severe psoriasis: indirect comparison. J Clin Pharm Ther. 2013;38(2):121–30.
123. Feagan BG, Rutgeerts P, Sands BE, Hanauer S, Colombel JF, Sandborn WJ, et al. Vedolizumab as induction and maintenance therapy for ulcerative colitis. N Engl J Med. 2013;369(8):699–710.
124. Sandborn WJ, Feagan BG, Rutgeerts P, Hanauer S, Colombel JF, Sands BE, et al. Vedolizumab as induction and maintenance therapy for Crohn's disease. N Engl J Med. 2013;369(8):711–21.
125. Loftus EV Jr, Feagan BG, Panaccione R, Colombel JF, Sandborn WJ, Sands BE, et al. Long-term safety of vedolizumab for inflammatory bowel disease. Aliment Pharmacol Ther. 2020;52(8):1353–65.
126. Sandborn WJ, Su C, Sands BE, D'Haens GR, Vermeire S, Schreiber S, Danese S, et al. Tofacitinib as induction and maintenance therapy for ulcerative colitis. N Engl J Med. 2017;376(18):1723–36.
127. Sandborn WJ, Ghosh S, Panes J, Schreiber S, D'Haens G, Tanida S, et al. Efficacy of upadacitinib in a randomized trial of patients with active ulcerative colitis. Gastroenterology. 2020;158(8):2139–49.
128. Ted A, Spiewak AP. User's guide to JAK inhibitors in inflammatory bowel disease. Curr Res Pharmacol Drug Discov. 2022;3:100096.
129. Ma C, Lee JK, Mitra AF, Teriaky A, Choudhary D, Nguyen TM, et al. Systematic review with meta-analysis: efficacy and safety of oral Janus kinase inhibitors for inflammatory bowel disease. Aliment Pharmacol Ther. 2019;50(1):5–23.
130. Argollo M, Furfaro F, Gilardi D, Roda G, Allocca M, Peyrin-Biroulet L, et al. Modulation of sphingosine-1-phosphate in ulcerative colitis. Expert Opin Biol Ther. 2020;20(4):413–20.
131. Sandborn WJ, Feagan B, D'Haens G, Wolf DC, Jovanovic I, Hanauer SB, et al. Ozanimod as induction and maintenance therapy for ulcerative colitis. N Engl J Med. 2021;385(14):1280–91.
132. Bernstein CN, Blanchard JF, Rawsthorne P, Yu N. The prevalence of extraintestinal diseases in inflammatory bowel disease: a population-based study. Am J Gastroenterol. 2001;96(4):1116–22.
133. Stawarski A, Iwańczak B, Krzesiek E, Iwańczak F. Intestinal complications and extraintestinal manifestations in children with inflammatory bowel disease. Pol Merkur Lekarski. 2006;20(115):22–5.
134. Smale S, Natt RS, Orchard TR, Russell AS, Bjamason I. Inflammatory bowel disease and spondylarthropathy. Arthritis Rheum. 2001;44(12):2728–36.
135. Vavricka SR, Brun L, Ballabeni P, Pittet V, Prinz Vavricka BM, Zeitz J, et al. Frequency and risk factors for extraintestinal manifestations in the Swiss inflammatory bowel disease cohort. Am J Gastroenterol. 2011;106(1):110–9.
136. Requena L, Yus ES. Erythema nodosum. Dermatol Clin. 2008;26(4):425–38.
137. DeFilippis EM, Feldman SR, Huang WW. The genetics of pyoderma gangrenosum and implications for treatment: a systematic review. Br J Dermatol. 2015;172(6):1487–97.
138. Callen JP. Pyoderma gangrenosum. Lancet. 1998;351:581–5.
139. Su CG, Judge TA, Lichtenstein GR. Extraintestinal manifestations of inflammatory bowel disease. Gastroenterol Clin N Am. 2002;31(1):307–27.
140. Horn CL, Ta AV. Gunn NT current and emerging treatments for non-alcoholic steatohepatitis. Curr Hepatology Rep. 2020;19:391–401.

141. Cohen ME, Parakkal D, Khanna G, Samson CM. Evaluation of nonalcoholic fatty liver disease in pediatric patients with inflammatory bowel disease. J Pediatr Gastroenterol Nutr. 2021;72(4):574–8.
142. McHenry SSY, Tirath A, et al. Crohn's disease is associated with an increased prevalence of nonalcoholic fatty liver disease: a cross-sectional study using magnetic resonance proton density fat fraction mapping. Clin Gastroenterol Hepatol. 2019;17:2816–8.
143. Gaspar RBC, Macedo G. Liver manifestations and complications in inflammatory bowel disease: a review. World J Hepatol. 2021;13(12):1956–67.
144. Annunziato RA, Emre S, Shneider B, Barton C, Dugan CA, Shemesh E. Adherence and medical outcomes in pediatric liver transplant recipients who transition to adult services. Pediatr Transplant. 2007;11(6):608–14.
145. Hersh AO, Pang S, Curran ML, Milojevic DS, von Scheven E. The challenges of transferring chronic illness patients to adult care: reflections from pediatric and adult rheumatology at a US academic center. Pediatr Rheumatol Online J. 2009;7:13.
146. Sebastian S, Jenkins H, McCartney S, Ahmad T, Arnott I, Croft N, et al. The requirements and barriers to successful transition of adolescents with inflammatory bowel disease: differing perceptions from a survey of adult and paediatric gastroenterologists. J Crohns Colitis. 2012;6(8):830–44.
147. Reid GJ, Irvine MJ, McCrindle BW, Sananes R, Ritvo PG, Siu SC, et al. Prevalence and correlates of successful transfer from pediatric to adult health care among a cohort of young adults with complex congenital heart defects. Pediatrics. 2004;113(3):e197–205.
148. McDonagh JE, Southwood TR, Shaw KL, British Paediatric Rheumatology Group. Unmet education and training needs of rheumatology health professionals in adolescent health and transitional care. Rheumatology (Oxford). 2004;43(6):737–43.
149. Trivedi I, Keefer L. The emerging adult with inflammatory bowel disease: challenges and recommendations for the adult gastroenterologist. Gastroenterol Res Pract. 2015;2015:260807.
150. Gawron LM, Hammond C, Keefer L. Documentation of reproductive health counseling and contraception in women with inflammatory bowel diseases. Patient Educ Couns. 2014;94(1):134–7.
151. Longobardi T. Work losses related to inflammatory bowel disease in the United States results from the National Health Interview Survey. Am J Gastroenterol. 2003;98(5):1064–72.
152. Sawicki GS, Whitworth R, Gunn L, Butterfield R, Lukens-Bull K, Wood D. Receipt of health care transition counseling in the national survey of adult transition and health. Pediatrics. 2011;128(3):e521–9.

# 33 Intellectual Disability

Erin Hickey and Kamala Gullapalli Cotts

## Outpatient Case Presentation

Mr. C.B. is a 52-year-old African American male with a history of diplegic cerebral palsy and intellectual disability. He has lower extremity weakness and has been using a wheelchair since early childhood, has a left-hand contracture, and experiences rare urinary tract infections. He is obese with a body mass index (BMI) of 35 kg/m$^2$. He has severe dysarthria. History is negative for decubiti. His family history is significant for hypertension and myocardial infarction (at age 58) in his father. He recently moved from the east coast to live with his brother in Chicago. He had not been to see a physician in almost 3 years as his mother was progressively more ill and was unable to care for him.

Mr. C.B. completed high school at age 18 and has not had further education. He requires help with all activities of daily life including feeding, dressing, and toileting due to his contractures. He is not able to perform math but knows how much a plane trip costs and that he can buy two airplane tickets with his monthly Supplemental Security Income. Although he is not able to call the doctor's office and make an appointment, he is able to converse on the telephone about sporting events and television shows. He had been living with his mother until her recent death. He becomes tearful as he talks about his mother's death. He misses his former neighbors who used to visit frequently. He has difficulty falling asleep at least twice a week, but when he does fall asleep, he does not wake early. He reveals that his wheelchair is nearly 10 years old. Over the course of the next several months, he is diagnosed with and treated for hypertension, diabetes mellitus, and hyperlipidemia. His brother asks about resources to care for Mr. C.B. while he is at work. On a subsequent visit, his brother states that he has recently had a colonoscopy and asks if Mr. C.B. should have a colonoscopy as well.

## Case Discussion

After surviving elderly parents, Mr. C.B. has moved to a different state. Although he is a middle-aged individual, he still requires transitional assessment. While he is able to participate in the medical decision-making process, he requires help. He is unable to make financial decisions. Information should be provided about the physician certification form and local affordable or volunteer legal services to establish

E. Hickey
Department of Academic Internal Medicine and Department of Pediatrics, University of Illinois Chicago, Chicago, IL, USA
e-mail: ehicke9@uic.edu

K. G. Cotts (✉)
Department of Internal Medicine, University of Chicago Medicine, Chicago, IL, USA
e-mail: kcotts@medicine.bsd.uchicago.edu


A. A. Kuo et al. (eds.), *Care of Adults with Chronic Childhood Conditions*,
https://doi.org/10.1007/978-3-031-54281-7_33

guardianship. Formal neuropsychiatric testing is often performed when an individual is receiving special education under the age of 18 years and is often updated as one transitions to adulthood. As he has moved here from another state, such information is not readily available. An office assessment of his intellectual disability and adaptive functioning may be sufficient. The family requires information for local Pre-Admission Screening (PAS) Agencies, the agencies that determine eligibility for state services, to obtain information about finding local supports required for his degree of adaptive functioning. Often, these agencies require formal neuropsychological testing in order to establish the need for the services. Referral to a social worker may be helpful to receive information regarding local resources such as the local department of rehabilitation and vocational services as well as homemaker services. Additionally, he requires counseling services and resources within the community.

Mr. C.B. requires subspecialty referral to multiple health-care providers. He should be evaluated by orthopedic surgery given his chronic contractures as well as physical and occupational therapy assessments and referrals for durable medical equipment needs, including braces and a new wheelchair. In addition to providing general medical care for his newly diagnosed hypertension, diabetes, and hyperlipidemia, his health maintenance needs must be addressed. At subsequent visits, he may require referrals for vision, hearing, and dental evaluation. His vaccinations should be reviewed and updated. Finally, screening procedures such as colonoscopy and bone mineral density assessment, which are recommended by the United States Preventive Services Task Force (USPSTF) guidelines, should be reviewed with Mr. C.B. and his brother.

## Background

The term intellectual disability (ID) refers to a condition in which an individual has significant limitations in both cognitive functioning and adaptive behavior [1]. The diagnosis of ID requires formal psychometric testing to assess the intelligence quotient (IQ) and adaptive functioning. ID initially presents in early childhood and by definition must manifest in the developmental period [1]. In adulthood, ID impacts the ability to live independently, find employment, and obtain healthcare and also influences the need for federal—and state-based supportive services. Medical care of individuals with ID requires delivering general medical care, screening for comorbid conditions, treating behavioral symptoms, continuing transitional special education, and providing variable degrees of community-based support. Adults with ID are living longer as a result of improved medical care, environmental conditions, and technology [2]. As these individuals live longer, they require primary care that is both general and that targets the associated health condition that led to their initial impairment in intellectual functioning, such as Fetal Alcohol Syndrome or Down syndrome. Complications of these health conditions, such as decubitus ulcers and psychiatric disorders, occur at a higher frequency compared to the general population. In addition, patients with ID often have comorbid medical conditions that are neither caused by nor occur as a result of the ID, such as diabetes and hypertension. Adults with ID require the same considerations for improving quality of life and health screening as the general population, particularly in screening for cardiovascular disease and cancer. This chapter reviews the definition and epidemiology of ID as well as common medical conditions among and health maintenance screening guidelines for individuals with ID.

## Definition of Intellectual Disability

The definition of Intellectual Disability is relevant not only in the medical field but also in the domains of education and policy. The two leading definitions in the medical field are from the American Association of Intellectual and Developmental Disabilities (AAIDD) and the *Diagnostic and Statistical Manual of Mental Disorders,* fifth edition (DSM-5) criteria. These two definitions, as detailed below, are very similar and cohesive. The AAIDD defines intellectual disability as a disability acquired prior to the age of 22 years and characterized by significant limitations both in intellectual functioning and in adaptive behavior as expressed in conceptual, social, and practical adaptive skills [1]. The age of onset criterion was updated from 18 years to 22 years in the most recent 12th edition of the AAIDD definition. This change was based on more recent research that brain development continues into early in the third decade of life. Table 33.1 summarizes the diagnostic AAIDD criteria for intellectual disability [1]. The AAIDD definition of ID is mirrored in the DSM-5 criteria, although the DSM-5 does not specify an age of presentation but rather that the onset must be in the "developmental period" [3]. In addition, the DSM-5 defines severity of ID (mild, moderate, severe, and profound) based on adaptive functioning skills in comparison with population norms, as shown in Table 33.2 [3, 4]. Of note, the terminology used to refer to this population has evolved from idiocy to mental retardation to intellectual disability when the original medical terms lost their neutral meaning and became socially stigmatizing. The term intellectual disability more adequately describes complex individuals with a wide range of abilities, gifts, and supportive needs.

The AAIDD definition and diagnostic criteria emphasize several additional considerations. An individual's limitations in functioning are assessed within the context of the culture and community environment typical of the individual's peers. Assessments consider linguistic and cultural diversity as well as differences in communication, sensory, motor, and behavioral factors. Additionally, the AAIDD recognizes that limitations often coexist with strengths. An essential purpose of identifying limitations is to develop personalized supports that, over a sustained period of time, will improve an individual's level of life functioning.

Analogous to the medical definitions presented by the AAIDD and DSM-5, the Individuals with Disabilities Education Act (IDEA) defines intellectual disability in educational policy as "significantly sub-average general intellectual functioning, existing concurrently with deficits in adaptive behavior and manifested during the developmental period, that adversely affects a child's educational performance." Again, the two key components identified within this definition are a student's IQ and his or her capability to function independently, referred to as adaptive behavior. In 2010, the federal government enacted legislation changing the term "mental retardation" to "intellectual disabilities" in all federal laws. Most states have made this change in their legislation and documents [5].

An extensive multifaceted evaluation is essential to determine whether an individual has an intellectual disability and then to tailor individualized support plans. In line with the diagnostic criteria, the evaluation involves both an

**Table 33.1** Diagnostic criteria for intellectual disability

| | | |
|---|---|---|
| *Intellectual disability*: significant limitations in both intellectual functioning and adaptive behavior. Disability originates prior to the age of 22 years | | |
| *Intellectual functioning*: IQ score below the range of 70–75; 2 standard deviations (SD) below the population mean | | |
| *Limitations in adaptive skill areas*<br>Individuals cannot function adequately in their environment, assessed through standardized testing. Scores must fall 2 SD below the mean in one of these areas or on a combined score of all three of the following areas: | | |
| *Conceptual deficits* | *Social deficits* | *Practical deficits* |
| Receptive and expressive language, reading, writing, math, reasoning, knowledge and memory | Interpersonal communication skills, friendship, empathy, social judgment skills including gullibility, naiveté, following rules, obeying laws, avoiding victimization | Personal care activities including eating, dressing, bathing, meal preparation, telephone communication, transportation, and occupational skills including organizing school and work activities, money management, job duties |

*Source* The American Association of Intellectual and Developmental Disabilities (AAIDD) [1]

**Table 33.2** Classification of intellectual disability severity and required support

| Severity level | Intelligence quotient range | Adaptive functioning | Intensity of support needed in daily living activities |
|---|---|---|---|
| Mild | 55–70 (±5) | • Unskilled job capacity<br>• Income support<br>• Stable relationships<br>• Poor parenting skills<br>• Able to communicate by phone and in writing<br>• Decision-making: Able to make some medical, financial, and personal decisions | Intermittent:<br>Support on an as-needed basis; episodic or short-term |
| Moderate | 40–50 (±5) | • Supported employment<br>• Income support<br>• Residential supervision<br>• Help with shopping<br>• Vocabulary adequate for daily functioning<br>• Decision-making: help with medical decision-making in all areas: personal, medical, and financial | Limited:<br>Consistent over time, but time-limited |
| Severe | 25–35 (±5) | • Supervision in residential and day programs<br>• Decision-making:<br>– Unable to make most medical decisions<br>– Not capable of making financial decisions | Extensive:<br>Regular, consistent lifetime support. Regular support in at least 1 aspect such as work, home |
| Profound | Less than 20–25 | • 24-h support and supervision<br>• Nonverbal<br>• Dependent on self-care/hygiene<br>• Does not have decision-making capacity | Pervasive:<br>High intensity, across all environments, lifetime, and potentially life-sustaining |

*Sources*: DSM-5 [3]; Patel [4]

IQ test to measure intellectual functioning and a standardized test of adaptive behavior such as the Diagnostic Adaptive Behavior Scale [6]. The various levels of severity as detailed in Table 33.2 are defined on the basis of adaptive functioning, not IQ scores, because it is adaptive functioning that determines the level of support required [3, 7]. It is also important to recognize that IQ measures are less valid in the lower end of the IQ range [3]. In situations where it is difficult to assess the degree of ID, clinical judgment must be used to specify the severity.

## Etiology of Intellectual Disability

There are many diverse etiologies of intellectual disability, and this population is quite heterogenous. Conditions that result in an impairment of intellectual functioning may be related to a genetic abnormality, brain malformation, inborn errors of metabolism, or a brain injury occurring prenatally, perinatally, or in early childhood. Genetic disorders are the underlying etiology for the majority of individuals with ID. More than 500 different genetic defects have been associated with ID, and a genetic cause can be identified in more than 50% of individuals with ID referred for an evaluation [8]. The two most common genetic disorders leading to ID are Down syndrome and Fragile X Syndrome, with Down syndrome being the most commonly identified genetic cause of intellectual disability [9]. Nongenetic causes are less commonly the root of ID than genetic causes but are responsible for many of the cases of mild ID. Brain injuries resulting in impaired brain development include trauma, congenital infections, toxin exposures (i.e., maternal alcohol and polysubstance abuse), pediatric infections such as meningitis or encephalitis, or metabolic abnormalities such as congenital hypothyroidism. Fetal alcohol syndrome is the most common noninheritable cause of intellectual disability in Western countries [10]. Approximately 30–50% of children with cerebral palsy (CP) will have a concomitant intellectual disability [11].

The diagnostic evaluation to determine the etiology of ID typically occurs in childhood and fundamentally includes a review of the individual's medical and developmental history, a family history which includes construction and analysis of a pedigree with three generations, a physical and neurological evaluation, and a dysmorphology examination [12]. Based on these, the clinician may include genetic testing, other laboratory testing, imaging, or other consultations. There is debate regarding whether or not genetic testing should be offered to adults with ID who did not have the testing in childhood [13]. In one-third of individuals with ID, no underlying etiology is identified [14]. This scenario is more common in cases of mild ID given that in cases of severe ID, an etiology can be identified in greater than 75% of cases, whereas in cases of mild ID, an etiology is identified in less than 50% of cases [14]. Identification of an underlying etiology leads to improved survival and health status of individuals with ID as the healthcare and treatment are tailored to the underlying diagnosis [12]. Table 33.3 shows common etiologies of ID.

## Prevalence and Life Span

The increasing need for medical care for adults with intellectual disabilities is due to increased prevalence and increased survival to adulthood. Globally, the prevalence of intellectual disability is around 1% [15]. In the United States, the overall prevalence of ID was 0.93% in 2009–2011 and 1.17% in 2015–2017 according to results of the National Health Interview Survey [2]. The prevalence is higher among males compared to females [2, 15]. The majority of individuals with intellectual disability have mild ID, and the incidence of mild ID is higher in children of low socioeconomic status [2, 16]. The United States prevalence of ID is 11.4 per 1000 in children and 6.6 per 1000 in adults. There is a ninefold variation from state to state [1]. The number of adults with ID at 60 years and older is projected to nearly double from 641,860 in 2000 to 1.2 million by 2030 [17]. The population is growing due to increasing identification and diagnosis as well as improved survival rates related to improvements in neonatal and medical care, nutrition, and socioeconomic conditions [2, 17, 18].

The increasing life expectancy of individuals with ID follows similar trends in the general population. As with the general population, in which the average lifespan has increased from 66 years in 1950 to 78.8 years of age in 2019, the life expectancy for people with ID has increased from less than 30 in the 1930s to the mid-50 s for those with more severe disabilities or Down syndrome and to the early 70 s for adults with mild/moderate ID [19, 20]. Although the life expectancy of people with ID is increasing, it still remains lower than that of the general population; based on a study of the National Vital Statistics System 2005–2017 US Multiple Cause-of-Death Mortality files, the average age at death is 12.8 years lower than the general population for individuals with ID but without a comorbid developmental disability such as Down syndrome or cerebral palsy living in the United States [21]. As noted above, the increase in lifespan is in part attributed to improved services and living situations for people with disabilities, and as these services and resources differ among countries and between states within the USA, the average lifespan can be expected to vary greatly based on lived environment. Moreover, because adults with ID are a highly heterogeneous group, differing in degree and cause of impairment as well as biological, psy-

**Table 33.3** Intellectual disability of all etiologies [14]

| Known causes: 2/3 of individuals with ID | |
|---|---|
| Genetic causes:<br>1. Down syndrome<br>2. Fragile X syndrome<br>3. Rett syndrome<br>4. Williams syndrome<br>5. Prader–Willi<br>6. Phenylketonuria<br>7. Angelman syndrome<br>8. Other genetic causes | Nongenetic causes:<br>1. Fetal alcohol syndrome<br>2. Fetal or Neonatal Brain Injury<br>3. Infections: meningitis, rubella, etc.<br>4. Teratogenic causes<br>5. Traumatic brain injury<br>6. Autism (genetic component as well)<br>7. Seizure Disorder |
| Unknown causes: 1/3 of individuals with ID | |

chological, and social background, the life spans of those with ID are highly individualized [22]. Table 33.4 shows the prevalence and life expectancy of common etiologies of ID.

Aging starts earlier in persons with ID, and medical problems are related to the natural history of the original disability. There is a higher prevalence of some age-related diseases such as hypothyroidism, obesity, epilepsy, sensory deficits, behavioral/mental health problems, frailty, and early onset of dementia [9, 20, 23]. These medical conditions contribute to the higher rates of mortality in adults with ID. Causes of mortality are more easily identifiable if there is an underlying etiology of ID. Dementia seems to be the most important cause of morbidity and mortality in adults with Down syndrome [20]. In a study of older persons with Down syndrome, persons with a severe to profound level of ID had a higher death rate compared to those with mild to moderate ID, and those living in institutions had a higher death rate than those living in the community [24]. In adults with CP, there were higher death rates as a result of aspiration and pneumonia due to dysphagia [25]. A 2021 study utilizing the National Vital Statistics System data from 2005 to 2017 identified the most common causes of death for adults whose death certificate indicated ID and for those who did not have ID [21]. The results are detailed below in Table 33.5

**Table 33.4** Prevalence and life expectancy of common causes of intellectual disability (ID) [99–119]

| Etiology of ID | Prevalence in live births | Life expectancy (years) |
|---|---|---|
| Down syndrome | 1/700 | 47–58 (mean) |
| Cerebral palsy | 1/345 | 45–54 (median)[a] |
| Phenylketonuria | 1/10,000 | Same as the general population |
| Rett syndrome | 1/10,000–1/22,000 (females only) | 45 (median) |
| Angelman syndrome | 1/12,000–1/20,000 | Decreased by 10–15 years from the general population |
| Williams syndrome | 1/7500 | Normal to decreased based on cardiovascular or renal complications |
| Prader–Willi syndrome | 1/10,000–1/30,000 | 30–40 |
| Seizure disorder | 7.6/1000 (lifetime prevalence) | Decreased by 2–10 years compared to the general population |
| Fetal alcohol syndrome | 0.3–0.8/1000 | 34 |
| Fragile X syndrome | 1/7000 males | Same as the general population |

[a]Varies widely based on the severity of CP

**Table 33.5** Leading causes of death or people with intellectual disability (ID) compared to the general population [21]

| Leading cause of death | People with ID | General Population (%) |
|---|---|---|
| Heart disease | 15.61% | 24.61 |
| Pneumonitis due to solids and liquids | 8.86% | 0.72 |
| Influenza and pneumonia | 8.71% | 2.18 |
| Malignant neoplasms | 7.12% | 22.92 |
| Dementia/Alzheimer's | 5.07% | 7.37 |
| Choking—Aspiration, ingestion, or inhalation of gastric contents, food, or other objects | 4.68% | 0.18 |
| Cerebrovascular disease | 3.24% | 5.36 |
| Genitourinary diseases—Nephritis, nephrotic syndrome and nephrosis, urinary tract infection | 3.16% | 2.37 |
| Diabetes mellitus | 3.07% | 2.96 |
| Chronic lower respiratory diseases | 3.04% | 5.65 |
| Unknown/unspecified | 4.63% | 1.30 |

and show that the leading cause of death for both populations is heart disease; however, beyond that the causes diverge. Most important to point out is the increased risk of death from choking among adults with ID and pneumonitis/pneumonia. Recognition of this risk indicates that providers should be screening for aspiration, dysphagia and swallowing disorders in this population, making sure caregivers are aware of methods to mitigate the risk of choking. Moreover, awareness and monitoring of age-related and disease-associated risks provide opportunities to intervene and thus prolong the lives of those with ID.

Adults with intellectual disabilities are more likely to live in community-based settings rather than large institutions [26, 27]. More than 75% of adults with ID live with families with more than 25% of family care providers being over the age of 60 and 38% between the ages of 41 and 59 years [17, 28, 29]. There is an increasing need for medical care for aging adults with ID and for access to quality supports that address health and social changes [17].

## Health Status and Health Disparities in Adults with Intellectual Disabilities

Although there has been progress, adults with intellectual disabilities experience inequities in health status at a disproportionately higher rate than the general population. In 2006, AAIDD declared "there's a marked disparity of health between persons with intellectual and developmental disability and the general population" [30]. The etiology of these differences in health status for individuals with ID is multifactorial. Health disparities can be due to decreased life expectancy, increased morbidity, increased negative determinants of health such as poverty, and differences in health-care access or quality of services (see Box 33.1) [31]. These determinants highlight the impact of intersectionality on the health of this population.

**Box 33.1**
Determinants of health disparities in adults with intellectual disabilities

- Genetics.
- Social circumstances (i.e., poverty, lack of employment, and lack of social networks).
- Environmental conditions.
- Health promotion.
- Healthcare access.

Intersectionality is "a theoretical framework that posits that multiple social categories (e.g., race, ethnicity, gender, sexual orientation, socioeconomic status) intersect at the micro level of individual experience to reflect multiple interlocking systems of privilege and oppression at the macro, social-structural level (e.g., racism, sexism, heterosexism) [32]." Intersectionality plays into both the incidence of ID and the health outcomes for individuals with ID. Nongenetic risk factors for mild ID include low socioeconomic status and low maternal education [2]. These risk factors affect minority populations within the United States to a disproportionate degree due to structural racism. As far as outcomes, the average age of death for adults with ID differs based on race-ethnicity as it does in the general population, with the average age at death for non-Latinx Whites 62.7 years, non-Latinx Blacks 55.5 years, and Latinx 52.8 years [21]. These statistics highlight the intersection of disability status and race.

As previously discussed, although life expectancy in adults with ID has increased in recent years, it remains decreased compared to the general population. Individuals with ID are more likely to have certain comorbidities, such as epilepsy, psychiatric disorders, sensory impairment, poor dental hygiene, limited mobility, and gastrointestinal problems [33, 34]. Determinants of health include individual behavior, genetics, environmental exposures, and social circumstances (i.e., poverty, lack of employment opportunities and social networks, and access to healthcare) [35]. The barriers to accessing quality healthcare include a lack of formal training for health-care providers in the care of adults with ID, communication deficits between providers and patients, complex health-care-financing systems that limit access to necessary care, and health-care providers that lack awareness about the steps required to ensure that individuals with ID have access to appropriate, culturally competent care [36]. The medical complexity of adults with ID is itself a crucial barrier [37]. In 2001, "Closing the Gap: A National Blueprint to Improve the Health of Persons with Mental Retardation: report of the Surgeon General's Conference on Health Disparities and Mental Retardation" prioritized increasing sources of healthcare for people with ID [38].

It is important to distinguish three distinct types of health conditions experienced by people with ID; these conditions can all contribute to measured health disparities but reflect different points of entry along the cascade of disparities. *Associated health conditions* are medical conditions that are regarded as having led to the impairment in intellectual functioning [39]. For example, cerebral palsy, Down syndrome, fetal alcohol syndrome, and encephalitis are examples of associated health conditions leading to ID. *Secondary conditions* refer to those conditions that a person with a preexisting disability experiences at higher rates than the general population and are generally regarded as preventable [40]. For people with ID, these may include decubitus ulcers, bowel obstruction, and depression. *Comorbid conditions* refer to concomitant but unrelated pathological processes that have an adverse impact on health. Examples of comorbid conditions in individuals with ID are adverse health conditions such as cancer or hypertension. As adults with ID are living longer, all of these conditions must be addressed.

People with ID experience lower rates of preventive care and health promotion practices than the general population [40]. In order to address equity in healthcare for individuals with disabilities, the United Nations Convention on the rights of persons with disabilities was updated in 2006. Article 25 of the convention outlines that persons with disabilities have the right to the following:

1. The same quality of free or affordable healthcare as the general population.
2. Health services that are specific to their disabilities, including early identification and intervention, with services designed to minimize and prevent further disabilities.
3. Health services as close as possible to people's own communities.
4. Care of the same quality, including ethical considerations of informed consent by raising awareness of the human rights, dignity, autonomy, and needs of persons with disabilities through training.
5. The provision of health insurance and life insurance that is permitted by national law and shall be provided in a fair and reasonable manner [37, 41].

In summary, there have been significant efforts to address the health-care needs and status of people with intellectual disabilities across their life spans. Adults with ID more fully participate in their communities when they are not constrained by poor health and can access health-care resources to address conditions affecting their health status [42, 43].

## Common Medical Considerations in Providing Care for Adults with Intellectual Disabilities

Medical conditions in individuals with ID differ from those that occur in the general population with regard to prevalence, age of onset, rate of progression, degree of severity, and presentation. Additionally, they are likely to be multiple and complex conditions [44].

Primary care providers (PCPs) are essential for the care of individuals with ID in that they provide continuous health-care services, interact regularly with caregivers, integrate psychological and social factors, and coordinate subspecialty and interdisciplinary health services. Their role is critical for early detection, disease prevention, and chronic management [45].

Because the definition of ID is broad, the etiology of ID guides the management of chronic diseases as well as preventive services—for example, management of mobility issues, urinary tract infections, and dysphagia in patients with CP, or hypothyroidism in those with Down syndrome (for additional information, please see Chaps. 25 and 30). There are many conditions that are common to most people with intellectual disability. The revised Canadian Consensus Guidelines from 2011 summarize evidenced-based data in providing primary care for adults with intellectual disabilities [45]. Other resources for health maintenance guidelines are the Massachusetts DDS Health Screening Recommendations and the guidelines provided by AAIDD [1, 46].

## Communication

Effective communication is foundational to high-quality medical care for all patients and is legally required under the Americans with Disabilities Act, but poor communication can present an especially magnified barrier to the care for people with disabilities [47]. First, a note about language; as stated above, the preferred term to refer to people with a cognitive impairment is "intellectual disability." Many in the disability rights movement previously championed "person-first language," which prioritizes acknowledging the personhood of the individual in lieu of the diagnosis with the structure "person with a disability." However, in more recent years "identity-first language" has arisen with the goal of acknowledging the person's disability as being a permanent and important part of their identity and with the structure "disabled person." As with all shades of identity, it is important to ask the individual what they prefer.

Another important aspect of communication is clarifying to whom you should refer to during an encounter. It is important to always refer to the individual with the disability first, ask them who they are with, and clarify to whom the provider should direct their questions. Even if the patient does not communicate verbally, they may use alternative methods of communication to direct the conversation. Many individuals with disabilities report experiences where providers direct the questions to the support person who they have brought to the visit instead of the patient themselves, even though they are independent in medical decision-making [47]. Directly communicate with the adult with ID unless instructed otherwise. In the case discussed at the beginning of this chapter, Mr. C.B. has dysarthria and is difficult to understand. He reported that when he was seen in an urgent care setting for a urinary tract infection, the results of his urinalysis were given to his brother who accompanied him rather than directly to him. As with patients in the general population, the provider communicating directly with each patient is essential to developing mutual respect and trust. It is important not to assume and to clarify before directing questions and making medical decisions. As with patients in the general population, the provider communicating directly with each patient is essential to developing mutual respect and trust.

Providers often obtain information from individuals who accompany them to their appointments. However, these individuals may not be the primary caregivers and may not be able to provide essential information. Thus, each provider should know the identity of the caregiver accompanying the patient and know their relationship and depth of interaction. As individuals with ID have medically complex conditions, it is important to communicate with caregivers most familiar with the individual either during the span of a clinic visit or afterward.

Finally, it is important to make sure that the patient understands as much of the clinical encounter and medical decision-making as possible. For people with an intellectual disability, this may require explaining the situation in multiple different ways, using drawings or visual aids, or simplifying the scenario. While not all individuals with ID are able to make their own medical decisions, they should still be involved in the conversation as much as possible.

## Unique Considerations for the Office Visit

It is important to assess the *living situation* of the individual with ID during each visit. Individuals with ID live in a variety of settings with varying degrees of ability to care for themselves. They may live with family members, independently, or in shared-living situations with supervised help versus structured group homes. Changes in living situations are a common cause of upheaval that may impact well-being and behavior. Some additional social, physical, and behavior barriers to providing medical care for patients with ID are notable.

*Physical challenges* can affect both the adults with ID and the providers. For example, individuals who require wheelchairs may have difficulty in accessing a health-care facility or with gynecological exams. Additionally, *behavioral issues* may impact the quality of healthcare delivery for those with ID. Prior negative experiences with providers, clinics, and hospitals may engender fear and anxiety. Such emotions may negatively impact the individual's cooperation for exams, tests, or injections. With respect to the patient, a provider must be open to rescheduling or modifying a nonemergent procedure or test when a patient expresses anxiety.

In addition to the aforementioned challenges, barriers from the provider's perspective include lack of formal training in caring for adults with ID, time constraints, reduced reimbursement, and difficulty in obtaining informed consent [48, 49]. Providers may require a longer visit to examine contractures or evaluate for decubitus ulcers. Many patients with ID have insurance plans with reduced reimbursement schedules. In a busy clinical practice where revenue is a consideration, this provides a challenge. Strategies for providers to improve a clinic visit include a chart review prior to the visit and making goals for the visit. Some portions of the exam may need to be deferred to a future visit. Additionally, a short-acting benzodiazepine for anxiety may facilitate obtaining blood work or other testing [48, 49].

Providers should routinely assess the medication regimen. *Polypharmacy* is common for the ID population; many have numerous medications and they often are prescribed by multiple providers. Medication reconciliation at each visit helps to sort out medication use, capacity to follow the medication regimen, and provide assistance required to support medication compliance. A review of *vaccinations* at the initial visit is essential. Adults with ID receive vaccinations at a lower rate than the general population. Individuals in group homes typically have the highest rate of vaccination among adults with ID as they follow state-based regulations. Adults with ID living at home with family have the lowest rates of vaccination [50]. Individuals transitioning from pediatrics typically have extensive records. For individuals who do not have documentation, it is important to check titers and update accordingly [48].

## Medical Considerations

*Physical inactivity and obesity* are common among adults with ID and have been documented in multiple studies [50, 51]. Obesity in adults with ID is associated with adverse outcomes, such as cardiovascular disease, diabetes, osteoporosis, constipation, and early mortality [52]. It is crucial for primary care providers to monitor body mass index and to involve caregivers, regional service coordination agencies, and other health professionals to promote a healthy lifestyle [53].

*Vision impairments* are common in adults with ID. The most common cause of decreased vision in individuals with ID is refractive errors, including hyperopia (farsightedness), myopia (nearsightedness), and astigmatism [54]. Strabismus, cataracts, and keratoconus are also more common in individuals with ID than those without ID [54]. Individuals with ID should have annual vision screening in the office and be referred for vision assessments to detect glaucoma and cataracts every 5 years after the age of 45.

*Hearing impairments* are also much more prevalent in adults with ID. In adults with severe ID, changes in behavior and adaptive functioning may be clues to a worsening or a new hearing or vision impairment. Cerumen impaction is a common cause of decreased hearing sensation. Assess for cerumen impaction every 6 months. Referral should be made to audiology for hearing assessment if indicated by screening (change in behavior and decreased communication) and for age-related hearing loss every 5 years after the age of 45 [45].

*Oral health* problems such as dental caries, gingivitis, and periodontal disease are among the top 10 secondary conditions among individuals with ID that cause limitations in their daily activities [33]. Primary care providers should promote dental hygiene practices and referral to a dental professional. Cleaning is recommended every 6 months. Complicated dental procedures may require sedation, and it is important for the primary care provider to identify state-specific Department of Human and Health Services resources for dentists who provide services to adults with intellectual and developmental disabilities [46].

Even in those with the most severe impairment, maintaining *musculoskeletal health* is strongly linked to survival into adulthood [55]. Scoliosis, contractures, and spasticity occur frequently in individuals with ID and can lead to pain, reduced mobility, and adverse health outcomes including decreased quality of life [45, 55]. Additionally, osteoarthritis is becoming more prevalent as adults with ID are living longer and is a common cause of pain leading to behavioral changes [55]. The need for physical or occupational therapy services should be assessed annually and when there is functional decline. The need for durable medical equipment including a new wheelchair, modified seating plans, or orthotic devices should also be periodically assessed.

*Seizure disorders* are common among individuals with intellectual disability and can increase with the severity of the intellectual disability. Typically, individuals with seizure disorders are under the care of a neurologist. The role of the primary care provider is to monitor the effects of antiepileptic medications. This involves not only checking levels but also monitoring for bone loss/osteoporosis. Phenytoin, a common antiepileptic, can cause significant bone loss over time, at a much higher rate than phenobarbital or carbamazepine. It is important to screen for osteoporosis more frequently among individuals with ID compared to the general population [31].

*Cardiac considerations* include assessing for congenital heart disease when intellectual disability is associated with certain genetic conditions such as Down syndrome and Williams syndrome. Antibiotic prophylaxis may be required for those individuals who meet criteria [45, 56].

*Respiratory disorders* are common in adults with ID. These include dysphagia and aspiration. Dysphagia is prevalent in up to 5% of individuals with ID. Adults with CP have a high death rate as a result of aspiration pneumonia [25]. If the individual with ID has symptoms of coughing and choking with meals, a referral for a speech therapy evaluation should be provided.

*Gastrointestinal and feeding problems* are common as well. Adults with ID have an increased risk of poor nutrition. A retrospective study on individuals with severe to profound ID in the UK showed the importance of nutrition and the improvement in body weight as a result of dietetic referrals. Better nutrition also led to other improvements in medical conditions, including resolution of amenorrhea, improved diarrhea, increased balance and mobility, and improvement in pressure sores [57].

Gastroesophageal reflux disease due to upper gastrointestinal dysmotility is common among individuals with ID. It is more prevalent in individuals with gastrostomy tubes. As it is difficult to identify reflux symptoms in profound ID, providers must evaluate for changes in behavior or adaptive functioning. There is a higher frequency of *Helicobacter pylori* infection in adults with ID than those in the general population [58]. Screening for *H. pylori* infection is recommended in symptomatic or asymptomatic adults with ID who are in group homes at a frequency of every 3–5 years [58].

*Constipation* has been reported in up to 40% of individuals with ID, often exacerbated by immobility or a lack of exercise [59]. Medications with anticholinergic effects may be contributing as well. An aggressive bowel regimen is important in preventing and treating constipation and has been shown to reduce the incidence of impaction and intestinal obstruction. A necessary strategy is a daily regimen of fiber, increasing fluids, and stool softeners. Frequent laxatives may be necessary, and tolerance to stimulant laxatives is less of a concern than the complications of untreated constipation [60].

*Hypothyroidism* is common in adults with ID and occurs with a much higher frequency in associated conditions such as Down syndrome (see Chap. 30: Down syndrome). It also occurs more frequently in individuals taking lithium or atypical or second-generation antipsychotic medications [45]. For individuals taking these medications, a primary care provider should establish a baseline thyroid screening test and check annually.

*Osteoporosis* is more prevalent in adults with ID, including in premenopausal women and in men [61]. A review of women with ID highlighted risk factors for osteoporosis including inactivity, long-term anticonvulsant use, CP, and possibly Down syndrome [62]. Low vitamin D level is an additional risk factor [63]. Earlier screening than the general population is recommended; age 40 for individuals who are institutionalized and age 45 for individuals who live in the community [63].

## Sexual Health

A common bias among health care providers is to view people with ID as asexual. This bias has contributed to decreased screening for STIs and cervical cancer in this population and less discussion about sexuality and sexual health overall. Assessing sexual health and appropriate screenings need to be a regular part of the primary care visit. This is especially important because people with ID are at increased risk of sexual violence and abuse. Because most sexual abuse is perpetrated by individuals close to the victim, consider interviewing the patient alone without anyone else in the room when circumstances allow.

Providers uniformly agree on a variety of reasons to provide *contraception*. Multiple studies described that people with ID are sexually victimized more often than others who do not have a disability [64]. One study reported that 25% of girls and women with intellectual disability who were referred for birth control had a history of sexual violence [65]. Communication and behavioral disorders contribute to very high levels of risk, and having multiple disabilities (e.g., intellectual disability and behavior disorders) results in even higher risk levels [66]. Another reason for contraception is therapeutic amenorrhea to treat dysmenorrhea/menorrhagia or for individuals who are frightened or for whom hygiene issues are difficult.

Just as with the general population, some women with ID desire pregnancy and some will have unplanned pregnancies [67]. It is important to honor the desires and decisions of the adult with ID whenever possible, but this also requires very detailed discussions with the individual and everyone in their family about how parenthood would affect everyone involved. Although views on this topic within society and medicine have evolved considerably, the experience of forced or coerced sterilization among those with ID and other disabilities in the not-so-distant past underscores the importance of providers advocating for the sexual and reproductive health of their patients.

For those women with ID who are sexually active, providers must counsel and screen for sexually transmitted infections (STIs). As with the general population, women with ID should also undergo pelvic examinations as appropriate to evaluate symptoms such as menorrhagia, dysmenorrhea, and pelvic pain.

## Behavioral and Mental Health Considerations

Aggressive, challenging behavior is frequently reported in adults with ID. Antipsychotic medications are frequently used, although evidence for their benefit is limited. A 2002 study examined the quality of preventive and psychiatric services for intellectually disabled adults living in California in 1997 [50]. One-third of the individuals in their study received psychotropic medications, but only 24% of these individuals had received psychiatric consultations. Despite the polypharmacy of psychotropic medications, 36% of this group did not have an identifiable diagnosis. A randomized trial comparing risperidone, haloperidol, and placebo in the treatment of aggressive challenging behavior in patients with intellectual disability did not show any clinically significant differences among the three study groups [68]. The authors concluded that antipsychotic drugs should no longer be regarded as an acceptable routine treatment for aggressive challenging behavior in people with intellectual disabilities.

The role of primary care providers is to screen for new behavioral issues or worsening of a previously well-controlled behavior disorder at each clinic visit. If new or worsening behavior patterns are identified, the provider pursues an evaluation of underlying medical causes or associated conditions leading to behavioral changes. Pain and distress are common causes of behavioral changes and can be assessed with a caregiver's help as well as pain assessment tools adapted for adults with ID [69]. There are multiple primary care toolkits to assess behavior changes provided by the American Academy of Pediatrics and Got Transition. These assessments include evaluation of physical, environmental, and emotional factors. While not comprehensive, Table 33.6 describes components of a primary care checklist to evaluate behavioral/emotional concerns [69–71].

The primary care provider should also be routinely monitoring psychotropic medications for side effects such as weight gain and QT prolongation. Phenothiazines such as haloperidol and chlorpromazine are generally accepted to cause QT prolongation with an increased risk for reentrant tachycardias. Other commonly used antipsychotics that can possibly cause QT prolongation include risperidone, quetiapine, and lithium. Periodic electrocardiogram (EKG) monitoring is prudent [72]. Box 33.2 describes considerations during the initial and then subsequent visits for evaluating the individual with intellectual disability.

**Box 33.2**
Multidisciplinary care at initial visit and then annual updates

- Guardianship assessment.
- Residential environment:
  - Home with family.
  - Independent living with support.
  - Group home.
- Medical evaluation:
  - Management of associated, comorbid, and secondary conditions.
  - Health screening, vaccines.
  - Behavioral evaluation.
  - Sexual health.
- Assess for polypharmacy.
- Subspecialty evaluation:
  - Orthopedics: musculoskeletal issues such as contractures, scoliosis.

**Table 33.6** Primary care evaluation of agitation/behavioral changes in adults with ID [69]

| Physical | Environmental | Emotional |
|---|---|---|
| • Medical conditions leading to pain: Peptic ulcer disease, dental pain, musculoskeletal disorders, arthritis, spasticity<br>• Infections: e.g., pneumonia, urinary tract infection<br>• Medication adverse effects<br>• Constipation<br>• Sensory discomfort: New clothes, shoes<br>• New hearing/vision impairment<br>• Hypothyroidism | • Reduced supports; loss of staffing<br>• Change in residence<br>• Changes in routines<br>• Lack of adequate communication with family, friends, caregivers<br>• Lack of activities | Depression or anxiety due to:<br>• Addition of a new roommate or sibling<br>• Loss of a parent/ caregiver<br>• Social isolation |

  - Neurology: seizure disorders.
  - Psychiatry: behavior disorders.
- Dental evaluation.
- Ophthalmology/hearing evaluation.
- Occupational/physical/speech therapy needs.
- Durable medical equipment.
- Assess for caregiver stress.
- Need for respite services.
- Social services referral.

## Health Maintenance/Preventive Health

As individuals transition to adulthood, the American Academy of Pediatrics (AAP), American College of Physicians (ACP), and American Academy of Family Physicians (AAFP) recommend applying the same guidelines for primary and preventive care for all adolescents and young adults, including those with special health care needs. Examples of such guidelines include the American Medical Association's *Guidelines for Adolescent Preventive Services (GAPS)* and the US Public Health Service's Guidelines for Clinical Preventive Services (USPSTF) [38, 73].

Effective health screening requires that a disease must be serious and have important consequences, that early intervention will improve outcomes, that a preclinical phase has a long duration and can be easily identified by a screening test, and that the disease is prevalent in the screened population. In adults with ID, the prevalence of various diseases is often not known, and these individuals may have a longer preclinical phase since limitations in cognitive functioning can make it difficult to identify symptoms. Even if early intervention is possible, it may be difficult to implement treatment [74]. Additionally, there are often barriers to screening in adults with ID including anxiety, lack of understanding of the test, and requirements for additional family members or extra staff from residential facilities to accompany individuals for these procedures [49].

### Cardiovascular Screening

As with the general population, the leading cause of death for adults with ID is heart disease. However, while individuals with ID develop heart disease at rates similar to or higher than the general population, they are less likely to be prescribed guideline-based pharmacotherapy for heart failure and atherosclerotic disease [75, 76]. As previously discussed, among individuals with ID, there is a higher rate of overweight/obesity, which are individual risk factors for developing cardiovascular disease. According to a 2020 meta-analysis, more than one in five individuals with ID have metabolic syndrome [77]. There is also a higher incidence among adults with ID of gum disease, which has also been shown to increase the risk for CVD [78]. It is important to provide the same screenings for risk factors for cardiovascular disease including hypertension, hyperlipidemia, and diabetes as recommended by the USPSTF guidelines [79]. Blood pressure should be checked at each clinic visit and then annually, lipids assessed at approximately 18 years of age and then every 5 years depending on other risk factors, and glycosylated hemoglobin levels followed every 3 years beginning at 45 years of age—earlier if at higher risk [80]. As with the general population, smoking cessation should be encouraged [81]. Furthermore, engagement in structured exercise programs has been shown to improve CV risk factors as well as improve self-efficacy [82, 83].

### Cervical Cancer Screening

People with ID are significantly less likely than the general population to be up to date on Papaniculou (Pap) screening as recommended by the USPSTF guidelines [84]. The majority of cervical cancers are caused by the sexually transmitted human papilloma virus (HPV), and there have been studies in the past suggesting that women with ID have lower rates of sexual activity than the general population [85]. However, the sexual histories of people with ID may be less accurate due to physician biases expecting the asexuality of this population and communication barriers. Moreover, this population is at increased risk of sexual victimization, so pap smears are recommended for routine screening at the same intervals as for the general population [79]. Positioning may be difficult in obtaining a Pap smear or performing a pelvic exam for people with physical disabilities, please see Chap. 7 for augmented positioning. After obtaining the initial Papanicolaou test, additional screening should be individualized based on a woman's sexual history rather than her cognitive ability.

## Breast Cancer Screening

Primary care providers should obtain mammograms for women with ID at the same frequency as for the general population. In general, women with ID are less likely to have children and to breastfeed. These factors may increase their risk for breast cancer. Two studies from England and Australia showed that only one-third of eligible women with ID were screened due to low rates of physician referral [86]. A US study also found that women with ID were significantly less likely to be up to date on breast cancer screening compared to the general population [87]. As women with ID live longer, the primary care provider should make every effort to obtain mammograms at regular intervals. Providers may need to advocate for patients to make sure that mammograms are physically accessible for patients with disabilities. Similarly, studies show that women with disabilities face disparities in breast cancer treatment and survival compared to the general population; primary care doctors should be aware of this disparity and advocate for their patients [88].

## Colon Cancer Screening

Colorectal cancer incidence may be slightly higher in people with ID, and screening practices are underused in this population [89]. One factor that may contribute to both of these trends is that constipation is a common problem for adults with ID and this makes the onset of colon cancer symptoms difficult to evaluate. The recommendation to pursue colon cancer screening in adults with ID is the same as that for the general population. Some adults with ID may require general anesthesia for the colonoscopy.

## Sedation

Some adults with ID may require sedation for health screening procedures. In an ideal setting, primary care providers and subspecialty colleagues can coordinate services to perform multiple procedures such as routine phlebotomy, immunizations, dental examinations, and gynecologic exams while the patient is under sedation. As adults with ID are living longer, it is important to maintain the same screening guidelines to maintain the same quality of life as the general population.

## Ethical Considerations

For adults with ID, providers often consider the concept of quality of life when making treatment decisions regarding both management of chronic medical conditions as well as for performing health maintenance procedures. The quality of life (QOL) construct has been examined by several researchers. The key to self-report of quality of life among people with disabilities is accurate modified instrumentation [90]. Studies have shown that individuals with disabilities can accurately assess their quality of life [36, 90]. The public opinion of individuals with disabilities was described in one 2010 study as: "Non-disabled people believe that the quality of life of people who live with disabilities is extremely low… When disabled people report about their own QOL, they rate it as only slightly lower than when non-disabled people self-report their own QOL" [91]. Health-care professionals' opinion of QOL of people with disabilities is lower than both the opinion of the general public and the disabled individual's own opinion of QOL [91, 92]. Health-care professionals must be aware of this bias concerning individuals with intellectual disabilities when discussing treatment options for medical conditions as well as for preventive measures.

The informed consent and decision-making process varies depending on the degree of intellectual disabilities. Individuals with moderate to severe intellectual disabilities typically do not have the decision-making capacity to comply with the principles of informed consent. The substitute decision-maker is required to make a decision based on the best interest of the individual with ID. A "bonded" guardian is an individual who has a previous relationship with the patient, such as a parent or caregiver. A non-bonded guardian is typically someone appointed through the courts. Providers typically prefer bonded guardians as they are better able to incorporate a patient's wishes into the health-care decision-making process [93]. As with the general population, end-of-life issues should be addressed prior to the occurrence of a life-threatening event. ID alone should not be a reason to forgo medical treatments for complicated conditions such as end-stage renal disease requiring dialysis, cancer, or organ transplantation. For those with mild to moderate intellectual disability, it is important to remember that even if they are not capable of some aspects of decision-making (such as financial management), it does not mean that they are unable to participate in their health care decision-making process. Individuals with ID can still convey their wishes based on a lifetime pattern of expressing their needs to their caregivers, who, in turn, can make the best decision for the individual. Providers must take this into consideration when making treatment decisions to improve quality of life by maintaining health and prolonging life [93].

## Inpatient Considerations

### Inpatient Case Presentation

Mr. S is a 41-year-old man with DiGeorge syndrome, intellectual disability, diabetes mellitus, diastolic dysfunction, and ESRD status-post two kidney transplants (1995 and 2019) with recent worsening of kidney graft function presenting from his nursing home with increased work of breathing. In the emergency room, he is started on low-flow nasal cannula (LFNC) oxygen and diagnosed with COVID-19 pneumonia. The transplant team is consulted, and the patient is admitted to general medicine for management. Due to the worsening renal function, hemodialysis is initiated after admission. Mr. S is verbal but has difficulty describing his symptoms, so most of the history is taken by calling the nurse at his nursing home; she reports that his shortness of breath started 2 days prior to admission and was accompanied by fevers, decreased appetite, and malaise. He has been living at the nursing home for the last year after his brother and guardian were charged with neglect for failing to give Mr. S his anti-rejection medications, leading to worsening graft function. The day after admission, Mr. S is breathing comfortably on 2–5 liters of oxygen/minute per LFNC and is being treated with dexamethasone for COVID-19. During the admission, he intermittently removes the nasal cannula from his nose with accompanying desaturation, although he will quickly replace the cannula himself when asked to by the medical staff. The medical team is unable to contact his brother, and the nursing home does not have documentation of another power of attorney (POA) or surrogate decision-maker. The medical team tries to contact other family members but is unsuccessful, so they are working on obtaining a state-appointed guardian.

On the fourth day of admission, he points to his chest and says it hurts. The team orders an EKG and troponin levels that are both within normal limits. He is empirically started on a heparin drip due to concern for pulmonary embolism while a computerized tomography scan with contrast is deferred due to his worsening renal function. A chest radiograph is stable when compared to his admissions imaging. That evening he has an increased oxygen requirement and is started on high-flow nasal cannula (HFNC) oxygen. In the early morning, he has a prolonged episode of desaturation, and the nurse goes to his room to find him less responsive with the HFNC out of his nose. The HFNC is replaced, and he returns to baseline. Due to this "near-miss" event, the team asks for a sitter to remain in his room and make sure he keeps the HFNC in his nose until his oxygen requirement decreases. Over the next few weeks, his oxygen requirement decreases, and he is ultimately discharged back to the nursing home on LFNC.

## Case Discussion

This case brings to light many important issues including in-hospital monitoring of the Person with Disability (PWD), obtaining a baseline status for hospitalized individuals, communication, decision-making, and disparity in outcomes. As far as in-hospital monitoring, this patient may have benefited from closer monitoring and possibly a sitter from the outset of his admission. The patient needed frequent reminders to replace the HFNC in his nose, especially as he required higher and higher liters of oxygen flow. Sitters are a very limited resource in the hospital; however, this population in particular needs close monitoring for safety and compliance, and a sitter should be considered when compliance with treatment is so necessary.

Another common issue for inpatient care of PWDs is that the providers often do not know the individual patient's baseline abilities and communication skills. Providers will often assume that someone with a visible disability is nonverbal or unable to make their own decisions. For this patient, the emergency room providers did not talk to him at all because they did not think he was able to communicate verbally. When a PWD presents to the hospital, they may be very sick and not as interactive as they are at baseline, reinforcing these biases. Limiting these assumptions, checking biases, and talking to the patient and the people who know the patient best can lead to enhanced mutual respect and trust as well as improved health outcomes. If the inpatient provider had not learned that the patient was verbal and inquired about his preferred communication strategies, she would not have learned of his new onset chest pain. Even when PWDs are not verbal or are limitedly verbal, their family members and caregivers can often give advice on how to read the person's expressions and nonverbal cues to learn when something is bothering them versus when they are comfortable.

The other difficult thing about this case was decision-making and guardianship. Providers should always be observant of the abuse and neglect of PWD as they are especially at risk. Because of the existence of neglect in this case, it was very difficult to find a surrogate decision-maker since the patient was not consentable. The nursing home had been functioning without a surrogate decision-maker. This is not a tenable situation, and the process to find an appropriate decision-maker should have been initiated when they assumed his care. The process for identifying a surrogate decision-maker varies by state, but if one cannot be identified, a state guardian needs to be appointed. This is a long process and often requires the help of social work.

Finally, this case highlights how PWDs have been disproportionately affected by the COVID-19 pandemic. People with ID have a higher risk of mortality from COVID-19 than the general population, even when controlling for comorbidities. This may be in part due to the structural vulnerabilities that this population faces, including congregate living and lack of preventive healthcare as previously reviewed. However, ableism may also contribute, as providers may offer less aggressive care to people with disabilities if they assume they have lower health status and poorer quality of life at baseline [94]. This theory is supported by studies showing people with an intellectual disability and COVID-19 were less likely to have care escalated by being admitted to the ICU [95]. The first step to combatting ableism is for providers to recognize their biases. It may prove beneficial to engage the family, caregivers, and primary care doctors in helping to paint a picture of how the PWD enjoyed life prior to the hospitalization and to make sure medical care offered is not affected by the patient's disability status.

## Inpatient Management

Individuals with ID experience high rates of hospitalization for ambulatory-sensitive conditions and high rates of hospitalizations in general, even when in formal community care systems [96]. During these more frequent hospitalizations, people with intellectual disabilities often have poor hospital experiences [97]. Some ways to improve hospital experiences and outcomes include optimizing communication, addressing biases, frequently engaging caregivers, and carefully monitoring medications.

When first meeting a person with ID, it can be very difficult for a provider to discern the patient's ability to communicate their history and symptoms. It is important for providers to avoid making assumptions about the ability to communicate and intellectual functioning based on the person's appearance and initial presentation; such assumptions can lead to the provider addressing a personal assistant instead of the patient or to the provider concluding that a person with a communication disability also has an intellectual disability when they do not. As previously mentioned in the section on Communication, providers should always address the person who is the patient first and ask clarifying questions to them and those around them to clearly ascertain who they prefer to speak to and what their preferred communication strategies include. Once these preferences are clarified, they should be clearly documented in the patient's chart and all consulting providers should be made aware of whom they should talk to and how they can make the patient most comfortable.

In addition to considering the previously discussed bias of ableism, it is also important for the inpatient provider to consider contact bias. Contact bias may result when the provider has not had sustained contact with the PWD so they are just meeting them for the first time and by virtue of seeing a patient only when they are hospitalized, they are seeing the patient at their worst. It can be difficult for an inpatient provider to picture what any person was like prior to the hospitalization when they were well, but that may be especially true when encountering PWDs because they have such diverse life experiences. Inpatient providers may find themselves thinking that PWDs do not have a rich and engaged life because of their disability and because they look so ill on presentation. These assumptions may lead them to treat the PWD as though they are elderly or closer to the end of life and thus suggest more comfort care measures than aggressive care. Providers can check these biases by asking the patient and their caregivers about what kinds of activities the PWD enjoys in their regular life and getting a better picture of their life outside of the hospital. Providers should also engage the patient, their caregivers, and the primary care physician in the treatment decisions and any discussions of goals of care.

A person with ID may behave much differently when hospitalized than they do outside of the hospital given that part of their condition includes difficulty with adaptive behavior. As a result, they have a much harder time adjusting to the unknown and often stress-invoking environment of the hospital. This may lead to difficult behaviors such as not complying with treatments. As mentioned previously, if compliance with treatment like keeping an oxygen cannula in place is imperative, it is recommended to consider a sitter when family members cannot be present. It may be beneficial to closely engage family members and caregivers in the inpatient management and ask them how to make the individual more comfortable in the hospital, such as whether they like certain music or movies. Sedatives and restraints should be avoided as these can worsen behavior and may be unnecessarily cruel. Providers should consider involving care services such as Child Life, as they may have distracting toys and methods to employ, especially during painful or long procedures.

Lastly, specific issues regarding medication use in this population should be reviewed. As already mentioned, some people with ID are on psychotropic medications. It is especially important to double-check and continue all home medications for this population, as sudden changes in these doses may cause a severe worsening in symptoms and behaviors. Moreover, care should be taken when initiating any new medications as their metabolism may be different in PWDs than among the general population.

## Community Resources

The 1999 Supreme Court ruling in Olmstead vs L.C. held that the unjustified institutionalization of individuals with disabilities is a form of discrimination under the Americans with Disabilities Act of 1990 [27]. This paved the way for an increase in state funding for community resources that support individuals with disabilities. The Developmental Disabilities Assistance and Bill of Rights Act of 2000, or "DD Act," is the law that provides financial assistance and structure for state-by-state resources for individuals with disabilities and their families. This law authorizes three programs that operate in each state and territory: the Developmental Disabilities Council, the University Centers for Excellence in Developmental Disabilities, and the Protection and Advocacy Systems. All of these agencies work together to "assure that individuals with developmental disabilities and their families participate in the design of and have access to needed community services, individualized supports, and other forms of assistance that promote self-determination, independence, productivity, and integration and inclusion in all facets of community life." [98] Providers can find their state's agencies and information on local resources, services, advocacy, and legislation at https://www.aucd.org. In addition, olmsteadrights.org organizes resources for individuals with disabilities by state.

Each adult with an ID should register with their state's Department of Human Services section or division that supports adults with intellectual or developmental disabilities. These offices can help the individual apply for and receive Long-Term Support Services (LTSS) through Home and Community-Based Services (HCBS) waivers so that they can best maintain independence and thrive in community living. These waivers provide services such as homemakers, home health aides, adult day programs, and respite care through Medicaid funding. The wait-list for these services varies by state but on average is 2.5 years, so it is important to sign up as soon as possible. Each state also has an Aging and Disability Resource Center (ADRC) ( https://www.adrc-tae.acl.gov ), which is a database of community resources broken down by area.

## Conclusions

Adults with intellectual disabilities have complex medical conditions differing from the general population. Aging starts earlier in persons with ID, and medical problems are related to the natural history of the original disability ("Appendix"). It is essential to screen for medical conditions that occur at an equal or higher prevalence than in the general population to avoid morbidity complications and premature death. As adults with intellectual disabilities are living longer due to improved medical care, technology, and environmental conditions, they require the same considerations for improving quality of life, improving access to health care, and health screening as the general population. The goal is to provide the same quality of healthcare for adults with intellectual disability by raising awareness of the human rights, dignity, autonomy, and needs of persons with disabilities through training and implementation of ethical standards for public and private healthcare.

## Appendix

<table>
<tr><th colspan="3">Intellectual disability (ID) condition fact sheet</th></tr>
<tr><td>Definition</td><td colspan="2">Intellectual disability (ID) is a lifelong neurodevelopmental condition characterized by the following:<br>IQ score below the range of 70–75; 2 standard deviations (SD) below the mean<br>Limitations in adaptive skill areas; 2 SD below the mean in 1 of these areas or in combination of all 3 areas:<br>• Conceptual deficits: Receptive and expressive language, reading, writing, math, reasoning, knowledge, and memory<br>• Social deficits: Interpersonal communication skills, friendship, empathy, social judgment skills including gullibility, naiveté, following rules, obeying laws, avoiding victimization<br>• Practical deficits: Personal care activities including eating, dressing, bathing, meal preparation, telephone communication, transportation, and occupational skills including organizing school and work activities, money management, job duties<br>These limitations must be present prior to the age of 18 years</td></tr>
<tr><td>Epidemiology</td><td colspan="2">• Prevalence of ID is estimated at ~1% of the population in the U.S. and Western European countries.<br>• Although the life expectancy of people with ID is increasing, it is still lower than that of the general population, with an average age at death of ~66 years<br>• Many individuals with ID have an underlying etiology; genetic and nongenetic causes<br>• Aging starts earlier in persons with ID and medical problems are related to the natural history of the original disability<br>• More than 75% of adults with ID live with families<br>• More than 25% of family care providers are over the age of 60<br>• Increasing need for medical care for aging adults with ID and their families and for access to quality supports that address health and social changes</td></tr>
<tr><td rowspan="2">Special considerations</td><td colspan="2">Individuals with intellectual disability have a higher prevalence of physical and mental health conditions, including the following:</td></tr>
<tr><td>• Physical inactivity/obesity<br>• Vision impairments: Refractive errors, hyperopia, myopia<br>• Hearing impairments<br>• Oral health problems: Dental caries, gingivitis, and periodontal disease<br>• Musculoskeletal problems<br>• Seizure disorder</td><td>• Congenital heart disease<br>• Respiratory conditions: Dysphagia, aspiration<br>• Gastrointestinal problems: Gastroesophageal reflux disease, H. Pylori infection<br>• Osteoporosis<br>• Anxiety and depression</td></tr>
<tr><td>Recommended preventive screening</td><td colspan="2">• Vision: Annually, glaucoma, and cataract screening every 5 years after age 45<br>• Hearing exams: Age-related reduced hearing every 5 years after age 45<br>• Cerumen impaction; assess every 6 months<br>• Dental evaluation: Cleaning every 6 months<br>• Osteoporosis screening: Age 40 in a group home, 45 if in the community, modify based on condition, e.g., cerebral palsy and anticonvulsant therapy.<br>• Cardiovascular screening: Same as USPSTF guidelines<br>Hypertension: BP each visit, annually<br>Diabetes: Glycosylated hemoglobin every 3 years >45, if risk factors, start <45<br>BMI: Counsel regularly<br>Lipids: Initial 18+, then every 5 years<br>• Thyroid function: At the initial visit, if on psychotropic medications, annually, modify based on conditions, e.g., down syndrome<br>Cancer screening:<br>• Breast cancer: Same as in the USPSTF guidelines<br>• COLON cancer: No modifications from USPSTF guidelines<br>• Cervical cancer: After the initial Papanicolaou smear, modify based on sexual history</td></tr>
</table>

## References


1. Schalock RL, Luckasson R, Tasse MJ. An overview of intellectual disability: definition, diagnosis, classification, and systems of supports. Am J Intellect Dev Disabil. 2021;126(6):439–42.
2. Zablotsky B, Black LI, Maenner M, Schieve LA, Danielson ML, Bitsko RH, et al. Prevalence and trends of developmental disabilities among children in the United States: 2009-2017. Pediatrics. 2019;144(4):e20190811.
3. Diagnostic and statistical manual of mental disorders. DSM-5™, 5th ed, in diagnostic and statistical manual of mental disorders: DSM-5™. 5th ed. Arlington, VA: American Psychiatric Publishing, Inc.; 2013. p. xliv, 947.
4. Patel D, Merrick J. In: Patel D, et al., editors. Intellectual disability, in neurodevelopmental disabilities: clinical care for children and young adults. New York, New York: Springer; 2011.
5. U.S. Department of Education. Individuals with disabilities education ACT (ACT). Washington, DC: US. Department of Education; 2004. https://sites.ed.gov/idea. Accessed 27 Jun 2022.
6. American Association on Intellectual and Developmental Disabilities. Diagnostic adaptive behavior scale. Silver Spring, MD: American Association on Intellectual and Developmental Disabilities; 2018. https://www.aaidd.org/education/events/2018/05/24/default-calendar/introducing-the-diagnostic-adaptive-behavior-scale. Accessed 27 Jun 2022.
7. Tassé MJ, Luckasson R, Schalock RL. The relation between intellectual functioning and adaptive behavior in the diagnosis of intellectual disability. Intellect Dev Disabil. 2016;54(6):381–90.
8. Moeschler JB. Genetic evaluation of intellectual disabilities. Semin Pediatr Neurol. 2008;15(1):2–9.
9. Coppus AMW. People with intellectual disability: what do we know about adulthood and life expectancy? Dev Disabil Res Rev. 2013;18(1):6–16.
10. Joya X, Garcia-Algar O, Salat-Batlle J, Pujades C, Vall O. Advances in the development of novel antioxidant therapies as an approach for fetal alcohol syndrome prevention. Birth Defects Res A Clin Mol Teratol. 2015;103(3):163–77.
11. Stadskleiv K. Cognitive functioning in children with cerebral palsy. Dev Med Child Neurol. 2020;62(3):283–9.
12. Moeschler JB, Shevell M, Committee on Genetics. Comprehensive evaluation of the child with intellectual disability or global developmental delays. Pediatrics. 2014;134(3):e903–18.
13. Baker K, Raymond FL, Bass N. Genetic investigation for adults with intellectual disability: opportunities and challenges. Curr Opin Neurol. 2012;25(2):150–8.
14. Shapiro BK, O'Neill ME. Developmental delay and intellectual disability. In: Kliegman RM, St. Geme JW, editors. Nelson textbook of pediatrics. 21st ed. Philadelphia: Elsevier; 2020. p. 283–93.
15. Maulik PK, Mascarenhas MN, Mathers CD, Dua T, Saxena S. Prevalence of intellectual disability: a meta-analysis of population-based studies. Res Dev Disabil. 2011;32(2):419–36.
16. Patel DR, Apple R, Kanungo S, Akkal A. Intellectual disability: definitions, evaluation and principles of treatment. Pediatr Med. 2018;1:11–20.
17. Impact. Feature Issue on Aging and People with Intellectual and Developmental Disabilities. 2010. 23(1). https://publications.ici.umn.edu/impact/23-1/cover. Accessed 27 Jun 2022.
18. Cooper SA, Melville C, Morrison J. People with intellectual disabilities. BMJ. 2004;329(7463):414–5.
19. Murphy SL, Kochanek KD, Xu J, Arias E. Mortality in the United States, 2020. NCHS Data Brief. 2021;427:1–8.
20. Janicki MP, Dalton AJ, Henderson CM, Davidson PW. Mortality and morbidity among older adults with intellectual disability: health services considerations. Disabil Rehabil. 1999;21(5–6):284–94.
21. Landes SD, Stevens JD, Turk MA. Cause of death in adults with intellectual disability in the United States. J Intellect Disabil Res. 2021;65(1):47–59.
22. Landes SD, Stevens JD, Turk MA. Heterogeneity in age at death for adults with developmental disability. J IntellectDisabil Res. 2019;63(12):1482–7.
23. Evenhuis H, Henderson CM, Beange H, Lennox N, Chicoine B. Healthy ageing—adults with intellectual disabilities: physical health issues. J Appl Res Intellect Disabil. 2001;14(3):175–94.
24. Coppus AMW, Evenhuis HM, Verberne G-J, Visser FE, Oostra BA, Eikelenboom P, et al. Survival in elderly persons with down syndrome. J Am Geriatr Soc. 2008;56(12):2311–6.
25. Strauss D, Cable W. Shavelle R causes of excess mortality in cerebral palsy. Dev Med Child Neurol. 1999;41(9):580–5.
26. Luckasson R, Borthwick-Duffy S, Buntinx WHE, Coulter DL, Craig EM, Reeve A, et al. Mental retardation: definition, classification, and systems of supports. 10th ed. Washington, DC: American Association on Mental Retardation; 2002.
27. MACPAC. Twenty Years Later: Implications of Olmstead v. L.C. on Medicaid's Role in Providing Long-Term Services and Supports. 2019. https://www.macpac.gov/wp-content/uploads/2019/07/Twenty-Years-Later-Implications-of-Olmstead-on-Medicaids-Role-in-LTSS.pdf. Accessed 27 Jun 2022.
28. THE ARC, AIDD, AUCD, UCP, NACDD, and SABE. Fact Sheet: developmental disabilities assistance and bill of rights act (D.D. Act). 2011. http://www.thearc.org/wp-content/uploads/forchapters/factsheet_DD-Act2.pdf. Accessed 27 Jun 2022.

29. Braddock D, Hemp R, Rizzolo MC. State of the states in developmental disabilities: 2004. Ment Retard. 2004;42(5):356–70.
30. Ervin DA, Hennen B, Merrick J, Morad M. Healthcare for persons with intellectual and developmental disability in the community. Front Public Health. 2014;2:83.
31. Kerr M, Scheepers M, Arvio M, Beavis J, Brandt C, Brown S, et al. Consensus guidelines into the management of epilepsy in adults with an intellectual disability. J Intellect Disabil Res. 2009;53(8):687–94.
32. Bowleg L. The problem with the phrase women and minorities: intersectionality—an important theoretical framework for public health. Am J Public Health. 2012;102(7):1267–73.
33. Traci MA, Seekins T, Szalda-Petree A, Ravesloot C. Assessing secondary conditions among adults with developmental disabilities: a preliminary study. Ment Retard. 2002;40(2):119–31.
34. Scheepers M, Kerr M, O'Hara DO, Baindbridge D, Cooper SA, Davis R, et al. Reducing health disparity in people with intellectual disabilities: a report from health issues special interest research group of the International Association for the Scientific Study of intellectual Disabilities1. J Policy Pract Intellect Disabil. 2005;2(3–4):249–55.
35. McGinnis JM, Williams-Russo P, Knickman JR. The case for more active policy attention to health promotion. Health Aff. 2002;21(2):78–93.
36. Finlay WM, Lyons E. Methodological issues in interviewing and using self-report questionnaires with people with mental retardation. Psychol Assess. 2001;13(3):319–35.
37. Ervin DA, Williams A, Merrick J. Primary care: mental and behavioral health and persons with intellectual and developmental disabilities. Front Public Health. 2014;2:76.
38. Office of the Surgeon General. National Institute of Child Health and Human Development; Centers for Disease Control and Prevention. Closing the gap: a National Blueprint to improve the health of persons with mental retardation. Washington, DC: US Department of Health and Human Services; 2002.
39. Centers for Disease Control and Prevention. Prevalence of Disabilities and Associated Health Conditions Among Adults—United States, 1999. Morb Mortal Wkly Rep. 2001;50(7):120–5.
40. Krahn GL, Hammond L, Turner A. A cascade of disparities: health and health care access for people with intellectual disabilities. Mental Retard Dev Disabil Res Rev. 2006;12(1):70–82.
41. United Nations Department of Economic and Social Affairs. Article 25—health. New York, NY: United Nations; 2006.
42. Rubin IL, Crocker AC. Medical care for children and adults with developmental disabilities, Rubin IL, Crocker AC (Eds). Baltimore: Paul H. Baltimore: Brookes Publishing Co; 2006.
43. Marks B, Sisirak J, Heller T. Health matters for people with developmental disabilities: creating a sustainable health promotion program. Baltimore, MD: Paul H Brookes Publishing Co.; 2010.
44. Haveman M, Heller T, Maaskant M, Shooshtari S, Lee L, Strydom A. IASSID special interest research group on ageing in intellectual disabilities. Report on the state of science on health risks and ageing in people with intellectual disabilities. Dortmund, Germany: University of Dotrmund; 2009.
45. Sullivan WF, Berg JM, Bradley E, Cheetham T, Denton R, Heng J, et al. Primary care of adults with developmental disabilities: Canadian consensus guidelines. Can Fam Physician. 2011;57(5):541–53.
46. Massachusetts Department of Developmental Services. Preventive health recommendations for adults with intellectual disabilities. Worester, MA: Massachusetts Department of Developmental Services; 2019. https://shriver.umassmed.edu/wp-content/uploads/2020/07/MA-DDS-health-screening-brochure_2019_final.pdf. Accessed 27 Jun 2022.
47. Agaronnik N, Campbell EG, Ressalam J, Iezzoni LI. Communicating with patients with disability: perspectives of practicing physicians. J Gen Intern Med. 2019;34(7):1139–45.
48. Messinger-Rapport BJ, Rapport DJ. Primary care for the developmentally disabled adult. J Gen Intern Med. 1997;12(10):629–36.
49. Doostan D, Wilkes M. Treating the developmentally disabled. West J Med. 1999;171(2):92–6.
50. Lewis MA, Lewis CE, Leake B, King BH, Lindeamann R. The quality of health care for adults with developmental disabilities. Public Health Rep. 2002;117(2):174–84.
51. Merrick J, Davidson PW, Morad M, Janicki MP, Wexler O, Henderson CM. Older adults with intellectual disability in residential care centers in Israel: health status and service utilization. Am J Ment Retard. 2004;109(5):413–20.
52. Rimmer JH, Braddock D, Fujiura G. Prevalence of obesity in adults with mental retardation: implications for health promotion and disease prevention. Ment Retard. 1993;31(2):105–10.
53. Bhaumik S, Watson JM, Thorp CF, Tyrer F, McGrother CW. Body mass index in adults with intellectual disability: distribution, associations and service implications: a population-based prevalence study. J Intellect Disabil Res. 2008;52(Pt 4):287–98.
54. Owens PL, Kerker BD, Zigler E, Horwitz SM. Vision and oral health needs of individuals with intellectual disability. Ment Retard Dev Res Rev. 2006;12(1):28–40.
55. Blair E, Watson L, Badawi N, Stanley FJ. Life expectancy among people with cerebral palsy in Western Australia. Dev Med Child Neurol. 2001;43(8):508–15.
56. Wilson W, Taubert KA, Gewitz M, Lockhart PB, Baddour LM, Levison M, American Heart Association Rheumatic Fever, Endocarditis, and Kawasaki Disease Committee; American Heart Association Council on Cardiovascular

Disease in Young; American Heart Association Council on Clinical Cariology; American Heart Association Council on Cardiovascular Surgery and Anesthesia; Quality of Care and Outcomes Research Interdisciplinary Working Group, et al. Prevention of infective endocarditis: guidelines from the American Heart Association: a guideline from the American Heart Association rheumatic fever, endocarditis, and Kawasaki disease Committee, council on cardiovascular disease in the young, and the council on clinical cardiology, council on cardiovascular surgery and anesthesia, and the quality of care and outcomes research interdisciplinary working group. Circulation. 2007;116(15):1736–54.

57. Jolly C, Jamieson JM. The nutritional problems of adults with severe learning disabilities living in the community. J Hum Nutr Diet. 1999;12(1):29–34.
58. Wallace R, Schluter PJ, Duff M, Oullette-Kuntz H, Webb PM, Scheepers M. A review of the risk factors for, consequences, diagnosis, and management of helicobacter pylori in adults with intellectual disabilities. J Policy Pract Intellect Disabil. 2004;1(3–4):147–63.
59. Mathew R, Attarha BO, Kallumkal G, Cribbin M, Izzo C, Edwards L, et al. A primary care approach to constipation in adults with intellectual and developmental disabilities. Advances in Medicine. 2021;2021:3248052.
60. Kozma AJ, Mansell J, Beadle-Brown J. Outcomes in different residential settings for people with intellectual disability: a systematic review. Am J Intellect Dev Disabil. 2009;114(3):193–222.
61. Tyler CV Jr, Snyder CW, Zyzanski S. Screening for osteoporosis in community-dwelling adults with mental retardation. Ment Retard. 2000;38(4):316–21.
62. Schrager S. Epidemiology of osteoporosis in women with cognitive impairment. Ment Retard. 2006;44(3):203–11.
63. Dreyfus D, Lauer E, Wilkinson J. Characteristics associated with bone mineral density screening in adults with intellectual disabilities. J Am Board Fam Med. 2014;27(1):104–14.
64. Furey EM. Sexual abuse of adults with mental retardation: who and where. Ment Retard. 1994;32(3):173–80.
65. Sobsey D. Violence and abuse in the lives of people with disabilities: the end of silence acceptance? Baltimore. MD: Paul H Brookes Publishers; 1994.
66. Sullivan PM, Knutson JF. The association between child maltreatment and disabilities in a hospital-based epidemiological study. Child Abuse Negl. 1998;22(4):271–88.
67. Iezzoni LI, Mitra M. Transcending the counter-normative: sexual and reproductive health and persons with disability. Disabil Health J. 2017;10(3):369–70.
68. Tyrer P, Oliver-Africano P, Ahmed Z, Bouras N, Cooray S, Deb S, et al. Risperidone, haloperidol, and placebo in the treatment of aggressive challenging behaviour in patients with intellectual disability: a randomised controlled trial. Lancet. 2008;371(9606):57–63.
69. Vanderbilt Kennedy Center for Research on Human Development; University of Tennessee Boling Center for Developmental Disabilities; Tennessee Department of Intellectual and Developmental Disabilities. Health care for adults with intellectual and developmental disabilities: toolkit for primary care providers. Nashville, TN: Vanderbilt Kennedy Center; 2014. Adapted from the developmental disabilities primary care initiative in Ontario, Canada. https://ddprimarycare.surreyplace.ca/tools-2/. https://iddtoolkit.vkcsites.org. Accessfved 27 Jun 2022.
70. American Academy of Pediatrics; American Academy of Family Physicians; American College of Physicians; Transitions Clinical Report Authoring Group, Cooley WC, Sagerman PJ. Supporting the health care transition from adolescence to adulthood in the medical home. Pediatrics. 2011;128(1):182–200.
71. Got Transition®. Transitioning to an adult approach to health care without changing clinicians. Washington, DC: Got Transition; 2020. https://gottransition.org/6ce/?staying-overview. Accessed 27 Jun 2022.
72. Nielsen J, Graff C, Kanters JK, Toft E, Taylor D, Meyer JM. Assessing QT interval prolongation and its associated risks with antipsychotics. CNS Drugs. 2011;25(6):473–90.
73. Elster AB, Kunzets NJ, editors. AMA guidelines for adolescent preventive services: recommendations and rationale. Baltimore, MD: Williams & Wilkins; 1994.
74. Aschengrau A, Seage GR. Essentials of epidemiology in public health. 4th ed. Sudbury, MA: Jones and Bartlett Publishers; 2020.
75. de Winter CF, van den Berge APJ, Schoufour JD, Oppewal A, Evenhius HM. A 3-year follow-up study on cardiovascular disease and mortality in older people with intellectual disabilities. Res Dev Disabil. 2016;53-54:115–26.
76. Erickson SR, Basu T, Dorsch MP, Kamdar N. Disparities in the use of guideline-based pharmacotherapy exist for atherosclerotic cardiovascular disease and heart failure patients who have intellectual/developmental disabilities in a commercially insured database. Ann Pharmacother. 2020;54(10):958–66.
77. Vancampfort D, Schuch F, Van Damme T, Firth J, Suetani S, Stubbs B, et al. Metabolic syndrome and its components in people with intellectual disability: a meta-analysis. J Intellect Disabil Res. 2020;64(10):804–15.
78. Hsieh K, Murthy S, Heller T, Rimmer JH, Yen G. Reported gum disease as a cardiovascular risk factor in adults with intellectual disabilities. J Intellect Disabil Res. 2018;62(3):187–98.
79. U.S. Preventive Services Task Force. A and B Recommendations. United States Preventive

Services Taskforce. Rockville, MD: USPSTF. https://www.uspreventiveservicestaskforce.org/uspstf/recommendation-topics/uspstf-a-and-b-recommendations. Accessed 27 Jun 2022.
80. Schroeder EC, DuBois L, Sadowsky M, Higlenkamp TIM. Hypertension in adults with intellectual disability: prevalence and risk factors. Am J Prev Med. 2020;58(5):630–7.
81. Wallace RA, Schluter P. Audit of cardiovascular disease risk factors among supported adults with intellectual disability attending an ageing clinic. J Intellect Develop Disabil. 2008;33(1):48–58.
82. Calders P, Elmahgoub S, de Mettelinge TR, Vandenbroeck C, Dewandele I, Rombaut L, et al. Effect of combined exercise training on physical and metabolic fitness in adults with intellectual disability: a controlled trial. Clin Rehabil. 2011;25(12):1097–108.
83. Jo G, Rossow-Kimball B, Lee Y. Effects of 12-week combined exercise program on self-efficacy, physical activity level, and health related physical fitness of adults with intellectual disability. J Exerc Rehabil. 2018;14(2):175–82.
84. Xu X, Mann JR, Hardin JW, Gustafson E, McDermott SW, Deroche CB. Adherence to US preventive services task force recommendations for breast and cervical cancer screening for women who have a spinal cord injury. J Spinal Cord Med. 2017;40(1):76–84.
85. Servais L, Jacques D, Leach R, Conod L, Hoyois P, Dan B, Roussaux JP. Contraception of women with intellectual disability: prevalence and determinants. J Intellect Disabil Res. 2002;46(Pt 2):108–19.
86. Sullivan SG, Hussain R, Threlfall T, Bittles AH. The incidence of cancer in people with intellectual disabilities. Cancer Causes Control. 2004;15(10):1021–5.
87. Xu X, McDermott SW, Mann JR, Hardin JW, Deroche CB, Carroll DD, et al. A longitudinal assessment of adherence to breast and cervical cancer screening recommendations among women with and without intellectual disability. Prev Med. 2017;100:167–72.
88. McCarthy EP, Ngo LH, Roetzheim RG, Chirikos TN, Donglin L, Drews RE, et al. Disparities in breast cancer treatment and survival for women with disabilities. Ann Intern Med. 2006;145(9):637–45.
89. Willis D, Samalin E, Satgé D. Colorectal cancer in people with intellectual disabilities. Oncology. 2018;95(6):323–36.
90. Cummins R. Self-rated quality of life scales for people with an intellectual disability: a review. J Appl Res Intellect Disabil. 2010;10:199–216.
91. Amundson R. Quality of life, disability, and hedonic psychology: quality of life, disability, and hedonic psychology. J Theory Soc Behav. 2010;40(4):374–92.
92. Albrecht GL, Devlieger PJ. The disability paradox: high quality of life against all odds. Soc Sci Med (1982). 1999;48(8):977–88.
93. Veatch RM. Limits of guardian treatment refusal: a reasonableness standard. Am J Law Med. 1984;9(4):427–68.
94. Chicoine C, et al. Ableism at the bedside: people with intellectual disabilities and COVID-19. J Am Board Fam Med. 2022;35(2):390–3.
95. Gleason Jonathan, et al., The devastating impact of Covid-19 on individuals with intellectual disabilities in the United States. EJM Catal Innov Care Deliv, 2021.
96. Ailey SH, et al. Hospitalizations of adults with intellectual disability in academic medical centers. Intellect Dev Disabil. 2014;52(3):187–92.
97. Iacono T, et al. A systematic review of hospital experiences of people with intellectual disability. BMC Health Serv Res. 2014;14(1):505.
98. Administration for Community Living. History of the DD Act. 2017.; https://acl.gov/about-acl/history-dd-act. Accessed 27 Jun 2022.
99. Centers for Disease Control and Prevention. Data and statistics on Down syndrome. Atlanta, GA: CDC; 2020. https://www.cdc.gov/ncbddd/birthdefects/downsyndrome/data.html. Accessed 27 Jun 2022.
100. Presson AP, Partyka G, Jensen KM, Devine OW, Rasmussen SA, McCabe LL, et al. Current estimate of down syndrome population prevalence in the United States. J Pediatr. 2013;163(4):1163–8.
101. Glasson E, Sullivan SG, Hussain R, Petterson BA, Montgomery PD, Bittles AH. The changing survival profile of people with Down's syndrome: implications for genetic counselling. Clin Genet. 2002;62(5):390–3.
102. Centers for Disease Control and Prevention. Data and statistics for cerebral palsy. Atlanta, GA: CDC; 2020. https://www.cdc.gov/ncbddd/cp/data.html. Accessed 27 Jun 2022.
103. Duruflé-Tapin A, Colin A, Niclas B, Lebreton C, Dauvergne F, Gallien P. Analysis of the medical causes of death in cerebral palsy. Ann Phys Rehabil Med. 2014;57(1):24–37.
104. Loeber JG. Neonatal screening in Europe; the situation in 2004. J Inherit Metab Dis. 2007;30(4):430–8.
105. Vockley J, Andersson HC, Antshel KM, Braverman NE, Burton BK, Frazier DM, et al. American College of Medical Genetics and Genomics Therapeutics Committee. Phenylalanine hydroxylase deficiency: diagnosis and management guideline. Genet Med. 2014;16(2):188–200.
106. Ghidoni BBZ. Rett Syndrome. Child Adolesc Psychiatr Clin N Am. 2007;16(3):723–43.
107. Kirby RS, Lane JB, Childers J, Skinner SA, Annese F, Barrish JO, et al. Longevity in Rett syndrome: analysis of the north American database. J Pediatr. 2010;156(1):135–138.e1.
108. Pearson E, et al. Communication in Angelman syndrome: a scoping review. Deve Med Child Neurol. 2019;61(11):1266–74.

109. Williams CA, Driscoll DJ, Dagli AI. Clinical and genetic aspects of Angelman syndrome. Genet Med. 2010;12(7):385–95.
110. Strømme P, Bjømstad PG, Ramstad K. Prevalence estimation of Williams syndrome. J Child Neurol. 2002;17(4):269–71.
111. Cleveland Clinic. Williams Syndrome, Williams Beuren syndrome: causes, symptoms & treatment. Cleveland, OH: Cleveland Clinic; 2022. https://my.clevelandclinic.org/health/diseases/15174-williams-syndrome. Accessed 27 June 2022.
112. Cassidy SB, Schwartz S, Miller JL, Driscoll DJ. Prader-Willi syndrome. Genet Med. 2012;14(1):10–26.
113. Butler MG, Manzardo AM, Forster JL. Prader-Willi syndrome: clinical genetics and diagnostic aspects with treatment approaches. Curr Pediatr Rev. 2016;12(2):136–66.
114. Fiest KM, Sauro KM, Wiebe S, Patten SB, Dwon C-S, Dykeman J, et al. Prevalence and incidence of epilepsy: a systematic review and meta-analysis of international studies. Neurology. 2017;88(3):296–303.
115. Gaitatzis A, Johnson AL, Chadwick DW, Shorvon SD, Sander JW. Life expectancy in people with newly diagnosed epilepsy. Brain. 2004;127(Pt 11):2427–32.
116. Denny L, Coles SM, Blitz R. Fetal alcohol syndrome and fetal alcohol spectrum disorders. Am Fam Physician. 2017;96(8):515–22.
117. Thanh MX, Jonsson E. Life expectancy of people with fetal alcohol syndrome. J Popul Ther Clin Pharmacol. 2016;23(1):e53–9.
118. Centers for Disease Control and Prevention. Data and Statistics on Fragile X Syndrome. Atlanta, GA: CDC; 2022. https://www.cdc.gov/ncbddd/fxs/data.html. Accessed 27 Jun 2022.
119. National Center for Advancing Translational Sciences, Genetic and Rare Diseases Information Center. Fragile X syndrome. Gaithersburg, MD: Genetic and Rare Diseases Information Center (GARD); 2021. https://rarediseases.info.nih.gov/diseases/6464/fragile-x-syndrome. Accessed 27 Jun 2022.

# Juvenile Idiopathic Arthritis

# 34

Tova Ronis and Patience H. White

## Case Presentation

Tina is an 18-year-old female with a history of polyarticular juvenile idiopathic arthritis (JIA). She will be starting college at a university near your practice and presents to the internal medicine office with her parents to establish care. Tina recently graduated high school and will be studying engineering at a local university that is a 4-hour drive from her home.

Tina reports that she was diagnosed with arthritis when she was 3 years of age. Her arthritis has involved her knees, ankles, wrist, and temporomandibular joint (TMJ). She has been followed regularly by an ophthalmologist and never had any eye complications. She was treated initially with intra-articular corticosteroid injections of the affected joints as well as naproxen and methotrexate when she was younger and was able to wean off of all her medications by the time she was 9. She then had a flare of wrist arthritis when she was 14 and is currently being treated with methotrexate, folic acid, and adalimumab injections, which she administers independently. She was recently treated with antibiotics for a urinary tract infection and continued her arthritis medications at that time. She has regular menstrual periods. On dietary history, she notes no restrictions but does not like drinking milk. She has no other health problems and her immunizations are up to date. There is no family history of autoimmune disease. Her father and maternal grandfather have coronary artery disease.

On musculoskeletal exam, you notice that Tina has micrognathia and a decreased oral aperture. Wrist range of motion is mildly decreased in both flexion and extension. Otherwise, the remainder of her musculoskeletal and general exam is normal. Gait evaluation reveals a 1.5 cm leg-length discrepancy. She compensates for this by wearing a shoe lift on the shorter side.

Recently, labs showed borderline elevated cholesterol and a negative rheumatoid factor (RF) and anticitrullinated cyclic peptide (CCP).

Tina is excited to be starting university. She graduated from a public high school where she had a 504 plan that provided accommodations for her physical limitations, such as the use of a computer to type notes in class and additional time to take tests if her wrists were in pain. She will be living in campus housing. At this initial appoint-

T. Ronis (✉)
Division of Rheumatology, Department of Pediatrics, Children's National Hospital, Washington, DC, USA

Got Transition, The National Alliance to Advance Adolescent Health, Washington, DC, USA
e-mail: tronis@childrensnational.org

P. H. White
Department of Medicine and Pediatrics, George Washington University School of Medicine and Health Sciences, Washington, DC, USA
e-mail: PWhite@thenationalalliance.org


A. A. Kuo et al. (eds.), *Care of Adults with Chronic Childhood Conditions*,
https://doi.org/10.1007/978-3-031-54281-7_34

ment, her mother raises concern about her immunocompromised state and the risk of exposure to infections in the school dormitory. She will still be covered under her parents' medical insurance plan. She will be responsible for getting her medications while at college. Additionally, she needs to have screening labs for methotrexate toxicity every 3 months.

## Case Discussion

This case demonstrates a typical course of polyarticular RF negative JIA and raises several issues that are faced by patients with JIA as they graduate from high school and enter college. In the United States, the Americans with Disabilities Act (ADA) states that postsecondary schools cannot deny enrollment based on the presence of physical or mental disabilities. The U.S. Department of Education shares that "academic adjustments may include auxiliary aids and modifications to academic requirements as are necessary to ensure equal educational opportunity" [1] (see more at: https://www2.ed.gov/about/offices/list/ocr/transition.html). College applications cannot ask about health conditions and prospective students do not need to disclose a health condition on applying. Most colleges and universities have an office for students with disabilities where students like Tina can register. This office can help provide accommodations now or at any time during the school year such as extra test time and excused absences for doctor's appointments or acute illness. If patients are significantly immunocompromised, this office can also help them find single rooms without a roommate to reduce the exposure to infections. However, this is not always necessary and college life should be normalized as much as possible. Students need to register with this office with documentation from their physician each year and, if not complete, the student can be denied any accommodation due to their condition. (For additional information on education among adults with chronic childhood conditions, please see Chap. 60 of this book.)

Because Tina will be living in a dormitory, she may be at higher risk of infection. Immunizations should be reviewed and patients on immunosuppressive medications should not be given live virus vaccines including intranasal flu, measles mumps rubella, varicella, and zoster vaccines. She will need a yearly injectable influenza vaccine and should have received both pneumococcal 13-valent conjugate (PCV13) and pneumococcal polysaccharide (PPSV23) as she is immunocompromised. She should also be given the meningitis MenACWY vaccine as she will be living in campus housing [2]. Additionally, she should be vaccinated for HPV and should have regular gynecologic care.

Often, immunosuppressive therapies will be temporarily held if a patient gets a serious infection such as a urinary tract infection requiring antibiotics. In this case, Tina should be counseled to stop her methotrexate and adalimumab if this happens again. Corticosteroids are usually continued despite infection given the risk for adrenal insufficiency if they are stopped abruptly.

A challenge faced by many teenagers and young adults at this phase is adherence. Since Tina will be responsible for getting and administering her own medications, she is at risk of having poor adherence. It is normal for adolescents and young adults to want to appear like their peers at this developmental stage. Patients with no outwardly apparent chronic diseases may not want to disclose to their peers that they have a health condition. If their arthritis has been asymptomatic, they may have some denial about their illness and stop taking their medications. There are web-based tools and applications (apps) to help patients remember to take their medications that may be helpful. (Free apps are available on both the Apple iTunes and Google Play stores.)

Additionally, many adolescent and young adult patients do not have experience in managing their own chronic disease if their care has been previously coordinated by their parents. Research has demonstrated that mature decision-making often does not emerge until the middle of the third decade of life [3]. You may need to assess Tina's knowledge of her disease and her skills in managing her health care in the adult care system. An American College of Rheumatology self-care assessment tool is available online for this pur-

**Table 34.1** American College of Rheumatology recommendations for follow-up laboratory monitoring intervals for complete blood count, liver transaminase levels, and serum creatinine levels for patients receiving DMARDs. Modified with permission obtained from [5]

| Medication | Monitoring interval based on duration of treatment[a] | | |
|---|---|---|---|
| | <3 months[b] | 3–6 months | >6 months |
| Hydroxychloroquine | None after baseline | None | None |
| Methotrexate (weeks) | 2–4 | 8–12 | 12 |
| Leflunomide (weeks) | 2–4 | 8–12 | 12 |
| Sulfasalazine (weeks) | 2–4 | 8–12 | 12 |

[a]Patients with comorbidities, abnormal laboratory results, and/or multiple therapies may require more frequent laboratory testing than what is generally recommended

[b]More frequent monitoring is recommended within the first 3 months of therapy or after increasing the dose

pose [4]. If she is accustomed to her parents ordering her medications and taking her to have her regular labs done, this may be difficult for her at first. Logistically, Tina is still covered under her parents' insurance plan but she will be responsible for managing her disease at college. It may be helpful to find a mail order pharmacy that can deliver her medications if there is no pharmacy close to her dormitory. She needs a plan for needle disposal on campus. She will also need to find a location to have her regular labs drawn (see schedule for lab tests for methotrexate screening in Table 34.1) [5]. Sometimes this can be done at a campus student health office, and she should find out where that is located on campus and make arrangements to have the results sent to the office. She should have access to a portable summary of her disease and her current medications at all times, which she can store in her cell phone (see patient guide for how to set up a Medical ID for iPhone and Android here: https://www.gottransition.org/resource/?setting-up-medical-id-smartphones). Young adults are familiar with electronic communication, and Tina should be encouraged to sign up for the office electronic portal, if available. It is also important to have a discussion with Tina about what is the best way to communicate with her about her appointments (e.g., text reminders) and for her to communicate with the office and her primary care physician about her questions. Young adults ages 18–25 years are one of the biggest users of the emergency room under the age of 75 in the United States and are poorly connected to primary care.

Now that Tina is 18, her medical information is protected under the Health Insurance Portability and Accountability Act (HIPAA). This includes confidentiality from her parents. If Tina wants her parents to continue to receive her medical information, she should be asked to sign a HIPAA waiver granting them this right. As she is a young adult, she should be interviewed without her parents present for at least part of the visit. Ideally, she has been seen alone for part of her visits to her pediatrician for the past few years so asking her parents to step out during the visit will not be a surprise. Parents are usually willing to step out of the room once their medical concerns about their child have been expressed. Methotrexate is a teratogenic medication with risk of hepatotoxicity, and Tina should be counseled about safe sexual practices and alcohol. Two simultaneous forms of contraception are recommended for patients who are sexually active and taking teratogenic medications (e.g., barrier methods and hormonal birth control). The latter is safe to use in young adults with JIA.

Medically, this case illustrates the deformities that can occur due to arthritis in a growing joint. Some joints such as the knee will grow faster when inflamed, resulting in leg-length discrepancy. Leg lengths should be measured along with a scoliosis assessment. If quadriceps muscle bulk is asymmetric due to disuse of the arthritic knee, physical therapy can assist with strengthening. When the TMJ is involved, this can lead to micrognathia and decreased range of motion of the jaw.

This patient will also need referrals to specialty care. She will need an adult rheumatologist, an ophthalmologist (see later section on "Uveitis"), a dentist, and a gynecologist (if gynecological care is not provided at the primary care provider's office). Tina may also be at higher risk of dyslipidemia and cardiac disease given her history of JIA and family history and this would require special consideration (see later section on "Cardiovascular disease"). Tina's diet may be low in calcium and vitamin D and she is at increased risk of osteoporosis (see "Bone health" section later). She should be counseled to increase her intake of calcium and vitamin D.

## Epidemiology and Outcome

JIA is not rare, but the incidence and prevalence vary around the world. Incidence rates of childhood arthritis range from 1 to 20 per 100,000 in various studies [6]. Prevalence ranges from below 10 to 400 per 100,000 [6]. In reports from North America, Australia, and Europe, there is at least a 2:1 female-to-male ratio. Boys are more often affected in reports from Asia [6]. There are geographic and ethnic differences in rates of subtypes of arthritis. Specific data for the individual JIA subtypes were summarized previously. A substantial number of JIA patients continue to have active arthritis into adulthood. The disease course can be characterized by periods of remission and flare with the accumulation of more joint involvement over time.

## Definition and Subgroups

The International League of Associations for Rheumatology (ILAR) classification of JIA (Table 34.2) replaces previous terms juvenile rheumatoid arthritis (JRA) and juvenile chronic arthritis (JCA) [6–8]. JIA is an autoimmune disease defined by arthritis occurring for greater than 6 weeks in a child younger than 16. Even as they enter adulthood, patients retain the diagnosis of JIA and their diagnosis does not change to rheumatoid arthritis. Most forms of JIA exhibit clinical and genetic similarity to adult-onset arthritis [9, 10]. There are several subtypes of JIA and the characteristic features of each of these subtypes will be discussed in this section.

**Table 34.2** ILAR classification of JIA

| Characteristic | Clinical features |
|---|---|
| Age at onset | <16 years old |
| Minimum duration | ≥6 weeks |
| Subtypes: | |
| Systemic | Arthritis<br>2 weeks of daily fever<br>Presence of at least one of: Rash, lymphadenopathy, organomegaly, or serositis<br>Risk of macrophage activation syndrome |
| Oligoarticular | Up to four involved joints in the first 6 months<br>*Persistent*—No more than four joints involved<br>*Extended*—More than four joints involved after first 6 months |
| Polyarticular | Involves five or more joints in the first 6 months<br>Rheumatoid factor negative or positive |
| Enthesitis-related arthritis | Arthritis and enthesitis, or arthritis or enthesitis with at least two of the following:<br>Sacroiliac joint tenderness and/or inflammatory back pain<br>HLA-B27 antigen positive<br>Onset of arthritis in a male over 6 years old<br>Acute (symptomatic) anterior uveitis<br>Family history of ankylosing spondylitis or HLA-B27-positive-related disease in first-degree relative |
| Psoriatic arthritis | Arthritis and psoriasis or arthritis and at least two of:<br>Dactylitis<br>Nail pitting or onycholysis<br>Psoriasis in a first-degree relative |
| Undifferentiated | Arthritis that meets none of the above categories or two or more categories |

Adapted from [7]

## Systemic Arthritis

This form of childhood arthritis is analogous to adult-onset Still's disease and accounts for 5–15% of all children with JIA. Diagnosis requires the presence of arthritis, 2 weeks of daily fevers, plus 1 of the following: classic evanescent rash, generalized lymphadenopathy, hepatomegaly or splenomegaly, or serositis [6]. This type of arthritis can occur at any age and affects males and females equally [6]. Patients can be very ill at the time of diagnosis. Systemic features including fevers and elevated inflammatory markers are common early in the course of disease; however, arthritis can predominate later in the course and can affect any number of both large and small joints [6]. This is a diagnosis of exclusion and has a broad differential diagnosis. Malignancy often needs to be excluded. Treatment for systemic arthritis depends on severity of disease and may include nonsteroidal anti-inflammatory drugs (NSAIDs); systemic or intra-articular corticosteroids; disease modifying antirheumatic agents (DMARDs), such as methotrexate; and biologic agents, particularly blockade of interleukin (IL)-1 (anakinra, canakinumab) or IL-6 (tocilizumab) [6]. Prognosis depends on the response to therapy and the amount of joint involvement. Patients can have long-term morbidity due to protracted use of systemic corticosteroids. The arthritis in this subtype can be destructive and lead to general growth abnormalities. Some patients eventually require joint replacement.

A rare and sometimes fatal complication seen with systemic JIA is macrophage activation syndrome (MAS). See MAS description below.

## Oligoarthritis

This is a chronic inflammatory arthritis lasting for at least 6 weeks involving 4 or fewer joints. It is called *persistent-oligoarthritis* if no more than four joints are involved throughout the disease course and *extended-oligoarthritis* if more than four joints become affected in the period following the initial 6 months [6]. Oligoarthritis is the most common subtype of childhood arthritis, affecting 50–80% of all children with chronic arthritis. The peak incidence is between the ages of 1–3 years and is more common in girls [6]. These patients should not have psoriasis or a family history of psoriasis, ankylosing spondylitis, or inflammatory bowel disease are not systemically ill and are rheumatoid factor (RF) negative. Large joints of the lower extremities are most commonly involved [6]. Patients are at risk for developing asymptomatic uveitis, which can be present at onset and can affect up to 20% of oligoarthritis patients [6] (see the "Uveitis" section). They are at risk for growth abnormalities from persistent inflammation, most commonly leg-length discrepancy from unilateral knee arthritis. Treatment includes NSAIDs, intra-articular corticosteroid injections, and physical therapy. DMARDs and biologic therapies are occasionally required [6]. Patients require regular slit lamp exams for screening for uveitis, and the frequency of recommended eye exams varies based on the presence of positive antinuclear antibody (ANA), age at disease onset, and duration of disease [11].

## Polyarthritis (Rheumatoid Factor Negative)

Polyarthritis accounts for approximately 20% of all JIA patients and Tina, the case presented earlier in this chapter, has this form of JIA [6]. This is a chronic arthritis affecting five or more joints within the first 6 months after disease onset [8]. Approximately 85% of polyarthritis patients test negative for RF. This is defined as a separate entity than those who test positive for RF. There is a biphasic age of onset with 1 peak at age 1–3 and another peak in later childhood and adolescence. It is 4 times more common in females [6]. Articular disease predominates, though some patients also have systemic features such as fatigue, growth failure, and elevated inflammatory markers. The onset is usually insidious and patients have significant morning stiffness and gelling after inactivity. Wrists and ankles are the most commonly affected joints. Small joint involvement of hands and feet may also occur. This subtype of patients is more likely to have TMJ involvement, which can eventually lead to micrognathia. The cervical spine can be involved, leading to loss of neck extension. Up to 15% of these patients develop uveitis, which, like oligoarticular arthritis, tends to occur in patients with younger age of onset and positive ANA. [6] This is a chronic disease that can last into adulthood. Arthritis can persist into adulthood and functional disability can be seen.

## Polyarthritis (Rheumatoid Factor Positive)

This is also a chronic arthritis affecting five or more joints within the first 6 months after disease onset. RF is positive on two occasions at least 3 months apart [8]. This subtype has similar features to adult seropositive rheumatoid arthritis [6]. It occurs in approximately 3% of patients with JIA and is much more common in females. The mean age of onset is 9–11 years of age [6]. Patients often test positive for anticitrullinated protein (CCP) antibodies [12], and up to 56% of patients have a positive ANA [13]. This form of arthritis is often symmetric and can involve upper and lower extremities, small joints, as well as the TMJ and cervical spine. Early limitation of the wrist can progress to substantial deformity and debility. Erosive joint disease often occurs. Systemic manifestations include fatigue and weight loss with active disease. Rheumatoid nodules may occur. The presence of CCP antibodies is often associated with a more severe disease course [14]. This subtype has a poor articular prognosis and early aggressive medical therapy is indicated in both forms of polyarthritis[6, 10]. These patients may have increased disability with chronic active disease that persists into adulthood [15].

## Enthesitis-Related Arthritis

This subtype of arthritis is defined as patients having arthritis and enthesitis (defined as inflammation at the sites of attachment of ligament, tendon, fascia, or capsule to bone). Alternatively, patients can have either arthritis or enthesitis with at least two of the following: sacroiliac joint tenderness and/or inflammatory spine pain; the presence of HLA-B27; family history in at least one first—or second-degree relative with HLA-B27 associated disease; anterior uveitis associated with pain, redness, or photophobia; or the onset of arthritis in a boy after 6 years of age [6]. This subtype affects the joints of the lower extremities and axial skeleton. There is a strong association with HLA-B27, which is positive in 90% of patients. Autoantibodies such as ANA and RF are characteristically absent [6]. Peripheral joint disease can precede axial involvement by years. Many patients eventually evolve to resemble adult ankylosing spondylitis (AS); however, the characteristic features of AS are usually absent in childhood. Up to 10% of patients with JIA have enthesitis-related arthritis. Up to 11% of patients with adult AS had their disease onset in childhood [16]. Onset typically occurs in late childhood or adolescence and is more common in males with a male-to-female ratio of 7:1 [6]. This form of arthritis may resemble that found in inflammatory bowel disease, which should be included on the differential diagnosis. This disease is often progressive, and symptoms persist into adulthood [17].

## Juvenile Psoriatic Arthritis

Clinical features of patients with psoriatic arthritis overlap with those of the other subtypes. The diagnostic criteria include patients with arthritis for 6 weeks associated with either psoriasis or at least two of the following: dactylitis (defined as swelling of a digit that extends beyond the borders of the joints), nail pitting or onycholysis, or psoriasis in a first-degree relative [8]. Development of psoriasis can lag behind arthritis in about half of children. The proportion of patients with JIA who have psoriatic arthritis is approximately 7%. The age of onset is biphasic, with a first peak occurring around 2–3 years and a second peak in late childhood. It is more common in females. Clinical manifestations are heterogeneous. Younger children are often females, can have a positive ANA, and are at risk for developing uveitis. Older children have a tendency to develop enthesitis and axial disease. RF is frequently absent. Patients often present with asymmetric monoarticular or oligoarticular disease. The highly destructive arthritis mutilans seen in adults is rare in children [6]. Long-term outcome is not well defined, however, up to 33% of patients continued to require DMARD therapy at 15 years of follow-up in one study [18].

## Undifferentiated Arthritis

Patients who have onset of inflammatory arthritis before the age of 16, which fits multiple categories or no category, are classified as undifferentiated JIA [8].

## Pathophysiology

The etiology of JIA is largely unknown but is believed to be multifactorial with genetic and environmental influences and differs among subtypes. Autoantibodies are common in oligoarthritis (ANA) and in RF-positive polyarthritis (IgM rheumatoid factor and anticitrullinated protein antibodies), suggesting the role of the humoral immune system in the pathophysiology of JIA. Other subtypes are associated with polymorphisms at the histocompatibility locus, but familial arthritis is rare. Systemic JIA is not associated with antibodies or a strong genetic signal and has been considered an autoinflammatory disease [6]. In all subtypes, T-cells and macrophages are involved in pathogenesis and lead to synovial inflammation.

## Clinical Manifestations

Clinical manifestations include pain, stiffness, and joint inflammation with swelling, tenderness, warmth, and limitation. Tenosynovitis is common. Children who are growing also have extra-articular manifestations of JIA such as abnormal growth and physical development due to the direct effect of disease, systemic inflammation, or medications. Localized growth disturbances of affected joints can be striking and lead to limb inequality and micrognathia. Puberty and sexual maturation are often delayed.

## Uveitis

Patients with JIA are at risk of developing the ocular complication of uveitis that is more common in patients with a positive ANA who present at a younger age, usually before the age of 7 years. The risk of developing uveitis diminishes over time but it can persist into adulthood. If untreated, uveitis can cause significant visual impairment and blindness. This complication is usually asymptomatic, and therefore patients are screened with slit lamp exams routinely according to generally accepted guidelines, with frequency varying depending on the JIA subtype and the ACR has developed criteria for screening for uveitis [11, 19]. Older patients, especially those with enthesitis-related arthritis, tend to have symptomatic uveitis.

## Therapy

All forms of JIA require a multifaceted approach to treatment. Mainstays in management include early anti-inflammatory treatment and physical and occupational therapy. Healthy lifestyle, including diet and physical activity, should be promoted. Medical management generally begins with NSAIDs unless contraindicated. In patients with a limited number of joints involved, intra-articular corticosteroid injections may be beneficial. Systemic corticosteroids are rarely used other than in systemic arthritis. DMARDs including methotrexate, leflunomide, and sulfasalazine are often required, and many patients have an excellent response. In those who do not, biologic therapies including tumor necrosis factor (TNF)-antagonists and others have been shown to be very effective. There is little to no role for opiate analgesia, a class of agents that will not address the underlying inflammatory problem and also has an adverse side effect profile as well as risk for dependency and addiction. Novel therapies are being studied in this condition. JAK inhibitors (tofacitinib) were recently approved for the treatment of polyarticular JIA [10] and studies in systemic JIA are ongoing. Treatment for systemic JIA was previously summarized.

The Childhood Arthritis and Rheumatology Research Alliance (CARRA) has published consensus-based treatment plans for new onset systemic [20, 21]and polyarticular JIA [22] as well as JIA-associated uveitis [23]. The American

College of Rheumatology (ACR) revised the guidelines for the treatment of JIA patients with nonsystemic polyarthritis, sacroiliitis, and enthesitis [24] as well as uveitis [19] in 2019.

The overall goal of therapy is to achieve disease remission quickly and to maintain remission with medications. There is no consensus to the approach, but if remission occurs, medications can be tapered. The aim is to prevent flares since chronic involvement with active arthritis can cause irreversible joint destruction.

Periodic monitoring labs are indicated. For patients taking daily NSAIDs, complete blood count, serum creatinine, liver enzymes, and urinalysis are recommended approximately twice yearly [18]. ACR guidelines for laboratory monitoring frequency in patients taking DMARD therapies from 2015 are summarized in Table 34.1 [5]. Basic labs should be assessed at the baseline. Tuberculosis (TB) testing should be performed before starting patients on biologic therapies and tofacitinib [5]. Hepatitis B and C serologies should be assessed before initiating biologic therapies in high-risk populations. For patients taking TNF-antagonists, labs should be checked every 3–6 months [25].

If an adult patient with JIA presents with acute pain, other causes such as trauma or amplified pain syndromes should be excluded. Arthritis flares may be addressed with local corticosteroid injection, escalation of therapy, or switching medications in conjunction with a rheumatologist.

Patients are not usually admitted for inpatient care unless they are being hospitalized for infection in the setting of an immunocompromised host. Some patients with systemic arthritis are hospitalized for their initial diagnosis. JIA is typically treated in an outpatient setting and if a patient with JIA is admitted with unexplained symptoms, more common etiologies should be ruled out.

Most medications used in JIA can be given safely over a long period. Long-term corticosteroids, however, should be avoided due to their multiple side effects. Risks of long-term immunosuppressive therapy include infection. Patients taking chronic corticosteroids have higher incidences of hospitalized bacterial infections [26]. The risk of TB remains a concern in patients taking biologic medications. While patients with JIA may have an increased risk of developing malignancy, this risk seems to be independent of DMARD and biologic therapy [27].

Methotrexate and leflunomide are teratogenic (pregnancy category X), and TNF-antagonist biologics are pregnancy category B drugs. A screening pregnancy test should be considered before recommending teratogenic medications to a young adult with arthritis. Teratogenic medications should be discontinued in the face of unplanned pregnancy. Patients on leflunomide require cholestyramine washout therapy prior to planning a pregnancy or in the event of an unplanned pregnancy. Methotrexate should be discontinued ≥1 ovulatory cycle before planning a pregnancy.

## Common Adult Conditions in the JIA Population

### Arthritis and Musculoskeletal Abnormalities

The most common adult condition in this population of patients is persistent arthritis in adulthood either due to ongoing disease that is refractory to treatment or flare of previously controlled arthritis. Patients are at risk of developing early secondary osteoarthritis due to joint damage from prior joint inflammation. This can lead to chronic pain and the need for arthroplasty. If present prior to cessation of growth, local growth abnormalities such as leg-length discrepancies, bony fusions, and TMJ involvement can lead to functional difficulties. TMJ arthritis, in particular, can lead to long-term consequences in oral health such as decreased chewing ability, malocclusion (in 66% of patients), and micrognathia (in 30% of patients). [28] Treatment of TMJ arthritis includes escalation of systemic therapy but despite this, some patients require corrective surgery. Patients who have had cervical spine arthritis may have ankylosis, erosions, and narrowing of cranio-cervical junction [29] and be at risk for atlanto-axial subluxation, which should be noted prior to any surgical procedure requiring anesthesia.

### Ocular Complications

Patients who had significant uveitis may have visual morbidity with low vision due to the disease itself or cataract formation as a result of treatment with topical glucocorticoids.

### Cardiovascular Disease

As in adult RA, there is evidence that patients with JIA may be at increased risk for premature atherosclerosis or accelerated cardiovascular disease [30, 31]. One study showed increased rates of heart disease in women with JIA [32]. Another study showed no increase in cardiovascular events in patients with JIA 29 years following disease onset when compared to the general population [33]. One study reported that 18% of patients with JIA were obese. Obesity was not associated with disease activity [34]. Patients with systemic JIA with prolonged exposure to corticosteroids may have dyslipidemia, hypertension, and diabetes. The long-term risk of cardiovascular disease for individuals with JIA remains unclear and there are no guidelines on cholesterol-lowering treatment in JIA patients currently available. Research has shown increased mortality risk among adult RA patients [35], and given the potential for longer disease duration in people with JIA, mortality risk in this group might be increased, especially if a family history of cardiovascular disease is present. Therefore, one might consider aggressive management of elevated cholesterol in a patient such as the clinical vignette presented previously in this chapter.

### Oral Health

There have been rare reports of secondary Sjögren's syndrome occurring years after diagnosis of JIA [36]. Good oral hygiene is important especially for those on immunosuppressive treatment or with Sjögren's symptoms.

## Special Issues that Arise in Patients with Juvenile Idiopathic Arthritis

### Arthritis Flares

If a patient has an arthritis flare, adherence should be assessed. Monoarthritis is rare in adults and should raise the question of infectious arthritis due to sexually transmitted infections or Lyme disease in endemic areas. If the pain is acute, other causes should be excluded.

### Macrophage Activation Syndrome

Macrophage activation syndrome (MAS) is a potentially fatal complication most commonly associated with systemic JIA but can also be seen in other forms of autoimmune disease. It is due to hemophagocytosis by macrophages, which can occur in the bone marrow and liver. This can be triggered in the setting of infections such as with mononucleosis. Patients appear unwell and can be febrile. Viral serologies should be checked. Labs show cytopenias, elevated liver enzymes, low erythrocyte sedimentation rate (ESR), hyperferritinemia, elevated triglycerides, elevated D-dimers, and low serum fibrinogen levels. Patients can have hepatic dysfunction, seizures, and can worsen rapidly. MAS is an indication for hospitalization. Diagnostic criteria for MAS in patients with systemic JIA were published in 2016 [37] and a diagnostic scoring tool for the identification of MAS in patients with systemic JIA was developed and validated in 2019 [38]. Patients with suspected MAS should be treated promptly with corticosteroids and biologics [41] in conjunction with rheumatology.

### Bone Health

Many children with arthritis do not develop adequate bone mineralization. A failure to undergo the normal increase in bone mass during puberty is common and patients are therefore less able to achieve an adequate peak skeletal mass [39]. These patients may then be at an increased risk for fractures in adulthood and for an earlier onset of osteoporosis [40]. There are no recommendations for regular bone densitometry screening exams. The recommended daily allowance (RDA) of calcium for 14–18 years old is 1300 mg/day, decreasing to 1000 mg/day for ages 19–30. RDA for vitamin D is 600 IU/day [41]. It is preferable that this come from dietary intake rather than supplements. Treatment may be indicated for poor bone health in this patient population at risk for steroid-induced osteoporosis [42].

## Psychosocial Function

There have been multiple studies investigating the long-term social outcomes of patients with JIA. Young adults with rheumatic diseases reported challenges with job absenteeism, disruptions, and loss of productivity [43]. A meta-analysis found that in general, young adults with a history of JIA were less likely to be employed when compared with healthy peers. This was associated with worse disease, less educational attainment, and female sex [44]. Adults with JIA may have more pain, depression, and anxiety than their peers without a chronic condition [45]. Having a comorbid depression was associated with poor adherence in youth with SLE [46]. A German study found that adults with JIA who completed a health-related quality of life (HRQOL) questionnaire were more likely to report depression and anxiety symptoms compared to healthy controls (28 vs 4%) as well as more pain symptoms (56 vs 28%) [47]. Another study of youth with JIA and SLE suggests an association between symptoms of depression and anxiety and disease-related outcomes, including HRQOL[48]. Screening tools are freely available [45] and addressing the behavioral health issues with early intervention by working closely with a mental health clinician will improve long-term clinical and psychological outcomes of youth and young adults with rheumatic disease conditions.

## Reproductive Health

Women with inflammatory arthritis may have lower fertility rates than the general population [48]. Patients with JIA can have normal healthy children. Special issues related to medication toxicity are discussed above (see “Therapy” section). The use of oral contraceptive pills is considered safe in women with rheumatoid arthritis. There is a theoretical concern about increased risk of pelvic infection with intrauterine devices (IUDs); however, this has not been reported in other immunocompromised patients. ACR guidelines for the management of reproductive health in rheumatic disease recommend all modalities of contraception for this patient population though preferentially recommends IUDs or progestin implants over other hormonal contraceptives [49].

## Pain

Some patients may continue to have pain despite clinical improvement of their arthritis. Arthritis pain is typically associated with morning stiffness and improvement with activity. If the history shows increased pain with activity, osteoarthritis, injury, or other mechanical causes should be considered. Pain syndromes are also seen in this population and JIA and fibromyalgia can coexist in the same patient. Pain syndromes should be considered if a patient’s reported symptoms are not congruent with their physical exam findings [43]. If a pain syndrome is diagnosed, the mainstays of treatment are physical therapy, psychotherapy, and ensuring adequate sleep [44]. There is a limited role for opiate analgesics in the treatment of JIA or pain syndromes and they should be used sparingly given the risk of dependency and addiction.

## Immunizations

If patients are taking immunosuppressive medications, then live vaccines (varicella, zoster, MMR, nasal influenza) are contraindicated. Patients should receive a yearly injectable influenza vaccine, pneumococcal vaccines, and routine adult vaccinations [2]. Vaccinations against SARS-CoV-2 infections are well tolerated in this patient population. Data have shown that the vaccine does not result in increased flares [50, 51]. Recommendations for vaccination in this patient population and the medication management are frequently updated on the ACR website [52].

## Healthcare Transition

Another important area to manage is the transition from pediatric to adult health care [53]. This time between ages 12 and 25 poses risks of increased morbidity and mortality especially for those with chronic conditions often coming from poor preparation in the pediatric system and lost to follow-up in the adult health care system [54]. Gaps in care can result in poor outcomes, disease flares, and hospitalizations [55]. Transition involves planning, transfer, and integration into adult care. Having a structured process has demonstrated improved medication adherence, improved patient satisfaction and utilization of health care [56]. The AAP, AAFP and ACP put together consensusguidelines that suggests utilizing the structured 6 Core Elements of healthcare transition approach [57]. There are tools and guides available at www.gottransition.org and the ACR website https://www.rheumatology.org/Practice-Quality/Pediatric-to-Adult-Rheumatology-Care-Transition. This approach has been demonstrated to improve outcomes in pediatric rheumatology settings [58]. During the COVID pandemic when many clinic visits were virtual and adolescents felt more isolated, the risks of a poor outcome were intensified [58]. Adult providers have guidance available on how to increase engagement of young adults in their care using a WELCOME mnemonic [59] that goes through areas to assist the newly transferred young adult to feel more comfortable in the adult provider's new clinic and the adult health care system.

## Conclusion

JIA is a chronic autoimmune condition, and arthritis can persist into adulthood. The goal of therapy is to eliminate inflammation, prevent joint destruction, and minimize the undesirable effects of the disease on the youth/young adults' growth and development. Patients are at risk for long-term consequences of growth disturbance and joint abnormalities. They may suffer from comorbid conditions such as vision loss and chronic pain. They are at risk for associated conditions such as cardiovascular disease and osteoporosis. They may have other concerns related to transition care, employment, and reproductive health. Adult providers need to be aware of the wide range of issues related to patients with JIA ("Appendix").

## Appendix

| Juvenile Idiopathic Arthritis (JIA) condition fact sheet | |
|---|---|
| Definition | JIA is an autoimmune disease defined by arthritis occurring for greater than 6 weeks in a child younger than 16<br>• Subtypes of JIA include systemic, oligoarticular, polyarticular (rheumatoid factor positive or negative), enthesitis-related arthritis, psoriatic arthritis, and undifferentiated<br>• Each subtype of JIA has a different presentation |
| Epidemiology | • Prevalence of JIA ranges from 10 to 400 per 100,000 around the world<br>• There is overall a 2:1 female-to-male ratio<br>• Oligoarthritis is the most common subtype of childhood arthritis affecting 50–80% of all children with chronic arthritis<br>• A substantial number of JIA patients continue to have active arthritis into adulthood |

<table>
<tr><th colspan="3">Juvenile Idiopathic Arthritis (JIA) condition fact sheet</th></tr>
<tr><td rowspan="3">Special considerations</td><td colspan="2">Individuals with JIA are at risk for comorbid physical and mental health conditions, including</td></tr>
<tr><td>• Persistent arthritis<br>• Growth abnormalities<br>• Ocular complications<br>• Medication toxicity including Infection, teratogenic risk</td><td>• Anxiety and depression<br>• Macrophage activation syndrome<br>• Chronic pain</td></tr>
<tr><td colspan="2">Individuals are at heightened risk for chronic conditions, including<br>• Uveitis<br>• Atherosclerosis and coronary heart disease<br>• Osteoporosis and fractures<br>• Osteoarthritis<br>• Malignancy<br>• Need for joint replacement surgery<br>• Sjögren's syndrome</td></tr>
<tr><td>Recommended screening</td><td colspan="2">Patients may require lab screening for medication side effects</td></tr>
</table>

### Suggested Reading List

- Petty RE, Laxer RM, Lindsley CB, Wedderburn L, Fuhlbrigge RC, Mellins ED (eds). Textbook of pediatric rheumatology, Eighth edition. Philadelphia, PA: Elsevier. 2020.
- Espinosa M, Gottlieb BS. Juvenile Idiopathic Arthritis. Pediatr. Rev. 2012;33, 303–313.
- Coulson EJ, Hanson HJM, Foster HE. What does an adult rheumatologist need to know about juvenile idiopathic arthritis? Rheumatol Oxf Engl. 2014 Dec;53(12):2155–66.

### Patient/Caregiver/Provider Resources

- Arthritis Foundation: http://www.kidsgetarthritistoo.org
- Getting Accommodations for Juvenile Arthritis at College: https://www.youtube.com/watch?v=ctuj0nXkey0
- Transition and Secondary School Issues Resources: http://www.gottransition.org

## References


1. U.S Department of Education. Students with disabilities preparing for postsecondary education. US Department of Education (ED); 2020. https://www2.ed.gov/about/offices/list/ocr/transition.html.
2. Center for Disease Control. In: CDC, editor. Adult immunization schedule by vaccine and age group; 2024. https://www.cdc.gov/vaccines/schedules/hcp/imz/adult.html.
3. Cauffman E, Steinberg L. (Im)maturity of judgment in adolescence: why adolescents may be less culpable than adults. Behav Sci Law. 2000;18(6):741–60.
4. American College of Rheumatology. Juvenile Idiopathic Arthritis (JIA). ACP High Value Care. 2016; https://www.acponline.org/sites/default/files/documents/clinical_information/high_value_care/clinician_resources/pediatric_adult_care_transitions/rheumatology/acr_self_assessment_young_adults.docx
5. Singh JA, Saag KG, Bridges SL, Akl EA, Bannuru RR, Sullivan MC, et al. American College of Rheumatology guideline for the treatment of rheumatoid arthritis. Arthritis Rheumatol. 2016;68(1):1–26.
6. Petty RE, Laxer RM, Lindsley CB, Wedderburn L, Fuhlbrigge RC, Mellins ED, editors. Textbook of pediatric rheumatology. 8th ed. Philadelphia: Elsevier; 2020.
7. Coulson EJ, Hanson HJM, Foster HE. What does an adult rheumatologist need to know about juvenile idiopathic arthritis? Rheumatol Oxf Engl. 2014;53(12):2155–66.
8. Petty RE, Southwood TR, Manners P, Baum J, Glass DN, Goldenberg J, et al. International league of associations for rheumatology classification of juvenile idiopathic arthritis: second revision, Edmonton, 2001. J Rheumatol. 2004;31(2):390–2.
9. Nigrovic PA, Colbert RA, Holers VM, Ozen S, Ruperto N, Thompson SD, Wedderburn LR, Yeung RSM, Martini A. Biological classification of childhood arthritis: roadmap to a molecular nomenclature. Nat Rev Rheumatol. 2021;17(5):257–69.
10. Debrach AC, Rougelot A, Beaumel A, Cabrera N, Belot A, Duquesne A, Aubry-Rozier B, Hofer M, Couret M, Larbre JP, Coury F. Comparison of paediatric and adult classification criteria in juvenile idiopathic arthritis during the transition from paediatric to adult care. Joint Bone Spine. 2021;88(1):105047.
11. Heiligenhaus A, Niewerth M, Ganser G, Heinz C, Minden K. German uveitis in childhood study group. Prevalence and complications of uveitis in juvenile idiopathic arthritis in a population-based nation-wide study in Germany: suggested modification of the current screening guidelines. Rheumatol Oxf Engl. 2007;46(6):1015–9.
12. Tebo AE, Jaskowski T, Davis KW, Whiting A, Clifford B, Zeft A, et al. Profiling anti-cyclic citrullinated peptide antibodies in patients with juvenile

idiopathic arthritis. Pediatr Rheumatol Online J. 2012;10(1):29.
13. Saurenmann RK, Rose JB, Tyrrell P, Feldman BM, Laxer RM, Schneider R, et al. Epidemiology of juvenile idiopathic arthritis in a multiethnic cohort: ethnicity as a risk factor. Arthritis Rheum. 2007;56(6):1974–84.
14. Farragher TM, Lunt M, Plant D, Bunn DK, Barton A, Symmons DPM. Benefit of early treatment in inflammatory polyarthritis patients with anti-cyclic citrullinated peptide antibodies versus those without antibodies. Arthritis Care Res. 2010;62(5):664–75.
15. Packham JC, Hall MA. Long-term follow-up of 246 adults with juvenile idiopathic arthritis: functional outcome. Rheumatol Oxf Engl. 2002;41(12):1428–35.
16. Gomez KS, Raza K, Jones SD, Kennedy LG, Calin A. Juvenile onset ankylosing spondylitis—more girls than we thought? J Rheumatol. 1997;24(4):735–7.
17. Hersh A, von Scheven E, Yelin E. Adult outcomes of childhood-onset rheumatic diseases. Nat Rev Rheumatol. 2011;7(5):290–5.
18. Flatø B, Lien G, Smerdel-Ramoya A, Vinje O. Juvenile psoriatic arthritis: longterm outcome and differentiation from other subtypes of juvenile idiopathic arthritis. J Rheumatol. 2009;36(3):642–50.
19. Beukelman T, Patkar NM, Saag KG, Tolleson-Rinehart S, Cron RQ, DeWitt EM, et al. American College of Rheumatology recommendations for the treatment of juvenile idiopathic arthritis: initiation and safety monitoring of therapeutic agents for the treatment of arthritis and systemic features. Arthritis Care Res. 2011;63(4):465–82.
20. Ruperto N, Brunner HI, Synoverska O, Ting TV, Mendoza CA, Spindler A, Vyzhga Y, Marzan K, Grebenkina L, Tirosh I, Imundo L, Jerath R, Kingsbury DJ, Sozeri B, Vora SS, Prahalad S, Zholobova E, Butbul Aviel Y, Chasnyk V, Lerman M, Nanda K, Schmeling H, Tory H, Uziel Y, Viola DO, Posner HB, Kanik KS, Wouters A, Chang C, Zhang R, Lazariciu I, Hsu MA, Suehiro RM, Martini A, Lovell DJ, Paediatric Rheumatology International Trials Organisation (PRINTO) and Pediatric Rheumatology Collaborative Study Group (PRCSG). Tofacitinib in juvenile idiopathic arthritis: a double-blind, placebo-controlled, withdrawal phase 3 randomised trial. Lancet. 2021;398(10315):1984–96.
21. Consensus treatment plans for new-onset systemic Juvenile Idiopathic Arthritis, EM DW, Kimura Y, Beukelman T, Nigrovic PA, Onel K, Prahalad S, Schneider R, Stoll ML, Angeles-Han S, Milojevic D, Schikler KN, Vehe RK, Weiss JE, Weiss P, Ilowite NT, Wallace CA. Juvenile idiopathic arthritis disease-specific research Committee of Childhood Arthritis Rheumatology and Research Alliance. Arthritis Care Res (Hoboken). 2012;64(7):1001–10.
22. Kimura Y, EM DW, et al. Adding canakinumab to the childhood arthritis and rheumatology research Alliance consensus treatment plans for systemic juvenile idiopathic arthritis. Arthritis Care Res (Hoboken). 2014;66(9):1430–1.
23. Ringold S, Weiss PF, Colbert RA, EM DW, Lee T, Onel K, Prahalad S, Schneider R, Shenoi S, Vehe RK, Kimura Y. Childhood arthritis and rheumatology research Alliance consensus treatment plans for new-onset polyarticular juvenile idiopathic arthritis. Arthritis Care Res (Hoboken). 2014;66(7):1063–72.
24. Angeles-Han S, et al. Childhood arthritis and rheumatology research Alliance consensus treatment plans for juvenile idiopathic arthritis-associated and idiopathic chronic anterior uveitis. Arthritis Care Res (Hoboken). 2019;71(4):482–91.
25. Ringold S, Angeles-Han ST, Beukelman T, Lovell D, Cuello CA, Becker ML, Colbert RA, Feldman BM, Ferguson PJ, Gewanter H, Guzman J, Horonjeff J, Nigrovic PA, Ombrello MJ, Passo MH, Stoll ML, Rabinovich CE, Schneider R, Halyabar O, Hays K, Shah AA, Sullivan N, Szymanski AM, Turgunbaev M, Turner A, Reston J. 2019 American College of Rheumatology/Arthritis Foundation guideline for the treatment of juvenile idiopathic arthritis: therapeutic approaches for non-systemic polyarthritis, Sacroiliitis, and Enthesitis. Arthritis Care Res (Hoboken). 2019;71(6):717–34.
26. Beukelman T, Xie F, Chen L, Baddley JW, Delzell E, Grijalva CG, et al. Rates of hospitalized bacterial infection associated with juvenile idiopathic arthritis and its treatment. Arthritis Rheum. 2012;64(8):2773–80.
27. Beukelman T, Haynes K, Curtis JR, Xie F, Chen L, Bemrich-Stolz CJ, et al. Rates of malignancy associated with juvenile idiopathic arthritis and its treatment. Arthritis Rheum. 2012;64(4):1263–71.
28. Ringold S, Cron RQ. The temporomandibular joint in juvenile idiopathic arthritis: frequently used and frequently arthritic. Pediatr Rheumatol. 2009;7(1):11.
29. Hospach T, Maier J, Müller-Abt P, Patel A, Horneff G, von Kalle T. Cervical spine involvement in patients with juvenile idiopathic arthritis—MRI follow-up study. Pediatr Rheumatol Online J. 2014;4(12):9.
30. Bohr AH, Fuhlbrigge RC, Pedersen FK, de Ferranti SD, Müller K. Premature subclinical atherosclerosis in children and young adults with juvenile idiopathic arthritis. A review considering preventive measures. Pediatr Rheumatol Online J. 2016;14:3.
31. Coulson EJ, Ng W-F, Goff I, Foster HE. Cardiovascular risk in juvenile idiopathic arthritis. Rheumatology. 2013;52(7):1163–71.
32. Feldman DE, Vinet É, Bérard A, Duffy C, Hazel B, Meshefedjian G, et al. Heart disease, hypertension, gestational diabetes and pre-eclampsia/eclampsia in mothers with juvenile arthritis: a nested case-control study. Arthritis Care Res. 2017;69(2):306–9.
33. Anderson JH, Anderson KR, Aulie HA, Crowson CS, Mason TG, Ardoin SP, et al. Juvenile idiopathic arthritis and future risk for cardiovascular disease: a multicenter study. Scand J Rheumatol. 2016;8:1–5.
34. Pelajo CF, Lopez-Benitez JM, Miller LC. Obesity and disease activity in juvenile idiopathic arthritis. Pediatr Rheumatol Online J. 2012;12(10):3.

35. Pincus T, Gibson KA, Block JA. Premature mortality: a neglected outcome in rheumatic diseases? Arthritis Care Res. 2015;67(8):1043–6.
36. Bouayed K, Alyanakian M-A, Cordonnier C, Caillat-Zucman S, Testelin S, Lambrey G, et al. Sjögren syndrome: an unexpected disease occurring fourteen years after oligoarticular onset juvenile idiopathic arthritis. Rheumatology. 2002;41(10):1190–3.
37. Ravelli A, Minoia F, Davì S, Horne A, Bovis F, Pistorio A, Aricò M, Avcin T, Behrens EM, De Benedetti F, Filipovic L, Grom AA, Henter JI, Ilowite NT, Jordan MB, Khubchandani R, Kitoh T, Lehmberg K, Lovell DJ, Miettunen P, Nichols KE, Ozen S, Pachlopnik Schmid J, Ramanan AV, Russo R, Schneider R, Sterba G, Uziel Y, Wallace C, Wouters C, Wulffraat N, Demirkaya E, Brunner HI, Martini A, Ruperto N, Cron RQ, Paediatric Rheumatology International Trials Organisation; Childhood Arthritis and Rheumatology Research Alliance; Pediatric Rheumatology Collaborative Study Group; Histiocyte Society. 2016 classification criteria for macrophage activation syndrome complicating systemic juvenile idiopathic arthritis: a European league against rheumatism/American College of Rheumatology/ Paediatric rheumatology international trials organisation collaborative initiative. Ann Rheum Dis. 2016;75(3):481–9.
38. Minoia F, Bovis F, Davì S on behalf of the Pediatric Rheumatology International Trials Organization, the Childhood Arthritis & Rheumatology Research Alliance, the Pediatric Rheumatology Collaborative Study Group and the Histiocyte Society, et al. Development and initial validation of the MS score for diagnosis of macrophage activation syndrome in systemic juvenile idiopathic arthritis. Ann Rheum Dis. 2019;78:1357–62.
39. Cassidy JT, Hillman LS. Abnormalities in skeletal growth in children with juvenile rheumatoid arthritis. Rheum Dis Clin N Am. 1997;23(3):499–522.
40. Zak M, Hassager C, Lovell DJ, Nielsen S, Henderson CJ, Pedersen FK. Assessment of bone mineral density in adults with a history of juvenile chronic arthritis: a cross-sectional long-term followup study. Arthritis Rheum. 1999;42(4):790–8.
41. Ross AC, Taylor CL, Yaktine AL, Del Valle HB, editors. Committee to review dietary reference intakes for vitamin D and calcium; food and nutrition board; Institute of Medicine. Dietary reference intakes for calcium and vitamin D. Washington, DC: National Academies Press; 2011.
42. Buckley L, Guyatt G, Fink HA, Cannon M, Grossman J, Hansen KE, Humphrey MB, Lane NE, Magrey M, Miller M, Morrison L, Rao M, Byun Robinson A, Saha S, Wolver S, Bannuru RR, Vaysbrot E, Osani M, Turgunbaev M, Miller AS, McAlindon T. 2017 American College of Rheumatology Guideline for the prevention and treatment of glucocorticoid-induced osteoporosis. Arthritis Care Res (Hoboken). 2017;69(8):1095–110. Erratum in: Arthritis Care Res (Hoboken). 2017 Nov;69(11):1776.
43. Jetha A, Badley E, Beaton D, Fortin PR, Shiff NJ, Gignac MAM. Unpacking early work experiences of young adults with rheumatic disease: an examination of absenteeism, job disruptions and productivity loss. Arthritis Care Res. 2015;67(9):1246–54.
44. Jetha A. The impact of arthritis on the early employment experiences of young adults: a literature review. Disabil Health J. 2015;8(3):317–24.
45. Treemarcki EB, Danguecan AN, Cunningham NR, Knight AM. In: Kimura Y, Schanberg L, editors. Mental Health in Pediatric Rheumatology inPediatrc Rheumatology Comes of Age: Part II. Rheumatic Disease Clinics; 2022. p. 67–90.
46. Davis AM, Graham TB, Zhu Y. Depression and Medication non adherence in childhood onset systemic lupys erythematosis. Lupus. 2018;27:1532–41.
47. Barth S, Haas J-P, Schlichtiger J, Molz J, Bisdorff B, Michels H, et al. Long-term health-related quality of life in German patients with juvenile idiopathic arthritis in comparison to German general population. PLoS One. 2016;11(4):e0153267.
48. Donneely C, Cunningham N, Jones JT, et al. Fatique and depression predict reduced health-relate quality of like in childhood onset lupus. Lupus. 2018;27:124–33.
49. Sammaritano LR, Bermas BL, Chakravarty EE, Chambers C, Clowse MEB, Lockshin MD, Marder W, Guyatt G, Branch DW, Buyon J, Christopher-Stine L, Crow-Hercher R, Cush J, Druzin M, Kavanaugh A, Laskin CA, Plante L, Salmon J, Simard J, Somers EC, Steen V, Tedeschi SK, Vinet E, White CW, Yazdany J, Barbhaiya M, Bettendorf B, Eudy A, Jayatilleke A, Shah AA, Sullivan N, Tarter LL, Birru Talabi M, Turgunbaev M, Turner A, D'Anci KE. 2020 American College of Rheumatology Guideline for the Management of Reproductive Health in rheumatic and musculoskeletal diseases. Arthritis Rheumatol. 2020;72(4):529–56.
50. Machado PM et al. Safty of Vaccination against SARS-COV2 in people with rheumatic and musculoskeletal diseases: results from the EULAR Coronovirus Vaccine (COVAX) reported physician Registry Annals Rheum Disease 2021.
51. Curtis J, et al. American College of Rheumatology Guidance for COVID-19 vaccination in patients with rheumatic and musculoskeletal diseases: version 3. Arthritis Rheumatol. 2021;73(10):e60–75.
52. Mikuls TR, Johnson SR, Fraenkel L, Arasaratnam RJ, Baden LR, Bermas BL, et al. American College of Rheumatology Guidance for the Management of Rheumatic Disease in adult patients during the COVID-19 pandemic: version 3. Arthritis Rheumatol. 2021;73(2):e1–e12. https://doi.org/10.1002/art.41596.
53. Tang S, Li S, Zheng S, Ding Y, Zhu D, Sun C, Hu Y, Qiao J, Fang H. Understanding of cytokines and targeted therapy in macrophage activation syndrome. Semin Arthritis Rheum. 2021 Feb;51(1):198–210.
54. Lebrun-Harris L, McManus M, Ilango SM, Cyr M, McLellan SB, Mann MY, White PH. Transition

planning among youth with and without special health care needs in the United States. Pediatrics. 2018;142(4):1–11.

55. Moreno MA. JAMA pediatric patient page. JAMA Pediatr. 2013;167:684.
56. Schmidt A, Ilango SM, McManus M, Rogers K, White PH. Outcomes of pediatric to adult health care transition interventions: an updated systematic review. J Pediatr Nurs. 2020;51:92–107.
57. White PH, Cooley WC, Transitions Clinical Authoring Group. American Academy of Pediatrics, American Academy of family physicians, American College of Physicians. Supporting the health care transition from adolescence to adulthood in the medical home. Pediatrics. 2018;142:85–104.
58. McDonagh JE, Tattersall R, Clinch J, Swan J, Foster HE, McCann L. Developmentally appropriate transitional care during the Covid-19 pandemic for young people with juvenile-onset rheumatic and musculoskeletal diseases: the rationale for a position statement. Pediatr Rheumatol Online J. 2021 Aug 25;19(1):136.
59. Sadun RE, Covert LT, Lawson RF. Transitioning to adulthood with a rheumatic disease inPediatric rheumatology comes of age: part II Eds Yukiko Kimura and Laura Schanberg rheumatic disease clinics; 2022. p. 141–56.

# Muscular Dystrophy 35

Lekha M. Rao and Elba Y. Gerena Maldonado

## Case Presentation

Luis Antonio is a pleasant 21-year-old male with Duchenne muscular dystrophy (DMD), who presents with his mother to establish care at the primary care clinic. A review of his medical records from his pediatrician and several specialists at the local children's hospital reveals that he was being treated for cardiomyopathy, restrictive lung disease, low bone density, and his limited functional status given his severe muscle weakness.

One of the main concerns that his mother brings up during the appointment is his recent unplanned weight loss. While obtaining his vital signs, the clinic medical assistant was unable to obtain his current body weight because she could not transfer him from his power wheelchair to the exam table. On examination, the patient has tetraplegia with a trace pincer grasp, which he uses to move the joystick of the wheelchair. He is also using a "Sip-n-Puff" machine that is mounted on the back of the power wheelchair. At one point during the appointment, the mother states that she misses the multidisciplinary clinics at the children's hospital and that the family is having a hard time transitioning from the pediatric system into the adult healthcare system.

During the interview process, the patient is able to provide most of his history and is cooperative and agreeable; however, his mother tends to interrupt the patient's answers. While speaking to Luis alone, he reveals that his career goal is to finish a teaching degree in a community college and start working. A close friend of Luis, who also had DMD, has recently died, and he is wondering about life and death and what measures he should start taking at this moment.

## Case Discussion

The story of Luis Antonio is a typical case of a young adult with DMD, which is a rapidly progressive neuromuscular disease with multisystemic involvement. For these patients and their families, the transition period from pediatric to adult healthcare systems is a challenging one. As they are often dealing with numerous changes simultaneously, many of these patients and their families tend to feel overwhelmed and unsupported by the adult healthcare system. Although efforts are being made by most pediatric hospitals to prepare and aid patients and their families

L. M. Rao (✉)
Division of Neurology, Department of Pediatrics, David Geffen School of Medicine at UCLA, Los Angeles, CA, USA
e-mail: lrao@mednet.ucla.edu

E. Y. Gerena Maldonado
Montana Providence Health and Services, Montana Spine and Pain Center, Missoula, MT, USA
e-mail: elba.gerenamaldonado@providence.org


A. A. Kuo et al. (eds.), *Care of Adults with Chronic Childhood Conditions*,
https://doi.org/10.1007/978-3-031-54281-7_35

in the transition process, it is still a taxing period for all those involved.

A 2012 study conducted in the United Kingdom, in which patients with DMD older than 15 years of age and their family members were interviewed, it was self-reported that these patients were more likely to receive fewer healthcare services and were less satisfied with their current health care compared to when they were children [1]. This period of transition to the adult healthcare system has been associated with a decline in health outcomes not only among the muscular dystrophy population but also among patients with many other chronic conditions of childhood [2]. It is for this reason that most experts in the care of individuals with Duchenne muscular dystrophy urge that transition not be thought of as a single event but as a continuing process of increased choices and autonomy [3].

For adult primary care providers (PCPs), the initial evaluation of a new patient with multiple comorbidities associated with a rare progressive disease can be an overwhelming process. The focus should be to organize multidisciplinary care, even when the providers are not in the same location. This process can be carried out in the adult healthcare system by having clear and open communication between the cardiologist, pulmonologist, endocrinologist, neuromuscular specialist, and PCP. Current guidelines emphasize the need for coordination among all adult specialists as the key to providing successful care to these patients [4, 5].

This case also illustrates the need to improve the architectural barriers that are still present in most adult practices. There is a growing population of patients who will need proper wheelchair access, special weighing scales that can accommodate wheelchairs or beds with integrated weighing systems, and Hoyer or ceiling lifts for safe transfers. Although these patients are likely going to establish care with an adult cardiologist and pulmonologist, it will be the PCP who will likely monitor the patient's weight, skin integrity, and nutrition.

Furthermore, adult healthcare providers need to reinforce the autonomy that these patients have while being respectful to the family dynamics. Among the discussions that should take place include sexual health, advance directives, physician orders for life-sustaining treatment (POLST) forms (as appropriate), and death and dying. These are important topics for discussion since many patients with DMD are now surviving into their fourth and fifth decade of life, and some parents might not have wanted these issues previously addressed with their children [6]. However, given the multiple comorbidities associated with this condition, patients with DMD are at a higher risk for rapid and serious complications from pneumonia, cardiac arrhythmia, and other life-threatening events. Therefore, it is imperative that patients are aware of the POLST forms and resources that might be needed as their condition progresses.

Optimal care for patients with DMD should maximize function and quality of life. Early involvement of palliative care specialists as part of the multidisciplinary team is theorized to likely improve the quality of life for these patients. The main goal is to help these young men attain the necessary skills to manage their personal needs and health care. It is important that they become effective self-advocates and be able to pursue their own interests. (For additional information on palliative care for adults with chronic childhood conditions, please see Chap. 45 of this book.)

## Definition

Muscular dystrophies encompass a diverse group of primarily muscle disorders, all of which fall under the category of orphan (rare) diseases. Most of the muscular dystrophies can be linked back to a genetic mutation, each with its own clinical course and expression [7, 8]. The most common symptom is muscle weakness that worsens with time. Some of these conditions have a rapid progressive course and tend to lead to an early death in childhood, whereas others are not immediately evident and manifest an "adult-onset" phenotype.

## Prevalence

DMD, myotonic dystrophy, and facioscapulohumeral muscular dystrophy are among the most common muscular dystrophies [9–11]. Duchenne muscular dystrophy is an X-linked disorder that has an estimated worldwide prevalence of about 1–2 per 10,000 males or 1 per 3500–5000 live births [12, 13]. Myotonic dystrophy type 1 and type 2 have a combined prevalence of 1 in 8000 (12.5/100,000), based on clinical ascertainment [14]. Facioscapulohumeral muscular dystrophy (FSHD) is the third most common form of muscular dystrophy, with a prevalence of approximately 1 in 15,000–20,000 [9, 15].

## Pathophysiology

The underlying molecular abnormalities in the muscular dystrophies involve structural proteins. DMD is clinically manifested when there is an absence of dystrophin, a key component of the sarcolemma of the skeletal muscle cell. Dystrophin is involved in the stabilization of the muscle cell membrane during contraction and relaxation and acts as a link between the intracellular cytoskeleton and extracellular matrix [16, 17]. Dystrophin also plays a role in the ability of muscle fibers to differentiate and may play a role in the organization of the postsynaptic membrane [18]. Loss or abnormal dystrophin destabilizes the sarcolemma, making the muscle fibers susceptible to contraction injury [19]. The repeated process of injury and necrosis eventually leads to the replacement of muscles by fat and connective tissue that is clinically manifested as progressive muscle weakness [20]. Dystrophin not only exists in the sarcolemma of skeletal muscle but also exists as a number of other tissue-specific isoforms, some exclusively or predominantly expressed in the brain, heart, and/or in other tissues [21].

The responsible gene, *DMD*, is located on the short arm of the X chromosome at locus Xp21 [22, 23]. Approximately two-thirds of cases are associated with a detectable deletion or duplication of segments within the *DMD* gene [24]. There is a variable phenotypic expression that generally correlates with the type of mutation found on this gene. Milder allelic variants of Duchenne muscular dystrophy include Becker muscular dystrophy, X-linked dilated cardiomyopathy, and manifesting female carriers. In Becker muscular dystrophy, the abnormal dystrophin preserves enough function to slow down the progression of the illness. Therefore, these patients tend to preserve ambulation well into their late teens or early 1920s. However, in Duchenne muscular dystrophy, the absence of dystrophin is characterized by a progressive muscular weakness that leads to loss of ambulation early in childhood, usually before 12 years of age. In X-linked dilated cardiomyopathy, dystrophin has a different expression or function in cardiac rather than skeletal muscle.

About 10% of all the female carriers will manifest with some muscle weakness, mostly in cognitive and/or cardiac function [25]. This is thought to be the result of skewed X inactivation.

In patients with DMD, death usually results from either cardiac or respiratory failure. However, the implementation of better respiratory care has improved survival in these patients with a current estimated life expectancy of 25–31.7 years [6, 26, 27].

## Treatment

### Glucocorticoids

The natural history of muscular dystrophy has changed in the last few decades due to the widespread use of corticosteroids as a pharmacological intervention for muscle strength and function [4, 28]. Glucocorticoids, such as prednisone and deflazacort, have been shown to prolong walking by transiently increasing and then slowing the decline in muscle strength and improving pulmonary measures by decreasing the progression of scoliosis [28, 29]. Due to the latter, many experts continue the use of glucocorticoids long after the patient has lost the ability to ambulate. This treatment has to be coupled with a comprehensive physiotherapy program that includes regular stretching exercises for the upper and lower limbs with the goal to avoid and/or minimize contractures.

Most often, boys are started on corticosteroids between 5 and 7 years of age, before they start to lose motor milestones. However, some specialists favor starting as early as 3–4 years of age. This practice introduces these patients to the consequences of long-term use of glucocorticoids, including behavioral issues, fracture risk, and obesity. Those patients who are not treated with corticosteroids have about a 90% chance of developing progressive scoliosis [30]. Depending on the rate of progression of the scoliosis, the patients might be eligible for spinal fusion surgery. Bone health is an important part of the lifelong care of patients with Duchenne muscular dystrophy, and awareness of potential problems and means to assess these problems are preferably done by the PCP in conjunction with bone health specialists. Experts recommend that these patients have their serum 25-hydroxy vitamin D levels monitored (at least annually) and undergo an assessment for nutritional intake of calcium and vitamin D, with appropriate supplementation of vitamin D and calcium, if needed. Patients are also encouraged to have physical activity (including standing) and exposure to sunshine as well as an endocrine consultation if no pubertal signs are present by 14 years of age. In regard to imaging studies to aid in the screening process, it is recommended that a baseline lumbar spine dual energy X-ray absorptiometry (DEXA) is obtained at 3 years of age or when the patient is started on glucocorticoids and subsequently repeated at 12–24 monthly intervals [31, 32]. If back pain is present, a spine radiograph should be obtained to assess for vertebral fractures [33].

Due to the high rate of complications related to long-term glucocorticoid treatment, alternate anti-inflammatory steroidal therapies are under investigation, including vamorolone, a synthetic compound that binds to corticosteroid receptors but lacks the 11-carbon oxygen group that is 1 of 5 molecular contacts with the glucocorticoid receptor, potentially leading to fewer adverse effects such as stunting of growth and decreased bone density [34].

### Gene Modulation Therapies

Emerging evidence is arising that gene therapy for DMD may be effective in slowing the course of disease and/or prolonging survival, whether via exon-skipping with antisense oligonucleotides or promotion of ribosomal read-through of premature termination codons. For patients with exon 51 deletions, which accounts for about 13% of patients, eteplirsen has been found to increase dystrophin production, attenuate the decline of forced vital capacity in nonambulatory patients, and show a slower decline in ambulation, leading to its FDA approval in 2016 [35–37]. Similarly, for the approximately 8% of DMD patients with an exon 53 deletion, golodirsen was approved in 2019 after initial studies showed an increase in dystrophin production, although a trial to prove clinical benefit is still underway [38]. Viltolarsen was also approved in 2020 for patients with an exon 52 deletion, which accounts for approximately 8% of all DMD patients, and for an additional approximately 8% of patients with an exon 45 deletion, casimersen was approved in 2021 [39, 40]. These medications are administered intravenously once a week and are generally well tolerated with a low rate of adverse events. Ataluren, which is available as an oral formulation in Europe, increases dystrophin production by promoting read through of nonsense mutations of the stop codon, which accounts for approximately 13% of DMD patients.

## Management of Comorbidities

### Respiratory

DMD is associated with progressive loss of respiratory muscle strength and a high risk for respiratory complications due to ineffective cough, nocturnal hypoventilation, sleep-disordered breathing, and daytime respiratory failure. There have been several published guidelines for respiratory management in DMD [41]. The proactive approach to respiratory management with the use of assisted cough and nocturnal ventilation has been shown to prolong survival [6]. Nevertheless, there has previously been controversy among experts regarding the best method of assisting ventilation, that is, whether to choose noninvasive ventilation or ventilation via tracheostomy. The currently favored method is the use of noninvasive ventilation in almost all clinical situations [42].

In patients who have not yet started glucocorticoids, idebenone has been shown to be a potentially beneficial adjunct treatment in reducing the loss of respiratory function in a small European trial. Idebenone is a short-chain benzoquinone which is an antioxidant and inhibitor of lipid peroxidation and which may stabilize peak expiratory flow as percentage predicted (a marker of expiratory muscle strength) [43].

## Cardiac

Cardiac disease in DMD manifests most often as a dilated cardiomyopathy and/or cardiac arrhythmia [44]. Patients with DMD should be followed by a cardiologist for regular monitoring with electrocardiogram (ECG), Holter monitor, and echocardiography. Published guidelines recommend a baseline assessment of cardiac function should be done at diagnosis or by the age of 6 years, especially if this can be done without sedation [44, 45]. It should be done every 2 years until the age of 10, at which time it should be done annually. Angiotensin-converting enzyme (ACE) inhibitors, beta-blockers, and other cardioprotective agents are currently used to reduce progression and can improve ventricular function [46]. A retrospective cohort study published in 2013 sought to determine the impact of steroid therapy on cardiomyopathy and mortality in patients with DMD. The study found that steroid therapy was associated with a considerably lower all-cause mortality rate, due largely to a significant reduction in heart failure-related deaths. Steroid-treated patients experienced a much lower incidence of new-onset cardiomyopathy [47].

## Gastrointestinal

Gastrointestinal and nutritional issues become more prominent in later stages of the disease. Older patients with DMD have progressive pharyngeal weakness that eventually leads to dysphagia, which can result in severe weight loss and the need to consider enteral tube feeding [48]. Other gastrointestinal complications that have been reported include gastric and intestinal dilatation related to air swallowing due to ventilator use and delayed gastric emptying or ileus. For motility issues, stool softeners, laxatives, and stimulants can be used [5]. There is limited published data on recommendations for gastrointestinal issues in the DMD population. Nevertheless, access to a dietitian or nutritionist, a swallowing/speech and language therapist, and a gastroenterologist is of importance as the condition progresses.

## Neurologic/Psychiatric

Cognitive involvement is common in patients with DMD. Of patients with DMD, about 30% have intellectual disability [49]. A recent large, multicenter, international cohort study reported cognitive function being lower in DMD patients as compared to the general population. It also reported that 21% of DMD males scored above the threshold for autism spectrum disorder (ASD), 24% for hyperactivity, and 44% for inattention. Similarly, 19% of patients with Duchenne/Becker muscular dystrophies met the criteria for ASD using the Autism Diagnostic Interview—Revised [50].

DMD is a multisystem disease. As these patients age and reach young adulthood, physicians might encounter issues with emotional adjustment and depression. Anxiety might also be an issue and can be exacerbated by cognitive deficits in mental flexibility and adaptability (i.e., overly rigid thought processes) [50]. Increased rates of depression in parents of children who have DMD underscore the need for assessment and support of the entire family [51]. Recommendations are to have a comprehensive neuropsychological assessment at or near the time of diagnosis and prior to entering formal schooling [4].

## Inpatient Considerations

In the setting of severe illness, trauma, or major surgery, patients on chronic glucocorticoid therapy require stress dosing to prevent acute adrenal insufficiency. Stress dosing is usually calculated based on body-surface area, rather than weight, with hydrocortisone 500–100 mg/m$^2$ per day being administered. Patients on noninvasive ventilation at home will require continued respiratory support in the hospital, along with a pulmonary toilet to prevent atelectasis. Care should be taken with transfers so as to not cause occult fractures in patients with reduced bone density.

Given the increasing mortality with age, involvement of palliative care may be beneficial early in the course of hospitalization, particularly for those on the older end of the expected survival age and those with significant cardiac and/or respiratory compromise.

## Preoperative/Anesthesia

The risks of anesthesia depend on the type of muscular dystrophy present. Patients with *DMD* and *RYR1* mutations are at a higher risk of malignant hyperthermia-like reactions and rhabdomyolysis with exposure to inhalational anesthetic agents, such as halothane and isoflurane [52]. For this reason, it is strongly recommended that intravenous anesthetic techniques be used for DMD patients. Other agents, such as depolarizing muscle relaxants, are contraindicated in this population due to the risk of fatal reactions.

In the preoperative setting, it is recommended that patients with DMD have an echocardiogram and electrocardiogram before general and/or local anesthesia. Preoperative training in the use of manual and assisted cough techniques is necessary, and the use of noninvasive ventilation is strongly recommended for patients with a baseline forced vital capacity below 50% of the predicted value [53].

## Palliative Care

Palliative care is a field with an inherent interdisciplinary nature that is now recognized as a medical subspecialty. As described by the American Academy of Hospice and Palliative Medicine, the focus of palliative care includes the relief of suffering for patients with life-threatening or serious debilitating illness. The intent of palliative care is to neither hasten nor postpone death but instead to offer a support system to help patients live as fully as possible through the integration of medical, psychosocial, and spiritual aspects of patient care [54].

Palliative care services are often provided initially as part of an acute care hospital stay and may be organized around an interdisciplinary consultation service with or without an acute inpatient palliative care ward. However, in the setting of severely progressive neuromuscular diseases, such as DMD, palliative care services are ideally first introduced as part of the multidisciplinary team that will be involved in the patient's care.

There is still a prevalent underutilization of these services, likely due to the existing misconceptions or lack of knowledge about this specialty by both providers and families alike. A 2011 study of 34 families of patients with DMD demonstrated that most families (85%) had never heard the term "palliative care," regardless of their socioeconomic status. The same study also reported that there was a low receipt of other important services, such as pastoral care (27%), respite care (18%), pain management (12%), and hospice care (6%). Only 8 respondents (25%)

reported having any type of directive document in place [55]. All of these services are an integral part of the services provided by the palliative care team.

Unlike hospice, palliative care is applicable earlier in the course of illness, in conjunction with other therapies that may indeed prolong life. The key to effective palliative care is communication. This enables the patient to feel empowered to make informed choices regarding their future care. Progressive conditions such as DMD pose medical and ethical challenges for the patient, the family, and the healthcare staff who are involved in their care. These patients often have high symptom burdens, and the patients and their families must make complex medical decisions regarding the potential use of life-prolonging therapies, such as mechanical ventilation. A significant portion of the impact may be felt by family caregivers who are simultaneously struggling with physical, emotional, and financial stressors associated with the disease [56]. Palliative care can provide the support that family-caregivers and PCPs need to aid in the process of taking care of these medically complex patients.

It is important to remember that optimal care should maximize function and quality of life for patients with muscular dystrophy. Expert multidisciplinary care may improve both the quality and length of life of patients with this type of progressive disease. Coordination and partnerships with hospice programs are major features in which palliative care can aid as the patient continues across the trajectory of their disease. The depth of support available from each palliative care program varies from institution to institution [57]. Therefore, PCPs should reach out to the local palliative care services and agencies and know the resources that are available for them and their patients.

## Conclusion

Patients with muscular dystrophies, in particular DMD, are surviving well into their fourth and fifth decade of life, in part due to early detection and adequate management of their cardiac and pulmonary complications ("Appendix"). Nevertheless, there is still a disparity in regard to the medical care that these patients experience in the pediatric setting compared to the adult healthcare system. It is for this reason that the adult healthcare system needs to continue its efforts in modifying its infrastructure to accommodate the needs of these patients. As part of the team of providers taking care of these patients, the role of the PCP is of the utmost importance, as they are at the center of this objective of maintaining adequate continuity of care. The ultimate goal is to be able to allow these patients to achieve the quality of life that they deserve.

## Appendix

| Muscular dystrophy condition fact sheet | | |
|---|---|---|
| Definition | *Muscular dystrophies are a heterogeneous group of neurodegenerative diseases characterized by:*<br>• Genetic inheritance<br>• Progressive muscle weakness as the primary symptom<br>• Onset of symptoms in either the pediatric or adult setting | |
| Epidemiology | • In the United States, the most common forms of muscular dystrophy are Duchenne muscular dystrophy (DMD), myotonic dystrophy, and facioscapulohumeral muscular dystrophy (FSHD)<br>• DMD is an X-linked disease, whereas myotonic dystrophy and FSHD are autosomal dominant<br>• Newborn screening for DMD places the incidence closer to 1:5000 live male births<br>• The worldwide prevalence of myotonic dystrophy lies in the 5–20 per 100,000 range<br>• The myotonic dystrophies afflict mostly people of European heritage, with lesser frequencies among those of Asian heritage and a virtual absence of disease among those of sub-Saharan African heritage<br>• FSHD has a prevalence of approximately 1:15,000–1:20,000 | |
| Special considerations | *Individuals with muscular dystrophies have high rates of co-morbid physical and mental health conditions, including:* | |
| | • Loss of ambulation<br>• Joint contractures<br>• Cardiomyopathy<br>• Osteopenia/osteoporosis<br>• Gastrointestinal problems | • Sleep disorders<br>• Autism spectrum disorders<br>• Anxiety and depression<br>• Respiratory failure<br>• Dysphagia |
| Recommended screening | • *Cardiac*: ECG, echocardiogram annually after the age of 10 years old<br>• *Respiratory*: Spirometry every 6 months and polysomnography if presenting with nocturnal hypercapnia<br>• *Dysphagia*: Weight and nutritional assessment at every office visit<br>• *Bone health*: Serum 25-hydroxy vitamin D levels at every visit, and DEXA scan every 1–2 years | |

*ECG* electrocardiogram, *DEXA* dual energy X-ray absorptiomtry.

### Suggested Reading List

- Guidelines for diagnosis and management of Duchenne Muscular Dystrophy (Lancet Neurology): https://www.parentprojectmd.org/care/care-guidelines/
- Guidelines for evaluation, diagnosis, and management of facioscapulohumeral muscular dystrophy (American Academy of Neurology and the American Association of Neuromuscular and Electrodiagnostic Medicine): http://www.neurology.org/content/85/4/357.full.pdf+html
- Guidelines for diagnosis and treatment of Limb-Girdle and Distal Muscular Dystrophies (American Academy of Neurology and the American Association of Neuromuscular and Electrodiagnostic Medicine): https://www.aan.com/Guidelines/home/GetGuidelineContent/672

### Patient/Caregiver Resources

- Family Guide for the diagnosis and management of Duchenne Muscular Dystrophy: https://www.parentprojectmd.org/wp-content/uploads/2018/09/CareGuideForFamilies_2018.pdf
- Family Guide for the diagnosis and management of Myotonic Muscular Dystrophy: https://www.myotonic.org/myotonic-dystrophy-start-your-journey-here
- Family Guide for the diagnosis and management of FSHD: https://www.aan.com/Guidelines/Home/GetGuidelineContent/702

## References


1. Abbott D, Carpenter J, Bushby K. Transition to adulthood for young men with Duchenne muscular dystrophy: research from the UK. Neuromuscul Disord NMD. 2012;22(5):445–6.
2. Goodman DM, Hall M, Levin A, Watson RS, Williams RG, Shah SS, et al. Adults with chronic health conditions originating in childhood: inpatient experience in children's hospitals. Pediatrics. 2011;128(1):5–13.
3. Schrans DG, Abbott D, Peay HL, Pangalila RF, Vroom E, Goemans N, et al. Transition in Duchenne muscular dystrophy: an expert meeting report and description of transition needs in an emergent patient population: (parent project muscular dystrophy transition expert meeting 17–18 June 2011, Amsterdam, The Netherlands). Neuromuscul Disord NMD. 2013;23(3):283–6.
4. Bushby K, Finkel R, Birnkrant DJ, Case LE, Clemens PR, Cripe L, et al. Diagnosis and management of Duchenne muscular dystrophy, part 1: diagnosis, and pharmacological and psychosocial management. Lancet Neurol. 2010;9(1):77–93.
5. Bushby K, Finkel R, Birnkrant DJ, Case LE, Clemens PR, Cripe L, et al. Diagnosis and management of Duchenne muscular dystrophy, part 2: implementation of multidisciplinary care. Lancet Neurol. 2010;9(2):177–89.
6. Eagle M, Baudouin SV, Chandler C, Giddings DR, Bullock R, Bushby K. Survival in Duchenne muscular dystrophy: improvements in life expectancy since 1967 and the impact of home nocturnal ventilation. Neuromuscul Diso NMD. 2002;12(10):926–9.
7. Wicklund MP. The muscular dystrophies. Continuum (Minneap Minn). 2013;19(6 Muscle Disease):1535–70.
8. Griggs RC, Amato AA. Muscular dystrophies. Preface. Handb Clin Neurol. 2011;101:9.
9. Flanigan KM, Coffeen CM, Sexton L, Stauffer D, Brunner S, Leppert MF. Genetic characterization of a large, historically significant Utah kindred with facioscapulohumeral dystrophy. Neuromuscul Disord NMD. 2001;11(6–7):525–9.
10. Parsons EP, Bradley DM, Clarke AJ. Newborn screening for Duchenne muscular dystrophy. Arch Dis Child. 2003;88(1):91–2.
11. Mathieu J, Allard P, Potvin L, Prevost C, Begin P. A 10-year study of mortality in a cohort of patients with myotonic dystrophy. Neurology. 1999;52(8):1658–62.
12. Romitti PA, Zhu Y, Puzhankara S, James KA, Nabukera SK, Zamba GKD, et al. Prevalence of Duchenne and Becker muscular dystrophies in the United States. Pediatrics. 2015;135(3):513–9.
13. Mendell JR, Rodino-Klapac LR, Sahenk Z, Roush K, Bird L, Lowes LP, et al. Eteplirsen for the treatment of Duchenne muscular dystrophy. Ann Neurol. 2013;74:637–47.
14. Harper PS, van Engelen BG, Eymard B, Rogers M, Wilcox D. 99th ENMC international workshop: myotonic dystrophy: present management, future therapy. 9–11 November 2001, Naarden, The Netherlands. Neuromuscul Disord NMD. 2002;12(6):596–9.
15. Padberg G, Eriksson AW, Volkers WS, Bernini L, Van Loghem E, Meera Khan P, et al. Linkage studies in autosomal dominant facioscapulohumeral muscular dystrophy. J Neurol Sci. 1984;65(3):261–8.
16. Berthier C, Blaineau S. Supramolecular organization of the subsarcolemmal cytoskeleton of adult skeletal muscle fibers. A review Biol Cell. 1997;89(7):413–34.
17. Koenig M, Kunkel LM. Detailed analysis of the repeat domain of dystrophin reveals four potential hinge segments that may confer flexibility. J Biol Chem. 1990;265(8):4560–6.
18. Cacchiarelli D, Martone J, Girardi E, Cesana M, Incitti T, Morlando M, et al. MicroRNAs involved in molecular circuitries relevant for the Duchenne muscular dystrophy pathogenesis are controlled by the dystrophin/nNOS pathway. Cell Metab. 2010;12(4):341–51.
19. Petrof BJ, Shrager JB, Stedman HH, Kelly AM, Sweeney HL. Dystrophin protects the sarcolemma from stresses developed during muscle contraction. Proc Natl Acad Sci USA. 1993;90(8):3710–4.
20. Blake DJ, Weir A, Newey SE, Davies KE. Function and genetics of dystrophin and dystrophin-related proteins in muscle. Physiol Rev. 2002;82(2):291–329.
21. Muntoni F, Torelli S, Ferlini A. Dystrophin and mutations: one gene, several proteins, multiple phenotypes. Lancet Neurol. 2003;2(12):731–40.
22. Kunkel LM, Beggs AH, Hoffman EP. Molecular genetics of Duchenne and Becker muscular dystrophy: emphasis on improved diagnosis. Clin Chem. 1989;35(7 Suppl):B21–4.
23. Mandel JL. Dystrophin. The gene and its product Nature. 1989;339(6226):584–6.
24. Monaco AP, Bertelson CJ, Liechti-Gallati S, Moser H, Kunkel LM. An explanation for the phenotypic differences between patients bearing partial deletions of the DMD locus. Genomics. 1988;2(1):90–5.
25. Hoffman EP, Arahata K, Minetti C, Bonilla E, Rowland LP. Dystrophinopathy in isolated cases of myopathy in females. Neurology. 1992;42(5):967–75.
26. Passamano L, Taglia A, Palladino A, Viggiano E, D'Ambrosio P, Scutifero M, et al. Improvement of survival in Duchenne muscular dystrophy: retrospective analysis of 835 patients. Acta Myol. 2012;31(2):121–5.
27. Broomfield J, Hill M, Guglieri M, Crowther M, Abrams K. Life expectancy in Duchenne muscular dystrophy. Neurology. 2021;97:e2304–e231.
28. Biggar WD, Harris VA, Eliasoph L, Alman B. Long-term benefits of deflazacort treatment for boys with Duchenne muscular dystrophy in their second decade. Neuromuscul Disord NMD. 2006;16(4):249–55.
29. King WM, Ruttencutter R, Nagaraja HN, Matkovic V, Landoll J, Hoyle C, et al. Orthopedic outcomes of long-term daily corticosteroid treatment in Duchenne muscular dystrophy. Neurology. 2007;68(19):1607–13.

30. Smith AD, Koreska J, Moseley CF. Progression of scoliosis in Duchenne muscular dystrophy. J Bone Joint Surg Am. 1989;71(7):1066–74.
31. Quinlivan R, Shaw N, Bushby K. 170th ENMC international workshop: bone protection for corticosteroid treated Duchenne muscular dystrophy. 27–29 November 2009, Naarden, The Netherlands. Neuromuscul Disord NMD. 2010;20(11):761–9.
32. Leung DG, Germain-Lee EL, Denger BE, Wagner KR. Report on the second endocrine aspects of Duchenne muscular dystrophy conference December 1–2, 2010, Baltimore, Maryland, USA. Neuromuscul Disord NMD. 2011;21(8):594–601.
33. McDonald DG, Kinali M, Gallagher AC, Mercuri E, Muntoni F, Roper H, et al. Fracture prevalence in Duchenne muscular dystrophy. Dev Med Child Neurol. 2002;44(10):695–8.
34. Smith EC, Conklin LS, Hoffman EP, Clemens PR, Mah JK, Finke RS, et al. Efficacy and safety of vamorolone in Duchenne muscular dystrophy: An18-month interim analysis of a non-randomized open-label extension study. PLoS Med. 2020;17(9):1–18.
35. Cirak S, Arechavala-Gomeza V, Guglieri M, Feng L, Torelli S, Anthony K, et al. Exon skipping and dystrophin restoration in patients with Duchenne muscular dystrophy after systemic phosphorodiamidate morpholino oligomer treatment: an open-label, phase 2, dose-escalation study. Lancet. 2011;378:595–605.
36. Mendell JR, Khan N, Sha N, Eliopoulos H, McDonald NG, Mercuri E, et al. Comparison of long-term ambulatory function in patients with Duchenne muscular dystrophy treated with eteplirsen and matched natural history controls. Journal of Neuromuscular Diseases. 2021;8:469–79.
37. Mendell JR, Goemans N, Lowes LP, Alfano LN, Berry K, Shao J, et al. Longitudinal effect of eteplirsen versus historical control on ambulation in Duchenne muscular dystrophy. Ann Neurol. 2016;79:257–71.
38. Frank DE, Schnell FJ, Akana C, El-Husayni SH, Desjardins CA, Morgan J, et al. Increased dystrophin production with golodirsen in patients with Duchenne muscular dystrophy. Neurology. 2020;94:e2270–82.
39. Clemens PR, Rao VK, Connolly AM, Harper AD, Mah JK, Smith EC, et al. Safety, tolerability, and efficacy of viltolarsen in boys with Duchenne muscular dystrophy amenable to exon 53 skipping: a phase 2 randomized clinical trial. JAMA Neurol. 2020;77(8):982–91.
40. Wagner KR, Kuntz NL, Koenig E, East L, Upadhyay S, et al. Safety, tolerability, and pharmacokinetics of casimersen in patients with Duchenne muscular dystrophy amenable to exon 45 skipping: a randomized, double-blind, placebo-controlled, dose-titration trial. Muscle Nerve. 2021;64:285–92.
41. Finder JD, Birnkrant D, Carl J, Farber HJ, Gozal D, Iannaccone ST, et al. Respiratory care of the patient with Duchenne muscular dystrophy: ATS consensus statement. Am J Respir Crit Care Med. 2004;170(4):456–65.
42. Birnkrant DJ, Bushby KM, Amin RS, Bach JR, Benditt JO, Eagle M, et al. The respiratory management of patients with Duchenne muscular dystrophy: a DMD care considerations working group specialty article. Pediatr Pulmonol. 2010;45(8):739–48.
43. Buyse GM, Voit T, Schara U, Straathof CSM, D'Angelo MG, Bernert G, et al. Efficacy of idebenone on respiratory function in patients with Duchenne muscular dystrophy not using glucocorticoids (DELOS): a double-blind randomised placebo-controlled phase 3 trial. Lancet. 2015;385:1748–57.
44. American Academy of Pediatrics section on cardiology and cardiac surgery. Cardiovascular health supervision for individuals affected by Duchenne or Becker muscular dystrophy. Pediatrics. 2005;116(6):1569–73.
45. Bushby K, Muntoni F, Bourke JP. 107th ENMC international workshop: the management of cardiac involvement in muscular dystrophy and myotonic dystrophy. 7th–9th June 2002, Naarden, The Netherlands. Neuromuscul Disord NMD. 2003;13(2):166–72.
46. Hunt SA, Abraham WT, Chin MH, Feldman AM, Francis GS, Ganiats TG, et al. ACC/AHA 2005 guideline update for the diagnosis and management of chronic heart failure in the adult: a report of the American College of Cardiology/American Heart Association task force on practice guidelines (writing committee to update the 2001 guidelines for the evaluation and management of heart failure): developed in collaboration with the American College of Chest physicians and the International Society for Heart and Lung Transplantation: endorsed by the Heart Rhythm Society. Circulation. 2005;112(12):e154–235.
47. Schram G, Fournier A, Leduc H, Dahdah N, Therien J, Vanasse M, et al. All-cause mortality and cardiovascular outcomes with prophylactic steroid therapy in Duchenne muscular dystrophy. J Am Coll Cardiol. 2013;61(9):948–54.
48. Jaffe KM, McDonald CM, Ingman E, Haas J. Symptoms of upper gastrointestinal dysfunction in Duchenne muscular dystrophy: case-control study. Arch Phys Med Rehabil. 1990;71(10):742–4.
49. Hendriksen JG, Vles JS. Neuropsychiatric disorders in males with Duchenne muscular dystrophy: frequency rate of attention-deficit hyperactivity disorder (ADHD), autism spectrum disorder, and obsessive–compulsive disorder. J Child Neurol. 2008;23(5):477–81.
50. Ricotti V, Mandy WP, Scoto M, Pane M, Deconinck N, Messina S, et al. Neurodevelopmental, emotional, and behavioural problems in Duchenne muscular dystrophy in relation to underlying dystrophin gene mutations. Dev Med Child Neurol. 2016;58(1):77–84.
51. Daoud MSA, Dooley JM, Gordon KE. Depression in parents of children with Duchenne muscular dystrophy. Pediatr Neurol. 2004;31(1):16–9.
52. Yemen TA, McClain C. Muscular dystrophy, anesthesia and the safety of inhalational agents revisited; again. Paediatr Anaesth. 2006;16(2):105–8.
53. Birnkrant DJ, Panitch HB, Benditt JO, Boitano LJ, Carter ER, Cwik VA, et al. American College of Chest

Physicians consensus statement on the respiratory and related management of patients with Duchenne muscular dystrophy undergoing anesthesia or sedation. Chest. 2007;132(6):1977–86.

54. Carter GT, Joyce NC, Abresch AL, Smith AE, VandeKeift GK. Using palliative care in progressive neuromuscular disease to maximize quality of life. Phys Med Rehabil Clin N Am. 2012;23(4):903–9.
55. Arias R, Andrews J, Pandya S, Pettit K, Trout C, Apkon S, et al. Palliative care services in families of males with Duchenne muscular dystrophy. Muscle Nerve. 2011;44(1):93–101.
56. Nozoe KT, Moreira GA, Hachul H, Tufik S, Andersen ML. The strength beyond the muscle. J Palliat Med. 2014;17(11):1280–1.
57. Grant M, Elk R, Ferrell B, Morrison RS, von Gunten CF. Current status of palliative care—clinical implementation, education, and research. CA Cancer J Clin. 2009;59(5):327–35.

# Sickle Cell Disease

# 36

Jennifer Jones, Nabil Abou, Linda S. Overholser, Kathryn Hassell, and Tiffiny Diers

## Case Presentation

A 20-year-old Black woman presents to an adult medical practice for a new patient appointment. She has just started classes at the local community college where she is a freshman living in the dorms. In providing her health history, she reports that she has a diagnosis of hemoglobin SS (HbSS) sickle cell disease (SCD). She is single and lives with a roommate.

At the age of 10 years, she had an abnormal transcranial doppler (TCD) screening and has since received regular blood transfusions, which she was told would help reduce the risk of having a stroke. Because of the transfusions, she was also prescribed a medication to help minimize the buildup of iron in her blood, although she reports that it tastes bad, and she frequently skips doses. She would like to continue transfusion therapy as an adult. However, she has concerns about how to arrange for this therapy with her specialist who is now located remotely and whether the local blood supply will be a match for her. She has heard about a medicine called hydroxyurea (HU) that might be an option. However, she has also heard that she should not get pregnant while taking this medicine. Though she does not currently desire pregnancy, she would like to be in a relationship and to understand the risks associated with HU and sexual activity. Moreover, she would like to know what her options are for contraceptive therapy.

She confirms that at 3 years of age, she had to have her spleen removed. As far back as she can remember, she had frequent hospitalizations, up to 5 times a year, and twice she was told that she had a "chest crisis." This pattern continued until she started chronic transfusion therapy at age 10 years. Her sickle cell crisis frequency improved and then remained stable until she

J. Jones (✉)
Transfusion Medicine and Hematology, Department of Pathology and Department of Medicine at the University of Michigan, Ann Arbor, MI, USA
e-mail: jonjm@med.umich.edu

N. Abou
Biological Sciences Division, Section of General Internal Medicine, University of Chicago, Chicago, IL, USA
e-mail: naboubaker@bsd.uchicago.edu

L. S. Overholser
Department of General Internal Medicine, University of Colorado Denver/University of Colorado Health, Aurora, CO, USA
e-mail: linda.overholser@cuanschutz.edu

K. Hassell
Division of Internal Medicine/Hematology, University of Colorado Denver/University of Colorado Health, Aurora, CO, USA
e-mail: kathryn.hassell@cuanschutz.edu

T. Diers
Department of Internal Medicine, University of Cincinnati College of Medicine, Cincinnati, OH, USA
e-mail: dierstl@ucmail.uc.edu


A. A. Kuo et al. (eds.), *Care of Adults with Chronic Childhood Conditions*,
https://doi.org/10.1007/978-3-031-54281-7_36

started her menses at around age 13 years. With her menstrual cycles, she has an increase in her pain, and she also has developed pain in both of her hips that she was told was because of her sickle cell disease. Her pain is severe enough that at times she requires doses of opioid pain medications, and about 3–4 times each year she must go to the hospital for a brief stay to control her symptoms. She has been told to avoid medications such as ibuprofen because it could be bad for her kidneys. Though the adult medical practice is in a major metropolitan area, and she is excited to attend college, she has expressed anxiety about the move and her medical care.

## Case Discussion

This case highlights the complexity of care for young adults with SCD, especially those transitioning from pediatric to adult care. Both hospitalization and mortality rates increase in transition-aged individuals with SCD [1–4]. The reasons for these poor outcomes are likely multifactorial. Patients with SCD experience accelerated aging and accumulation of chronic complications over time. Adult patients experience poor access to sickle cell hematologic care due to a general lack of benign hematologists and primary care doctors who are comfortable caring for patients with SCD. Since most patients with SCD survive to adulthood, it is imperative that the adult health care workforce, and in particular the adult primary care workforce, be prepared to anticipate needs and coordinate care for these individuals. This chapter will focus on major themes that highlight the unique needs for young adults with SCD transitioning into adult care.

This case discussion focuses on a young woman who is attending community college for the first time at age 20 years. It is notable that she is slightly older than the typical college-age freshman. Children diagnosed with SCD are at risk for frequent acute sickle cell crises requiring intensive medical intervention that may begin in infancy. As they age and schooling begins, these episodes can result in missed days of school that accumulate over time. Progressive vascular changes in the brain can lead to stroke, estimated to affect up to 10% of children with HbSS or Hemoglobin S$\beta^0$ thalassemia, with onset beginning in the first few years of life [5]. Additionally, this underlying process may manifest as silent cerebral infarction, with a clinical presentation that may be subtle but that can affect brain function nonetheless [6, 7]. For individuals who have already had or who are at an increased risk of neurological complications, there is a significant risk of new events, progression, and cumulative cognitive and physical impairment unless long-term treatment to address the underlying SCD pathophysiology is undertaken. The management of neurologic complications of SCD will be discussed later in this chapter.

Young adults with chronic conditions often hesitate to transfer care from a pediatric specialty setting to primary care, for fear that their adult primary care provider (PCP) may lack familiarity with SCD. Surveys of providers support that there are variable levels of comfort caring for patients with SCD [8]. This may be especially true for individuals with less prevalent and lifelong medical conditions such as SCD, where care is often dependent upon an ongoing relationship with a specialist. In this case, with the requirement for frequent blood transfusions and a diagnosis of one of the most severe forms of SCD, coordination of care with a hematologist is crucial. Likewise, while guidelines now exist for primary care management of hydroxyurea (HU), initiation in most settings still involves coordination with hematology [9]. Over time, coordination may also need to occur with other adult subspecialists as chronic medical conditions arise. To capitalize on the gains that have been made in SCD survival, it is prudent for adults with SCD to have a primary care medical home where routine health maintenance, general medical care, and care coordination can occur. Support for accessing primary care and for care coordination within the medical home through community health workers or patient navigators has been helpful in SCD care [10].

## Overview of Sickle Cell Disease

### Definition and Epidemiology

Sickle cell disease comprises a heterogeneous group of blood disorders with a spectrum of clinical severity. All SCD conditions result from a point mutation in the β globulin gene, resulting in the formation of hemoglobin S. However, the paired allele determines the patient's clinical course. HbSS and hemoglobin (Hb) S$\beta^0$ thalassemia produce the most severe phenotype and are often referred to as "sickle cell anemia," though, in this chapter, we will refer to all sickle cell genotypes as "SCD." The average life expectancy for patients diagnosed with HbSS and HbS$\beta^0$ thalassemia is 42 years for men and 48 years for women, 25–30 years shorter than unaffected African Americans [11]. Hemoglobin SC disease (HbSC) and hemoglobin (Hb) S$\beta^+$ thalassemia are considered milder, and affected patients can expect a longer life expectancy, 60 years for men and 68 years for women. The hemoglobin S gene paired with less common abnormal hemoglobins (e.g., Lepore, $O_{arab}$, and D) may also produce a sickling disorder and should be treated in proportion to clinical severity. Patients with one hemoglobin S and one unmutated hemoglobin A have "sickle cell trait." Patients with sickle cell trait experience a slightly increased risk of venous thromboembolism, proteinuria, chronic kidney disease (CKD), and rhabdomyolysis during times of intense physical exertion compared to peers but otherwise have a clinically silent phenotype and normal life expectancy [12, 13].

Symptoms of SCD do not manifest clinically until at least 6 months of life due to a natural hemoglobin switching phenomenon. Prior to birth, all humans produce fetal hemoglobin, a hemoglobin with greater oxygen affinity than adult hemoglobin A, to support the metabolic needs of the fetus. Following birth, fetal hemoglobin production ceases and is slowly replaced by production of hemoglobin A, or hemoglobin S in patients with SCD. Due to national universal newborn screening, we can diagnose SCD and start hydroxyurea therapy prior to the onset of symptoms. Approximately 1 in 2474 live births in the United States are of children diagnosed with SCD [2, 14]. Improvements in pediatric sickle cell care, such as the introduction of prophylactic penicillin, implementation of transcranial doppler screening, use of blood transfusion as a therapeutic measure, initiation of iron chelation therapy, and administration of hydroxyurea, have resulted in 94% of children with SCD and 99% of children with HbSC disease and HbS$\beta^+$ thalassemia living to adulthood [15].

### Pathophysiology

The clinical manifestations of SCD result from complex interactions between red blood cells (RBC), the blood vessel endothelium, the coagulation cascade, and the immune system. Under physiologic stress, deoxygenated hemoglobin S polymerizes to form rod-like structures within the RBC, which distorts the membrane into the pathognomonic "sickle" shape. These cells can cause microvascular obstruction, leading to downstream tissue ischemia and, eventually, reperfusion injury. However, sickled RBCs also demonstrate enhanced adhesion to the blood vessel endothelium which can trigger inflammation, platelet activation, and hypercoagulability. Furthermore, due to membrane fragility, the sickled RBCs experience shortened survival in circulation and may undergo both intravascular and extravascular hemolysis. Release of free hemoglobin following intravascular hemolysis causes further endothelial activation and nitric oxide scavenging, causing vasoconstriction and end-organ ischemia. These processes lead to chronic anemia, repeated vaso-occlusive crises, and end-organ damage (described below) [16, 17].

## Disease-Modifying Therapy

### Hydroxyurea

Since gaining FDA approval in 1998, hydroxyurea (HU) has been the first-line disease-modifying therapy for SCD [18]. HU promotes the production of fetal hemoglobin, which prevents

RBC sickling, and reduces circulating white blood cells, which may lessen the inflammatory effects of SCD [16] The Multicenter Study of Hydroxyurea in Sickle Cell Anemia, the largest clinical trial of HU use in sickle cell anemia (HbSS patients) to date, showed that HU reduces annual pain crisis frequency and incidence of acute chest syndrome [19]. Subsequent analysis has shown that HU also confers a survival benefit to patients with sickle cell anemia [20, 21]. The National Heart, Lung, and Blood Institute (NHLBI) has published guidelines outlining the use of HU therapy for individuals with SCD [9]. Indications for initiation of HU in patients with sickle cell anemia (HbSS disease) include:

- 3 or more acute pain episodes in a year
- pain that is severe enough to impair quality of life or daily functioning
- recurrent severe episodes of acute chest syndrome
- severe anemia

It should be noted that only HbSS patients were included in the Multicenter study. Consultation with a hematologist is recommended prior to initiating HU in patients with SCD other than HbSS. HU therapy can be prescribed and managed in primary care settings, ideally in partnership with an adult hematology specialist. When considering candidates for HU, it is critical to educate patients about the indications for and goals of therapy as well as the need for long-term monitoring for complications of therapy, including low white blood cell (WBC) and platelet counts. Monitoring includes baseline assessment of the complete blood count (CBC) with differential, reticulocyte count, fetal hemoglobin measurement, and kidney and liver function, as well as pregnancy testing for women [9]. The initial dose of hydroxyurea is 15 mg/kg/day (rounded to the nearest 500 mg). The daily dose should be adjusted by 500 mg/day every 2 weeks until a maximally tolerated dose (MTD) is reached. For an adult, MTD is defined as an absolute neutrophil count of 2000–4000/mm$^3$, platelet count >80,000/mm$^3$, hemoglobin >5.3 g/dL, and absolute reticulocyte count >95,000/mm$^3$ if the hemoglobin is <9 g/dL. A CBC with differential and reticulocyte counts should be checked every 2 weeks prior to each dose adjustment. Once the patient is on a stable dose, laboratory studies should be repeated every 2–3 months. Dosages may need to be adjusted for renal dysfunction. Therapy can be temporarily held if needed for recovery of abnormally low blood cell parameters, as described in the NHLBI guidelines [9]. Hydroxyurea should be continued during hospital stays when hematologic parameters are met. Adherence may be challenging, especially for transition patients, who may be newly responsible for their own medical care; however, adherence should be strongly encouraged. Patients should be reminded frequently that the benefits of hydroxyurea are seen in the long term with longer life expectancy and fewer crises per year.

Prior to initiation of HU, a discussion regarding family planning should occur between the patient and provider. HU is a category D medication and has shown evidence of teratogenicity in animal studies. Therefore, women are advised against pregnancy when taking HU. NHLBI guidelines suggest discontinuing HU therapy if a woman becomes pregnant and in women who are breastfeeding [9, 22]. Contraceptive options should be offered to women who express a desire to avoid pregnancy (see below for additional recommendations regarding contraception in patients with SCD). Lastly, an emerging literature has suggested a correlation between decreased ovarian reserve and sperm count in women and men with SCD, respectively, taking hydroxyurea. These studies are in the early stages and are not a justification for fertility preservation in teenagers with SCD [23, 24]. Further studies are underway to determine if HU has a definitive effect on fertility, since this would be an important consideration in the risk–benefit discussion prior to initiation.

## Therapeutic Blood Transfusion

Chronic transfusion therapy (CTT) is often-utilized for primary and secondary prevention of end-organ complications of SCD. Indications for

CTT include recurrent episodes of acute chest syndrome or severe vaso-occlusive crisis despite treatment with HU, history of stroke, and history of multiorgan failure syndrome. Patients on CTT may require simple or exchange transfusions every 3–4 weeks to maintain hemoglobin S% < 30 and hemoglobin at 9 g/dL. These standard goals can be adjusted by the transfusion medicine physician and/or hematologist based on the specific patient or indication. Since this is a resource-intensive therapy, it is often used as second-line unless specifically indicated for severe complications such as a stroke. When possible, RBC units should be ABO, Rh, and Kell matched to avoid alloimmunization. For patients who have become alloimmunized, collaboration must occur with transfusion medicine to supply RBC units with extended red cell antigen matching to avoid acute and delayed hemolytic transfusion reactions. This process can be time-consuming and expensive. Therefore, alloimmunization should be avoided as often as possible.

Urgent or acute simple blood transfusions may be required for specific indications. These include:

- Symptomatic anemia
- Moderate and severe acute chest syndrome
- Acute stroke
- Acute intrahepatic cholestasis
- Acute hepatic sequestration crisis
- Acute splenic sequestration
- Multisystem organ failure syndrome

Patients with severe end-organ complications will benefit from an exchange transfusion over a simple transfusion. Decisions regarding appropriateness of exchange transfusions should be made by the assessing provider, hematologist, transfusion medicine physician, and apheresis service. If exchange transfusion is deemed necessary but unavailable at the admitting institution, prompt transfer to an exchange transfusion-capable institution should be made.

Of note, patients with SCD often experience a decline in hemoglobin during hospitalization for vaso-occlusive crisis. In the absence of other listed indications, there is no current recommendation for simple or exchange transfusion to treat anemia during an uncomplicated vaso-occlusive crisis [25]. Primary care providers can play a key role in alerting acute care facilities to the unique transfusion needs of their SCD patients. Reduction of unnecessary, intermittent blood transfusions will reduce the risk for alloimmunization and iron overload in the long term.

## Iron Chelation Therapy

Transfusion-related iron overload is common among all adults with SCD and may result in the development of end-organ complications such as cirrhosis and cardiomyopathy [26–28]. Conservative transfusion practices should be observed in all patients with SCD to reduce iron loading. However, in patients who are diagnosed with iron overload and who are not eligible for phlebotomy, iron chelation therapies are available to treat iron overload prior to the development of irreversible tissue damage. Primary care providers may play a key role in monitoring iron overload and toxicities from iron chelation therapy. In chronically transfused patients, the American Society of Hematology (ASH) and the NHLBI recommend screening for hepatic iron overload with magnetic resonance imaging (MRI) T2* (an MRI technique to quantify tissue iron) every 1–2 years, rather than relying on serum ferritin as a marker of iron overload. However, if the serum ferritin is <1000 ng/mL, hepatic imaging may be deferred. Routine cardiac MRI T2* testing may be reserved for patients with high hepatic iron overload (>15 mg/g dry weight) [9, 25]. For patients diagnosed with iron overload, there are three iron chelators available in the United States: deferoxamine (subcutaneous or intravenous), deferiprone (oral), or deferasirox (oral, two formulations available). All patients initiating chelation therapy should have baseline serum ferritin, complete blood count, comprehensive metabolic panel, urine protein/creatinine ratio, baseline audiology, and ophthalmology evaluations. All lab work should be repeated monthly and prior to dose increases.

Audiology and ophthalmology screening should be performed annually.

Non-adherence to iron chelation due to poor taste, abdominal pain, and other symptoms is the most common reason for treatment failure [26, 29]. Therefore, it is important to develop a feasible treatment plan with the patient, reassess at every visit, and change strategy when necessary. All patients, including the patient in the case, must be reminded that although the effects of iron chelation are not physically apparent, they are beneficial in the long term.

## New Therapies

Since 2017, the FDA has approved three new pharmaceutical therapies for the treatment of sickle cell disease. The first of these, L-glutamine, is a pharmaceutical-grade amino acid product, which is taken daily as a 10 to 30 g powder in divided doses based on body weight. The supplement is thought to support the RBC antioxidant properties that resist hemolytic stressors. The phase 3 clinical trial leading to its approval showed a modest improvement in per-year pain crises (3.9 to 3.2) in patients with sickle cell anemia [30]. In practice, this therapy may be a useful adjunct for patients over the age of 5 years who suffer from multiple vaso-occlusive pain events. Crizanlizumab gained approval in 2019. This infused monoclonal antibody inhibits P-selectin, a protein necessary for chemotaxis, or rolling of the leukocytes along the endothelium of the blood vessels. It is thought that impairing chemotaxis will result in reduction of inflammation at sites of microvascular damage due to sickling and downstream ischemic injury. Like L-glutamine, crizanlizumab reduced the number of crises per year in study participants; however, unlike in the L-glutamine trials, the crizanlizumab trials included patients with hemoglobin SC and $S\beta^+$ thalassemia [31]. Ten days following approval of crizanlizumab, another therapy, voxelotor, received FDA approval for treatment of anemia in sickle cell disease. Voxelotor increases the oxygen binding affinity of hemoglobin S, thereby preventing intracellular polymerization and ultimately hemolysis. In the phase 3 HOPE trial, individuals who received voxelotor experienced a >1 g/dL hemoglobin increase and a reduction in hemolysis markers at 6 months as compared to controls, though no improvement was seen in clinical benchmarks such as pain crises [32]. Patients are thought to benefit in the long term from maintaining higher hemoglobin values, though these data are not yet available. Studies are ongoing to evaluate novel combinations of these therapies with hydroxyurea and chronic transfusion therapy. A summary of SCD pharmacologic therapies can be found in Table 36.1.

**Table 36.1** Sickle cell disease therapies

| Disease-modifying therapies | | |
|---|---|---|
| Name | Indication | Administration instructions |
| Hydroxyurea | • 3 or more pain crises per year<br>• Pain severe enough to impair quality of life or daily functioning<br>• Recurrent severe episodes of acute chest syndrome<br>• Severe anemia | Initial dose of 15 mg/kg/day with titration to maximally tolerated dose[a] over several weeks |
| L-glutamine (Endari®)[b] | Multiple pain crises per year | 10–30 g daily in divided doses based on body weight |
| Crizanlizumab (Adakveo®)[b] | Multiple pain crises per year | Infusion of 5 mg/kg every 2 weeks for 2 doses followed by 5 mg/kg every 4 weeks |
| Voxelotor (Oxbryta®)[b] | Hemoglobin ≤10.5 g/dL | 1500 mg per day with or without food |
| *Adjunctive medications* | | |
| Deferoxamine[b] | Systemic iron overload | Continuous subcutaneous or intravenous infusion 40–50 mg/kg/day |

**Table 36.1** (continued)

| Disease-modifying therapies | | |
|---|---|---|
| Name | Indication | Administration instructions |
| Deferasirox[b] | Systemic iron overload | **Exjade**<br>20–40 mg/kg/day titrated to ferritin response<br>**Jadenu**<br>14–28 mg/kg/day titrated to ferritin response |
| Deferiprone [b,c] | Systemic iron overload | Initial dose of 45 mg/kg as BID or TID divided daily doses and uptitrated to 75 mg/kg/day as divided doses |
| Erythropoietin<br>Darbepoietin | Anemia due to renal failure | Traditional non-hemodialysis vs dialysis dosing<br>**American Society of Hematology recommends use in combination with low-dose hydroxyurea |

[a]For an adult, maximally tolerated dose is defined as an absolute neutrophil count of 2000–4000/mm$^3$, platelet count >80,000/mm$^3$, hemoglobin >5.3 g/dL, and absolute reticulocyte count >95,000/mm$^3$ if the hemoglobin is <9 g/dL
[b]Restricted to Hematology/Oncology providers
[c]Black box warning for development of neutropenia and agranulocytosis

Curative therapies for SCD are available, though it is beyond the scope of this chapter to discuss in detail bone marrow transplant (BMT) or gene therapy in SCD. Matched sibling BMT can be performed as a standard of care in children with SCD who have suffered a stroke or other severe end-organ complications. BMT with any other donor type should only be performed as part of a clinical trial. Two cell-based gene therapies received FDA approval in 2023 for patients with SCD over the age of 12 years and who have suffered vaso-occlusive events. Curative therapies are most successful for patients under the age of 20 years; however, any patient with a history of severe sickle-cell-related end-organ dysfunction should discuss the risks and benefits of curative therapy with a specialist [33–36].

## Common Clinical Issues for Adults with Sickle Cell Disease

SCD is a lifelong medical condition, the clinical manifestations of which begin shortly after birth as protective levels of fetal hemoglobin decline. Infants and young children present with acute complications of SCD in an episodic fashion. However, as individuals age, these episodic presentations lead to cumulative damage to the organ systems most affected by the vascular pathology of SCD. In addition to treating acute complications such as pain crises and acute chest syndrome, chronic organ system disease must be managed just as it would be for those individuals without SCD. A multidisciplinary team approach and involvement of multiple specialists becomes increasingly important over time. The role of the adult primary care provider, particularly as it pertains to addressing adult preventive care recommendations, is central to the coordination of this care. This section will review several of the most prevalent issues observed among the young adult population of individuals living with SCD.

### Pulmonary Issues

SCD can cause devastating acute and chronic pulmonary complications. Acute pathologies include acute chest syndrome (ACS), pneumonia, and pulmonary emboli. ACS is a potentially life-threatening event defined by acute vaso-occlusion within the microvasculature of the lung, resulting in capillary leak and ischemia. The diagnostic criteria for ACS are intentionally broad and include an infiltrate on chest imaging plus fever or other respiratory symptoms, such as dyspnea or hypoxia. Treatment for ACS often consists of antibiotics, blood transfusions, and pain management and should occur in the inpatient setting [9]. Pneumonia often resembles ACS and occurs commonly in patients with SCD due to functional or anatomic asplenia. All patients presenting with concern for pneumonia should be treated with antibiotic therapy and monitored closely for clinical deterioration [9]. Lastly, pulmonary emboli occur more frequently in patients with SCD compared to African American controls due to intrinsic hypercoagulability and provoking factors, such as hospitalization, surgery, or indwelling central catheters [37, 38]. Hypercoagulability in SCD is discussed below.

Pulmonary hypertension (PH) is a significant chronic pulmonary comorbidity of SCD. About 6–11% of adults with SCD will develop PH, though the pathophysiology is unclear [39]. The American Society of Hematology (ASH) and the American Thoracic Society (ATS) have written diagnostic and management guidelines for PH in SCD [39]. Initial screening should include a careful history, physical examination, echocardiography, 6-Minute Walk Test, and serum N-terminal pro-brain natriuretic peptide (NT-pro-BNP) levels. An elevated tricuspid regurgitant jet velocity (TRV) > 2.5 m/s on echocardiogram is associated with an increased risk of early mortality, even in the absence of pulmonary hypertension. Patients with concerning findings on noninvasive evaluation should undergo right heart catheterization to confirm the diagnosis. The ATS guidelines recommend the initiation of HU therapy for individuals diagnosed with PH, although there is no direct evidence that HU reduces mortality [39]. Chronic transfusion therapy can also be considered. Initial diagnosis of PH should prompt an evaluation for sleep disordered breathing (SDB), an under-recognized comorbidity in SCD. Lastly, asthma occurs commonly in patients with SCD and can compound other pulmonary complications, such as ACS and PH. Studies suggest that asthma in SCD is an independent risk factor for mortality and should be managed aggressively [2].

For the primary care provider focused on preventive health, it is critical to assess smoking status, treat nicotine dependence, and ensure that appropriate preventive measures are taken to reduce overlapping pulmonary morbidity from non-SCD causes such as asthma, infection with influenza virus or pneumococcal infection, or SDB.

## Renal Issues

SCD, like other vascular disorders, may affect the kidney. The kidney is highly metabolically active, and the local environment of the kidney may predispose this organ system to RBC adhesion, endothelial activation, intermittent ischemia, and reperfusion injury, resulting in a cycle of renal hypoperfusion [40]. This can initially result in glomerular hyperfiltration or "hyposthenuria" and can lead to glomerulopathies over time. Albuminuria is the most common clinical manifestation of chronic SCD kidney damage, and hypertension can be comorbid. In youth under the age of 21 years, the prevalence of albuminuria may be as high as 26%, and in older adults, the prevalence is higher [40]. The NHLBI guidelines recommend yearly screening for albuminuria from age 10 years onward. The ASH Cardiopulmonary and Renal guidelines suggest angiotensin-converting enzyme inhibitors and angiotensin receptor blockers for patients who develop albuminuria due to sickle nephropathy [40]. Additionally, it is important to appropriately manage hypertension because uncontrolled hypertension may compound renal dysfunction. Management principles are similar to the general population with hypertension, though care should be taken to avoid dehydration due to diuretic medications. Progressive sickle nephropathy, like other renal injuries, can lead to end-stage renal disease over time if not monitored or treated. Though renal transplant is an option, death from renal disease can occur prior to evaluation, listing, or transplant surgery. It is important to refer all patients diagnosed with sickle-cell-related renal disease to a nephrologist for management.

## Brain-Related Issues

SCD can have devastating effects on the central nervous system. The risk of overt or clinically apparent stroke is highest among children with SCD under 20 years of age but remains elevated throughout the lifespan [41, 42]. Ischemic or hemorrhagic cerebral vascular accidents can leave patients with lifelong physical and cognitive disabilities. One of the major therapeutic advances of the last few decades has been the ability to predict risk of overt strokes in children using transcranial doppler (TCD) imaging, permitting an opportunity for primary prevention [43]. It is now recommended that children with sickle cell anemia (HbSS disease) begin annual TCD screening at age 2 years and continue until age 16 years [9]. Patients with an abnormal TCD should be referred to both hematology and neurology for additional work up and initiation of chronic transfusion therapy (CTT), the current first-line standard of care [9]. Following one year of CTT, patients with a history of an abnormal TCD and no radiographic evidence of cerebral vasculopathy may be eligible to transition to HU therapy based on the results of the recent TWiTCH trial [44]. This option could be presented to the young woman in the case above. For patients with a history of overt stroke, CTT is the mainstay of therapy; however, these patients may be eligible for a BMT as mentioned previously.

More insidious than overt strokes are silent cerebral infarcts (SCIs). SCIs do not produce focal neurologic deficits but are associated with lower intelligence quotient (IQ) scores and cognitive deficits. SCIs are common in both children and adults and may result in poor academic and work performance [6, 7, 45]. It is not known from the above case if the patient has sustained any silent neurologic injury. In children and adults with HbSS or HbS$\beta^0$ thalassemia, ASH recommends screening for SCI with MRI at least once and surveillance for cognitive impairment [46]. Formal neuropsychological testing may provide specific evaluation of all cognitive domains and determine if confounding psychological factors, such as depression, are present. In the case above, vocational and educational counseling may be available to support the patient if she displays cognitive impairment or difficulty adjusting socially.

## Ophthalmologic Complications

The visual manifestations of SCD are varied and depend on the area of the orbital blood supply that is affected. Presentations can range from conjunctival vessel dilation, orbital cellulitis, atrophy or irregularity of the iris, retinal artery occlusion, glaucoma, angioid streaks, and proliferative sickle retinopathy (PSR) [47]. PSR has been well described and can lead to both vitreous hemorrhage and retinal detachment, which are the primary mechanisms of vision loss [47]. PSR and other eye diseases associated with SCD can be identified by an eye specialist and treated with available therapies. SCD patients should complete an eye exam with ophthalmology yearly.

## Infectious Disease Considerations

Impaired immunity from functional asplenia occurs in the first 1–2 years of life in children with HbSS/S$\beta^0$ thalassemia or later in young adulthood for patients with HbSC and HbS$\beta^+$ thalassemia. Invasive bacterial infections have historically caused significant morbidity and mortality in infants and young children with SCD. However, implementation of prophylactic penicillin until age 5 or beyond in patients with a history of severe infection have markedly reduced life-threatening infections and improved childhood survival in SCD [48]. Despite these advances, fever in a patient with SCD should still prompt clinical evaluation [48]. Vaccinations have also served a pivotal role in preventing infection in patients with SCD. The Centers for Disease Control publishes up-to-date vaccination schedules for children and adults with SCD (in the section for patients with asplenia). For vaccine-naïve adults, vaccination against encapsulated organisms (e.g., pneumococcus, haemophilius B, and meningococcus) and viral infections (e.g., hepatitis A and B) should be prioritized.

Like our case patient, many patients with SCD will require splenectomy in childhood or adulthood. Splenectomy results in a more abrupt, though similar, immunodeficiency to patients who experience functional asplenia as a result of splenic autoinfarction. If performed electively, patients can receive immunizations against encapsulated organisms, influenza, and COVID-19 before the procedure. If performed emergently, immunizations should be provided as soon as possible after the procedure. All adults should receive prophylactic antibiotics for at least 1 year post-splenectomy [9].

Greater exposure to blood products also poses unique risks to patients with SCD. Although enhanced screening techniques have significantly reduced the prevalence of viral infections in the donor pool and the risk of transfusion-associated infection is low, all patients with SCD on chronic transfusion therapy or who receive frequent acute transfusions should receive yearly screening for HIV, hepatitis B, and hepatitis C [9, 49]. Fever in patients who receive frequent blood transfusions should prompt an extended infectious work up.

## Hypercoagulability

Venous thromboembolism (VTE) is common in patients with SCD. Traditional risk factors, such as frequent hospitalizations, indwelling catheters, joint replacement surgeries for avascular necrosis, and pregnancy increase the risk for VTE in patients with SCD; however, patients also exhibit intrinsic hypercoagulability. Though the pathophysiology of hypercoagulability in SCD is incompletely understood, chronic hemolysis, endothelial injury, and inflammation are thought to increase expression of prothrombotic factors and decrease expression of anticoagulant factors, such as protein C and S [50–53]. Approximately 11–12% of patients with SCD will experience a VTE prior to the age of 40 years, with a higher incidence among patients with more severe disease (>3 hospitalizations per year). Patients with SCD also have a high rate of recurrent VTE, about 20–30% [37, 54, 55]. Despite the high prevalence of VTE in patients with SCD, there are no clinical trials to inform population-specific VTE treatment recommendations. Therefore, patients should receive treatment according to the most up-to-date general VTE treatment guidelines [56] Of note, monitoring d-dimer values is not reliable in patients with SCD due to baseline elevation and well described fluctuation due to complications such as vaso-occlusive crisis and infection [50, 57, 58]. Decisions regarding long term and prophylactic anticoagulation for VTE should be individualized and take into consideration the patient's personal and family history of VTE, modifiable VTE risk factors, and bleeding risk.

## Reproductive Counseling and Pregnancy

Discussion of family planning is an integral component of transitional care, especially for patients with SCD. For female patients desiring contraception, NHLBI guidelines note that all forms of contraception can be considered, including estrogen-containing contraceptives. However, if there is a history of stroke or other thrombosis, estrogen-containing contraception should be avoided. Some female patients may receive additional benefits such as reduced vaso-occlusive crises while using contraception [59, 60]. For patients desiring pregnancy, providers should provide pre-conception counseling regarding the unique physiology of SCD in pregnancy, risk of SCD or sickle cell trait inheritance, and options for pre-implantation genetic therapy. Patients desiring further discussion of family planning and pre-implantation genetic options should be referred to reproductive endocrinology.

Women with HbSS or HbS$\beta^0$ thalassemia have higher rates of pregnancy complications and may experience increased episodes of sickle cell pain, especially in those who must interrupt their chronic hydroxyurea therapy [61]. For those who experience an increase in sickle-cell-related pain during pregnancy, chronic transfusion therapy may improve their symptoms [62]. These high-risk pregnancies should be co-managed by maternal fetal medicine, hematology, and other specialty providers if the patient has chronic end-organ sickle cell complications.

## Mental Health

It is important to assess the mental health of all patients on a regular basis. This practice may be of particular importance in patients with chronic conditions such as SCD. This patient population carries a high prevalence of major depressive disorder and generalized anxiety disorder [63, 64]. Instruments validated in adolescents and young adults, such as the Patient Health Question-9 and Generalized Anxiety Disorder-7, should be used for psychological assessment. Notably, high rates of comorbid mental health diagnoses have been reported in the chronic pain population, especially among those prescribed opioids [65].

## Pain Management

Pain is a hallmark of SCD. Acute pain episodes, such as vaso-occlusive crises, are a classic presentation of SCD. Specifically, the pain pattern experienced in infants and children can evolve into a chronic pain syndrome, which may continue into adulthood. Complications such as avascular necrosis, arthritis, chronic skin ulceration, peripheral neuropathy, bony infarctions, or opioid hypersensitivity can cause chronic pain. Inadequate pain management can significantly impact a patient's quality of life and contribute to mortality [11]. Communication between pediatric and adult providers is essential to ensure individualized pain management plans enacted in the pediatric clinic continue following transition. These individualized pain plans should describe the patient's acute pain management plan when pain is managed at home. More comprehensive plans also describe the patient's emergency department and inpatient pain management strategies.

The management of adolescent and young adult patients with chronic pain presents special challenges for primary care providers. Chronic pain in SCD is defined by the American Pain Society as persistent pain for most days over the past 6 months either in a single location or in multiple locations with evidence of tenderness on exam, decreased range of motion due to pain or weakness, skin ulceration, organ damage, or bone damage [66]. There are 3 main subtypes of chronic SCD pain:

1. Chronic pain without contributory disease complication
2. Chronic pain with contributory disease complication
3. Chronic pain with mixed types

Chronic pain in adolescents and young adults increases with age, with females reporting more frequent and severe pain than males [67]. Common sites of pain include headaches, abdominal pain, limb pain, and back pain, with many adolescents reporting pain at multiple sites [68]. Adolescents report that living with chronic pain affects multiple aspects of life, including school, play, and sleep [68–70]. Parents are also affected, with increased rates of mood disorders and stress of parenting adolescents with chronic pain [71, 72].

### Assessment

Standardized pain assessment instruments such as pain intensity self-report scales, including the visual analog scale and the Faces Pain Scale-Revised, as well as pain questionnaires such as the Varni/Thompson Pediatric Pain Questionnaire, are well established and recommended for use in the adolescent age group [73]. In an effort to improve pain management, functional pain assessments specifically for SCD exist, such as the Youth Acute Pain Functional Ability Questionnaire [74]. This is particularly important as the opioid epidemic has led to a need for limiting opioids due to overprescribing [75–77]. SCD patients have been negatively affected due to a decrease in opioid prescription rates, resulting in inadequate pain management. Patients with SCD are not the major cause of the opioid epidemic, and opioid overdose is not a major cause of death in patients with SCD [78, 79]. However, tools exist to evaluate patients for opioid use disorder—for example, the Opioid Risk Tool or Brief Risk Assessment [80, 81].

## Management

While HU, L-glutamine, and crizanlizumab can reduce the frequency of acute complications and hospitalizations, they are not indicated for the treatment of chronic pain. Treatment of chronic pain can be difficult for the patient and the provider, given the need for trial and error of different therapeutic modalities and the likelihood that the patient's pain may improve but not resolve completely. Despite these adjunctive medications, some patients will continue to have debilitating daily pain.

A multimodal treatment strategy that addresses the multiple impacts of chronic pain on the lives of adolescents and young adults is often needed. Best results are achieved with a multidisciplinary (MD) approach, although access to MD team members is often limited in primary care settings [82]. Collaborative decision-making with patients and families can improve adherence to treatment plans and self-management. Education and support for behavioral changes in lifestyle habits that affect pain—such as sleep, exercise, diet, and stress management—are critical but may not be provided at home by parents or in the office by providers. Innovative approaches to self-management incorporating technology and tailored to adolescents and young adults may increase effectiveness [84, 85]. Psychological therapies including cognitive behavioral therapy, relaxation training, and biofeedback have also been found effective in adolescents and young adults with chronic pain [86]. These modalities may prove useful in managing causes of pain that might be directly due to a SCD complication and could be multifactorial in nature.

Medication use can be guided by the type of pain being experienced, comorbid conditions, especially mood disorders, and effectiveness of nonpharmacologic therapies. Not all patients require one, however, many would benefit from having an individualized pain plan. This is a document created in concert with the patient that delineates the patient's pain protocol. ASH recommends using multimodal nonopioid medication to manage pain in this patient population, including nonsteroidal anti-inflammatory drugs (for example, ibuprofen), serotonin and norepinephrine reuptake inhibitor (for example, duloxetine), tricyclic antidepressants (for example, amitriptyline), and gabapentinoids (for example, gabapentin). A patient may also use common medications such as oral acetaminophen and topical medications such as lidocaine and diclofenac gel for additional pain relief. Nonpharmacologic and complimentary medicine treatments exist, in addition to therapy, such as distraction, heat, massage, and acupuncture. An overview of pain management modalities is presented in Table 36.2. It should be noted that prevention of pain is a management strategy as well. Patients should attempt to determine their specific past triggers of pain, for example cold and dehydration, and focus on avoiding triggers if possible, staying well hydrated, eating a balanced diet, and obtaining regular exercise.

Opioids have little long-term role in the management of chronic non-malignant pain in adolescents and young adults. Opioid medications should be reserved for patients who have severe refractory pain that limits their function. Thus, it is vital that functional goals are established when chronic opioid therapy (COT) is in use. It is also generally accepted that clinics have opioid use agreements between the patient and provider with provisions to minimize multiple prescribers of opioids. Patients should be well educated regarding the benefits and risks of taking chronic opioids such as opioid hyperalgesia, dependence, tolerance, respiratory depression, and death. Naloxone education and prescription should be given to all patients requiring an oral morphine milligram equivalent (MME) greater than 50 [87]. Patients with SCD on COT with a high MME may find controlling their pain more challenging due to opioid hyperalgesia. Improvements in functional status and pain management may

**Table 36.2** Pain management modalities

| Pain management | Example treatments | Secondary management use |
|---|---|---|
| Oral nonsteroidal anti-inflammatory (NSAID) | Ibuprofen, naproxen, ketorolac, celecoxib, etoricoxib | Fever |
| Serotonin and norepinephrine reuptake inhibitor (SNRI) | Duloxetine, milnacipran, venlafaxine, desvenlafaxine | Major depressive disorder, migraines |
| Gabapentinoids | Gabapentin, pregabalin | Neuropathic pain, seizure disorder |
| Tricyclic antidepressants (TCA) | Amitriptyline, nortriptyline | Major depressive disorder |
| Non-NSAIDs | Acetaminophen | Fever |
| Topical agents | Lidocaine and diclofenac gel | None |
| Nonpharmacologic | Acupuncture, distraction, heat, massage, yoga, transcutaneous electrical nerve stimulation (TENS), guided audiovisual relaxation, virtual reality | None |
| Adjuvant therapy | Physical therapy, occupational therapy, biofeedback, cognitive behavioral therapy, relaxation training | Gross motor skills, fine motor skills, major depressive disorder, generalized anxiety disorder |
| Opioids | Tramadol, codeine, morphine, oxycodone, hydromorphone, hydrocodone, fentanyl | None |

necessitate down titration of the COT dosage. Weaning of COT should be done in conjunction with an MD team and the patient to ensure improved outcomes and patient satisfaction.

## Bias in SCD

SCD is historically an illness that has been subjected to systematic structural issues such as being under-researched and underfunded and having limited access to care [88]. To compound these issues, many publications have documented a bias against patients with SCD by health care professionals [89, 90]. Studies have demonstrated that medical professionals may attribute negative qualities, such as “over-reporting of pain” and “drug-seeking behavior,” to patients with SCD [91–93]. Attitudes like these can affect patient care and lead to greater pain burden and lower quality of life [90]. It is important to counteract biases in our health care system to improve care for these patients [94].

## Conclusion

Sickle cell disease is a lifelong, chronic disease that may affect nearly every organ system in the body while greatly impacting a patient's quality of life and limiting the typical life expectancy. Care of patients with SCD is best managed by a multidisciplinary team to utilize the expertise of all those involved, including the primary care physician, hematologist, therapists, and other team members. Patients with SCD are particularly vulnerable during the transition period from adolescence to adulthood due to the complications highlighted in this chapter.

# Appendix

<table>
<tr><th colspan="3">Sickle cell disease (SCD) fact sheet</th></tr>
<tr><td>Definition</td><td colspan="2">Sickle cell disease (SCD) is a group of blood disorders characterized by the presence of hemoglobin S (HbS) instead of normal HbA due to a point mutation in the hemoglobin β-globin gene. Disease classification depends upon the specific combinations of abnormal hemoglobin present:<br>• The most severe forms of SCD are HbSS (sickle mutation in both β-globin genes) and HbS$\beta^0$thalassemia (sickle mutation in one gene and absent β-globin production due to inactivation of the other gene). These are also referred to as “sickle cell anemia”<br>• Less severe forms of SCD include HbSC (sickle mutation in 1 gene and another mutation causing abnormal “C” hemoglobin in the other gene) and HbS$\beta^+$thalassemia (sickle mutation in 1 gene and underproduction of β-globin due to mutation of the other gene)</td></tr>
<tr><td>Prevalence</td><td colspan="2">SCD disproportionately affects individuals of African or Mediterranean descent and occurs in approximately 1 in 2474 live births in United States<br>• SCD can rarely occur in Latino/Hispanic and White populations<br>• demographic shifts affect local prevalence<br>• > 90% of children with SCD survive to adulthood</td></tr>
<tr><td>Pathophysiology</td><td colspan="2">Disease manifestations result from polymerization of the deoxygenated, sickle hemoglobin within the red blood cell (RBC) during times of stress. This conformation results in:<br>• “sickling” of the RBC<br>• shortened RBC survival due to membrane fragility and chronic hemolysis<br>• increased vascular adhesion<br>• continuous cascade of inflammation, activation of white blood cells, platelets, and endothelial cells through complex biochemical processes that affect microvascular blood flow<br>• tissue injury via ischemia-reperfusion cycles and end-organ damage over time</td></tr>
<tr><td>Symptoms</td><td colspan="2">SCD causes acute and chronic systemic complications:</td></tr>
<tr><td></td><td>Acute:<br>• vaso-occlusive pain crisis<br>• acute chest syndrome<br>• acute ischemic or hemorrhage stroke<br>• sepsis<br>• splenic sequestration crisis (not discussed)<br>• acute hepatobiliary complications (not discussed)<br>• fat embolization syndrome (not discussed)<br>• multiorgan failure syndrome (not discussed)</td><td>Chronic:<br>• chronic pain syndromes<br>• pulmonary hypertension<br>• chronic kidney disease and hypertension<br>• silent cerebral infarctions, cognitive dysfunction<br>• proliferative sickle retinopathy and visual loss<br>• systemic iron overload<br>• depression and mood disorders<br>• avascular necrosis (not discussed)<br>• leg ulcers (not discussed)</td></tr>
<tr><td>Challenges in transition</td><td colspan="2">• the transition from pediatric to adult phase of life is associated with increased SCD complications and mortality<br>• the use of disease-modifying therapies to manage SCD complications may also be underutilized in affected adolescents and young adults<br>• there are not enough adult SCD care specialists, and many adult primary care providers are unfamiliar with the care of those living with SCD<br>• stigma and lack of trust are key issues, especially for chronic pain management</td></tr>
</table>

| Sickle cell disease (SCD) fact sheet | |
|---|---|
| Helpful resources | • American Society of Hematology clinical practice guidelines for sickle cell disease: https://www.hematology.org/education/clinicians/guidelines-and-quality-care/clinical-practice-guidelines/sickle-cell-disease-guidelines<br>• National Heart, Lung, and Blood Institute sickle cell disease guidelines: http://www.nhlbi.nih.gov/health-pro/guidelines/sickle-cell-disease-guidelines http://www.nhlbi.nih.gov/health-pro/guidelines/sickle-cell-disease-guidelines<br>• Sickle Cell Trait toolkit (resource for patients and family members with sickle cell trait): https://www.cdc.gov/ncbddd/sicklecell/toolkit.html<br>• Sickle Cell Disease Association of America (resources for patients and family members; may include local chapters in communities throughout the US): http://www.sicklecelldisease.org<br>• Sickle Cell Adult Provider Network (resources for health care providers; includes links to connect with SCD experts): http://www.scapn.net/ohana<br>• Chest VTE guidelines for sickle cell disease: https://journal.chestnet.org/article/S0012-3692(21)01507-5/fulltext |

## References


1. Hamideh D, Alvarez O. Sickle cell disease related mortality in the United States (1999–2009): sickle cell disease-related mortality. Pediatr Blood Cancer. 2013;60(9):1482–6.
2. Kanter J, Kruse-Jarres R. Management of sickle cell disease from childhood through adulthood. Blood Rev. 2013;27(6):279–87.
3. Hemker BG, Brousseau DC, Yan K, Hoffmann RG, Panepinto JA. When children with sickle-cell disease become adults: lack of outpatient care leads to increased use of the emergency department. Am J Hematol. 2011;86(10):863–5.
4. Blinder MA, Vekeman F, Sasane M, Trahey A, Paley C, Duh MS. Age-related treatment patterns in sickle cell disease patients and the associated sickle cell complications and healthcare costs. Pediatr Blood Cancer. 2013;60(5):828–35.
5. Helton KJ, Adams RJ, Kesler KL, Lockhart A, Aygun B, Driscoll C, et al. Magnetic resonance imaging/angiography and transcranial Doppler velocities in sickle cell anemia: results from the SWiTCH trial. Blood. 2014;124(6):891–8.
6. DeBaun MR, Armstrong FD, McKinstry RC, Ware RE, Vichinsky E, Kirkham FJ. Silent cerebral infarcts: a review on a prevalent and progressive cause of neurologic injury in sickle cell anemia. Blood. 2012;119(20):4587–96.
7. Kawadler JM, Clayden JD, Clark CA, Kirkham FJ. Intelligence quotient in paediatric sickle cell disease: a systematic review and meta-analysis. Dev Med Child Neurol. 2016;58(7):672–9.
8. Mainous AG, Tanner RJ, Harle CA, Baker R, Shokar NK, Hulihan MM. Attitudes toward Management of sickle cell disease and its complications: a National Survey of academic family physicians. Anemia. 2015;2015:1–6.
9. Yawn BP, Buchanan GR, Afenyi-Annan AN, Ballas SK, Hassell KL, James AH, et al. Management of sickle cell disease: summary of the 2014 evidence-based report by expert panel members. JAMA. 2014;312(10):1033.
10. Sickle Cell Disease Treatment Demonstration Program. NICHQ—National Institute for Children's Health Quality. [cited 2022 Oct 4]. Available from: https://www.nichq.org/project/sickle-cell-disease-treatment-demonstration-program
11. Platt OS, Brambilla DJ, Rosse WF, Milner PF, Castro O, Steinberg MH, et al. Mortality in sickle cell disease—life expectancy and risk factors for early death. N Engl J Med. 1994;330(23):1639–44.
12. Nelson DA, Deuster PA, Kurina LM. Sickle cell trait and rhabdomyolysis among U.S. Army Soldiers. N Engl J Med. 2016;375(17):1695–6.
13. Naik RP, Smith-Whitley K, Hassell KL, Umeh NI, de Montalembert M, Sahota P, et al. Clinical outcomes associated with sickle cell Trait: a systematic review. Ann Intern Med. 2018;169(9):619.
14. Therrell BL, Hannon WH. National evaluation of US newborn screening system components. Ment Retard Dev Disabil Res Rev. 2006;12(4):236–45.
15. Hassell KL. Population estimates of sickle cell disease in the U.S. Am J Prev Med. 2010;38(4):S512–21.
16. Sundd P, Gladwin MT, Novelli EM. Pathophysiology of sickle cell disease. Annu Rev Pathol Mech Dis. 2019;14(1):263–92.
17. Kato GJ, Steinberg MH, Gladwin MT. Intravascular hemolysis and the pathophysiology of sickle cell disease. J Clin Invest. 2017;127(3):750–60.
18. Ault A. US FDA approves first drug for sickle-cell anaemia. Lancet. 1998;351(9105):809.
19. Charache S, Terrin ML, Moore RD, Dover GJ, Barton FB, Eckert SV, et al. Effect of hydroxyurea on the frequency of painful crises in sickle cell anemia. N Engl J Med. 1995;332(20):1317–22.
20. Steinberg MH, Barton F, Castro O, Pegelow CH, Ballas SK, Kutlar A, et al. Effect of hydroxyurea on mortality and morbidity in adult sickle cell anemia: risks and benefits up to 9 years of treatment. JAMA. 2003;289(13):1645.

21. Steinberg MH, McCarthy WF, Castro O, Ballas SK, Armstrong FD, Smith W, et al. The risks and benefits of long-term use of hydroxyurea in sickle cell anemia: a 17.5 year follow-up. Am J Hematol. 2010;85:403.
22. Walsh KE, Cutrona SL, Kavanagh PL, Crosby LE, Malone C, Lobner K, et al. Medication adherence among pediatric patients with sickle cell disease: a systematic review. Pediatrics. 2014;134(6):1175–83.
23. Berthaut I, Bachir D, Kotti S, Chalas C, Stankovic K, Eustache F, et al. Adverse effect of hydroxyurea on spermatogenesis in patients with sickle cell anemia after 6 months of treatment. Blood. 2017;130(21):2354–6.
24. Pecker LH, Hussain S, Mahesh J, Varadhan R, Christianson MS, Lanzkron S. Diminished ovarian reserve in young women with sickle cell anemia. Blood. 2022;139(7):1111–5.
25. Chou ST, Fasano RM. Management of Patients with sickle cell disease using transfusion therapy. Hematol Oncol Clin North Am. 2016;30(3):591–608.
26. Coates TD, Wood JC. How we manage iron overload in sickle cell patients. Br J Haematol. 2017;177(5):703–16.
27. Pack-Mabien A, Brown B, Herbert DE, Haynes J. Iron overload in adults with sickle cell disease who have received intermittent red blood cell transfusions. J Am Assoc Nurse Pract. 2015;27(10):591–6.
28. Wilson SR, Sears M, Williams E, Drapekin J, Sivakumar I, Padrino S, et al. Gaps in the diagnosis and management of iron overload in sickle cell disease: a 'real-world' report from the GRNDaD registry. Br J Haematol. 2021;195(5):e157. https://doi.org/10.1111/bjh.17762.
29. Oyedeji CI, Crawford RD, Shah N. Adherence to iron chelation therapy with Deferasirox formulations among patients with sickle cell disease and β-thalassemia. J Natl Med Assoc. 2021;113(2):170–6.
30. Niihara Y, Smith WR, Stark CW. A phase 3 trial of l -glutamine in sickle cell disease. N Engl J Med. 2018;379(19):1879–80.
31. Ataga KI, Kutlar A, Kanter J, Liles D, Cancado R, Friedrisch J, et al. Crizanlizumab for the prevention of pain crises in sickle cell disease. N Engl J Med. 2017;376(5):429–39.
32. Vichinsky E, Hoppe CC, Ataga KI, Ware RE, Nduba V, El-Beshlawy A, et al. A phase 3 randomized trial of Voxelotor in sickle cell disease. N Engl J Med. 2019;381(6):509–19.
33. Eapen M, Brazauskas R, Walters MC, Bernaudin F, Bo-Subait K, Fitzhugh CD, et al. Effect of donor type and conditioning regimen intensity on allogeneic transplantation outcomes in patients with sickle cell disease: a retrospective multicentre, cohort study. Lancet Haematol. 2019;6(11):e585–96.
34. Bernaudin F, Socie G, Kuentz M, Chevret S, Duval M, Bertrand Y, et al. Long-term results of related myeloablative stem-cell transplantation to cure sickle cell disease. Blood. 2007;110(7):2749–56.
35. Fitzhugh CD, Walters MC. The case for HLA-identical sibling hematopoietic stem cell transplantation in children with symptomatic sickle cell anemia. Blood Adv. 2017;1(26):2563–7.
36. Gragert L, Eapen M, Williams E, Freeman J, Spellman S, Baitty R, et al. HLA match likelihoods for hematopoietic stem-cell grafts in the U.S. registry. N Engl J Med. 2014;371(4):339–48.
37. Naik RP, Streiff MB, Haywood C, Nelson JA, Lanzkron S. Venous thromboembolism in adults with sickle cell disease: a serious and under-recognized complication. Am J Med. 2013;126(5):443–9.
38. Stein PD, Beemath A, Meyers FA, Skaf E, Olson RE. Deep venous thrombosis and pulmonary embolism in hospitalized patients with sickle cell disease. Am J Med. 2006;119(10):897.e7–897.e11.
39. Klings ES, Machado RF, Barst RJ, Morris CR, Mubarak KK, Gordeuk VR, et al. An official American Thoracic Society clinical practice guideline: diagnosis, risk stratification, and Management of Pulmonary Hypertension of sickle cell disease. Am J Respir Crit Care Med. 2014;189(6):727–40.
40. Ataga KI, Derebail VK, Archer DR. The glomerulopathy of sickle cell disease. Am J Hematol. 2014;89(9):907–14.
41. Ohene-Frempong K, Weiner SJ, Sleeper LA, Miller ST, Embury S, Moohr JW, et al. Cerebrovascular accidents in sickle cell disease: rates and risk factors. Blood. 1998;91(1):288–94.
42. Balkaran B, Char G, Morris JS, Thomas PW, Serjeant BE, Serjeant GR. Stroke in a cohort of patients with homozygous sickle cell disease. J Pediatr. 1992;120(3):360–6.
43. Adams RJ, McKie VC, Hsu L, Files B, Vichinsky E, Pegelow C, et al. Prevention of a first stroke by transfusions in children with sickle cell anemia and abnormal results on transcranial Doppler ultrasonography. N Engl J Med. 1998;339(1):5–11.
44. Ware RE, Davis BR, Schultz WH, Brown RC, Aygun B, Sarnaik S, et al. Hydroxycarbamide versus chronic transfusion for maintenance of transcranial doppler flow velocities in children with sickle cell anaemia—TCD with transfusions changing to hydroxyurea (TWiTCH): a multicentre, open-label, phase 3, non-inferiority trial. Lancet. 2016;387(10019):661–70.
45. Kassim AA, Pruthi S, Day M, Rodeghier M, Gindville MC, Brodsky MA, et al. Silent cerebral infarcts and cerebral aneurysms are prevalent in adults with sickle cell anemia. Blood. 2016;127(16):2038–40.
46. DeBaun MR, Jordan LC, King AA, Schatz J, Vichinsky E, Fox CK, et al. American Society of Hematology 2020 guidelines for sickle cell disease: prevention, diagnosis, and treatment of cerebrovascular disease in children and adults. Blood Adv. 2020;4(8):1554–88.
47. Elagouz M, Jyothi S, Gupta B, Sivaprasad S. Sickle cell disease and the eye: old and New concepts. Surv Ophthalmol. 2010;55(4):359–77.
48. Gaston MH, Verter JI, Woods G, Pegelow C, Kelleher J, Presbury G, et al. Prophylaxis with Oral penicillin in children with sickle cell anemia. N Engl J Med. 1986;314(25):1593–9.

49. Dodd RY, Crowder LA, Haynes JM, Notari EP, Stramer SL, Steele WR. Screening blood donors for HIV, HCV, and HBV at the American red Cross: 10-year trends in prevalence, incidence, and residual risk, 2007 to 2016. Transfus Med Rev. 2020;34(2): 81–93.
50. Hagger D, Wolff S, Owen J, Samson D. Changes in coagulation and fibrinolysis in patients with sickle cell disease compared with healthy black controls. Blood Coagul Fibrinolysis. 1995;6(2):93–9.
51. Westerman MP, Green D, Gilman-Sachs A, Beaman K, Freels S, Boggio L, et al. Antiphospholipid antibodies, proteins C and S, and coagulation changes in sickle cell disease. J Lab Clin Med. 1999;134(4):352–62.
52. Noubouossie D, Key NS, Ataga KI. Coagulation abnormalities of sickle cell disease: relationship with clinical outcomes and the effect of disease modifying therapies. Blood Rev. 2016;30(4):245–56.
53. Bayazit AK, Kilinc Y. Natural coagulation inhibitors (protein C, protein S, antithrombin) in patients with sickle cell anemia in a steady state. Pediatr Int. 2001;43(6):592–6.
54. Brunson A, Lei A, Rosenberg AS, White RH, Keegan T, Wun T. Increased incidence of VTE in sickle cell disease patients: risk factors, recurrence and impact on mortality. Br J Haematol. 2017;178(2):319–26.
55. Naik RP, Streiff MB, Haywood C, Segal JB, Lanzkron S. Venous thromboembolism incidence in the cooperative study of sickle cell disease. J Thromb Haemost. 2014;12(12):2010–6.
56. Stevens SM, Woller SC, Kreuziger LB, Bounameaux H, Doerschug K, Geersing GJ, et al. Antithrombotic therapy for VTE disease. Chest. 2021;160(6):e545–608.
57. Ataga KI, Moore CG, Hillery CA, Jones S, Whinna HC, Strayhorn D, et al. Coagulation activation and inflammation in sickle cell disease-associated pulmonary hypertension. Haematologica. 2008;93(1):20–6.
58. Shah N, Thornburg C, Telen MJ, Ortel TL. Characterization of the hypercoagulable state in patients with sickle cell disease. Thromb Res. 2012;130(5):e241–5.
59. de Abood M, de Castillo Z, Guerrero F, Espino M, Austin KL. Effect of depo-Provera® or Microgynon® on the painful crises of sickle cell anemia patients. Contraception. 1997;56(5):313–6.
60. Manchikanti Gomez A, Grimes DA, Lopez LM, Schulz KF. Steroid hormones for contraception in women with sickle cell disease. Cochrane Fertility Regulation Group, editor. Cochrane Database Syst Rev. 2007;2012(1) https://doi.org/10.1002/14651858.CD006261.pub2.
61. Rogers DT, Molokie R. Sickle cell disease in pregnancy. Obstet Gynecol Clin N Am. 2010;37(2):223–37.
62. Koshy M, Burd L, Wallace D, Moawad A, Baron J. Prophylactic red-cell transfusions in pregnant patients with sickle cell disease. N Engl J Med. 1988;319(22):1447–52.
63. Moody KL, Mercer K, Glass M. An integrative review of the prevalence of depression among pediatric patients with sickle cell disease. Soc Work Public Health. 2019;34(4):343–52.
64. Osunkwo I, Andemariam B, Minniti CP, Inusa BPD, El Rassi F, Francis-Gibson B, et al. Impact of sickle cell disease on patients' daily lives, symptoms reported, and disease management strategies: results from the international sickle cell world assessment survey (SWAY). Am J Hematol. 2021;96(4):404–17.
65. Richardson LP, Russo JE, Katon W, McCarty CA, DeVries A, Edlund MJ, et al. Mental health disorders and long-term opioid use among adolescents and young adults with chronic pain. J Adolesc Health. 2012;50(6):553–8.
66. Dampier C, Palermo TM, Darbari DS, Hassell K, Smith W, Zempsky W. AAPT diagnostic criteria for chronic sickle cell disease pain. J Pain. 2017;18(5):490–8.
67. Keogh E, Eccleston C. Sex differences in adolescent chronic pain and pain-related coping. Pain. 2006;123(3):275–84.
68. Roth-Isigkeit A, Thyen U, Stöven H, Schwarzenberger J, Schmucker P. Pain among children and adolescents: restrictions in daily living and triggering factors. Pediatrics. 2005;115(2):e152–62.
69. Roth-Isigkeit A, Thyen U, Raspe HH, Stöven H, Schmucker P. Reports of pain among German children and adolescents: an epidemiological study. Acta Paediatr. 2004;93(2):258–63.
70. Palermo TM, Kiska R. Subjective sleep disturbances in adolescents with chronic pain: relationship to daily functioning and quality of life. J Pain. 2005;6(3):201–7.
71. Jordan AL, Eccleston C, Osborn M. Being a parent of the adolescent with complex chronic pain: an interpretative phenomenological analysis. Eur J Pain. 2007;11(1):49–56.
72. Eccleston C, Crombez G, Scotford A, Clinch J, Connell H. Adolescent chronic pain: patterns and predictors of emotional distress in adolescents with chronic pain and their parents. Pain. 2004;108(3):221–9.
73. Cohen LL, Lemanek K, Blount RL, Dahlquist LM, Lim CS, Palermo TM, et al. Evidence-based assessment of pediatric pain. J Pediatr Psychol. 2008;33(9):939–55.
74. Zempsky WT, O'Hara EA, Santanelli JP, New T, Smith-Whitley K, Casella J, et al. Development and validation of the youth acute pain functional ability questionnaire (YAPFAQ). J Pain. 2014;15(12):1319–27.
75. Makary MA, Overton HN, Wang P. Overprescribing is major contributor to opioid crisis. BMJ. 2017;359:j4792.
76. Clark DJ, Schumacher MA. America's opioid epidemic: supply and demand considerations. Anesth Analg. 2017;125(5):1667–74.
77. Zhang H, Kilaru AS, Meisel ZF, Bao Y. Prescription drug monitoring program mandates and opioids dispensed following emergency department encounters for patients with sickle cell disease or cancer with bone metastasis. JAMA. 2021;326(3):274.

78. Ballas SK, Kanter J, Agodoa I, Howard R, Wade S, Noxon V, et al. Opioid utilization patterns in United States individuals with sickle cell disease. Am J Hematol. 2018;93(10):E345–7.
79. Ballas SK. Opioids are not a major cause of death of patients with sickle cell disease. Ann Hematol. 2021;100(5):1133–8.
80. Webster LR, Webster RM. Predicting aberrant behaviors in opioid-treated patients: preliminary validation of the opioid risk tool. Pain Med. 2005;6(6):432–42.
81. Jones PDT, Lookatch MAS, Moore PDT. Validation of a new risk assessment tool: the brief risk questionnaire. J Opioid Manage. 2015;11(2):171–83.
82. Bodenheimer T. Transforming practice. N Engl J Med. 2008;359(20):2086–9.
83. Eccleston C, Clinch J. Adolescent chronic pain and disability: a review of the current evidence in assessment and treatment. Paediatr Child Health. 2007;12(2):117–20.
84. Stinson JN, McGRATH PJ, Hodnett ED, Feldman BM, Duffy CM, Huber AM, et al. An internet-based self-management program with telephone support for adolescents with arthritis: a pilot randomized controlled trial. J Rheumatol. 2010;37(9):1944–52.
85. Stinson JN, Lalloo C, Harris L, Isaac L, Campbell F, Brown S, et al. *iCanCope with pain* ™: user-Centred Design of a web- and Mobile-Based Self-Management Program for youth with chronic pain based on identified health care needs. Pain Res Manage. 2014;19(5):257–65.
86. Palermo TM, Eccleston C, Lewandowski AS, de C. Williams AC, Morley S. Randomized controlled trials of psychological therapies for management of chronic pain in children and adolescents: an updated meta-analytic review. Pain. 2010;148(3):387–97.
87. Dowell D, Haegerich TM, Chou R. CDC guideline for prescribing opioids for chronic pain—United States, 2016. JAMA. 2016;315(15):1624.
88. Lee L, Smith-Whitley K, Banks S, Puckrein G. Reducing health care disparities in sickle cell disease: a review. Public Health Rep. 2019;134(6):599–607.
89. Haywood C, Beach MC, Lanzkron S, Strouse JJ, Wilson R, Park H, et al. A systematic review of barriers and interventions to improve appropriate use of therapies for sickle cell disease. J Natl Med Assoc. 2009;101(10):1022–33.
90. Wakefield EO, Pantaleao A, Popp JM, Dale LP, Santanelli JP, Litt MD, et al. Describing perceived racial bias among youth with sickle cell disease. J Pediatr Psychol. 2018;43(7):779–88.
91. Haywood C, Lanzkron S, Hughes MT, Brown R, Massa M, Ratanawongsa N, et al. A video-intervention to improve clinician attitudes toward patients with sickle cell disease: the results of a randomized experiment. J Gen Intern Med. 2011;26(5):518–23.
92. Anderson D. Barriers and resident attitudes surrounding care of patients with sickle cell disease. Blood 2020;136:21–22 [cited 2022 Oct 4]. Available from: https://ash.confex.com/ash/2020/webprogram/Paper142986.html
93. Freiermuth CE, Haywood C, Silva S, Cline DM, Kayle M, Sullivan D, et al. Attitudes toward patients with sickle cell disease in a multicenter sample of emergency department providers. Adv Emerg Nurs J. 2014;36(4):335–47.
94. Sukhera J, Watling C. A framework for integrating implicit bias recognition into health professions education. Acad Med. 2018;93(1):35–40.

# Solid Organ Transplantation 37

Ruchi Gupta Mahajan, Sheila Quinn, Eva Waite, and Heather Stewart

## Case Presentation

D.M. is a 19-year-old patient, presenting for a routine monthly transplant follow-up appointment. D.M recently transitioned from a pediatric to an adult kidney transplant division within the same hospital system. She had end-stage kidney disease (ESKD) secondary to nephronophthisis and is status post deceased donor renal transplant (DDRT) done at age 9 years. She has a history of dilated cardiomyopathy with resolved ventricular dysfunction after her renal transplant. She also has a history of cytomegalovirus (CMV) viremia and asthma. She was being followed by endocrinologists given a history of elevated hemoglobin A1c (HgA1c), was initially started on metformin and later switched to insulin as she was diagnosed with diabetes mellitus. Her family history is negative for hypertension and kidney disease.

D.M. was admitted 2 years prior due to concerns for continued elevation in her serum creatinine. Transplant biopsy performed at that time demonstrated Banff 1B rejection. She received anti-thymocyte globulin (ATG) and corticosteroids, after which her serum creatinine transiently stabilized at 1.11 mg/dL before increasing again to 2.0 mg/dL 6 months later. She has had ongoing issues with non-compliance with her immunosuppressive regimen and was noted to have low serum tacrolimus levels during multiple recent admissions. In the last year, she was admitted three times for an episode of acute kidney injury (AKI) and has had two additional kidney biopsies. Her hemoglobin was also noted to be 7.5 g/dL during the last admission and she was started on an erythropoietin-stimulating agent. She did not collect the medication from the pharmacy for 2 weeks and presented to the emergency department 4 months prior with fatigue and shortness of breath and required admission. Her hemoglobin was noted to be 6.6 g/dL, and she received two units of packed red blood cells. Her serum tacrolimus level was again noted to be low. Her serum creatinine after that admission increased to

R. G. Mahajan (✉)
Division of Nephrology, Department of Pediatrics, University of Minnesota, Masonic Children's Hospital, Minneapolis, MN, USA
e-mail: mahaj104@umn.edu

S. Quinn
Division of General Internal Medicine, University of Pennsylvania School of Medicine, Philadelphia, PA, USA
e-mail: sheila.quinn@pennmedicine.upenn.edu

E. Waite
Department of General Internal Medicine, Mount Sinai Medical Center, New York, NY, USA
e-mail: eva.waite@mssm.edu

H. Stewart
Department of Pediatrics, Dwaine & Cynthia Willet Children's Hospital of Savannah, Savannah, GA, USA
e-mail: Heather.Stewart3@hcahealthcare.com


A. A. Kuo et al. (eds.), *Care of Adults with Chronic Childhood Conditions*,
https://doi.org/10.1007/978-3-031-54281-7_37

3.2 mg/dL. D.M. was again admitted 3 months ago after being diagnosed with COVID-19 infection, neutropenia, and another episode of AKI. Her serum creatinine was noted to be increased to 4.5 mg/dL during this admission. She also reported not taking her asthma inhalers or her short-acting insulin for the past month. She received granulocyte colony-stimulating factor (G-CSF) during this admission for neutropenia. She was discharged and followed up the following month. She has been closely followed by psychiatry and has been diagnosed with moderate episode of recurrent major depressive disorder for the past 2 years. D.M. missed her last two appointments with psychiatry as well. D.M.'s mother also shared that her D.M.'s boyfriend recently broke up with her and D.M. has been quite upset and heartbroken since.

Today, D.M. is accompanied by her mother who reports that D.M. has lost 8 pounds in the last 2–3 months. D.M. states that she has trouble sleeping and has been feeling occasionally dizzy. She denies dysuria, fever, hematuria, edema, vomiting, and diarrhea.

Her physical exam is remarkable in that she appears pale but otherwise alert and communicative. Her blood pressure (BP) is elevated at 143/88 and body mass index (BMI) is 22.2 kg/m$^2$. Her skin exam is normal with a few healed surgical scars but no abnormal nevi. Her labs are remarkable for a hemoglobin of 6.6 g/dL, potassium of 6.1 meq/L, blood urea nitrogen of 45 mg/dL, and serum creatinine of 5.49 mg/dL. She is admitted for further management and to assess the need for dialysis and failure of her kidney transplant.

## Case Discussion

In caring for a patient with a solid organ transplant in the adolescent age group, adherence becomes a very important issue. Not being able to fully comprehend the consequences of their actions, risk-taking behavior, social pressure to conform, experimentation with drugs and alcohol, and avoidance of parental advice and supervision all make adolescence a difficult time period. Apart from the usual stressors associated with adolescence, having a chronic disease makes adolescents more liable to feel socially isolated, less likely able to participate in sports/gym activities or plan for college and future careers, and unable to eat like their peers. In general, anxiety and depression are predominant in children with chronic diseases. Given the immunocompromised state of transplant patients, it is often necessary for them to socially isolate for long time period, which can contribute to the development of mental health issues.

With the COVID-19 pandemic, at-risk adolescents have further been restricted to home and been unable to meet with friends/support personnel in person to share their concerns. The impact on mental health has been extreme due to feelings of uncertainty, lack of daily routines, lack of access to health services provided through schools, and lack of advanced emotional development to cope with all these changes. Due to stay-at-home orders, school closures, or new at-home learning methods, students are seeking ways to connect and to socialize in manners that may not be productive for optimal health. The result of these behaviors can be smartphone and internet addiction. It has been noted that adolescents have increased their use of alcohol and cannabis to cope with stress during the pandemic period.

D.M. is one example of the many patients who struggle with the challenges associated with complex chronic medical conditions that require timely medications and scheduled follow-up appointment with multiple providers while also dealing with issues at a personal level. It is important to incorporate mental health screening as a routine part of follow up, identifying productive application of smartphones (such as applications for listing and taking their medications and online support group), foster family and social support, connecting patients of similar age group going through similar situations to help share their feelings. Despite the uncertainty of the current crisis, it is important that adolescents receive the physical and mental care that they need to develop, grow, and thrive.

## Overview

### Prevalence and Epidemiology

The optimal treatment for eligible patients with ESKD that offers improved patient survival, reduced morbidity, improved quality of life, and economic savings compared to dialysis is kidney transplantation. Pediatric kidney disease affects children of all ages, and with a number of available renal replacement therapies, including dialysis and transplantation, these patients are expected to survive into adulthood. Advances in the medical and surgical care of kidney transplant recipients including the judicious use of antibiotics, the improved understanding of the immunobiology of rejection and the advances in immunomodulatory medications for the treatment of rejection, and use in maintenance immunosuppression have undoubtedly played a role in the success of patient and allograft survival. In the United States, the incidence and prevalence of the ESKD in children has been slowly decreasing. As of 2017, there were 9684 children between the ages of 0 and 21 years with ESKD [1]. Of these children, kidney transplant was the most common modality of renal replacement therapy (5485 [72.9%]), followed by an essentially equal distribution of hemodialysis (1138 [15.1%]) and peritoneal dialysis (899 [12%]). The number of pediatric patients living with a kidney transplant has more than doubled since 1988, with 7082 children transplanted in 2017.

The first-year deceased-donor (DD) and living-donor (LD) transplant outcomes have steadily improved over the last 20 years. In the most recent reporting year of 2016, the first-year graft failure and mortality rates for both DD (probability of graft failure 2.7% and death 0.9%) and LD (probability of graft failure 1.3% and death 0.4%), pediatric transplant recipients were better for LD transplants as compared to DD [1]. Kidney transplantation is not a cure. The Organ Procurement and Transplantation Network (OPTN)/Scientific Registry of Transplant Recipients Annual Data Report notes that the proportions of living donor and deceased donor recipients from 2018 with an estimated glomerular filtration rate (eGFR) 90 mL/mi/1.73 $m^2$ or higher at 12 months post-transplant were 26.7% (increased from 19.7% in 2008) and 31.9% (increased from 22.3%), respectively [2]. Overall, the number of pediatric kidney transplants peaked in 2005 at 899 and has remained steady at approximately 736 since 2019 [2]. Since 2006, the number of DD transplants has exceeded the number of LD transplants; in 2019, there were 519 DD transplants and 244 LD transplants [2]. This is partly due to the implementation of an allocation policy known as Share 35. This policy was implemented in September 2005 and awarded pediatric priority for donors less than 35 years of age.

### Pathophysiology, Risk Factors, and Transplantation Complications

The major indications for kidney transplantation in childhood are congenital abnormalities of the kidney and urinary tract (CAKUT), congenital nephrotic syndrome, polycystic disease, and neonatal kidney injury/cortical necrosis due to thrombosis.

More than one-third of pediatric patients with ESKD have comorbidities, including cerebral palsy, heart disease, chromosomal abnormalities, a syndromic diagnosis, and developmental delay, all of which may adversely impact the patient's quality of life and overall prognosis following kidney transplant [1].

Post-transplantation patients are at an increased risk of allograft dysfunction, rejection, infection, metabolic bone problems, cardiovascular disease (CVD), dyslipidemia, type II diabetes mellitus, growth delay, malignancies, alteration in neurocognitive development, poor adherence to medication, and decreased quality of life. The major cause of graft loss is patient death, mainly due to complications related to cardiovascular disease, infection, and malignancy. The patient's transplant status and long-term immunosuppression can impact routine primary care issues and recommended algorithms.

## Conditions Associated with Solid Organ Transplant

### Hypertension

Hypertension (HTN) is quite common in kidney transplant recipients and is associated with an increased risk of graft failure. Epidemiological studies indicate that the prevalence of hypertension has generally increased over time. Overall prevalence of post-transplant HTN has ranged from 24% to 90% [3]. Most recipients require two or more antihypertensive medications to achieve target BP goals. The major goals of antihypertensive therapy after transplant are to preserve kidney function and to decrease cardiovascular risk. After kidney transplantation, poorly controlled BP has been shown to be an independent risk factor for cardiovascular disease (CVD) and is also associated with an increased risk of graft failure [4]. Kidney Disease Outcomes Quality Initiative (KDOQI) clinical practice guidelines on hypertension and antihypertensive agents in chronic kidney disease (CKD) recommend reduction to target BP in kidney transplant patients to less than 130/80 [5]. Post-transplantation hypertension arises from a variety of factors. Some of these factors may have originated pre-transplant while others are related to immunosuppressive medication effects or post-transplant complications. Pre-transplant factors include increased vascular stiffness and vascular calcification. Dialysis patients have functional and structural alterations in their arterial walls leading to increased vascular stiffness. Vascular calcifications also develop in the ESKD population due to deranged calcium–phosphorus metabolism and secondary renal hyperparathyroidism. Post-transplant factors include delayed or poor allograft function, volume overload, presence of native kidneys, and transplant renal artery stenosis (TRAS). Delayed graft function (DGF) is a risk factor for post-transplant HTN. DGF results in the kidney's decreased ability to excrete sodium, which contributes to a lag in daily sodium excretion, salt and water retention, rightward shift of the pressure natriuresis curve, and an increase in blood pressure [6, 7]. Native kidneys induce HTN via renin secretion or through increased sympathetic nerve activity. The overall prevalence of HTN associated with native kidneys is unknown. Studies have noted that bilateral native nephrectomies in patients with resistant HTN can lead to the improvement in BP control in most but not all patients. Native nephrectomies are not commonly performed in the recent decades, likely due to improved antihypertensive drug therapies [6, 7]. Transplant renal artery stenosis (TRAS) increases BP by activation of the renin-angiotensin-aldosterone system (RAAS), leading to systemic vasoconstriction and increase in sodium and water retention. Significant TRAS can be refractory to medical management and can contribute to unexplained worsening of allograft function [6, 7].

The immunosuppressive medications most often used in transplant, especially calcineurin inhibitors (CNIs) and prednisone, can potentiate HTN. CNIs, the mainstay in the prevention of allograft rejection, cause widespread arterial vasoconstriction, thereby increasing systemic vascular resistance. CNIs also cause vasoconstriction of the afferent arteriole leading to a reduction in GFR, thereby leading to an increase in tubular sodium reabsorption. Prednisone-induced HTN has been attributed to the activation of free mineralocorticoid receptor, promoting sodium and water retention.

All classes of antihypertensive agents can be used to lower blood pressure in kidney transplant patients. Short-term randomized-controlled trials (RCTs) suggest a beneficial effect of calcium channel blockers (CCB), as compared with either placebo or angiotensin-converting enzyme inhibitors (ACE-Is), with regard to level of kidney function. In addition, a recent meta-analysis of RCTs indicated that the use of CCB, versus placebo or no treatment, was associated with a 25% lower rate of graft loss and a higher GFR. KDIGO recommends that a dihydropyridine CCB or an angiotensin II receptor blocker (ARB) be used as the first-line antihypertensive agent in adult kidney transplant recipients [8]. When selecting a particular class of antihypertensive as the initial treatment of post-transplant hypertension, it is practical to consider the presence or absence of proteinuria, diabetes mellitus, allograft dysfunction, volume overload, and risk factors for cardiovascular events. It is also important to become familiar with the interactions between antihypertensive and immunosuppressive agents. While CCBs are useful, it is important to avoid the non-dihydropyridine group, such as diltiazem and verapamil. These drugs are potent inhibitors of the cytochrome p450 system and increase CNI levels. The dihydropyridine class, nifedipine XL, amlodipine, and isradipine, are often used since they do not affect GFR or electrolyte balances. They can, however, potentiate gum hyperplasia. ACE-Is and ARBs are useful if a patient has proteinuria, but renal function and electrolytes must be monitored as they can decrease GFR and cause significant hyperkalemia. The evidence review found that ACE-Is, alpha blockers, beta blockers, and mineralocorticoid receptor antagonists (MRAs), compared to placebo or no treatment, had no significant effect on mortality, graft loss, or CV event [8]. Beta blockers such as labetalol and carvedilol can be useful in diminishing headaches caused by CNIs. Diuretics are particularly effective in volume-dependent HTN and can be useful in the setting of hyperkalemia. Alpha blockers are less commonly used due to problems with hypotension. Centrally acting agents, such as clonidine, can be used as a second-line therapy, especially when compliance may be improved with the form of a weekly transdermal patch [9].

## Post-Transplant Diabetes Mellitus

Post-transplant diabetes Mellitus (PTDM) refers to the recognition of diabetes in persons after organ transplantation. PTDM occurs in an estimated 10–40% of patients within the first 3 years after solid organ transplantation. The majority of PTDM cases appear during the first 6 months after transplantation, when patients are treated with high doses of immunosuppression. As immunosuppression is weaned in the first 3 months post-transplant, 30% of patients will continue to have hyperglycemia and meet criteria for diabetes. For this reason, it is recommended to screen for diabetes at least once each year, indefinitely. International Consensus Guidelines on PTDM were published in 2003, recommending that PTDM be diagnosed based on the American Diabetes Association (ADA) criteria for type 2 diabetes [10]. Criteria are namely HgA1c ≥6.5%; or fasting plasma glucose of ≥126 mg/dL; or 2-h plasma glucose level of ≥200 mg/dL after an oral load of 75 g of anhydrous glucose; or random plasma glucose level of ≥200 mg/dL plus the presence of symptoms.

PTDM is associated with increased morbidity, mortality, and healthcare costs. Besides the traditional risk factors for type 2 diabetes mellitus (age, obesity, family history, and ethnicity), hepatitis C virus infection, and the exposure to immunosuppressive agents, specifically CNIs and corticosteroids, increase the risk for diabetes [11]. Recipients that develop PTDM are not only at risk for the complications associated with diabetes itself but they are also at an increased risk for graft-related complications such as rejection, graft loss, infection, and vascular complications [4, 11, 12]. Current immunosuppressive regimens rely heavily on the use of agents that have been identified as being diabetogenic, such as corticosteroids, CNIs, and mammalian target of rapamycin inhibitors (mTOR) [4]. Corticosteroids increase hepatic gluconeogenesis, the development of insulin resistance, and defective insulin secretion. CNIs, which have been shown to be superior to prednisone in regard to patient and graft-survival, impose a higher risk of promoting the development of diabetes in solid organ transplant recipients. CNIs reduce glucose-stimulated insulin release in a dose-related and reversible manner, without affecting insulin resistance. Data also suggest that CNIs are directly toxic to the pancreatic β (beta)-cells [13, 14]. It should be noted that mTOR inhibitors are also diabetogenic, especially if combined with CNIs [15]. Although the mechanism is not yet completely understood, the use of mTOR inhibitors leads to hypertriglyceridemia-related peripheral insulin resistance and impaired pancreatic β (beta)-cell response [16]. Based on animal and human data, rapamycin appears to induce an insulin secretion defect and impairs β (beta)-cell survival and proliferation [17].

The management of a transplant recipient with PTDM is best accomplished with a multidisciplinary team approach among the primary care provider (PCP), transplant subspecialist, endocrinologist, and dietician. The targets for treatment are the same as for all diabetic patients with sufficiently intensive treatment to maintain normal or near-normal glycemia with an HgA1c lower than 7.0%. The choice of glucose-lowering agent should consider the desired level of glucose control, potential drug–drug interactions, and renal function. It is important to note that the majority of kidney transplant recipients with a well-functioning allograft have some degree of CKD. A stepwise approach to the treatment of PTDM is recommended. In consultation with the transplant subspecialist, consideration should be given to modifying the patient's immunosuppressive regimen to reverse or ameliorate diabetes, after weighing the potential adverse effects including the risk of rejection. It is also critical to address modifiable risk factors including weight control, diet, and exercise. For those patients still not at target after such interventions, it is appropriate to initiate medical therapy—initially monotherapy with insulin or an oral hypoglycemic agent taking into account patient-specific factors, renal function, side effects, and potential drug–drug interactions with the patient's immunosuppressive regimen. If monotherapy is insufficient in achieving glucose control, one should proceed to combination therapy, adding another hypoglycemic agent with different mechanisms of action. When oral hypoglycemic medications fail to reach glycemic control targets, insulin therapy should be considered.

When selecting the medications used to treat PTDM, it is always important to consider the patient's renal and hepatic function and assess for possible drug interactions with the patient's immunosuppressant and other medical therapies. Concern for lactic acidosis has limited the use of metformin in kidney transplant recipients. However, there are recent reports suggesting benefits from metformin therapy in patients with mild to moderate CKD. Caution is recommended in using metformin with appropriate dose adjustment based on the eGFR and close laboratory monitoring of renal function and electrolytes. There are various recommendations regarding metformin dosing in renal impairment. The proposes are the following: for those patients whose renal function has decreased below an eGFR of 45 mL/min/1.73 $m^2$, metformin initiation must be avoided and that other classes of oral agents should be considered; for those with an eGFR greater than 45 mL/min/1.73 $m^2$, metformin can be used but renal function must be monitored close with the interval depending on the level of renal dysfunction. Metformin should be discontinued when the eGFR is <30 mL/min/1.72 $m^2$ [9, 18]. Of the sulfonylureas, glipizide is the preferred agent in patients with impaired renal function; it is primarily converted to inactive metabolites and less likely to cause hypoglycemia than other sulfonylureas.

Thiazolidinediones (TZDs) such as pioglitazone and rosiglitazone can be used without need for renal clearance adjustment. However, they must be avoided in patients with heart failure. In addition, TZDs have been linked to decreased bone formation, accelerated bone loss, and increased risk for fractures. They must be used with caution in patients with CKD and metabolic bone disease. Other agents such as α (alpha)-glucosidase inhibitors, amylin analogs, and meglitinides can be used at somewhat lower levels of renal function but have less potent blood sugar-lowering effect.

Newer classes of hypoglycemic agents, such as dipeptidyl peptidase 4 (DDP-4) inhibitors, can be used in adjusted doses for patients with eGFR < 30 mL/min/1.73 $m^2$. Linagliptin can be used with no renal or hepatic adjustment.

Glucagon-like peptide (GLP)-1 agonists have become more popular due to their associated weight loss and cardioprotective effects. Liraglutide (daily injection), dulaglutide (weekly injection), and semaglutide (oral or injectable) offer increasing flexibility for diabetes control. They are currently not listed as having recommendations for either renal or hepatic adjustment. However, when combined with CNIs, they have the potential to increase risk of renal toxicity [9].

Sodium-glucose co-transporter 2 (SGLT2) inhibitors ("flozins") have indications for diabetes as well as cardiovascular and renal disease. Empagliflozin (indications for cardiovascular disease and heart failure), canagliflozin (indications for CVS and renal disease), and dapagliflozin (indications for congestive heart failure and renal disease) can be used cautiously. This class of drug can cause significant diuresis with volume loss and renal hypoperfusion, especially in patients also on ARBs, ACE-Is, or diuretics. Their use needs to be monitored carefully and discussed with transplant service. It is not recommended to start SGLT2 inhibitors in patients with an eGFR < 45 mL/min/1.73 $m^2$.

Finally, one should remember that insulin is the safest of the medications used for transplant, associated diabetes with the fewest drug interactions [9, 19].

## Cardiovascular Disease and Dyslipidemia

Atherosclerotic cardiovascular disease is the leading cause of mortality and death-censored graft loss after transplantation. The annual rate of fatal or nonfatal CVD events is 3.5–5.0% in kidney transplant recipients, a rate 50-fold higher than the general population [8]. Kidney transplantation is known to reduce mortality compared with dialysis; studies suggest that this effect may be due to the reduction in cardiovascular risk associated with the improvement in kidney function. The reason for this observation is unknown. Specific risk factors for post-transplantation CVD include age, male gender, hypertension, cardiovascular event prior to transplantation, longer pre-transplant time on dialysis, post-transplant diabetes mellitus, use of corticosteroids, lower serum albumin post-transplant, and higher triglyceride levels post-transplant [20].

Dyslipidemia is often a complication of the use of immunosuppressive drugs. Patients treated with corticosteroids and CNIs can have adverse lipid profiles with elevated LDL and reduced HDL. Sirolimus can also contribute to moderate-to-severe hypercholesterolemia and hypertriglyceridemia. Dyslipidemia can contribute to the patient's preexisting elevated cardiovascular risk profile. In 2009, the KDIGO Working Group did not find new guidelines or systematic reviews since the KDOQI Dyslipidemia Guidelines were published in 2004 [21]. Therefore, the KDIGO working group recommendations include screening with a serum lipid panel for all adult and adolescent kidney transplant recipients 2–3 months after transplantation, 2–3 months after change in treatment or with the onset of other conditions known to cause dyslipidemia, and at least annually thereafter. The KDIGO guidelines for lipid management recommend statin therapy in all kidney transplant patients, designating renal transplant as a coronary artery disease (CAD) risk equivalent [22]. The working group further recommends treating adults to a goal LDL <100 mg/dL and non-HDL <130 mg/dL and adolescents to a goal LDL <130 mg/dL and non-HDL <160 mg/dL.

HMG-CoA reductase inhibitors (statins) are widely used in kidney transplant recipients given their established benefits in the general population. A 2009 systematic review noted that among kidney transplant recipients statins did not decrease all-cause mortality but were associated with a significant reduction in total cholesterol, low-density lipoprotein (LDL) cholesterol, and triglycerides levels [23]. Although there are drug–drug interactions that must be monitored in kidney transplant recipients, the use of statins is generally safe. All statins appear to be effective in lowering LDL and total cholesterol with little evidence to support recommending one agent over another. Atorvastatin, simvastatin, pravastatin, and fluvastatin have all been used in studies of kidney transplant recipients. In the assessment of fluvastatin in renal transplantation (ALERT) study, a large placebo-controlled trial, fluvastatin effectively lowered LDL cholesterol to a goal of <100 mg/dL and also demonstrated a 30% decreased risk in fatal and nonfatal cardiac events [24].

Certain drug interactions should be taken into consideration when using statins in kidney transplant recipients. The hepatic metabolism of statins is affected by concurrent use of CNIs, which increases the risk of rhabdomyolysis. Simvastatin, lovastatin, and atorvastatin are the statins most likely to adversely interact with CNIs, with cyclosporine (CsA) being the most problematic [22]. It is important to remain mindful of additional medications that can increase CNI levels (azole antifungals, macrolides, and diltiazem) and magnify the risk of liver toxicity and rhabdomyolysis. Serum transaminase levels and CNI drug levels should be monitored closely when initiating a statin and serially monitored once stable drug dosing has been achieved. Finally, if adequate lipid lowering is not achieved, ezetimibe and PCSK9 inhibitors (alirocumab, inclisiran, or evolucamab) can be used, with no current evidence of drug interaction with CNIs or prednisone.

## Bone Mineral Density and Osteoporosis

While many complications of ESKD may be reversed by transplantation, bone and mineral disturbances may persist.

Bone disease is common in transplant recipients with multiple factors involved in its pathogenesis. Rates of bone loss are greatest in the first 6–18 months after kidney transplantation and range from 4% to 9% at the spine and 5% to 8% at the hip [25]. There are numerous contributing factors, but the main factors are pre-existing renal osteodystrophy at the time of renal transplantation, transplant-specific therapies, and reduced GFR. In kidney recipients, osteopenia can also be influenced by long-term hemodialysis, age, heredity, gender, exercise habits, and the presence of diabetes mellitus.

Chronic kidney disease-mineral and bone disorder (CKD-MBD) is the most complex pre-transplant bone disease. One or more types of bone disease may be present including low turnover bone disease (osteomalacia or adynamic bone disease), osteitis fibrosa cystica due to secondary hyperparathyroidism, osteoporosis, and mixed bone disease [26].

Bone biopsy studies have revealed that the low turnover bone disease states of osteomalacia and adynamic bone disease are the two most common bone disorders seen in kidney transplant recipients (Table 37.1).

**Table 37.1** Different types of bone disease seen in kidney transplant recipients

| Type of bone disease | Characteristics |
|---|---|
| *Low turnover* | |
| Adynamic | Reduced bone volume and mineralization is paralleled by a decrease in bone formation<br>Few osteoid seams and few osteoblasts<br>Osteoclasts can be low, normal, or high |
| Osteomalacia | Accumulation of unmineralized matrix<br>Decrease in mineralization precedes or is more pronounced than the inhibition of collagen deposition |
| *High turnover* | |
| Hyperparathyroid | Marked increase in bone turnover<br>Irregularly shaped trabecules with numerous abnormal remodeling sites<br>Unusually high number of bone cells with irregular arrangement and shape |
| Mixed renal osteodystrophy | Caused by defective mineralization with or without increased bone formation and increased parathyroid hormone (PTH) activity in bone<br>Bone volume is variable and depends on dominant pathogenic cause<br>Increased numbers of heterogeneous remodeling sites<br>Typically an increase in osteoclasts |

References utilized in the construction of table: KDIGO [8], Danovitch 2010 [42], UpToDate 2022

The risk for fracture after kidney transplant is approximately 2–3% per patient per year with 7–10% of all renal transplant patients suffering one or more fractures over their lifetime [27, 28]. Hypercalcemia is also common post-kidney transplant and is considered to result from parathyroid (PTH)-induced osteoclast activation and bone resorption. The dominant clinical adverse bone events following transplantation include bone loss, fractures, osteonecrosis, and bone pain. A 2009 analysis of 68,814 patients reported to the United States Renal Data System (USRDS) revealed that 22.5% kidney transplant recipients developed a fracture within 5 years [29]. Given the extent of the problem, various screening tools have been suggested to mitigate risk. Strategies include routine measurement of PTH, 25-hydroxy vitamin-D, and bone mineral density (BMD) by dual-emission x-ray absorptiometry (DEXA).

BMD screening with DEXA is currently recommended for all women who are older than 65-years-of-age and postmenopausal women who are younger than 65-years-of-age with one or more additional risk factors for osteoporosis. Densitometry testing is recommended for transplant recipients on the basis of the assumption that data from the general population are pertinent to this cohort. Fractures resulting from osteoporosis typically involve the lumbar spine or hip. However, fractures in the transplant population frequently include the non-axial skeleton (hips, long bones, ankles, and feet), supporting the hypothesis that post-transplant bone disease is not a simple form of osteoporosis.

The KDIGO Working Group summarizes key observations about the utility of various screening strategies. KDIGO notes: (1) no randomized clinical trials in kidney transplant recipients have examined bone-specific therapies on patient-level outcomes, including mortality or fractures; (2) low bone mineral density in non-kidney transplant recipients predicts fractures but data are scant for kidney transplant recipients; (3) there are insufficient data to suggest any bone-specific therapies after the first year of transplant; (4) treatment with calcium, calcitriol, or vitamin D analogs and/or bisphosphonates has been suggested to improve bone density in kidney transplant recipients; (5) reports of the use of bisphosphonates indicate therapy is associated with improvements in bone density without being adequately powered to note improvements in patient survival or fracture risk [8].

A major factor in the pathogenesis of post-transplant bone disease is immunosuppressive therapy. Glucocorticoids are commonly used in most maintenance immunosuppressive regimens and in the event of allograft rejection. The highest glucocorticoid-associated rates of bone loss are in the first 6 months after transplantation. Glucocorticoids reduce bone formation by decreasing osteoblast replication and differentiation as well as increasing apoptosis. They also promote osteopenia and calcium loss. Additional mechanisms include reduced gonadal hormone production, decreased calcium absorption from the gut, decreased insulin-like growth factor (IGF)-1 production, diminished PTH sensitivity, and increased osetoclastogenesis [30–33]. The CNIs CsA and tacrolimus have also been linked to osteoporosis. Both direct and indirect effects of these medications influence bone resorption. CsA is thought to cause bone loss through direct effects on osteoclasts and by indirectly acting on T-cell function. Tacrolimus inhibits T-cell activation and proliferation and cytokine gene expression. Rat studies have demonstrated that tacrolimus leads to bone loss; however, skeletal effects in humans are not well studied [34]. Less intense bone loss has been noted in patients on tacrolimus, probably due to the fact that tacrolimus allows for lower doses of glucocorticoids.

Therapeutic options for post-transplantation bone disease focus on glucocorticoid avoidance or withdrawal as well as use of vitamin-D analogs, calcium supplementation, calcimemetics, and bisphosphonates. The rational for minimizing glucocorticoid use relates to its established risks of osteoporosis and avascular necrosis. Studies have noted beneficial effects on BMD after early tapering of prednisolone. A 2012 study analyzed both the USRDS and SRTR databases to assess whether early corticosteroid withdrawal after kidney transplant would result in lower fracture risk [35]. With adjustment for multiple covariates, the investigators found that corticosteroid withdrawal was associated with a 31% fracture risk reduction and observed that fractures requiring hospitalization were also significantly reduced. For patients with persistent hyperparathyroidism, options include use of vitamin-D analogs or calcimimectics such as cinacalcet as well as surgery. PTH levels usually decline rapidly during the first 3–6 months post-transplantation due to the reduction in functional parathyroid gland mass. Persistently elevated levels of serum PTH can lead to complications such as soft tissue calcification, hypophosphatemia, and hypercalciuria. During the first months following transplantation, 1,25-dihydroxy vitamin D levels are low due to the action of glucocorticoid-induced reduction of 1-alpha-hydroxylase activity. In this case, it is recommended to administer cholecalciferol to replace the substrate for calcitriol. Cinacalcet is a calcimimetic drug licensed for the treatment of secondary hyperparathyroidism in patients with ESKD. It is often used off label in patients with persistent hyperparathyroidism after transplantation. A few small studies indicate that this drug is effective in mitigating high PTH levels post-kidney transplantation with no adverse effects on renal function. One such study published in 2008 reported a favorable effect of cinacalcet on BMD in kidney transplant patients [36]. An earlier 2004 blinded study demonstrated that the use of calcium and the vitamin D analog calcitriol attenuated bone loss and increase BMD compared to transplant patients who received calcium alone [37]. There was also no hypercalcemia or decrease in renal function. However, there was no evaluation of the beneficial or harmful effects of therapy on fracture rate, hospitalization, or mortality. Numerous studies have shown that bisphosphonates are effective in preventing bone loss when used early after transplantation. They may also help improve bone density when used late in the setting of established bone loss. Despite the positive effect on bone density, there are concerns with the use of bisphosphonates, particularly given the issues regarding renal safety, the unknown effects on fracture rates, and the potential exacerbation or induction of adynamic bone disease. Most transplant nephrologists agree that bisphosphonate therapy should be limited to patients who have a particularly high risk of fracture. Ideally in these kidney transplant patients, adynamic bone disease should be excluded by bone biopsy prior to the administration of bisphosphonate therapy. Monoclonal antibodies against the receptor activator of nuclear factor kappa-B ligand (RANKL) are also increasingly being considered in the kidney transplant population, as it is not cleared renally, averting any issue for those patients with lower GFR. Although patients with transplants have largely been excluded from the trials investigating optimal treatment protocols for these medications, emerging studies are showing promising results for increased BMD when compared to bisphosphonates [38, 39]. Although the more common gastrointestinal side effects associated with bisphosphonates are avoided with RANKL inhibitors, patients must be monitored for hypocalcemia. Overall, an individualized approach is necessary for the prevention of post-transplantation bone loss.

## Hyperuricemia and Gout

In the general population, hyperuricemia is defined as a serum uric acid level > 6 mg/dL. The risk of developing gout increases twofold for every incremental increase in serum uric acid of 1 mg/dL. Because of gender differences and the absence of detailed information in kidney transplant recipients, KDIGO defines hyperuricemia as >6 mg/dL in women and > 7 mg/dL in men. Monitoring and management of hyperuricemia in kidney transplant patients is important due to the increased incidence of gout in addition to the association with loss of kidney function and cardiovascular disease. It is important to be aware of drug interactions with immunosuppressive medications in this particular patient population.

Hyperuricemia is a common metabolic problem in kidney transplant recipients and is exacerbated by the use of CNIs that impair renal uric acid secretion, use of diuretics, and impaired renal function. Among the CNIs, cyclosporine has the highest risk of hyperuricemia and gout. The annual incidence of gout is 0.5% for patients with hyperuricemia (7–8.9 mg/dL) and increases exponentially to 4.9% for patients with serum uric acid levels of >9 mg/dL [40]. The American College of Rheumatology (ACR) guidelines recommend a target serum uric acid level of <6 mg/dL at a minimum in all patients and < 5 mg/dL in more severe or complicated cases [41]. KDIGO guidelines reiterate the recommendation of a treatment threshold of <5 mg/dL in kidney transplant patients. This is in part due to their risk factors, prior history of hyperuricemia/gout, existence of comorbid conditions, higher BMI, older age, use of diuretics, and complex drug regimen. In the general population, there is evidence that modifications that decrease risk include weight loss, adherence to a low purine diet (reduced meat and alcohol consumption), and avoidance of diuretics. Some antihypertensive drugs such as amlodipine and losartan are reported to have a uricosuric effect.

Treatment of asymptomatic hyperuricemia is not generally recommended in the general population or in kidney transplant recipients; however, it is advocated in patients with recurrent symptomatic episodes of gout, tophi, uric acid stones, or radiographic changes of gout.

Options for treatment include:

*Xanthine Oxidase Inhibitors: allopurinol and febuxostat*. These drugs reduce the production of uric acid by inhibiting xanthine oxidase. *Allopurinol* dosing is dependent on renal function and should *not* be used in conjunction with azathioprine due to the risk of severe myelotoxicity. This potentially life-threatening adverse drug–drug interaction results from an increase in concentration of 6-mercaptopurine (the active metabolite of azathioprine) which is metabolized by xanthine oxidase [40]. If used concomitantly with allopurinol, azathioprine dosing should be reduced by at least 50% and frequent complete blood counts should be used to monitor the interaction. *Febuxostat* has the same mechanism of action as allopurinol. However, since it is a nonpurine analog, it can be used in patients who have had hypersensitivity reactions to allopurinol [40]. While febuxostat does not require renal dose adjustment, caution is advised when used in the presence of severe renal dysfunction (eGFR < 30 mL/min/1.73 m$^2$) or hepatic disease.

*Uricosuric Agents: probenecid and sulfinpyrazone*. These drugs are not recommended in transplant recipients due to their ineffectiveness in patients with poor renal function (eGFR < 30 mL/min/1.73 m$^2$) and reports of drug–drug interactions with cyclosporine and mycophenolate mofetil. They are also contraindicated in patients with a history of renal calculi and low urine volume < 1500 mL/day.

*Non-steroidal anti-inflammatory drugs (NSAIDs) and cyclooxygenase-2 inhibitors* are effective agents during acute attacks; however, high doses of these agents are required for uricosuric effect. At high doses, these agents can lead to impaired glomerular perfusion, hyperkalemia, and increased sodium retention contributing to hypertension. In conjunction with CNIs, there can be additional escalation in acute kidney injury, hyperkalemia, and hypertension due to vasoconstriction.

*Colchicine* is an effective and rapidly acting anti-inflammatory agent. However, it may be poorly tolerated due to the increased likelihood of diarrhea when used in conjunction with immunosuppressant drugs. Toxic effects on muscle tissue have been reported in patients with decreased renal function <50 mL/min/1.73 m$^2$. Without dose adjustment, kidney transplant recipients are at high risk of experiencing adverse drug effects of colchicine, including myelotoxic effect as well as myopathy in patients receiving a combination of cyclosporine and colchicine [40]. Serum levels of colchicine are increased by several drugs such as clarithromycin, voriconazole, fluconazole, diltiazem, verapamil, ritonavir, and cyclosporine as well as grapefruit juice.

*Corticosteroids* primary anti-inflammatory mechanism of action is the inhibition of nuclear factor xB (NF-xB) via tumor necrosis factor TNF-a (TNF-alpha) or interleukin 1beta (IL-1beta) [40]. Corticosteroids are commonly used in kidney disease and kidney transplant patients for the treatment of acute gout attacks. Issues to consider when using them are exacerbation of hypertension and hyperglycemia, impaired wound healing, and rebound gout attack when tapering down to prior maintenance immunosuppressive dose.

The American College of Rheumatology recommends the use of NSAIDs, colchicine, or corticosteroids for acute gout in patients without significant renal impairment [41]. These agents are to be used cautiously in kidney transplant patients. Acute gout flares respond to increased doses of oral steroids and colchicine.

As a result of overproduction and undersecretion of uric acid, hyperuricemia and gout are common conditions in the kidney transplant population. Important considerations in the implementation of treatment are impaired organ function and the numerous drug interactions. It is reasonable to consider implementing treatment for asymptomatic hyperuricemia with a serum uric acid level > 9 mg/dL. However, the standard prophylactic regimen recommended by the ACR utilizing NSAIDs and colchicine may not be feasible in kidney transplant recipients. The choice of prophylaxis and treatment regimens should be made in consultation with the patient's transplant nephrologist.

## Special Transplant Drug Interactions and Long-Term Adverse Effects

During the first year post-transplant, a typical drug regimen for a recipient consists an average of 8–10 medications. The necessity for polypharmacy increases the potential for serious drug interactions. Interactions affecting drug metabolism are common and typically involve the cytochrome P-450 system. With the increasing number of new agents on the market, it remains challenging for physicians to recognize potential drug interactions without the assistance of pharmacists. Therefore, the information in this section should by no means be considered all inclusive. We recommend the provider consider discussing the addition of any new medication in a transplant recipient with the transplant center (Table 37.2).

A number of drugs interact with immunosuppressants either pharmacodynamically or pharmacokinetically, potentially altering the efficacy and safety of immunosuppressive drugs. Drugs that induce or compete with the cytochrome P450 enzyme system can dramatically increase or decrease the blood concentrations of immunosuppressants. Such alterations place the transplant recipient at risk of under-immunosuppression and rejection or enhanced side effects due to drug toxicity (Table 37.3).

## Reproductive Health and Fertility

Most female patients have a rapid recovery of normal menstrual cycles and fertility after receiving their solid organ transplant, and if transplanted during childhood, most have normal

**Table 37.2** Common maintenance immunosuppressive medications in transplantation

| Class | Agent | Mechanism of action | Adverse side effects |
|---|---|---|---|
| Calcineurin Inhibitors (CNI) | Tacrolimus, cyclosporine | Inhibit calcineurin phosphatase and T-cell activation<br>*Metabolized by cytochrome P450 IIA (CYP3A)* | *Tacrolimus*: Pancreatic islet cell toxicity, neurotoxicity (insomnia, tremor, delirium), alopecia, hyperkalemia, hypomagnesemia<br>*Cyclosporine*: Gingival hyperplasia, hirsutism, tremor, hypertension, hypercholesterolemia, hyperkalemia, hypomagnesemia, hyperuricemia/gout |
| Mammalian target of Rapamycin (mTOR) Inhibitors | Sirolimus, Everolimus | Inhibit IL-2-induced T-cell proliferation<br>*Metabolized by cytochrome P450 IIA (CYP3A)* | Nephrotoxicity when used in combination with CNIs; *de novo* proteinuria, impaired wound healing and dehiscence, hypertriglyceridemia, mucositis, leukoencephalopathy, embryotoxic and fetotoxic |
| Antimetabolites | Mycophenolate mofetil (MMF), Mycophenolic acid (MPA), Azathioprine (AZA) | Prevents proliferation of both T and B cells | *MMF and MPA*: Diarrhea, Leukopenia, Teratogenic (REMS)<br>*AZA*: Myelosuppression, hepatic dysfunction, pancreatitis |
| Co-stimulatory blocker | Belatacept | Modulates T cell activation | Patient must be negative for Epstein–Barr virus (EBV)<br>HTN, edema, alteration in potassium and magnesium<br>Only used in kidney transplant |

References utilized in the construction of table: Danovitch 2010 [42], Lexicomp Online [9], Padiyar 2008 [11], Pedraza 2014 [4], UpToDate 2022

**Table 37.3** Selected medications and their interactions with calcineurin inhibitors and mTOR inhibitors

| Class | Agent | Major interactions | Side effects |
|---|---|---|---|
| Calcineurin inhibitors (CNI) | Tacrolimus, cyclosporine | Drugs that increase blood levels by inhibition of cytochrome P450:<br>• Antibiotics: clarithromycin, erythromycin, azithromycin[a]<br>• Antifungals: ketoconazole, fluconazole, itraconazole, voriconazole<br>• Antiretrovirals: protease inhibitors especially ritonavir<br>• Calcium channel blockers: Verapamil, diltiazem, nicardipine, nifedipine, amlodipine[a]<br>• Histamine blockers: ranitidine, cimetidine<br>• Hormones: Oral contraceptives, anabolic steroids, testosterone analogs, danazol<br>• Others: Amiodarone, allopurinol, bromocriptine, carvedilol, cisapride, conivaptan, HMG-CoA reductase inhibitors, metoclopromide, theophylline<br>• Herbals: grapefruit juice, goldenseal, herbal teas (e.g., chamomile), pomegranate juice, schisandra<br>Drugs that decrease blood levels by induction of cytochrome P450:<br>• Antibiotics: cephalosporins, imipenem<br>• Antituberculosis drugs: rifabutin, rifampin, oxcarbazepine, isoniazid<br>• Anticonvulsants: barbiturates, carbamazepine, phenytoin<br>• Others: bosentan, cholestyramine, cinacalcet, sevelamer, ticlopidine<br>• Herbals: St. John's Wort | Acute Kidney Injury<br>Hypertension<br>Vasoconstriction<br>Thrombotic microangiopathy (TMA)<br>Sodium retention<br>Edema<br>Hyperkalemia<br>Hypomagnesemia<br>Hyperuricemia<br>Hyperlipidemia<br>New-onset diabetes<br>Alopecia<br>Gingival hyperplasia<br>Rhabdomyolysis/Myotoxicity when used in conjunction with HMG-CoA reductase inhibitors |
| Mammalian target of rapamycin (mTOR) Inhibitors | Sirolimus, everolimus | Use of the following are contraindicated:<br>clarithromycin, ketoconazole, mifepristone, rifabutin, rifampin, voriconazole<br>Share the same metabolism by CYP450 system as CNIs; therefore, mTORs have similar interactions with calcium channel blockers, antifungals, anticonvulsants, antituberculosis agents as noted above. | Potentiation of CNI nephrotoxic effects<br>De novo proteinuria/nephrotic syndrome<br>Impaired healing<br>Hypertriglyceridemia<br>Interstitial pneumonia<br>Teratogenic |
| Antimetabolites | Mycophenolate mofetil (MMF), mycophenolic acid (MPA) | Major interactions:<br>• Hematologic/myelosuppressive–azathioprine (hematologic toxicity), hydroxychloroquine, acyclovir, ganciclovir<br>• Increase drug level of MMF and MPA—Amoxicillin<br>• Reduce absorption of MMF and MPA—Antacids, cholestyramine, Sevelamer | Diarrhea<br>Nausea / emesis<br>Leukopenia<br>Progressive multifocal leukoencephalopathy (PML)<br>Congenital malformations |
| | Azathioprine (AZA) | Major interactions:<br>Hematologic/myelosuppressive—allopurinol | Myelosuppression<br>Nausea/emesis<br>Hepatic dysfunction<br>Pancreatitis |

References utilized in the construction of table: Danovitch 2010 [42], Lexicomp Online [9], Padiyar 2008 [11], Pedraza 2014 [4]

Cautions: This table is not a complete list of potential drug interactions. Interaction data refers to systemic drug forms as immunosuppressants. Refer to drug references and transplant pharmacist for assistance on specific agents and for further details on potential interactions

[a]Note: the interaction with these medications is usually minimal

menarche, barring any other substantial growth or pubertal delays. Thus, it is important to engage in pre-conception and contraception counseling options early on in a patient's reproductive life.

## Contraception

When selecting contraceptive methods, it is important to consider the effectiveness of the method, relative contraindications due to the patient's transplant and any other comorbidities such as hypertension, and bleeding or clotting disorders. If pregnancy is not desired, patients should receive comprehensive, patient-centered, and non-judgmental contraceptive counseling, just like patients without transplants. Although some methods are more effective than others, patients are likely to be adherent to a method with which they feel most comfortable. In addition to efficacy of pregnancy prevention, one must consider menstrual profiles that accompany each choice; for example, a copper intrauterine device (IUD) is highly effective in birth control but will likely result in heavier menses, which may be unacceptable to some patients.

When discussing the safety of a contraceptive method, it is often helpful to compare the method to the risks of an unplanned pregnancy. One can refer to the Centers for Disease Control 2016 United States Medical Eligibility Criteria for Contraceptive Use (USMEC), which includes recommendations for solid organ recipients [43–45]. The guidelines were developed in four different categories based on the balance of potential risk of pregnancy and benefits of contraception (Table 37.4).

**Table 37.4** United States medical eligibility criteria for contraceptive use

| | |
|---|---|
| Category 1 | Condition for which there is no restriction for the use of contraceptive method |
| Category 2 | A condition for which the advantage of using the method generally outweighs theoretical or proven risks |
| Category 3 | A condition for which the theoretical or proven risks usually outweighs the advantages of using the method |
| Category 4 | A condition that represents an unacceptable risk if the contraceptive method is used |

Reference utilized in the construction of table as noted in the preceding text: Krajewaki [43], Josephson [44], and Krajewski [45]

For people with uncomplicated transplants, every contraceptive method is a Category 2, indicating the benefits of contraception generally outweigh the risks [45]. A complicated transplant (defined as graft failure, graft rejection, or cardiac allograft vasculopathy) places the patient in the higher risk Category 4. For these people, estrogen-containing contraceptives that increase the risk of coagulation and thromboembolism are effectively contraindicated. IUD initiation is considered a Category 3 (largely based on very little and inconsistent data from case reports) whereas continuation of an IUD is considered Category 2 and can remain safely in place. Estrogen-containing methods remain contraindicated in such conditions as venous thromboembolic disease, hypertension, or diabetic nephropathy. In these conditions progesterone-only containing options are likely the safest choice.

Previous concerns about IUD being contraindicated in transplant patients have been disproven. In addition, concerns about increased risk for infection due to IUD have not been born out with other immunocompromised populations, such as women with human immunodeficiency virus (HIV) infection.

Depot medroxyprogesterone acetate (DMPA) carries a black box warning concerning the bone effects of DMPA with long-term use. When counseling patients with kidney transplant regarding DMPA, the benefits of decreased bleeding and contraceptive efficacy should be balanced with the decrease in BMD (reversible upon discontinuation of DMPA) and individual ramifications of an unplanned pregnancy.

Included in comprehensive contraceptive counseling is the option for emergency contraception. In the United States, FDA-approved options currently include oral levonorgestrel or ulipristal as well as a copper IUD inserted within 5 days after unprotected sex, all of which are considered safe options for patients with solid organ transplants.

Finally, medication interactions must be considered when providing contraceptive counseling for individuals with organ transplants. For example, mycophenolate mofetil may decrease serum progestin levels, so additional methods may need to be employed if pregnancy is not considered safe or desired. Both ethinyl estradiol and some progestins can increase tacrolimus or cyclosporine levels, necessitating more judicious monitoring for possible nephro- or cardiotoxicities, as well as worsening hypertension.

With careful attention to a patient's reproductive and menstrual goals, concurrent medical conditions and medications, clinicians should be able to offer a number of contraceptive options to people with solid organ transplants.

## Pregnancy

The recommended time interval between transplant surgery and conception should be at least 12 months and individualized according to the patient's general health, completion of anti-viral prophylaxis, and establishment of stable immunosuppression level and graft function [44]. Patients should ideally stop teratogenic medications such as mycophenolate or leflunomide before conception if at all possible. Although pregnancies in patients who have received transplants are generally successful, outcomes differ from the general population in terms of prematurity and low birthweight, indicating that these pregnancies remain high risk in spite of good allograft function [46]. For patients with lung or cardiac transplants, the risk of pre-eclampsia was 18%, significantly higher than the 7% in healthy nulliparous women. A number of associated factors such as age, parity, chronic hypertension, or renal disease determines the risk of pregnancy complications, including miscarriage and gestational diabetes, and are probably more important than the type of transplant [46]. Patients should establish high-risk obstetrical care as early as possible in their pregnancy.

## Cancer

Solid organ transplant recipients have a twofold to threefold increased risk of developing cancer compared to the general population [47]. The risk of developing cancer is most likely multifactorial due to the type of organ transplanted, the immunosuppressant regimen, exposure to oncogenic viruses—Epstein–Barr virus (EBV), human papillomavirus (HPV), and human herpesvirus-8 (HHV-8)—and environmental factors. There are three proposed oncogenic mechanisms by which immunosuppression can increase cancer risk: direct pro-oncogenic property of the immunosuppressant, increased risk of oncoviral-driven malignancy, and impaired immune surveillance of neoplastic cells. Cyclosporine, tacrolimus, and azathioprine exert direct effects on cells that promote cancer while mTOR inhibitors and MMF show anti-proliferative effect and decrease cancer risk [47].

Post-transplant cancers can be arbitrarily divided into de novo, donor-related, and recurrent cancers. De novo cancers include non-melanoma skin cancer, post-transplant lymphoproliferative disorder (PTLD), and anogenital cancers, as they are new tumors that develop away from the transplanted organ. Donor-related cancers may be transmitted by the donor organ or may originate within the transplant graft. Recurrent cancers recur from pre-transplant malignancies such as hepatocellular carcinoma or cholangiocarcinoma [47].

Non-melanoma skin cancer is the most common post-transplant malignancy, with an increased incidence up to 250-fold compared to non-transplanted individuals [47]. Squamous cell carcinoma (SCC) is the most common, followed by basal cell, Merkel cell, and Kaposi sarcoma. Post-transplant SCCs are biologically aggressive and often multi-centric with a tendency to recur locally in >10% of patients and leading to metastatic disease in 5% of patients.

PTLD is the second most common malignancy in adults. It is predominantly B cell in origin, accounting for 85–90% of cases, with many of these being associated with EBV. The remaining 10–15% are T cell in origin and are usually EBV negative [47]. The greatest risk is in the first-year post-transplant and is affected by host risk factors such as degree of immunosuppression, viral infections, age of the recipient, and type of allograft. PTLD is highest among individuals receiving intestinal transplants (20%) and lowest for individuals receiving liver/kidney transplants (1–5%).

The relative risk of non-Hodgkin lymphoma (NHL) is elevated eightfold compared to the general population. It can be divided into early disease (a gift from the donor) or late disease, which occurs beyond the second year of transplant. Use of cyclosporine and azathioprine increases risk for NHL. Hodgkin lymphoma is raised fourfold in transplant recipients. Both Hodgkin lymphoma and NHL are more aggressive than in immunocompetent patients [48].

The next most common group of cancers are the anogenital cancers, which make up <3% of cancers but again are 100-fold more common in the immunosuppressed population. They are twice as common in females as male patients and have about a 7-year latency from transplant. HPV-related lesions can arise despite a pretransplant HPV-negative status. HPV-positive renal transplant recipients have 14-fold higher risk for cervical cancer, 50-fold higher risk for vulvar cancer, and 100-fold greater risk for anal carcinoma [47].

Patients with predisposing chronic conditions are at increased risk for developing cancer. Patients with primary sclerosing cholangitis and ulcerative colitis with liver transplants are at an increased risk for cholangiocarcinoma and colon cancer. Patients with renal, liver, and heart transplants are at greater risk of developing renal cell carcinoma, though they are typically small asymptomatic lesions with a favorable surgical prognosis.

Due to the significant increased risk of skin and anogenital cancers, it is recommended that transplant patients have annual skin examinations. Immunosuppressed females should have cervical/pelvic examination at least every 3 years, with close attention to following up detected abnormalities and HPV status [45].

Except for patients with history of ulcerative colitis, there is no change in the recommendations for screening for breast, colon, or prostate cancer in the transplant population. Despite patients with immunosuppression having worse outcomes when cancers are detected, there are no changes to the current cancer screening guidelines. Although early cancer diagnosis may improve cancer outcomes, the reduced life expectancy and multiple comorbidities that exist make cancer screening controversial [49]. Thus, although lung cancer is increased by 1.4- to 5.4-fold in transplant patients compared to the general population, there is currently no change in the selection criteria of patients to screen for lung cancer. Breast, lung, prostate, and colon cancer screening adhere to the same guidelines as for non-immunosuppressed patients.

## Infection

One of the factors that have allowed transplantation to progress has been the advances in approach to infectious disease in the transplant patient [50]. "Prevention of infection whenever possible with prophylactic or preemptive antimicrobial therapy and prompt diagnosis and aggressive treatment of invasion when invasion fails are key pillars." It is useful to segregate the risk for infection based on a timetable in the care of the post-transplant patient. The key periods are divided into **early:** up to the first month post-transplant; **intermediate**: from 1 month to 6 months after transplant; and **late**: greater than 6 months after transplant. Interestingly, during the first month post-transplant, the patient is not at high risk for opportunistic infections but rather those infections stemming from complications of the surgical procedures (wound infection), donor-derived infections (viral reactivation or colonization or contamination), or healthcare-associated infections (urinary tract infections, line or catheter infections, *C. difficile* colitis, and pneumonia). The **intermediate** period is marked by lingering infections secondary to anatomic or technical abnormalities; viral infections, either reactivations or de novo infections (CMV, EBV, human herpesvirus 6, hepatitis B virus, hepatitis C virus, and HIV); and the beginning of opportunistic infections like *Pneumocystis jirovecii* pneumonia and aspergillosis. These infections are made possible by the sustained treatment with immunosuppressive agents and the effects of the co-infecting viruses [50, 51]. Prevention requires disease-specific prophylaxis and recognition and control of CMV and EBV replication and invasion. Herpes simplex, HBV, HCV, human T-lymphocyte virus type II (HTLV-II), and polyomaviruses may also manifest. Opportunistic infections can include *Pneumocystis jirovecii* pneumonia, nocardia, mycobacteria, fungi, and protozoal infections [51].

In the **later** time period, greater than 6 months post-transplant, as immunosuppression is tapered, infections tend to be more typical of those in the community. By this time period, 80% of infections are in those with normal functioning grafts with community-acquired respiratory infections, 10% with recurrence of hepatitis B or C virus, and 10% or less among those with poorly functioning grafts who are at highest risk for opportunistic infection [50]. It is important to remember, however, that transplanted patients may present indolently, without classic symptoms such as high fevers and cell count elevations, but then progress rapidly.

When treating infections in the post-transplant patient, it is often necessary to use empiric therapy. These regimens depend on the clinical syndrome (pneumonia, urinary tract infection, bacteremia), the timing after transplant, and antibiotic-resistance patterns of the local treatment site [50]. One should first ascertain if the patient has a therapeutic emergency with emphasis on immediate clinical assessment and resuscitation of the patient followed by obtaining appropriate cultures and initiating broad-spectrum bactericidal therapy. Once the patient is stable and improving, reassessment and narrowing of regimens can be done [51].

### Vaccinations

It is ideal if the patient can receive the majority of their primary vaccination series pre-transplant, due to decreased efficacy in the immunosuppressed patient. Unfortunately, some patients have not been able to receive all vaccinations due to ill health and uncertainty of the timing of the transplant. Usually, live vaccines are not given within 2–4 weeks of the transplant, with this determination complicated by the uncertainty as to when a patient will actually receive an organ. Vaccination of patients can be resumed post-transplant after 3 months (earlier for influenza, which can be given after 1 month). Typically, the patient will have been tapered off the highest dose of steroids and be reaching a more stable level of immunosuppression by this time. In 2019, The American Society of Transplantation Infectious Diseases Community of Practice (AST IDCOP) published updated guidelines for the vaccination of solid organ transplant candidates and recipients [52]. Per these guidelines, it is not necessary to restart any vaccine series that was already initiated pre-transplant. Further, killed and component vaccines are generally safe to give to the post-transplant patient. These vaccines include: formulations of the diphtheria, tetanus, and acellular pertussis vaccine; *Haemophilus influenza* type B vaccine; HBV vaccine; hepatitis A virus vaccine; inactivated polio vaccine (IPV); pneumococcal vaccines (both the 23-valent pneumococcal polysaccharide vaccine and the 10-, 13-, 15-, and 20-valent pneumococcal conjugate vaccine); meningococcal vaccines (both the meningococcal conjugate vaccines and the serogroup B meningococcal vaccines); and the human papilloma virus (HPV) vaccines.

While vaccines have been shown to be less immunogenic in patients with lowered immune systems, it is not customary to assess for immunity post vaccination for most vaccines with the exception of hepatitis B vaccine, and more recently after the Covid-19 mRNA vaccines. Evidence and recommendations for checking and re-boosting patients for the hepatitis B vaccine come mostly from the hemodialysis literature. Patients found to have waning protective antibody levels to hepatitis B surface antibody benefited from booster vaccination. The need for booster doses for coronavirus vaccination among transplant patients has been demonstrated in one systematic review and meta-analysis [53].

It is important to remember to not give live vaccines to the post-transplant patient. These include measles, mumps, and rubella (whether singly or as the MMR) vaccines, varicella vaccines, the oral polio vaccine (which is no longer routinely given in the United States), the live-attenuated influenza vaccine (given via the nasal route), yellow fever vaccines, or oral typhoid or cholera vaccines. Patient's family members should receive all live-virus vaccines (if they are not already immune) to help protect the transplant patient. It is useful to know the transplant patient's titers to assess what infections they might still be susceptible to and avoid exposure. This is done universally pre-transplant at centers in the United States and can often be obtained from the transplant specialist. If not available, it is reasonable to check these titers to know to what organisms the patient is susceptible and offer immediate post-exposure prophylaxis as indicated. Letters of medical waiver should be given to schools or work as appropriate to avoid receipt of live vaccines.

Recommendations for "travel vaccinations" in the post-solid-organ transplant patient can also be reviewed in the 2019 AST IDCOP guidelines [54]. It is not common to need to decide if your patient should be offered protection prior to traveling outside the United States. Recommendations can be viewed on the cdc.gov/travel website based on the country of travel. It is usually strongly recommended that the patient be up to date on routine adult vaccinations with emphasis on local risk factors listed for each country. These may include hepatitis A virus vaccination, Japanese encephalitis, rabies, and parenteral typhoid and cholera vaccines, if indicated. They should not, however, receive oral typhoid vaccine, oral cholera vaccines, oral polio, or yellow fever vaccine, as previously noted. Under no circumstances should a patient receive the Bacilli Calmette-Guérin (BCG) vaccine. In some circumstances, administration of immune globulin may be administered for short-term protection of non-immune transplant patients at high risk of exposure to measles, hepatitis A, and even varicella [54]. Letters of medical waiver should be given to the patient in lieu of contraindicated vaccines. The need for malaria prophylaxis should be reviewed and offered while also carefully assessing for possible interactions with the patient's transplant regimen. Advice regarding measures to avoid contaminated food, water, and mosquito/tick/vector-borne diseases should be emphasized. In addition, it is important to give your patient a summary letter of their medical condition and a list of medications. It is, unfortunately, not common for travelers to lose their medication abroad, and this can sometimes necessitate their emergent replacement.

## Conclusion

Solid organ transplant recipients represent a growing population of medically complex patients for whom outcomes are optimized through a well-coordinated plan of care delivered by a multidisciplinary team ("Appendix"). Though much of this care is directed by transplant subspecialists, PCPs have several critical roles to fulfill. PCPs should be familiar with the diagnosis and treatment goals of common comorbid conditions associated with solid organ transplant as well as commonly used immunosuppressive agents and their associated toxicities and drug–drug interactions. PCPs should also address the sexual and reproductive health of patients and be familiar with cancer screening guidelines for transplant patients. Finally, PCPs should help support young adults with solid organ transplants navigate challenges while transitioning to adult-centered care systems.

## Appendix

| Solid organ transplant fact sheet | |
|---|---|
| Definition | The replacement of a nonfunctioning solid organ such as kidney, liver, or heart with an organ obtained by donation from another individual. It can be either cadaveric or living donor. The individual must remain on immunosuppressant regimen in order to avoid rejecting the organ |
| Epidemiology | The number of pediatric patients living with a kidney transplant has more than doubled since 1988 with 7082 children transplanted in 2017. The first-year deceased- and living-donor transplant outcomes have steadily improved over the last 20 years |

| Solid organ transplant fact sheet | |
|---|---|
| Pathophysiology | The type of solid organ, and whether it is a first or second transplant, often predicates the intensity of the immunosuppressant regimen used<br>The immunosuppressants are from several classes:<br>Calcineurin inhibitors (tacrolimus, cyclosporine)<br>mTOR inhibitors (Sirolimus, Everolimus)<br>Corticosteroids (prednisone)<br>Anti-metabolite (mycophenolic acid, mycophenolate, and azathioprine)<br>Costimulatory blocker (Belatacept)—kidney transplantation only |
| Sequelae of original disease | Poor growth<br>Metabolic bone disease<br>Association with syndromes affecting other organ systems:<br>Alagille syndrome<br>Alport syndrome<br>May have some degree of developmental delay associated with underlying disease or complicated treatment course<br>Recurrence of original disease (systemic lupus erythematosus) |
| Sequelae of immunosuppressant regimen | Infection<br>Increase risk of metabolic disorders:<br>Diabetes<br>Hyperlipidemia<br>Gout<br>Osteoporosis<br>Hypertension<br>Increased risk for cardiovascular disease<br>Increased risk for kidney dysfunction<br>Increased risk for cytopenias<br>Increased for malignancies:<br>Dermatologic<br>Aero-digestive<br>Vulvar<br>Post-transplant lymphoproliferative disorder |
| Medication interaction | Must always adjust for decreased function of the transplanted organ<br>Always evaluate interaction with immunosuppressant regimen |
| Challenges in transition | Some centers have reported increased risk of graft rejection and loss when transitioning from pediatric to adult providers<br>Adult providers are less familiar with some of the underlying pediatric syndromes |
| Helpful Resources | CDC contraception 2010 application (app) download for smartphones |

*CDC* Centers for disease control

## References


1. US Renal Data System (USRDS). 2021 USRDS Annual Report: Atlas of Chronic Kidney Disease and End Stage Renal Disease in the United States. Bethesda, MD: National Institutes of Health, National Institute of Diabetes and Digestive and Kidney Diseases; 2021.
2. Hart A, Lentine KL, Smith JM, Miller JM, Skeans MA, Prentice M, et al. OPTN/SRTR 2019 annual data report: kidney. Am J Transplant. 2021;21(S2):21–137.
3. Tantisanttomao E, Molnar MZ, Ho BT, et al. Approach and management of hypertension after kidney transplantation. Front Med (Lausanne). 2020;7:229. Published 2020 June
4. Pedraza F, Roth D. Medical management of the kidney transplant recipient. Prim Care Clin Office Pract. 2014;41(4):895–906.
5. Kidney Disease Outcomes Quality Initiative. K/DOQI clinical practice guidelines on hypertension and antihypertensive agents in chronic kidney disease. Am J Kidney Dis. 2021;43:S1–S290.
6. Lakkis J, Weir MR. Treatment-resistant hypertension in the transplant recipient. Semin Nephrol. 2014;34(5):5360.70.
7. Wadei HM, Textor SC. Hypertension in the kidney transplant recipient. Transplant Rev. 2010;24:105–20.
8. Kidney Disease: Improving Global Outcomes (KDIGO) Transplant Work Group. KDIGO Clinical Practice Guideline for the care of kidney transplant recipients. Am J Transplant. 2009;9(Suppl. 3):S1–S157.
9. Lexicomp Online®. Lexicomp online database. Hudson, OH: Lexi-Comp, Inc. Wolters Kluwer; 2022.

10. Davidson J, Wilkinson A, Dantal J, Dotta F, Haller H, Hernandez D, Kasiske B, et al. International Expert Panel. New-onset diabetes after transplantation: 2003 international consensus guidelines. Proceedings of an international expert panel meeting Barcelona, Spain, 19 February 2003. Transplantation. 2003;75(Suppl. 10):SS3–SS24.
11. Padiyar A, Akoum FH, Hricik DE. Management of the kidney transplant recipient. Prim Care Clin Office Pract. 2008;35(3):433–50.
12. Schaefer HM. Long-term management of the kidney transplant recipient. Blood Purif. 2012;33:205–11.
13. Soleimanpour SA, Crutchlow MF, Ferrari AM, Raum JC, Groff DN, Rankin MM, et al. Calcineurin signaling regulates human islet (beta)-cell survival. J Biol Chem. 2010;285:40050–9.
14. Ajabnoor MA, El-Naggar MM, Elayat AA, Abdulrafee A. Functional and morphological study of cultured pancreatic islets treated with cyclosporine. Life Sci. 2007;80:345–55.
15. Flechner SM, Glyda M, Cockfield S, Grinyó J, Legendre C, Russ G, et al. The ORION study: comparison of two sirolimus-based regimens versus tacrolimus and mycophenolate mofetil in renal allograft recipients. Am J Transplant. 2011;11:1633–44.
16. Galindo RJ, Fried M, Breen T, Tamler R. Hyperglycemia management in patients with post-transplantation diabetes. Endocr Pract. 2016;22(4):454–65.
17. Barlow AD, Nicholson ML, Herbert TP. Evidence for rapamycin toxicity in pancreatic β-cells and a review of the underlying mechanisms. Diabetes. 2013;62:2674–82.
18. Lipska KJ, Bailey CJ, Inzucchi SE. Use of metformin in the setting of mild-to-moderate renal insufficiency. Diabetes Care. 2011;34(6):1431–7.
19. Ghisdal L, Van Laecke S, Abramowicz MJ, VanHolder R, Abramowicz D. New-onset diabetes after renal transplantation: risk assessment and management. Diabetes Care. 2012;35(1):181–8.
20. Vanrenterghem YF, Claes K, Montagnino G, Fieuws S, Maes B, Villa M, et al. Risk factors for cardiovascular events after successful renal transplantation. Transplantation. 2008;85:209–16.
21. Kasiske B, Cosio FG, Beto J, Bolton BM, Chavers R, Grimm R, Levin A, et al. Clinical practice guidelines for managing dyslipidemias in kidney transplant patients: a report from the managing dyslipidemias in chronic kidney disease work group of the national kidney foundation kidney disease outcomes quality initiative. Am J Transplant. 2004;4(Suppl. 7):13–53.
22. Warden B, Duell B. Management of dyslipidemias in adult solid organ transplant recipients. J Clin Lipidol. 2019;13(2):231–45.
23. Navaneethan SD, Perkovic V, Johnson DW, Nigwekar SU, Craig JC, Strippoli GF. HMG CoA reductase inhibitors (statins) for kidney transplant recipients. Cochrane Database Syst Rev. 2009;2:CD005019.
24. Holdaas H, Fellstrom B, Jardine AG, Holme I, Nyberg G, Fauchald P, Gonhagen-Riska C, et al. Effect of fluvastatin on cardiac outcomes in renal transplant recipients: a multicenter, randomized, placebo-controlled trial. Lancet. 2003;361(9374):2024–31.
25. Ebeling PR. Approach to the patient with transplantation-related bone loss. J Clin Endocrinol Metab. 2009;94:1483–90.
26. Ebeling PR. Transplantation osteoporosis. Curr Osteoporos Rep. 2007;5:29–37.
27. Nisbeth U, Lindh E, Ljunghall S, Backman U, Fellstrom B. Increased fracture rate in diabetes mellitus and females after renal transplantation. Transplantation. 1999;67(9):1218–22.
28. Abbott KC, Ogelsby RJ, Hypolite IO, Kirk AD, Ko CW, Welch PG, et al. Hospitalizations for fractures after renal transplantation in the United States. Ann Epidemiol. 2001;11(7):450–7.
29. Nikkel LE, Hollenbeak CS, Fox EJ, Uemura T, Ghahramani N. Risk of fractures after renal transplantation in the United States. Transplantation. 2009;87(12):1846–51.
30. Canalis E, Mazziotti G, Giustina A, Bilezikian JP. Glucocorticoid-induced osteoporosis: pathophysiology and therapy. Osteoporos Int. 2007;18(10):1319–28.
31. Kuroki Y, Kaji H, Kawano S, Kanda F, Takai Y, Kajiwaka M, et al. Short-term effects of glucocorticoid therapy on biochemical markers of bone metabolism in Japanese patients: a prospective study. J Bone Miner Metab. 2008;26(3):271–8.
32. Guistani A, Mazziotti G, Canalis E. Growth hormone, insulin-like growth factors, and the skeleton. Endocr Rev. 2008;29(5):535–9.
33. Mazziotti G, Giustina A. Glucocorticoids and the regulation of growth hormone secretion. Nat Rev Endocrinol. 2013;9(15):265–76.
34. Epstein S. Post-transplantation bone disease: the role of immunosuppressive agents and the skeleton. J Bone Miner Res. 1996;11(1):1–7.
35. Nikkel LE, Mohan S, Zhang A, McMahon DJ, Boutroy S, Dube G, et al. Reduced fracture risk with early corticosteroid withdrawal after kidney transplant. Am J Transplant. 2012;12:649–59.
36. Bergua C, Torregrosa JV, Fuster D, Gutierrez-Dalmau A, Oppenheimer F, Campistol JM. Effect of cinacalcet on hypercalcemia and bone mineral density in renal transplanted patients with secondary hyperparathyroidism. Transplantation. 2008;86:413–7.
37. Josephson MA, Schumm LP, Chiu MY, Marshall C, Thistlethwaite JR, Sprague SM. Calcium and calcitriol prophylaxis attenuates post transplant bone loss. Transplantation. 2004;78:1233–6.
38. McKee, et al. Comparison of the clinical effectiveness and safety between the use of denosumab vs. Bisphosphonates in renal transplant patients. Osteoporosis Int. 2020;31(5):973–80.
39. Affi MK, Kenawy AS, Demellawy HH, Azouz AA, Al-Otaibi T, Gheith O, Elmonem MA, AbdElhalim MS, Hussein RRS. Optimization of osteoporosis and osteopenia management among renal transplant

recipients. Future J Pharm Sci. 2021;7:230. https://doi.org/10.1186/s43094-021-00378-1.
40. Sullivan PM, William A, Tichy EM. Hyperuricemia and gout in solid-organ transplant: update in pharmacological management. Prog Transplant. 2015;25(3):263–70.
41. Khanna D, Fitzgerald JD, Khanna PP, Bae S, Singh MK, Neogi T, Pillinger MH, et al. 2012 American College of Rheumatology guidelines for the management of gout. Arthritis Care Res. 2012;64(10):1431–61.
42. Danovitch GM. Handbook of kidney transplantation. 5th ed. Philadelphia: Lippincott Williams & Wilkins; 2010.
43. Krajewski CM, Geetha D, Gomez-Lobo V. Contraceptive options for women with a history of solid-organ transplantation. Transplantation. 2013;95(10):1183–6.
44. Josephson MA, McKay DB. Women and Transplantation: fertility, sexuality, pregnancy, contraception. Adv Chronic Kidney Dis. 2013;20(5):433–40.
45. Krajewski C, Sucato G. Reproductive health care after transplantation. Best Pract Res Clin Obstet Gynaecol. 2014;28:1222–34.
46. Brosens I, Brosens J, Benagiano G. The risk of obstetrical syndromes and solid organ transplantation. Best Pract Res Clin Obstet Gynaecol. 2014;28:1211–21.
47. Katabathina V, Menias CO, Pickhardt P, Lubner M, Prasad S. Complications of immunosuppressive therapy in solid organ transplantation. Radiol Clin North Am. 2016;54:303–19.
48. Grulich AE, Vajdic CM. The epidemiology of cancers in human immunodeficiency virus infection and after organ transplantation. Semin Oncol. 2015;42(2):247–57.
49. Acuna SA, et al. Cancer screening recommendations for solid organ transplant recipients: a systematic review of clinical practice guidelines. Am J Transplant. 2017;17(1):103–4.
50. Marty FM, Rubin RH. The prevention of infection post transplant: the role of prophylaxis, preemptive and empiric therapy. Transpl Int. 2006;19(1):2–11.
51. Zhong D, Liang S. Approach to transplant infectious diseases in the emergency department. Emer Med Clin NA. 2018;36(4):811–22.
52. Danziger-Isakov L, Kumar D. Vaccination of solid organ transplant candidates and recipients: Guidelines from the American Society of Transplantation infectious Disease community of practice. Clin Transpl. 2019;33(9):e13563. 1–10
53. Manothummetha K, Chuleerux N, Sanguankeo A, Kates OS, Hirankarn N, Thongkam A, et al. Immunogenicity and risk factors associated with poor humoral response of SARS-CoV-2 vaccines in recipients of solid organ transplant: a systematic review and meta-analysis. JAMA Netw Open. 2022;5(4):e226822.
54. Buchan CA, Kotton CN. Travel medicine, transplant tourism and the solid organ transplant recipient—Guidelines from the American Society of Transplantation Infectious Diseases community of practice. Clin Transpl. 2019;33(9):e13529. p. 1–16

# 38 Spina Bifida

Ellen Fremion, Natalia Hernandez, Rose Khavari, Julie Stewart, and Jonathan Tolentino

## Case Presentation

Roxanne is a 19-year-old Latinx female with mid-lumbar spina bifida (SB), a ventriculoperitoneal (VP) shunt placed at birth without revision, and neurogenic bowel and bladder who presents to establish primary adult care. She uses a manual wheelchair in the community and crawls at home. She was previously cared for by a pediatric SB multi-subspecialty clinic and general pediatrician. For neurogenic bladder care, her mother performs clean intermittent catheterization (CIC) through the urethra. Roxanne lacks dexterity to catheterize independently. Despite CIC every 4 h, she has urinary incontinence. She was hospitalized for a urinary tract infection (UTI), elevated blood pressure, and acute kidney injury (AKI) 6 months prior. Her bowel regimen is to have timed bowel movements on the toilet every 2–3 days. Her stools are hard, and she has fecal incontinence 1–2 times per week. Roxanne graduated from high school but is not attending college nor working. During high school, her grades were borderline passing, and she had particular difficulty with math and reading comprehension. She has undergone adult disability determination and receives supplemental social security income and Medicaid. She dresses and bathes independently, but she needs help with cooking, household chores, money management, and transportation. She is often anxious and worries about discrimination in future job environments because she has difficulty with her bowel and bladder continence. She has never dated or been sexually active, but she would like to be married, have children, and live independently.

E. Fremion (✉)
Department of Medicine, Baylor College of Medicine, Houston, TX, USA
e-mail: ellen.fremion@bcm.edu

N. Hernandez · R. Khavari · J. Stewart
Department of Urology, Houston Methodist Hospital, Houston, TX, USA
e-mail: nhernandez2@houstonmethodist.org; rkhavari@houstonmethodist.org; jnstewart2@houstonmethodist.org

J. Tolentino
Departments of Medicine and Pediatrics, University of Miami Miller School of Medicine, Miami, FL, USA
e-mail: jxt1084@med.miami.edu

**Box 38.1 Patient Laboratory and Imaging Studies upon Establishment of Care**

**Serum chemistry**

Sodium: 138 mEq/L, potassium: 5.0 mEq/L, chloride: 110 mEq/L, bicarbonate: 18 mEq/L, blood urea nitrogen: 13 mg/dL, creatinine: 0.9 mg/dL (previous baseline of 0.5 mg/dL a year ago)


A. A. Kuo et al. (eds.), *Care of Adults with Chronic Childhood Conditions*,
https://doi.org/10.1007/978-3-031-54281-7_38

**Ultrasound of kidneys, ureters, and bladder**

Left kidney length of 7.8 cm, with decreased echogenicity and hydronephrosis; right kidney length of 9.8 cm with normal echogenicity; bladder was small sized with a thickened wall; debris and a possible stone were seen in the bladder.

**Video urodynamics**

Small bladder capacity 100 mL (typical adult capacity is 400–500 mL), detrusor overactivity, high bladder pressures >40 cm $H_2O$, stress urinary incontinence, and severe vesicoureteral reflux to the left kidney

## Case Discussion

Roxanne's elevated blood pressure and recent AKI are concerning. Individuals with SB have a higher prevalence of prehypertension and hypertension than the general population due to renal scarring, obstructive uropathy, and obesity [1–3]. Thus, patients with SB presenting with hypertension should have: (1) review of their bladder management including medications and catheterization regimens; (2) serum chemistry and renal function labs; (3) an ultrasound of the kidneys, ureters, and bladder to evaluate the renal size as well as monitor for hydronephrosis and nephrolithiasis; and (4) a urology evaluation including urodynamics to measure bladder pressure and evaluate for vesicoureteral reflux.

Upon review of Roxanne's labs (see Box 38.1), she has a high-normal serum potassium level and an elevation in her serum creatinine from baseline. These lab findings along with the finding of hydronephrosis and decreased size of the left kidney are concerning for acute-on-chronic obstructive uropathy leading to renal damage. Because urodynamics showed small bladder capacity, high-pressure bladder, and severe vesicoureteral reflux, she is considered high risk per the American Urologic Association (AUA)/Society of Urodynamics, Female Pelvic Medicine & Urogenital Reconstruction (SUFU) 2021 Neurogenic Lower Urinary Tract Dysfunction Guidelines [4]. Therefore, reconstructive surgery such as bladder augmentation may be indicated (see section "Bladder and Pelvic Floor Concerns" below). Given her difficulty with self-catheterization due to dexterity and mobility impairment, a catheterizable abdominal channel for bladder management and Malone antegrade colonic enema (MACE) procedure would be options to consider increasing her independence and urinary continence.

Depression and anxiety are common in adults with SB, with an incidence > 40 % for both [5, 6]. Studies have found that urinary tract dysfunction and family support correlate with these mental health concerns [5, 6]. Roxanne felt nervous around new people because she had often been bullied at school about her physical impairments and incontinence. Roxanne should be referred to counseling and occupational therapy to help her gain confidence and independent living skills. Once Roxanne's acute medical needs are addressed and she is better able to manage her bowel and bladder regimens, referral to vocational rehabilitation to assess her vocational abilities and help with job placement would be beneficial. This referral would enable her to learn about her rights in the workplace as a person with a disability afforded to her by the Americans with Disabilities Act, including her right to have wheelchair-accessible facilities and the necessary modifications to perform her self-care at work. She would have the opportunity to practice how to communicate her needs with her employer and coworkers with a family and vocational coach. (For additional information regarding disability rights, please see Chap. 13 in section "Disability Policy: Shaping the Neurodiversity Landscape".)

The most common diagnoses requiring admission among adults with SB are urinary tract infections (UTIs), complications of devices, grafts, and implants, skin ulcers, and osteomyelitis [7]. Given her history of UTIs and kidney disease, Roxanne is at risk for urosepsis. While shunt revisions are less common in adults than in children, shunt malfunctions can still occur [8].

Thus, a computed tomography (CT) scan of the head and shunt series should be done if a patient exhibits symptoms of increased intracranial pressure, new onset seizures, and/or altered mental status to evaluate for shunt obstruction. If she were to have a peritoneal infection or require abdominal surgery, neurosurgery should be available to evaluate for any shunt complications. Finally, due to scoliosis (particularly common among those with thoracic SB), body habitus, midbrain elongation, and the presence of Chiari II malformation, individuals with SB have an increased risk for central and obstructive sleep apnea, restrictive lung disease, and possibly sudden death [9–11]. Thus, pulmonary function evaluation and/or sleep study should be considered preoperatively, and those with significant obstructive/restrictive lung disease should be monitored closely for respiratory failure in the setting of sepsis.

## Overview

SB is the most common neural tube defect (NTD) and is due to failure of the spinal neural tube to close at 25–28 days post-conception [12]. An estimated 1500–2000 babies with SB are born in the United States annually with the highest incidence in the Latinx population [13]. The disproportionate burden on self-identified Latinx patients is likely due to structural factors such as less formal education, public health campaigns not targeted to certain populations, and subsequent decreased rates folic acid supplementation [14]. Approximately 166,000 people in the United States have SB, with the majority being adults [15]. There are three SB types: (1) *occulta*, in which there is a cleft in the vertebral bodies with closed skin; (2) *meningocele*, where the meninges protrude through the vertebral cleft with no neural elements; and (3) *myelomeningocele* (MMC), in which the spinal cord and neural elements are exposed through the vertebral cleft. Spina bifida occulta requires no repair and rarely has associated neuromuscular deficits. Meningoceles often can be repaired without neurologic complications. MMCs are the most common lesion and most often referred to as "spina bifida" [15]. MMCs are repaired a few days after birth, though increasingly some pediatric centers also offer prenatal repairs. Depending on pre- or post-natal repair, approximately 40–80% of infants with MMC have hydrocephalus and require a ventricular shunt placement [16, 17]. The majority of individuals with SB have gait impairment and bladder and bowel dysfunction [18] While most individuals with MMC do not have an intellectual disability, many have weakness in processing skills and executive functioning compared to verbal skills [19, 20]. The degree of impairment usually correlates with MMC spinal level and especially with the presence of hydrocephalus [21]. Other spinal dysraphisms with similar sequelae that are often followed by SB-specialists include: caudal regression/sacral agenesis, lipomyelomeningoceles, lipomyeloceles, and congenital tethered cord. SB is classified by functional level using the Hoffer Scale: *thoracic* (flaccid lower extremities), *high-lumbar* (hip flexion present), *mid-lumbar* (knee extension present), *low-lumbar* (dorsiflexion present), and *sacral* (foot plantar flexion present) [22]. The level of function guides expectations for neurocognitive, motor, and organ system comorbidities. About 75% to 94% of people with SB survive to adulthood [8]. Common causes of death for adults with SB include sepsis, renal failure, cardiopulmonary failure, and shunt complications [7, 23].

## Etiology

The etiology of SB as with all NTDs is multifactorial, having both genetic and environmental components. Defects in genes regulating neuropore closing, the folic acid metabolic pathway, nucleotide synthesis, and deoxyribonucleic acid (DNA) repair are thought to be responsible for NTDs, but the exact mechanism is not known. Prenatal screening for methylenetetrahydrofolate reductase (MTHFR*)* mutations has become more widely available and utilized, as mothers who are homozygous for the C677T allele coding for *MTHFR*, an enzyme regulating the intracellular folate, have a twofold increased risk for having a child born with SB [24]. Additional risk factors for having a baby with SB include maternal hyperthermia, environmental exposure (e.g., pesticides, contaminated water, hazardous waste), nutritional factors (e.g., folic acid deficiency, maternal obesity, and high intake of high-glucose foods), lower socioeconomic status, and fetal exposure to folic acid antagonists (e.g., valproic acid, carbamazepine, and methotrexate) [25]. Women who are at high risk for NTDs (those who themselves have a NTD, have had a child with a NTD, or have a family history of NTD) are recommended to take at least 4 mg of folic acid daily beginning 2–3 months prior to conception, throughout pregnancy, and for 4–6 weeks postpartum or while breastfeeding [26].

## Transition from Pediatric to Adult Care for SB

A multi-subspecialty clinic associated with an urban academic hospital is the most common model of care for pediatric patients with SB, but adult clinics that specialize in SB care are rare [27]. Research regarding best practices for adults with SB is limited. Young adults with SB need: (1) adult providers who are welcoming and familiar with the management of their condition; (2) care coordination to ensure insurance coverage, subspecialty care, supplies, and equipment; (3) support for self-management and community engagement (education, employment, transportation, independent living, and day activities); (4) general adult health care; and (5) chronic SB management [28]. To facilitate these care needs, patients may require the following adult providers: neurosurgery (to establish care and address acute concerns), pulmonology (for sleep apnea or restrictive lung disease evaluation), urology (preferably a neuro-urologist for neurogenic bladder management,), physical medicine and rehabilitation/physiatry (for equipment selection, spasticity, pain, and mobility management), orthopedics (as needed for scoliosis and limb deformity), obstetrics and gynecology (for pelvic floor health and well-woman care), and social work (for community, funding, and vocational resources). Other care needs include equipment (e.g., wheelchairs, orthotics, crutches, lifts, and shower chairs) and supplies (e.g., catheters, bowel management equipment, and protective undergarments).

## Office Visit Considerations

Given the various degrees of ambulation among people with SB, it is important to standardize height, weight, and body mass index (BMI) measurement. For those patients who are ambulatory, height should be measured with a standiometer with shoes/braces off. For non-ambulatory individuals, arm length should be measured using a meter/yard stick from middle fingertip to opposite middle fingertip across the laryngeal prominence (Adam's apple) [29]. An estimate of patient height can then be made using arm span-to-height ratio formulas, multiplying by 0.95 for individuals with mid-lumbar SB and 0.90 for those with high-lumbar/thoracic SB. If the patient is able to stand unsupported, weight should be measured without orthotics on a regular scale. For those who are wheelchair-dependent, the patient should be weighed in the wheelchair on a wheelchair-accessible scale and then have the measured wheelchair weight subtracted [29]. As many people with SB are allergic to latex, latex-free exam gloves should be used. A large exam room and an exam table that can lower to the ground are helpful for patients who use wheelchairs. Extra pillows for the exam table can help make positioning more comfortable, especially if severe scoliosis is present. Patients should be asked for both permission and guidance before they are assisted during a visit with any needs pertaining to wheelchair or exam table positioning, transfers, and clothing adjustments that will facilitate the examination.

## Specific Care Considerations for Adults with SB by Organ System

Adults with SB should have general adult screenings for: (1) reproductive function and sexually transmitted infections; (2) metabolic syndrome (including hypertension, elevated blood sugar, obesity, and abnormal serum cholesterol); (3) mental health; and (4) cancer based on age and risk factors [30]. In addition to these general health needs, patients with SB have condition-specific care needs as will be reviewed in this section.

## Neurocognitive Concerns

While there is a spectrum of cognitive abilities for individuals with SB, most individuals do not have intellectual disability (IQ < 70) and the neurocognitive profile of individuals with MMC has some unique features [21, 31]. Individuals with MMC tend to have stronger verbal skills than processing skills and difficulty with executive function (i.e., comprehension, computation, problem solving, and planning) [19, 20]. While individuals with MMC may have difficulty with planning and initiating new tasks, they have relative strengths in carrying out routines once established. School concerns may include reading comprehension and math learning disabilities [32]. Higher MMC lesions and hydrocephalus are associated with more anomalous brain development and thus more cognitive deficit [21, 33]. Knowing the neurocognitive tendencies for people with SB can help providers develop strategies for patient self-management and care plans. It is important to remember that language fluency may mask deficits in comprehension, thus checking for understanding is helpful. Simple written instructions, phone alarm reminders, follow-up calls, patient teaching by nursing and/or home health providers, and frequent follow-up appointments can facilitate engagement in care and plan implementation. Intellectual ability, adaptive function, and executive function testing can help direct decision-making, educational, employment, and independent living choices [32, 34]. However, adult insurances may not cover neurocognitive testing, but vocational rehabilitation programs may be able to provide testing or results of previous testing may be obtained from high school records. If available in their state, supported decision-making may be a good option for individuals who need some assistance with decisions [35].

## Neurological Concerns

Unique neurological co-morbidities for SB include ventricular shunts, tethered cord, Chiari II malformations (CM II), and syringomyelia/hydromyelia [36].

### Ventricular Shunts

Ventriculoperitoneal shunts drain cerebral spinal fluid (CSF) into the peritoneal cavity. Shunts may also be placed as ventriculopleural or ventriculoatrial (right atrium) shunts if there are contraindications for placing the tubing in the peritoneal space. Programmable shunts may be used to control the flow of CSF. If patients have a programmable shunt, then neurosurgery should be consulted to manage the shunt before and after magnetic resonance imaging (MRI) is performed as changes in shunt settings for some shunt types may result from the magnet in the MRI scanner. Shunt revisions are more common during childhood, but shunt malfunctions can occur in adulthood and may result in catastrophic complications if not emergently managed [37]. Symptoms of shunt malfunction include severe headache, fever, vomiting, visual changes, lethargy, and new onset seizures. More subtle findings include decreased concentration, decreased work or school performance, and changes in lower extremity or urologic function. If there is a concern for shunt malfunction, an emergent head CT scan without contrast and shunt series x-ray should be performed. If dilated ventricles are found, immediate neurosurgery evaluation is required. Some individuals with shunt malfunctions may have no change in ventricular size. If symptoms are not otherwise explained, a neurosurgeon familiar with shunt management should be consulted. Neurosurgery should also be consulted if an individual with a ventriculoperitoneal shunt has abdominal surgery complications or peritoneal infection.

### Tethered Cord

Clinically significant cord tethering is less common in adulthood but can occur. Tethered cord is due to scar tissue or lipomeningocele causing tension on the spinal cord, usually at the level of the SB repair. Triggers for tethered cord include trauma, heavy lifting, and vaginal childbirth. Signs of tethered cord include severe back pain, worsening lower extremity weakness and/or decreased sensation, worsening neurogenic bladder symptoms with resultant urodynamic changes, and rapidly progressive scoliosis or foot deformity. If these clinical findings are present, an MRI spine (with and without contrast) should be ordered and neurosurgery consulted. After untethering, pain symptoms often improve (seen in >75%) [38]. While usually there is motor function stabilization (80–90%), there is variable improvement in motor function (25–80%) postoperatively [38]. Also, surgical complications can occur, including CSF leak, infection, worsening bowel/bladder or neurological function, and decreased mobility [39]. If tethered cord is seen on imaging but the patient is asymptomatic, watchful monitoring may be an acceptable approach, but neurosurgical evaluation is recommended.

### Chiari II Malformation

CM II is the downward displacement of cerebellar and brainstem structures into the foramen magnum. Varying degrees of CM II are almost universally present in patients with MMC, but many may be asymptomatic [36]. CM II compression symptoms include occipital headache, neck pain, diplopia, nystagmus, dysphagia/aspiration, dysphonia, stridor, apnea, upper-limb paresis and hypertonia, loss of dexterity, and gait instability. The onset can be a rapid deterioration over a few days or an insidious decline. Patients can have recurrent symptoms after cervical decompression due to abnormal hindbrain brain development. Other diagnoses can present with CM II symptoms such as shunt malfunction, hydromyelia, syringomyelia, and tethered cord. MRI is the best study to evaluate CM II, but if MRI is not possible, high-resolution CT scan with sagittal reconstructions can be used.

### Syringomyelia and Hydromyelia

Syringomyelia (cystic cavitation in the spinal cord parenchyma) and hydromyelia (enlargement of the central spinal canal) occur in 25–45% of patients with SB, and of these, 60% may be symptomatic [40]. Syringomyelia/hydromyelia symptoms are similar to tethered cord and can coexist with tethered cord. Syringobulbia is a cavity in the cervicomedullary junction and can present with symptoms similar to CM II. If clinical suspicion exists, it is recommended to obtain a MRI of the spine for evaluation and correlate imaging with clinical findings. Symptomatic patients should be referred promptly for neurosurgery consultation.

## Ophthalmologic Concerns

Eye findings associated with SB include strabismus, nystagmus, and optic atrophy [41]. These abnormalities are predominately seen in individuals with hydrocephalus, higher MMC lesions, and multiple shunt revisions. Annual dilated eye exams and assessment of strabismus are recommended [30]. New onset strabismus or nystagmus are concerning for shunt malfunction with resultant hydrocephalus or CM II compression. In these instances, imaging of the brain should be performed.

## Cardiopulmonary Concerns

Congenital heart defects are not associated with SB, but many adults have risk factors for cardiovascular disease including hypertension, obesity, and metabolic syndrome. Prehypertension and hypertension are associated with diabetes, previous bladder procedures, and renal dysfunction [1]. General adult guidelines for screening and management of CVD risk factors should be followed [30].

Pulmonary complications associated with SB are likely under described [11]. Decreased pulmonary function and respiratory muscle weakness are associated with higher lesions and more severe scoliosis. Even with reduced vital capacity, many individuals may be functionally asymptomatic [10]. Individuals with SB are at risk for central or obstructive sleep apnea as well as central hypoventilation syndrome due to CM II, diminished respiratory muscle function, kyphoscoliosis, and obesity [9, 42]. Sleep-disordered breathing (SDB) symptoms such as breathing difficulties and apnea may be more common than snoring or daytime sleepiness. Positive-pressure therapy can improve central and obstructive apnea and hypopnea. Patients with significant central apnea may warrant CM II decompression. Patients with SB are more likely to have respiratory complications, pneumonia, respiratory insufficiency, prolonged mechanical ventilation, and pulmonary embolism post-operatively [7, 43]. Thus, preoperative screeningd for SDB and restrictive lung symptoms is recommended. Consider ordering sleep studies and pulmonary function tests for patients with severe CM II, thoracic SB, severe kyphoscoliosis, or general population risk factors, especially preoperatively. Caution should be taken with sleep aids, benzodiazepines, and pain medications that may suppress respiratory function.

## Gastrointestinal Concerns

Neurogenic bowel concerns include: (1) constipation due to impaired peristalsis and infrequent voiding, (2) difficulty evacuating stool due to impaired rectal reflex, and (3) incontinence due to impaired anal sphincter tone and voluntary control. Fecal incontinence is a major barrier to quality of life and socialization [44]. With regimen compliance, 70–90% of patients have bowel accidents less than once per month, (see Table 38.1) [45, 46]. Most bowel regimens start with oral laxatives, fiber (goal of 25–30 g per day), and/or a rectal-stimulating agent with timed toileting [47]. Secondly, retrograde colonic enema (RCE) using a cone enema or anal irrigation system (Peristeen®) may be used. A cone enema is a plastic cone tip attached with tubing to a bag of fluid with approximately 20 mL/kg of water or saline (maximum amount is 600 mL) [48]. The cone is held in the rectum while the fluid fills the colon. The cone is then removed, allowing the patient to evacuate into the toilet. Patients with thoracic or high-lumbar lesions may have difficulty holding the cone in place and balancing on the toilet. An anal irrigation system (Peristeen®) may offer patients more independence and continence, as it has a balloon that inflates around a catheter inserted into the rectum, similar to the cone enema. However, cost and insurance coverage and clinical support may be prohibitive to using a Peristeen® system. Additionally, if the rectal vault is dilated, patients may not be able to use a RCE due to difficulty forming a seal around the cone or balloon, in which case surgical options may be pursued. Surgical options include creation of a stoma for Malone antegrade continence enema (MACE) or colostomy. A MACE offers 90% continence and independence [49]. For a MACE, a reconstructive urologist or colorectal surgeon creates a continent channel from the terminal ileum or the appendix that connects the cecum and abdominal wall. To perform the MACE evacuation, a catheter attached to a 1000 mL kangaroo bag with water or saline (approximately 600–1000 mL) is inserted in the stoma while the individual sits on the toilet. The bowel is flushed from the cecum to the rectum, a process that takes approximately 30–45 min and needs to be repeated every 1–2 days in order to achieve continence. Alternatively, interventional radiology may be able to insert a pig-tail Chait tube into the cecum which can also be used as an antegrade enema.

## Bladder and Pelvic Floor Concerns

Neurologic lesions associated with SB bladder innervation can impact bladder storage and emptying. Urologic problems in SB include: (1) UTIs, (2) urinary retention, (3) urolithiasis, (4) urinary incontinence, (5) deterioration of renal function, (6) pelvic organ prolapse, and (7) sexual dysfunction [51, 52]. Preservation of renal function, sexual function, continence, infection prevention, and independent management are the goals of urologic care [51].

### Monitoring and Evaluation

The most recent AUA/SUFU 2021 Neurogenic Lower Urinary Tract Dysfunction Guidelines have provided a new perspective on approach to these patients [4]. Risk stratification is now the

**Table 38.1** Neurogenic bowel assessment and management for individuals with SB [47, 50]

| Assessment | Considerations | Treatment options |
|---|---|---|
| Stool amount | Approximately 12–18 in. of stool per day is needed for adequate emptying | Use fiber (25–30 g per day), sufficient water (2 L per day or more), ± an osmotic agent (polyethylene glycol or lactulose), ± motility agent (senna, bisacodyl), and/or rectal-stimulating agent (suppository, mini-enema, digital stimulation) |
| Stool consistency Goal = Smooth and soft, like a sausage (Bristol 4) | Hard balls (Bristol 1) = slow motility | – Bowel prep cleanout may be needed prior to starting regimen if inadequate BMs for >5 days.<br>– Increase water intake, fruits and vegetables, fiber (25–30 g/day), and/or add osmotic agent (polyethylene glycol, lactulose)<br>– May need a motility agent like bisacodyl or senna |
| | Liquid (Bristol 6–7) = increased motility and/or need for bulking | – Consider bulking agent such as fiber (methylcellulose may cause less gas than other agents, titrate fiber by 5 g every 3–5 days for tolerance).<br>– Decrease foods that increase motility: greasy, spicy, some fruit/vegetables, and beans<br>– Evaluate for constipation as leaking can occur around impaction<br>– Anti-diarrheal agents can be used temporarily |
| Anal sphincter tone | If good tone, likely to respond to rectal-stimulating agent | – Docusate mini-enema can help to initiate a BM in 10–20 min, though some patients may prefer suppository or RCE |
| | If poor tone, may be difficult to attain fecal continence without 1–2 BMs daily. May be difficult to use RCE | – Schedule toileting 1–2 times daily with mini-enema<br>– If failure to achieve continence refer for MACE or Chait-tube evaluation.<br>– Colostomy may be preferred for some patients, particularly if ischial/sacral skin ulcers or difficulty with accessing an adaptive toilet |
| Bowel timing | Timed BMs decrease accidents, improve compliance with regimen. Ideal regimen duration is 30–45 min maximum | – Toilet timing 15–30 min post-prandial may maximize gastro-colonic reflex<br>– Schedule toileting in relationship to routine activities such as showering<br>– Bowel motility and rectal-stimulating agents may shorten duration |
| Mobility | Review ability to enter bathroom, transfer, and balance on the toilet | – Consider ordering a bedside commode, bath chair to put around toilet, or recommending installing handles around toilet |
| Difficulties with antegrade enemas (MACE/Chait tube) | (1) Constipation or taking too long to evacuate?<br>(2) Leaking?<br>(3) MACE stoma stricture?<br>(4) Chait-tube obstruction? | (1) Add a tablespoon of mineral oil, glycerin, or baby shampoo to the irrigation water or prior to instilling water. Also, add oral laxatives to regimen.<br>(2) From stoma, evaluate for constipation. If still leaking, order a barium cecostomy study to evaluate for stricture/backup in the cecum From anus, evaluate for constipation/incomplete emptying. Consider fiber to bulk stool or stand up/sit down to try to evacuate more<br>(3) Either use a smaller catheter with lubricant, or consider using a placeholder catheter (L-stent) with steroid cream between irrigation<br>(4) Use warm water to clear the obstruction. If pig-tail chait, contact IR to replace if leaking/obstructed |

**Table 38.1** (continued)

| Assessment | Considerations | Treatment options |
|---|---|---|
| Supplies for MACE | Straight catheter, syringes, or feeding bag with extension tubing | (1) Straight catheter-hydrophilic or non-hydrophilic with lubricant (usually 10–12 French, 30 per month)<br>(2) Feeding bag with extension tubing to attach to the catheter (1 per month)<br>(3) Syringes (if used in place of the feeding bag, 60 mL with loop handle, 1–2 per month) |
| Goals for bowel regimen | (1) BM every 1–2 days of adequate amount<br>(2) Maximize independence and compliance<br>(3) Goal regimen time 30–45 min or less<br>(4) Minimize unpredictable accidents | – Start with fiber and water +/- stool softener +/- motility agent with timed toileting<br>– May need to start with rectal medication to initiate BMs.<br>– If not at goal with titrating oral and rectal medications and timing, consider RCE or referral for MACE/Chait.<br>– May need to start with a bowel clean out (magnesium citrate or sodium sulfate, potassium sulfate and magnesium sulfate) before initiating a bowel routine if very constipated |

*BM* bowel movement, *RCE* retrograde colonic enema, *MACE* Malone antegrade continence enema, *IR* interventional radiology

cornerstone of the initial evaluation such that evaluation and follow up is determined by categorizing patients as either low risk or unknown risk. Patients stratified into unknown risk need further investigation including renal function, post-void residual (PVR), urinary tract imaging, and urodynamics in order to properly stratify them [4]. Individuals able to spontaneously void and who have normal renal function and stable bladder function are considered low risk and do not require regular surveillance unless they report a change in symptoms (e.g., difficulty voiding, renal dysfunction, or UTIs) [4]. As most individuals with SB already have voiding dysfunction and require intermittent catheterization, they would be categorized as moderate or high risk depending on their renal function and urodynamics. Urodynamic testing provides the urologist with useful information regarding urine storage and emptying that guides further management and follow up in these patients. Urodynamic studies evaluate urinary storage phase by measuring bladder compliance and capacity, presence or absence of detrusor overactivity or underactivity, and bladder neck competence as well as providing a comprehensive evaluation of the emptying or voiding phase by evaluating detrusor pressure, presence or absence of detrusor sphincter dyssynergia, and urinary flow and post-void residual. Individuals in moderate- or high-risk categories require at least annual serum creatinine assessment and ultrasound of the kidneys, ureters, and bladder every 1–2 years to monitor for hydronephrosis, urolithiasis, and upper urinary tract concerns [4, 51]. Urodynamic evaluations (preferably a video urodynamic study to also assess for vesicoureteral reflux and evaluate bladder contour) are recommended for initial evaluation and then as clinically indicated based on new concerns (e.g., renal function changes, hydronephrosis, increased UTIs, urolithiasis, or worsening incontinence) [4, 51]. Patients with poor bladder compliance and/or detrusor pressures more than 40 cm $H_2O$ without leakage during bladder filling are at risk for vesicoureteral reflux and upper tract deterioration and thus require medical or procedural intervention [53]. Patients who were initially classified in the low-risk category but present with new-onset UTI, urolithiasis, or upper tract deterioration require reevaluation and repeat risk stratification [4].

## Medical Management of Neurogenic Bladder

Neurogenic bladder management often involves clean intermittent catheterization (CIC) and anticholinergic and/or beta-3 agonist medication. CIC allows for timely bladder emptying, decreased incontinence, prevention of UTIs and urolithiasis, lower bladder storage volumes, and safer pressures to protect renal function. CIC complications (urethral injury, epididymitis, and meatitis) occur in less than 30% [53]. Anticholinergics and beta-3 agonists are used to improve capacity and compliance by relaxing the detrusor smooth muscle during storage phase [54, 55]. Side effects to monitor for include dry mouth, constipation, and blurred vision for anticholinergics and hypertension, tachycardia, palpitations, and angioedema for beta-3 agonists [54, 55]. If anticholinergics fail to increase bladder capacity and decrease pressure, intravesical botulinum toxin A injections can help decrease incontinence, increase capacity, decrease filling pressures, and increase quality of life for a mean duration of 6–7 months [56].

## Surgical Management of Neurogenic bladder

When maximal medical management fails to prevent urinary upper tract deterioration or improve urinary incontinence, surgical reconstruction is recommended [53]. Common reconstructive surgeries for SB include bladder augmentation (usually ileocecoplasty), creation of a CIC, ileovesicostomy, and bladder outlet procedures. Ileocecoplasty (reconfigured portion of terminal ileum attached to the bladder) is the most common augmentation and improves compliance and capacity, preserves renal function, and minimizes incontinence. A continent catheterizable channel allows for easier access to the bladder and more CIC independence as the individual cath through an abdominal stoma rather than the urethra. A continent channel is constructed from the appendix (Mitrofanoff appendicovesicostomy procedure), a transverse ileal tube (Yang-Monti), tapered ileum implant, or ileocecal valve (ileocecocystoplasty) [57, 58]. Complications are not common but may include stomal leakage or stenosis. Patients with augmentation may have a slightly higher risk for bladder cancer long term [59]. Some neurologists recommend regular cystoscopy surveillance starting at 10 years post-augmentation, but this recommendation may lead to over-monitoring. It is reasonable to obtain cystoscopy evaluation for previously augmented patients with persistent hematuria, chronic UTIs, or new upper tract dilation [59]. A continent catheterizable channel may be preferred in patients who would have difficulty with CIC due to dexterity or adherence to a catheterization schedule. Lastly, bladder outlet procedures (bladder slings, formal bladder neck closures, or artificial urinary sphincter devices) treat refractory stress urinary incontinence or urethral tract strictures and fistulae [60].

## Bladder Complications: UTIs and Urolithiasis

UTIs are the most common diagnosis for acute care utilization and hospital readmission among adults with SB [7, 61]. In cohort studies of adults with SB, approximately 30%–40% experience one or more UTIs per year [62, 63]. However, asymptomatic bacteriuria occurs in 70% [64]. The frequent use of antibiotics for UTI treatment or prophylaxis in the SB population poses an increased risk for multi-drug resistant (MDR) organism colonization [65]. Investigators in a 2016 systematic review defined three criteria for the diagnosis of UTIs in patients with SB: (1) two or more symptoms among fever > 38 °C, new back or abdominal pain, malaise, increased spasticity, new/worse incontinence, dysuria, and new/worse malodorous or new/worse cloudy urine; (2) > 10 white blood cells per high-power field on urine microscopy from a clean catch or catheterized specimen; and (3) > 100,000 colony-forming units (CFU)/mL of at least one organism on urine culture [66]. Thus, it is recommended to obtain a urinalysis to evaluate for UTI only if there are noted symptoms. Empiric antibiotic therapy can be initiated if there are severe symptoms or if the patient is at higher risk for urosepsis; otherwise, it is recommended to await culture results. Recurrent UTIs defined as ≥2 UTIs in 6 months or ≥3 UTIs in 1 year warrant evaluation for adherence to bladder management routines and further urological evaluation for urolithiasis, ureter reflux, and urodynamic changes [4, 67]. Regarding UTI prevention, adherence to routine catheterization regimens and hydration is recommended (single-use and hydrophilic catheters may be better); oral prophylactic antibiotics are not routinely recommended in non-pregnant individuals; intravesical gentamicin instillation for 3–6 months may be considered; and there is insufficient evidence to support oral supplement for UTI prevention (e.g., probiotics and cranberry supplements) [68, 69].

Bladder stones are ten times more common in adults with SB than in the general population [70]. Those who have undergone bladder augmentation and who have recurrent UTIs are particularly susceptible to bladder stones [70]. For those who have undergone augmentation, routine bladder irrigation with water or saline may help decrease bladder stone formation [71]. Bladder irrigation is performed by catheterizing the bladder and then using a 60-mL syringe to insert approximately 180 mL water or saline into the bladder and aspirating the fluid out with the syringe. This can be repeated until the aspirate is clear. Hydration is also important and may help to prevent stones and UTIs. Most adults should be educated to drink 2–3 L of water per day and monitor for clear/light yellow urine [72].

### Pelvic Organ Prolapse

Pelvic Organ Prolapse (POP) is likely a more common problem in women with SB than in the general population [73]. POP is the symptomatic descent of the vaginal walls, the apex (cervix/uterus), and/or the vaginal vault and is staged from stage 0 (normal) to stage IV (complete prolapse) [74]. POP affects functional status, continence, and sexual function. Women with SB may present with POP at a younger age (mean age 25 years), with more severe prolapse, and with symptoms including vaginal bulge, difficult intercourse, and difficult catheterization [75, 76]. Management options include observation, pessary device, sacrocolpopexy, uterosacral ligament suspension, or sacrospinous suspension.

Primary care clinicians should monitor chronic bladder management including catheterization regimens and incontinence, identify and initiate work up for complications such as difficulty performing catheterization and UTIs, and coordinate care with urology including visits and supplies. Patients should see urology annually and additionally for complications including recurrent UTIs (three or more per year), difficulty performing catheterization, increased incontinence, urolithiasis, new/worsening hydronephrosis, and/or POP [51, 77].

## Sexual/Reproductive Health

An estimated 24–68% of adolescent and young adults with SB (AYASB) are sexually active [78, 79]. Many report having had some sex education from school or parents, but physician-directed sex education is uncommon [80]. Most AYASB report inadequate reproductive and sexual knowledge as issues of physical impairment, fertility, and heredity of SB are rarely addressed [80]. Many AYASB desire sexual relationships and plan to get married. About 50% of sexually active AYASB report being satisfied with their sexual relationships [78]. Wheelchair dependence and incontinence are barriers to satisfactory sexual relationships. Individuals with lesions at or above the lumbar 2 (L2) level are more likely to have decreased genital sensation and decreased likelihood of engaging in sexual activity, but those with lower lumbar and sacral lesions can also have sexual dysfunction [79, 81]. It is also important to note that individuals with disability are at higher risk for sexual abuse and inter-partner violence. Routine well care for adults with SB should include annual genital/gynecological exams, evaluation of sexual function, and individualized sexual education [82].

### Men's Health

Sexual dysfunction and infertility concerns for men with SB include difficulties with ejaculation, low sperm counts, and erectile dysfunction (ED) and are more common in high-lumbar or thoracic MMC [51]. Most men can achieve ejaculation and orgasm, but sometimes ejaculate may be minimal and not associated with orgasm. Failure of spermatogenesis may be due to prostatitis, increased testicular temperatures, cryptorchidism, or medications such as chronic antibiotics and tricyclic antidepressants. ED has been reported in up to 70 – 75% of men with SB,

**Table 38.2** Complications in pregnancy among individuals with SB [69, 83]

| Concern | Management | Notes |
|---|---|---|
| Urinary incontinence | • Increase CIC | • Anti-muscarinic agents (oxybutynin, solifenacin, etc.) are classified as Pregnancy Category B; animal studies have not shown definitive evidence of harm to the fetus, but safety has not been established for women who are or may become pregnant<br>• OnabotulinumtoxinA is classified as a Pregnancy Category C drug; animal reproduction studies have demonstrated an adverse effect on the fetus, but no formal studies have been performed on pregnant women to determine the risks |
| Recurrent urinary tract infections | • Increase frequency of CIC<br>• Consider antibiotic prophylaxis | • Management of recurrent UTIs can assist in preventing miscarriage, prematurity, and low birth weight |
| Neurogenic bowel dysfunction | • Increase fiber, fluids, and exercise<br>• Emollient laxatives (mineral oil, glycerin)<br>• Osmotic laxatives for refractory constipation<br>• Glycerin suppository or water enemas can be safely used for stool evacuation | |

*CIC* clean intermittent catheterization, *UTI* urinary tract infection

especially for lesions above the thoracic 10 (T10) level, and contributes to a lack of confidence, poor body image, and difficulty maintaining intimate relationships [81]. ED treatments include phosphodiesterase type 5 inhibitors (sildenafil 50 mg is most effective), intracavernous self-injection with papaverine or prostaglandin E1, use of a vacuum constriction device, and prostheses [52]. Neuro-urology or urologists who specialize in male sexual function can help with management.

## Women's Health

Gynecologic concerns for women with SB include early menarche (on average 10–11 years of age); congenital reproductive tract anomalies; orthopedic abnormalities of the pelvis, spine, and lower limbs; and POP [77]. Women with SB are recommended to take folic acid 4 mg daily before and during pregnancy to reduce the risk of having a baby with a NTD, although dose-related outcomes have not been studied [83]. Genetic counseling should be offered, and early management by a high-risk obstetrician can yield the best outcomes. Live births occur in 70–80% of pregnancies in women with SB [84, 85]. Nevertheless, pregnancy complications occur including shunt problems, UTIs, problems with bowel and bladder conduits, incontinence, and constipation (see Table 38.2) [69, 84, 85]. Cesarean sections are common due to small pelvis size, hip bone abnormalities, contractures, severe kyphosis, and vertebral anomalies. Ambulatory women are more likely to have successful vaginal deliveries compared to non-ambulatory patients [84, 85].

## Osteoporosis

Fracture prevalence in the pediatric population of SB is estimated to be approximately 30%, but studies in adults are limited [86, 87]. Medical co-morbidities (urinary diversion, kidney disease, and use of anti-epileptics), higher MMC lesions, wheelchair use, hypercalciuria, high body fat levels, contractures, and previous fractures are significant osteoporosis risk factors ([86, 87]. The distal femur is the most common fracture site [86, 87].

Concluding from sparse studies, a baseline dual energy x-ray absorptiometry (DEXA) with serum and urine calcium as well as serum 25-hydroxy vitamin D, phosphorus, and parathyroid hormone levels may be considered in patients with a previous fracture or risk factors [86, 87]. Limitations to using DEXA in this population include positioning due to scoliosis and/or contractures and the use of DEXA software that measures bone density of the wrists, lumbar spine, and hips when the most vulnerable sites among this population are the long bones. Treatment for osteoporosis in adults with SB has not been well studied. Clinicians should encourage patients to take 1000 mg of calcium daily and 800 units of vitamin D daily (more may be required for deficiencies) and engage in physical activity to promote bone health.

## Skin/Soft Tissue concerns

Impaired ambulation, decreased sensation, and skeletal abnormalities increase the risk of pressure ulcers in individuals with SB [88, 89]. Risk factors are listed in Box 38.2, with the highest risks being wheelchair use and thoracic lesion level. The most common sites for pressure ulcers are the foot, ankle, and buttocks [86, 87]. Infected decubitus ulcers are common reasons for emergency room visits and hospital admission [7, 90].

**Box 38.2 Patients at Highest Risk for Pressure Ulcer [86, 87]**

| | |
|---|---|
| • Higher lesion level<br>• Wheelchair use<br>• Improper wheelchair seating<br>• Urinary incontinence<br>• Shunt presence<br>• Arnold-Chiari malformation<br>• Above-the-knee orthopedic surgery | • Recent surgery<br>• Male sex<br>• Prior ulcerations<br>• Poorly fitting orthotics<br>• Obesity<br>• Inadequate nutrition<br>• Difficulty with transfers |

Clinicians should assess for risk factors, regularly examine high risk areas of decreased sensation, and refer to wound care practitioners for early-stage ulcers [91]. Patients and/or families should regularly check skin for pressure changes and sores, especially on the buttocks, back, lower extremities, angulation areas, and skin folds. Infected, chronic, or stage IV decubitus ulcers increase the risk for osteomyelitis. Symptoms often include increased warmth, tenderness, fever, and bone pain. However, many patients with SB may not have or recognize symptoms due to decreased sensation. If concern for osteomyelitis is present, an erythrocyte sedimentation rate, a C-reactive protein level, a white blood cell count, and blood cultures should be obtained. X-ray imaging may show bony changes consistent with osteomyelitis, but MRI is more sensitive especially if low bone density is present. If osteomyelitis is present on imaging, it is necessary to consult surgery to obtain bone cultures and infectious disease to coordinate plans for appropriate antibiotic regimens.

## Musculoskeletal Issues

### General Mobility and the Use of Assistive Devices

Overall, 57 – 60% of individuals with SB use a wheelchair [92]. Individuals with lesions above L2, hydrocephalus, and/or hip dislocation are likely to be wheelchair dependent. In individuals with lower lumbar and sacral lesions, approximately 35% require braces and 23% require walking aides such as walkers, forearm crutches, or canes [33, 92]. While most adults with SB already use assistive devices, mobility may continue to deteriorate with age due to obesity, fractures, and other long-term non-musculoskeletal consequences. Physiatrists, physical therapists, and wheelchair clinics can help determine which assistive technology best suits an individual patient's mobility needs (see Box 38.3) [93].

**Box 38.3 Considerations for Assistive Technology Evaluation**

- Equipment needed and date of last new supplies
- Insurance coverage or other funding sources to cover equipment
- Patient's functional goals for home, education, employment, and community
- Physical and functional assessment by physical therapist and/or physiatrist.
- Documentation and diagnoses association needed (contact equipment company to clarify)

## Musculoskeletal Pain

Pain is a common concern for adults with SB. In one national survey, 46.9% of respondents reported pain within the last week [63]. In general, and among the SB population, wheelchair use is associated with increased musculoskeletal pain, in the shoulders most commonly, followed by the neck, elbow, wrist, hand, and low back [63, 94]. Initial intervention recommendations include equipment adjustments, physical therapy, exercise, non-steroidal inflammatory medications (use with caution with those who have underlying kidney disease), and topical pain medications [94]. Imaging and surgical consultation may be warranted for severe or unremitting pain.

## Orthopedic Concerns

Orthopedic problems and musculoskeletal deformities are common in SB and affect function, preclude lower extremity bracing, and contribute to skin breakdown and chronic pain [95]. Spinal deformities such as scoliosis and kyphosis are more severe in higher SB levels and present management challenges. Scoliosis usually progresses until age 15 years, and thus few adults undergo scoliosis surgery. However, individuals may have had prior spinal fusion to maximize height and mobility, decrease pain, and improve forced vital lung capacity [96]. Non-operative care including trunk balance exercises, upper extremity manipulation, and orthotics may improve or maintain seating function. Surgery may be considered for scoliosis more than 50°, curvature with pain, or restrictive lung disease, but post-operative complications occur in 50%, so risks and benefits should be weighed carefully [97]. Individuals with lumbar 4 (L4) level or higher lesions and severe scoliosis often have hip dislocation, which can cause chronic pain and limited mobility [95]. Hip reduction surgery is often not effective and may lead to stiffness, contractures, hyperlordosis, and decreased function [95]. Foot deformities are more common at the lumbosacral level, and various types of foot deformities correlate with various SB levels [98]. Orthotics are often used to facilitate ambulation and gait, whereas surgical intervention may be considered if orthotics do not fit well, for recurrent skin ulcers, or for inadequately managed pain [97].

## Obesity

Up to 35 to 50% AYASB are obese [2, 28]. These patients tend to have lower aerobic fitness, eat less healthy diets, and be more sedentary than their peers, putting them at greater risk for obesity, metabolic syndrome, cardiovascular disease, chronic wounds, and lymphedema [99]. Exercise regimens and physical therapy reduce pain, increase efficiency in wheelchair propulsion, and improve physical activity and balance [99]. Barriers to physical activity need to be addressed, including lack of motivation and time, fatigue, body image concerns, lack of knowledge about adaptive exercise, lack of facilities and programs, and weather/environmental limitations [100]. Motivation to stay healthy, improving physical appearance, maintaining physical skills, and social support promote engagement in physical activity [29, 100].

## Quality of Life

People with SB have lower quality of life (QOL) scores than the general population in regard to physical functioning, general health, vitality, pain, and social functioning [101]. For adults, the level of lesion, full-time wheelchair use, hydrocephalus, pain, depression, and bowel and bladder incontinence have been associated with reduced QOL. Self-efficacy, personal hope and coping skills, parental hope, psychological stress, and pain have been found to more strongly correlate with QOL than physical deficits [102–107]. Thus, QOL for people with SB can be best supported by: (1) engaging them in emerging adult activities (education, employment, recreation, and relationships); (2) supporting them in adaptive skills; (3) promoting self-efficacy and a positive outlook; and (4) addressing pain, mental health, and continence concerns [107].

## Conclusion

With more than three-fourths of children born with SB surviving into adulthood, chronic condition management and preventive care for adults with SB will increasingly need to be facilitated by the adult clinician. Adult clinicians must be prepared to manage the psychosocial as well as the medical needs of adults with SB. Adult practices planning to manage this population should prepare for facility accessibility; care coordination with adult subspecialists such as neurosurgeons, physiatrists, physical therapists, wound care specialists, and urologists familiar with the co-morbidities associated with SB; health care funding support; and community resources to support adaptive living. The adult inpatient and outpatient clinician should be comfortable recognizing shunt complications; managing complications of neurogenic bowel and bladder and skin/soft tissue breakdown/ulceration; adapting general health guidelines to individual with SB; and facilitating care coordination and self-management to optimize health and promote quality of life for adults with SB.

## Parent/Caregiver Resources

Spina Bifida Association: http://spinabifidaassociation.org/adults/

Center for Disease Control—Spina Bifida: http://www.cdc.gov/ncbddd/spinabifida/adult.html

International Federation for Spina Bifida and Hydrocephalus: http://www.ifglobal.org/en/

National Institute of Neurological Disorders and Stroke/NIH: https://www.ninds.nih.gov/health-information/disorders/spina-bifida

| Spina Bifida (SB) condition sheet | | |
|---|---|---|
| Definition | • SB is the most common neural tube defect (NTD) and is due to failure of the spinal neural tube to close at 25–28 days post-conception.<br>• SB is classified by Hoffer functional level: *thoracic* (flaccid lower extremities), *high lumbar* (hip flexion present), *mid lumbar* (knee extension present), *low lumbar* (dorsiflexion present), and *sacral* (foot plantar flexion present). | |
| Epidemiology | • An estimated 1500–2000 babies with SB are born in the United States annually with the highest incidence in the Latino population.<br>• Approximately 166,000 people in the United States have SB, with the majority being adults.<br>• Primary prevention for SB is 4 mcg folic acid for women without SB and no family history of SB and 4 mg for women with SB or who have a family history of SB. | |
| Special considerations | **Adults with SB may have following co-occurring conditions:** | |
| | • Shunted hydrocephalus<br>• Neurocognitive impairment/Executive function<br>• Neurogenic bladder/UTIs<br>• Neurogenic bowel/constipation<br>• Skin ulcers | • Musculoskeletal concerns: scoliosis, varying levels of paralysis, contractures, foot deformities, pain, disuse osteoporosis<br>• Central/obstructive sleep apnea<br>• Latex allergy |
| | **Adults with SB have increased risk of:** | |
| | • Obesity<br>• Hypertension | • Anxiety/depression<br>• Impairment of sexual function |

| Spina Bifida (SB) condition sheet | |
|---|---|
| Recommended screening and prevention | • Neurogenic bladder risk stratification based on the AUA/SUFU guidelines and then surveillance based on risk (usually annual): basic metabolic panel chemistry, renal/bladder ultrasound, urodynamics, and urology follow up.<br>• Regular skin exams<br>• Routine evaluation of bowel and bladder regimens<br>• Routine evaluation of mobility impairment and adaptive equipment need<br>• Routine preventative adult health care (e.g., cardio/metabolic prevention, reproductive health care, and mental health care)<br>• Routine evaluation of adaptive supports for vocation and independent living |

## References


1. Stepanczuk BC, Dicianno BE, Webb TS. Young adults with spina bifida may have higher occurrence of prehypertension and hypertension. Am J Phys Med Rehabil. 2013;92(11):1–7.
2. Dosa NP, Foley JT, Eckrich M, Woodall-Ruff D, Liptak GS. Obesity across the lifespan among persons with spina bifida. Disabil Rehabil. 2009;31(11):914–20.
3. Kanaheswari Y, Mohd Rizal AM. Renal scarring and chronic kidney disease in children with spina bifida in a multidisciplinary Malaysian centre: renal outcomes in spina bifida children. J Paediatr Child Health. 2015;51(12):1175–81.
4. Ginsberg D, Boone T, Cameron A, Gousse A, Kaufman MR, Keays E, et al. The AUA/SUFU Guideline on adult neurogenic lower urinary tract dysfunction panel. J Urol. 2021;206:1106.
5. Showen A, Copp HL, Allen IE, Baradaran N, Liaw A, Hampson LA. Characteristics associated with depression, anxiety, and social isolation in adults with spina bifida. Urology. 2021;149:255–62.
6. Bellin MH, Zabel TA, Dicianno BE, Levey E, Garver K, Linroth R, et al. Correlates of depressive and anxiety symptoms in young adults with spina bifida. J Pediatr Psychol. 2010;35(7):778–89.
7. Dicianno BE, Wilson R. Hospitalizations of adults with spina bifida and congenital spinal cord anomalies. Arch Phys Med Rehabil. 2010;91(4):529–35.
8. Bowman RM, McLone DG, Grant JA, Tomita T, Ito JA. Spina bifida outcome: a 25-year prospective. Pediatr Neurosurg. 2001;34:114–20.
9. Jernigan SC, Berry JG, Graham DA, Bauer SB, Karlin LI, Hobbs NM, et al. Risk factors of sudden death in young adult patients with myelomeningocele. J Neurosurg Pediatr. 2012;9(2):149–55.
10. Crytzer TM, Cheng Y-T, Bryner MJ, Wilson R III, Sciurba FC, Dicianno BE. Impact of neurological level and spinal curvature on pulmonary function in adults with spina bifida. J Pediatr Rehabil Med. 2019;11(4):243–54.
11. Kirk VG, Morielli A, Brouillette RT. Sleep-disordered breathing in patients with myelomeningocele: the missed diagnosis. Dev Med Child Neurol. 1999;41(1):40–3.
12. Manning SM, Jennings R, Madsen JR. Pathophysiology, prevention, and potential treatment of neural tube defects. Ment Retard Dev Disabil Res Rev. 2000;14:6–14.
13. Parker SE, Mai CT, Canfield MA, Rickard R, Wang Y, Meyer R, et al. Updated national birth prevalence estimates for selected birth defects in the United States, 2004–2006. Birth Defects Res Part A. 2010;88:1008–16.
14. Boulet SL, Yang Q, Mai C, Kirby RS, Collins JS, Robbins JM, et al. Trends in the postfortification prevlaence of spina bifida and anencephaly in the United States. Birth Defects Res A Clin Mol Teratol. 2008;82(7):527–32.
15. NINDS. Spina Bifida fact sheet. [cited 2018 Jun 6]. Available from: https://www.ninds.nih.gov/Disorders/Patient-Caregiver-Education/Fact-Sheets/Spina-Bifida-Fact-Sheet.
16. Adzick NS. Fetal myelomeningocele: natural history, pathophysiology, and in-utero intervention. Bone Semin Fetal Neonatal Med. 2010;15(1):9–14.
17. Rintoul NE, Sutton LN, Hubbard AM, Cohen B, Melchionni J, Pasquariello PS, et al. A new look at myelomeningoceles: functional level, vertebral level, shunting , and the implications for fetal intervention. Pediatrics. 2002;109(3):409–13.
18. Sawin KJ, Liu T, Ward E, Thibadeau J, Schechter MS, Soe MM, et al. The National Spina Bifida Patient Registry: profile of a large cohort of participants from the first 10 clinics. J Pediatr. 2015;166(2):444–450.e1.
19. Hampton LE, Fletcher JM, Cirino P, Blaser S, Kramer LA, Dennis M. Neuropsychological profiles of children with aqueductal stenosis and spina bifida myelomeningocele. J Int Neuropsychol Soc. 2013;19(2):127–36.
20. Dennis M, Landry SH, Barnes M, Fletcher JM. A model of neurocognitive function in spina bifida over the life span. J Int Neuropsychol Soc. 2006;12(2):285–96.
21. Fletcher JM, Copeland K, Frederick JA, Blaser SE, Kramer LA, Northrup H, et al. Spinal lesion level in spina bifida: a source of neural and cognitive heterogeneity. J Neurosurg. 2005;102(Suppl. 3):268–79.
22. Hoffer M, Feiwell E, Perry R, Perry J, Bonnett C. Functional ambulation in patients with myelomeningocele. J Bone Joint Surg Am. 1973;55(1):137–48.
23. Dicianno B, Sherman A, Roehmer C, Zigler C. Comorbidities associated with early mortality in adults with spina bifida. Am J Phys Med Rehabil. 2018;97(12):861–5.

24. Botto L, Yang Q. 5,10-Methylenetetrahydrofolate reductase gene variants and congenital anomalies: a HuGE review. Am J Epidemiol. 2000;151(9):862–77.
25. Donnan J, Walsh S, Sikora L, Morrissey A, Collins K, MacDonald D. A systematic review of the risks factors associated with the onset and natural progression of spina bifida. Neurotoxicology. 2017;61:20–31.
26. Douglas Wilson R, Audibert F, Brock JA, Carroll J, Cartier L, Gagnon A, et al. Pre-conception folic acid and multivitamin supplementation for the primary and secondary prevention of neural tube defects and other folic acid-sensitive congenital anomalies. J Obstet Gynaecol Can. 2015;37(6):534–49.
27. Thibadeau J, Walker WO, Castillo J, Dicianno BE, Routh JC, Smith KA, et al. Philosophy of care delivery for spina bifida. Disabil Health J. 2020;13(2):100883.
28. Dicianno BE. 21st century challenges to the provision of health care to adults with spina bifida: a rehabilitation approach. Arch Phys Med Rehabil. 2014;95(9):1601–2.
29. McPherson AC, Chen L, O'Neil J, Vanderbom KA. Nutrition, metabolic syndrome, and obesity: guidelines for the care of people with spina bifida. J Pediatr Rehabil Med. 2020;13(4):637–53.
30. Fremion E, Kanter D, Turk M. Health promotion and preventive health care service guidelines for the care of people with spina bifida. J Pediatr Rehabil Med. 2020;13(4):513–23.
31. Dennis M, Barnes MA. The cognitive phenotype of spina bifida meningomyelocele. Dev Disabil Res Rev. 2010;16(1):31–9.
32. Queally JT, Barnes MA, Castillo H, Castillo J, Fletcher JM. Neuropsychological care guidelines for people with spina bifida. J Pediatr Rehabil Med. 2020;13(4):663–73.
33. Verhoef M, Barf HA, Post MWM, van Asbeck FWA, Gooskens RHJM, Prevo AJH. Functional independence among young adults with spina bifida, in relation to hydrocephalus and level of lesion. Dev Med Child Neurol. 2006;48(2):114–9.
34. Fremion EJ, Dosa NP. Spina bifida transition to adult healthcare guidelines. J Pediatr Rehabil Med. 2019;12(4):423–9.
35. National Resource Center for Supported Decision-Making. National Resource Center for supported decision-making. [cited 2021 Nov 5]. Available from: http://www.supporteddecisionmaking.org/
36. Blount JP, Bowman R, Dias MS, Hopson B, Partington MD, Rocque BG. Neurosurgery guidelines for the care of people with spina bifida. J Pediatr Rehabil Med. 2020;13(4):467–77.
37. Protzenko T, Salomão JFM, Junior SCG, Bellas AR. Myelomeningocele: long-term neurosurgical treatment and follow up in 231 patients. Childs Nerv Syst. 2017;33(10):1831. Available from: http://www.embase.com/search/results?subaction=viewrecord&from=export&id=L618558120
38. Lew SM, Kothbauer KF. Tethered cord syndrome: an updated review. Pediatr Neurosurg. 2007;43(3):236–48.
39. Tseng JH, Kuo MF, Kwang TY, Tseng MY. Outcome of untethering for symptomatic spina bifida occulta with lumbosacral spinal cord tethering in 31 patients: analysis of preoperative prognostic factors. Spine J. 2008;8(4):630–8.
40. Tsitouras V, Sgouros S. Syringomyelia and tethered cord in children. Childs Nerv Syst. 2013;29(9):1625–34.
41. Gaston H. Ophthalmic complications of spina bifida and hydrocephalus. Eye. 1991;5(3):279–90.
42. Patel DM, Rocque BG, Hopson B, Arynchyna A, Bishop ER, Lozano DBJ. Sleep-disordered breathing in patients with myelomeningocele. J Pediatr Neurosurg. 2015;15:30–5.
43. Wang H, Wiener J, Ferrandino M. Complications of surgical management of upper tract calculi in spina bifida patients: analysis of nationwide data. J Urol. 2015;193:1270–4.
44. Verhoef M, Lurvink M, Barf H, Post M, van Asbeck F, Gooskens R, et al. High prevalence of incontinence among young adults with spina bifida: description, prediction and problem perception. Spinal Cord. 2005;43(6):331–40.
45. Velde SV, Biervliet SV, Bruyne RD, Winckel MV. A systematic review on bowel management and the success rate of the various treatment modalities in spina bifida patients. Spinal Cord. 2013;51(12):873–81.
46. Imai K, Shiroyanagi Y, Kim WJ, Ichiroku T, Yamazaki Y. Satisfaction after the Malone antegrade continence enema procedure in patients with spina bifida. Spinal Cord. 2014;52(1):54–7.
47. Beierwaltes P, Church P, Gordon T, Ambartsumyan L. Bowel function and care: guidelines for the care of people with spina bifida. J Pediatr Rehabil Med. 2020;13(4):491–8.
48. Mombelli G, Chiarulli EF, Rossini M, Sentina M, Tagliabue A, Fuse A, et al. Reduction of urinary tract infections related to trans-anal irrigation (TAI): results on long term in a single centre. Neurourol Urodyn. 2017;36:S51. Available from: http://www.embase.com/search/results?subaction=viewrecord&from=export&id=L617217973
49. Neal D. Efficacy and complications of total continence surgery. Urology. 2012;80(3):S340. Available from: http://www.embase.com/search/results?subaction=viewrecord&from=export&id=L70900161
50. Leibold SR. Achieving Continence with a Neurogenic Bowel. Pediatr Clin North Am. 2010;57(4):1013–25.
51. Joseph DB, Baum MA, Tanaka ST, Frimberger DC, Misseri R, Khavari R, et al. Urologic guidelines for the care and management of people with spina bifida. J Pediatr Rehabil Med. 2020;13(4):479–89.
52. Wiener JS, Frimberger DC, Wood H. Spina bifida health-care guidelines for men's health. Urology. 2018;116:218–26.
53. Snow-Lisy DC, Yerkes EB, Cheng EY. Update on urological management of spina bifida from prenatal diagnosis to adulthood. J Urol. 2015;194(2):288–96.
54. Kessler TM, Bachmann LM, Minder C, Löhrer D, Umbehr M, Schünemann HJ, et al. Adverse event assessment of antimuscarinics for treating overactive

bladder: a network meta-analytic approach. PLoS One. 2011;6(2):e16718.
55. Park JS, Lee YS, Lee CN, Kim SH, Kim SW, Han SW. Efficacy and safety of mirabegron, a β3-adrenoceptor agonist, for treating neurogenic bladder in pediatric patients with spina bifida: a retrospective pilot study. World J Urol. 2019;37(8):1665–70.
56. Kaviani A, Pande R, Boone TB, Khavari R. Outcomes of intradetrusor onabotulinumtoxinA injection in adults with congenital spinal dysraphism at a tertiary transitional urology clinic. Urol Pract. 2019;6(2):112–6.
57. Monti P, Lara R, Dutra M, Al E. New techniques for construction of efferent conduits based on the Mitrofanoff principle. Urology. 1997;49:112–5.
58. Mitrofanoff P. Trans-appendicular continent cystostomy in the management of the neurogenic bladder. Chir Pediatr. 1980;21:297–305.
59. Mühlbauer J, Stein R, Younsi N. Bladder cancer in patients with spina bifida: a serious risk. World J Urol. 2021;39(5):1531–7.
60. Veenboer PW, de Kort LMO, Chrzan RJ, de Jong TPVM. Urinary considerations for adult patients with spinal dysraphism. Nat Rev Urol. 2015;12(6):331–9.
61. Armour BS, Ouyang L, Thibadeau J, Grosse SD, Campbell VA, Joseph D. Hospitalization for urinary tract infections and the quality of preventive health care received by people with spina bifida. Disabil Health J. 2009;2(3):145–52.
62. Werhagen L, Gabrielsson H, Westgren N, Borg K. Medical complication in adults with spina bifida. Clin Neurol Neurosurg. 2013 Aug;115(8):1226–9.
63. Morley CP, Struwe S, Pratte MA, Clayton GH, Wilson PE, Dicianno BE, et al. Survey of U.S. adults with spina bifida. Disabil Health J. 2020;13(2):100833.
64. Sturm R, Johnson E, Halline C, Meyer T, Snow-Lisy D, Rosoklija I, et al. Predictors of bacteriuria and antibiotic resistance in asymptomatic children using CIC for bladder management. J Urol. 2018;199(4):e929–30. Available from: http://www.embase.com/search/results?subaction=viewrecord&from=export&id=L621737615
65. Friedman ND, Temkin E, Carmeli Y. The negative impact of antibiotic resistance. Clin Microbiol Infect. 2016;22(5):416–22.
66. Madden-Fuentes RJ, McNamara ER, Lloyd JC, Wiener JS, Routh JC, Seed PC, et al. Variation in definitions of urinary tract infections in spina bifida patients: a systematic review. Pediatrics. 2013;132(1):132–9.
67. Gupta K, Trautner B. Diagnosis and management of recurrent urinary tract infections in non-pregnant women. BMJ. 2013;346:f3140. Available from: http://www.embase.com/search/results?subaction=viewrecord&from=export&id=L369047037%5Cn
68. Tradewell M, Pariser JJ, Nimeh T, Elliott SP. Neurogenic Bladder Research Group. Systematic review and practice policy statements on urinary tract infection prevention in adults with spina bifida. Transl Androl Urol. 2018;7(Suppl 2):S205–19.
69. Fremion E, Bustillos P, Khavari R. Contemporary management considerations of urinary tract infections for women with spina bifida. Int Urogynecol J. 2022;33(3):493–505.
70. Veenboer PW, Ruud Bosch JLH, van Asbeck FWA, de Kort LMO. Urolithiasis in adult spina bifida patients: study in 260 patients and discussion of the literature. Int Urol Nephrol. 2013;45(3):695–702.
71. Zhang H, Yamataka A, Koga H, Kobayashi H, Lane GJ, Miyano T. Bladder stone formation after sigmoidocolocystoplasty: statistical analysis of risk factors. J Pediatr Surg. 2005;40(2):407–11.
72. Institute of Medicine. Dietary reference intakes for water, potassium, sodium, chloride and sulfate. Washington, DC: National Academies Press; 2005. 73 p. Available from: http://scholar.google.com/scholar?hl=en&btnG=Search&q=intitle:DIETARY+REFERENCE+INTAKES#5
73. Palm SJ. Pelvic organ prolapse comorbids: intersect that complicates care. Female Pelvic Med Reconstr Surg. 2018;24(5):S154. Available from: http://www.embase.com/search/results?subaction=viewrecord&from=export&id=L627772672
74. Hendrix SL, Clark A, Nygaard I, Aragaki A, Barnabei V, McTiernan A. Pelvic organ prolapse in the Women's Health Initiative: gravity and gravidity. Am J Obstet Gynecol. 2002;186(6):1160–6.
75. Liu JS, Vo AX, Doolittle J, Hamoui N, Lewicky-Gaupp C, Kielb SJ. Characterizing pelvic organ prolapse in adult spina bifida patients. Urology. 2016;97:273–6.
76. Khavari R, Tokaz MC, Stewart JN, Boone TB. Pelvic organ prolapse in female patients presenting to transitional urology care clinic. J Urol. 2015;194(6):1654–8.
77. Berndl A, Nosek M, Waddington A. Women's health guidelines for the care of people with spina bifida. J Pediatr Rehabil Med. 2020;13(4):655–62.
78. Choi EK, Kim SW, Ji Y, Lim S-W, Han SW. Sexual function and quality of life in women with spina bifida: are the women with spina bifida satisfied with their sexual activity? NeurourolUrodyn. 2018;37(5):1785–93.
79. Gamé X, Moscovici J, Guillotreau J, Roumiguié M, Rischmann P, Malavaud B. Sexual function of young women with myelomeningocele. J Pediatr Urol. 2014;10(3):418–23.
80. Cardenas DD, Topolski TD, White CJ, McLaughlin JF, Walker WO. Sexual functioning in adolescents and young adults with spina bifida. Arch Phys Med Rehabil. 2008;89(1):31–5.
81. Gamé X, Moscovici J, Gamé L, Sarramon JP, Rischmann P, Malavaud B. Evaluation of sexual function in young men with spina bifida and myelomeningocele using the International Index of Erectile Function. Urology. 2006;67(3):566–70.
82. Tong CMC, Tanaka ST. Let's talk about sex: special considerations in reproductive care and sexual edu-

cation in young women with spina bifida. Urology. 2021;151:79–85.
83. Sivarajah K, Relph S, Sabaratnam R, Bakalis S. Spina bifida in pregnancy: A review of the evidence for preconception, antenatal, intrapartum and postpartum care. Obstet Med. 2019;12(1):14–21. Available from: http://www.embase.com/search/results?subaction=viewrecord&from=export&id=L622315615
84. Shepard CL, Yan PL, Kielb SJ, Wittmann DA, Quint EH, Kraft KH, et al. Complications of delivery among mothers with spina bifida. Urology. 2019;123:280–6.
85. Arata M, Grover S, Dunne K, Bryan D. Pregnancy outcome and complications in women with spina bifida. J Reprod Med Obstet Gynecol. 2000;45(9):743–8.
86. Trinh A, Wong P, Brown J, Hennel S, Ebeling PR, Fuller PJ, et al. Fractures in spina bifida from childhood to young adulthood. Osteoporos Int. 2017;28(1):399–406.
87. Marreiros H, Marreiros HF, Loff C, Calado E. Osteoporosis in paediatric patients with spina bifida. J Spinal Cord Med. 2012;35(1):9–21.
88. Cai B, McDermott S, Wang YD, Royer JA, Mann JR, Hardin JW, et al. Skin ulcers and mortality among adolescents and young adults with spina bifida in South Carolina during 2000–2010. J Child Neurol. 2016;31(3):370–7.
89. Kim S, Ward E, Dicianno BE, Clayton GH, Sawin KJ, Beierwaltes P, et al. Factors associated with pressure ulcers in individuals with spina bifida. Arch Phys Med Rehabil. 2015;96(8):1435–41.e1.
90. Mann JR, Royer JA, Turk MA, McDermott S, Holland MM, Ozturk O, et al. Inpatient and emergency room visits for adolescents and young adults with spina bifida. PM R. 2015;7(5):499–511.
91. Beierwaltes P, Munoz S, Wilhelmy J. Integument: guidelines for the care of people with spina bifida. J Pediatr Rehabil Med. 2020;13(4):543–8.
92. Dicianno BE, Gaines A, Collins DM, Lee S. Mobility, assistive technology use, and social integration among adults with spina bifida. Am J Phys Med Rehabil. 2009;88:533–41.
93. Wilson PE, Mukherjee S. Mobility guidelines for the care of people with spina bifida. J Pediatr Rehabil Med. 2020;13(4):621–7.
94. Liampas A, Neophytou P, Sokratous M, Varrassi G, Ioannou C, Hadjigeorgiou GM, et al. Musculoskeletal pain due to wheelchair use: a systematic review and meta-analysis. Pain Ther. 2021;10(2):973–84.
95. Conklin MJ, Kishan S, Nanayakkara CB, Rosenfeld SR. Orthopedic guidelines for the care of people with spina bifida. J Pediatr Rehabil Med. 2020;13(4):629–35.
96. Ollesch B, Brazell C, Carry PM, Georgopoulos G. Complications, results, and risk factors of spinal fusion in patients with myelomeningocele. Spine Deform. 2018;6(4):460–6.
97. Mummareddy N, Dewan MC, Mercier MR, Naftel RP, Wellons JC, Bonfield CM. Scoliosis in myelomeningocele: epidemiology, management, and functional outcome. J Neurosurg Pediatr. 2017;20(1):99–108.
98. Gunay H, Sozbilen MC, Gurbuz Y, Altinisik M, Buyukata B. Incidence and type of foot deformities in patients with spina bifida according to level of lesion. Childs Nerv Syst. 2016;32(2):315–9.
99. Buffart LM, van den Berg-Emons RJ, Burdorf A, Janssen WG, Stam HJ, Roebroeck ME. Cardiovascular disease risk factors and the relationships with physical activity, aerobic fitness, and body fat in adolescents and young adults with myelomeningocele. Arch Phys Med Rehabil. 2008;89(11):2167–73.
100. Buffart LM, van den Berg-Emons RJG, van Mechelen W, van Meeteren J, van der Slot W, Stam HJ, et al. Promoting physical activity in an adolescent and a young adult with physical disabilities. Disabil Health J. 2010;3(2):86–92.
101. Cope H, McMahon K, Heise E, Eubanks S, Garrett M, Gregory S, et al. Outcome and life satisfaction of adults with myelomeningocele. Disabil Health J. 2013;6(3):236–43.
102. Parekh AD, Trusler LA, Pietsch JB, Byrne DW, DeMarco RT, Pope JC, et al. Prospective, longitudinal evaluation of health related quality of life in the pediatric spina bifida population undergoing reconstructive urological surgery. J Urol. 2006;176:1878–82.
103. Liptak GS, Kennedy JA, Dosa NP. Youth with spina bifida and transitions: health and social participation in a nationally represented sample. J Pediatr. 2010;157(4):584–8. 588.e1
104. Bellin MH, Dicianno BE, Osteen P, Dosa N, Aparicio E, Braun P, et al. Family satisfaction, pain, and quality-of-life in emerging adults with spina bifida: a longitudinal analysis. Am J Phys Med Rehabil. 2013;92(1):641–55.
105. Lemelle JL, Guillemin F, Aubert D, Guys JM, Lottmann H, Lortat-Jacob S, et al. Quality of life and continence in patients with spina bifida. Qual Life Res. 2006;15(9):1481–92.
106. Barf HA, Post MWM, Verhoef M, Gooskens RHJM, Prevo AJH. Is cognitive functioning associated with subjective quality of life in young adults with spina bifida and hydrocephalus? J Rehabil Med. 2010;42(1):56–9.
107. Sawin KJ, Brei TJ, Houtrow AJ. Quality of life: guidelines for the care of people with spina bifida. J Pediatr Rehabil Med. 2020;13(4):565–82.

## Suggested Reading

Guidelines for the Care of People with Spina Bifida (n.d.) https://www.spinabifidaassociation.org/guidelines/

# Inherited Metabolic Disorders 39

Jordan Kemere, Claudia Soler-Alfonso,
and Lindsay Burrage

## Case Presentation

A 20-year-old female with a history of phenylketonuria (PKU), anxiety, depression, obesity, and irregular menses comes to clinic for a health prevention visit. Her PKU was diagnosed by the state newborn screening program in infancy, and she was followed by a metabolic physician for many years. However, her last visit with a metabolic physician or dietitian was at 17 years of age. Since that time, she was lost to follow-up because of a lack of insurance. She has been consuming an unrestricted diet, and she has not monitored her phenylalanine or tyrosine levels in the last 3–4 years. Her anxiety and depression were diagnosed two years ago, but she is no longer taking medication or seeing a therapist. Given that she has not had a period for more than 3 months, a urine pregnancy test is performed and is positive.

J. Kemere (✉)
Department of Internal Medicine, Baylor College of Medicine, Houston, TX, USA
e-mail: kemere@bcm.edu

C. Soler-Alfonso · L. Burrage
Department of Molecular & Human Genetics, Baylor College of Medicine, Houston, TX, USA

## Case Discussion

Phenylketonuria (PKU) is an inborn error of metabolism due to deficiency of phenylalanine hydroxylase, the enzyme responsible for converting phenylalanine to tyrosine. As a result of enzyme deficiency, phenylalanine levels are elevated, and tyrosine levels are low. When untreated, PKU is associated with intellectual disability, decreased skin and hair pigmentation, abnormal odor, and eczema. However, early initiation and maintenance of a phenylalanine-restricted diet prevent the sequelae of the disorder [1]. As a result, newborn screening was introduced to facilitate early diagnosis and therapy for infants with this diagnosis. The maintenance of phenylalanine levels within the target range of 2–6 mg/dL is recommended throughout the lifespan. Relaxation of the diet and secondary, chronic elevations in phenylalanine levels are associated with neuropsychiatric complications in adulthood (e.g., depression, anxiety, attention issues, and tremors), [1] and adherence to dietary restrictions can be very challenging for individuals with PKU. In addition, phenylalanine is a teratogen and levels above the target range in females during pregnancy can lead to increased risk for intellectual disability, intrauterine growth restriction, microcephaly, and cardiac defects in their unaffected infants. Thus, phenylalanine levels in the target range are recommended prior to and throughout pregnancy. Individuals with PKU are


A. A. Kuo et al. (eds.), *Care of Adults with Chronic Childhood Conditions*,
https://doi.org/10.1007/978-3-031-54281-7_39

at high risk of being lost to follow-up in the adolescent and early adult years [1] due to a variety of factors including a paucity of adult metabolic providers, insurance issues, and challenges with adherence to therapy. As a result, patients may discontinue dietary restrictions and phenylalanine level monitoring. Moreover, these individuals are unable to take advantage of new dietary and medical therapies that are introduced in the intervening years, and opportunities for genetic counseling and caution regarding maternal PKU risks are missed. In the presented case, untreated PKU is the most likely contributor to her anxiety and depression. Her pregnancy is at high risk for the sequelae of maternal PKU. Thus, a phenylalanine level should be checked as soon as possible, and she should be referred to a metabolic physician and dietitian for management. If the patient is not under the care of a metabolic specialist, contacting the newborn screening state lab can be the initial step to receive guidance on treatment and referrals. In addition, counseling regarding the risks for maternal PKU and recurrence risks for PKU should be provided, and she should be referred to maternal–fetal medicine given that the pregnancy is at high risk for congenital anomalies, including cardiac defects. An introduction to a PKU family support group and available financial resources for dietary management may be helpful including an immediate social work consultation.

## Overview of Inborn Errors of Metabolism

Inborn errors of metabolism are a group of more than 1400 inherited disorders that typically affect either an enzyme, transporter, or other protein involved in a biochemical pathway [2]. Although individual inborn errors of metabolism are rare, estimates suggest an overall prevalence of ~1:1000 to ~1:2000 live births [3]. The presentation for these disorders varies, and the age of onset ranges from infancy to adulthood. In the last several decades, the development of expanded newborn screening and increased utilization of molecular and biochemical testing have led to improved recognition and diagnosis of these disorders. Although treatment for some inborn errors of metabolism is limited to supportive care, a growing list of therapies including nutritional therapies, enzyme replacement, pharmaceuticals, and even organ transplantation are available for a subset of these disorders. Moreover, as these disorders are associated with a variety of inheritance patterns, genetic counseling is important for individuals with inborn errors of metabolism as they approach reproductive age. Thus, as a growing population of individuals with inborn errors of metabolism is entering adulthood, an awareness of these disorders by adult providers is necessary.

## Major Categories of Inborn Errors of Metabolism

The inborn errors of metabolism can affect a wide variety of biochemical pathways. To date, there are >20 different groups of inborn errors of metabolism [2] with a subset of the most common groups of disorders presented in Table 39.1. Some inborn errors, such as urea cycle disorders and organic acidemias can present with an acute, life-threatening metabolic intoxication phenotype whereas others are associated with more chronic complications. Many of these disorders have late-onset forms that may not be recognized and diagnosed until a patient reaches adulthood. Moreover, individuals with a subset of disorders require surveillance for age-related complications such as tumors in adulthood or monitoring for complications during pregnancy. Thus, a successful transition to providers familiar with their diagnosis is necessary to prevent poor morbidity and mortality associated with these disorders.

**Table 39.1** Common inborn errors of metabolism

| Disorder category | Common disorders (inheritance pattern) | Therapeutic strategies |
|---|---|---|
| Urea cycle disorders | Ornithine transcarbamylase deficiency (XL)<br>Citrullinemia Type 1 (AR)<br>Argininosuccinic aciduria (ASL deficiency)<br>Arginase deficiency (AR) | Protein-restricted diet, nitrogen scavenging agents, amino acid supplementation, liver transplantation |
| Amino acid disorders | Phenylketonuria (AR) | Phenylalanie-restricted diet, Glycomacropeptide, Sapropterin,<br>enzyme substitution therapy (Pegvaliase, adults only) |
| | Homocystinuria (AR) | Vitamin supplementation, protein-restricted diet, Betaine |
| | Maple syrup urine disease (AR) | Branched-chain amino acid-restricted diet, Isoleucine + Valine supplementation (if needed), liver transplantation |
| | Tyrosinemia (AR) | Nitisinone, low tyrosine diet, liver transplantation |
| Organic acidemias | Propionic acidemia (AR)<br>Methylmalonic acidemia (AR) | Protein-restricted diet, levocarnitine, vitamin supplementation (if responsive), antibiotic therapy. Liver transplantation, kidney transplantation (in some cases for MMA only) |
| Vitamin disorders | Biotinidase deficiency | Biotin supplementation |
| | Cobalamin disorders | Hydroxocobalamin, betaine, and other vitamin supplementation |
| Fatty acid oxidation disorders | Medium-Chain Acyl-CoA Dehydrogenase Deficiency (MCAD) | Heart healthy diet. Avoid prolonged fasting. Carnitine supplementation |
| | Very-Long-Chain Acyl-CoA Dehydrogenase Deficiency (VLCAD) | Low long chain fat diet. Medium Chain Triglycerides supplementation or triheptanoin. Avoidance of prolonged fasting and severe exercise. |
| | Carnitine palmitoyltransferase II deficiency | High carbohydrate, low fat diet<br>+/- Levocarnitine supplementation. Medium Chain Triglycerides or triheptanoin. Avoidance of prolonged fasting. |
| Transport disorders | Primary carnitine deficiency | Levocarnitine supplementation |
| Lysosomal storage disorders | Gaucher disease | Enzyme replacement therapy, substrate reduction therapy |
| | Fabry disease | Enzyme replacement therapy, chaperone therapy |
| | Morquio syndrome | Enzyme replacement therapy (Morquio A) |
| | Marateaux-Lamy syndrome | Enzyme replacement therapy |
| Mitochondrial disorders | Various mt-DNA-encoded (e.g. MELAS) and nuclear-encoded disorders | Supportive therapy, vitamin supplementation. Citrulline/arginine supplements (MELAS) |
| Carbohydrate disorders | Galactosemia | Galactose and Lactose-restricted diet |
| | Glycogen storage disorder Type 1a | Frequent feeds, corn starch and modified corn starch products. Sucrose/Fructose/Galactose avoidance |
| Congenital disorders of glycosylation | PMM2-CDG | Supportive Care |
| | MPI-CDG | Mannose |

A list of a select inborn errors of metabolism that may be encountered in adulthood is provided. This list is not comprehensive but includes a sampling of disorders to highlight the diverse subtypes of inborn errors of metabolism and various therapeutic strategies that may be used

## Expanded Newborn Screening

Newborn screening was introduced when Dr. Robert Guthrie developed an inexpensive, reliable, biochemical screening assay that could detect elevated phenylalanine, the offending metabolite in PKU, using whole blood spots from infants [4]. This simple biochemical assay served as the basis for population screening of newborns for this disorder to facilitate early diagnosis and initiation of dietary therapy in the presymptomatic period. With the success of PKU screening, additional individual disorders were added to the newborn screening panel over the next several decades. In the early 2000s, tandem mass spectrometry revolutionized newborn screening allowing the detection of multiple metabolites simultaneously. As a result, state newborn screening panels now include >30 disorders with new disorders continuing to be added each year. As therapies are available for many of these disorders, the individuals who have benefited from expanded newborn screening are entering adulthood.

## Therapies for Inborn Errors of Metabolism

### Nutritional Therapy

Nutritional interventions are a common therapeutic strategy for many inborn errors of metabolism [5]. These interventions may include dietary restriction of a toxic metabolite or supplementation with deficient metabolites. In some cases, special medical formulas may be used to ensure adequate nutritional intake while preventing excess consumption of toxic metabolites. To prevent malnutrition, special low-protein medical foods are available for patients who require a low protein diet. As vitamins serve as cofactors for various enzymes, vitamin supplementation may also be used in some disorders. When nutritional interventions are used, patients are carefully monitored by metabolic dietitians to prevent nutritional or vitamin deficiencies and to monitor micronutrient and macronutrient intake. As adherence to restricted diets can be challenging as patients grow into adulthood due to the cost and availability of foods and medical formulas, education about the necessity of the nutritional therapy should begin early, and resources (e.g., financial) to facilitate adherence should be provided.

### Pharmaceutical Therapy

An increasing number of pharmaceutical agents are available for various inborn errors of metabolism. These therapies may include synthetic cofactors for enzymes that promote enzyme activity, scavenging therapies that prevent accumulation of toxic metabolites, enzyme replacement therapies, and substrate reduction therapies. With the increasing number of clinical trials in rare metabolic disorders, the number of FDA-approved therapies for this group of disorders is expected to grow. Continuity of care in these disorders is led by medical geneticists with further training in inborn errors of metabolism available in metabolic clinics. This allows adults to be made aware of any new or emerging therapeutic agents that become available for their diagnosis.

### Transplantation

Solid organ transplantation or hematopoietic stem cell transplantation are increasingly used as therapeutic strategies in several inborn errors of metabolism [6]. For instance, liver transplantation eliminates the risk for hyperammonemia from urea cycle dysfunction secondary to urea cycle disorders [7]. Likewise, liver ± kidney transplantation has been associated with a reduced number of episodes of metabolic decompensation in organic acidemias [8, 9] Liver transplantation prevents metabolic decompensations associated with elevated leucine in maple syrup urine disease [10]. Liver transplantation has also been used in tyrosinemia type 1 and glycogen storage disorders, typically in the setting of liver adenomas given the increased risk for hepatocellular carcinoma or failure of medical management [11, 12]. Hematopoietic stem cell transplantation is beneficial in a subset of lysosomal storage disorders and X-linked adrenoleukodystrophy [13]. It is important to recognize that transplantation does not necessarily lead to amelioration of all phenotypes associated with inborn errors of metabolism and thus, routine follow-up for long-term complications may be necessary in addition to routine post-transplantation management.

## Special Considerations

### Neuropsychiatric Illness and Neurocognitive Effects

Neuropsychiatric illness and neurocognitive deficits are common features of many inherited metabolic disorders as approximately 85% primarily affect the nervous system [14]. Some conditions can cause developmental delays, intellectual disability, and/or neurodegeneration [15] whereas others may cause neurocognitive impairments, such as deficits in executive function, processing speed, visuospatial functions, and language [16–19]. A subset of inherited metabolic conditions can initially present in adolescence or adulthood with psychiatric symptoms, such as adrenoleukodystrophy, Neimann Pick type C disease, maple syrup urine disease, or certain urea cycle disorders [20]. In individuals with certain inherited metabolic disorders, optimal medical management is necessary to prevent worsening of psychiatric and neurological symptoms.

### Emergency Management

A subset of disorders, such as the urea cycle disorders and organic acidemias, are associated with an increased risk for acute metabolic intoxication in the setting of catabolic stress, intercurrent illness, or dietary non-adherence. Similarly, individuals with glycogen storage disorders may be at risk for life-threatening hypoglycemia during illness or inadequate intake, while strenuous physical activity can elevate the risk of rhabdomyolysis in certain fatty acid oxidation disorders. These episodes of metabolic decompensation can occur at any age. Depending on the disorder, the patient may present with nausea and vomiting, poor appetite, lethargy, altered mental status, muscle pain, seizures, or coma. Laboratories may show severe acidosis, hypoglycemia, hyperammonemia, lactic acidosis, elevated creatine kinase (CK), or acute kidney or liver failure. Individuals with metabolic disorders associated with acute metabolic decompensation are encouraged to wear an emergency bracelet and are encouraged to carry an emergency letter that outlines an initial approach to their resuscitation and care including medications to avoid, if relevant. This emergency letter should also contain emergency contact information for their metabolic providers who can provide consultation regarding management. If surgery is necessary, precautions may be needed to prevent catabolic stress and associated metabolic decompensation in the perioperative period. Thus, consultation with the metabolic provider is recommended prior to admission to the inpatient ward or intensive care unit and prior to all emergent or planned procedures for appropriate management recommendations. Table 39.2 provides examples of considerations during hospitalization for individuals with inborn errors of metabolism. Furthermore, primary care providers should have a written care plan in place in advance of any hospitalization for unique needs during a hospital stay. These care plans should be formed in collaboration with a geneticist, the patient, and the patient's supporters.

### Sexual Health and Contraception

Sexual health is an important aspect of long-term follow-up in individuals with chronic conditions as well as those with intellectual disabilities (IDD). Young people with chronic conditions including intellectual disability may engage in consensual romantic relationships and should discuss these relationships with their physicians. In addition, prevalence rates of sexual abuse in individuals with IDD range from 7% to 34% in adults [21]. Discussion regarding sexual health as well as contraception if desired should begin prior to healthcare transition to adulthood and should continue in the adult healthcare setting on a regular basis. Age-appropriate screening for sexually transmitted infections and cervical cancer should be discussed with individuals and their supporters to assess for desire for screening and understanding of test procedures (e.g., Pap smear).

**Table 39.2** Considerations during hospitalization for select inborn errors of metabolism

| Diagnosis | Hospital consideration |
|---|---|
| Phenylketonuria (PKU) | Avoid aspartame-containing medications. Continue specialized metabolic formula. |
| Maple syrup urine disease (MSUD) | Avoid prolonged fast; Monitor for elevated plasma leucine. Monitor sodium closely. |
| Homocystinuria | Increased risk for thromboembolism (especially in setting of elevated homocysteine). |
| Methylmalonic acidemia and propionic acidemia | Risk for metabolic acidosis and hyperammonemia; Avoid fasting. At risk of acute basal ganglia injury. |
| Glycogen storage disorder type 1a | Risk for life-threatening hypoglycemia; Strict adherence to dietary plan; Avoid fasting; Avoid abrupt discontinuation of fluids and/or feeds. |
| Glycogen storage disorder Type V | Avoid medications associated with malignant hyperthermia; Low threshold for evaluation for rhabdomyolysis. |
| Very long chain Acyl CoA dehydrogenase deficiency and carnitine Palmitoyltransferase II deficiency | Risk for rhabdomyolysis and cardiomyopathy. |
| Urea cycle disorders | Risk for hyperammonemia; Avoid corticosteroids (if possible) and valproic acid; Avoid skipped medication doses and precautions prior to procedures should be discussed with metabolic team; Avoid prolonged fast. |
| Mitochondrial disorders | Avoid valproic acid and other medications with mitochondrial toxicities; If on ketogenic diet, intravenous fluids should be discussed with metabolic team prior to initiation; Precautions prior to surgery. |

Examples of considerations during hospitalizations for select inborn errors of metabolism. This list is not all inclusive and consultation with the metabolic specialist is recommended for all individuals with inborn errors of metabolism

## Pre-conception Genetic Counseling and Pregnancy

While pre-conception genetic counseling is recommended for all women and their partners, such counseling is strongly advised for individuals with inborn errors of metabolism. Comprehensive genetic counseling will facilitate a review of the inheritance pattern associated with the genetic diagnosis, provide information about the associated recurrence risks, and provide an opportunity for questions. In addition, carrier screening can be offered, if relevant. For some inborn errors of metabolism, risks during pregnancy, childbirth, and/or the post-partum period should also be reviewed with the patient so that appropriate care can be provided before, during, and after pregnancy.

Dietary requirements change throughout pregnancy and may necessitate diet modifications in individuals with inherited metabolic disorders. Exacerbations of certain metabolic conditions may also masquerade as common symptoms of pregnancy (e.g., fatigue and nausea/vomiting) and thus require additional evaluation beyond supportive care that may be typically offered in pregnancy. Finally, certain conditions require changes in management (e.g., medication changes) during pregnancy and have higher risks of complications during pregnancy [22]. Depending on the condition, risks to the fetus may also exist. Many women may require a maternal-fetal medicine specialist to assist in the care along with their metabolic geneticist.

## Self-Management in Transition Age Adolescents and Adults

### Understanding Diagnosis

With increases in newborn screening and genetic testing in early childhood, many individuals received their diagnosis as infants or young children. As patients age into their teens, many have a limited understanding of their diagnosis and rationale for certain therapies/diet modifications.

In the early teen years, a review of the diagnosis is recommended in a setting that allows for patients and family members to ask questions and check understanding of the diagnosis and proposed treatments. An understanding of the diagnosis is critical for the development of self-management skills as well as understanding how to recognize emergency situations.

## Self-Management of Diet and Medication

Many young patients have had caregivers perform the daily management of their condition for their entire lives, including administering all medications and monitoring dietary intake and supplements. It is appropriate for individuals with inborn errors of metabolism to begin to learn how to manage their condition at a young age so that they can learn in a supervised environment. As with many other chronic conditions from childhood, individuals with metabolic conditions are less likely to be adhere to their care plan in adolescence [23] and are at increased risk of exacerbations of their medical disorder once they assume care of their condition independently. Self-management should be discussed and practiced many years before the transfer of that responsibility. Talking directly with adolescents at their routine visits and checking their own understanding and management is an important part of their medical visits. For those individuals who will always need significant caregiver support in care planning, it is also important that more than one individual understands and facilitates the plan in the event of emergencies or inevitable life changes.

## Decision-Making

Individuals with inborn errors of metabolism have a wide range of intellectual ability and decision-making capacity. While some disorders may be associated with intellectual disability, others may have no impact on cognitive development especially in the setting of optimal medical management or mild disease. In addition, where there are cognitive impacts, the deficits in some individuals may be mild and primarily impacting executive functioning and attention. However, in disorders associated with intoxication, decision-making during metabolic decompensation may be impacted even if the individual has minimal, if any, deficits at baseline.

Discussion about whether guardianship or a supportive decision-making agreement is appropriate should occur with physicians prior to the age of majority. For individuals who make decisions independently, establishing medical power of attorney once they reach adulthood is important as they may have fluctuations in their capacity with exacerbations of their illness.

## Insurance Considerations

Another important aspect of transition to adult healthcare is changes in health insurance. For individuals with inherited metabolic disorders, there are several unique concerns. Most patients regardless of age receive care from a metabolic geneticist working in a pediatric hospital [24] which may not be in network/accept some adult insurance plans resulting in a barrier to care. Even for patients with pediatric insurance, not all medical foods (such as modified low-protein foods) and supplements are covered by insurance and significant out of pocket costs exist for many families [25]. Some supplements that were covered by pediatric insurance are no longer covered under adult insurance, creating another barrier to receiving care.

## Resources

### Family Groups and Patient Groups

With improved genetic testing, the number of individuals receiving a genetic diagnosis is rapidly growing. As these disorders are rare, patients may find few other individuals with the same diagnosis in their own community. However, international diagnosis-specific family groups provide a source of community and wealth of resources that many families find helpful. These groups often have an online presence and may host online or in person conferences that allow for networking among families.

## Fact Sheets

Fact sheets are brief, disorder-specific sources of information directed at healthcare providers. These can be particularly helpful for rare diseases, offering healthcare providers basic details of a condition along with important nuances such as medications to avoid or additional screening recommendations. If possible, patients should carry a disease-specific fact sheet with them to new doctor's visits or emergency room visits. There are some fact sheets accessible online or metabolic geneticists can create their own fact sheets for their patients.

### Rare Disease Information

Finally, it is important to know where to find reliable information. In addition to condition-specific review papers, websites such as NIH GeneReviews (https://www.ncbi.nlm.nih.gov/books/NBK1116/) and National Organization of Rare Disorders (NORD, https://rarediseases.org/) are helpful resources for adult providers to learn aboutrare genetic diagnoses.

**Facts sheets**

| Inherited metabolic disorders condition fact sheet | |
|---|---|
| Definition | Inherited metabolic disorders are a group of >1400 inherited disorders that typically affect either an enzyme, transporter, or other protein involved in a biochemical pathway.<br>• The presentation for these disorders varies as there are >20 different groups of inborn errors of metabolism. Some of the more common inherited metabolic disorders can be found in Table 39.1.<br>• Some inherited metabolic disorders can present with an acute, life-threatening metabolic intoxication phenotype whereas others are associated with more chronic complications.<br>• Individuals may or may not have co-occurring intellectual disability<br>• Therapy options are growing and include nutritional therapies, enzyme replacement, pharmaceuticals, and organ transplantation for a subset of these disorders. |
| Epidemiology | Estimates suggest an overall incidence of 1:1000–1:2000 live births<br>• The age of onset ranges from infancy to adulthood, and many disorders have late-onset forms that may not be recognized and diagnosed until an individual reaches adulthood.<br>• State newborn screening panels now include >30 disorders with more being added.<br>• Life expectancy varies with different disorders and their comorbidities. |
| Challenges in Transition | • Many teens and young adults have a poor understanding of their diagnosis and rationale for certain therapies/diet modifications.<br>• Many individuals have exacerbations of their disorder as they takeover self-management of therapies and diet.<br>• Specialized therapies and supplements are harder to access as an adult if that individual is uninsured or under-insured. |
| Special considerations | Individuals with inherited metabolic conditions can have a variety of comorbid physical and mental health conditions depending on the condition.<br>• Neuropsychiatric illness and neurocognitive deficits are common features of many inherited metabolic disorders as approximately 85% primarily affect the nervous system.<br>• For those disorders that can have acute metabolic intoxication which is life-threatening, patients are encouraged to wear emergency bracelets and carry emergency letters to aid emergency room and hospital physicians in the unique needs of that patient. Metabolic geneticists should be consulted when patients present to the hospital with acute exacerbations.<br>• Sexual health should be regularly discussed with individuals that have inherited metabolic disorders. Contraception, if pregnancy is not desired, should be offered to patients.<br>• Pre-conception genetic counselling should be offered to all individuals with inherited metabolic disorders.<br>• Some disorders may require close monitoring as well as changes in management during pregnancy, necessitating a maternal-fetal medicine specialist and close consultation with a metabolic geneticist. |

## References


1. Vockley J, Andersson HC, Antshel KM, Braverman NE, Burton BK, Frazier DM, Mitchell J, Smith WE, Thompson BH, Berry SA. American College of Medical Genetics and Genomics Therapeutics Committee. Phenylalanine hydroxylase deficiency: diagnosis and management guideline. Genet Med. 2014;16(2):188–200.
2. Ferreira CR, Rahman S, Keller M, Zschocke J, ICIMD Advisory Group. An international classification of inherited metabolic disorders (ICIMD). J Inherit Metab Dis. 2021;44(1):164–77.
3. Waters D, Adeloye D, Woolham D, Wastnedge E, Patel S, Rudan I. Global birth prevalence and mortality from inborn errors of metabolism: a systematic analysis of the evidence. J Glob Health. 2018;8(2):021102.
4. Guthrie R. Blood screening for phenylketonuria. JAMA. 1961;178(8):863.
5. Boyer SW, Barclay LJ, Burrage LC. Inherited metabolic disorders: aspects of chronic nutrition management. Nutr Clin Pract. 2015;30(4):502–10.
6. Sirrs S, Hannah-Shmouni F, Nantel S, Neuberger J, Yoshida EM. Transplantation as disease modifying therapy in adults with inherited metabolic disorders. J Inherit Metab Dis. 2018;41(5):885–96.
7. Yu L, Rayhill SC, Hsu EK, Landis CS. Liver transplantation for urea cycle disorders: analysis of the united network for organ sharing database. Transplant Proc. 2015;47(8):2413–8.
8. Zhou GP, Jiang YZ, Wu SS, Kong YY, Sun LY, Zhu ZJ. Liver transplantation for propionic acidemia: evidence from a systematic review and meta-analysis. Transplantation. 2021;105(10):2272–82.
9. Jiang YZ, Zhou GP, Wu SS, Kong YY, Zhu ZJ, Sun LY. Safety and efficacy of liver transplantation for methylmalonic acidemia: a systematic review and meta-analysis. Transplant Rev (Orlando). 2021;35(1):100592.
10. Ewing CB, Soltys KA, Strauss KA, Sindhi R, Vockley J, McKiernan P, Squires RH, Bond G, Ganoza A, Khanna A, Mazariegos GV, Squires JE. Metabolic Control and "Ideal" outcomes in liver transplantation for Maple syrup urine disease. J Pediatr. 2021;237:59–64.e1.
11. Arnon R, Annunziato R, Miloh T, Wasserstein M, Sogawa H, Wilson M, Suchy F, Kerkar N. Liver transplantation for hereditary tyrosinemia type I: analysis of the UNOS database. Pediatr Transplant. 2011;15(4):400–5.
12. Ziogas IA, Tasoudis PT, Serifis N, Alexopoulos SP, Montenovo MI, Shingina A. Liver transplantation for hepatic adenoma: a UNOS database analysis and systematic review of the literature. Transplant Direct. 2022;8(2):e1264.
13. Tan EY, Boelens JJ, Jones SA, Wynn RF. Hematopoietic stem cell transplantation in inborn errors of metabolism. Front Pediatr. 2019;7:433.
14. Mochel F, Sedel F. Inborn errors of metabolism in adults: a diagnostic approach to neurological and psychiatric presentations. In: Saudubray JM, Baumgartner MR, Walker J, editors. Inborn metabolic diseases. Germany: Springer-Verlag GmbH; 2016. p. 71–89.
15. Saudubray JM, Garcia-Cazorla A. An overview of inborn errors of metabolism affecting the brain: from neurodevelopment to neurodegenerative disorders. Dialogues Clin Neurosci. 2018;20(4):301–25.
16. Blundell J, Frisson S, Chakrapani A, Kearney S, Vijay S, MacDonald A, Olson A. Markers of cognitive function in patients with metabolic disease: Morquio syndrome and tyrosinemia type III. Cogn Neuropsychol. 2018;35(3-4):120–47. https://doi.org/10.1080/02643294.2018.1443913.
17. De Felice S, Romani C, Geberhiwot T, MacDonald A, Palermo L. Language processing and executive functions in early treated adults with PKU. Cogn Neuropsychol. 2018;35(3-4):148–70.
18. Potter NL, Lazarus JAC, Johnson JM, Steiner RD, Shriberg LD. Correlates of language impairment in children with galactosaemia. J Inherited Metab Dis. 2008;31:524–32.
19. Heitz C, Epelbaum S, Nadjar Y. Cognitive impairment profile in adult patients with Niemann pick type C disease. Orphanet J Rare Dis. 2017;12:16.
20. Walterfang M, Bonnot O, Mocellin R, Velakoulis D. The neuropsychiatry of inborn errors of metabolism. J Inherit Metab Dis. 2013;36(4):687–702.
21. Lin L-P, Yen C-F, Kuo F-Y, Jia-Ling W, Lin J-D. Sexual assault of people with disabilities: results of a 2002–2007 national report in Taiwan. Res Dev Disabil. 2009;30(5):969–75.
22. Preece MA, Green A. Pregnancy and inherited metabolic disorders: maternal and fetal complications. Ann Clin Biochem. 2002;39(Pt 5):444–55.
23. MaCdonald A, van Rijn M, Feillet F, Lund AM, Bernstein L, Bosch AM, Gizewska M, van Spronsen FJ. Adherence issues in inherited metabolic disorders treated by low natural protein diets. Ann Nutr Metab. 2012;61(4):289–95.
24. Gold JI, Gold NB, Strong A, Tully E, Xiao R, Schwartz LA, Ficicioglu C. The current state of adult metabolic medicine in the United States: results of a nationwide survey. Genet Med. 2022;24(8):1722–31. S1098-3600(22)00747-X
25. Berry SA, Kenney MK, Harris KB, Singh RH, Cameron CA, Kraszewski JN, Levy-Fisch J, Shuger JF, Greene CL, Lloyd-Puryear MA, Boyle CA. Insurance coverage of medical foods for treatment of inherited metabolic disorders. Genet Med. 2013;15(12):978–82.

# 40 Endocrine Disorders

Courtney N. Sandler and Kaitlyn R. Shank

## Introduction

Endocrinology is a subspecialty rich in the breadth of diagnoses for which patients are managed across their lifespan. As diabetes mellitus, cancer survivorship, and transgender management are addressed elsewhere in this guide, this chapter focuses on more widely encountered endocrine conditions with unique aspects related to the management of young adults: congenital adrenal hyperplasia (CAH) with additional discussion on how to treat adrenal insufficiency from any etiology; Turner syndrome (TS); hypothyroidism and hyperthyroidism with a particular focus on pregnancy and conception counseling related to these disorders; and polycystic ovary syndrome (PCOS).

C. N. Sandler (✉)
Division of Endocrinology, Diabetes, and Hypertension, Brigham and Women's Hospital, Boston, MA, USA
e-mail: cnsandler@bwh.harvard.edu

K. R. Shank
Departments of Medicine and Pediatrics, Brigham and Women's Hospital, Boston, MA, USA
e-mail: kshank@bwh.harvard.edu

## Congential Adrenal Hyperplasia

### Case Presentation

Sara, age 25, and Brian, age 23, are siblings with salt-wasting CAH due to 21-hydroxylase deficiency. Sara was diagnosed when she was found to have ambiguous genitalia at birth, with work-up notable for elevated 17-hydroxyprogesterone and genetic testing consistent with a mutation in CYP21A2; Brian received a prenatal diagnosis through chorionic villus sampling. While both were treated from infancy with hydrocortisone and fludrocortisone, since early adolescence adherence has been a challenge for which they were transitioned to prednisone given its longer half-life compared to hydrocortisone. More recently, Brian has spurts of adherence alternating with non-adherence and routinely misses his evening prednisone dose. Sara has been diligent in her dosing since moving out of their family home for college at age 18, particularly as she achieved better control of bothersome symptoms of acne and hirsutism on optimized treatment. While Brian's recent visits have focused on medication adherence, Sara, who identifies as cisgender, has newly begun to explore the possibility of clitoral reduction and labioplasty, procedures deferred by her parents during Sara's infancy to allow her ownership regarding surgical decision-making in adulthood. She has a supportive sexual partner but has anxiety about the appearance of



A. A. Kuo et al. (eds.), *Care of Adults with Chronic Childhood Conditions*,
https://doi.org/10.1007/978-3-031-54281-7_40

her genitalia and thus has avoided routine gynecologic care including Papanicolaou smears.

## Case Discussion

Adherence can be a significant challenge faced by patients with CAH, both with respect to medication administration and medical follow-up [1–4]. Patients with classic CAH have underlying glucocorticoid and mineralocorticoid insufficiency from 21-hydroxylase deficiency, such that steroids are life-sustaining therapy. During periods of illness, failure to take adequate stress-dose steroids can result in hospitalization and mortality. Many young adults with CAH have not been adequately educated regarding the life-threatening nature of their diagnosis and the appropriate administration of stress dose-steroids, as these topics may have been primarily discussed with their caregivers in early life [5]. This is particularly concerning, given that loss to follow-up with endocrinology is well documented in studies of the young adult CAH population [2–4]. Primary care providers (PCPs) may therefore take on the roles of prescribing medications and educating on adrenal sick-day plans. In addition to adrenal replacement, steroids are necessary for preventing shifts to adrenal androgen production. Undertreatment may result in bothersome acne, hirsutism, and ongoing masculinization of external genitalia in female patients. Steroids are likewise important in preventing the development of adrenal rest tumors in testes and ovaries, tumors which can result in hypogonadism and infertility [6, 7]. Lack of adherence can therefore have significant adverse health effects for patients such as Brian.

In Sara's case, anxiety about the appearance of her genitalia has adversely affected her mental health and prevented her from getting routine health screening. In the past, surgical management of ambiguous genitalia often began in infancy. More recently, patient and family advocacy groups as well as individual medical centers have advocated policies of holding surgical management until patients can meaningfully participate in discussion, provided anatomical differences place no threat to physical health. This is currently an area of controversy in CAH management [6, 8].

### CAH Prevalence, Underlying Pathophysiology, and Diagnosis

CAH defines a set of autosomal recessive disorders caused by defects in adrenal steroidogenesis, with an incidence of 1:14,000–1:18,000 births. Ninety-five percent of cases are caused by a mutation in the 21-hydroxylase enzyme encoded by the CYP21A2 gene [6]. Less common subtypes of CAH, such as 11-hydroxylase and 17-hydroxylase deficiency, likewise cause defects in steroidogenesis and/or ambiguous genitalia but will not be explored further in this chapter. Enzymatic defects in 21-hydroxylase result in ineffective synthesis of cortisol and aldosterone from their precursors, while ongoing adrenal stimulation by the hypothalamic and pituitary axis leads to diversion of cortisol precursors into androgen biosynthesis. Depending on the degree of enzymatic malfunction, CAH severity can therefore range in presentation from the most to least severe forms ranging from classic salt-wasting to simple virilizing to nonclassical. Patients with classic CAH have lifetime glucocorticoid and mineralocorticoid requirement. Female infants with classic CAH will have virilization of external genitalia at birth, while male infants who are not salt-wasting may not be diagnosed until they are noted to have signs of advanced skeletal maturation or premature adrenarche in childhood. Patients with nonclassical CAH (NCAH) tend to have intact glucocorticoid and mineralocorticoid axes and are diagnosed later in life. In childhood, this diagnosis may arise due to evidence of premature adrenarche and advanced skeletal maturation in both sexes. In post-pubertal females, evidence of hyperandrogenism, irregular menses, and/or infertility may lead to a diagnosis of NCAH or misdiagnosis as PCOS [6, 9].

### Management of Steroid Replacement in CAH and General Adrenal Insufficiency

Adult patients with classic CAH require lifelong daily glucocorticoid replacement both for physiologic replacement of adrenal insufficiency and for androgen suppression. Balancing the need for androgen suppression with the risk of glucocorticoid over-replacement can be challenging. Oral hydrocortisone divided in to 2–3 doses per day is the preferred treatment due to its shorter half-life and therefore diminished risk of steroid over-replacement. Guidelines for hydrocortisone use in CAH do not specify fractionation of dosing, although dosing tends to be more evenly distributed to suppress overnight adrenocorticotropic hormone (ACTH) stimulation of androgens. This is distinct from the use of hydrocortisone for adrenal insufficiency outside of CAH, in which higher doses are recommended in the early morning with sequential dose decreases during the day to mimic the circadian rhythm of endogenous cortisol production. Longer-acting steroids in place of hydrocortisone can be useful to help with adherence in adults with CAH who have completed linear growth, including twice-daily prednisone or prednisolone, or daily dexamethasone [6, 10]. While dexamethasone requires the least dose frequency and may be most effective in androgen suppression, it may be associated with the lowest bone mineral density scores and highest body mass index (BMI) [11]. Of note, pregnant women with CAH should avoid dexamethasone, as it crosses the placenta. Another difference in glucocorticoid management in CAH versus adrenal insufficiency includes the fact that total daily doses are higher in CAH for the purposes of androgen blockade in both sexes (see Table 40.1). Most patients with classic CAH also require fludricortisone replacement in doses of 0.05–0.2 mg dosed one to two times per day, doses akin to recommendations for adults with adrenal insufficiency from other causes [6, 10, 11].

**Table 40.1** Adult glucocorticoid physiologic replacement for adrenal insufficiency [6, 12]

| Corticosteroid | Total daily dose (mg/day) for CAH | Total daily dose (mg/day) for adrenal insufficiency not due to CAH |
|---|---|---|
| Hydrocortisone | 15–25 throughout day | 15–25 with highest dose in early day |
| Prednisone[a] | 5–7.5 | 3–5 mg |
| Prednisolone | 4–6 | 3–5 |
| Dexamethasone | 0.25–0.5 | Not recommended |

*CAH* congenital adrenal hyperplasia
[a]Note: Prednisone is not preferred per Endocrine Society guidelines as it is a precursor steroid needing hepatic activation before exerting biological activity

To reduce the risk of over-exposure to glucocorticoid while likewise improving hyperandrogenism, many women with both classic and nonclassical CAH require non-glucocorticoid therapy to reduce androgen synthesis and bind free androgens. This management is comparable to treatment used in women with PCOS and may include oral contraceptive therapy and/or treatment with androgen receptor antagonists. Of note, spironolactone is not recommended for patients with salt-wasting CAH to avoid mineralocorticoid antagonism and volume depletion [6]. While patients with NCAH typically do not require glucocorticoid therapy in adulthood, it may be used in the treatment of women with severe clinical symptoms of hyperandrogenism. Glucocorticoids may also be used in women with both classic and nonclassical forms of CAH struggling with infertility to restore ovulation (except for dexamethasone, which crosses the placenta). Doses are adjusted by monitoring follicular phase progesterone to reach levels of <0.6 ng/mL [6, 12].

Monitoring the appropriateness of glucocorticoid and mineralocorticoid doses in patients with adrenal insufficiency of any cause includes routine assessment of weight, blood pressure, serum electrolytes, and physical exam for signs of glucocorticoid excess (violaceous striae, moon facies, dorsocervical fat pad, easy bruising, central adiposity, muscle wasting). Additional labs specific for patients with CAH include monitoring of androstenedione, 17-hydroxyprogesterone (17-OHP), and plasma renin activity (PRA) [6, 12]. Androstenedione levels should be targeted in the normal range, whereas normal range values of 17-OHP suggests steroid over-replacement and should be avoided [12]. While there is no generalized recommendation for timing of these analyses, blood draws should be timed consistently for each individual patient, either always before or after a specific dose of glucocorticoid. This allows for each patient to serve as their own control in assessing fluctuations in laboratory levels over time [6, 10]. For those in whom there is cod over-replacement, routine bone mineral density monitoring is recommended [4].

All patients with adrenal insufficiency of any cause require stress-dose steroids during illness defined by fever, gastroenteritis with dehydration, surgery accompanied by anesthesia, or major trauma. Home dosing suggestions to prevent adrenal crisis vary from double to triple a patient's typical daily dose regimen, or 25 mg of hydrocortisone equivalent every 6 h. Stress dosing should continue until 24–48 h after the stressor prompting initiation of stress dosing has ceased. Supportive care, including maintenance of adequate hydration, is likewise important. All patients are recommended to have a glucocorticoid emergency injection kit at home in case of intolerance to oral steroids and to wear a medical alert identifying their diagnosis of adrenal insufficiency and need for emergency replacement glucocorticoids. Should a patient be intolerant to oral steroids, a dose of injectable glucocorticoid should be administered at home. Ongoing oral intolerance after initial injection or inability to inject should prompt emergency room care for intravenous hydrocortisone and fluids. Teaching adrenal stress-dose rules is important for patients at every visit where time allows, ideally in both verbal and written forms. This is particularly crucial for young adults, as prior education may have been offered to parents and caregivers. Failure to give appropriate steroid dose increases during times of physical stress, especially illnesses leading to volume loss such as gastrointestinal illnesses, can lead to life-threatening adrenal crisis marked by hypotension, volume depletion, and electrolyte abnormalities [6, 10].

While insufficient steroid dosing for adrenal insufficiency increases risk of morbidity and mortality, inadequate glucocorticoid treatment to suppress hyperandrogenism in patients with CAH has additional consequences. Men who are inadequately treated may develop testicular adrenal rest tumors (TARTs). If left untreated, these can lead to hypogonadism and infertility. As TARTs are infrequently detectable by palpation on physical exam, screening testicular ultrasounds are recommended starting in early adolescence and then every 1–2 years in asymptomatic males. Ancillary signs of poor control in men with CAH may also be followed to include: (1) testosterone-to-androstenedione ratio greater than two; (2) low morning testosterone with elevated luteinizing hormone (LH) suggesting Leydig cell dysfunction; (3) elevated follicle-stimulating hormone (FSH) suggesting Sertoli cell dysfunction; and (4) azoospermia on semenalysis [6, 7, 9]. TARTs can be treated by restoring suppressive doses of glucocorticoid but occasionally require surgical management. Patients should be counseled that even surgical management may not restore previously impaired fertility, which is why early detection and management of TARTs is important [7]. Inadequate glucocorticoid treatment in female patients may lead to virilization, irregular menses, and infertility. Women are likewise at risk for ovarian rest tumors, although these can be difficult to diagnose as there is no easily accessible routine imaging. Elevated follicular phase progesterone and irregular menses may be a sign of impaired fertility in women with CAH [6, 9].

## Additional Aspects of Care in Patients with CAH

### Pregnancy

As discussed, glucocorticoids are necessary for suppressing androgens, preventing adrenal rest tumors, and promoting fertility in both men and women with CAH. Recall that follicular phase progesterone is a potential target for glucocorticoid dosing in those seeking conception. Studies of fertility in women with CAH show that those on appropriate maintenance therapy have intact fertility. However, there are lower pregnancy and live birth rates in women with CAH compared to age-matched controls. Women having difficulty conceiving with both classical and nonclassical CAH should be referred to reproductive endocrinology [6, 13].

Once pregnant, women with underlying adrenal insufficiency should be followed closely by an endocrinologist comfortable in glucocorticoid management in pregnancy. Women may remain on their pre-pregnancy doses of glucocorticoid in early pregnancy but often require increased dosing as pregnancy progresses, particularly into the second and third trimesters. A stress-dose steroid plan should be pre-planned for labor and delivery and outlined both to the patient and their obstetrician [6]. Women with CAH may require scheduled delivery by cesarean section, particularly if they have a history of surgical genitoplasty [13].

For patients with CAH, preconception counseling should be used to understand the risk of CAH transmission. In the past, women at risk of carrying a fetus with CAH were advised to take high-dose dexamethasone in early pregnancy (ideally before week 7 of gestation) to prevent virilization of external genitalia. However, this is no longer recommended by professional societies. First, CAH cannot be diagnosed until near the end of the first trimester and only 1 in 8 fetuses would benefit from treatment (1 in 4 affected, half of those female) thus exposing the majority to unnecessary therapy. Additionally, the safety of high-dose dexamethasone is poorly understood, with potential teratogenicity and long-term risks to cardiometabolic, cognitive, and behavioral health [6, 13, 14].

#### Genitoplasty

For women with virilized genitalia, vaginoplasty with urogenital mobilization and neurovascular-sparing clitoroplasty are the recommended procedures if desired. The timing of surgical management of virilized genitalia recently has become controversial. Patient and physician proponents of early surgery cite the risks of stigmatization and psychological trauma and prevention of urinary tract infections as indications for management early in life. Proponents of later surgery impute value on the importance of the individual patient's ability to participate in shared decision-making following affirmation of gender identity and personal knowledge of surgical risks and benefits. Potential complications related to surgical management may include cosmetic concerns, urinary incontinence, urethral-vaginal fistulae, vaginal stenosis, and impaired sexual function/clitoral sensation. While the timing of surgery remains controversial, a multidisciplinary, patient- and family-centered approach in shared decision-making is widely recommended. Conversations should include details regarding surgical approach, cosmetic expectations, postoperative sexual function, and potential complications. A multidisciplinary approach involving urology, gynecology, plastic surgery, and pelvic floor physical therapy can also be quite beneficial where available [6, 8].

#### Mental Health

Mental health support plays an important role in the lives of patients with CAH, both at the time of diagnosis for families and ongoing throughout adulthood. Special concerns for patients with CAH include quality of life, particularly given the chronicity of their condition resulting in the need for multiple daily doses of medication, worry about emergent situations requiring stress doses, and frequent medical follow-up. CAH has been associated with mood disorders, postulated by some to be due to the influence of androgens, excess glucocorticoids, or elevated corticotrophin-releasing hormone (CRH)-to-ACTH ratios leading to changes in brain structure and function. High-dose glucocorticoids have likewise been implicated in mood disorders as well as cognitive and learning disabilities. Finally, counseling addressing sexual health is important, as women with CAH have been found to have delays in dating and sexual activity compared to their peers and may be less likely to engage in relationships. This is postulated to relate to insecurity related to genital appearance or concerns with sexual function (with or without genitoplasty). For women with CAH, further exploration of gender role and gender identities may be warranted [6, 15–18]. A multidisciplinary approach to healthcare including mental health support is therefore important for these patients. Likewise, meeting others with CAH may be helpful for patients through engagement in patient groups or advocacy societies.

## Turner Syndrome

### Case Presentation

Erica is a 30-year-old female with Turner syndrome (TS) presenting to establish new primary care. Erica was diagnosed with TS at age 12 following referral to pediatric endocrinology for short stature given height below the third percentile despite having parents of average height. Work-up revealed TS with 46X,iX(q10) karyotype. She did enter puberty on her own at age 11, but puberty subsequently stalled. She followed with an endocrinologist regularly for growth hormone therapy and pubertal induction with transdermal estrogen. Once linear growth stopped and she started on regular doses of oral contraceptive pills (OCPs) for estrogen replacement, she ceased care with endocrinology. She previously saw a primary care doctor every few years to continue her OCP refills when pressed, although admits she has been successful obtaining refills with infrequent interval appointments. She has not followed consistently with a provider, which she attributes to time constraints from her pursuit of an advanced degree and the later demands of her early career. Recently, she developed significant fatigue and has found herself thirty pounds above her weight from the time of college graduation. She now seeks to resume routine medical follow-up to optimize her health, as she and her husband would like to expand their family in the next 3 years, although she admits that they are not familiar with their options to achieve this goal given Erica's TS diagnosis.

## Case Discussion

Patients with TS often have a close relationship with their pediatric endocrinologist due to their need for frequent visits to monitor growth hormone therapy and pubertal induction. Studies across several European registries have shown that loss to follow-up of these patients is a common occurrence once adult stature and secondary sexual characteristics have been achieved. This lapse in care is of particular concern for TS patients who may have congenital anomalies and/or are at risk for multiple physical and mental health complications throughout their lifespan that require routine screening. Some of these complications may already be occurring for Erica, who has manifested new symptoms that may have a variety of etiologies common for patients with TS necessitating work-up [19–22]. Obesity is of particular concern for her given higher rates of cardiovascular mortality in women with TS. Typically, a multidisciplinary approach involving several subspecialists is necessary for health maintenance. In addition to careful surveillance for medical complications, women with Turner syndrome require counseling for family planning. While women with TS are unlikely to achieve pregnancy spontaneously, donor oocytes may be considered for the patient who wishes to carry a pregnancy. All women with TS are at higher risk of eclampsia and pregnancy complications, which should be part of counseling regarding options for motherhood.

### Background

The incidence of TS is 1 in 2000–2500 female births. Diagnosis is made with a karyotype of one X chromosome and either complete or partial deletion of the second X chromosome [23]. Historically, there have been delays in TS diagnosis. Infant diagnoses have largely been made with observation of neonatal lymphedema or neck webbing, while other TS patients are diagnosed in later childhood or adolescence with evidence of linear growth failure, failure to enter puberty, halted puberty, or primary amenorrhea. Of note, approximately one-third of TS women will have spontaneous thelarche, and less than 10% will have regular menses (mostly in patients with mosaic karyotypes). Delayed diagnosis may lead to a delay in growth hormone treatment and thus compromised adult height, missed opportunity for detection of other congenital disorders associated with TS, and onset of ovarian failure limiting ability to harvest oocytes or ovarian tissue [23–25]. More recently, monosomy can be detected on first trimester cell-free DNA testing, although the positive predictive value of this screening is low and confirmatory testing with amniocentesis for pregnancy counseling is recommended [26]. Any prenatal suspicion of TS requires post-natal karyotype testing to confirm genotype [23].

### Health Complications

Patients with TS may have a number of congenital abnormalities. These include but are not limited to short stature, external ear deformities, cystic hygroma, micrognathia, low posterior hairline, webbed neck, broad chest, cubitus valgus, short fourth metacarpal, Madelung deformity, nail dysplasia, renal abnormalities (horseshoe kidney, abnormally positioned or duplicated renal pelvis/ureters, renal aplasia, among others), and cardiac abnormalities (bicuspid aortic valve, coarctation of the aorta, aortic valve stenosis, aortic dilatation, among others). Finally, as many as 10% of patients with TS have Y chromosome material necessitating gonadectomy due to a resulting higher risk of gonadoblastoma [23].

Patients with TS are at higher risk of additional health complications that can occur throughout their lifespan requiring ongoing surveillance by multiple subspecialists. Guidelines therefore suggest close medical follow-up with routine screenings every 1–5 years to assess these conditions (see Table 40.2). These tests are typically ordered by the patient's PCP and/or endocrinologist [23, 27].

Adult endocrinology visits are warranted for the management of primary ovarian insufficiency, although this may also be managed by gynecology. Controversy exists as to the ideal method of sex steroid replacement from the standpoint of optimal cardiovascular and skeletal health benefits. Acceptable options include transdermal or oral estradiol plus progesterone (as oral pill or intrauterine device [IUD]) for uterine protection; or combined oral contraceptive therapy. Therapy should be continued until the typical age of menopause and can be tapered to prevent estrogen withdrawal symptoms and optimize skeletal health [6, 28]. Patients with TS are at high risk of low bone density, which is further impetus for ongoing estradiol treatment. In addition to bone density monitoring, patients should receive counseling on adequate calcium and vitamin D intake as well as weight-bearing exercise. They should be treated for low bone density as would be recommended in the general population, with acknowledgment that dual-energy X-ray absorptiometry (DEXA) may underestimate the bone density in TS patients due to short stature compared to age- and ethnicity-matched controls [6, 29]. In addition to the management of sex steroid replacement and skeletal health, endocrinology may be involved in the care of TS patients given their increased risk of autoimmune endocrinopathies including Type 1 diabetes mellitus, hypothyroidism, and hyperthyroidism for which symptom and laboratory screening is warranted. Finally, patients with TS are also more prone to obesity, dyslipidemia, dysglycemia, and Type 2 diabetes mellitus as part of an overall increased propensity toward metabolic syndrome. Atherosclerotic cardiovascular disease is a known significant contributor to mortality in these patients. Weight management counseling involving optimal nutrition and physical activity from an early age may be beneficial for patients with TS. Likewise, they should be carefully monitored for the develop-

**Table 40.2** Recommended tests by frequency for adults with Turner syndrome [23, 27]

| Annually | Initially then every 1–5 years as indicated | As indicated |
|---|---|---|
| Weight/body mass index | Electrocardiogram<br>2D-echocardiogram<br>Cardiac magnetic resonance imaging | Psychosocial screen |
| Blood pressure | Otolaryngology<br>Audiology | Celiac screen |
| Blood urea nitrogen<br>Serum creatinine | Celiac screen | |
| Liver function tests | Papanicolaou smear | |
| Thyroid stimulating hormone<br>Free thyroxine (T4) | Bone densitometry | |
| Fasting serum glucose or Glycosylated hemoglobin (HgA1c) | 25-hydroxy Vitamin D | |
| Serum lipid profile | | |
| Complete blood count | | |

ment of dysglycemia or dyslipidemia. Treatment of these conditions is akin to recommendations for the general population [23, 30].

Cardiologists are of utmost importance in the management of patients with TS. Twenty-five to 50% of women with TS may be born with some degree of congenital cardiac disease. In addition, women with TS are at higher risk of acquired cardiac disease including early-onset hypertension, life-threatening aortic dissection and/or rupture, and atherosclerosis leading to higher risk of early ischemic cardiac disease or stroke. Counseling on the signs/symptoms of these conditions may be important for early detection, particularly in the case of aortic dissection, which occurs at an average age of 35 years. It is important to note that cardiovascular disease is the leading cause of mortality in women with TS [23, 31, 32].

Additional subspecialty care may be required. Visits to otolaryngology and audiology are recommended due to higher risk of hearing defects as well as middle ear infections. Ophthalmology screening includes monitoring for strabismus and nearsightedness. Gastroenterology may become involved due to increased risks among TS patients of celiac disease, inflammatory bowel disease, and elevated liver enzymes with a six-time higher risk of cirrhosis than the general population [6, 23, 33]. Lymphedema may be managed by cardiovascular surgeons, rehabilitation medicine, and/or physical therapy. Due to higher risk of pigmented nevi, dermatology surveillance may be warranted. Dermatology may also be necessary due to higher risk of vitiligo and alopecia, going along with increased propensity toward autoimmunity. Kyphosis and scoliosis occur more commonly in patients with TS necessitating orthopedic attention. Lastly, dental issues are more common prompting establishment of care with dentistry and orthodontics [23].

Finally, although the majority of TS patients have normal an intelligence quotient (IQ), they are known to be at higher risk for neurocognitive and psychological diagnoses. Screening for neurocognitive issues such as dyscalculia, visuospatial impairment, and attention deficits should occur in childhood to allow for ideal educational adaptations [23, 25]. Mood disorders including depression and social anxiety can be seen in patients with TS perhaps related to differences in physical appearance, delayed development, and challenges with social interaction [34]. Women with TS also are at double the risk of schizophrenia than the general population [35].

### Fertility, Pregnancy, and Motherhood Counseling

Women with TS are likely to have premature ovarian insufficiency, with declining fertility in early life. Patients should be counseled that their chances of having spontaneous pregnancy is unlikely. Rates of spontaneous pregnancy in TS are about 5–7.5%, unfortunately with a higher accompanying rate of miscarriage than the general population as well as higher risk of fetal malformation or chromosomal abnormality such as TS or Down Syndrome [23, 36, 37] For patients with TS and evidence of ovarian function after age 12, ovarian hyperstimulation may be used. Successful retrieval of mature oocytes in patients with mosaic TS has been published, as well as one study on in vitro fertilization in women with mosaic TS which found an 8.6% pregnancy rate and 5.7% live birth rate [23, 37, 38]. Ovarian tissue cryopreservation for girls with evidence of ovarian reserve but who are too young to undergo stimulation is theoretically possible, although outcomes of this approach are yet unknown [37]. Most women with TS therefore require donated oocytes to achieve pregnancy. Pre-pregnancy counseling and evaluation with maternal-fetal medicine and cardiology is necessary, given the higher risk of pre-existing hypertension, pre-eclampsia, aortic dissection, and cardiovascular complications in women with TS. Given a higher risk for cardiovascular morbidity and mortality in pregnancy with TS, alternative means to pursue motherhood, including the possibility of using a gestational carrier or adoption, should also be discussed [37].

## Thyroid Disease

While a comprehensive review of the diagnosis and management of thyroidal illness is well beyond the scope of this chapter, this section focuses on the aspects of autoimmune thyroid disease relevant to the young adult population with specific attention to preconception management and pregnancy. The management of subclinical hypothyroidism and hyperthyroidism is also briefly addressed, as these diagnoses are most often addressed in the primary care setting.

## Case Presentation

Emily is a 24-year-old female with Hashimoto's hypothyroidism who presents to her PCP at 9 weeks gestation for her annual visit. She was initially diagnosed with thyroid autoimmunity at age 12 during a work-up for fatigue. She was found to be positive for anti-thyroperoxidase (TPO) and anti-thyroglobulin (TG) antibodies but was clinically euthyroid for which treatment initiation was deferred. She was managed off hormone replacement until age 19, when she developed worsening fatigue and constipation and was found to have subclinical hypothyroidism with a thyroid-stimulating hormone (TSH) of 7.3 mIU/L and free thyroxine (T4) at the lower end of the normal range. She was initiated on 50 micrograms (mcg) levothyroxine daily which alleviated her symptoms and remains her current dose. She endorses mild fatigue, ankle swelling, and weight gain, but feels that all symptoms can be attributed to her pregnancy. Her PCP checks thyroid function tests (TFTs) and finds her TSH to be 4.5 mIU/L with free T4 of 1.1. She wonders if her dose of levothyroxine needs to be adjusted.

## Case Discussion

The treatment of subclinical hypothyroidism is an area of investigation. As occurred in Emily's case at age 19, many clinicians will offer a trial of treatment for those patients with subclinical hypothyroidism and symptoms potentially attributable to hypothyroidism, particularly in the presence of positive thyroid antibodies. This treatment had been effective for Emily, who now requires careful monitoring of her thyroid axis in pregnancy. TFTs during pregnancy must be interpreted by a separate reference range that accounts for the interaction of β-human chorionic gonadotropin (hCG) on TSH. Since the upper limit of normal TSH during the first trimester is 2.5 mIU/L (compared to 4–5 mIU/L in non-pregnant patients), gestational hypothyroidism is often under-diagnosed (see Table 40.3). Given the risk of adverse maternal and fetal outcomes, subclinical hypothyroidism is more readily treated in pregnancy, especially in patients who are anti-TPO positive. In this case, even if she were asymptomatic, Emily's dose of levothyroxine should be increased with repeat TFTs in 4–6 weeks.

**Table 40.3** Trimester-specific reference intervals for TSH

| Trimester | Thyroid stimulating hormone[a] (mIU/L) |
|---|---|
| Non-pregnant | 0.5–5.0 |
| First trimester | 0.1–2.5 |
| Second trimester | 0.2–3.0 |
| Third trimester | 0.3–3.0 |

[a]According to the American Thyroid Association (2011) and the Endocrine Society (2012)

### Subclinical Hypothyroidism

Up to 8 of every 1000 Americans have overt hypothyroidism, with a 16-times higher prevalence (130/1000) of subclinical hypothyroidism, defined as an elevated TSH with normal thyroxine levels [39]. There is little consensus among professional societies regarding the frequency of screening and indications for treatment of subclinical hypothyroidism. Autoimmune thyroiditis is the most common cause of primary hypothyroidism, but nearly 50% of cases of autoimmune thyroiditis resolve spontaneously within 2 years of diagnosis [40]. Those that do not resolve often present with TSH > 7 mIU/L and have a 33–55% of converting to overt hypothyroidism in 10–20 years from onset. This risk is significantly increased in the presence of positive TPO antibodies [40]. Identifying those at high risk for progression to overt hypothyroidism and who could benefit from early initiation of hormone replacement is important, as subclinical hypothyroidism has been associated with adverse metabolic, cardiovascular, neuromuscular , and cognitive outcomes [41]. At the same time, the risk of unnecessary treatment should be thoughtfully considered, as levothyroxine's narrow therapeutic window and long half-life can predispose a patient to the adverse effects of over-replacement.

Multiple professional societies have created guidelines for the frequency of screening for hypothyroidism. They focus on early screening for those at highest risk of disease including patients with personal or family history of thyroid disease, prior neck radiation, prior partial thyroidectomy, dyslipidemia, atrial fibrillation, history of autoimmune disease, or hyperprolactinemia [40]. The most clearly delineated screening guidelines from the American Thyroid Association (ATA) recommend the initiation of TSH and free T4 screening beginning at age 35 with repeat testing every 5 years in patients who have no signs or symptoms of hypothyroidism, and more frequently in those who do [40, 42]]. The guideline excludes patients who already warrant more frequent screening such as those with other autoimmune diagnoses (such as autoimmune diabetes) or known TPO-antibody positivity from childhood [40, 42].

Treatment for subclinical hypothyroidism has been a controversial topic among professional clinical societies for many years. The primary impetus for consideration of early treatment has been the association of hypothyroidism with cardiovascular disease (CVD) risk factors such as dyslipidemia and hypertension [43–45]. To this end, ATA guidelines from 2012 recommended treatment initiation at TSH > 10 mIU/L or at TSH > 4.5–10 mIU/L in the presence of CVD risk factors [45, 46] This recommendation does not come risk-free, however, as a study in 2018 unveiled an increased risk of mortality for older patients (age > 65 years) treated for subclinical hypothyroidism with initial TSH < 10 mIU/L [47]. Based on a systemic review of 21 trials that showed no clinically relevant benefit, the 2019 British clinical practice guidelines recommended hormone replacement for subclinical hypothyroidism only for TSH >20 mIU/L, excluding patients with other indications for treatment including age < 30 or pregnant women [48]. This remains quite controversial, however, and the decision to initiate treatment should be made in a shared decision-making process individualized to each patient based on factors such as TSH level, age, comorbidities, and antibody status. A useful clinical tool that encompasses these factors collectively was published in 2017 and can be used to help guide these decisions (see Fig. 40.1) [49].

## Administration of Levothyroxine

The goal of levothyroxine treatment is to provide resolution of potential symptoms of hypothyroidism, normalize TSH while improving thyroxine levels, and avoid over-replacement. Determining the appropriate dose of thyroid hormone is based upon weight, age, pregnancy status, degree of TSH elevation, and TSH goal as determined by the patient's overall clinical status [50]. Dosing may be complicated by the interaction profile of levothyroxine related to decreased absorption or alterations in transport by thyroxine binding globulin (TBG), conversion to triiodothyronine (T3), or hepatic metabolism. Given the risk of changes to levothyroxine pharmacokinetics in patients taking other therapies, medication lists should be assessed for potential interference with levothyroxine and dosing adjusted accordingly. As many substances interfere with absorption (particularly antacids, iron, calcium, or soy), levothyroxine is ideally taken in the mornings on an empty stomach, at least 60 min prior to eating or at bedtime (3 h after the evening meal) and ideally dosed at least 4 h from medications that may interfere with absorption [50]. With a half-life of nearly 7 days, supratherapeutic doses will linger. As it takes 4–8 weeks to see changes to TSH with dose adjustment, it is important to give clear guidance on proper administration of the medication upon prescribing it.

Levothyroxine monotherapy is currently the only ATA-recommended treatment for hypothyroidism. The ATA recommends the use of synthetic levothyroxine over other thyroid extracts due to lack of data on long-term safety and lack of superiority studies in the latter. The concurrent use of combination levothyroxine and liothyronine is likewise not routinely recommended. Of note, the use of brand preparations or ensuring consistency with a specific generic formulation may be advisable where available to maintain

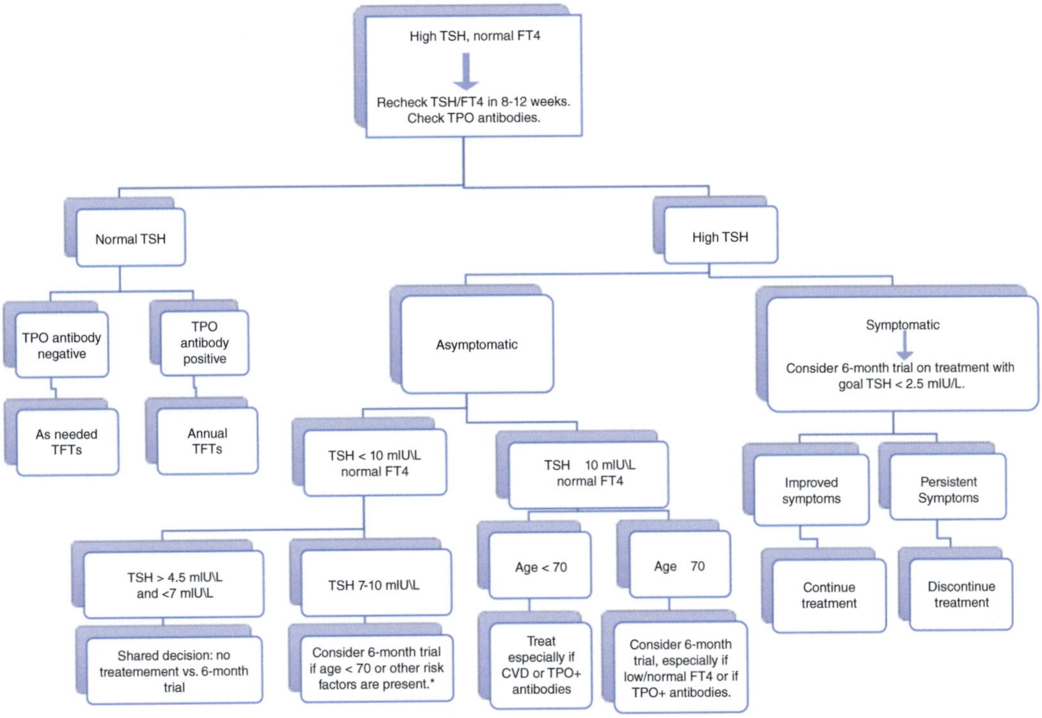


**Fig. 40.1** Treatment algorithm for subclinical hypothyroidism in the non-pregnant patient
Adapted from Peeters et al. [49]
*TSH* thyroid stimulating hormone, *FT4* Free thyroxine, *TPO* thyroid peroxidase, *TFTs* thyroid function tests, *CVD* cardiovascular disease

*Other risk factors include cardiovascular disease, TPO antibodies, pregnancy, and presence of goiter

steady levels [50]. More recently, studies have suggested that soft gel or liquid formulations of levothyroxine may be useful in patients with gastric or intestinal disorders and/or a history of bariatric surgery as well as those who are taking medications affecting levothyroxine absorption to more effectively reach TSH targets [51].

## Hypothyroidism in Pregnancy

The most common thyroid gland dysfunction during pregnancy is hypothyroidism. An estimated 12.4% of pregnant women experience subclinical hypothyroidism without any known preexisting thyroid dysfunction. Of these women, roughly 1 in 4 will go on to have residual thyroid dysfunction postpartum [52]. Gestational subclinical hypothyroidism carries increased risk for pregnancy complications including preeclampsia, placental abruption, preterm delivery, increased neonatal mortality, and impaired growth and development of the fetus [52]. Universal thyroid function testing in pregnant women remains a widely debated topic with insufficient existing evidence. However, it is generally accepted that women with known increased risk for thyroid dysfunction such as strong family or personal history of autoimmunity, prior thyroid surgery, or current hormone replacement therapy benefit from screening.

An important aspect of screening for hypothyroidism in pregnancy is to understand how normal thyroid hormone ranges are affected by pregnancy. β-hCG is structurally very similar to TSH, with a nearly identical alpha subunit that nonspecifically binds to TSH receptors on the thyroid. This phenomenon results in a relatively suppressed TSH that is most pronounced in the first trimester. It is important, therefore, to recognize that the upper limit of normal for TSH in the first trimester is 2.5 mIU/L, as compared to 5.0 mIU/L in the non-pregnant iodine-replete female (see Table 40.3) [53]. Failing to adjust these reference ranges for pregnancy can lead to under-diagnosis of hypothyroidism and over-diagnosis of hyperthyroidism in the gestational period. This is especially true given the fact that free T4 can be unreliable in pregnancy due to pregnancy-modified plasma proteins interfering with the accuracy of the assays [54].

Because of the risk for adverse maternal and fetal outcomes, there is a low threshold to treat subclinical hypothyroidism in pregnancy. Levothyroxine therapy is advised for TSH levels greater than 2.5 mIU/L in the first trimester and greater than 3.0 mIU/L in the second and third trimesters, especially in the presence of TPO antibodies [40]. Of note, there is a higher risk for progression to overt hypothyroidism in TPO-positive pregnant women in the postpartum period, even if TSH remains within reference range throughout their pregnancy [52]. These patients should be monitored closely.

## Hyperthyroidism—Treatment of Graves' Disease

Similar to hypothyroidism, one of the most common causes of primary hyperthyroidism is autoimmunity. Graves' disease is characterized by thyroid goiter formation secondary to unregulated overstimulation of the thyroid gland by thyroid-stimulating immunoglobulin (TSI), also known as anti-TSH-receptor antibodies (TRAb). Diagnostic testing for patients presenting with hyperthyroid symptoms should include serum TRAb levels. It may also include thyroid ultrasound to evaluate for discrete toxic nodules versus diffuse gland involvement, or iodine uptake scan. The ultimate goal of treatment is to reduce the conversion of T4 to its active metabolite T3. Acutely, glucocorticoids can effectively suppress this conversion, but long-term they carry several undesired side effects such as hypertension, hyperglycemia, and impaired bone mineral density [42] For this reason, the mainstay treatments for thyrotoxicosis secondary to Graves' disease include anti-thyroid medications, surgical removal of thyroid gland, and radioactive iodine (RAI) with iodium-131. The choice for therapy is based on severity of thyrotoxicosis, age, goiter size, availability of agents, prior response to treatment, and other comorbidities [42].

For a generally healthy, young, non-pregnant patient with mild goiter, the gold standard treatment is anti-thyroid hormone (ATH). Three options currently exist worldwide, including propylthiouracil (PTU) and the mercaptoimidazolines methimazole (MMI) and carbimazole (MMI), with carbimazole being only available in select countries. By slightly different mechanisms, both drug classes inhibit iodine utilization by the thyroid gland to prevent formation of thyroxine. Both medications have notable side effect profiles. A study comparing safety and efficacy of these drugs in Graves' disease suggested that MMI was a more suitable treatment modality, with low-dose MMI (up to 15 mg/d) as a suitable option for mild and moderate Graves' disease and high-dose MMI (30 mg/d or above) advised for severe cases [55]. PTU has largely fallen out of favor given reports of a four-times higher incidence of fulminant hepatotoxicity compared to MMI treatment, as well as increased risk of agranulocytosis [56]. MMI should be initiated on diagnosis and continued for a minimum of 12–18 months, with discontinuation based on normalization of TSH and TRAb serum levels or desire to pursue definitive surgical or ablative therapy [42].

## Subclinical Hyperthyroidism

Subclinical hyperthyroidism is a condition marked by subnormal TSH levels with normal thyroxine and triiodothyronine levels. Endogenous causes of this condition include Graves' disease, single or multiple autonomous nodules, and silent or post-partum thyroiditis [57–60]. It may also be seen more commonly in thyroid-deficient regions, where there may be a higher tendency toward thyroid autonomy [59]. Prior to making the diagnosis of subclinical hyperthyroidism, the clinician must first rule out other causes of low TSH such as iatrogenic (levothyroxine administration or other drug effects), central pituitary or hypothalamic hypothyroidism, euthyroidal illness, and pregnancy [57–60].

In the asymptomatic patient, evaluation generally includes repeating TSH, free T4, and total T3 after 2–6 weeks in patients deemed at high risk of complications of potential hyperthyroidism (such as those aged 65 years or older or with known heart disease), or otherwise in 3–6 months after initial lab assessment to assess either for persistence of lab abnormalities or progression to frank hyperthyroidism [60]. If subclinical hyperthyroidism proves persistent, TRab antibody levels should first be obtained to work-up for indolent Graves' disease. Alternatively, a thyroid uptake scan can be done to assess for diffuse uptake suggesting Graves' disease or irregular uptake suggesting toxic nodular disease [59]. The reason to pursue said work-up is that it can be difficult to predict when indolent Graves' disease will progress to frank hyperthyroidism, necessitating more frequent monitoring in patients with TRab positivity or diffuse uptake on thyroid uptake scan [58, 59]. Alternatively, this information can prove useful as subclinical hyperthyroidism related to Graves' disease may remit spontaneously while patients with single or multiple toxic adenomas are more likely to have persistent disease. In those patients with negative TRab and/or uptake scans, subclinical hyperthyroidism has a low rate of progression to frank hyperthyroidism, particularly if TSH is >0.1 mUI/L [59–61]. Generally, those patients with TSH levels <0.1 mIU/L are at highest risk of progression to frank hyperthyroidism [57–61]. For patients who have resolution of subclinical hyperthyroidism without treatment, repeat thyroid function tests can be delayed 1–2 years or may be drawn sooner should signs and/or symptoms of hyperthyroidism occur. In patients with ongoing, persistent subclinical hyperthyroidism, it would be reasonable to consider reassessment every 3–12 months [58].

Subclinical hyperthyroidism has been associated with an increased risk of atrial fibrillation, heart failure, and cardiovascular mortality as well as worsening in bone mineral density scores with increased fracture risk, especially in postmenopausal women [57–60]. Given these risks, professional societies generally recommend treatment only for levels <0.1 in patients over the age of 65 or in younger patients with hyperthyroid symptoms, underlying cardiovascular disease and/or osteoporosis. Treating patients with TSH in the range of 0.1–0.4 mIU/mL is not recommended for asymptomatic patients under the age of 65 who do not have the aforementioned comorbidities; treatment for those in this range can otherwise be considered but is not universally recommended [57, 59, 60]. For patients with untreated subclinical hyperthyroidism, avoiding exposure to high doses of iodine in contrast dyes, certain foods, or supplements is important to prevent precipitation of frank hyperthyroidism [57].

### Gestational Hyperthyroidism

Hyperthyroidism in pregnancy can be challenging both to identify and to treat. Transient thyrotoxicosis has been reported in a number of women with hyperemesis gravidarum and is often self-limited without treatment. Pregnancy itself, however, can be a trigger for the onset of autoimmunity (i.e., Graves' disease) or a trigger for functional thyrotoxic nodules. As such, the prevalence of gestational hyperthyroidism is approximately 2/1000 pregnancies. If left untreated, hyperthyroidism in pregnancy can lead to significant adverse outcomes to both the mother (life-threatening thyrotoxicosis, postpartum thyrotoxicosis) and to the neonate (fetal hyperthyroidism, spontaneous abortion, fetal demise) [62, 63].

The treatment of gestational thyrotoxicosis is complicated by the high risk of fulminant hepatotoxicity from PTU and the teratogenicity associated with MMI (aplasia cutis congenital, choanal atresia, tracheoesophageal fistula, omphalocele) [62]. Given higher rates of teratogenicity with MMI, PTU is the preferred agent in the first trimester during embryogenesis, but patients should be switched to MMI in the second and third trimesters to mitigate risk for fulminant hepatitis [62, 64]. Therapeutic response should be monitored with regular TSH and free T4 surveillance (see Table 40.4). Given adjusted physiologic TSH ranges in pregnancy (see Table 40.3) and the fact that antithyroid hormone crosses the placenta to affect the neonatal thyroid, the goal of suppressive therapy is not to normalize TSH but rather to target the upper limit of normal of free T4 [65]. The minimum dose of antithyroid hormone should therefore be used to achieve this. For many women with mild to moderate Graves' disease, their thyrotoxicosis resolves as the autoimmune response is dampened during pregnancy, and many women may be able to stop treatment during pregnancy [62].

**Table 40.4** Screening and treatment guidelines for gestational hyperthyroidism [63]

| | First trimester (weeks 1–12) | Second trimester (weeks 13–27) | Third trimester (weeks 28–40+) |
|---|---|---|---|
| Screening labs | TSH if HR[a] or Symptomatic[b] | TRAb (20–24 weeks) if history of Graves' disease | |
| Surveillance labs | TSH/FT4 every 2-6 weeks after treatment initiation | TSH/FT4 every 2-6 weeks after treatment initiation | TSH/FT4 every 2-6 weeks after treatment initiation |
| FDA-approved Treatment | PTU | MMI | MMI |
| Treatment Target | Upper limit of normal for FT4 (not TSH normalization) | | |

*TSH* thyroid stimulating hormone, *TRAb* thyrotropin receptor antibodies, *FT4* free thyroxine (T4), *FDA* United States Food and Drug Administration, *PTU* propylthiouracil, *MMI* methimazole

[a]HR = high risk for thyroid disease = past medical history/family history of thyroid disease, autoimmunity, neck radiation, etc.

[b]Symptomatic of thyroid dysfunction

### Contraception and Preconception Planning

In light of the teratogenic potential for gold standard antithyroid medications, it is paramount that contraception and preconception planning be discussed at the time of diagnosis and initiation of therapy for women with hyperthyroidism. Upon initiation of MMI, the patient should concurrently be initiated on at least one form of birth control to prevent unexpected pregnancy. If indicated, thyroidectomy and thyroid ablation with RAI may be excellent therapeutic options for a patient planning future pregnancy to minimize exposure to potentially teratogenic medications. When coupled with post-therapy levothyroxine, these treatments can be a safe and effective means for achieving a euthyroid sate prior to conception. Of note, although women may be euthyroid at the time of conception following preconception thyroidectomy or RAI, they may still have positive thyroid antibodies that should be assessed during pregnancy to effectively stratify the risk of neonatal Graves' disease [66].

## Polycystic Ovary Syndrome (PCOS)

### Case Presentation

Joanna is a 23-year-old female with a history of PCOS, diagnosed 7 years ago after several years of unwanted weight gain, poorly controlled acne on multiple therapies, and irregular periods. She was started on OCPs at age 16 for irregular menstrual cycles. She and her fiancé have recently discussed a timeline for having children, and Joanna wonders what her fertility will be like once she stops taking "the pill." She also worries about her risk for developing diabetes, as this runs in her family.

### Case Discussion

The defining diagnostic criteria for PCOS are currently an area of controversy, with risk of false diagnosis when made in adolescence. As PCOS has significant implications for cardiometabolic health, fertility, and cosmesis, verifying this diagnosis for Joanna will be important for future management and counseling.

### PCOS Prevalence and Diagnosis

PCOS is a heterogenous condition in women that exists at the intersection of androgen excess and ovarian dysfunction and is often a diagnosis of exclusion. Though the most common clinical signs are oligomenorrhea, hirsutism, and obesity, the presentation and associated comorbidities can vary widely [67] Despite this, PCOS is the most common endocrine disorder in reproductive-aged women, with prevalence of 5–15% depending on diagnostic criteria used [68]. The pathophysiology of the syndrome is still poorly understood and is multigenic in nature, with ongoing identification of new culprit epigenetic and environmental triggers [69]. Nearly half of affected women have features of metabolic syndrome including insulin resistance, which in turn promotes ongoing androgen production [68]. Women with PCOS and metabolic syndrome are therefore at increased risk for cardiovascular disease [68]. As cardiovascular disease is the leading cause of death for women, it is crucial that primary care providers are familiar with the diagnostic criteria and available treatments for PCOS.

The diagnostic criteria for PCOS have long been debated, and its defining characteristics continue to be an area of controversy. The 2003 Rotterdam Criteria is the most commonly adopted definition of PCOS in the United States. Following the exclusion of any other conditions that may explain hyperandrogenism and menstrual irregularities, the Rotterdam Criteria states that two of three of the following must be met for the diagnosis of PCOS: (1) Clinical or biochemical evidence of hyperandrogenism; (2) Menstrual irregularities (<9 cycles/year or > 35 days between cycles); (3) Polycystic ovaries visualized on transvaginal ultrasound (>12 antral follicles in one ovary or ovarian volume >10 $cm^3$) [68, 70, 71].

The limitations of these criteria are perhaps most pronounced in the adolescent population, as the non-hyperandrogenism criteria can be present in normal puberty. For example, multi-follicular ovaries can be found in approximately 26% of adolescents, and menstrual dysfunction is quite common in reproduction maturation [70, 72]. It has been suggested that ovarian ultrasound should be avoided in patients who are less than 8 years post-menarche due to a higher rate of false positives related to the physiologic polycystic nature of pubescent ovaries [71, 73]. Likewise, oligomenorrhea may be a less specific diagnostic criteria in the adolescent population. The label should not be applied to adolescents unless they are at least 2 years post-menarche [71, 73]. The persistence of oligomenorrhea in the latter half of teen years (ages 14–19) has been shown to be a predictor for ongoing menstrual irregularities in young adulthood (ages 20–28), which in turn is associated with increased risk of impaired glucose tolerance, obesity, and diabetes [73]. Therefore, clinicians may consider labeling adolescent patients who present with persistent irregular menses (ages 14–19) without clinical or biochemical hyperandrogenism as "at risk" for PCOS and its associated metabolic complications [73].

### Clinical Manifestations in the Diagnosis of PCOS

Since the diagnosis of PCOS relies heavily on clinical suspicion and physical exam, understanding how to identify manifestations of androgen excess is paramount to the diagnosis. The signature features of hyperandrogenism include acne, alopecia, and hirsutism. Because each element also exists along a spectrum of physiologic pubertal changes, there are guidelines designed to help providers differentiate. For instance, in adolescents, given the prevalence of acne in physiologic pubertal changes, only severe acne refractory to common topical and oral therapies should be included in the diagnostic criteria [73, 74]. Hirsutism, or excessive growth of terminal hair in androgen-dependent areas of the body, is perhaps the most sensitive way to clinically evaluate for hyperandrogenism [75]. To quantify, the modified Ferriman-Gallwey (mFG) score should be used, which evaluates excessive hair growth in nine androgen-specific locations [71]. Prior to mFG assessment, providers must ask about self-removal of hair. It is important to recognize that there is significant ethnic variation in clinical androgen expression that is not necessarily accounted for in the mFG scale, although some have proposed alternate scoring by ethnicity [71, 76]. Generally, a score of 8 or greater is considered positive for hirsutism, though a direct correlation between the extent of hirsutism on exam and elevation in androgen levels has not been found [75].

The onset, timing, and distribution of symptoms should direct the diagnostic labs and imaging pursued for PCOS work-up. The clinical manifestations marking the onset of PCOS tend to occur peripubertally and progress in a gradual manner [77]. Rapidly progressive virilizing symptoms, especially outside the peripubertal window, should induce high suspicion for an androgen-secreting tumor as well as prompt work-up, including an adrenal computerized tomography (CT) scan or magnetic resonance imaging (MRI) and ovarian transvaginal ultrasound [77]. In the absence of this presentation, however, with high suspicion for PCOS, laboratory work-up may be obtained.

## Laboratory Recommendations for PCOS Diagnosis

First, as PCOS is a diagnosis of exclusion, alternative etiologies for oligomenorrhea and/or hirsutism should be assessed including:

(a) A urine or serum pregnancy test should be obtained in all patients with prolonged oligomenorrhea, regardless of reported history of sexual activity.
(b) 17-OHP to assess for nonclassical congenital adrenal hyperplasia (ideally drawn before 9 AM, in the follicular phase) [67].
(c) TSH and free T4 to assess for hypothyroidism [67].
(d) Prolactin to assess for hyperprolactinemia [67].
(e) Dehydroepiandrosterone-sulfate (DHEA-S): while elevated levels can be consistent with PCOS, levels two times the upper limit of normal should raise concern for an adrenal tumor and therefore further work-up [78].
(f) Gonadotropins (LH/FSH) and estradiol should be assessed in prolonged oligomenorrhea to assess for premature ovarian insufficiency [78].
(g) In cases of high suspicion for Cushing syndrome, consider referral to endocrinology, as a random serum cortisol level is often uninformative, and formal testing will be required for the diagnosis which may include dexamethasone suppression testing, midnight salivary testing, and/or 24-h urine free cortisol depending on other patient clinical factors [79].

To assess for hyperandrogenism, testosterone levels including total and free testosterone should be assessed, the latter of which may be measured directly or calculated by obtaining a serum sex hormone-binding globulin (SHBG) and a total testosterone level [67, 80]). It is not imperative to test LH and FSH levels for the diagnosis of PCOS, but an elevated LH: FSH ratio supports the diagnosis [67, 72]. It is important to recognize that while biochemical evaluation of hyperandrogenism is an important aspect in the work-up for PCOS, it is insufficient in isolation, especially as there are several subtypes of PCOS that do not manifest with elevated androgen levels (see Table 40.5) [74, 81]. Clinicians therefore should be familiar with the constellation of clinical manifestations and laboratory findings defining this condition. There are several promising studies investigating the role of anti-Mullerian hormone (AMH) levels as a surrogate marker for ovarian follicle counts given the limitations of transvaginal ultrasound screening, particularly in adolescents. Although high AMH levels suggest a diagnosis of PCOS, the test is not currently recommended as part of diagnostic work-up due to lack of standardization of assays [81].

**Table 40.5** Phenotypes of PCOS based on Rotterdam Criteria

| Phenotype. | Androgen Excess | Ovulatory dysfunction | Ultrasound findings |
|---|---|---|---|
| A | X | X | X |
| B | X | X | |
| C | X | | X |
| D | | X | X |

*Adapted from Hoeger *et al.*, JCEM 2021 [74]

## Management of PCOS

Currently no single universal treatment for PCOS exists given the variability in its manifestations, and therefore management is largely tailored to the individual's symptoms [77]. The therapies that do exist are primarily focused on menstrual regulation, cosmesis, fertility optimization, and risk mitigation for cardiometabolic comorbidities.

### Management of Hyperandrogenism

Pharmacologic systemic therapy is often utilized in the management of hyperandrogenism in PCOS. Recommended treatments for hirsutism include combined oral contraceptives, spironolactone, finasteride, or topical eflornithine (for facial hirsutism). Combination OCPs tend to be first-line treatment as they treat hyperandrogenism in addition to offering menstrual regulation and contraception. In the management of hyperandrogenism, oral estradiol increases hepatic production of SHBG, which in turn binds circulating androgens, decreasing their bioavailability and resultant effects on acne and unwanted hair growth [82–84]. Additionally, OCPs have been shown to decrease adrenal androgen production [85]. It is generally advised that patients with PCOS avoid OCPs containing first- and second-generation progestins (norethindrone and noregestrel/levonorgestrel) as these have higher androgenic effects [86]. While studies unequivocally demonstrate the benefit of combination OCP in treatment for hirsutism [84, 87], the guidelines on secondary agent choice are less clearly delineated. Antiandrogen monotherapy with finasteride and spironolactone were found to be equally effective, and each showed augmented effect when combined with OCPs [87]. Similarly, oral insulin-sensitizer agents such as metformin and rosiglitazone were shown to be equally effective when paired with OCPs but notably suboptimal when used as monotherapy [87, 88]. Systemic therapies should be trialed for a minimum of 6 months to fully assess the efficacy of the treatment given the length of the hair growth cycle [76]. It is important to note the teratogenic potential of antiandrogenic therapies, however, and to ensure that reliable birth control therapies are in place prior to medication initiation [89].

Cosmetic treatments for the symptoms of hirsutism, alopecia, and acne may also be utilized, although expense may be a barrier for many patients. The most common non-systemic treatments for hirsutism management include shaving, waxing, bleaching, plucking, chemical treatments, laser hair removal, photoepilation, and electrolysis [77, 90]. Similarly, for alopecia, patients rely heavily on cosmetic solutions for symptom relief, notably through hair additions, hair styling, or in extreme cases, hair transplants [91]. Topical minoxidil is sometimes found to be effective, but patients should be warned that hair loss would most likely abruptly recur once the medication is discontinued [77]. Newer stem-cell-based therapies are available, but there are sparse evidence-based data behind these, and the procedures often incur high out-of-pocket costs [92, 93] As far as acne treatment, laser or light therapy can be considered for severe, scarring acne, but most women pursue topical or oral medications first, often requiring oral antibiotics or retinoid agents [93].

### Menstrual Regulation to Reduce Cancer Risk and Fertility

Menstruation irregularity for women with PCOS carries more sobering implications than simply the inconvenience of period planning. Women with PCOS are nearly three times more likely to develop endometrial cancer and additionally carry an increased risk for the development of ovarian cancer [94–96]. The major factor contributing to these increased malignancy risks is prolonged exposure to unopposed estrogen in the setting of anovulation [94]. The diagnosis of PCOS does not independently increase breast cancer risk, though notably obesity and metabolic syndrome are well-established risk factors for breast cancer and are highly associated with PCOS [94, 95].

The goal for women with PCOS should be to have a menstrual cycle at least every 3 months in order to reduce endometrial hyperplasia and to suppress gonadotropins to reduce ovarian cancer risk [95, 97]. This can be achieved through the use of OCPs or monthly to every 3-month dosing of progesterone to stimulate withdrawal bleeding, per patient preference [98]. In patients who wish to have more steady contraception and avoid menses, a progesterone-containing intrauterine device (IUD) may likewise offer protection against uterine hyperplasia [99].

Approximately 80% of women with anovulatory infertility also carry the diagnosis of PCOS [100]. It is important for women with PCOS to know that the diagnosis does not automatically assign them a fate of infertility. Even in the setting of irregular menstruation pregnancy is possible, and contraception use is imperative if pregnancy is undesired. Though menstrual irregularity does unequivocally complicate the ability to conceive, pharmacologic ovulation induction (through medications such as clomiphene citrate or letrozole) or *in vitro* fertilization with gonadotropin-releasing hormone (GnRH) antagonists can improve pregnancy rates [100]. Weight reduction is also among the most significantly effective treatment for improving fertility and pregnancy outcomes [101]. Obese women have been shown to have poorer fertility outcomes regardless of the mode of conception used [102–104]. Primary care providers should provide counsel on lifestyle modifications as well as discuss initiation of insulin-sensitizing medications to assist in weight loss, as described below. Metformin, specifically, has been shown to increase the ovulation rate in PCOS compared to placebo, although it is not first line given higher efficacy of agents specific for ovulation induction [105]. Women who have been trying to conceive unsuccessfully for 6 months with a diagnosis of PCOS should be referred to reproductive endocrinology.

### Obesity, Impaired Glucose Tolerance, and Cardiovascular Disease Risk

PCOS is highly associated with metabolic and cardiovascular comorbidities including gestational diabetes, metabolic syndrome, impaired-glucose tolerance, type 2 diabetes mellitus, and cardiovascular disease [61]. Screening labs include hemoglobin A1c, fasting glucose, oral glucose tolerance test, lipid panel, and liver function tests [73, 74, 106]. Of note, obtaining total fasting insulin levels has low yield. Insulin resistance in PCOS promotes increased ovarian androgen production while simultaneously driving many metabolic derangements that worsen cardiovascular health [61, 62]. Women with PCOS demonstrate intrinsic insulin resistance, even in the absence of obesity [107]. Insulin resistance has therefore become an important target in PCOS therapy.

Metformin was the first insulin-sensitizing drug used in the treatment of PCOS and was shown by investigators in a 1994 published study to improve menstrual regularity, circulating androgen levels, and weight loss [103]. Several studies have since shown that the direct effect of metformin on ovarian steroidogenesis is less clear but corroborated its benefit in reducing circulating insulin levels, leading to weight loss, improved fertility, and reduced risk of cardiovascular disease [104, 108, 109]. Given its otherwise low side effect profile, low cost, and ease of administration, metformin should be the first-line therapy for women with PCOS, used in conjunction with lifestyle modifications [110]. Treatment should be started with a low dose (500 mg daily) and taken 10–15 min before a meal on an empty stomach so as to maximize drug absorption [111]. The dose should be increased by 500 mg each week as tolerated to a target goal of up to 2500 mg/day for maximal effect [112]. At higher doses, patients may benefit from the extended-release formulation to mitigate adverse gastrointestinal effects of the drug [111].

Therapies that decrease insulin resistance while simultaneously targeting weight reduction are increasing in popularity for treatment of this condition. Glucagon-like peptide-1 (GLP-1) agonists as monotherapy or in conjunction with metformin have shown significant weight reduction, testosterone level reduction, and decreased risk of non-alcoholic fatty liver disease in patients with PCOS [101, 113].

## Conclusion

Care of the patient with chronic endocrine diagnoses is best achieved through multidisciplinary care, with a key role played by the PCP. While some aspects of pediatric disease management remain unchanged into adulthood, the transition can introduce new challenges to the care of each endocrine disorder through aspects such as pregnancy, stress, mental health, and acquired comorbidities. Ensuring proper management of these conditions starting in young adulthood can set patients up for optimized symptom management, reduced morbidity and mortality, attainment of reproductive goals, and lifelong maintenance of health.

## References

1. Jenkins-Jones S, Parviainen L, Porter J, Withe M, Whitaker MJ, Holden SE, et al. Poor compliance and increased mortality, depression and healthcare costs in patients with congenital adrenal hyperplasia. Eur J Endocrinol. 2018;178:309–20.

2. Gleeson H, Davis J, Jones J, O'Shea E, Clayton PE. The challenge of delivering endocrine care and successful transition to adult services in adolescents with congenital adrenal hyperplasia: experience in a single centre over 18 years. Clin Endocrinol. 2013;78:23–8. https://doi.org/10.1111/cen.12053. John Wiley & Sons, Ltd
3. Arlt W, Willis DS, Wild SH, Krone N, Doherty EJ, Hahner S, et al. Health status of adults with congenital adrenal hyperplasia: a cohort study of 203 patients. J Clin Endocrinol Metab. 2010;95:5110–21. Available from: https://pubmed.ncbi.nlm.nih.gov/20719839
4. Bachelot A. Transition of care from childhood to adulthood: congenital adrenal hyperplasia. Endocr Dev. 2018;33:17–33. https://doi.org/10.1159/000487523.
5. Ekbom K, Strandqvist A, Lajic S, Hirschberg AL, Falhammar H, Nordenström A. Assessment of medication adherence in children and adults with congenital adrenal hyperplasia and the impact of knowledge and self-management. Clin Endocrinol. 2021;94:753–64.
6. Speiser PW, Arlt W, Auchus RJ, Baskin LS, Conway GS, Merke DP, et al. Congenital adrenal hyperplasia due to steroid 21-hydroxylase deficiency: an endocrine society* clinical practice guideline. J Clin Endocrinol Metab. 2018;103:4043–88.
7. Claahsen-van der Grinten HL, Hermus ARMM, Otten BJ. Testicular adrenal rest tumours in congenital adrenal hyperplasia. Int. J Pediatr Endocrinol. 2009;2009:1–8.
8. Hebenstreit D, Ahmed SF, Krone N, Krall C, Bryce J, Alvi S, et al. Surgical practice in girls with congenital adrenal hyperplasia: an international registry study. Sex Dev. 2021;15:229–35. https://doi.org/10.1159/000517055.
9. Turcu AF, Auchus RJ. Adrenal steroidogenesis and congenital adrenal hyperplasia. Endocrinol Metab Clin N Am. 2015;44:275–96. Available from: https://pubmed.ncbi.nlm.nih.gov/26038201
10. Bornstein SR, Allolio B, Arlt W, Barthel A, Don-Wauchope A, Hammer GD, et al. Diagnosis and treatment of primary adrenal insufficiency: An endocrine society clinical practice guideline. J Clin Endocrinol Metab Endocrine Soc. 2016;101:364–89.
11. Whittle E, Falhammar H. Glucocorticoid Regimens in the Treatment of congenital adrenal hyperplasia: a systematic review and meta-analysis. J Endocr Soc Endocrine Soc. 2019;3:1227–45. Available from: https://pubmed.ncbi.nlm.nih.gov/31187081
12. Auchus RJ. Management of the adult with congenital adrenal hyperplasia. Int J Pediatr Endocrinol. 2010;2010:614107. https://doi.org/10.1155/2010/614107.
13. Pereira N, Lin-Su K, Ronald O, Perelman C. Reproductive function and fertility in women with congenital adrenal hyperplasia. EMJ Reprod Health. 2018;4(1):101–7.
14. McCann-Crosby B, Placencia FX, Adeyemi-Fowode O, Dietrich J, Franciskovich R, Gunn S, et al. Challenges in prenatal treatment with dexamethasone. Pediatr Endocrinol Rev. 2018;16:186–93. Available from: https://pubmed.ncbi.nlm.nih.gov/30371037
15. Falhammar H, Butwicka A, Landén M, Lichtenstein P, Nordenskjöld A, Nordenström A, et al. Increased psychiatric morbidity in men with congenital adrenal hyperplasia due to 21-hydroxylase deficiency. J Clin Endocrinol Metabol. 2014;99:E554–60. https://doi.org/10.1210/jc.2013-3707.
16. Strandqvist A, Falhammar H, Lichtenstein P, Hirschberg AL, Wedell A, Norrby C, et al. Suboptimal psychosocial outcomes in patients with congenital adrenal hyperplasia: epidemiological studies in a nonbiased national cohort in Sweden. J Clin Endocrinol Metabol. 2014;99:1425–32. https://doi.org/10.1210/jc.2013-3326.
17. Malouf MA, Inman AG, Carr AG, Franco J, Brooks LM. Health-related quality of life, mental health and psychotherapeutic considerations for women diagnosed with a disorder of sexual development: congenital adrenal hyperplasia. Int J Pediatr Endocrinol. 2010;2010:253465. https://doi.org/10.1155/2010/253465.
18. Zucker KJ, Bradley SJ, Oliver G, Blake J, Fleming S, Hood J. Psychosexual development of women with congenital adrenal hyperplasia. Horm Behav. 1996;30:300–18.
19. Bondy C, Bakalov VK, Lange ED, Ceniceros I. Deficient medical care for adults with the Turner syndrome. Ann Internal Med. 2006;145:866–7. https://doi.org/10.7326/0003-4819-145-11-200612050-00020.
20. Freriks K, Timmermans J, Beerendonk CCM, Verhaak CM, Netea-Maier RT, Otten BJ, et al. Standardized multidisciplinary evaluation yields significant previously undiagnosed morbidity in adult women with Turner syndrome. J Clin Endocrinol Metabol. 2011;96:E1517–26. https://doi.org/10.1210/jc.2011-0346.
21. Verlinde F, Massa G, Lagrou K, Froidecoeur C, Bourguignon JP, Craen M, et al. Health and psychosocial status of patients with Turner syndrome after transition to adulthood: the Belgian experience. Horm Res Paediatr. 2004;62:161–7. https://doi.org/10.1159/000080099.
22. Devernay M, Ecosse E, Coste J, Carel J-C. Determinants of medical care for young women with Turner syndrome. J Clin Endocrinol Metabol. 2009;94:3408–13. https://doi.org/10.1210/jc.2009-0495.
23. Gravholt CH, Andersen NH, Conway GS, Dekkers OM, Geffner ME, Klein KO, et al. Clinical practice guidelines for the care of girls and women with Turner syndrome: proceedings from the 2016 Cincinnati International Turner Syndrome Meeting. Eur J Endocrinol. 2017;177:G1–70.

24. Sävendahl L, Davenport ML. Delayed diagnoses of Turner's syndrome: proposed guidelines for change. J Pediatr. 2000;137:455–9. Available from: https://www.sciencedirect.com/science/article/pii/S0022347600374340
25. Stochholm K, Juul S, Juel K, Naeraa RW, Højbjerg GC. Prevalence, incidence, diagnostic delay, and mortality in Turner syndrome. J Clin Endocrinol Metabol. 2006;91:3897–902. https://doi.org/10.1210/jc.2006-0558.
26. Bianchi DW. Turner syndrome: New insights from prenatal genomics and transcriptomics. Am J Med Genet Part C: Semin Med Genet. 2019;181:29–33. https://doi.org/10.1002/ajmg.c.31675.
27. Bondy CA. Care of girls and women with Turner syndrome: A guideline of the Turner syndrome study group. J Clin Endocrinol Metabol. 2007;92:10–25. https://doi.org/10.1210/jc.2006-1374.
28. Klein KO, Rosenfield RL, Santen RJ, Gawlik AM, Backeljauw PF, Gravholt CH, et al. Estrogen replacement in Turner syndrome: literature review and practical considerations. J Clin Endocrinol Metabol. 2018;103:1790–803.
29. Faienza MF, Ventura A, Colucci S, Cavallo L, Grano M, Brunetti G. Bone fragility in Turner syndrome: mechanisms and prevention strategies. Front Endocrinol. 2016;7:34.
30. Collett-Solberg PF, Gallicchio CT, da Silva Coelho SC, Siqueira RA, de Figueiredo Alves ST, Guimarães MM. Doenças endócrinas, perspectivas e cuidados na síndrome de turner. Arq Bras Endocrinol Metabol. 2011;55(8):550–8.
31. Silberbach M, Roos-Hesselink JW, Andersen NH, Braverman AC, Brown N, Collins RT, et al. Cardiovascular health in Turner syndrome: a scientific statement from the American heart association. Circulation. 2018;11:e000048. https://doi.org/10.1161/HCG.0000000000000048.
32. Bondy CA. Aortic dissection in Turner syndrome. Curr Opin Cardiol. 2008;23:519–26. Available from: https://pubmed.ncbi.nlm.nih.gov/18839441
33. Roulot D. Liver involvement in Turner syndrome. Liver Int. 2013;33:24–30.
34. Morris LA, Tishelman AC, Kremen J, Ross RA. Depression in Turner syndrome: a systematic review. Arch Sex Behav. 2020;49:769–86. Available from: https://pubmed.ncbi.nlm.nih.gov/31598804
35. Björlin Avdic H, Butwicka A, Nordenström A, Almqvist C, Nordenskjöld A, Engberg H, et al. Neurodevelopmental and psychiatric disorders in females with Turner syndrome: a population-based study. J Neurodev Disord. 2021;13:51. https://doi.org/10.1186/s11689-021-09399-6.
36. Hagman A, Källén K, Barrenäs M-L, Landin-Wilhelmsen K, Hanson C, Bryman I, et al. Obstetric outcomes in women with Turner karyotype. J Clin Endocrinol Metabol. 2011;96:3475–82. https://doi.org/10.1210/jc.2011-1421.
37. Oktay K, Bedoschi G, Berkowitz K, Bronson R, Kashani B, McGovern P, et al. Fertility preservation in women with Turner syndrome: a comprehensive review and practical guidelines. J Pediatr Adolesc Gynecol. 2016;29:409–16. Available from: https://pubmed.ncbi.nlm.nih.gov/26485320
38. Doğer E, Çakıroğlu Y, Ceylan Y, Ulak E, Özdamar Ö, Çalışkan E. Reproductive and obstetric outcomes in mosaic Turner's Syndrome: a cross-sectional study and review of the literature. Reprod Biol Endocrinol. 2015;13:59. https://doi.org/10.1186/s12958-015-0055-7.
39. The Endocrine Society. Endocrine facts and figures. Thyroid. 2015; First edition
40. Azim S, Nasr C. Subclinical hypothyroidism: when to treat. Cleve Clin J Med. 2019;86:101. Available from: http://www.ccjm.org/content/86/2/101.abstract
41. Baumgartner C, Blum M, Rodondi N. Subclinical hypothyroidism: summary of evidence in 2014. Swiss Med Wkly. 2014;144(5152):w14058.
42. Azizi F, Malboosbaf R. Long-term antithyroid drug treatment: a systematic review and meta-analysis. Thyroid. 2017;27:1223–31.
43. Jabbar A, Pingitore A, Pearce SHS, Zaman A, Iervasi G, Razvi S. Thyroid hormones and cardiovascular disease. Nat Rev Cardiol. 2017;14:39–55.
44. Razvi S, Jabbar A, Pingitore A, Danzi S, Biondi B, Klein I, et al. Thyroid hormones and cardiovascular function and diseases. J Am Coll Cardiol. 2018;71:1781–96.
45. Sue LY, Leung AM. Levothyroxine for the treatment of subclinical hypothyroidism and cardiovascular disease. Front Endocrinol (Lausanne). 2020;11:591588.
46. Garber JR, Cobin RH, Gharib H, Hennessey JV, Klein I, Mechanick JI, et al. Clinical practice guidelines for hypothyroidism in adults: cosponsored by the American Association of Clinical Endocrinologists and the American Thyroid Association. Endocr Pract. 2012;18:988–1028.
47. Grossman A, Feldhamer I, Meyerovitch J. Treatment with levothyroxin in subclinical hypothyroidism is associated with increased mortality in the elderly. Eur J Intern Med. 2018;50:65–8.
48. Bekkering GE, Agoritsas T, Lytvyn L, Heen AF, Feller M, Moutzouri E, et al. Thyroid hormones treatment for subclinical hypothyroidism: a clinical practice guideline. BMJ. 2019;365:l2006.
49. Peeters RP. Subclinical hypothyroidism. N Engl J Med. 2017;376:2556–65.
50. Jonklaas J, Bianco AC, Bauer AJ, Burman KD, Cappola AR, Celi FS, et al. Guidelines for the treatment of hypothyroidism: prepared by the American thyroid association task force on thyroid hormone replacement. Thyroid. 2014;24:1670–751. Available from: https://pubmed.ncbi.nlm.nih.gov/25266247
51. Virili C, Brusca N, Capriello S, Centanni M. Levothyroxine therapy in gastric malabsorptive disorders. Front Endocrinol. 2021;11:621616.

52. Garg A, Vanderpump MPJ. Subclinical thyroid disease. Br Med Bull. 2013;107:101–16. https://doi.org/10.1093/bmb/ldt024.
53. Springer D, Jiskra J, Limanova Z, Zima T, Potlukova E. Thyroid in pregnancy: from physiology to screening. Crit Rev Clin Lab Sci. 2017;54:102–16. https://doi.org/10.1080/10408363.2016.1269309.
54. Lee RH, Spencer CA, Mestman JH, Miller EA, Petrovic I, Braverman LE, et al. Free T4 immunoassays are flawed during pregnancy. Am J Obst Gynecol. 2009;200:260.e1–6.
55. Nakamura H, Noh JY, Itoh K, Fukata S, Miyauchi A, Hamada N. Comparison of methimazole and propylthiouracil in patients with hyperthyroidism caused by Graves' disease. J Clin Endocrinol Metabol. 2007;92:2157–62.
56. Liaw Y-F. Hepatic injury during propylthiouracil therapy in patients with hyperthyroidism: a cohort study. Ann Intern Med. 1993;118:424.
57. Wartofsky L. Management of subclinical hyperthyroidism. J Clin Endocrinol Metabol. 2011;96:59–61.
58. Santos Palacios S, Pascual-Corrales E, Galofre JC. Management of subclinical hyperthyroidism. Int J Endocrinol Metab. 2012;10:490–6.
59. Donangelo I, Suh SY. Subclinical hyperthyroidism: when to consider treatment. Am Fam Physician. 2017;95:710–6.
60. Ross DS, Burch HB, Cooper DS, Greenlee MC, Laurberg P, Maia AL, et al. 2016 American Thyroid Association Guidelines for diagnosis and management of hyperthyroidism and other causes of thyrotoxicosis. Thyroid. 2016;26:1343–421.
61. Woeber KA. Observations concerning the natural history of subclinical hyperthyroidism. Thyroid. 2005;15:687–91.
62. Foulds N, Walpole I, Elmslie F, Mansour S. Carbimazole embryopathy: an emerging phenotype. Am J Med Genet A. 2005;132A:130–5.
63. Cooper DS, Laurberg P. Hyperthyroidism in pregnancy. Lancet Diab Endocrinol. 2013;1:238–49.
64. U.S Food & Drug Administration. FDA Drug Safety Communication: new boxed warning on severe liver injury with propylthiouracil. 2018.
65. Alexander EK, Pearce EN, Brent GA, Brown RS, Chen H, Dosiou C, et al. 2017 Guidelines of the American Thyroid Association for the diagnosis and management of thyroid disease during pregnancy and the postpartum. Thyroid. 2017;27:315–89.
66. van der Kaay DCM, Wasserman JD, Palmert MR. Management of neonates born to mothers with Graves' disease. Pediatrics. 2016;137(4):e20151878.
67. Escobar-Morreale HF. Polycystic ovary syndrome: definition, aetiology, diagnosis and treatment. Nat Rev Endocrinol. 2018;14:270–84.
68. Rosenfield RL, Ehrmann DA. The pathogenesis of polycystic ovary syndrome (PCOS): The hypothesis of PCOS as functional ovarian hyperandrogenism revisited. Endocr Rev. 2016;37:467–520.
69. Escobar-Morreale HF, Luque-Ramírez M, San Millán JL. The molecular-genetic basis of functional hyperandrogenism and the polycystic ovary syndrome. Endocr Rev. 2005;26:251–82.
70. Bridges NA, Cooke A, Healy MJR, Hindmarsh PC, Brook CGD. Standards for ovarian volume in childhood and puberty**Presented at the 12th meeting of the British Endocrine Societies, Liverpool, United Kingdom March 29 to April 1, 1992. Fertil Steril. 1993;60:456–60. Available from: https://www.sciencedirect.com/science/article/pii/S0015028216561603
71. Khan A, Karim N, Ainuddin JA, Faheem MF. Polycystic ovarian syndrome: correlation between clinical hyperandrogenism, anthropometric, metabolic and endocrine parameters. Pak J Med Sci. 2019;35(5):1227–32.
72. Rosenfield RL, Ghai K, Ehrmann DA, Barnes RB. Diagnosis of the polycystic ovary syndrome in adolescence: comparison of adolescent and adult hyperandrogenism. J Pediatr Endocrinol Metab. 2000;13(Suppl 5):1285–9.
73. Glueck CJ, Woo JG, Khoury PR, Morrison JA, Daniels SR, Wang P. Adolescent oligomenorrhea (age 14–19) tracks into the third decade of life (age 20–28) and predicts increased cardiovascular risk factors and metabolic syndrome. Metabolism. 2015;64:539–53.
74. Hoeger KM, Dokras A, Piltonen T. Update on PCOS: Consequences, challenges, and guiding treatment. J Clin Endocrinol Metabol. 2021;106:e1071–83.
75. Aswini R, Jayapalan S. Modified Ferriman–Gallwey score in hirsutism and its association with metabolic syndrome. Int J Trichology. 2017;9:7.
76. Martin KA, Anderson RR, Chang RJ, Ehrmann DA, Lobo RA, Murad MH, et al. Evaluation and treatment of hirsutism in premenopausal women: an Endocrine Society* Clinical Practice Guideline. J Clin Endocrinol Metab. 2018;103:1233–57.
77. Witchel SF, Burghard AC, Tao RH, Oberfield SE. The diagnosis and treatment of PCOS in adolescents: an update. Curr Opin Pediatr. 2019;31:562–9.
78. Rosenfield RL. The diagnosis of polycystic ovary syndrome in adolescents. Pediatrics. 2015;136:1154–65.
79. Nieman LK. Diagnosis of Cushing's syndrome in the modern era. Endocrinol Metab Clin N Am. 2018;47:259–73.
80. Rosner W, Auchus RJ, Azziz R, Sluss PM, Raff H. Utility, limitations, and pitfalls in measuring testosterone: an endocrine society position statement. J Clin Endocrinol Metabol. 2007;92:405–13.
81. Casadei L, Madrigale A, Puca F, Manicuti C, Emidi E, Piccione E, et al. The role of serum anti-Müllerian hormone (AMH) in the hormonal diagnosis of polycystic ovary syndrome. Gynecol Endocrinol. 2013;29:545–50.
82. Westhoff CL, Petrie KA, Cremers S. Using changes in binding globulins to assess oral contraceptive compliance. Contraception. 2013;87:176–81.
83. Plymate SR, Hoop RC, Jones RE, Matej LA. Regulation of sex hormone-binding globu-

lin production by growth factors. Metabolism. 1990;39:967–70.
84. Maier PS, Mattiello SS, Lages L, Spritzer PM. 17-hydroxysteroid dehydrogenase type 5 gene polymorphism (−71A/G HSD17B5 SNP) and treatment with oral contraceptive pills in PCOS women without metabolic comorbidities. Gynecol Endocrinol. 2012;28:606–10.
85. Rosenfield RL. Hirsutism. N Engl J Med. 2005;353:2578–88.
86. Oguz SH, Yildiz BO. An update on contraception in polycystic ovary syndrome. Endocrinol Metab (Seoul). 2021;36:296–311.
87. Barrionuevo P, Nabhan M, Altayar O, Wang Z, Erwin PJ, Asi N, et al. Treatment options for hirsutism: a systematic review and network meta-analysis. J Clin Endocrinol Metabol. 2018;103:1258–64.
88. Costello MF, Shrestha B, Eden J, Johnson N, Moran LJ. Insulin-sensitising drugs versus the combined oral contraceptive pill for hirsutism, acne and risk of diabetes, cardiovascular disease, and endometrial cancer in polycystic ovary syndrome. Cochrane Database Syst Rev. 2007;(1):CD005552.
89. Paparodis R, Dunaif A. The Hirsute woman: challenges in evaluation and management. Endocr Pract. 2011;17:807–18.
90. Escobar-Morreale HF, Carmina E, Dewailly D, Gambineri A, Kelestimur F, Moghetti P, et al. Epidemiology, diagnosis and management of hirsutism: a consensus statement by the Androgen Excess and Polycystic Ovary Syndrome Society. Hum Reprod Update. 2012;18:146–70.
91. Dinh QQ, Sinclair R. Female pattern hair loss: current treatment concepts. Clin Interv Aging. 2007;2:189–99.
92. Yuan A-R, Bian Q, Gao J-Q. Current advances in stem cell-based therapies for hair regeneration. Eur J Pharmacol. 2020;881:173197.
93. Acmaz G, Cınar L, Acmaz B, Aksoy H, Kafadar YT, Madendag Y, et al. The effects of oral isotretinoin in women with acne and polycystic ovary syndrome. Biomed Res Int. 2019;2019:2513067.
94. Dumesic DA, Lobo RA. Cancer risk and PCOS. Steroids. 2013;78:782–5.
95. Chittenden BG, Fullerton G, Maheshwari A, Bhattacharya S. Polycystic ovary syndrome and the risk of gynaecological cancer: a systematic review. Reprod Biomed Online. 2009;19:398–405.
96. Barry JA, Azizia MM, Hardiman PJ. Risk of endometrial, ovarian and breast cancer in women with polycystic ovary syndrome: a systematic review and meta-analysis. Hum Reprod Update. 2014;20:748–58.
97. Harris HR, Titus LJ, Cramer DW, Terry KL. Long and irregular menstrual cycles, polycystic ovary syndrome, and ovarian cancer risk in a population-based case-control study. Int J Cancer. 2017;140:285–91.
98. Sharts-Hopko NC. Depo-Provera. MCN Am J Matern Child Nurs. 1993;18:128.
99. Karimi-Zarchi M, Dehghani-Firoozabadi R, Tabatabaie A, Dehghani-Firoozabadi Z, Teimoori S, Chiti Z, et al. A comparison of the effect of levonorgestrel IUD with oral medroxyprogesterone acetate on abnormal uterine bleeding with simple endometrial hyperplasia and fertility preservation. Clin Exp Obstet Gynecol. 2013;40:421–4.
100. Balen AH, Morley LC, Misso M, Franks S, Legro RS, Wijeyaratne CN, et al. The management of anovulatory infertility in women with polycystic ovary syndrome: an analysis of the evidence to support the development of global WHO guidance. Hum Reprod Update. 2016;22:687–708.
101. Cena H, Chiovato L, Nappi RE. Obesity, polycystic ovary syndrome, and infertility: a new avenue for GLP-1 receptor agonists. J Clin Endocrinol Metab. 2020;105(8):e2695–709.
102. Talmor A, Dunphy B. Female obesity and infertility. Best Pract Res Clin Obstet Gynaecol. 2015;29:498–506.
103. Velazquez EM, Mendoza S, Hamer T, Sosa F, Glueck CJ. Metformin therapy in polycystic ovary syndrome reduces hyperinsulinemia, insulin resistance, hyperandrogenemia, and systolic blood pressure, while facilitating normal menses and pregnancy. Metabolism. 1994;43:647–54.
104. Lashen H. Review: role of metformin in the management of polycystic ovary syndrome. Ther Adv Endocrinol Metab. 2010;1:117–28.
105. Penzias A, Bendikson K, Butts S, Coutifaris C, Falcone T, Fossum G, et al. Role of metformin for ovulation induction in infertile patients with polycystic ovary syndrome (PCOS): a guideline. Fertil Steril. 2017;108:426–41.
106. Wild RA, Carmina E, Diamanti-Kandarakis E, Dokras A, Escobar-Morreale HF, Futterweit W, et al. Assessment of cardiovascular risk and prevention of cardiovascular disease in women with the polycystic ovary syndrome: a consensus statement by the Androgen Excess and Polycystic Ovary Syndrome (AE-PCOS) Society. J Clin Endocrinol Metabol. 2010;95:2038–49.
107. Kakoly NS, Khomami MB, Joham AE, Cooray SD, Misso ML, Norman RJ, et al. Ethnicity, obesity and the prevalence of impaired glucose tolerance and type 2 diabetes in PCOS: a systematic review and meta-regression. Hum Reprod Update. 2018;24:455–67.
108. Tang T, Norman RJ, Balen AH, Lord JM. Insulin-sensitising drugs (metformin, troglitazone, rosiglitazone, pioglitazone, D-chiro-inositol) for polycystic ovary syndrome. In: Tang T, editor. Cochrane database of systematic reviews. Chichester, UK: John Wiley & Sons, Ltd; 2003.
109. Arlt W, Auchus RJ, Miller WL. Thiazolidinediones but not metformin directly inhibit the steroidogenic enzymes P450c17 and 3β-hydroxysteroid dehydrogenase. J Biol Chem. 2001;276:16767–71.

110. Diamanti-Kandarakis E, Economou F, Palimeri S, Christakou C. Metformin in polycystic ovary syndrome. Ann N Y Acad Sci. 2010;1205:192–8.
111. Genazzani AD, Ricchieri F, Lanzoni C. Use of metformin in the treatment of polycystic ovary syndrome. Womens Health (Lond). 2010;6:577–93.
112. Bruno RV, de Avila MAP, Neves FB, Nardi AE, Crespo CMS, Sobrinho ATC. Comparison of two doses of metformin (2.5 and 1.5 g/day) for the treatment of polycystic ovary syndrome and their effect on body mass index and waist circumference. Fertil Steril. 2007;88:510–2.
113. Tzotzas T, Karras SN, Katsiki N. Glucagon-Like Peptide-1 (GLP-1) receptor agonists in the treatment of obese women with polycystic ovary syndrome. Curr Vasc Pharmacol. 2017;15:218–29.

# Part VII

# Other Clinical Considerations in the Care of Adults with Chronic Childhood Conditions

# Respiratory Care of Adults with Chronic Pulmonary Disease and Assisted Ventilation

41

Tara Lynn Barto

## Introduction

The last 30 years have seen a shift in the care of chronic pulmonary disease, owing in large part to the advancements in medicine and technology. Comprehensive chronic disease management, as demonstrated in cystic fibrosis (CF) and muscular dystrophy (MD), has led to improved survival and quality of life for children diagnosed with previously fatal conditions, such that now these patients are living well into adulthood. The care of patients with chronic respiratory failure (CRF) has followed suit with this changing landscape of chronic disease management. CRF is defined as a condition persisting for greater than 1 month and requiring mechanical ventilation for part (at least 6 h) or all of the day to provide adequate ventilation [1]. Previously, children with CRF would be confined to a hospital with personnel trained in respiratory care and ventilator management, with patients and their families choosing home only for palliative or hospice care. Today, patients are offered multiple options for the management of respiratory failure at home, albeit requiring significant education, family commitment, and medical community support.

T. L. Barto (✉)
Division of Pulmonary, Critical Care and Sleep Medicine, Baylor College of Medicine, Houston, TX, USA
e-mail: tara.barto@bcm.edu

Like many changes in medicine, the initial impetus to move toward home care for patients with CRF was financial in origin. However, what seems to have grown out of this movement is a paradigm for managing complex medical patients safely while improving survival and quality of life. Integral to these improvements has been the development of programs supporting the care of chronically-ventilated patients with CRF at home as well as multi-disciplinary teams knowledgeable in the care of these patients. In addition to these changes, the trends in parental expectations of long-term survival in children with chronic respiratory failure have led to more parents, initially taking on the long-term responsibility for these patients.

## Chronic Respiratory Failure

CRF can be divided into three categories, each with different expectations of progression and need for lifelong mechanical ventilation. The first is CRF related to ventilatory muscle weakness, for example, neuromuscular diseases such as Duchenne's muscular dystrophy or quadriplegia. As home care for CRF was gaining popularity, these patients comprised more than 50% of patients offering home mechanical ventilation (HMV), although reports reviewing the trends in HMV have shown that patients with other categories of CRF are more often being offered home


A. A. Kuo et al. (eds.), *Care of Adults with Chronic Childhood Conditions*,
https://doi.org/10.1007/978-3-031-54281-7_41

care options as well [2]. Because these conditions are typically chronic and progressive, it is unlikely that once a patient requires mechanical ventilatory support, they would be able to successfully wean from such support.

The second category of CRF is related to disorders of the lung parenchyma and airways, which in turn cause an increase in the work of breathing. Examples include patients with bronchopulmonary dysplasia, interstitial lung disease, and chest wall deformities. As children with such conditions age and grow, their respiratory mechanics may improve, allowing them to be potentially weaned from ventilation.

The final category of CRF is related to disorders that cause a failure of neurologic control of breathing, examples are post-encephalitis, brain trauma, or rarer conditions such as congenital central hypoventilation syndrome (CCHS). These conditions typically require lifelong ventilation, although in certain conditions, such as CCHS, ventilation may only be required at night.

## Mechanical Ventilation

Home mechanical ventilation (HMV) can be described in different ways: positive versus negative pressure ventilation, invasive versus non-invasive ventilation (NIV), and mode of ventilation, to name a few. As a primary care provider (PCP), it is most important to understand the difference between the invasive and non-invasive mechanical ventilation and possible complications of each. The initiation of HMV should be accomplished in coordination with a specialist in pulmonary disease. Furthermore, the ventilator settings, regardless of whether invasive or non-invasive ventilation is being employed, should first be established with inpatient titration and monitoring, typically during a sleep study. Optimal ventilation is achieved once the partial pressure of carbon dioxide ($PaCO_2$) normalizes. If a patient remains hypoxemic at this point, then oxygen supplementation is added. Oxygen should not be used until adequate ventilation is maintained, as it can mask cyanosis, worsen hypercapnia, and delay the initiation of ventilatory support [3]. The chronic management of mechanically-ventilated patients employs monitoring carbon dioxide levels, typically with venous blood gases and intermittent sleep studies to ensure appropriate ventilation. Such monitoring may be required more frequently in children, as they tend to grow and require more frequent changes in their settings than adults do.

The goals of initiating HMV are to improve quality of life, improve mobility and rehabilitation potential, and improve growth and development. Qualitative data on patients' experiences before and after the initiation of mechanical ventilation are limited but suggest that patients' improvement in dyspnea directly impacts their quality of life. Though a minority of patients report negative social impacts and low self-esteem, these outcomes do not negate the reported improvement in quality of life due to relief of dyspnea [4]. The standard outcome measure of quality of life in children has been the patient's ability to reintegrate into the school system [5–7]. In order to accomplish the goals of HMV, ventilators must be small, lightweight, portable, durable, and able to be powered by a battery. As technology is advancing, these devices are becoming more portable and user friendly [8]. Recently, home ventilators have been equipped with the ability to wirelessly transmit usage and performance data, allowing more efficient remote monitoring. The implications of this technology are yet undetermined, but the expectation is decreased in emergency room visits and hospitalizations [9].

Non-invasive ventilation (NIV) employs a simpler device and is accomplished using a mask or nasal pillows, making this device less cumbersome. The success of NIV is highly dependent on the patient's ability to tolerate the masks. These devices exert pressure on the face to maintain the seal and reduce air leak potential, leading to a risk of midface hypoplasia in children or pressure ulcers in adults. Regular monitoring of the site of contact of the mask and face is important. Additionally, NIV cannot meet high flow demands of certain patients, causing dyssynchrony between the patient and the ventilator which the patient would perceive as dyspnea. As such, certain patients may not be comfortably ventilated with this type of ventilator.

Invasive mechanical ventilation is accomplished with a traditional home ventilator through a tracheostomy. This type of ventilator is a more cumbersome machine but can provide more sophisticated modes of ventilation, allowing for improved patient comfort. Despite placement of a tracheostomy, most patients will still be able to vocalize.

The decision to use invasive or non-invasive ventilation should be made only after discussion among the patient, family, pulmonologist, and, if desired, the PCP. Traditionally, if a patient requires mechanical ventilation for 24 h per day, then the invasive modality is recommended. However, in children, even those requiring ventilation for 24 h per day, non-invasive ventilation is often initiated until there is failure to adequately ventilate, failure to tolerate the mask, high risk of ongoing aspiration due to changes in bulbar function, or ineffective management of airway secretions [3, 5, 10].

## Tracheostomy

A tracheostomy tube is surgically placed in the neck extending into the trachea to allow for adequate ventilation, both assisted and non-assisted. These tubes require special attention and care to ensure proper cleaning and use. Typically, tracheostomy care is coordinated with an otolaryngologist (ENT), the surgeon that most commonly places these devices. Once the decision is made to pursue invasive mechanical ventilation, a tracheostomy tube is placed. The choice of the type of tube to use is made based on many factors. The two most common types of tracheostomies are plastic and metal. Plastic tubes are more flexible and typically smaller in nature. They are comprised of an outer cannula and an inner removable or disposable cannula. They come in standard sizes, although custom tubes can be made if a patient needs to have a longer portion entering the trachea, for example, in individuals with significant redundant neck tissue. Metal tubes are less flexible but more easily cleaned and therefore are used when patients have thick tenacious secretions or if they frequently obstruct their plastic tube. Tubes can also be uncuffed or cuffed, meaning that there is a cuff on the distal intra-tracheal limb that is used to prevent air leaks in patients requiring mechanical ventilation. It is important to know that cuffs, if not managed properly, can cause damage as high pressure over extended periods of time can cause tracheal scarring. Tracheostomy tube cuffs are designed to be a high-volume, low-pressure system, cuffs should only be inflated enough to prevent air leaks during mechanical ventilation, as over inflation can cause tracheal damage over time. Tracheostomy tube cuffs should not be inflated above a maximum pressure of 20 cm of water ($cmH_2O$).

Patients and caregivers will need training in tracheostomy care, which should be performed once a day. This typically involves changing the dressings and tracheostomy ties as well as cleaning the inner cannula. Plastic tubes must also be removed, and a new one is placed periodically. The ENT physician changes the tube the first time, typically 1–2 weeks after placement. There are no well-established guidelines on how often chronic tracheostomy tubes need to be changed thereafter, but recommendations range from every 2 weeks to every 3–4 months. This decision is best made in consultation with the ENT physician [11].

Complications of tracheostomy tubes are categorized into early and late. Early complications are those complications most commonly occurring up until the first tube change. They can be directly related to placement, for example, development of a false tract or pneumothorax, or local complications including infection, bleeding, or obstruction. The tracheostomy tube is sutured in place until the first change, so decannulation is uncommon. Late complications also include infection, obstruction, and bleeding, the most concerning of which would be an innominate artery fistula, typically occurring in the first 3 weeks after placement. This is exhibited by recurrent bleeding from the tracheostomy tube site. Chronic tracheostomy tube placement can result in other complications over time including recurrent tracheitis, granulation tissue formation, which would lead to recurrent obstruction, and permanent tracheocutaneous fistula. Routine monitoring for the development of these complications is mandatory. Some patients will develop chronic or recurrent tracheitis, as such they should routinely have tracheal cultures performed to determine the nature of the bacterial flora in their airway in the event of an infection or an exacerbation.

## Airway Clearance and Humidification

Patients with CRF due to any number of reasons often have difficulty managing respiratory secretions. For example, muscle weakness in patients with MD, increased secretion production in individuals with CF, and loss of cough reflex in those with central neurologic conditions can all pose challenges in the handling of respiratory secretions. To assist patients in managing these secretions, additional respiratory therapies should be administered 2–4 times daily. These therapies include inhaled airway hydration, mechanical airway clearance techniques, and frequent suctioning. There are multiple forms of airway clearance techniques including chest physiotherapy (CPT), high frequently chest wall compression (HFCWC), and intrapulmonary percussive ventilation, all of which can be used with both invasive and non-invasive mechanical ventilation. Consultation with the pulmonologist should be sought to determine if the patient would benefit from these therapies.

Heated humidification is the delivery of air, with or without supplemental oxygen, that has been heated and passed over sterile water to increase the humidity. Heated humidification is mandatory for all patients who use invasive mechanical ventilation. Its benefits include prevention of tracheal mucosa dryness, preventing infection; prevention of inspissated secretions by increasing hydration; decreasing the risk of hypothermia; and increasing patient comfort. Care must be taken to ensure proper cleaning of the humidifier and use of sterile water.

## Emergency Action Plans

Emergency action plans should be devised early in the planning of mechanical ventilation with input from the pulmonologist, ENT, and PCP. Key topics to include would be which physician should be contacted for an acute illness or particular issue and who is responsible for ordering specific equipment and supplies. Families should be provided with the appropriate equipment in the event of an emergency. For example, they should have equipment and training to perform manual ventilation in the event of power outages and extra tracheostomy tubes for placement in the event of an accidental decannulation.

## Weaning from Ventilation

Patients will ask if weaning off the ventilator is an option. This often is not possible if the condition requiring mechanical ventilation is a chronic progressive condition. However, for children who are placed on mechanical ventilation due to bronchopulmonary dysplasia or tracheobronchomalacia, it is possible that, as they grow, their respiratory mechanics may improve such that HMV is no longer required. If weaning is a potential option, after consultation with the pulmonologist, patients are usually liberated from the ventilator for progressively longer periods of time rather than adjusting ventilator settings. Careful monitoring of vital signs and assessment of patient tolerance of being off the ventilator are critical. The final steps of weaning from a ventilator at night should be done in a monitored setting, such as an inpatient stay or during sleep study.

## Caregivers

Caregivers are the most integral part of the care of a ventilated patient. It has been suggested that it is not the education level of the caregiver that predicts success but rather the commitment and dedication to appropriate home care [8]. It is a lot of time consuming physically and mentally rigorous undertaking to be a caregiver for a patient requiring mechanical ventilation. The role of home health care services is to provide the caregiver a reprieve to allow them to rest and care for themselves as well as to provide support for certain patient activities such as bathing, respiratory treatments, and tracheostomy care. Prior to a mechanically-ventilated patient being discharged to home, the caregivers must go through extensive education to learn tracheostomy care, understand the ventilator, coordinate emergency action plans, and be instructed in basic life support, among many other things (see Table 41.1).

**Table 41.1** Caregiver education checklist

| | |
|---|---|
| General | Understanding of underlying disease<br>Concerning signs and symptoms<br>Inhaled therapies/airway clearance techniques<br>Emergency care/CPR<br>Emergency call number<br>Medical history document |
| Oxygen therapy | Understand why it is necessary<br>Oxygen source<br>Care/maintenance of equipment<br>Flow rate of oxygen<br>Complications of oxygen therapy |
| Tracheostomy care | Understand why it is necessary<br>Safe activities of daily living<br>Communication and speech<br>Cleaning and sterilization of equipment<br>Suctioning techniques and equipment<br>Tube and ties change<br>Accidental decannulation plan<br>In home safety<br>Transportation safety |
| Ventilator care | How the ventilator works<br>Understanding alarms/complications<br>Problem solving ventilator malfunction<br>Check ventilator and humidifier<br>Mask/tracheostomy tube interface<br>Cleaning and sterilization of equipment<br>In home safety<br>Battery and power supply<br>Manual bag mask ventilation |

Adapted from Preutthipan A. Indian J of Pediatr 2015:82(9):852–9

Experience has shown that, with a multidisciplinary approach to care and dedicated family and caregivers, HMV is a viable option that can improve both quality of life and survival among individuals with CRF. A number of support systems have been established to assist in these endeavors.

## References


1. Adams AB, Whitman J, Marcy T. Surveys of long term ventilatory support in Minnesota: 1986 and 1992. Chest. 1993;103(5):1463–9.
2. Chatwin M, Tan HL, Bush A, Rosenthal M, Simonds AK. Long term non-invasive ventilation in children: impact on survival and transition to adult care. PLoS One. 2015;10(5):e0125839.
3. Hull J, Aniapravan R, Chan E, et al. British Thoracic Society Guideline for respiratory management of children with neuromuscular weakness. Thorax. 2012;67:i1–40.
4. Noyes J. Health and quality of life of ventilator-dependent children. J Adv Nurs. 2006;56(4):392–403.
5. Amin R, Fitton C. Tracheostomy and home ventilation in children. Semin Neonatol. 2003;8:127–35.
6. Gilgoff IS, Kahlstrom E, Maclaughlin E, Keens TG. Long-term ventilatory support in spinal muscular atrophy. J Pediatr. 1989;115(6):904–9.
7. Marcus CL, Jansen MT, Poulson MK, Keens SE, Nield TA, Lipsker LE, et al. Medical and psychosocial outcome of children with congenital central hypoventilation syndrome. J Pediatr. 1991;119(6):888–95.
8. Preutthipan A. Home mechanical ventilation in children. Indian J Pediatr. 2015;82(9):852–9.
9. Ackrivo J, Elman L, Hansen-Flaschen J. Telemonitoring for home—assisted ventilation: a narrative review. Ann Am Thorac Soc. 2021;18(11):1761–72.
10. Nixon GM, Edwards EA, Cooper D et al. Ventilatory support at home for children. A consensus statement from the Australian Paediatric Respiratory Group. February 2008. APRG Working. Available from http://www.thoracicorgau/documents/papers/aprg-homeventilationguideline.pdf.
11. White AC, Kher S, O'Connor H. When to change a tracheostomy tube. Respir Care. 2010;55(8):1069–75.

# Nutritional Support

# 42

Susan Hunt, Dana Topper, and Deonna C. Monnahan

## Introduction

As children move into adolescence and young adulthood, their nutritional goals transition from weight gain and linear growth to weight maintenance. For young adults with chronic childhood conditions (YACCC), this transition may be complicated by changes in caloric needs over time as severity of illness or functional ability changes and thus requires special attention from their adult providers. Some YACCC may already be receiving nutrition support while others may need to have these issues addressed anew. The assessment of ongoing needs in both groups is needed to prevent malnutrition or overweight and obesity. Involvement of a dietitian may be advisable in complex situations, but medical providers should have a working understanding of potential nutritional issues such as malnutrition and overnutrition as well as types of nutritional support and their potential complications.

S. Hunt (✉)
Departments of General Internal Medicine and Pediatric Medicine, University of Washington Medical Center and Seattle Children's Hospital, Seattle, WA, USA
e-mail: hunts1@uw.edu

D. Topper · D. C. Monnahan
Department of Nutrition, Seattle Children's Hospital, Seattle, WA, USA
e-mail: dana.topper@seattlechildrens.org; deonna.monnahan@seattlechildrens.org

## Malnutrition

Malnutrition is common in YACCC. Although the diversity of conditions makes general estimates impossible, children with cerebral palsy, as one example, may have rates of 29–46%, with prevalence increasing with age [1]. Malnutrition is associated with increased morbidity and mortality, more frequent hospital admissions and longer length of stay, and decreased quality of life [2]. Nutritional deficits may be multifactorial in origin and type, depending on the young adult's underlying medical condition. For example, in cystic fibrosis (CF), patients may have calorie deficit, fatty acid deficiency, and vitamin deficiency as a result of the multisystem effects of their underlying disorder [3, 4]. Causes of caloric and nutrient deficits in CF further demonstrate the major categories of malnutrition in transition patients:

1. Normal nutritional intake but increased needs due to medical condition.
2. Inadequate nutritional intake due to oral feeding difficulties or restrictions.
3. Malabsorption, feeding intolerance, and other gastrointestinal (GI) issues that cause nutritional losses.

Increased caloric needs are hypothesized as a common cause of undernutrition in chronic illness, but this is often difficult to quantify due to


A. A. Kuo et al. (eds.), *Care of Adults with Chronic Childhood Conditions*,
https://doi.org/10.1007/978-3-031-54281-7_42

complexity of measuring resting energy expenditure (REE) and total energy expenditure in real-life situations. CF provides a well-studied example of this issue. While initial speculation suggested the underlying genetic defect of CF as the source of increased requirements, studies in children with CF show that REE does not differ from that of healthy controls [5]. In adults with preserved lung function, REE is also unchanged. However, as lung function declines, exacerbations become more frequent and secondary complications such as diabetes and liver disease manifest, resulting in an increase in REE, placing patients at risk of caloric deficiency [4]. Another condition where the complications of the disorder cause increased REE is cerebral palsy, where the subset of patients with athetosis, or continuous involuntary movements, have increased caloric needs [6, 7].

Inadequate oral intake, regardless of REE, is the most frequent cause of undernutrition in YACCC. In CF, for example, appetite may decrease due to nausea associated with recurrent pulmonary exacerbations or gastroparesis resulting from CF-related diabetes. Selective eating patterns can also lead to inadequate intake and are common in patients with developmental disability, with some studies indicating prevalence of up to 80% in children, although rates may show some improvement with age [8]. In children with autism, for example, approximately 60% have “strong food preferences,” often related to texture (up to 70% of preferences) or restricted food choices, placing them at increased nutritional risk [9]. Iatrogenic limitations on intake resulting from admissions for illness or planned procedures with provider-ordered held nutrition can have a higher impact on YACCC who start in a tenuous nutritional state. Finally, dysphagia can be a factor in multiple disorders including central neurologic disorders such as hypoxic-ischemic injury with resultant cerebral palsy, degenerative muscular disorders such as Duchenne muscular dystrophy (DMD), or genetic anomalies with physical variations causing poor oropharyngeal coordination, such as Pierre Robin sequence [10–12].

A subset of underlying conditions impairs adequate absorption from the gastrointestinal tract or leads to increased losses. CF patients may have both insufficient absorption of fats and vitamins, even when symptoms of pancreatic insufficiency are clinically well controlled, as well as sugar loss due to glycosuria from CF-related diabetes [3]. Conditions such as inflammatory bowel disease (IBD) and celiac disease can cause poor absorption during disease flares. Children with Crohn’s disease, for example, have high rates of growth failure, up to 56% in some studies [13]. Young adults with prior intestinal resections, such as those with a history of necrotizing enterocolitis or IBD, may have decreased absorptive intestine or ostomies, which further complicate nutritional status.

## Overnutrition

In addition to conditions predisposing to undernutrition, YACCC, like the general population, can also suffer from overnutrition, overweight, and obesity. In cerebral palsy and spina bifida, for example, energy needs are significantly linked to physical activity, and patients who have progressive loss of ambulatory ability due to worsening contractures or weakness may have decreased energy requirements, placing them at risk of weight gain and obesity if feeding is not adjusted [7, 14]. Genetic conditions may predispose to obesity, such as Prader-Willi syndrome, with associated hyperphagia, and trisomy 21 (Down syndrome), due to poor impulse management and carryover dietary habits from childhood [12]. Obesity can have short-term morbidity costs, such as decreased ambulatory ability and caregiver difficulty lifting and transferring non-ambulatory patients, as well as the typical long-term costs associated with obesity in adult populations, such as metabolic syndrome and cardiovascular disease.

## Assessing Nutritional Status in YACCC

This section covers basic nutritional concepts and common situations that a PCP may encounter when caring for YACCC. These include the assessment of weight goals, accurate diagnosis of nutritional status, and gathering a dietary history from a patient with intellectual or developmental disability. Familiarity with these fundamentals will allow PCPs to adequately address the basic nutritional health of most YACCC. In certain instances, though, consultation with a dietitian may be necessary.

## Consultation with a Dietitian

For those patients not meeting their nutritional goals after assessment and intervention by the PCP, consideration should be given to involving a registered dietitian, who can complete a thorough evaluation of the patient's nutritional intake and status and help the patient set nutrition goals based on specialized medical needs and lifestyle. A dietitian should be involved in most decisions about initiation or adjustment of enteral and parenteral nutrition. Additional specific conditions may require a dietitian analysis of specific nutrients; for example, a patient with chronic kidney disease (CKD) who struggles to decrease their potassium or phosphorus levels, or a patient with a very low caloric intake who may be at risk for nutrient deficiencies. Some common instances of these conditions and appropriate use of a dietitian's services are highlighted throughout the following sections, although a comprehensive list is beyond the scope of this text.

## Assessing Weight Goals

Identifying appropriate caloric intake and weight goals is a foundational step of nutritional assessment. Adult providers are likely to be familiar with the body mass index (BMI) as an indicator of total body fat, with 18.5–24.9 kg/m$^2$ considered a healthy range for men and women. BMI < 18.5 kg/m$^2$ indicates underweight, >25 kg/m$^2$ overweight, and >30 kg/m$^2$ obese [15]. There are many equations that can be used to calculate ideal body weight but little research to support their validity. A BMI of 22 kg/m$^2$ is associated with the lowest rate of mortality for those between the age of 30 and 59 years and so may be an appropriate goal for healthy adults [16]. However, BMI should not be used alone as the primary measure to assess nutritional status, since it is not a good indicator of body composition and does not consider the patient's underlying condition [17].

When assessing YACCC, weight goals should be individualized, taking into consideration the patient's medical condition, weight history, body type, and degree of muscle mass. For example, in patients with lower muscle mass, a BMI at the low end of normal may be appropriate, such as those who are non-ambulatory with hypotonic cerebral palsy or Down syndrome. In addition, BMI is only useful if the weight and height are accurately measured, and obtaining an accurate height can be difficult in patients with contractures or who are unable to stand. For wheelchair users, recumbent length gives the most accurate measurement [18]. For those who are unable to safely transfer to a flat table or have contractures, the next best approach is the knee height method or self-report [18].

## Diagnosis of Nutritional Status

Correctly diagnosing malnutrition is important for heightened focus on the nutritional status of the patient and targeted interventions, as well as for accurate coding, billing, and research purposes. Clinical indicators of malnutrition can be identified by a thorough medical history, assessment of nutritional intake, physical signs of nutrient deficiencies, anthropometrics, and possibly hand grip strength (see Table 42.1) [2]. Additional elements that can elucidate increased risk for malnutrition include mental health history, psychosocial factors, and lab results, in particular markers of inflammation [2]. Historically, albumin and prealbumin have been used as biomarkers of nutritional status [19]. However, more recently, albumin in particular has been criticized due to the lack of specificity as it can be influenced by underlying disease and inflammation [19]. When malnutrition is confirmed, the PCP should address the etiology/etiologies of the mal-

**Table 42.1** Diagnosing malnutrition

| Clinical characteristic | Acute illness or injury | | Chronic illness (≥3 months) | | Social or environmental circumstances | |
|---|---|---|---|---|---|---|
| | Moderate malnutrition | Severe malnutrition | Moderate malnutrition | Severe malnutrition | Moderate malnutrition | Severe malnutrition |
| Energy intake | <75% estimated energy requirement for >7 days | ≤50% estimated energy requirement for ≥5 days | <75% estimated energy requirement for ≥1 month | <75% estimated energy requirement for ≥1 month | <75% estimated energy requirement for ≥3 months | ≤50% estimated energy requirement for ≥1 month |
| Weight loss | 1–2% in 1 week, 5% in 1 month, or 7.5% in 3 months | >2% in 1 week, >5% in 1 month, or > 7.5% in 3 months | 5% in 1 month, 7.5% in 3 months, 10% in 6 months, 20% in 1 year | >5% in 1 month, >7.5% in 3 months, >10% in 6 months, >20% in 1 year | 5% in 1 month, 7.5% in 3 months, 10% in 6 months, 20% in 1 year | >5% in 1 month, >7.5% in 3 months, >10% in 6 months, >20% in 1 year |
| Body fat loss | Mild | Moderate | Mild | Severe | Mild | Severe |
| Muscle loss | Mild | Moderate | Mild | Severe | Mild | Severe |
| Fluid accumulation | Mild | Moderate to Severe | Mild | Severe | Mild | Severe |
| Reduced grip strength | N/A | Reduced | N/A | Reduced | N/A | Reduced |

At least two characteristics are recommended for the diagnosis of moderate or severe malnutrition. The table is created using data from White JV *et al.* [2]
There is inadequate evidence to define mild malnutrition [2]

nutrition, develop an intervention with the patient or caregiver, and confirm a plan for routine monitoring and adjustment of the intervention until the malnutrition is resolved. Basic initial interventions for malnutrition typically include encouraging consumption of high-calorie, high-protein foods and addressing barriers to doing so, starting a multivitamin and mineral supplement, and providing any additional supplements indicated by lab abnormalities. For malnourished patients, an appropriate rate of weight gain is 1–2 pounds per week toward ideal body weight. Further information on how to support patients who are unable to increase their oral intake to meet their needs will be discussed in subsequent sections of this chapter.

The clinical assessment for overweight and obese patients includes the same factors as for malnutrition. For overweight patients, an appropriate weight loss goal is 0.5–1 pounds per week toward achieving 10% body weight loss over a 6-month period [20]. Regular follow-up is essential to support patient centered goals and ensure healthy weight trends. Dietitian support should be considered if the patient weight goals are unclear, goals are not being met, or patient and/or caregivers would benefit from additional counseling.

## Gathering a Diet History from a Patient with Intellectual or Developmental Disability

The high prevalence of underweight and overweight among adults with intellectual or developmental disabilities makes nutritional evaluation a valuable part of their clinical assessment [21]. Adults with intellectual or developmental disabilities may not be able to provide an accurate diet history, and unfortunately, currently there is no validated approach to completing a dietary intake assessment for this population [21]. A proxy reporter may be able to provide accurate information if they are consistent with the patient during eating opportunities [21]. There are many strategies to assess dietary intake, such as retrospective food record, 24-hour recall, food frequency questionnaire, food checklists, and direct observation. There is no evidence to support prospective methods being more accurate than retrospective or vice versa, and no gold standard method using the patient report has been established [22]. Underreporting intake is a common reporter bias [22]. Of the various methods, the 24-hour recall can be the fastest approach to assessing a patient's intake. This method requires the patient to report all the foods and beverages consumed the day prior, and if time allows including portion sizes. Patients are often more accurate in their reporting if they are prompted to recall the previous day in a sequential order. These principles can be applied to caregiver histories as well. Other comorbidities affecting intake should be noted in the initial nutritional history, such as dysphagia, GI problems, and sensory issues that limit food choices. This information will also help inform a dietary consultant if your history does not reveal causes for weight imbalance.

### Psychosocial Factors in Dietary History

When assessing dietary intake, composition, and quality in YACCC, psychosocial factors such as food insecurity and access to healthy food options should be explored. In general, food insecure adults take in fewer fruits, vegetables, and dairy products than those who are food secure and can have reduced intake of essential vitamins and minerals including calcium, magnesium, and zinc [23]. YACCC may be at increased risk of food insecurity; for example, a survey of the US young adults found higher rates of food insecurity in those with intellectual and developmental disabilities than those without, even controlling for poverty [24]. Young adults just leaving a school environment are particularly vulnerable as the nutritional supports provided in public school settings are lost. Limitations on food assistance, such as work-requirements in place in some US states to qualify for the Supplemental Nutrition Assistance Program (SNAP), can also limit access to remedies for food insecurity; while not intended to apply to people with disabilities, in practice these requirements reduce use by patients with disabilities and also disproportionately affect non-White participants [25]. In situations where food insecurity or monetary factors are severely impacting nutrition, social work consultation should be considered.

As with all patients, assessing cultural differences in food preferences or restrictions and food associations with cultural practices, such as fasting or food-focused religious holidays, should be included in a dietary history. Nutritional recommendations should be adapted to cultural factors whenever possible to increase adherence.

## Common Nutritional Considerations

### Bone Health

Growth and bone health are a major focus of medical nutrition therapy for children with chronic disease. Patients will no longer be growing in height by the time they transition to adult care, so this focus should shift to maintaining bone health. Young adults with intellectual or developmental disabilities are at higher risk for poor bone health compared to those who are typically developed [21]. Patients who are non-ambulatory are at greater risk for lower bone density [26].

Adequate calcium and phosphorus intake are crucial for bone health, as they make up 80–90% of bone mineral content. Vitamin D, given its role in promoting calcium absorption and decreased bone turnover, is also a critical nutrient [27]. Dietary phosphorus is typically less of a focus when counseling patients, likely because national surveys have shown that calcium intake is low whereas phosphorus intake is greater than recommended among adults in the United States [27].

At 19 years of age, the recommended dietary allowance (RDA) for calcium decreases from 1300 mg to 1000 mg of elemental calcium daily [28]. The National Osteoporosis Foundation has a guide to quickly assess your patient's calcium intake [29]. Notably, multivitamins and mineral supplements typically do not contain significant amounts of calcium, so separate supplementation is often warranted. Food sources of calcium include dairy products, sardines, spinach, kale, broccoli, bok choy, soybeans, tofu, and fortified breakfast cereals and fruit juices [30].

The RDA for vitamin D intake remains 15 mcg (600 IU) daily in adulthood, although higher intake is necessary for repletion in those with preexisting vitamin D deficiency or insufficiency [28]. Vitamin D deficiency is common among young adults, with the primary causes being inadequate exposure to sunlight and very few foods rich in vitamin D [31, 32]. Food sources of vitamin D include fatty fish, fish liver oil, beef liver, egg yolk, and mushrooms [33, 34]. In addition, some dairy products, including cow's milk and plant milk alternatives, have been fortified with vitamin D [33, 34]. Screening for vitamin D deficiency should be considered in YACCC, particularly those at high risk such as patients on anticonvulsant therapy and those with dark skin due to lower rates of synthesis in response to the sun [33, 35]. The Endocrine Society recommends adults on anticonvulsant medications, glucocorticoids, antifungals, and medications used to treat human immunodeficiency virus (HIV) infection/acquired immunodeficiency syndrome (AIDS) receive 2–3 times the RDA for vitamin D, since these medications increase the catabolism of vitamin D [33].

Additional nutrients essential for bone health include protein, magnesium, zinc, copper, iron, fluoride, and vitamins A, C, and K [27].

## Iron Deficiency

Providers should be aware of common vitamin and mineral deficiencies among YACCC, including iron deficiency anemia (IDA), which is the most common cause of anemia worldwide [36]. Groups at particularly high risk of iron deficiency include infants, young children, women of reproductive age, and pregnant women. Additionally, YACCC may be at risk for IDA if they have a condition resulting in malabsorption, such as celiac disease, or inflammation of the gastrointestinal tract, such as in IBD [37]. Other risk factors for iron deficiency in this population include poor intake, feeding difficulties, limited diet variety, and food insecurity.

Signs and symptoms of IDA may include fatigue, pallor of the conjunctiva and skin, shortness of breath, tachycardia, restless leg syndrome, koilonychias (spoon-shaped nails), angular stomatitis, glossitis, and pica [38]. In the absence of inflammation, a serum ferritin level is one of the most cost-effective and efficient indicators to assess iron status [37]. Other lab indicators suggestive of iron deficiency include low serum iron, elevated total iron binding capacity (TIBC), and low transferrin saturation [36]. A complete blood count (CBC) may also reveal a microcytic anemia, with low hemoglobin and low mean corpuscular volume (MCV), although this is not a sensitive nor specific indicator for IDA [36, 37].

Oral iron therapy is the first-line approach to treating IDA [38]. To promote optimal absorption, iron supplements should be taken with a source of vitamin C and apart from tea, coffee, and calcium containing foods/beverages or supplements [37]. In those patients that cannot tolerate oral/enteral iron supplementation, or if there are concerns for malabsorption, an intravenous iron infusion can be considered [37].

In addition, promoting iron-rich food sources is important for the prevention of iron deficiency. From ages 19–50 years, the RDA for iron is 8 mg daily for males and 18 mg daily for females [39]. Iron is present in food in two forms, heme iron, which is more readily absorbed, and non-heme iron. Food sources of heme iron include meat, poultry, and seafood. Sources of non-heme iron include legumes, nuts, green leafy vegetables, tofu, whole grains, and iron-fortified cereal.

## Drug–Nutrient/Food Interactions

Drug–nutrient and drug–food interactions can have significant impact on patient health and must be evaluated as a part of medication review. Some medications can alter the patient's nutritional status or lead to nutrient deficiencies, and conversely some foods can alter the drug effect [40]. Table 42.2 outlines common drug–nutrient/food interactions that may be seen with YACCC.

**Table 42.2** Drug–nutrient, drug–food interactions

| | |
|---|---|
| Anticonvulsants | Can increase need for vitamins D, K, C, B12, folate, and calcium with long-term use associated with low carnitine levels |
| Corticosteroids | Decreased bone mineral density; ensure adequate intake of calcium and vitamin D |
| Diuretics | Increased losses of sodium, potassium, chloride, calcium, magnesium, and zinc |
| Immunosuppressants | Grapefruit can increase drug concentration<br>Increased losses of magnesium and potassium<br>Special attention to food safety to avoid food-borne illness |
| Statins | Grapefruit can increase drug concentration<br>May decrease absorption of fat-soluble vitamins (A, D, E, and K), vitamin B12, folic acid, and calcium |
| Anticoagulants (warfarin) | Vitamin K decreases anticoagulation effect (keep vitamin K intake consistent for best results). Licorice, vitamin E, fish oil, mango, and grapefruit may increase anticoagulation effect |
| Monoamine oxidase inhibitors | Interaction with tyramine in food can cause severe hypertension |
| Proton pump inhibitors | May impair absorption of calcium, magnesium, iron, zinc, folic acid, and B12<br>May increase risk of bone fractures; ensure adequate intake of calcium and vitamin D |
| Calcium channel blockers | Grapefruit can increase drug concentration<br>Large amount of natural licorice can increase blood pressure |
| Beta blockers | Large amount of natural licorice can increase blood pressure |

Additionally, some medications may affect appetite, such as certain psychiatric medications including antidepressants and antipsychotics as well as stimulants for attention disorders, and their potential contribution should be assessed in patients with weight management issues.

## Nutrition for Wound Healing

Patients with malnutrition and unintentional weight loss are at risk for delayed wound healing and infection [41]. Losing more than 15% lean body mass will delay wound healing, and losing more than 30% will actually promote the development of wounds [42]. Ideally, all patients with pressure ulcers or who are at risk for pressure ulcers, such as malnourished young adults with immobility from spina bifida or cerebral palsy, should have a formal nutrition assessment by a dietitian [43]. Wounds create a catabolic state that significantly increases calorie and protein requirements. Therefore, PCPs should encourage their patients with a wound to increase their calorie and protein intake [42].

Oral nutrition supplements and a multivitamin and mineral supplement are recommended for those with abnormal weight status or poor nutritional intake [41]. Enteral nutrition support is indicated for those unable to maintain adequate oral intake, either temporarily or chronically. Patients who are underweight or overweight can have micronutrient deficiencies that further impede healing. Vitamin C and zinc deficiencies are associated with poorly healing wounds, and patients with deficiencies benefit from supplementation and repeat labs every 2 weeks until replete [41]. Research has shown no benefit to supplementation when there is no evidence of a vitamin C or zinc deficiency [41].

## Types of Nutrition Support

For YACCC whose complex condition includes malnutrition, nutrition support may be indicated [44]. Some transitioning young adults will already have nutrition support in place, with adult practitioners assuming supervising responsibility from their pediatric colleagues. Primary management of nutrition support in pediatric-centered care is often the responsibility of subspecialty medical homes. Conversely, in adult care systems, the primary care provider often assumes this role with support from subspecialists and dietitians. Modes of nutritional support include oral supplementation, enteral nutrition, and parenteral nutrition. Each method has risks and benefits and should be weighed carefully based on the underlying condition and patient and family needs.

## Oral Supplementation

### Formula Supplements

Commercial oral nutrition supplements can be of significant value for patients who are struggling to meet their nutrition needs with traditional foods alone. Some young adults rely on oral supplements as an exclusive source of nutrition; for example, the patient with autism who has severe food selectivity, or the patient with cerebral palsy who has inadequate muscle tone to coordinate solids but can take liquids safely by mouth. If a patient is taking all or the majority of their nutrition from an oral supplement, the PCP must ensure that it is nutritionally complete to prevent nutrient deficiencies (i.e., not missing any essential vitamins or minerals). Manufacturers use wording such as "sole-source nutrition" or "appropriate for tube feeding" in their descriptions to indicate nutritionally complete formulations. However, when in doubt, the PCP should consult with a dietitian to review the appropriateness of the oral supplement for the patient.

Insurance coverage for oral supplements typically changes as young adults reach transition age, raising concerns for patients using them as a main source of nutrition. The Department of Health and Human Services (DSHS) will cover the oral formula cost for children and adolescents through a home health company after prior authorization, though this coverage may end at the age of 21 years [45]. Continued insurance coverage, if possible, may require prior authorization and medical justification by the provider, but this varies by state. Addressing this issue prior to reaching the limiting age is recommended to avoid possible gaps in supply.

Paying out of pocket for oral supplements can be quite costly. Therefore, for those patients who cannot obtain insurance coverage, a dietitian can explore other options such as homemade high-calorie shakes and smoothies, though these options may not be a realistic or feasible substitute for caregivers.

### Vitamin and Mineral Supplements (VMS)

Patients who are lacking variety in their diet, are malnourished, or have hypocaloric calorie needs may benefit from a multivitamin and mineral supplement (VMS). For example, a VMS may be indicated for the patient who is tube fed and receives less than 1400 calories per day, since this amount of formula may not meet their protein, vitamin, and mineral requirement. Over-the-counter supplements can vary from incomplete to excessive dosing with the risk for toxicity and should therefore be reviewed carefully. Some supplements contain herbs that could have drug interactions or pose other health risks to the chronically ill, further highlighting the importance of reviewing ingredients with the patient. VMS are commonly recommended supplements; however, their use in YACCC requires special consideration. As noted previously in the section on "Bone Health," VMS do not contain significant amounts of calcium or phosphorus. YACCC with swallowing difficulty, intellectual disability, or those who are tube fed may use alternative forms of VMS, such as liquid or gummy formulations. Liquid VMS are typically not nutritionally complete and specifically often do not contain folic acid, vitamin K, calcium, phosphorus, magnesium, and selenium. Gummy VMS do not contain iron, thus requiring separate supplementation in patients with iron deficiency. VMS may contain higher than recommended doses of some vitamins and minerals posing risk in certain populations, including those with chronic liver or renal disease.

## Enteral Nutrition Support

Enteral nutrition (EN) support typically refers to nutrition delivered via feeding tube and is appropriate for patients unable to take adequate oral intake, as highlighted previously. Though comanagement of EN typically occurs with the support of gastroenterologists and dietitians, PCPs should be familiar with commonly used enteral access devices and their maintenance, available enteral formulas, and the presentation and management of the complications of EN.

### Enteral Access Devices

While short-term EN via the nasal route is common in inpatient and acute care settings, young adults with chronic feeding difficulties typically require long-term EN and have more permanent enteral access. Basic knowledge of long-term enteral tube options, placement methods, management, and potential complications are important for clinicians caring for these complex patients. Distinctions between tube types include terminus location (prepyloric versus postpyloric), placement method (endoscopic, radiology guided, or laproscopic/open surgical procedure), and external extension type (standard versus low-profile "button").

The most clinically significant distinction between tube types is prepyloric (gastric) versus postpyloric (jejunal) terminus location (see Fig. 42.1a, b). In general, prepyloric tubes are

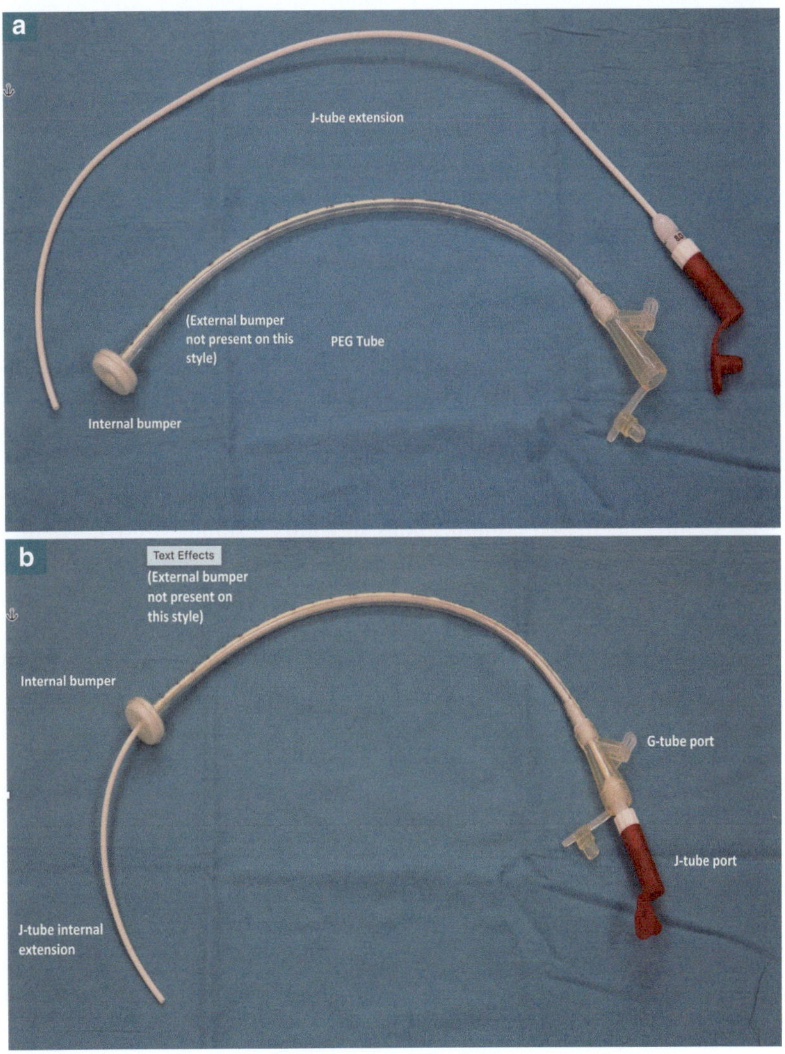


**Fig. 42.1** (a) PEG tube length compared with J-tube extension length. This tube style does not have a built-in external bumper, text indicates where this item would be located. (b) PEG tube with J-tube extension in place

preferred because of increased ease of placement, decreased risk of reprocedure (for tube repositioning and replacement), and because they allow for more physiologic feeding regimens (bolus feeding). Postpyloric tubes may be indicated in patients with severe gastroesophageal reflux disease (GERD) or recurrent vomiting, gastric dysmotility or outlet obstruction and gastric anomalies (congenital or postsurgical) [46]. Postpyloric tubes are also often recommended for patients with feeding-related aspiration, although aspiration pneumonias from oral secretions can still occur [47]. Postpyloric tubes can be placed through an existing gastrostomy site, known as a percutaneous endoscopic gastrostomy with jejunal extension (PEG-J) tube, or directly into the jejunum, referred to as a direct percutaneous endoscopic jejunostomy (DPEJ) tube [47]. Patients with postpyloric tubes often also have a gastric port, which can be used to drain gastric contents, termed "venting," or to give certain medications that may be differentially absorbed in the small intestine. Drawbacks of jejunal tubes include requirement for continuous tube feeding, which may limit patient lifestyle, frequent retrograde dislodgements requiring replacement, and increased risk for tube clogging due to smaller caliber of tube [46, 47].

Initial placement of a long-term enteral access device may be percutaneous, laparoscopic, or surgical. Complication rates between these approaches in pediatric patients are comparable, with slightly decreased complications in adults with nonsurgical techniques [48]. Tubes are secured by an internal bolster, typically a balloon or bumper, and an external bolster. Following initial placement, tract maturation takes approximately 4 weeks, after which replacement can be accomplished either at the bedside (in clinic or at home) or by interventional radiology (IR), depending on the type of bolster and tube, with J-tubes typically requiring IR. Following tract maturation, some patients opt for transition to a low-profile "button" connection, which lies flush with the skin and is less visible under clothing but requires a connector for feeding (see Fig. 42.2a, b).

Frequency of tube exchange varies by tube type and use. Prepyloric tubes have the longest life, with routinely used PEG tubes lasting up to 2 years [47]. Low-profile "button" tubes have a shorter lifetime, typically requiring exchange every 6 months, though exchanges can often be done by patient or caregiver at home. Postpyloric tubes usually need to be exchanged more often due to the frequency of retrograde dislodgement and obstruction or mechanical failure related to the small caliber of the tube. Typically, IR recommends exchange every 3–4 months for postpyloric tubes, although the mean functional use of postpyloric tubes is actually around 55 days in adults due to the complications noted above, with the possibility of shorter duration [48].

Important information to document about the patient's enteral access device includes type, length, frequency of recommended replacement, and method of replacement (bedside by clinician or IR-guided). Patients should have an extra tube at home in case of dislodgement, either for home replacement or to bring with them to the office or emergency department to speed replacement. In the absence of an appropriate tube, a Foley catheter with a balloon can typically be placed in the short term to maintain the tract while awaiting definitive tube replacement.

Acute complications of long-term enteric tube devices should be addressed with the team who initially placed the tube. PCPs should, however, be familiar with the common complications seen in chronic enteral access and their management, summarized in Table 42.3 [47–49]. Additional less common but severe complications of enteric tubes include fistulous tracts, which are typically related to procedure complications or occur in patients with prior abdominal surgery. Work-up and treatment of fistulae should involve consultation with gastroenterology and surgical colleagues.

## Enteral Formulas

The four major categories of enteral formulas are polymeric (standard), partially hydrolyzed/semi-elemental, elemental, and blended food, summarized in Table 42.4. The formula types can vary in protein, fat, and carbohydrate composi-

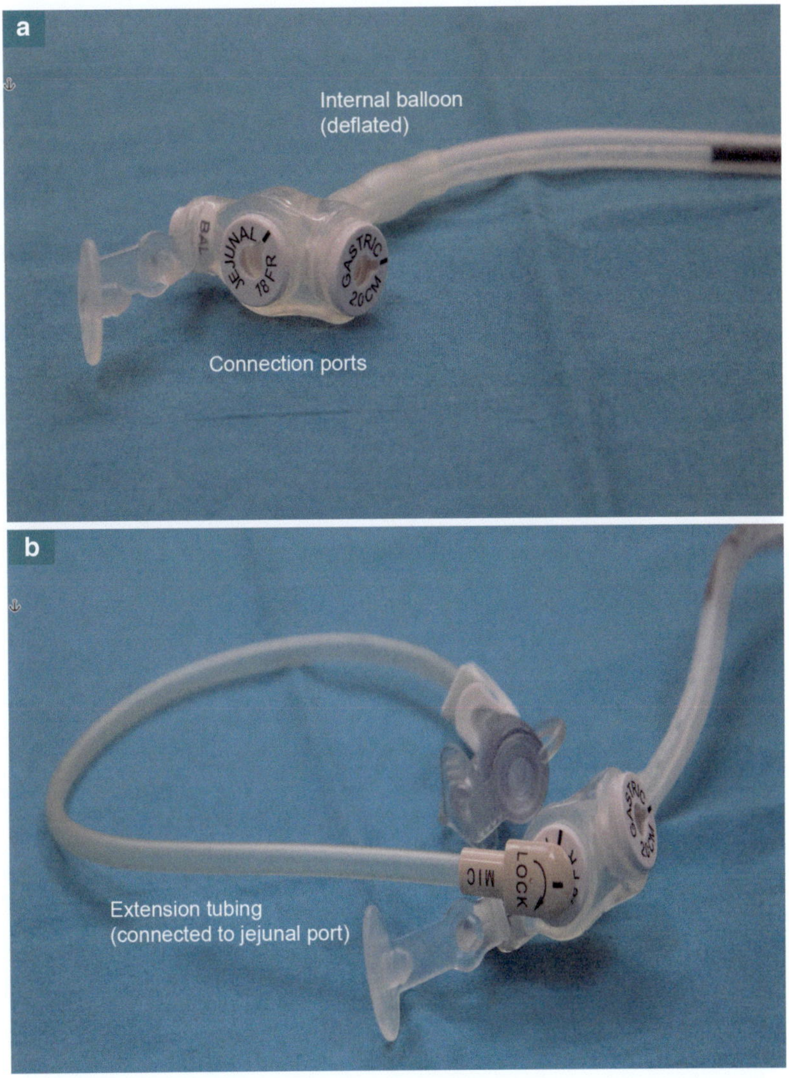


**Fig. 42.2** (**a**) A low-profile tube set up. (**b**) A low-profile tube with connected extension tubing

tion, and PCPs should have a basic understanding of these differences as well as available special formulas and transitioning from pediatric to adult formulas.

Polymeric and blended food formulas contain complete proteins, while in partially hydrolyzed formulas, the protein is enzymatically hydrolyzed to small peptides and amino acids. Partially hydrolyzed formulas are typically used with the treatment of feeding intolerance, GI dysfunction, short bowel syndrome, malabsorption, pancreatic insufficiency, and intractable diarrhea—although there is conflicting evidence on whether these formulas improve diarrhea [50]. Due to limited evidence supporting the use of hydrolyzed formulas, the American Society of Parenteral and Enteral Nutrition (ASPEN) and the European Society of Parenteral and Enteral Nutrition make no recommendations on the use of these formulas [50]. Elemental formulas contain proteins that are completely broken down into amino acids. These formulas are indicated for severe food allergies as well as all of the same indications as partially hydrolyzed formulas. Drawbacks of elemental formulas include increased cost, more time spent preparing feeds since elemental formulas are powder based, and higher risk of contamination since powdered formulas are not

**Table 42.3** Common complications associated with chronic enteric tube access. Compiled from [47–49]

| Complication | Incidence | Symptoms | Risk factors | Prevention | Treatment |
|---|---|---|---|---|---|
| Peristomal wound infection | 4–30% | Erythema<br>Swelling<br>Fever<br>Pain | Immunosuppression<br>Diabetes<br>Obesity or malnutrition | Avoid excessive traction on tube<br>Pre-procedure antibiotics | Antibiotics |
| Clogged tube | 23–35% (higher occurrence among those with postpyloric tubes) | Inability to flush<br>Inability to aspirate | Small caliber tube<br>Crushed medications<br>Use of bulking agents | Avoid gastric residual aspiration<br>Dissolve all medications<br>Frequent water flushes | Pancreatic enzymes mixed with bicarbonate<br>Mechanical clearing<br>Tube replacement |
| Dislodged tube | 1.6–4.4% (likely higher in practice) | Removed tube | Developmental disability | Low-profile tube<br>Abdominal binder/cover | Replacement with Foley to maintain tract<br>New tube placement by parent, provider or in IR |
| Peristomal leakage | 1–2% reported (likely higher in practice) | Formula leakage<br>Gastric content leakage<br>Skin irritation | Infection<br>Gastric hypersecretion<br>Traction on tube site | PPI for hypersecretion | Barrier cream<br>Consider replacement or convert to G-J tube<br>Do NOT upsize tube |
| Buried bumper syndrome (internal bolster migrates) | 2–6% (usually late complication) | Immobile tube<br>Increased resistance to flushes<br>Tube leakage<br>Tube occlusion<br>Abdominal pain | Excessive traction between bumpers | Allow 1.5 cm between skin and external bolster<br>Mobilize PEG every other day | Consult IR regarding removal and new tube placement |
| Bleeding (delayed) | | Anemia<br>Gastroccult positive | Buried bumper<br>GERD (esophagitis is most common cause) | PPI | PPI<br>Consider endoscopic evaluation |

*IR* interventional radiology, *PPI* proton pump inhibitor, *PEG* percutaneous endoscopic gastrostomy, *GERD* gastroesophageal reflux disease

sterile. Therefore, elemental formula is typically reserved for those situations when partially hydrolyzed formulas are not tolerated.

The majority of enteral formulas contain fats in the form of medium-chain triglycerides (MCTs), which do not require pancreatic enzymes or bile to be absorbed and which bypass the lymph system directly into portal circulation. MCTs are essential to promote fat absorption for patients with cholestasis or bile salt malabsorption such as with short gut syndrome. Formulas also contain some long-chain triglycerides (LCTs) because MCTs do not provide essential fatty acids.

Carbohydrate source varies by formula but all pediatric and adult formulas are lactose free. Standard caloric concentration is 30 calories per ounce, but many formulas are also available in 36

**Table 42.4** Categories of enteral formulas

| | Polymeric/standard | Partially hydrolyzed/ semi-elemental | Elemental | Blended food |
|---|---|---|---|---|
| Ingredients | Complete cow's milk protein and/or soy protein, corn syrup/maltodextrin/ sugar, MCT, and LCT (oral supplements do not contain MCT), vitamins, and minerals<br>With or without fiber | Hydrolyzed whey and/ or casein, maltodextrin/ sugar, MCT, and LCT<br>With or without fiber | Amino acids, maltodextrin/ modified cornstarch, MCT, and LCT | Highly varied<br>Food contains fiber |
| Indications | Standard formula for normal GI function | Feeding intolerance, GI dysfunction, short bowel syndrome, malabsorption, pancreatic insufficiency | Same indications as partially hydrolyzed formula and severe food allergies | Commercially sterile and convenient alternative for homemade blenderized tube feeding |
| Examples | Boost, Ensure, Nutren, Jevity, Osmolite | Peptamen, Vital | Vivonex (low fat), Tolerex (very low fat, not for long-term use) | Compleat, Liquid Hope, Real Food Blends, Kate Farms |

*MCT* medium-chain triglycerides, *LCT* long-chain triglycerides, *GI* gastrointestinal

and 45 calories per ounce preparations. Other variations include those with high protein concentrations, with or without fiber, and with prebiotics. Prebiotics are a form of fiber that is fermented in the ileum and colon by bacteria, thereby stimulating growth and/or activity of gut microbiota [50].

Blended tube feeding (BTF) is growing in popularity due to a desire to provide whole foods and minimize artificial sugar and additives. BTF includes both commercially-prepared blended food formulas and home blended preparations. Some blended food formulas are nutritionally complete with added vitamins and minerals, and some contain only a few foods per packet with minimal or incomplete vitamin, mineral, or electrolyte supplementation. Some caregivers will prepare their own home BTF Challenges with home BTF include extensive preparation time, increased risk of tube occlusion due to viscosity, food safety concerns, and ensuring nutritional adequacy [51]. In addition, home BTF requires a very powerful and typically expensive commercial grade blender, although some blender companies will give discounts if the device will be used to prepare tube feeding. Home BTF should be monitored by a dietitian to ensure adequate fluid and nutrient intake as well as food safety.

Explanation of the wide variety of disease-specific formulas is beyond the scope of this chapter, but the PCP should know that specialized options exist for conditions such as renal failure, liver failure, diabetes mellitus, pancreatitis, and specific pulmonary diagnoses; for patients requiring immune-modulating therapy or critical care; for patients with chylous effusions or who have undergone bariatric surgery; and for ketogenic diets used for seizure control. It is worth noting that if a patient on a ketogenic diet requires changes to medications or supplements, the provider should collaborate with a dietitian specializing in the ketogenic diet. Many medications, especially liquid formulations, contain sugars which shift ketogenesis and can increase risk of seizures in these patients.

Some transitioning patients who are tube fed may still be receiving a pediatric formula when they reach adult care. Compared to pediatric formulas, adult formulas typically have more protein, more fiber, less calcium and phosphorus, and a variable content of other vitamins and minerals. An adult patient receiving all or the majority of their nutrition from a pediatric formula may be receiving an inadequate or, in some cases, an excess amount of certain nutrients, in particular calcium. Poor feeding tolerance with other formula trials may lead to ongoing use of pediatric formulas, and an adequate history and possible consultation with prior providers should be considered prior to suggesting changes. For those patients who would benefit from a detailed nutrient analysis or change in formula, consultation with a dietitian is appropriate.

## Adjusting Enteral Nutrition

Determination of an appropriate feeding schedule is patient-specific and depends on multiple factors, including the type of tube, amount of formula and fluid needed, and the patient's lifestyle. A general comparison of the two methods is outlined in Table 42.5 [52, 53]. Prepyloric tubes allow either feeding type, whereas postpyloric tubes require continuous feeding due to inability to handle volume required for boluses.

In active patients without gastrointestinal contraindications, bolus feeding is usually preferred as it is more physiological and allows for an intermittent schedule. In patients who still take some nutrition orally, bolus feeding or overnight continuous feeding with disconnection during the day can facilitate hunger cues. In patients with high aspiration risk, continuous feeding is often recommended due to presumed decreased aspiration risk, although most studies demonstrating this decreased risk were conducted in critically ill patients [52, 53]. With continuous feeding, caution must be exercised about overnight feeding as risk of aspiration may be increased with sleep. Proper positioning and prevention of tube dislodgement are important factors to consider.

**Table 42.5** Comparison of bolus and continuous feeding methods

| Feeding type | Bolus feeding | Continuous feeding |
|---|---|---|
| What | Periodic, moderate volume | Continuous slow infusion |
| Frequency | Up to 6 times per day | 12–24 h/day |
| How | By syringe, gravity, or over a pump | Pump |
| Benefits | Physiologic "meals"<br>Ample disconnected time | Improved tolerance for those with poor GI motility<br>May reduce aspiration risk [39, 40] |
| Drawbacks | Sometimes requires tolerance to large bolus volumes<br>Not possible with postpyloric tubes | Requires pump<br>Prolonged connected time |

When assessing a patient's tube feeding regimen, nutrition and fluid needs should be assessed separately, as the volume of formula intake may not match fluid requirement. Fluid requirements for adults is generally 30–40 mL/kg per day or 1–1.5 mL/kcal expended, although it should be individualized based on clinical assessment [44]. For example, patients with chronic constipation may benefit from a formula that contains fiber and a fluid intake above their maintenance fluid requirement to promote regularity. Additionally, acute illnesses can change fluid needs, particularly if the illness involves vomiting, diarrhea, or increased sweating, temporarily requiring an increase in fluid intake.

When a patient who is tube fed has chronic unintentional weight loss or gain, a conservative first step is to modify their caloric intake by 10–15%, keeping in mind weight goals noted earlier in this chapter. If the patient is having rapid weight gain or loss, a more aggressive approach may be necessary with a 20–30% change in caloric intake. When reducing formula intake, one needs to consider whether the volume should be replaced with water to meet their fluid requirement and whether the decreased formula intake will still meet their protein, vitamin, and mineral requirements. Patients receiving less than 1400 calories per day are at increased risk of inadequate nutrient intake, as noted previously. When uncertainty exists, a dietitian should be consulted for a thorough nutrient analysis. Interval assessments of weight with tube feeding adjustments should be considered every 2–3 weeks to monitor changes and tolerance issues.

## Enteral Nutrition Complications and Feeding Intolerance

EN is often associated with changes in gastrointestinal function, with the most common being diarrhea, followed by nausea and constipation [47]. The evaluation of feeding intolerance symptoms by the PCP should follow a stepwise approach.

Stool consistency in exclusively tube fed individuals should be soft to mushy, and 2–3 bowel movements per day may be normal. Watery stools or higher frequency may constitute diarrhea. Initial assessment should include review of formula type, any recent changes in formula or medications, evidence of malabsorption, and risk assessment for intestinal infections. Hospitalized patients receiving enteral tube feeding have been shown to have a ninefold increased risk of developing *Clostridium difficile* infections [47]. Whether this risk extends to chronic EN is unclear, but new onset of diarrhea in a patient receiving long-term EN should prompt increased clinical suspicion.

Treatment of noninfectious enteral feeding-related diarrhea can include adjustment of formula type or addition of fiber [54]. Such changes may be guided by a dietitian. In theory, fiber may decrease diarrhea due to soluble fiber increasing fluid absorption and insoluble fiber slowing transit time. However, there has been conflicting evidence on whether adding fiber to tube feeding decreases diarrhea [50]. Adding probiotics may be of some help in slowing diarrhea, with minimal risk in otherwise stable patients [55]. The use of antidiarrheal medications such as loperamide should be reserved for refractory cases.

Constipation can also occur and may be more prevalent in patients with extended time on EN [47]. In YACCC, constipation may be compounded by the underlying condition that resulted in need for nutritional support, such as neurogenic bowel in patients with cerebral palsy or spina bifida. Treatment and prevention of constipation is frequently managed with a stable bowel regimen that may include increased fluid flushes, stool softeners, such as colace, and promotility agents, such as senna and miralax. Addition of fiber has not shown consistent benefit for constipation in enterally fed patients and is not recommended as first-line therapy [47].

In addition to diarrhea and constipation, feeding intolerance may present as nausea, vomiting, abdominal distention, or discomfort. As with constipation and diarrhea, the patient's clinical status and whether medications, infection, inflammation, or constipation could be causing intolerance should be assessed. When these variables have been addressed or eliminated from consideration, one should look to overfeeding, rapid infusion time, infusion of very cold formula, any recent changes in formula type or fiber intake, or bacterial contamination of enteral feeds as potential causes of the feeding intolerance [50].

If the infusion rate is a concern and the patient is receiving gravity bolus feeds, the rate can be decreased by lowering the height of the syringe or feeding bag or by controlling the rate with a feeding pump. High-osmolality formulas rarely cause diarrhea, but this can occur if these formulas are infused too quickly [50]. Osmolality increases with formula caloric density, and elemental and low-fat formulas have a higher osmolality than polymeric formulas.

If the infusion rate is ruled out as causative, one might consider a change in formula, such as a trial of partially hydrolyzed formula for the patient not tolerating a polymeric formula or adjustment of fiber content, either with a modified formula or powdered supplement.

## Parenteral Nutrition Support

Parenteral nutrition (PN) is an intravenous infusion comprised of dextrose, amino acids, lipids, electrolytes, vitamins, minerals, and trace elements. It may also contain other additives depending on the patient's needs, including acid suppressing medications, such as famotidine, and insulin for those with diabetes. PN is most commonly used in the acute care setting for patients who are unable to tolerate EN [56]. Adult providers are likely most familiar with its use in this short-term setting. However, in rare cases, young adults may receive chronic PN support. Clinical conditions in young adults that may warrant PN include short gut syndrome (due to resections from necrotizing enterocolitis, inflammatory bowel disease, or recurrent bowel obstructions), malabsorption syndromes (such as severe IBD or celiac disease), high-output gastric fistulas or severe intestinal dysmotility with inability to tolerate EN [44].

Monitoring and prescribing PN requires the close involvement of a dietitian and pharmacist who work with a home infusion company. The PCP is typically responsible for ordering laboratory testing and communicating with the dietitian and infusion company for periodic adjustment of PN orders, typically on a monthly basis. As nutrition goals shift from growth to maintenance in young adults, adjustments are usually less dramatic than in childhood.

PN has multiple risks including those associated with the long-term central intravenous access (IV) required for administration and the nutrition itself. Young adults with long-term central IV access are at risk for line malfunction and catheter-related blood stream infections, a risk that is amplified in the setting of daily access for PN [44]. PN can also cause liver dysfunction, termed parenteral nutrition-associated liver disease (PNALD), which is typically cholestatic and can range from mild to severe liver failure. PNALD risk is also associated with an increased frequency of line infections [57].

In addition to increased medical risks, PN is significantly more expensive than enteral options. Insurance companies typically require strict documentation of the clinical indication for PN in order to provide coverage of PN. This documentation typically needs to be resubmitted periodically to ensure ongoing coverage [44].

## Inpatient Considerations in Nutritional Supplementation

YACCC receiving enteral or parenteral nutritional support at baseline often need adjustments during acute illness and hospitalization due to change in nutritional needs or need to hold enteral feeds associated with the underlying reason for admission, such as in bowel obstruction or other GI illnesses. In addition, YACCC may use specialized formulas not easily available in the inpatient setting, requiring a change in product during their acute stay. Consultation with an inpatient dietician in conjunction with the patient and their caregiver supports is recommended prior to making any changes or adjustments. YACCC with enteral feeding may also have altered bowel motility, such as in patients with cerebral palsy, so when restarting feeds after a break, providers may want to start at lower than the goal rate (or on continuous feeding for those who use bolus feeds) to ensure tolerance with steady advance to full feeds.

## Conclusion

YACCC are at increased nutritional risk, and the management of nutritional needs is an essential part of primary care for this population. The assessment of nutritional status includes determining caloric and weight goals as well as vitamin and mineral needs. Nutritional needs may vary based on underlying condition, disease progression, and medications, requiring periodic assessment by the PCP. A PCP should have a basic understanding of nutritional support options, including oral, enteral, or parenteral support with additional aid of a dietician in complex cases.

## References

1. Marchand V, Motil KJ, NASPGHAN Committee on Nutrition. Nutrition support for neurologically impaired children: a clinical report of the North American society for pediatric gastroenterology, hepatology, and nutrition. J Pediatr Gastroenterol Nutr. 2006;43(1):123–35.
2. White JV, Guenter P, Jensen G, Malone A, Schofield M, Academy of Nutrition and Dietetics Malnutrition Work Group; A.S.P.E.N. Malnutrition Task Force, A.S.P.E.N. Board of Directors. Consensus statement of the academy of nutrition and dietetics/American society for parenteral and enteral nutrition: characteristics recommended for the identification and documentation of adult malnutrition (undernutrition). J Acad Nutr Diet. 2012;112(5):730–8.

3. Sinaasappel M, Stern M, Littlewood J, Wolfe S, Steinkamp G, Heijerman HGM, et al. Nutrition in patients with cystic fibrosis: a European consensus. J Cyst Fibros. 2002;1(2):51–75.
4. Pencharz PB, Durie PR. Pathogenesis of malnutrition in cystic fibrosis. Clin Nutr. 2000;19(6):387–94.
5. Marin VB, Velandia S, Hunter B, Gattas V, Fielbaum O, Herrera O, et al. Energy expenditure, nutrition status, and body composition in children with cystic fibrosis. Nutrition. 2004;20:181–6.
6. Johnson RK, Goran MI, Ferrara MS, Poehlman ET. Athetosis increased resting metabolic rate in adults with cerebral palsy. J Am Diet Assoc. 1996;96:145–8.
7. Johnson RK, Hildreth HG, Contompasis SH, Goran MI. Total energy expenditure in adults with cerebral palsy as assessed by doubly labeled water. J Am Diet Assoc. 1997;97:966–70.
8. Mari-Bauset S, Zazpe I, Mari-Sanchis A, Llopis-Gonzalez A, Morales-Suarez-Varela M. Food selectivity in autism spectrum disorders: a systematic review. J Autism Dev Disord. 2014;29(11):1554–61.
9. Kerwin ML, Eicher PS, Gelsinger J. Parental report of eating problems and gastrointestinal symptoms in children with pervasive developmental disorders. Child Health Care. 2005;34:217–34.
10. Fung EB, Samson-Fang L, Stallings VA, Conaway M, Liptak G, Henderson RC, et al. Feeding dysfunction is associated with poor growth and health status in children with cerebral palsy. J Am Diet Assoc. 2002;102(261–368):373.
11. van den Engel-Hoek L, Erasmus CE, Hendriks JC, Geurts AC, Klein WM, Pillen S, et al. Oral muscles are progressively affected in Duchenne muscular dystrophy: implications for dysphagia treatment. J Neurol. 2013;260(5):1295–303.
12. Cooper-Brown L, Copeland S, Dailey S, Downey D, Peterson MC, Stimson C, et al. Feeding and swallowing dysfunction in genetic syndromes. Dev Disabil Res Rev. 2008;14:147–57.
13. Abraham BP, Mehta S, El-Serag HB. Natural history of pediatric-onset inflammatory bowel disease: a systematic review. J Clin Gastroenterol. 2012;46(7):581–9.
14. Bell KL, Samson-Fang L. Nutritional management of children with cerebral palsy. Eur J Clin Nutr. 2013;67(suppl 2):S13–6.
15. Centers for Disease Control and Prevention. About adult BMI. 2015. http://www.cdc.gov/healthyweight/assessing/bmi/adult_bmi/index.html.
16. Tokunaga K, Matsuzawa Y, Kotani K, Keno Y, Kobatake T, Fujioka S, et al. Ideal body weight estimated from the body mass index with the lowest morbidity. Int J Obes. 1991;15(1):1–5.
17. Calcatera V, Pelizzo G, Cena H. BMI is a poor predictor of nutritional status in disabled children. What is the most recommended method for body composition assessment in this pediatric population? Front Pediatr. 2019;7:226.
18. Froehlich-Grobe K, Nary DE, Van Sciver A, Lee J, Little TD. Measuring height without a stadiometer: empirical investigation of four height estimates among wheelchair users. Am J Phys Med Rehabil. 2011;90(8):658–66.
19. Keller U. Nutritional laboratory markers of malnutrition. J Clin Med. 2019;8(6):775.
20. NHLBI Obesity Education Initiative Expert Panel. Clinical guidelines on the identification, evaluation, and treatment of overweight and obesity in adults. Obes Res. 1998;6(Suppl. 2):51S–209S.
21. Humphries K, Traci MA, Seekins T. Nutrition and adults with intellectual or developmental disabilities: systematic literature review results. Intellect Dev Disabil. 2009;47(3):163–85.
22. Trabulsi J, Schoeller DA. Evaluation of dietary assessment instruments against doubly labeled water, a biomarker of habitual energy intake. Am J Physiol Endocrinol Metab. 2001;281(5):E891–9.
23. Hanson K, Connor L. Food insecurity and dietary quality in US adults and children: a systematic review. Am J Clin Nutr. 2014;100(2):684–92.
24. Brucker D, Nord D. Food insecurity among young adults with intellectual and developmental disabilities in the United States: evidence from the national health review survey. Am J Intellect Dev Disabil. 2016;121(6):520–32.
25. Brantley E, Pillai D, Ku L. Association of work requirements with supplemental nutrition assistance program participation by race/ethnicity and disability status, 2013–2017. JAMA Netw Open. 2020;3(6):e205824.
26. Chad KE, McKay HA, Zello GA, Bailey DA, Faulkner RA, Snyder RE. Body composition in nutritionally adequate ambulatory and non-ambulatory children with cerebral palsy and a healthy reference group. Dev Med Child Neurol. 2000;42(5):334–9.
27. Ilich JZ, Kerstetter JE. Nutrition in bone health revisited: a story beyond calcium. J Am Coll Nutr. 2000;19(6):715–37.
28. Institute of Medicine of the National Academies. Report brief November 2010. Dietary reference intakes for calcium and vitamin D. http://iom.nationalacademies.org/~/media/Files/Report%20Files/2010/Dietary-Reference-Intakes-for-Calcium-and-Vitamin-D/Vitamin%20D%20and%20Calcium%202010%20Report%20Brief.pdf.
29. International Osteoporosis Foundation. Calcium calculator. https://www.osteoporosis.foundation/educational-hub/topic/calcium-calculator
30. National institute of health office of dietary supplements: calcium fact sheet for professionals. https://ods.od.nih.gov/factsheets/Calcium-HealthProfessional/
31. Tangpricha V, Pearce EN, Chen TC, Holick MF. Vitamin D insufficiency among free-living healthy young adults. Am J Med. 2002;112(8):659–62.
32. Holick MF, Chen TC. Vitamin D deficiency: a worldwide problem with health consequences. Am J Clin Nutr. 2008;87(4):1080S–6S.
33. Holick MF, Binkley NC, Bischoff-Ferrari HA, Gordon CM, Hanley DA, Heaney RP, et al. Endocrine society. Evaluation, treatment, and prevention of

vitamin D deficiency: an endocrine society clinical practice guideline. J Clin Endocrinol Metab. 2011;96(7):1911–30.
34. National institute of health office of dietary supplements: Vitamin D fact sheet for professionals. https://ods.od.nih.gov/factsheets/VitaminD-HealthProfessional
35. Clemens TL, Adams JS, Henderson SL, Holick MF. Increased skin pigment reduces the capacity of skin to synthesise vitamin D3. Lancet. 1982;1(8263):74–6.
36. Power J, Buchanan GR. Disorders of iron metabolism: new diagnostic and treatment approaches to iron deficiency. Hematol Oncol Clin North Am. 2019;33(3):393–408.
37. DeLoughery TG. Iron deficiency anemia. Med Clin North Am. 2017;101(2):319–32.
38. Clark SF. Iron deficiency anemia. Nutr Clin Pract. 2008;23(2):128–41.
39. National institute of health office of dietary supplements: Iron fact sheet for professionals. https://ods.od.nih.gov/factsheets/Iron-HealthProfessional/#h6
40. Boullata JI, Hudson LM. Drug–nutrient interactions: a broad view with implications for practice. J Acad Nutr Diet. 2012;112(4):506–17.
41. Thompson KL, Leu MG, Drummond KL, Popalisky J, Spencer SM, Lenssen PM. Nutrition interventions to optimize pediatric wound healing an evidence-based clinical pathway. Nutr Clin Pract. 2014;29(4):473–82.
42. Demling RH. Nutrition, anabolism, and the wound healing process: an overview. Eplasty. 2009;9:e9.
43. Dorner B, Posthauer ME, Thomas D, National Pressure Ulcer Advisory Panel. The role of nutrition in pressure ulcer prevention and treatment: national pressure ulcer advisory panel white paper. Adv Skin Wound Care. 2009;22(5):212–21.
44. ASPEN Board of Directors and the Clinical Guidelines Task Force. Guidelines for the use of parenteral and enteral nutrition in adult and pediatric patients. J Parenter Enter Nutr. 2002;26(Suppl. 1):1SA–138SA.
45. Washington State Department of Social and Health Services. Medicare Purchasing Administration (MPA). Enteral Nutrition Billing instructions. Chapter 388–554 WAC. 2010. http://www.hca.wa.gov/medicaid/billing/documents/guides/enteral_nutrition_biasof063011.pdf.
46. Gopalan S, Khanna S. Enteral nutrition delivery technique. Curr Opin Clin Nutr Metab Care. 2003;6:313–7.
47. Blumenstein I, Shastir YM, Stein J. Gastroenteric tube feeding: techniques, problems and solutions. World J Gastroenterol. 2014;20(26):8505–24.
48. ASGE Technolgy Committee, Kwon RS, Banerjee S, Desilets D, Diehl DL, Farraye FA, Kaul V, et al. Enteral nutrition access devices. Gastrointest Endosc. 2010;72(2):236–48.
49. Lynch CR, Fang JC. Prevention and management of complications of percutaneous endoscopic gastrostomy (PEG) tubes. Pract Gastroenterol. 2004;28:66–76.
50. Mueller CM, McClave SA, Kuhn JM. The ASPEN adult nutrition support core curriculum. 2nd ed. Silver Spring, MD: American Society for Parenteral and Enteral Nutrition; 2012.
51. Weeks C. Home blenderized tube feeding: a practical guide for clinical practice. Clin Transl Gastroenterol. 2019;10(2):e00001.
52. Alkhawaja S, Martin C, Butler RJ, Gwadry-Sridhar F. Post-pyloric versus gastric tube feeding for preventing pneumonia and improving nutritional outcomes in critically ill adults. Cochrane Database Syst Rev. 2015;8:CD008875.
53. Wang D, Zheng SQ, Chen XC, Jiang SW, Chen HB. Comparisons between small intestinal and gastric feeding in severe traumatic brain injury: a systematic review and meta-analysis of randomized controlled trials. J Neurosurg. 2015;123:1194–201.
54. Whelan K, Schneider SM. Mechanisms, prevention, and management of diarrhea in enteral nutrition. Curr Opin Gastroenterol. 2011;27:152–9.
55. Whelan K, Myers CE. Safety of probiotics in patients receiving nutritional support: a systematic review of case reports randomized controlled trials, and nonrandomized trials. Am J Clin Nutr. 2010;91:687–703.
56. Zaloga GP. Parenteral nutrition in adult inpatients with functioning gastrointestinal tracts: assessment of outcomes. Lancet. 2006;367:1101–11.
57. Wales PW, Allen N, Worthington P, George D, Compher C, American Society for Parenteral and Enteral Nutrition, Teitelbaum D. ASPEN clinical guidelines: support of pediatric patients with intestinal failure at risk of parenteral nutrition-associated liver disease. J Parenter Enter Nutr. 2014;38(5):538–57.

# 43 Technology Dependence of the Nervous System

Vrunda Vithalani, Devesh Upadhya, and Cynthia Peacock

## Introduction

Numerous childhood medical conditions significantly impact the nervous system, including cerebral palsy, spina bifida, intracranial hemorrhage, and intractable epilepsy. With recent medical advances, the prevalence of these conditions has increased in the last 20 years. Based on data from 2010, one in every 345 children in the United States has cerebral palsy, making it the most common motor-impacting disability in childhood; there are an estimated one million adults living with cerebral palsy in the United States today [1, 2]. There are more individuals still with spastic diplegia or quadriplegia secondary to genetic conditions or post-traumatic brain injury. Spina bifida is estimated to occur in approximately 2.7–3.8 per 10,000 live births, with approximately 85% of these individuals surviving into adulthood [3–5]. Additionally, 1.2% of the U.S. population (approximately three million adults and ~ 500,000 children) have epilepsy [6]; approximately, one-third of these adults and 20-25% of children have intractable or drug-resistant epilepsy [7].

The impacts of these disease processes are wide-ranging and can affect motor function, spasticity, executive function, communication, and memory. Implantable devices designed for use in these individuals have been shown to improve both the quality and duration of life. While the devices themselves are often managed by neurosurgeons or neurologists, an understanding of their indications and function allows primary care physicians (PCPs) to refer patients for consideration of placement when appropriate as well as to recognize and assist in the early management of potentially fatal complications, including infection or failure of the devices.

## Intrathecal Baclofen Therapy

Intrathecal baclofen is an increasingly utilized tool for the management of spasticity. It may be used in the treatment of spasticity associated with cerebral palsy, those with traumatic brain injury, numerous genetic conditions that cause spasticity, and multiple sclerosis, amongst other conditions. Intrathecal delivery of baclofen decreases systemic side effects and improves response to therapy. This allows for better control of tone and spasms, thereby reducing pain and improving the functional capabilities of affected individuals.

V. Vithalani (✉) · D. Upadhya · C. Peacock (✉)
Department of Internal Medicine and Pediatrics, Baylor College of Medicine, Houston, TX, USA
e-mail: vrunda.vithalani@bcm.edu; upadhya@bcm.edu; cpeacock@bcm.edu


A. A. Kuo et al. (eds.), *Care of Adults with Chronic Childhood Conditions*,
https://doi.org/10.1007/978-3-031-54281-7_43

## Device

The primary device available for the delivery of baclofen is the Medtronic SynchroMed II [8]. The pump is placed underneath the anterior abdominal skin, typically in the right lower quadrant, with the catheter tunneled laterally to the spine. The device is a disc with a three-inch diameter and one-inch thickness; it has a peripheral catheter access port as well as a central port that allows access to the drug reservoir. The device is easily palpated subcutaneously on examination of the lower abdomen, with a small divot in the device indicating the central reservoir. Specific precautions following baclofen pump placement are available from the manufacturer but include the possibility of baclofen overdose and withdrawal (see section "Complications" below) [8]. Important issues to review at routine visits include regular pump refills, additional sedative medications, and pump alarms. The SynchroMed II has a one-tone alarm that sounds when the pump has an issue or when it requires a refill or replacement. There is a separate, two-tone alarm to indicate the discontinuation of baclofen infusion. Two-tone alarming is considered an urgent issue and requires prompt care by the managing provider or in the emergency room. While routine magnetic resonance imaging (MRI) can be safely performed, the physician managing the pump should be contacted before the imaging is done. Pump function should also be confirmed following exposure to MRI.

## Complications

Complications of baclofen pump therapy are managed in concert with the prescribing physical medicine and rehabilitation (PM&R) physician and may also require the involvement of a neurosurgeon. Device complications typically present as baclofen withdrawal or baclofen overdose.

Baclofen overdose is frequently iatrogenic or associated with pump refilling; less frequently, it is associated with pump malfunction. Patients may present with hypotension, hypotonia, flaccid paralysis, somnolence, delirium, respiratory depression, seizures, or cardiac abnormalities. There is no specific antidote for intrathecal baclofen overdose. Instead, supportive care involves resuscitation and mechanical ventilation when necessary. The physician managing the pump should be contacted to assist with urgent discontinuation of drug infusion. If necessary, there is an access port on the pump that can be aspirated to empty baclofen from the reservoir, and a lumbar puncture can be performed to drain baclofen from the intrathecal space [9].

Baclofen withdrawal is a potential medical emergency. It may be associated with delay in refilling the reservoir, catheter problems such as kinking or line disruption, device problems, or intentional discontinuation of the device by the treating physician. Patients may present with the recurrence of initial spasticity symptoms, tachycardia, hyperthermia, itching, irritability, or seizures. Less frequently, patients may exhibit neuropsychiatric symptoms, malignant hyperthermia, autonomic instability, rhabdomyolysis, disseminated intravascular coagulation, or multi-organ failure. The initial management includes the use of various sedative medications, including propofol, benzodiazepines, or, with more limited efficacy, and high-dose oral baclofen. Many patients will have oral baclofen available for emergency administration. Externalized intrathecal catheters have also been used for temporizing therapy. The definitive management requires device interrogation and assessment of catheter continuity and flow [9].

Other complications can be related to device placement or other components of the system [10–12]. Infection of overlying skin or the central nervous system (CNS) has been reported in 5–17% of patients. Catheter damage, tip migration, kinking, or blockage is seen in 15–20% of patients, and cerebrospinal fluid (CSF) leak is seen in 22% of patients. Standard abdominal anterior-posterior (AP) radiographs, lateral lumbar spine radiographs, and AP thoracic spine radiographs can help identify catheter problems. In the absence of visible catheter disruption, more advanced fluoroscopic and nuclear medicine techniques can aid in the diagnosis of catheter dysfunction [13]. Additional online resources are available for both providers as well as patients [14].

## Ventricular Shunts

Ventriculoperitoneal (VP) shunts are extensively used for the treatment of symptomatic hydrocephalus. They consist of an intraventricular portion, typically placed in the right lateral ventricle, a valve that regulates outflow of CSF based on intracranial pressure, and shunt tubing that travels along the lateral neck, across the clavicle and ribs, and into the peritoneum. The shunt is usually palpable subcutaneously at the right parietal scalp and down the lateral neck on physical exam. Although the preferred distal site for the shunt placement is the peritoneal space, less commonly used is the ventriculoatrial (VA) shunt, which has CSF flowing from the cerebral ventricular system to the atrium of the heart, or the ventriculopleural shunt, with CSF flowing to the pleural space. There can be many reasons to select these alternative sites, and these options should be discussed by neurosurgeons with patients and their families. The remainder of the discussion in this section will focus on the more commonly used VP shunts.

## Complications

Complications of VP shunts should be managed in concert with a neurosurgeon. Complications can include infection, obstruction, mechanical failure, over-drainage, loculations within the ventricular system, and abdominal pathology. The type of complication seen is often associated with the timing since shunt placement. Most patients with a VP shunt experience at least one shunt failure in their lifetime, often occurring years after the initial placement and into adulthood [15, 16]. One study suggests that the median time of shunt survival of a shunt placed in a child is almost two-thirds of that placed in an adult. Furthermore, patients who were less than 17 years of age at the time of their first shunt revision were 3.7 times more likely to require multiple revisions compared to those who were adults at the time of their first shunt failure [17].

Infection is most common in the period immediately after shunt placement, but risk persists throughout the lifetime of the shunt. In one retrospective analysis of adults with VP shunt infections, the most frequently presenting symptoms were fever (78%), neck stiffness (45%), and local signs of infection such as erythema over shunt tubing (49%) [18]. In this study, the CSF leukocyte count was elevated in 80% of patients, and cultures were positive in 66% of patients; yield was highest when the specimen was obtained by valve puncture. The peripheral white blood cell count was not a reliable indicator of infection. Intracranial imaging was of limited value, but intra-abdominal imaging was frequently abnormal when the intra-abdominal portion of the shunt was infected. Computed tomography (CT) scan was more useful than ultrasound in this regard; CT findings associated with infection included inflamed fat or muscle around the shunt, thickened gut wall, intra-abdominal abscess, and peritoneal cyst. Common etiologic agents are coagulase-negative staphylococci (CoNS), *Staphylococcus aureus*, and *Propionibacterium acnes*. Notably, infection with CoNS tends to be less symptomatic [19].

A variety of noninfectious shunt complications can occur. Shunt obstruction or mechanical failure can occur anywhere along the system. It usually manifests with signs of elevated intracranial pressure, including nausea, vomiting, headache, lethargy, irritability, decline in academic performance, change in vision, increase in seizure frequency, and ataxia [20]. A shunt series using plain radiographs can assist in the diagnosis of mechanical shunt failure, as may occur with cracks in shunt tubing or recession of the shunt tip out of the peritoneum. However, the majority of shunt failure happens in the absence of apparent mechanical failure on plain films. At times, even cross-sectional imaging may not provide definitive diagnosis, and in these cases, either further imaging (i.e., radionucleotide injection into the shunt reservoir) or surgery based on clinical suspicion may be undertaken [21]. Severe constipation has been a noted cause of VP shunt malfunction in children with one noted case report in an adult as well; management of the constipation resolved the symptoms of shunt malfunction in these patients [22, 23].

Over-drainage of CSF can result in the slit ventricle syndrome, with CT findings of very small, "slit-like" ventricles. This condition presents symptoms similar to shunt obstruction, although symptoms are often worse with the patient in the upright position. Within the abdomen, shunts can become obstructed by pseudocyst formation around the catheter tip. In this situation, patients typically present with abdominal distention. Rarely, distal shunt components can cause perforation of the bladder or intestines [24].

There remains a paucity of guidance around whether individuals with a ventriculoperitoneal or lumboperitoneal shunt can play organized sports. Based on a survey of pediatric neurosurgeons in 2004, notable sports-related shunt complications are rather uncommon; the most common of these complications is a broken or fractured catheter. The most commonly implicated sports in shunt complications included soccer and wrestling. Based on that same survey, most pediatric neurosurgeons did not restrict participation in non-contact sports. For contact sports, however, one-third of neurosurgeons restricted participation in all contact sports, one-third restricted participation in some specific sports, and one-third recommended no restrictions. The most commonly restricted sports included football, boxing, and wrestling. Some also suggest that patients with lumboperitoneal shunts should avoid sports that would result in twisting of the trunk [25].

Additional online information is available for providers and patients [26].

## Vagal Nerve Stimulator (VNS)

Vagal nerve stimulation is an evolving therapeutic modality. The VNS is U.S. Food and Drug Administration (FDA)-approved for the treatment of focal epilepsy in individuals 4 years of age and older, though it may be effective in management in generalized epilepsy as well [27]. It works by intermittently stimulating the vagus nerve at preset time intervals; a typical starting point is the stimulation of the vagus nerve for 30 s every 5 min [28]. This is believed to alter blood flow and neurotransmitters within the thalamus and thus control seizure activity; studies in rodents implicate increased norepinephrine concentration in the short-term and gamma-aminobutyric acid (GABA)-modulation in the long-term for improved seizure control [27, 28]. The VNS also has an acute impulse delivery mechanism, where providers or caregivers can swipe a magnet across the stimulator in the anterior chest wall during an active clinical seizure; this added impulse may help to abort the seizure or may reduce the duration of the postictal period [28]. Newer VNS models have an Automatic Stimulation Mode ("Autostim") feature, which delivers an added custom stimulation in response to a noted preprogrammed change in heart rate; this change in the heart rate acts as a surrogate for seizure activity, with the goal of aborting seizures mid-course. VNS devices allow for improved seizure control, though complete seizure freedom is not typical and most people will still require anti-seizure medications in addition to the VNS [27, 28].

Initially utilized for intractable epilepsy, the VNS is now indicated for treatment-resistant depression as well [29]. Notably, in the population of patients with chronic childhood conditions, it has also been observed to have a beneficial effect on disruptive behavior and obesity [29]. The VNS device is usually implanted on the left to avoid interference with innervation of the sinoatrial node, which receives its innervation from the right vagus nerve. The electrode is placed adjacent to the vagus nerve in the neck, within the neurovascular bundle containing the common carotid and internal jugular veins. The lead is tunneled subcutaneously to a pocket in the lateral chest, which can easily be palpated along the left anterior chest wall on physical exam.

### Complications

Several complications associated with VNS placement are procedure-related; the most common complication is superficial soft tissue infection, which can be seen in 3-6% of cases [30, 31]. Injury to the adjacent structures can also result in vocal cord palsy, swallowing difficulty, and neck pain [27, 30, 31]. Many notable side effects are related to stimulation of the vagus nerve, which can be relieved with the adjustment of VNS settings or with postural changes. Hoarseness is the most common of these stimulation-related side effects; it is the most noticeable at the initiation of VNS stimulation and with changes to VNS settings [27, 32]. Side effects including throat pain, cough, dyspnea, and headaches are the most noticeable around 3 months post-implant but decrease in intensity within a year of implantation and are uncommon 5 years post-implant [27]. The use of an external magnet with a programmable VNS allows individual testing for the correlation of symptoms [33]. Aspiration may occur in some patients, and causation can be investigated with the manipulation of device settings [33]. Sleep-disordered breathing, specifically obstructive and central sleep apneas, has been clinically reported; they can be treated either with the alteration of the VNS settings or treatment of the apnea (ex: positive airway pressure [PAP] therapy) [27, 28, 34]. Bradycardia and asystole are incredibly rare but should be monitored for [27].

## Special Considerations

The use of MRI is limited in patients with VNS due to concerns for heating the tip of the device lead; however, it has been safely performed with modified protocols [35] or by placing the device in safe mode (for newer models) [27]. Special notice is required if electrodes or leads from prior devices were left in place after a previous device removal [27].

Additional online information is available for providers and patients [36–38].

## Responsive Neurostimulation (RNS)

Responsive neurostimulation is an emerging therapeutic modality used to treat focal epilepsy. In individuals aged 18 years and older with refractory focal epilepsy involving one or two foci, an RNS may be a beneficial treatment modality. With an RNS, a neurostimulator placed under the scalp is attached to two leads which are placed at the identified epileptogenic focus or foci within the brain. The electrodes from these leads allow for intracranial electroencephalogram (EEG) monitoring. This EEG data is continuously monitored and recorded. Upon the identification of abnormal ictal patterns, an electrical stimulation impulse is sent to the area, aborting the imminent seizure prior to its onset. This closed-loop feedback system allows for real-time response and abortion of seizures in an effective manner, without potential side effects from more fixed-scheduled electrical impulses (as seen in the VNS). Recorded EEG data is uploaded by patients or caregivers for physician review, allowing for more customized settings and therefore individualized and improved seizure control. In some cases, long-term EEG data has provided more specific information about epileptic zones, illuminating the potential for ablation or surgical resection in some patients. It can also be used to help titrate anti-seizure medications more effectively [27, 28, 39]. A significant number of patients with an RNS report decreased seizure frequency and improved quality of life [27]. Some evidence suggests that the rates of sudden, unexpected death of someone with epilepsy (SUDEP) may also be lower in patients with an RNS compared to those without [39].

The most common complication from the placement of the RNS is intracranial hemorrhage, occurring in approximately 4.7% of patients; thus far, none of these hemorrhages have caused permanent neurologic deficits. The other significant complication from RNS placement is infection of the device or the leads; while conservative management with antibiotics is an option, device infection may necessitate lead and/or device replacement or complete removal [27]. Care is required with an MRI, as only certain models of the RNS are MRI-compatible; neurologists should be involved, and the RNS must be in MRI mode prior to imaging [40].

With an increased use of the RNS device, more long-term data involving complications and management is expected. Furthermore, it has thus far been used off-label in pediatrics for the management of focal epilepsy with some positive results and may be FDA approved for use in children in the future [41]. The primary device currently available in the United States is the NeuroPace. Additional online information is available for providers and patients [40–42].

## Conclusion

The use of implantable devices to treat neurological conditions is an evolving science, with new technology and improvements on existing technology designed for more targeted and customizable therapies and interventions. These advancing technologies promise significant improvement in both the quality of life and life expectancy for individuals in need of such therapies. As usage of these applications expands in both pediatric and adult populations, PCPs can serve as an ally to their patients by building and broadening their knowledge base around these technologies. In doing so, they can help guide their patients through the consideration, implantation, and ongoing management of these innovative devices and therapies.

## References

1. CDC: Centers for Disease Control and Prevention. Data and statistics for cerebral palsy. https://www.cdc.gov/ncbddd/cp/data.html. Accessed 16 September 2022.
2. Yi YG, Jung SH, Bang MS. Emerging issues in cerebral palsy associated with aging: a physiatrist perspective. Ann Rehabil Med. 2019;43(3):241–9.
3. CDC: Centers for Disease Control and Prevention. Data and statistics for cerebral palsy. https://www.cdc.gov/ncbddd/spinabifida/data.html. Accessed 17 September 2022.
4. Mukherjee S, Pasulka J. Care for adults with spina bifida: current state and future directions. Top Spinal Cord Inj Rehabil. 2017;23(2):155–67.
5. Spina Bifida Association. Guidelines for the care of people with spina bifida. 2018. https://www.spinabifidaassociation.org/wp-content/uploads/Guidelines-for-the-Care-of-People-with-Spina-Bifida-2018.pdf. Accessed 16 September 2022.
6. CDC: Centers for Disease Control and Prevention. Epilepsy data and statistics. https://www.cdc.gov/epilepsy/data/index.html. Accessed 17 September 2022.
7. Epilepsy Foundation. Drug resistant epilepsy. https://www.epilepsy.com/treatment/medicines/drug-resistant-epilepsy. Accessed 17 Sept 2022.
8. Medtronic. Medtronic for healthcare professionals: intrathecal baclofen therapy. http://professional.medtronic.com/pt/neuro/itb/index.htm#.Vv2w8pwrJhE. Accessed 14 September 2022.
9. Watve SV, Sivan M, Raza WA, Jamil FF. Management of acute overdose or withdrawal state in intrathecal baclofen therapy. Spinal Cord. 2012;50(2):107–11.
10. Motta F, Antonello CE. Analysis of complications in 430 consecutive pediatric patients treated with intrathecal baclofen therapy: 14-year experience. J Neurosurg Pediatr. 2014;13(3):301–6.
11. Dickey MP, Rice M, Kinnett DG, Lambert R, Donauer S, Gerber MA, et al. Infectious complications of intrathecal baclofen pump devices in a pediatric population. Pediatr Infect Dis J. 2013;32(7):715–22.
12. Overgard TM, Kjaersgaard-Hansen L, Soe M, Illum NO. Positive experience with intrathecal baclofen treatment in children with severe cerebral palsy. Dan Med J. 2015;62(1):A4999. Epub 2015/01/06
13. Miracle AC, Fox MA, Ayyangar RN, Vyas A, Mukherji SK, Quint DJ. Imaging evaluation of intrathecal baclofen pump-catheter systems. AJNR Am J Neuroradiol. 2011;32(7):1158–64.
14. Medtronic. Baclofen pump for ITB therapy. www.baclofenpump.com. Accessed 14 September 2022.
15. Reddy GK, Bollam P, Caldito G, Guthikonda B, Nanda A. Ventriculoperitoneal shunt surgery outcome in adult transition patients with pediatric-onset hydrocephalus. Neurosurgery. 2012;70(2):380–8. (discussion 8–9)
16. Stone JJ, Walker CT, Jacobson M, Phillips V, Silberstein HJ. Revision rate of pediatric ventriculoperitoneal shunts after 15 years. J Neurosurg Pediatr. 2013;11(1):15–9.
17. Kesava Reddy G, Bollam P, Caldito G, Guthikonda B, Nanda A. Ventriculoperitoneal shunt surgery outcome in adult transition patients with pediatric-onset hydrocephalus. Neurosurgery. 2012;70:380–9.
18. Conen A, Walti LN, Merlo A, Fluckiger U, Battegay M, Trampuz A. Characteristics and treatment outcome of cerebrospinal fluid shunt-associated infections in adults: a retrospective analysis over an 11-year period. Clin Infect Dis. 2008;47(1):73–82.
19. Prusseit J, Simon M, von der Brelie C, Heep A, Molitor E, Volz S, et al. Epidemiology, prevention and management of ventriculoperitoneal shunt infections in children. Pediatr Neurosurg. 2009;45(5):325–36.
20. Browd SR, Ragel BT, Gottfried ON, Kestle JR. Failure of cerebrospinal fluid shunts: Part I: Obstruction and mechanical failure. Pediatr Neurol. 2006;34(2):83–92.
21. O'Brien DF, Taylor M, Park TS, Ojemann JG. A critical analysis of 'normal' radionucleotide shuntograms in patients subsequently requiring surgery. Childs Nerv Syst. 2003;19(5–6):337–41.

22. Martinez-Lage J, Martos-Tello J, Ros-de-San Pedro J, Almagro M. Severe constipation: an under-appreciated cause of VP shunt malfunction: a case-based update. Childs Nerv Syst. 2008;24(4):431–5.
23. Nakamura L, Saito R, Kanamori M, Morita T, Tashiro R, Tominga T. A case of ventriculoperitoneal shunt dysfunction in an adult secondary to constipation. No Shinkei Geka. 2018;46(5):385–9.
24. Browd SR, Gottfried ON, Ragel BT, Kestle JR. Failure of cerebrospinal fluid shunts: Part II: Overdrainage, loculation, and abdominal complications. Pediatr Neurol. 2006;34(3):171–6.
25. Blount J, Severson M, Atkins V, Tubbs R, Smyth M, Wellons J, Grabb P, Oakes W. Sports and pediatric cerebrospinal fluid shunts: who can play? Neurosurgery. 2004;54(5):1190–6.
26. Association H. Shunt systems. http://www.hydroassoc.org/shunt-systems/. Accessed 14 September 2022.
27. Simpson H, Schulze-Bonhage A, Cascino G, Fisher R, Jobst B, Sperling M, Lundstrom B. Practical considerations in epilepsy neurostimulation. Epilepsia. 2022;00:1–16.
28. Ryvlin P, Rheims S, Hirsch L, Sokolov A, Jehi L. Neuromodulation in epilepsy: state-of-the-art approved therapies. Lancet Neurol. 2021;20:1038–47.
29. Ogbonnaya S, Kaliaperumal C. Vagal nerve stimulator: evolving trends. J Nat Sci Biol Med. 2013;4(1):8–13.
30. Kabir SM, Rajaraman C, Rittey C, Zaki HS, Kemeny AA, McMullan J. Vagus nerve stimulation in children with intractable epilepsy: indications, complications and outcome. Childs Nerv Syst. 2009;25(9):1097–100.
31. Kahlow H, Olivecrona M. Complications of vagal nerve stimulation for drug-resistant epilepsy: a single center longitudinal study of 143 patients. Seizure. 2013;22(10):827–33.
32. Ghanem T, Early SV. Vagal nerve stimulator implantation: an otolaryngologist's perspective. Otolaryngol Head Neck Surg. 2006;135(1):46–51.
33. Parhizgar F, Nugent K, Raj R. Obstructive sleep apnea and respiratory complications associated with vagus nerve stimulators. J Clin Sleep Med. 2011;7(4):401–7.
34. Lundgren J, Ekberg O, Olsson R. Aspiration: a potential complication to vagus nerve stimulation. Epilepsia. 1998;39(9):998–1000.
35. Rösch J, Hamer HM, Mennecke A, Kasper B, Engelhorn T, Doerfler A, et al. 3T-MRI in patients with pharmacoresistant epilepsy and a vagus nerve stimulator: a pilot study. Epilepsy Rev. 2015;110:62–70.
36. LivaNova. VNS therapy. https://www.livanova.com/epilepsy-vnstherapy/en-gb. Accessed 14 September 2022.
37. Epilepsy Foundation. Vagal nerve stimulation (VNS). http://www.epilepsy.com/learn/treating-seizures-and-epilepsy/devices/vagus-nerve-stimulation-vns. Accessed 14 September 2022.
38. Surgeons AAoN. Vagus nerve stimulation. http://www.aans.org/patient%20information/conditions%20and%20treatments/vagus%20nerve%20stimulation.aspx. Accessed 14 September 2022.
39. Skarpaas T, Jarosiewicz B, Morrell M. Brain-responsive neurostimulation for epilepsy (RNS System). Epilepsy Res. 2019;153:68–70.
40. Starnes K, Miller K, Wong-Kisiel L, Nils LB. A review of neurostimulation for epilepsy in pediatrics. Brain Sci. 2019;9(10):283.
41. Neuropace. RNS: The RNS system. https://www.neuropace.com/. Accessed 26 August 2022.
42. Epilepsy Foundation. Responsive neurostimulation (RNS). https://www.epilepsy.com/treatment/devices/responsive-neurostimulation. Accessed 26 August 2022.

# 44 Mobility Impairment

Jenny M. Lieberman and Miguel X. Escalon

## Patient Factors to Consider in Wheelchair Assessments

Many factors should be considered when evaluating patients for mobility devices as concerns for both functionality for the user as well as prevention of long-term complications. This section will review the most common patient variables that should be addressed when making a mobility device assessment.

## Supine Versus Seated Positioning

The effect of gravity on posture and functional mobility is an important consideration. The gravitational pull on a person changes when he or she is seated as opposed to being in the supine position. These forces can impact posture, tone, and skin integrity. For patients requiring mobility assistance, posture should be physically assessed when the patient is supine as well as seated to determine the asymmetrical pull of muscles from gravity, weakness, and spasticity.

J. M. Lieberman (✉)
Department of Rehabilitation Medicine, The Mount Sinai Hospital, New York, NY, USA
e-mail: jenny.lieberman@mountsinai.org

M. X. Escalon
Department of Rehabilitation Medicine, Icahn School of Medicine at Mount Sinai, New York, NY, USA
e-mail: miguel.escalon@mountsinai.org

## Pelvic and Spine Alignment

The pelvis is the base of support when an individual is seated, and in persons with disability, it serves as a stabilizing force on the spine. Pelvic asymmetry can thus lead to improper seating and mechanics, thereby resulting in long-term adverse outcomes such as skin breakdown and scoliosis. Pelvic asymmetry may be caused directly by the seating system or may be inherent to the individual and not accounted for the seating system. If the former is true and the asymmetry is flexible, it can be corrected in order to improve postural stability when the patient is seated. This is best confirmed by demonstrating that the patient's collapsed trunk can be straightened. Furthermore, pelvic asymmetry can be a result of spinal position with the pelvis achieving a more neutral position when the spinal asymmetry is encouraged and vice versa. This is an important consideration for function. Forward reach is more difficult when positioned with a posterior pelvic tilt and collapsed trunk and self-propulsion is more difficult when lateral flexion is encouraged.

## Upper and Lower Extremity Range of Motion

Lower extremity positioning is extremely important when considering the seated position in a wheelchair. Tight hamstrings and hip extensors


A. A. Kuo et al. (eds.), *Care of Adults with Chronic Childhood Conditions*,
https://doi.org/10.1007/978-3-031-54281-7_44

are the most common extremity derangement causing impaired skin integrity, and these conditions require unique seating considerations. For example, the use of elevating leg rests with tight hamstrings often results in the user sliding out of the seat, which can in turn lead to shear forces and increased pressure on the sacrum and bilateral ischial tuberosities. Likewise, forcing an individual to sit more upright than his or her hip extensors will allow results in the user sliding out of the seat, again encouraging negative shear forces. A common deformity in the lower extremities in those individuals with asymmetrical muscle pull is a windswept deformity in which both legs shift to a particular side. This position can sometimes extend into the trunk as well and thus impact the overall required seat width. Considerations for upper extremity range relate primarily to propulsion and joystick control. Adults with childhood disabilities have often developed contractures in their upper extremities, impacting wheel access and joystick control. Adjustments can be made in order to allow them better access to wheels and joystick controls, and referral to a specialized therapist to assist in the evaluation is essential.

## Muscle Tone and Reflexes

Spasticity, low tone, and abnormal reflexes are all very important considerations with this patient population, as each can directly impact posture and function. For example, some patients require spasticity (hyperreflexia) in order to maintain a seated posture, whereas for others, spasticity may be a hindrance to proper seating. Individuals with hypotonia face similar issues.

## Mobility Devices

Though a formal assessment of patients who require the assistance of a mobility device is typically done in consultation with a licensed clinical specialist, adult healthcare providers should be familiar with the various types of available devices.

This section will provide an overview of the indications for and limitations of the mobility devices most commonly utilized in clinical practice for young adults with childhood conditions.

## Walkers and Canes

Though not as frequently used by the young adult population, walking devices are a consideration for some individuals. There are various types of devices, determined by the number of supports that are used. Quad canes provide increased stability as compared to a standard cane. Some walkers have wheels while others must be lifted for forward movement. The devices that will best meet the individual's needs should be determined by a physical therapy assessment. For example, individuals with decreased balance from impaired motor control, such as in spastic diplegic cerebral palsy, would benefit from a device with a wider base of support and with wheels, so they do not have to lift it when walking. However, individuals with less controlled movements would not benefit from a wheeled walking device, as they could more easily lose control of this.

## Scooters

Due to their inability to provide postural support, a scooter is not a common mobility device used by young adults with mobility concerns. However, for individuals with slowly progressing debility and without significant neuromuscular impairment, such as those with emphysema or morbid obesity, a scooter can be an effective mobility device.

## Manual Wheelchairs

Wheelchairs are classified by categories, with their delineation dependent on axle position. A standard wheelchair and lightweight wheelchair do not have an adjustable axle. These should not be used as long-term mobility devices as they do not allow for an adequate hand-to-wheel ratio,

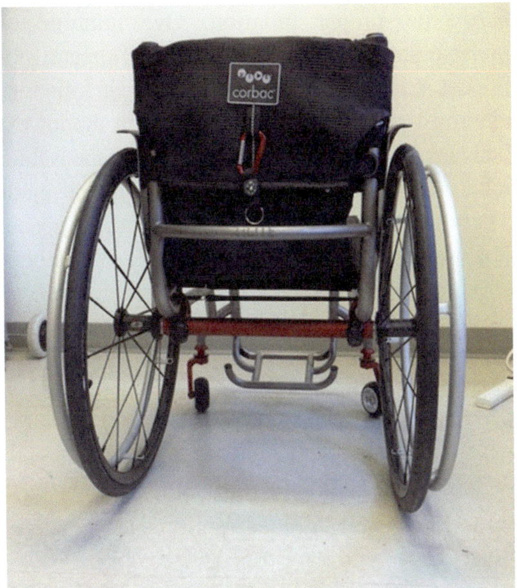

**Fig. 44.1** Ultra-lightweight wheelchair that allows adjustment of rear wheel position

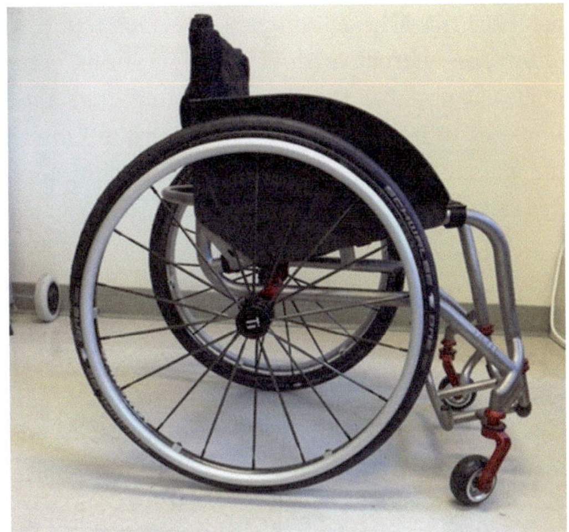

**Fig. 44.2** Ultra-lightweight wheelchair showing camber, where the distance between the base of the wheels is wider than the top

potentially leading to chronic shoulder and upper extremity issues. Ultra-lightweight wheelchairs do allow for an adjustment in the rear wheel position, allowing for the movement of the wheel forward and for a discrepancy between front and rear wheel position (as seen in Fig. 44.1). They also allow for camber, which is where the base of the wheel is wider than the top (as seen in Fig. 44.2). These adjustments create a healthy environment for upper extremity propulsion.

Another consideration when evaluating a patient for a manual wheelchair is foot propulsion. Some adults with cerebral palsy, for example, prefer propulsion with their feet in a manual wheelchair. This results in the need for a wheelchair that allows for a lower seat-to-floor height. The ideal, long-term manual wheelchair for this population is customized and requires referral to a proper seating clinic or therapist.

Reclining wheelchairs should not be used as full-time mobility devices since they encourage shear. Transitioning from a reclined to seated position results in sliding of the user down the seat, with shear created along the bony prominence of the pelvis and spine. As a short-term solution—for example, after a lower extremity orthopedic surgery—a reclining wheelchair is an effective mobility device. However, for patients who are dependent long term for mobility, the most appropriate device is a manual tilt-in-space wheelchair. This allows for proper position while allowing for the removal of gravity to promote good skin integrity and encourage improved alignment. A manual wheelchair is a dependent mobility device as it requires that someone else help propel the patient. There is also the option for a power tilt that adds on to a manual base for those who cannot mobilize themselves but would be able to shift their weight with assistance.

## Power Wheelchairs

Standard power wheelchairs can either include van seating or rehabilitation seating. The type of seat chosen is dependent upon the postural needs of the individual. Power wheelchairs allow for very basic adjustments to position and electronics, which is necessary for those with impaired upper extremity function.

Adults with childhood conditions often require external assistance for positional change. Power wheelchairs allow for the addition of power tilt, recline, elevating leg rests, and an elevating seat. Though not as frequently used, alternative options are lateral tilt, precline, and anterior tilt. These complex wheelchairs also allow for alternative drive configurations. This makes it possible for those with impaired hand function to use alternative body parts to control the wheelchair; for example, the head, chin, foot, and elbow.

## Wheelchair Seating Support Surfaces

Cushions are defined by their supportive and pressure-relieving capabilities. Full-time wheelchair users should avoid general-use standard cushions as they lack the ability to support postural asymmetry and do not promote good skin integrity. There are two principles of pressure relief to consider when selecting a seating support surface: immersion and suspension. Immersion refers to the amount of pressure and is equal to force over area. The better the immersion, the less force there is over the area (as the force or pressure is dispersed throughout the cushion) and the greater the pressure-relieving capabilities. For some individuals, no contact (suspension) is preferred over full contact to facilitate wound healing. This occurs with suspension of the bony prominence by weight bearing through larger support area surfaces.

The most common material used to fabricate cushions is foam. Viscosity determines the stability versus pressure-relieving capabilities. Some pressure-relieving cushions have a rigid foam base to provide stability, whereas others have softer conforming foam on top for pressure relief.

Gel cushions are a combination of chemicals that allow for a fluid substance that is a cross between water and gel. These cushions have fair to good immersion. This design requires maintenance with fluid moved back into the center of the cushion after each time the patient gets into or transfers out of the chair.

Air is considered the best support surface for skin integrity due to its ability to fully conform to the surface area. Air allows one to sink into the cushion, often with the lowest pressure gradient achieved. These cushions also require maintenance for proper inflation. Over-inflating or under-inflating these cushions will negatively impact skin integrity. To assess proper inflation, one must place their hand underneath the lowest bony prominence of the pelvis (usually the ischial tuberosity) and feel for the bottom of the cushion. There should only be a palms' width of space. For a demonstration, please refer to www.roho.com.

Back supports for wheelchairs can either be off-the-shelf or custom-molded types. Off-the-shelf back supports are distinguished by the extent of their lateral curve. The more aggressive the support needed, the deeper is the lateral wall.

For individuals with custom needs, the only option is custom-molded seating. For example, individuals with scoliosis and rotational spine deformities where there is greater risk for increased pressure or for those with trunk weakness, making it impossible to sit unassisted against gravity. This is very common with adults aging with a childhood disability. There are three different styles of custom-molded seat backs: subtle contour, thick aggressive support, and orthotic style. The seat back most appropriate for the individual should be assessed by the licensed specialist. The determining factor of one option over the other is due to several factors, including carryover by caretakers and mobility needs. Orthotic style systems require better carryover to ensure proper positioning and due to their narrower profile are better options for those attempting to propel or easily access a joystick in proximal position. The thicker options are better if there is need for support that is more highly padded as these consist of thicker foam.

## Consequences of Long-term Use of a Mobility Device

Long-term wheelchair use is associated with several adverse health outcomes. Adult healthcare providers should be familiar with the prevention, identification, and management of these adverse health outcomes, including the following:

## Decreased Bone Mineral Density

Prolonged wheelchair use has been shown to impact bone density. Individuals who use wheelchairs as their primary mode of mobilization do not bear weight often. Research has shown that bone density dramatically decreases the longer the period of non-weight bearing [1].

## Skin Integrity

Prolonged sitting without pressure relief places wheelchair users at high risk for impairment in skin integrity. Impairment in skin integrity results from pressure, shear, and force. For some individuals, decreased sensation and incontinence can further contribute to skin breakdown.

Peak pressures prevent blood from flowing to the area, resulting in tissue death. This situation arises when direct pressure is applied into one localized area and when bony prominences are not properly supported. Frequent weight shifts help to ensure that there are no prolonged, unsafe pressures. Research has identified that pressure reliefs need to be at least 3 min in order to reduce oxygen tension into tissues [2]. Research has also distinguished proper angles for weight shift, which is only able to be achieved with dynamic seating. The optimal positions are 35° of tilt and 100 of recline, or 15–25° of tilt and 120° of recline, with greater angles providing even greater pressure relief [3–5]. Therefore, weight shifts or change of position in chair, usually by a tilt backwards or lean, should occur every 30 min for a duration of at least 3 min per weight shift.

Shear is a mechanical force that acts on an area of skin in a direction parallel to the body's surface. Shear is affected by the amount of pressure exerted, the coefficient of friction between the materials contacting each other, and the extent to which the body makes contact with the support surface [6]. Shearing forces are a result of pulling or sliding of a person while the skin stays in place, leading to tearing of and lateral damage to the tissue. Deeper tissues, such as muscles, are particularly susceptible to shearing. Two common examples of shearing forces are (1) when a patient slides out of his or her seat and is then slid back into the seat and (2) when a patient slides along the tire of a wheelchair during transfers. Shearing ulcers are often difficult to heal due to the mechanism of injury and the fact that deep tissues are affected.

Force is a concept that is used to describe the effect on an object by an external influence. Force has a direction and a magnitude. Perpendicular forces cause pressure. The pressure at the junction between the skin and a support surface is often called "interface pressure." Pressure is defined as the amount of force applied perpendicular to a surface per unit area of application [7]. Force has been found to play a large role in impairment in skin integrity with the intensity of thrust into tissue, resulting in greater deforming effects.

To assist in the prevention and identification of impairment in skin integrity, routine healthcare visits should include skin integrity assessments for individuals who rely on a wheelchair for most of their mobility needs.

## Pelvic and Spinal Asymmetry

Prolonged sitting against gravity can lead to spinal and pelvic asymmetry, as mentioned previously. Dynamic seating is essential for the positional change of the adult with childhood conditions to provide gravity-assisted positioning [8–10]. Long-term wheelchair users are at very high risk of impairment of the joints of the upper extremities, either from propulsion or from the push-up style weight shift [11, 12]. For this reason, weight shifts and pressure reliefs are best performed by leaning forward or changing dynamic position of the chair.

## Pain

Many adults with childhood conditions experience pain, either from immobility, contracture, deformity, or impairment in skin integrity [13]. Many individuals who experience pain and who use power wheelchairs can benefit from proper device, seating, and cushion to decrease their complaints of pain [13]. An increase or change in pain patterns may be related to immobility issues and can require a referral to physical therapy for the evaluation of the wheelchair fit.

## Considerations for Specific Populations

Though a comprehensive discussion of all conditions that may necessitate the use of a mobility device is beyond the scope of this chapter, this section will review several of the more common childhood conditions that may warrant specific modifications to the mobility device.

## Cerebral Palsy

Individuals with cerebral palsy (CP) often have abnormal reflexes that might aid in their mobility such as seating that has deep lateral contours may be contraindicated. For example, some patients with CP utilize their abnormal tonic reflex pattern to access the joystick of a power wheelchair for independent mobility. Asymmetrical tonicity can result in dramatic deformity necessitating custom rehabilitation seating. An additional consideration for individuals with CP is foot propulsion versus powered mobility. Foot propellers generally propel backwards. However, the increased exertion required by foot propellers can increase the onset of spasticity worsening overall alignment. For those individuals in which self-propulsion is contraindicated and for whom there are no cognitive generated safety concerns, powered mobility is essential for increased function and participation in daily activities.

## Spina Bifida

Though upper spinal levels can be affected in individuals with spina bifida, the most common presentation resembles that of a low-level paraplegic. There are several considerations with this population. First, height is stunted in this population, predominantly due to scoliosis and poor bone growth. When considering seating with this population, trunk length is very important for good postural support. For individuals with a gibbus (short-segment structural thoracolumbar kyphosis), the extent of the gibbus determines the need for customization. More often than not, these individuals will require custom-molded seating to offload the gibbus.

## Osteogenesis Imperfecta

Due to the frequency of fracture with individuals with osteogenesis imperfecta, seating needs to be adjustable, allowing for both standard foot support as well as elevating leg rests in the event of fracture. A well-padded seating system can provide some additional protection to decrease the risk of fracture.

## Arthrogryposis Multiplex

There are several considerations with patients who have arthrogryposis multiplex, including stature, contracture, and limitations in the range of motion. Custom seating is necessary as the patient ages to support the spine and encourage elongation.

## Muscular Dystrophy

For patients with muscular dystrophy (MD), the subtype of MD determines mobility needs and type of equipment. Considerations should include respiratory function and the need for a ventilator, as well as spinal deformity and hand function. Custom seating is often required due to dramatic asymmetries that may be present. Alternative joystick access (head, finger, elbow, etc.) or joystick accessible to a caregiver may be necessary to power the wheelchair dependent on the individual's hand function. Multiple power seat functions are necessary for continuous mobility to manage discomfort and pain.

## Additional Considerations

### Referral to a Wheelchair Seating Clinic

Because many young adults with chronic childhood conditions must use a mobility device full time, they should not be provided with basic equipment. This population should be referred to a wheelchair seating clinic for the evaluation of their mobility needs whenever possible. A list of clinicians able to complete these assessments can be found at the Rehabilitation Engineering and Assistive Technology Society of America (RESNA) site, found in section "Helpful Resources" at the end of this chapter.

### Insurance Reimbursement

Medicare has specific requirements for the documentation of wheelchair needs (refer to the information in section "Helpful Resources"). Many insurance policies, including private and managed Medicare and Medicaid plans, follow Medicare guidelines. Requirements for insurance reimbursement of a wheelchair are that the individual must have a mobility limitation that significantly impairs his or her function in the "customary locations in the home." Additionally, the mobility limitation must prevent the individual from accomplishing his or her Mobility-Related Activities of Daily Living (MRADL), including toileting, feeding, dressing, grooming, and bathing. Finally, the mobility limitation must place the client at risk of morbidity or mortality when attempting to perform his or her MRADL or must prevent the client from completing his or her MRADL within a reasonable time frame.

If the individual is being considered for a standard K0001 wheelchair, a lightweight K0003 wheelchair, or a K0004 active duty lightweight wheelchair, then the individual must be unable to walk at all and requires a manual wheelchair to access the rooms in their home. To be considered for a K0005 ultra-lightweight wheelchair, the weight of the wheelchair must affect the individual's ability to propel the wheelchair, the individual's medical condition, and position of the rim in relation to the arm position (hand-to-wheel ratio) must be integral to the ability to self-propel the wheelchair, and the individual must have the cognitive ability to independently function in the lightweight wheelchair. Additionally, the individual's medical condition requires a frame with multiple adjustments that cannot be achieved with a less costly wheelchair.

To qualify for a tilt-in-space wheelchair, the individual must be dependent for transfers, and there must be in place a plan of care that identifies the need for frequent positional changes for medical reasons. To qualify for a powered wheelchair, an individual must not be able to safely or independently propel a manual wheelchair and/or scooter in his or her home for completion of his or her MRADLs.

In order to qualify for specialized mobility devices, a face-to-face visit between the patient and the provider is usually in order. If the individual is in the hospital, the doctor still needs to document a face-to-face evaluation in the medical record. The physician must clearly state the limitations the patient faces depending on the device selected. For example, in order to qualify for a power wheelchair, one must state that the client cannot walk and is unable to propel a manual wheelchair or control a scooter to complete his or her MRADLs. The physician must also document the patient's diagnostic history, physical exam, and functional assessment as well as the individual's willingness to utilize the equipment and cognitive and physical ability to safely and independently control the device. Many equipment companies are familiar with the documentation needed for the different wheelchair requirements and can help the physician understand these requirements.

## Conclusion

Many childhood conditions are associated with mobility impairments. With advances in medicine, an increasing number of individuals with these conditions are surviving well into adulthood and being cared for adult medical practices. In co-management with a licensed clinical specialist, such as occupational therapist or physical therapist, adult healthcare providers should be familiar with the indications for and limitations of the various available mobility devices. Additionally, providers should recognize appropriate prevention, screening, diagnosis, and management strategies for the most common adverse outcomes associated with long-term dependence on mobility devices. The information presented in this chapter is more of an overview and is meant only to serve as a guide. Additional information about wheelchairs and other mobility devices can be found in section "Helpful Resources" included at the end of this chapter.

## Helpful Resources

Rehabilitation Engineering and Assistive Technology Society of North America (RESNA) search engine to find certified professionals in users' area:

- https://www.resna.org/

Information sheet for physicians on insurance requirements:

- https://www.cms.gov/Outreach-and-Education/Medicare-Learning-Network-MLN/MLNProducts/downloads/pmd_DocCvg_FactSheet_ICN905063.pdf

Consumer support organizations:

- United Cerebral Palsy: www.cerebralpalsy.org
- Muscular Dystrophy Association: www.mda.org
- Spina Bifida: www.spinabifidaassociation.org
- Osteogenesis imperfecta foundation: www.oif.org
- Arthrogryposis Multiplex Congenita: www.amcsupport.org

## References


1. King W, Levin R, Schmidt R, Oestrich A, Heubi J. Prevalence of reduced bone mass in children and adults with spastic quadriplegia. Dev Med Child Neurol. 2003;45(1):12–6.
2. Jan YK, Liao F, Jones M, Rice LA, Tisdell T. Effect of durations of wheelchair tilt-in-space and recline on skin perfusion over the ischial tuberosity in people with spinal cord injury. Arch Phys Med. 2012;94(4):667–72.
3. Jan YK, Crane BA, Liao F, Woods JA, Ennis WJ. Comparison of muscle and skin perfusion over the ischial tuberosities in response to wheelchair tilt-in-space and recline angles in people with spinal cord injury. Arch Phys Med. 2013;94(10):1990–6.
4. Chen Y, Wang J, Liu L, Li S. Comparative effects of different posterior tilt sitting postures on buttock pressure in children. In: Paper presented at the 2010 3rd international conference on biomedical engineering and informatics (BMEI). 2010.
5. Sprigle S, Maurer C, Sorenblum SE. Load redistribution in variable position wheelchairs in people with spinal cord injury. J Spinal Cord Med. 2010;33(4):58–64.
6. Bergstrom N, Allman RM, Alvarez OM, Bennett MA, Carlson CE, Frantz RA, et al. Treatment of pressure ulcers guideline panel. Treatment of pressure ulcers. AHCPR clinical practice guidelines, no. 15. AHCPR publication no. 95-0652. Rockville: Agency for Health Care Policy and Research (AHCPR). 1994.
7. International Review. Pressure ulcer prevention: pressure, shear, friction and microclimate in context. A consensus document. London: Wounds International; 2010.
8. Bushby K, Finkel R, Birnkrant DJ, Case LE, Clemens PR, Cripe L, et al. Diagnosis and management of Duchenne muscular dystrophy, part 2: implementation of multidisciplinary care. Lancet Neurol. 2010;9(2):177–89.
9. Calhoun CL, Schottler J, Vogel LC. Recommendations for mobility in children with spinal cord injury. Top Spinal Cord Inj Rehabil. 2013;19(2):142–51.
10. Mcnamara L, Casey J. Seat inclinations affect the function of children with cerebral palsy: a review of the effect of different seat inclines. Disabil Rehabil Assist Technol. 2007;2(6):309–18.
11. Paralyzed Veterans of America. Consortium for Spinal Cord Medicine. Pressure ulcer prevention and treatment following spinal cord injury: a clinical practice guideline for health-care professionals, 2nd ed. 2014. https://pva.org/wp-content/uploads/2021/09/cpg_pressure-ulcer.pdf. Accessed 22 Sept 2022.
12. Reyes ML, Gronley JK, Newsam CJ, Mulroy SJ, Perry J. Electromyographic analysis of shoulder muscles of men with low-level paraplegia during weight relief raise. Arch Phys Med Rehabil. 1995;76:433–9.
13. Frank AO, De Souza LH, Frank JL, Neophytou C. The pain experiences of powered wheelchair users. Dis Rehabil. 2012;34:770–8.

# 45 Palliative Care and Hospice

Natasha Piracha, Kathleen Irby, and Jill Ann Jarrell

## Case Presentation

Wynton is a 22 year-old man with Duchenne Muscular Dystrophy (DMD), cardiomyopathy, and restrictive lung disease on night-time BiPAP via face mask. He uses an electric wheelchair and is known for zooming around his neighbourhood to visit friends. He also enjoys drinking Dr. Pepper and playing video games. He recently received a gastrostomy for medications and nutrition and was told he should not eat or drink by mouth as his dysphagia could cause aspiration. His elder brother, Ben, also had DMD and died last year in the hospital after having a tracheostomy and home ventilator support for many years.

During an outpatient appointment with you, Wynton acknowledges his decline, expresses sadness that he can no longer drink Dr. Pepper and that his ability to use the controls on his wheelchair and video games is diminishing. He says, "I'm tired of coming to a thousand doctors' visits every month. What's the point? We all know how this will end." His mother, Judy, who has been the primary caregiver of both Wynton and Ben, looks at you with tears in her eyes.

"I don't want to go out like Ben, I want to do things my own way," Wynton adds.

## Case Discussion

This case, based on real patients, highlights many aspects of palliative care that are unique in adults with chronic childhood conditions. Wynton is starting to have severe manifestations related to his life-limiting illness (cardiomyopathy and dysphagia), but the management of these issues may be compromising his quality of life. It is important to engage Wynton, and potentially his mother, in goals of care discussions.

Approaching goals of care and end-of-life discussions is particularly challenging with adults with chronic childhood illnesses, given the unique developmental and psychosocial issues seen in this population [1]. Previous studies have

N. Piracha (✉)
Pediatric Palliative Care, Department of Pediatrics, Columbia University Vagelos College of Physicians and Surgeons and New York-Presbyterian, New York, NY, USA

Adult Palliative Care, Department of Medicine, Columbia University Vagelos College of Physicians and Surgeons and New York-Presbyterian, New York, NY, USA
e-mail: np2775@cumc.columbia.edu

K. Irby
Department of Internal Medicine, Baylor College of Medicine, Houston, TX, USA

J. A. Jarrell
Division of Palliative Care, Department of Pediatrics, Texas Children's Hospital, Baylor College of Medicine, Houston, TX, USA
e-mail: jajarrel@texaschildrens.org


A. A. Kuo et al. (eds.), *Care of Adults with Chronic Childhood Conditions*,
https://doi.org/10.1007/978-3-031-54281-7_45

shown that this group understands that death may be an outcome of their disease, and most patients report a desire to discuss their wishes and worries with friends and/or family [2, 3]. Yet, end-of-life discussions often do not include the patient and frequently occur closer to death, which can lead to patient suffering and decisional regret among families [4, 5].

These discussions may be made more challenging by potential intellectual disability or other cognitive impairment of the patient and/or reliance on a surrogate caregiver for decision-making. In the above case, Wynton and his mother both need a psychological assessment for bereavement related to Ben's death and coping with Wynton's current decline.

## Palliative Care

### Definitions

Palliative care is an approach to caring for patients and families of patients with life-threatening illnesses that focuses on improving quality of life.

The word *palliate* comes from the Latin word *palliare*, which means "to cloak"; thus, palliative care is often associated with pain and other symptom mitigation. However, palliative care attempts to address and assist with facets of the patient and family's illness experience that may not only be physical, but also emotional, psychosocial, and spiritual.

In adults with chronic childhood conditions, it is important to consider aspects of pediatrics in implementing palliative care. The patient's physiology and psychosocial health as well as pertinent legal and ethical issues may be more pediatric in nature than what one is accustomed to in adult medicine or may be unique to this population, all together. The World Health Organization has similar but distinct definitions of adult and pediatric palliative care (Table 45.1) [6].

**Table 45.1** World Health Organization definitions of palliative care for adults and pediatrics

| *WHO definition of palliative care* |
|---|
| Palliative care is an approach to caring for patients and families facing life-threatening illnesses that improves the quality of life through the prevention and relief of suffering by means of early identification and impeccable assessment and treatment of pain and other problems that are physical, psychosocial, emotional, and spiritual. Palliative care: |
| Provides relief from pain and other distressing symptoms |
| Affirms life and regards dying as a normal process |
| Intends neither to hasten nor postpone death |
| Integrates the psychological and spiritual aspects of patient care |
| Offers a support system to help patients live as actively as possible until death |
| Offers a support system to help the patient and family cope during the illness and in bereavement |
| Uses a team approach to address the needs of patients and their families, including bereavement counseling |
| Will enhance quality of life, and may also positively influence the course of illness |
| Is applicable early in the course of illness and may be used in conjunction with other therapies that are intended to prolong life |
| *WHO definition of palliative care for children* |
| Palliative care for children is the active total care of the child's body, mind and spirit, and also involves giving support to the family |
| It begins when illness is diagnosed, and continues regardless of whether or not a child receives treatment directed at the disease |
| Health providers must evaluate and alleviate a child's physical, psychological, and social distress |
| Effective palliative care requires a broad multidisciplinary approach that includes the family and makes use of available community resources; it can be successfully implemented even if resources are limited |
| It can be provided in tertiary care facilities, in community health centers and even in children's homes |

Adapted from the World Health Organization. The WHO definition of palliative care and WHO Definition of Palliative Care for Children. https://www.who.int/health-topics/palliative-care

### Who Should Receive Palliative Care?

Palliative care is for patients of any age, and at any stage of illness, whether that illness is curable, chronic, or life threatening [7]. Patients do not have to be actively dying or near the end of life to receive palliative care.

There has been a conceptual shift away from identifying diagnoses appropriate for palliative care toward identifying patients with *unmet palliative care needs*. For example, the patient may have complex or refractory pain or other symptoms such as anxiety, depression, insomnia, dyspnea, secretions, or fatigue. Additionally, there may be nuanced aspects of the patient's care due to prognostic uncertainly, complex medical decision-making, need for care coordination or transitional services, psychosocial stressors, or spiritual concerns.

## When to Implement Palliative Care

Studies have shown that the earlier implementation of palliative care can not only improve patient's symptom control and decrease healthcare utilization, but also prolong life [8, 9].

The components of palliative care should be offered at the time of diagnosis of a life-threatening condition and continued throughout the course of the illness, whether the outcome is cure or death. Palliative care can be provided alongside efforts to cure illness and/or prolong life, as appropriate and desired [10].

Older models depict curative and palliative care as being at opposite ends of the care continuum. However, newer recommendations encourage incorporating aspects of palliative care early, alongside more traditional aspects of care to accommodate varying goals and to maximize patients' quality of life (Fig. 45.1) [11].

## Who Provides Palliative Care?

Every medical provider should practice palliative care to the extent of his/her abilities and comfort. *Primary palliative care* refers to basic skills and competencies required of all physicians and other healthcare professionals in areas such as pain management, guiding discussions regarding advance directives, and assisting in end-of-life decision-making.

*Secondary palliative care* refers to the specialist clinicians and organizations that provide consultation and specialty care. *Tertiary palliative care* refers to the academic medical centers where specialist knowledge for the most complex cases is practiced, researched, and taught.

Higher levels of palliative care are commonly accomplished through a multi- or trans-disciplinary palliative care team comprising nurses, physicians, social workers, chaplains, counselors, child life specialists, and volunteers with the patient and family at its center.

Utilizing primary palliative care skills can provide great benefit to adolescents and young adults with chronic childhood conditions. Providers well known to the patient and family, such as primary care providers or subspecialists central to care plan, can provide continuity and stability while patients are working with multiple subspecialists and transitioning from pediatric to adult providers. In particular, primary care providers often have a longitudinal relationship with patients and families and may be more accessible. There are easily-accessible educational and clinical practice tools available to equip clinicians with primary palliative care skills (Table 45.2).

In general, referral to a specialist or center for palliative care should occur when the limit of the primary provider has been reached. Table 45.3 provides referral criteria applicable to all conditions. For some specific populations, referral criteria have been published by specialty organizations or foundations. The Cystic Fibrosis Foundation has published guidelines for referral and the Muscular Dystrophy Association (MDA) website provides links to available guidelines for specific conditions.

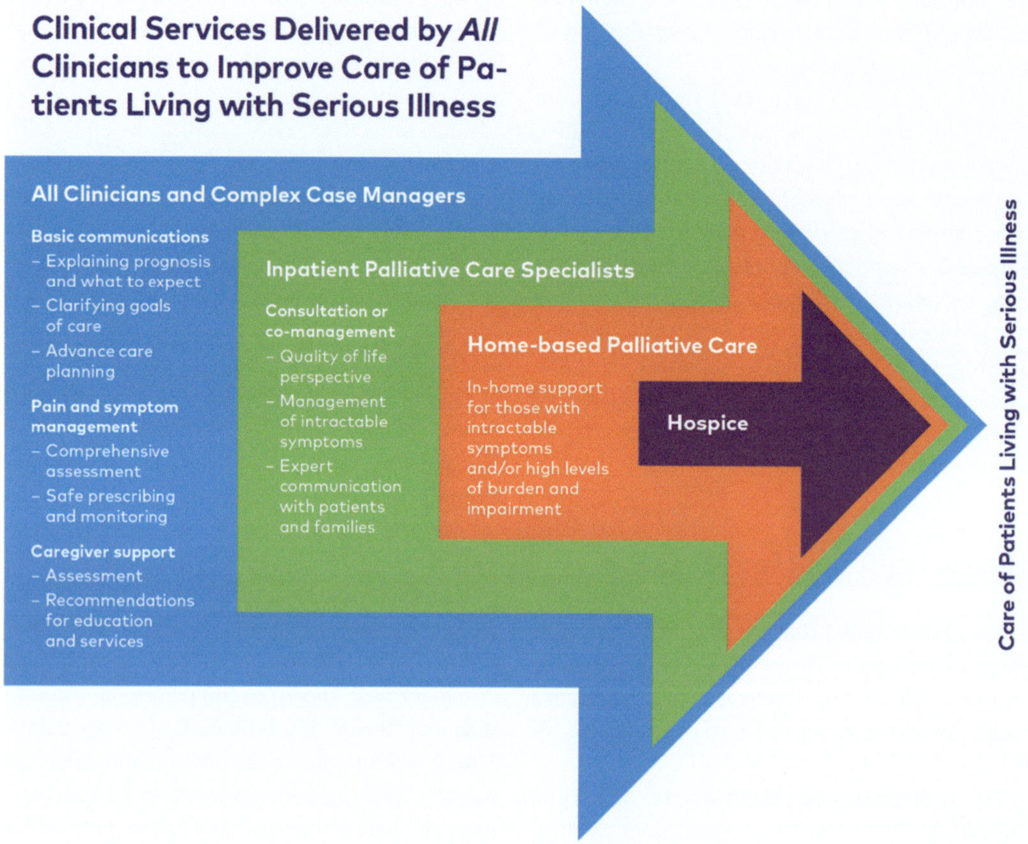

Clinical Services Delivered by All Clinicians to Improve Care of Patients Living with Serious Illness
All Clinicians and Complex Case Managers
Basic communications
- Explaining prognosis and what to expect
- Clarifying goals of care
- Advance care planning
Pain and symptom management
- Comprehensive assessment
- Safe prescribing and monitoring
Caregiver support
- Assessment
- Recommendations for education and services
Inpatient Palliative Care Specialists
Consultation or co-management
- Quality of life perspective
- Management of intractable symptoms
- Expert communication with patients and families
Home-based Palliative Care
In-home support for those with intractable symptoms and/or high levels of burden and impairment
Hospice
Care of Patients Living with Serious Illness


**Fig. 45.1** Clinical services to improve the care of patients living with serious illness. (Adapted from the Center to Advance Palliative Care, Case Study of Trinity Health System. www.capc.org)

**Table 45.2** Resources for building primary palliative care skills

| |
|---|
| Communication |
| – Vital Talk www.vitaltalk.org |
| – Serious Illness Conversation Gide www.ariadnelabs.org/wp-content/uploads/2017/05/SI-CG-2017-04-21_FINAL.pdf |
| Pain and Symptom Management |
| – Fast Facts www.mypcnow.org/fast-facts/ |
| – Center to Advance Palliative Care www.capc.org |
| Finding a palliative care or hospice team near you |
| – www.getpalliativecare.org |
| – www.nhpco.org/find-hospice |

## Where Does Palliative Care Take Place?

Primary palliative care can take place in the context of every provider–patient relationship, regardless of place. Consultative palliative care can take place in the hospital setting, clinic, home, or in other post-acute facilities. A growing number of hospitals and institutions have multidisciplinary palliative care services that serve patients at various places along the care continuum.

**Table 45.3** Recommendations for referral to or consultation with secondary or tertiary palliative care specialists and teams

| Palliative care referral criteria |
|---|
| Advanced pain or other symptom management |
| Functional decline; inability to complete activities of daily living |
| Patient, family or physician uncertainty regarding goals of care |
| Patient, family or physician uncertainty regarding prognosis |
| Establishing or interpreting advance directives |
| Complex medical decision-making (e.g., use of feeding tube in cognitively impaired or seriously ill patient) |
| Considering adding or changing supportive devices or technology (feeding tubes, respiratory support, etc.) |
| Assistance with end-of-life discussions |
| Guidance in end-of-life care |
| Assistance with hospice placement or other transitions in care |
| Multiple or lengthy hospitalizations |
| Multiple or lengthy intensive care unit (ICU) admissions |
| Limited social supports in the setting of a serious illness |
| Patient or family psychological or spiritual distress |

Adapted from www.getpalliativecare.org

## Hospice

### Definition

Hospice is a subset of palliative care focused on caring for patients at the end of life through interdisciplinary services and expert symptom management.

### Eligibility

In the United States, hospice is a benefit for terminally ill patients with a life expectancy of less than 6 months if the underlying illness runs its normal course. In patients >21 years of age, hospice includes foregoing any further disease directed therapy with curative or life-prolonging intent to maximize comfort and quality of life. Hospice patients who live beyond their expected prognosis of 6 months but demonstrate progressive clinical decline and hospice care needs may be recertified by the hospice physician for continuation of services, also known as benefit periods. Patients are eligible for an unlimited number of benefit periods with continued recertification.

Hospice is a benefit under Medicare Part A, the Department of Veterans Affairs, health maintenance organizations (HMOs), most private insurance plans and other managed care organizations. In most states, Medicaid also includes a hospice benefit, although individual eligibility criteria and services may vary. Hospice care can be provided at home/long-term care facility, assisted living or a dedicated hospice facility depending on patient and family care needs.

After enrolment, Medicare beneficiaries may continue to receive therapy for illnesses unrelated to their hospice diagnosis, billed separately via Medicare Part B.

### Services

As with all of palliative care, the hospice philosophy is interdisciplinary. In addition to medical providers, medications, and durable medical equipment, services most commonly include social work, chaplaincy, family support, limited home-health aide services, physical, occupational, and speech-language therapy. Hospice also provides families with 1 year of bereavement support.

Despite extensive services, the majority of a hospice patient's daily cares, including medication administration and device management, fall on the family/caregivers, with remote assistance available 24/7. Additional short-term support can be provided for uncontrolled symptoms (crisis care), caregiver respite, or to assist with transitioning to a new care setting (ex. skilled nursing facility).

### Concurrent Care for Pediatrics

Under the Patient Protection and Affordable Care Act of 2010, patients who are 21 years of age or younger, enrolled in a Medicaid or state

Children's Health Insurance Plan (CHIP), and eligible for and receiving hospice care may continue disease directed therapy related to their terminal illness with curative or life-prolonging intent. Patients must still meet hospice criteria, as outlined previously [12].

This concurrent care model allows patients and families to continue long-standing therapeutic and supportive relationships with primary and subspecialty providers while addressing previously identified barriers in pediatric hospice utilization.

## Advance Care Planning

### Definitions

Advance care planning is the process of clarifying and documenting an individual's wishes regarding their healthcare in the event of serious illness or end of life. Advance directives give guidance to family members, friends, and healthcare providers in what can be moments of crisis. Additionally, they can provide patients with increased autonomy regarding their future health care.

### Who Needs Advance Care Planning?

Advance care planning is not just for persons who are sick or dying. All adults, emancipated minors, and children with chronic illnesses are encouraged to discuss and document their wishes.

### Types of Advance Care Planning Documents

There are several types of advance care planning documents (Table 45.4). Specific documents are used during different stages and severity of illness, and documents vary by state. For example, most states recognize a Directive to Physicians (also known as a living will) as a legally binding document, but a few do not. It is important to be aware of the advance directives specific to the

**Table 45.4** Advance care planning documents and resources

| Document/Resource | Purpose | Recommended for |
|---|---|---|
| Directive to Physicians or Living Will | Provides direction for inpatient care in the event of sudden, severe illness, and inability to participate in decision-making; typically differentiates between aggressive and comfort care | General population |
| Medical Power of Attorney, Durable Power of Attorney for Healthcare, Healthcare Proxy | Designates surrogate decision maker for medical decision-making in the event of incapacity | General population |
| Durable Power of Attorney | Designates surrogate or proxy for financial/estate-related decision-making in the event if incapacity | General population |
| Organ Donation | Provides direction for organ and/or tissue donation | General population |
| Out of Hospital or Pre-Hospital Do Not Resuscitate (OOH DNR) | Provides direction to emergency response teams surrounding cardiopulmonary resuscitation | Patients with serious illness or frailty, for whom a healthcare professional would not be surprised if they died within 1 year |
| Physician Orders for Life-Sustaining Treatment (POLST), Medical Orders for Life-Sustaining Treatment | Direction to healthcare providers across care settings surrounding wishes for healthcare. Includes wishes surrounding cardiopulmonary resuscitation, hospital transfer, antibiotics and artificial nutrition | Patients with serious illness or frailty, for whom a healthcare professional would not be surprised if they died within a 1 year |

state in which an individual lives or seeks care. Some patients have advance directives in multiple states.

## How to Formalize Advance Care Plans

In most situations, advance directives can be accessed and completed in the privacy of one's own home or in a physician's office. Physicians and social workers can play an important role in initiating and guiding the advance care planning process as a routine part of care for all patients. Lawyers, while not necessary for the completion of advance directives, can also be helpful in some aspects of the advance care planning process.

The verification of advance care planning documentation also varies by state. Some states require two witnesses, some require notarization, and others require both witnesses and notarization.

## Resources

Social workers often have access to advance care planning forms. Useful Internet resources for obtaining state-specific advance care planning information and paperwork include www.caringinfo.org and individual states' Departments of Aging and Disability. State-specific organ donor registries and forms can be accessed via http://donatelife.net.

## Communication Regarding Advance Care Plans

Advance care plans should be discussed early between patients, their families and their healthcare teams. Copies of advanced directives should be given to physicians, put in the medical record, kept at home, and given to family and friends, especially those serving as surrogates. Conversations should be revisited regularly to explore changes a patient may have in his or her wishes.

Most states have laws to assign a surrogate decision maker for patients unable to assign a healthcare proxy. Laws may differ in surrogate hierarchy and the extent of surrogate decision-making ability. Some states also have statutes surrounding medical decision-making for adults with developmental or intellectual disability. Providers should refer to their individual state laws for further guidance.

## Palliative Care Issues Unique to Adults with Chronic Childhood Conditions

### Physical

Adults with chronic childhood illness may be small for their age and require pediatric or weight-based dosing of medications common in palliative care such as opioids or benzodiazepines. These patients may also require medical equipment that is more pediatric in nature due to its size, design, or function. For example, some adolescents and young adults (AYA) with chronic respiratory illnesses rely heavily on mechanisms more commonly used in children than in adults to maintain their comfort such as airway clearance devices or chest compression systems.

### Communication and Decision-Making

Some of the AYA population may be developmentally or intellectually delayed as a result of their underlying disease process. AYA who are cognitively intact may have communication and decision-making skills at a developmental level that is far below their chronological age due to the isolation of their protracted illness and dependence on proxy caregivers. It is important to use developmentally-appropriate communication strategies. Child life services may be useful even in a young adult patient who has cystic fibrosis or congenital heart disease, as an example, as they may have known the patient for many years and know the best ways of communicating with them.

Likewise, it is important to involve the AYA patient in decision-making to the extent of their ability and desire. Many adult patients with chronic disease of childhood do not wish to be involved in their own medical decision-making and defer such decisions to their parent or other trusted caregiver. This is ethically and legally permissible with the appropriate communication and documentation. Depending on the patient's illness and degree of disability, guardianship may be pursued for the patient or a Medical Power of Attorney can be completed.

## Coping

Because of the aforementioned developmental and communication considerations, assessing and assisting with patient coping in the adult patient with chronic childhood illnesses can be challenging. The patient may be unable to articulate fears and feelings, while others may engage in risky behaviors. Referral to a specialized palliative care team, child life services, or mental health professional such as a psychiatrist or psychologist with expertise in palliative care may be helpful in such cases [13].

Additionally, attention should be paid to the caregiver of the AYA patient as they may be experiencing caregiver fatigue and/or having coping difficulties. Screening for caregiver fatigue and collaborating with social work for appropriate supportive resources and referrals may be necessary.

## Advance Care Planning

The merits of advance care planning are well described; early discussions, including hypothetical conversations about end-of-life wishes, not only lead to better end-of-life care but also engender trust in clinicians, minimize psychological distress, improve quality of life, and facilitate hope [14–20]. Formalized pediatric advance care planning has been shown to increase families' appraisal of their care while not significantly burdening them with distress or strain [21].

Voicing My Choices is an advance care planning guide designed for AYA patients to help them communicate their end-of-life preferences to family, caregivers, and friends [22]. Voicing My Choices is not a legal document but a legacy document developed through research with AYA with cancer and human immunodeficiency virus (HIV) infection [23]. These guides can be found at agingwithdignity.org

Recommendations for advance care planning in AYA from this research include: that it be introduced by a trusted member of the healthcare team; when the patient's health is relatively stable and that the conversation evolve gradually over time, that the AYA's concerns and emotions be addressed throughout the advance care planning process, and that decisions regarding "life support" are best done with a healthcare professional [23].

## Systems-Based Issues

Pediatric hospitals, palliative care programs, and hospices may be ill-equipped to care for adults with chronic conditions of childhood due to lack of provider education, staff training and experience, and institutional policy [24]. For example, nurses at pediatric hospitals are usually only trained, licensed, and insured to care for children.

Similarly, adult hospitals, palliative care programs, and hospices may be lacking in infrastructure and resources to adequately address the psychosocial and familial needs of this patient population. This may result in the adult patient with a chronic childhood condition not having the robust interdisciplinary support, particularly the psychosocial elements, that they are accustomed to in pediatric palliative care.

Curricula and other educational offerings are being created to cross-train palliative care teams both ways [25]. Additionally, involving palliative care in the transition process is becoming best practice in multiple disciplines.

## References

1. Zebrack B, Isaacson S. Psychosocial care of adolescent and young adult patients with cancer and survivors. J Clin Oncol. 2012;30:1221–6.
2. Wiener L, Zadeh S, Battle H, et al. Allowing adolescents and young adults to plan their end-of-life care. Pediatrics. 2012;130:897–905.
3. Jacobs S, Perez J, Cheng YI, Still A, Wang J, Lyon ME. Adolescent end of life preferences and congruence with their parents' preferences: results of a survey of adolescents with cancer. Pediatr Blood Cancer. 2015;62:710–4.
4. Lyon ME, Jacobs S, Briggs L, Cheng YI, Wang J. Family-centered advance care planning for teens with cancer. JAMA Pediatr. 2013;167:460–7.
5. Mack JW, Joffe S, Hilden JM, et al. Parents' views of cancer-directed therapy for children with no realistic chance for cure. J Clin Oncol. 2008;26:4759–64.
6. World Health Organization. WHO definition of palliative care. www.who.int/cancer/palliative/definition/en/.
7. Palliative Doctors. http://palliativedoctors.org/.
8. Temel JS, Greer JA, Muzikansky A, et al. Early palliative care for patients with metastatic non-small-cell lung cancer. N Engl J Med. 2010;363(8):733–42.
9. Zimmermann C, Swami N, Krzyanowska M, et al. Early palliative care for patients with advanced cancer: a cluster-randomized controlled trial. Lancet. 2014;383(9930):1721–30.
10. American Academy of Pediatrics. Section on hospice and palliative medicine. 2016. http://www2.aap.org/sections/palliative/.
11. Carter B, Levetown M, Friebert S. Palliative care for infants, children, and adolescents. Baltimore: The Johns Hopkins University Press; 2011.
12. Center for Medicaid, CHIP and Survey and Certification. Hospice care for children in Medicaid and CHIP. 2010. https://downloads.cms.gov/cmsgov/archived-downloads/SMDL/downloads/SMD10018.pdf.
13. Rodin G, An E, Shnall J, et al. Psychological interventions for patients with advanced disease: implications for oncology and palliative care. J Clin Oncol. 2020;38:885–904.
14. Weiner L, Ballard E, Brennan T, et al. How I wish to be remembered: the use of an advance care planning document in adolescent and young adult populations. J Palliat Med. 2008;11(10):1309–13.
15. McDermott CL, Engelberg RA, Sibley J, et al. The association between chronic conditions, end-of-life health care use, and documentation of advance care planning among patients with cancer. J Palliat Med. 2020;23(10):1335–41. https://doi.org/10.1089/jpm.2019/0530.
16. Marron JM, Cronin AM, Kang TI, et al. Intended and unintended consequences: ethics, communication, and prognostic disclosure in pediatric oncology. Cancer. 2018;124:1232–41.
17. Wright AA, Zhang B, Ray A, et al. Associations between end-of-life discussions, patient mental health, medical care near death, and caregiver bereavement adjustment. JAMA. 2008;300:1665–73.
18. Smith TJ, Dow LA, Virago E, et al. Giving honest information to patients with advanced cancer maintains hope. Oncology (Williston Park). 2010;24:521–5.
19. Mack JW, Fisher L, Kushi L, Chao CR, Vega B, Rodrigues G, Josephs I, Brock KE, Buchanan S, Casperson M, Cooper RM, Fasciano KM, Kolevska T, Lakin JR, Lefebvre A, Schwartz CM, Shalman DM, Wall CB, Wiener L, Altschuler A. Patient, family, and clinician perspectives on end-of-life care quality domains and candidate indicators for adolescents and young adults with cancer. JAMA Netw Open. 2021;4(8):e2121888.
20. Rosenberg AR, Bradford MC, McCauley E, Curtis JR, Wolfe J, Baker KS, Yi-Frazier JP. Promoting resilience in adolescents and young adults with cancer: results from the PRISM randomized controlled trial. Cancer. 2018;124(19):3909–17. https://doi.org/10.1002/cncr.31666. Epub 2018 Sep 19. PMID: 30230531.
21. Thompkins JD, Needle J, Baker JN, Briggs L, Cheng YI, Wang J, et al. Pediatric advance care planning and families' positive caregiving appraisals: an RCT. Pediatrics. 2021;147(6):e2020029330.
22. Voicing My Choices. www.agingwithdignity.org/voicing-my-choices.php.
23. Weiner L, Zadeh S, Battles H, et al. Allowing adolescents and young adults to plan their end-of-life care. Pediatrics. 2012;130:1–9.
24. Humphrey L, Dell ML. Identifying unique aspects of adolescent and young adult palliative care: a case study to propel programmatic changes in pediatric hospitals. Semin Pediatr Neurol. 2015;22:166–71.
25. Weiner L, Weaver M, Bell C, et al. Threading the cloak: palliative care education for care providers of adolescent and young adults with cancer. Clin Oncol Adolesc Young Adults. 2015;5:1–18.

# Healthcare Procedures for Adults with I/DD

46

Dorothea Lerman, John C. Berens, Niraj Sharma, Julianna Rava, Ben F. Warner, Erin McElrath, Alice A. Kuo, and David F. Fray

## Abbreviations

| | |
|---|---|
| I/DD | Intellectual and developmental disability |
| SAS | Protective stabilization, general anesthesia, or intravenous sedative medications |

## Behavioral Interventions

Patient noncompliance and anxiety are commonly cited as barriers to providing adequate healthcare to those with I/DD. Research suggests that individuals with I/DD may engage in problem behavior to escape aversive medical and dental procedures and that healthcare professionals may exclude individuals with I/DD from their practice as a result of these behavioral difficulties [1]. Healthcare procedures also may evoke emotional responses that make it challenging for professionals to provide necessary care. Anxious and uncooperative behaviors can take a variety of forms, including crying, protesting, refusing to follow directions, running away, and hitting. Uncooperative behavior may lead to the use of restraints, sedation, or anesthesia during treat-

D. Lerman (✉)
Department of Clinical, Health, and Applied Sciences, University of Houston-Clear Lake, Houston, TX, USA
e-mail: Lerman@uhcl.edu

J. C. Berens
Department of Medicine, Section of Transition Medicine, Baylor College of Medicine, Houston, TX, USA
e-mail: john.berens@bcm.edu

N. Sharma
Department of Medicine, Brigham and Women's Hospital, Boston, MA, USA

Department of Pediatrics, Boston Children's Hospital, Boston, MA, USA

Harvard Medical School, Boston, MA, USA
e-mail: nsharma@bwh.harvard.edu

J. Rava
Department of Medicine, University of California, Los Angeles, Los Angeles, CA, USA
e-mail: JRava@mednet.ucla.edu

B. F. Warner
Department of General Practice and Dental Public Health, UTHealth Houston School of Dentistry, Houston, TX, USA
e-mail: Ben.F.Warner@uth.tmc.edu

E. McElrath
Department of Medicine, Brigham and Women's Hospital, Boston, MA, USA
e-mail: emcelrath@bwh.harvard.edu

A. A. Kuo
Division of Medicine-Pediatrics and Preventive Medicine, University of California, Los Angeles, CA, USA
e-mail: akuo@mednet.ucla.edu

D. F. Fray
Department of General Practice and Dental Public Health, School of Dentistry, University of Texas Health Science Center at Houston, Houston, TX, USA
e-mail: david.f.fray@uth.tmc.edu


A. A. Kuo et al. (eds.), *Care of Adults with Chronic Childhood Conditions*,
https://doi.org/10.1007/978-3-031-54281-7_46

ment [1–4]. Such procedures come with risks and may deter caregivers from seeking services for their family member [5].

A procedure called "tell-show-do" is one of the most common behavior management strategies implemented by medical and dental professionals [6]. For this strategy, the professional first describes the procedure to the patient (e.g., "I am going to place this cuff around your upper arm"). Next, the professional shows the patient the procedure (e.g., puts the blood pressure cuff on their own arm). Finally, the professional implements the procedure with the patient. Despite its popular use, tell-show-do is unlikely to promote cooperation in patients with I/DD when implemented as the sole intervention [7].

In light of the behavioral difficulties that often hinder access to healthcare services, training curricula for healthcare professionals should include more strategies for promoting cooperative behavior. Research has identified a number of evidence-based behavioral interventions that are effective for increasing cooperation or decreasing physiologic measures of fear during medical/dental procedures, such as X-rays, blood draws, physical exams, and magnetic resonance imaging [1]. Most interventions are based on a presumption that uncooperative behavior is maintained by escape or avoidance of aversive stimuli associated with medical procedures. Medical professionals could easily implement some of these interventions within the context of routine healthcare procedures or exams. These interventions include distraction, pairing of preferred items or activities with medical procedures [8], frequent breaks from the procedure [9], and reinforcement for cooperation [10–13].

To use distraction, the medical professional ensures that the patient has continuous access to some type of auditory, tactile, and/or visual stimulation, such as music, videos, toys, or projected lights [14]. Ideally, the patient enjoys engaging with the items or activities, as pairing preferred stimuli with medical procedures may reduce the aversiveness of the procedures. Providing the patient with frequent, short breaks during ongoing medical exams and procedures also can be highly effective in reducing uncooperative behavior [9]. For example, a physician might move away from the patient for 15 seconds at least once every minute during a physical exam. Finally, medical professionals can provide rewards, or reinforcers, for cooperation during medical exams. For example, a physician could give the patient an opportunity to watch their preferred movie for one minute each time they cooperate with a step in a routine physical exam (e.g., allow the physician to check their ears). This latter strategy requires the professional to obtain information about the patient's highly preferred items prior to the appointment or request that the patient brings these items to the appointment.

Other interventions typically require the expertise of behavior specialists, who work with the patients as an adjunct to their medical care. These interventions include graduated exposure [15–19] and escape prevention (i.e., escape extinction) [20, 21].

With graduated exposure, the therapist breaks down the medical/dental procedures into a series of steps and then introduces the steps gradually over time during mock healthcare appointments. For example, the therapist might initially just ask the patient to enter the exam room and sit down on the exam table while reinforcing any cooperative behavior. Once the patient consistently complies with these steps, the therapist introduces the next step in the physical exam (e.g., inspects the patient's left ear), again providing reinforcement for cooperation. The therapist continues to introduce new steps across repeated mock exams as long as the patient consistently complies with the earlier steps. For a specific medical procedure like a blood draw, the therapist might first ask the patient to place their arm in position. Once they are cooperative with this step, the therapist might move a mock needle closer and closer to the arm until it eventually touches the arm as long as the patient remains calm. Throughout the graduated exposure process, the patient receives reinforcement for tolerating or complying to the targeted steps.

Graduated exposure and reinforcement are sometimes combined with escape prevention, which can increase the likelihood of success [20]. For this procedure, the therapist continues to implement the medical or dental procedures even if the patient exhibits uncooperative behavior. For example, the therapist would continue to perform the steps of a physical or dental exam regardless of whether the patient is turning away, yelling, or resisting the procedure. This often requires the therapist to use physical guidance, blocking, or immobilization of body parts (e.g., holding the head still). The goal is to teach the patient that problem behavior will no longer lead to escape or avoidance of the medical procedure. Escape prevention should only be implemented by trained therapists after weighing the risks associated with the use of physical guidance/restraint and the undesirable side effects associated with escape prevention (e.g., escalation of problem behavior and increases in emotional responding) [22].

Once a patient begins to cooperate with therapist-implemented mock medical/dental procedures, the goal is to transfer this success to actual appointments with healthcare professionals. Meeting this goal requires collaboration between the therapist and the healthcare professional. For example, the therapist might initially accompany the patient to appointments and provide guidance to the healthcare professional for modifying their typical procedures to increase the likelihood of success.

Healthcare professionals who are interested in collaborating with behavior specialists to help their patients could search for qualified specialists in several ways. They could search for Board Certified Behavior Analysts® in their area by accessing the certificant registry at www.bacb.com. If practitioners are required to hold a license to practice behavior analysis in their state, healthcare professionals could contact the relevant state agency to obtain a list of licensed behavior analysts. After identifying credentialed and licensed behavior analysts in their area, healthcare professionals will need to identify those who have specialized training and experience in providing behavioral interventions to patients with I/DD during healthcare procedures. Healthcare professionals also could reach out to local and state affiliates of the Association for Behavior Analysis-International to inquire about members who might have expertise in assisting patients with I/DD.

## Dental Procedures

There is a growing body of evidence demonstrating the important effect that oral health has on overall health, and poor oral health has been shown to increase the risk of cardiovascular disease, diabetes and worsening glycemic control in persons with diabetes, and adverse pregnancy outcomes [23–26]. Oral health includes not only healthy teeth, but absence of oral pain, having functional teeth, and healthy gums and surrounding structures. Unfortunately, individuals with chronic childhood conditions—particularly individuals with intellectual and developmental disabilities (I/DD)—have relatively poorer oral health that includes higher rates of edentulism (tooth loss), periodontal disease, erosive dental disease, untreated dental caries and other orofacial infections, and lower rates of receiving dental treatment [27–31]. This perhaps is not surprising, given the relatively lower rates of other types of preventative care and other health disparities seen in adults with I/DD [32, 33].

The underlying reasons to explain this oral health disparity are complex and multifactorial. Several contributing factors, along with mitigation strategies for front-line clinicians, include:

1. Physical/cognitive limitations:

   People with developmental disabilities may experience limitations in their ability to perform adequate oral hygiene in the home. Optimal oral hygiene requires numerous physical skills—including gross and fine motor skills and coordination—as well as cognitive skills such as remembering to perform oral hygiene and being able to process and perform the numerous sequential steps required. Without sufficient supports, these limitations can lower the effectiveness of preventative oral health measures.

When discussing oral hygiene during a medical or dental encounter, it is important to review how the individual is completing oral care in the home. Depending on the individual's medical conditions and abilities, they may need various supports, such as concrete schedules/reminders, direct support (ranging from mere supervision to ensure adequate oral care to total oral care provided by a caregiver), and potentially modified equipment such as a special manual toothbrush [34].

2. Medication/disease effects:

Individuals with I/DD may be on medications that impact saliva production (particularly anticholinergics), and the resulting xerostomia (dry mouth) is a caries risk factor. There are other specific medications that may have side effects affecting oral health, such as gingival hyperplasia with phenytoin. Certain disease states confer increased oral health burden as well; for example, individuals who experience seizures may have dental trauma and oral soft tissue injuries following a seizure event [30, 35].

It is important for clinicians to be aware of the potential oral health-related consequences of certain medical conditions and medications. A thorough oral exam of all aspects of the dentition and soft tissues can identify many previously unrecognized pathologies and occlusion issues, especially if the individual cannot communicate unpleasant symptoms. For example, dental erosion of the posterior molars may be a sign of undiagnosed gastroesophageal reflux disease. For a review of oral manifestations of systemic disease, see Chi et al. (2010) [36].

3. Poor access to dental care:

Most adults with I/DD are eligible to receive Medicaid due to their disability and experience higher rates of poverty so would be less expected to have access to additional funding [29]. However, dental benefits associated with Medicaid plans are widely variable among states, and less than half cover comprehensive dental care, including the potential costs of intravenous sedation or general anesthesia. Even if there are dental benefits available, the percentage of dentists who accept Medicaid is low and widely variable among states [37]. While approximately 60% of dentists nationwide are enrolled with Medicaid, the percentage drops dramatically when measuring the number of dentists who treat any (i.e., more than one patient; median ~44% acceptance rate) or substantial (i.e., more than 100 patients; median ~20% acceptance rate) numbers of individuals with Medicaid annually [38]. In other words, coverage does not guarantee access.

Insurance coverage issues aside, not all dental providers treat adults with chronic childhood conditions. In 2019, the Commission on Dental Accreditation changed its code of ethics to require dental student training to include the assessment and management of vulnerable patients that include individuals with I/DD. Meaning, until the year 2019, this training was optional for dental schools, and there was no obligation for practicing dentists to be able to treat these individuals. The widespread lack of training within dental (and medical) school and the subsequent lack of competency has been documented [39]. It should not come as a surprise that in one large survey, dentists reported several perceived barriers to seeing individuals with disabilities, mostly commonly patient behavior, followed by the level of disability, level of disease, and level of training [40].

When counseling adult patients with I/DD and their families, it is important for the medical provider to be aware of these barriers and knowledgeable about the locally available resources. Becoming familiar with state-specific Medicaid dental benefits will allow for more accurate and timely information. In states where Medicaid does not provide comprehensive dental benefits, individuals can typically utilize home and community-based waivers as an additional source of funding if they have them. Identifying local dentists who accept Medicaid and those who have received positive reviews from persons with I/DD can also help individuals receive dental care more quickly and successfully. Looking forward, undergraduate dental and medical education needs to systematically include curriculum to train healthcare professionals capable of caring for this population.

4. Behavioral limitations:

   Being able to cooperate with the instructions provided by the dentist is a critical part of receiving safe, comprehensive dental care without the use of protective stabilization (also called restraint), general anesthesia, or intravenous sedative medications (SAS). While these methods can be effective and safe, they do carry an increased risk of complications [2, 41, 42] and higher costs that may lead to less frequent preventative dental care and eventually, decreased oral health. Not being able to follow instructions during dental care can make it challenging to complete the necessary procedures, and at worst, could result in physical harm.

   Non-compliance during the dental exam may have several causes. Cognitive and/or receptive speech impairments may make it difficult for an individual to understand the instructions. Individuals with neuromuscular disease, such as cerebral palsy, may not have sufficient control over the muscles in their face, head, and neck to follow the instructions even if they are understood. Some individuals, particularly those with autism, may be especially sensitive to physical, auditory, or olfactory stimuli present during dental care, evoking fear or anxiety that leads to non-compliance and/or an attempt to escape from the causative stimuli [43].

   As front-line medical providers, it is important not only to ask if adult patients with I/DD have access to preventative dental care, but if they are currently requiring SAS to receive it. A prior history of requiring these measures does not necessarily mean the need will be ongoing; assuming there are dentists in the community with experience in caring for adults with I/DD, giving the individual a chance to complete a dental exam without SAS should be considered. There is emerging evidence that a significant minority of adults with I/DD can participate in routine dental care with minimal supports, even if sedation or general anesthesia was previously utilized [44]. Even more adults with I/DD may be successful with behavioral training and there is a growing body of literature supporting their use [45]. It is important to be familiar with the local behavioral therapy experts and the coverage options required to access them.

## General Considerations for the Clinical Encounter

The guiding principles behind a patient-centered clinical encounter for an individual with a chronic childhood condition (particularly I/DD) should, in theory, not be significantly different from any other encounter. In practice, of course, there are numerous implications and nuances to be aware of when caring for a person with I/DD in a healthcare setting. There is no official or comprehensive guide, though there are various resources published by private organizations such as The Arc (many states have their own published document) and governmental agencies such as the Department of Homeland Security [46].

When interacting with a person with a disability in a clinical setting, it is important to respect the autonomy and dignity of the patient, regardless of their abilities. To this end, introductions should first be directed at the patient, and whenever possible, communication should go through the individual, utilizing supports from caregivers only as needed. Should an individual have limited verbal communication, the clinician can ask the caregivers about communication preferences, which may range from vocalizations/facial expressions to complete, independent communication using an augmented communication device. It is important to note that verbal communication may be incongruent with intellectual functioning—in one study, 9% of non-verbal individuals with cerebral palsy did not have an intellectual disability [47]. If an intellectual disability or other learning/cognitive disability is present or suspected, clinicians should strive to make their language accessible and rely more heavily on methods to ensure comprehension (such as read-back or asking the patient to repeat their understanding of the conversation).

On the topic of speech, there are a few points of etiquette worth mentioning. The preferred term is "intellectual disability," with "mental retardation" no longer accepted due to the stigma the term carries. For most medical conditions, person-first language is preferred. In other words, place the descriptor after the person, such as "person with diabetes/autism/disability" instead of "diabetic/autistic/disabled person". There are exceptions to this rule and some people prefer the opposite approach, especially when the condition is closely/positively linked to their identity, such as some Deaf individuals [48]. When in doubt, having a humble, open attitude and taking cues from the individual or their caregivers is a reasonable approach.

Communication goes beyond the spoken words. Getting on the same level of the patient can minimize the power dynamic that may evoke more anxiety if the clinician is towering over them. Spending extra time to build rapport and trust may be even more important when treating a person with I/DD; asking the individual about their favorite things might also help to identify items or activities that can be utilized during the clinical encounter to decrease anxiety and increase cooperation—see the behavioral therapy section for more detail. Clinicians should also consider their choice of attire as wearing a white coat may evoke a fear response if the patient has been conditioned to be fearful of such a stimulus. Speaking in calm, warm tones may also reduce anxiety even if the person does not comprehend the actual speech.

## Considerations for the Dental Encounter

In addition to the general considerations above, there are also elements more specific to the dental encounter when treating individuals with I/DD. In positioning the individual, the standard approach may need to be modified. If the person is in a wheelchair, it is possible that the wheelchair may recline; there are also specialty equipment that can recline the entire wheelchair if there is not a built-in mechanism to do so. Some individuals may be able to sit in a standard dental chair even if they arrived in a wheelchair, depending on their condition and the type of chair available. If none of these options are available, or if the patient does not want to sit in the exam chair, dental professionals may consider alternative options such as sitting in a regular chair, if possible, or even in a bean bag. The latter option is often a more comfortable option that allows for more optimal positioning compared to the head-on approach of a non-reclining chair.

Environmental modifications may need to be considered, particularly for individuals who have previously experienced difficulty completing the dental encounter. For some individuals, particularly with sensitivities to the sights, smells, and sounds of a dental office, a more isolated environment (e.g., a separate, closed off area) may decrease the severity of these cues. Otherwise, noise-cancelling headphones may help if a person has sensitivity to sound(s) or else a positive stimulus (preferred song or video) could be played to mask the other sounds. For smell sensitivity, a pleasant-smelling lip balm or other fragrant ointment could be applied below the nose. Sunglasses can help with light sensitivity, especially when overhead lights are used, and double as eye protection. In addition to masking existing environmental cues, it is important to consider small ways that might make the dental encounter more pleasant for the individual, particularly if they are anxious about the visit. Positive modifications could include having a loved one present, having a preferred item nearby (e.g., toy), or having other positive stimuli around (e.g., photo of favorite musical artist). For more specific details on oral health behavioral interventions to improve cooperation with the dental exam, refer to Lyons (2009) [45].

## Considerations for the Dental Treatment Planning and Delivery

Promoting regular dental visits is one of the cornerstones of preventive dentistry for all adults with or without chronic conditions of childhood

[49]. However, due to poor access to dental care due to the factors described above, dental visits for individuals with intellectual disabilities can be much less frequent than the typically recommended 3- to 6-month interval, which still may not be frequent enough for optimal prevention for some [50]. Combined with a higher likelihood of suboptimal oral hygiene at home, this leads to dental care that must focus more on restoration and less on prevention and prophylaxis. Improving this system of care will likely take a different approach that emphasizes more frequent encounters with the dental team, which will also help to overcome anxiety related to oral examination and dental treatment. More frequent interactions will likely require the utilization of technology-based platforms, i.e., teledentistry, a group of evidence-based strategies used to promote oral health and practice dentistry remotely [51].

When planning for dental treatment, it is especially important to consider the urgency of any recommendation when caring for an individual who may have difficulties cooperating with dental procedures. Certainly, there are conditions that need immediate intervention and may subsequently require more invasive means to achieve (i.e., SAS). At the other end of the spectrum, there is the absence of active disease and the opportunity to promote optimal oral health and prevent future disease. Here, it is important to strongly consider additional supports (e.g., behavioral therapy) for a more gradual approach to achieve cooperation with dental procedures over time. Reimbursement considerations aside, having a relaxed approach with no set expectations allows for trust-building and addressing the long-term goal of the individual feeling safe with dental procedures and in control as opposed to the short-term goal of completing a given procedure.

When triaging situational urgency, there are options for conditions that fall somewhere in the middle, such as active dental caries without a secondary complication (e.g., abscess). As part of a broader movement known as Minimally Invasive Dentistry [52], there exists a substance called silver diamine fluoride that can arrest active caries when applied topically [53]. This evidence-based intervention may be an excellent alternative for a patient who cannot cooperate with typical caries restoration procedures. It may also be an emerging option for individuals with poor access to dental care if more primary care medical providers are trained to apply it [54].

## Future Directions and Importance of Advocacy for Integrated Dental Health

Given the significant disparities in oral health, it is important to at least mention possible future directions and opportunities to advocate for more equitable health for individuals with I/DD and other childhood conditions. This sentiment has been echoed by multiple national bodies, such as the American Academy for Developmental Medicine and Dentistry [55] and the American Public Health Association. The latter released a policy statement in the year 2016 that called for a public health strategy integrating oral health with medical care for persons with I/DD through the implementation of evidence-based interdisciplinary models of care. This approach considers the effects that social determinants of health have on access to care. It pools the resources and knowledge of the entire interdisciplinary team to optimize overall health, identify resources, and execute care plans. Better access to care and the integration of medical and dental care make sense from an economic viewpoint as well [56, 57].

Taking an interdisciplinary, public-health approach to dental care has its barriers. Current undergraduate medical and dental education are poorly integrated, and the lack of education in caring for individuals with I/DD has been highlighted above. Healthcare systems are usually not designed to readily facilitate cross talk between different health disciplines (for a summary of existing medical/dental integration, see [55]). Reimbursement for medical and dental care does also not take into consideration the enhanced levels of service that are often needed to provide patient-centered, developmentally appropriate, safe care. Substantial changes to existing healthcare policy and insurance reimbursement models will be needed to carry out the strategies that have been highlighted by these, and other national organizations.

## Colonoscopies and Preventive Procedures

As mentioned above, there is an inequity for adults with Intellectual/Developmental Disabilities (I/DD) receiving preventive medicine and other required screenings and procedures. Existing research shows that individuals with I/DD are less likely than the general public to receive recommended preventive health screenings and procedures, such as colonoscopies and mammograms [58–60]. For example, patients with I/DD are 46% less likely to be up to date with colonoscopy screenings and 51% less likely to experience adequate bowel preparation than individuals living without I/DD [59, 61, 62]. Furthermore, procedures for patients with I/DD, such as a gynecological exams, are often delayed which can lead to delayed and missed diagnoses. These inequities are worse for individuals who are socioeconomically disadvantaged, live with complex healthcare conditions, have limited access to quality healthcare programs, or identify with other historically marginalized groups [63]. This section focuses on colonoscopies as an exemplar for preventive medicine procedures. Colorectal cancer is the second leading cause of national cancer mortality, and therefore, ensuring that high-risk patients receiving required screenings are paramount to their health.

### A Model for Colonoscopies

At our institution, we have developed a four-step process for patients who require a screening colonoscopy. This can serve as a model for other procedures such as mammograms and gynecological exams.

1. *Collect information and partners*

   The first step is to ensure that a protocol has been established in advance at your institution for the given procedure to collect important information and organizes the appropriate team members. For example, it will be important to determine the documentation that must either be written or collected in advance. This can include details about guardianship to determine who can make medical decisions for the patient. Also, paperwork should be written about the risks and benefits of the procedure at an appropriate reading level for the patient and caregiver.

   A protocol should be written with a decision tree for each step of the procedure. It can include, for example, when it would be appropriate to use conscious sedation versus general anesthesia for the colonoscopy. Finally, champions should be found for each procedure in the division responsible for it. Partnering with a specific gastroenterologist who has an interest and expertise with patients who have special needs is beneficial. It is also helpful to train administrative staff who understand the specific needs of this patient population to assist in steps such as ensuring guardianship is documented during registration and scheduling additional time for appointments. Their input and expertise in the nonclinical and administrative aspects will be invaluable in developing the protocol.

2. *Developing an ordering protocol for the procedure*

   An organization should develop a protocol for how to place the order for the procedure and specific questions that should be considered. For a colonoscopy, the first step could be asking the ordering provider if a non-invasive colorectal cancer screen, such as a fecal immunochemical test, would be an appropriate alternative. Additional questions to consider in the order set are the level of anesthesiology required, special equipment needs, if the procedure is best suited for an outpatient clinic or an operating room, and if the colonoscopy is best conducted by a gastroenterologist or a general surgeon.

3. *Steps prior to the procedure*

   Once the procedure has been ordered, there are processes that should be considered to improve the likelihood of success and the patient's overall experience. For a colonoscopy, a patient must complete a prep to clear out the colon to ensure the greatest visibility. A consideration would include where the prep should be done—at home alone by the patient, at a home with the assistance of visiting nursing, or in the hospital as a preplanned admission with the assistance of nursing. Hydration is an issue when doing bowel clean outs and providers/caregivers need to pay close attention to this aspect of the prep. Additional equipment or appropriate medications should be identified in advance to anticipate issues that may arise. Planning could also include ensuring that a supportive party is present, such as child-life or an equivalent team member, who can advocate for the patient and help them navigate the health system during the experience.

4. *Assessing the procedure*

   If the preceding steps are planned appropriately, then the procedure should go smoothly. This can also be an opportunity for quality improvement. In advance, the team should consider data that can be collected to measure success. This can include patient/caregiver satisfaction, the success of the colonoscopy, discussions with clinical and administrative staff to learn about any lessons learned, and additional equipment that could be used in the future. After the procedure, this information can be reviewed to improve the process for the next iteration.

Following these steps can ensure that the procedure is successfully completed to the satisfaction of the patient, caregiver, and medical team and can be improved upon for the future.

## Blood Draw Procedures

For children and adults with intellectual and developmental disabilities (I/DD), disparities in healthcare quality and health outcomes are a significant concern. People with I/DD are at increased risk for both physical and mental health challenges, including cardiovascular disease, diabetes, gastrointestinal disorders, depression, and other chronic conditions [64, 65]. Furthermore, research estimates over a third of deaths for people with I/DD are related to not receiving preventable healthcare interventions, leading to a lower life expectancy for this population [66, 67].

Limited physician knowledge on the healthcare needs and characteristics of I/DD is one reason for health disparities among people with I/DD [68]. Additionally, many physicians report biased views related to accessible, quality care for people with disabilities [69]. Unfortunately, lack of physician knowledge and competence leads many healthcare providers to refer patients to specialists for routine care procedures. This requires patients with I/DD to expend more time and costs than is necessary for health services; many patients would rather not seek further care. Ultimately, these barriers to care compromise healthcare quality and health outcomes for patients with I/DD.

In addition to physician knowledge, the physical structure of the healthcare environment and health systems' protocols are not designed to support people with I/DD. Many people with I/DD experience sensory overload related to bright lights, strong smells, and loud sounds in healthcare settings or have sensory sensitivities when healthcare providers or medical objects touch their skin [70, 71]. The sensory distress can inhibit their ability to communicate or proceed with examinations and tests [72, 73]. Additionally, healthcare processes are not adapted to the precise needs of people with I/DD—such as extensive wait times, brief appointments, and protocols limited to hospital settings [74, 75]. These barriers add to the low utilization rate of preventive health services among people with I/DD.

Primary care providers play a crucial role in providing accessible healthcare to patients with I/DD. An initial approach to improving care is understanding common barriers for this population and strategizing innovative methods to increasing utilization of preventive health measures. In doing so, we can hopefully begin to close the gap on health disparities for people with I/DD.

## Needle-Related Anxiety in Primary Care

Needle-related procedures, such as vaccinations and blood draws, are frequent occurrences in primary care practices and essential tools in providing preventive medical care. Although these procedures are necessary for maintaining optimal health, many children and adults experience overwhelming anxiety when needles are involved in care. It is estimated that nearly 10% of the general population has needle-related procedural anxiety (i.e., the fear of needles during a medical procedure) and 1–2% have needle phobia [76]. A fear of needles can cause physical distress and discomfort, leading some patients to skip doctor's appointments or refuse preventive services, ultimately putting their health at risk.

One primary care scenario that requires needles is diabetes management. An adult with diabetes that has needle-related anxiety may refuse to have their blood drawn on regular visits to check their A1C levels. To not distress the patient, a clinician may commit to irregular blood draws. However, this often leads to further complications down the road, including increased morbidity and lower quality of life.

## Needle-Related Anxiety for People with I/DD

While roughly 10% of the population experiences needle-related anxiety, it is three times as prevalence among individuals with intellectual and developmental disabilities (I/DD) [77–79]. This is a cause of concern, as individuals with I/DD experience less than excellent health outcomes compared to the general population. For those with I/DD and needle-related anxiety, the distress associated with a fear of needles can exacerbate already prevalent health disparities. For example, patients with I/DD that have needle-related anxiety may experience both sensory overload and fear of needles, leading to a traumatic procedural visit that makes them resistant to future doctor's appointments.

For patients with I/DD and needle phobia, they may not be able to receive routine needle-related medical procedures without being sedated. Deep sedation, or general anesthesia, requires an in-patient hospital visit to complete needle-related medical procedures. This is not a feasible solution to routine care and is also a significant financial burden on patients and their families. Ultimately, patients that experience needle phobia and require sedation receive limited preventive care services for their health needs.

Overall, patients with I/DD and needle-related anxiety or phobia are at increased risk of lower preventive care utilization and lower quality of life. Primary care providers need strategies to mitigate distress experienced by patients with I/DD and needle anxiety when performing routine needle-related medical care.

## Considerations for Your Clinic or Institution

Evidence-based behavioral interventions and pain management techniques are simple strategies that can be implemented in any primary care practice to improve needle-related medical procedures for individuals with I/DD (approaches are described below in the Three Tier Program). First, these approaches universally improve the patient-provider interaction—patients with or without needle anxiety benefit from these techniques to improve patient comfort and safety. Second, these strategies are low cost and can be utilized by any healthcare professional. Ultimately, there are little to no risks incorporating these interventions into a primary care clinic's current practice.

Each clinic needs to assess the feasibility of implementing a minimal sedation protocol in an outpatient setting for patients with anxiety related to routine needle-related medical procedures. Currently, there is no gold standard on how to implement minimal sedation techniques in the primary care setting. While there are novel guidelines developed for the UCLA Health's Needle

Anxiety Program, these may not be feasible for your practice [80]. Some of the challenges your practice may need to consider are the delivery and storage of temperature-regulated controlled substances at the outpatient clinic and having enough staff on site that can handle a potential high-level emergency, such as an overdose. If your clinic is part of a larger hospital system, you may need to go through added layers of safety approvals before you can integrate a minimal sedation protocol. However, if these challenges can be managed, there are significant benefits for patients and providers. Rather than relying on the emergency department for routine care procedures, which can be unreliable due to patient volume, or scheduling time through operating rooms (which incur steep medical bills), the minimal sedation protocol enables patients and providers to remain in the primary care setting, allowing flexibility of time, less stress, and less costs.

## Three-Tier Needle Anxiety Program

A Three-Tier Needle Anxiety Program was developed to remove barriers to routine needle-related medical procedures for children and adults with I/DD in the primary care setting [81]. While the main goal of the program is to increase uptake of preventive needle-related procedures among patients with I/DD and needle-related anxiety, additional aims include decreasing distress in the patient-provider interaction and improving patient & provider safety. Figure 46.1 displays the Three-Tier system; Tier 1) Train Nurses in Evidence-Based Behavioral Interventions, Tier 2) Distraction Devices & Pain Management, and Tier 3) Minimal Sedation. The Needle Anxiety Program is structured for the majority of patients to require noninvasive, low-risk, evidence-based practices to complete the needle-related procedure. It is expected that 90% of individuals will need Tier 1 techniques, 9% will need Tier 2 strategies, and 1% will need Tier 3 to complete the needle-related procedure. Based on this system, a limited number of individuals will need the innovative minimal sedation protocol.

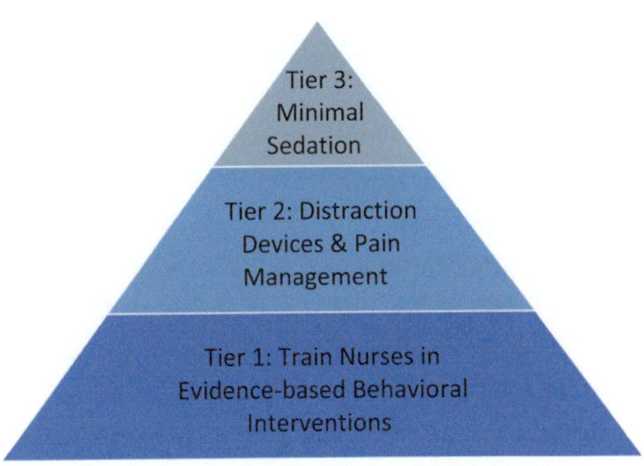


**Fig. 46.1** The Three-Tier Needle Anxiety Program [81]

Tier 1 strategies include training nursing staff in evidence-based behavioral modification practices. Incorporating behavioral intervention techniques minimize the discomfort for the patients during needle-related procedures. These strategies not only reduce distress for the patient but assist nurses in maintaining a safe environment for the patient and themselves. Evidence-based behavioral interventions include comfort positioning, modeling, systematic desensitization, and caregiver coaching [84–86]. When Tier 1 strategies are not effective at reducing distress, Tier 2 is initiated to complete the needle-related procedure. Tier 2 strategies include distraction devices and/or a numbing cream. At the appointment, patients may watch a preferred video to distract themselves during the procedure. Also, nurses may apply mechanical stimulation or a topical analgesic to reduce the painful sensation from the needle. Tier 2 strategies should be used in conjunction with Tier 1 behavioral techniques.

Tier 3 is suggested for patients that experienced unsuccessful attempts to complete needle-related medical procedures using the intervention strategies in Tier 1 and Tier 2. Tier 3 is a minimal sedation protocol that can be administered by a physician, registered nurse, or nurse practitioner in the primary care setting. Minimal sedation is considered a drug-induced state during which patients respond normally to verbal commands; cognitive function and physical coordination may be impaired; however, airway, reflexes, ventilatory, and cardiovascular functions are unaf-

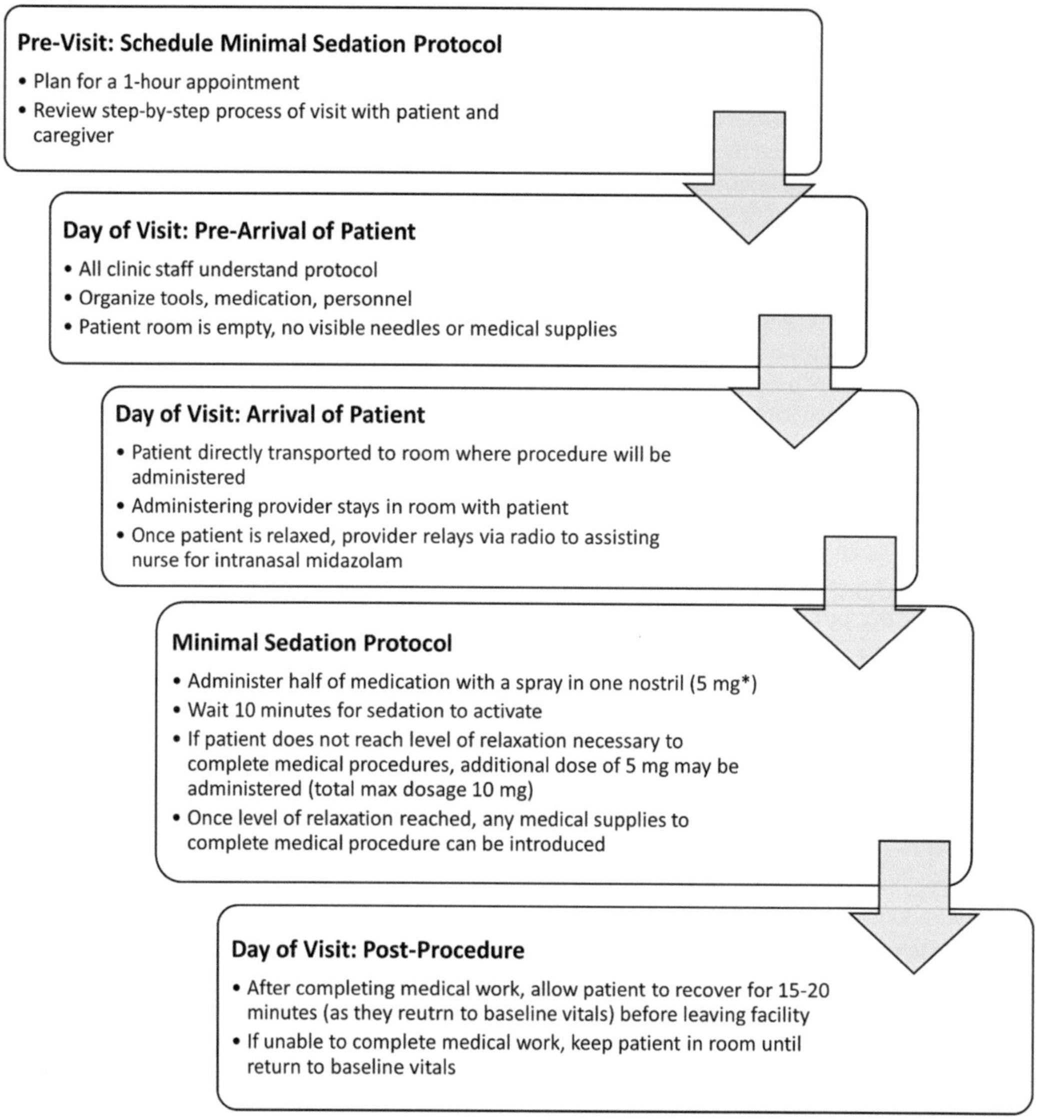


**Fig. 46.2** Medical visit procedure for minimal sedation protocol [81]

fected. Within the Needle Anxiety Program, Tier 3 uses an intranasal benzodiazepine to manually relax the patient before administering the needle-related medical procedure [80]. Figure 46.2 details how to prepare for a medical visit utilizing the minimal sedation protocol [81]. Although a more novel approach, a minimal sedation intervention is one strategy for patients with severe needle-anxiety or needle phobia to receive routine needle-related care in an outpatient setting, therefore reducing the amount of time, cost, and resources needed if more intensive strategies were utilized.

## Recommendations for Providers

There are many benefits to implementing a needle anxiety program at your primary care practice. For individuals with I/DD, needle-related anxiety interventions can reduce distress during medical visits and increase uptake of routine needle-related medical procedures. In turn, individuals with I/DD will receive appropriate routine preventive care, hopefully narrowing the gap in health disparities for this population. While some of the needle-related anxiety approaches discussed in this chapter may be novel and require further study before implementing on a large scale—most of the strategies can be incorporated into all primary care practices. Therefore, we recommend the following to reduce needle-related anxiety in primary care:

- *Train nursing staff in evidence-based behavioral interventions* to reduce distress during the patient visit. This includes removing non-evidence-based practices from use, such as restraint.
- *Plan ahead of time with your patient.* Discuss what strategies they prefer and the ways they can prepare ahead of the scheduled needle-related procedures.
- *Have your resources ready before the patient's arrival.* Make sure distraction devices and pain management interventions are ready before the patient arrives. You may need more than one nurse to complete the procedure.
- *Allow for flexibility in the appointment.* Patients may need additional time during their visit to get comfortable and reach a calm state. Do not rush the patient.
- *Do not force the completion of a needle-related medical procedure.* If the patient is not reaching a level of relaxation to complete the needle-related medical procedure, do not force it. This can traumatize the patient and can lead to the resistance of needle-related medical procedures in the future.

We hope these strategies help reduce patient discomfort and increase administration of routine needle-related medical procedures for individuals with I/DD. Additionally, the interventions identified in this section are low cost and easy-to-implement in any primary care setting. Most importantly, as a health equity issue, patients with I/DD should have the standard of care practiced for any health condition, the same as a patient without I/DD. Therefore, health systems need to develop interventions to help patients with I/DD overcome any challenges related to needles and minor procedures so that they, too, can have optimal health outcomes.

## References

1. Kupzyk S, Allen KD. A review of strategies to increase comfort and compliance with medical/dental routines in persons with intellectual and developmental disabilities. J Dev Phys Disabil. 2019;31(2):231–49.
2. Boynes SG, Moore PA, Lewis CL, Zovko J, Close JM. Complications associated with anesthesia administration for dental treatment in a special needs clinic. Spec Care Dentist. 2010;30(1):3–7.
3. Dougherty N. The dental patient with special needs: a review of indications for treatment under general anesthesia. Spec Care Dentist. 2009;29(1):17–20.
4. Kouo JL, Kouo TS, Gallogly J. Brief report: the experiences of families of children with an autism spectrum disorder when seeking patient-and family-centered care. J Autism Dev Disord. 2022;52(9):4172–80.
5. Kannikeswaran N, Mahajan PV, Sethuraman U, Groebe A, Chen X. Sedation medication received and adverse events related to sedation for brain MRI in children with and without developmental disabilities. Pediatr Anesth. 2009;19(3):250–6.
6. Allen KD, Stanley RT, McPherson K. Evaluation of behavior management technology dissemination in pediatric dentistry. Pediatr Dent. 1990;12(2):79–82.
7. Mah JW, Tsang P. Visual schedule system in dental care for patients with autism: a pilot study. J Clin Pediatr Dent. 2016;40(5):393–9.
8. Nordahl CW, Mello M, Shen AM, Shen MD, Vismara LA, Li D, et al. Methods for acquiring MRI data in children with autism spectrum disorder and intellectual impairment without the use of sedation. J Neurodev Disord. 2016;8(1):1–10.
9. O'Callaghan PM, Allen KD, Powell S, Salama F. The efficacy of noncontingent escape for decreasing children's disruptive behavior during restorative dental treatment. J Appl Behav Anal. 2006;39(2):161–71.
10. Allen KD, Loiben T, Allen SJ, Stanley RT. Dentist-implemented contingent escape for management of disruptive child behavior. J Appl Behav Anal. 1992;25(3):629–36.
11. Maguire KB, Lange B, Scherling M, Grow R. The use of rehearsal and positive reinforcement in the dental treatment of uncooperative patients with mental retardation. J Dev Phys Disabil. 1996;8(2):167–77.
12. Cavalari RNS, DuBard M, Luiselli JK, Birtwell K. Teaching an adolescent with autism and intellectual disability to tolerate routine medical examination: effects of a behavioral compliance training package. Clin Pract Pediatr Psychol. 2013;1(2):121–8.
13. Stuesser HA, Roscoe EM. An evaluation of differential reinforcement with stimulus fading as an intervention for medical compliance. J Appl Behav Anal. 2020;53(3):1606–21.
14. Isong IA, Rao SR, Holifield C, Iannuzzi D, Hanson E, Ware J, Nelson LP. Addressing dental fear in children with autism spectrum disorders: a randomized con-

trolled pilot study using electronic screen media. Clin Pediatr. 2014;53(3):230–7.
15. Carter L, Harper JM, Luiselli JK. Dental desensitization for students with autism spectrum disorder through graduated exposure, reinforcement, and reinforcement-fading. J Dev Phys Disabil. 2019;31(2):161–70.
16. Conyers C, Miltenberger RG, Peterson B, Gubin A, Jurgens M, Selders A, Dickinson J, Barenz R. An evaluation of in vivo desensitization and video modeling to increase compliance with dental procedures in persons with mental retardation. J Appl Behav Anal. 2004;37(2):233–8.
17. Cuvo A, Reagan A, Ackerlund Brandt J, Huckfeldt R, Kelly C. Training children with autism spectrum disorders to be compliant with a physical exam. Res Autism Spectr Disord. 2010;4:168–85.
18. Davit CJ, Hundley RJ, Bacic JD, Hanson EM. A pilot study to improve venipuncture compliance in children and adolescents with autism spectrum disorders. J Dev Behav Pediatr. 2011;32(7):521.
19. Grider B, Luiselli JK, Turcotte-Shamski W. Graduated exposure, positive reinforcement, and stimulus distraction in a compliance-with-blood-draw intervention for an adult with autism. Clin Case Stud. 2012;11(3):253–60.
20. McConnell KL, Sassi JL, Carr L, Szalwinski J, Courtemanche A, Njie-Jallow F, Cheney WR. Functional analysis and generalized treatment of disruptive behavior during dental exams. J Appl Behav Anal. 2020;53(4):2233–49.
21. Szalwinski J, Thomason-Sassi JL, Moore E, McConnell K. Effects of decreasing intersession interval duration on graduated exposure treatment during simulated routine dental care. J Appl Behav Anal. 2019;52(4):944–55.
22. Lerman DC, Iwata BA, Wallace MD. Side effects of extinction: prevalence of bursting and aggression during the treatment of self-injurious behavior. J Appl Behav Anal. 1999;32(1):1–8.
23. Kane SF. The effects of oral health on systemic health. Gen Dent. 2017;65(6):30.
24. Dietrich T, Sharma P, Walter C, Weston P, Beck J. The epidemiological evidence behind the association between periodontitis and incident atherosclerotic cardiovascular disease. J Clin Periodontol. 2013;40:S70.
25. Chapple ILC, Genco R. Diabetes and periodontal diseases: consensus report of the joint EFP/AAP workshop on periodontitis and systemic diseases. J Clin Periodontol. 2013;40:S106.
26. Ide M, Papapanou PN. Epidemiology of association between maternal periodontal disease and adverse pregnancy outcomes—systematic review. J Clin Periodontol. 2013;40:S181.
27. Anders PL, Davis EL. Oral health of patients with intellectual disabilities: a systematic review. Spec Care Dentist [Internet]. 2010;30(3):110–117.
28. Kancherla V, van Naarden BK, Yeargin-Allsopp M. Dental care among young adults with intellectual disability. Res Dev Disabil. 2013;34(5):1630.
29. Morgan JP, Minihan PM, Stark PC, Finkelman MD, Yantsides KE, Park A, et al. The oral health status of 4732 adults with intellectual and developmental disabilities. J Am Dent Assoc [Internet]. 2012;143(8):838–846.
30. Ward LM, Cooper SA, Hughes-McCormack L, Macpherson L, Kinnear D. Oral health of adults with intellectual disabilities: a systematic review. J Intellect Disabil Res. 2019;63:1359.
31. U.S. Department of Health and Human Services, National Institute of Dental and Craniofacial Research, National Institutes of Health. Oral health in America: a report of the surgeon general. 2000.
32. Havercamp SM, Scandlin D, Roth M. Health disparities among adults with developmental disabilities, adults with other disabilities, and adults not reporting disability in North Carolina. Public Health Rep. 2004;119(4):418.
33. Havercamp SM, Scott HM. National health surveillance of adults with disabilities, adults with intellectual and developmental disabilities, and adults with no disabilities. Disabil Health J. 2015;8(2):165.
34. Waldron C, Nunn J, Phadraig CMG, Comiskey C, Guerin S, van Harten MT, et al. Oral hygiene interventions for people with intellectual disabilities. Cochrane Database Syst Rev. 2019;2019:CD012628.
35. Aragon CE, Burneo JG. Understanding the patient with epilepsy and seizures in the dental practice. J Can Dent Assoc. 2007;73:71.
36. Chi AC, Neville BW, Krayer JW, Gonsalves WC. Oral manifestations of systemic disease. Am Fam Physician. 2010;82(11):1381–8.
37. Center for Health Care Strategies. Medicaid adult dental benefits coverage by state [Internet]. 2019 [cited 2021 Aug 15]. https://www.chcs.org/media/Medicaid-Adult-Dental-Benefits-Overview-Appendix_091519.pdf
38. Warder CJ, Edelstein BL. Evaluating levels of dentist participation in Medicaid: a complicated endeavor. J Am Dent Assoc. 2017;148(1):26.
39. Holder M, Waldman HB, Hood H. Preparing health professionals to provide care to individuals with disabilities. Int J Oral Sci. 2009;1(2):66.
40. Casamassimo PS, Seale NS, Ruehs K. General dentists' perceptions of educational and treatment issues affecting access to care for children with special health care needs. J Dent Educ. 2004;68(1):23.
41. Reed DD, Luiselli JK, Miller JR, Kaplan BA. Therapeutic restraint and protective holding in 2013.
42. Collado V, Faulks D, Nicolas E, Hennequin M. Conscious sedation procedures using intravenous midazolam for dental care in patients with different cognitive profiles: a prospective study of effectiveness and safety. PLoS One. 2013;8(8):e71240.
43. Altabet SC. Decreasing dental resistance among individuals with severe and profound mental retardation. J Dev Phys Disabil. 2002;14(3):297.
44. Berens JC, Tsami L, Lerman DC, Matteucci M, Fray DF, Warner BF, et al. Preliminary results of an inter-

disciplinary program improving dental care access for adults with intellectual/developmental disabilities. Intellect Dev Disabil. 2022;60:504.

45. Lyons RA. Understanding basic behavioral support techniques as an alternative to sedation and anesthesia. Spec Care Dentist. 2009;29(1):39.
46. U.S. Department of Homeland Security Office for Civil Rights and Civil Liberties. A guide to interacting with people who have disabilities [Internet]. [cited 2022 Apr 17]. https://www.dhs.gov/sites/default/files/publications/guide-interacting-with-people-who-have-disabilties_09-26-13_0.pdf.
47. Reid SM, Meehan EM, Arnup SJ, Reddihough DS. Intellectual disability in cerebral palsy: a population-based retrospective study. Dev Med Child Neurol. 2018;60(7):687.
48. Hauser PC, O'Hearn A, Mckee M, Steider A, Thew D. Deaf epistemology: deafhood and deafness. Am Ann Deaf. 2010;154(5):486.
49. Thomson WM, Williams SM, Broadbent JM, Poulton R, Locker D. Long-term dental visiting patterns and adult oral health. J Dent Res. 2010;89(3):307.
50. Altabet S, Rogers K, Imes E, Boatman IM, Moncier J. Comprehensive approach toward improving oral hygiene at a state residential facility for people with mental retardation. Ment Retard. 2003;41(6):440.
51. Fernández CE, Maturana CA, Coloma SI, Carrasco-Labra A, Giacaman RA. Teledentistry and mHealth for promotion and prevention of oral health: a systematic review and meta-analysis. J Dent Res. 2021;100:914.
52. Jingarwar MM, Bajwa NK, Pathak A. Minimal intervention dentistry—A new frontier in clinical dentistry. J Clin Diagn Res. 2014;8(7):ZE04–8.
53. Contreras V, Toro MJ, Eliás-Boneta AR, Encarnación-Burgos A. Effectiveness of silver diamine fluoride in caries prevention and arrest: a systematic literature review. Gen Dent. 2017;65:22.
54. Bernstein RS, Johnston B, Mackay K, Sanders J. Implementation of a primary care physician-led cavity clinic using silver diamine fluoride. J Public Health Dent. 2019;79(3):193.
55. Fenton SJ, Hood H, Holder M, May PB, Mouradian WE. The American Academy of Developmental Medicine and Dentistry: eliminating health disparities for individuals with mental retardation and other developmental disabilities. J Dent Educ. 2003;67(12):1337.
56. Simon L. Inequity along the medical-dental divide. AMA J Ethics. 2022;24(1):E3–5.
57. Fleming E, Frantsve-Hawley J, Minter-Jordan M. Health equity needs teeth. AMA J Ethics. 2022;24(1):E48–56.
58. Bradley VJ. Exploring health disparities among people with intellectual and developmental disabilities. 51.
59. Fischer LS, Becker A, Paraguya M, Chukwu C. Colonoscopy and colorectal cancer screening in adults with intellectual and developmental disabilities: review of a series of cases and recommendations for examination. Intellect Dev Disabil. 2012;50(5):383–90.
60. Deroche CB, McDermott SW, Mann JR, Hardin JW. Colorectal cancer screening adherence in selected disabilities over 10 years. Am J Prev Med. 2017;52(6):735–41.
61. Ouellette-Kuntz H, et al. Uptake of colorectal cancer screening among Ontarians with intellectual and developmental disabilities. PLoS One. 2015;10(2):e0118023.
62. Parungao JM, Reyes C, Jackson N, Roizen N, Piper M. Factors influencing the adequacy of bowel preparation in patients with developmental disabilities. Gastroenterology Res. 2018;11(6):416–21.
63. Bradley V. Exploring health disparities among people with intellectual disabilities. In: Presented at the: NASDDDS annual meeting; November 13, 2014.
64. Young-Southward G, Rydzewska E, Philo C, Cooper SA. Physical and mental health of young people with and without intellectual disabilities: cross-sectional analysis of a whole country population. J Intellect Disabil Res. 2017;61(10):984–93.
65. Croen LA, Zerbo O, Qian Y, et al. The health status of adults on the autism spectrum. Autism. 2015;19(7):814–23.
66. Lauer E, McCallion P. Mortality of people with intellectual and developmental disabilities from select US state disability service systems and medical claims data. J Appl Res Intellect Disabil. 2015;28:394–405.
67. Hirvikoski T, Mittendorfer-Rutz E, Boman M, Larsson H, Lichtenstein P, Bölte S. Premature mortality in autism spectrum disorder. Br J Psychiatry. 2016;208(3):232–8.
68. Pelleboer-Gunnink HA, Van Oorsouw W, Van Weeghel J, Embregts P. Mainstream health professionals' stigmatising attitudes towards people with intellectual disabilities: a systematic review. J Intellect Disabil Res. 2017;61(5):411–34.
69. Iezzoni LI, Rao SR, Ressalam J, et al. Physicians' perceptions of people with disability and their health care: study reports the results of a survey of physicians' perceptions of people with disability. Health Aff (Millwood). 2021;40(2):297–306.
70. Nicolaidis C, Raymaker DM, Ashkenazy E, McDonald KE, Dern S, Baggs AE, et al. "Respect the way I need to communicate with you": healthcare experiences of adults on the autism spectrum. Autism. 2015;19(7):824–31.
71. Bradshaw P, Pellicano E, van Driel M, Urbanowicz A. How can we support the healthcare needs of autistic adults without intellectual disability? Curr Dev Disord Rep. 2019;6(2):45–56.
72. Raymaker DM, McDonald KE, Ashkenazy E, Gerrity M, Baggs AM, Kripke C, et al. Barriers to healthcare: instrument development and comparison between autistic adults and adults with and without other disabilities. Autism. 2017;21(8):972–84.
73. Tint A, Weiss JA. A qualitative study of the service experiences of women with autism spectrum disorder. Autism. 2018;22(8):928–37.

74. Mason D, Ingham B, Urbanowicz A, Michael C, Birtles H, Woodbury-Smith M, Brown T, James I, Scarlett C, Nicolaidis C, Parr JR. A systematic review of what barriers and facilitators prevent and enable physical healthcare services access for autistic adults. J Autism Dev Disord. 2019;49:3387–400.
75. Shady K, Phillips S, Newman S. Barriers and facilitators to healthcare access in adults with intellectual and developmental disorders and communication difficulties: an integrative review. Rev J Autism Dev Disord. 2022:1–13.
76. Bienvenu OJ, Eaton WW. The epidemiology of blood-injection-injury phobia. Psychol Med. 1998;28(5):1129–36.
77. Evans DW, Canavera K, Kleinpeter FL, Maccubbin E, Taga K. The fears, phobias and anxieties of children with autism spectrum disorders and Down syndrome: comparisons with developmentally and chronologically age matched children. Child Psychiatry Hum Dev. 2005;36(1):3–26.
78. Leyfer OT, Folstein SE, Bacalman S, et al. Comorbid psychiatric disorders in children with autism: interview development and rates of disorders. J Autism Dev Disord. 2006;36(7):849–61.
79. Sukhodolsky DG, Scahill L, Gadow KD, et al. Parent-rated anxiety symptoms in children with pervasive developmental disorders: frequency and association with core autism symptoms and cognitive functioning. J Abnorm Child Psychol. 2008;36(1):117–28.
80. Rava J, Rosenau K, Wilkie K, Curcio E, Kuo AA. Implementation of a minimal sedation protocol for patients with developmental disabilities and needle phobia. Cureus. 2023;15(7):e42154. https://doi.org/10.7759/cureus.42154.
81. Rava J, Rosenau K, Wilkie K, Bernacki J, Curcio E, Kuo AA. The needle anxiety program: a patient-centered initiative for individuals with developmental disabilities. Cureus. 2023;15(7):e42253. https://doi.org/10.7759/cureus.42253.

# Part VIII

# Hospital Medicine

# 47 Preoperative Clearance

Eleanor Comfort, Lao-Tzu Allan-Blitz, Ahmet Uluer, and Niraj Sharma

Preoperative risk assessment is an area in which the hospitalist or general internist must pay particular attention to known chronic conditions and their expected sequelae. There are multiple excellent references available to guide the general pre-anesthesia assessment, so this chapter will focus exclusively on considerations unique to young adults with chronic childhood conditions. This population is not immune from the risks experienced by all patients undergoing surgery, so these standard areas of evaluation should not be overlooked.

The request for "surgical clearance" is commonly encountered by the generalist provider both inpatient and outpatient and can be an area of tension between the generalist and surgeon. The generalist is encouraged to think of this request as an opportunity to provide consultative recommendations for the management of risk factors both pre- and postoperatively, and to ensure that the patient's medical conditions are well-defined and optimized prior to a planned surgical procedure. Because the underlying childhood condition of an adult patient may not be familiar to an adult-focused operative team, the consultation can also be an opportunity to provide education around unique considerations specific to the underlying condition. The evaluator should consider avoiding the phrase "cleared for surgery" and instead provide an assessment of the level of risk to the patient and suggestions for mitigating risk when possible.

There is a paucity of literature detailing perioperative risk for this population, but that literature which is available suggests a general increased risk of poor outcomes in the perioperative period [1–4]. In addition, the existence of chronic childhood conditions can be expected to predispose affected patients to a variety of unique operative and perioperative risks, and some guidelines exist to guide medical optimization prior to surgery. This chapter will review overall recommendations for preoperative evaluation and planning for patients with chronic childhood conditions and will also address a variety of common childhood conditions individually.

Eleanor Comfort and Lao-Tzu Allan-Blitz contributed equally with all other contributors.

E. Comfort (✉)
Division of General Internal Medicine, University of Colorado Anschutz, Aurora, CO, USA
e-mail: eleanor.comfort@cuanschutz.edu

L.-T. Allan-Blitz · A. Uluer · N. Sharma
Department of Medicine, Brigham and Women's Hospital, Boston, MA, USA

Department of Pediatrics, Boston Children's Hospital, Boston, MA, USA

Harvard Medical School, Boston, MA, USA
e-mail: Lallan-blitz@partners.org; ahmet.uluer@childrens.harvard.edu; nsharma@bwh.harvard.edu


A. A. Kuo et al. (eds.), *Care of Adults with Chronic Childhood Conditions*,
https://doi.org/10.1007/978-3-031-54281-7_47

## Preoperative History Taking

A useful preoperative consultation requires extensive familiarity with the patient's medical and surgical history. For young adults with childhood chronic conditions, developing this familiarity is both more important and more difficult than for a patient with a less extensive medical history or one which has developed only in adulthood. The patient and/or family members are the most helpful source of information about historical features impacting perioperative risk. However, patients with a very extensive medical history or multiple past surgeries may not be aware of everything that is in their medical record. Additionally, important information is frequently lost in the transition from the pediatric to adult healthcare system. Pediatric records should be directly reviewed, particularly those pertaining to prior anesthesia events and operations, if time allows. A telephone consult from a member of the pediatric anesthesia team most familiar with the patient is often available and should be taken advantage of if the patient in question has an extensive operative history or reports a history of difficulty with intubation or anesthesia.

If the provider performing the risk assessment is not a primary care provider or primary specialist already familiar with the patient, the patient and provider should review the patient's documented problem list, past medical history, and past surgical history together. Modern electronic medical records systems permit patients to directly add, remove, or comment on listed problems, which should be performed by the patient or caregiver prior to the consultation if possible.

Any report of difficulties with past surgeries or anesthesia events should prompt a detailed search for contemporaneous medical documentation. Even if the provider performing the initial assessment is not an anesthesiologist, documentation in the consult note of prior reactions to anesthesia, prior difficulties with intubation, and size of prior endotracheal tubes if known can be helpful to the anesthesia team. Additionally, successful pre- or post-anesthesia techniques for behavior management in relevant patients should be documented.

The assessing provider should also consider direct consultation with primary specialists responsible for the underlying conditions, particularly if these are being managed in an outside healthcare system. Many specialists provide emergency letters or surgical plans if these are relevant to the underlying condition, and these should be sought if not readily available.

Adherence to medical treatment plans frequently declines during the young adult period, so careful assessment of the degree of adherence and identification of specific barriers to following medical recommendations is particularly important. A gentle, understanding approach which takes into consideration the difficulties inherent in the management of a chronic condition during the young adult years is most helpful in building rapport to ensure an accurate history. This approach will also help with patient-centered planning for the management of expected sequelae of surgical procedures and the increased burden of disease inherent in recovery from a procedure.

Patients with chronic childhood illnesses are more likely than the general population to be dependent on medical intervention and support in their daily routines (e.g., bowel and bladder management, feeding, airway clearance, etc.). These daily and sometimes hourly interventions are often forgotten or mismanaged in hospital, particularly with very complex regimens, and it can be extremely helpful to have this schedule documented in the preoperative evaluation to facilitate its continuance while inpatient. As many specifics as possible should be included, with an eye toward noting any devices or support equipment (properly sized catheters or other devices, specialty formula, etc.) that may not be available at the institution where the operation is to take place.

## Preoperative Physical Exam

In addition to including a general physical exam, the preoperative exam should be tailored to include investigation of organ systems known to be affected by underlying chronic conditions. It is particularly helpful to clearly document preoperative abnormalities and baseline level of functioning, so that the team managing the patient postoperatively can avoid concern or unnecessary testing provoked by undocumented preoperative abnormalities. This should include an explicit description of mental status and neurologic exam both for patients whose baseline is abnormal. It is worth noting that patients with physical disabilities, but normal mental status, are frequently assumed by unfamiliar providers to have altered mental status at baseline, so a note of normal level of functioning preoperatively can help avoid unrecognized neurologic injury postoperatively. The examining provider should carefully perform the remainder of the exam to evaluate for evidence of previously undiagnosed underlying conditions.

## Preoperative Laboratory Assessment

Although preoperative laboratory assessment is not recommended for otherwise-healthy adults undergoing planned lower-risk surgeries, patients with a chronic childhood condition are more likely to require preoperative laboratory tests. These should be tailored to the conditions in question.

As a general rule, metabolic, endocrinologic, renal, or gastrointestinal conditions require preoperative assessment of liver and kidney function. Hematologic and inflammatory conditions or those treated with immunosuppression require preoperative complete blood count and potentially evaluation of coagulation. For conditions where routine laboratory evaluation is required to monitor disease activity, the evaluating physician should review records to ensure that these labs are up to date and order updated testing as needed. See below for further disease-specific considerations.

Patients with significant behavioral conditions may not be able to tolerate routine laboratory assessment without sedation, making preoperative laboratory assessment difficult or impossible. Decision-making around the importance of preoperative labs should take into consideration the risk level of the procedure and its importance, known preexisting conditions, and the ability of the patient or caregivers to give a reliable history allowing for the exclusion of chronic symptoms and evaluation of functional status. If it is determined that the risk of the procedure is too high to proceed without obtaining testing, many patients who are not able to tolerate lab draws under typical circumstances can tolerate testing with the help of child life specialists, specialized pediatric phlebotomists, or nurses. These resources may be available in partnered pediatric institutions or affiliated neonatal intensive care units.

## Other Preoperative Testing

The patient with known conditions affecting specific organ systems must frequently undergo preoperative testing directed at the affected organ system (for example, EKG and echocardiogram for the patient with known heart disease). If possible, this testing should be ordered in conjunction with a specialist in the area in question.

For patients whose exercise capacity is not known (e.g., non-ambulatory patients or those with orthopedic conditions preventing maximal cardiovascular exertion), the threshold for ordering preoperative cardiac stress testing should be lower than in the typical adult patient.

## Formulation of Recommendations

The consultative report should include an evaluation of all chronic conditions, including any complications and current level of control. For those conditions which are not controlled, or which require changes in the management for the physiologic stress of surgery, the consultant should make recommendations regarding the optimization of condition preoperatively. Many childhood conditions can impact wound-healing and surgical recovery [5–7], so a preoperative assessment may also include recommendations for postoperative care.

## Considerations by Underlying Chronic Condition

This section contains an organ system-based overview of many common childhood conditions with potential ramifications of which the preoperative evaluator should be aware. Where possible, specialty-specific guidelines have been referenced, but these are available only for a subset of conditions discussed. The recommendations below are drawn from a combination of relevant guidelines, expert opinion, and generalization of pediatric guidelines.

### Neurologic Conditions

#### Epilepsy

People with epilepsy are at risk of worsening seizure control postoperatively and intraoperatively. Motor seizures during an operation can be extremely dangerous for the patient and the operative team. The preoperative assessment should include a description of types and frequencies of seizures, an assessment of degree of preoperative seizure control, and recommendations for seizure management intraoperatively and postoperatively. The outpatient seizure rescue plan should be reviewed and included in documentation.

#### Cerebral Palsy

Cerebral palsy can cause varying degrees of motor and cognitive impairment. Motor impairment is generally slowly progressive during adulthood, and surgical complications can become more common as patients age. Typical or desired operative positioning can be impossible due to longstanding contractures or neuromuscular scoliosis. The anesthesia team should be cautioned about expected motor limitations which may or may not improve with neuromuscular blockade. Baseline motor and cognitive functioning should be documented in as much detail as possible. This will prevent unnecessary diagnostic investigation for deficits which existed preoperatively, but which were not documented as such, and also help avoid delayed diagnosis of neurologic injury occurring during the procedure.

Cerebral palsy can also be associated with restrictive lung disease and cognitive impairment, discussed in more detail below.

#### Muscular Dystrophy

Muscular dystrophies are a heterogenous group of disorders with varying causes. The most commonly discussed issue related to anesthesia is the risk of rhabdomyolysis and hyperkalemia with succinylcholine and possibly inhaled anesthetics; consultation with an anesthesiologist should be obtained prior to surgery to plan for safe management.

Careful assessment of baseline respiratory status, function, and level of support is needed; if time allows PFT's including the assessment of cough and respiratory muscle strength is helpful to plan for support during induction of anesthesia and extubation. The management of respiratory status postoperatively requires careful monitoring for effects of pain, changes in position, and the operative procedure itself. Frequent respiratory therapist assessments and aggressive airway clearance measures are suggested [8].

Muscular dystrophies can also be associated with cardiomyopathies, particularly dilated cardiomyopathy. Consultation with the patient's cardiology team is recommended; baseline electrocardiogram and echocardiogram are helpful if not already available. However, a normal baseline EKG and echocardiogram should not be considered as reassuring against the possibility of postoperative cardiac complications or congestive heart failure. The postoperative team should be aware that troponin elevations may be present at baseline in muscular dystrophy patients (dependent on type of muscular dystrophy, degree of underlying cardiac involvement, and particular assay performed), so postoperative troponin elevations may not be an indicative of acute cardiac injury [9].

#### Neural Tube Defects

Patients with spina bifida and other neural tube defects have frequently undergone multiple surgeries in childhood and adolescence, so a complete surgical history is particularly important. If the patient is not already hospitalized during the preoperative assessment, a detailed discussion of daily routines particularly including bowel-bladder regimen, feeding considerations if any, and support devices can be helpful in planning for postoperative inpatient care. Early physical therapy consultation should be recommended postoperatively to facilitate return to preoperative levels of function as quickly as possible.

## Congenital Heart Disease

The patient with congenital heart disease ranges from the medically quite simple (repaired ventricular septal defect or patent ductus arteriosus) to the extremely complex (hypoplastic left heart, Tetralogy of Fallot, etc.). These patients can be more precisely classified using the ACC/AHA ACHD AP classification system [10]. Patients with a simpler history (AP class IA) can be easily evaluated by the hospitalist or primary care provider, with recommendations made regarding the need for (or more often lack of need for) prophylactic antibiotics and any straightforward preoperative testing. However, for patients with more complex congenital heart disease, a cardiologist must be involved in the preoperative evaluation, and guidelines recommend performing noncardiac surgery in a hospital with expertise in adult congenital heart disease [10].

If there is any lack of clarity regarding the nature of the congenital defect (for example, if the patient or caregiver cannot recall or give history and childhood records are not available), further testing including EKG and echocardiogram should be pursued preoperatively. For patients with a complex noncardiac history, a remote abnormal finding on echocardiography which was lost to follow-up is not uncommon. The evaluating physician should ask specifically about any history of heart problems, heart disease, or abnormal testing including EKG and echocardiogram. Any family history concerning for sudden cardiac death should be explored, as with the general population. For patients with rare genetic disorders, the evaluator should use available resources to investigate whether the known condition is associated with cardiac defects [11].

## Pulmonary Conditions

All patients with underlying pulmonary conditions should have a targeted history and chart review undertaken. Remote histories of lung disease (e.g., bronchopulmonary dysplasia stable on room air for many years) may not be readily evident in the chart or explicitly listed by the patient as a known medical condition. The examiner may find it helpful to ask specifically about any lifetime history of needing oxygen or seeing lung specialists [12, 13]. For all patients with underlying pulmonary conditions, both baseline and current oxygenation and ventilation status should be assessed [13]. The need for baseline respiratory support and airway clearance measures should be documented. If the patient has a "sick day plan" with a planned increase in respiratory support or airway clearance, this should be included in the preoperative assessment if possible. The evaluator should not neglect to collect information on smoking status, including vaping or use of e-cigarettes, which is unfortunately common in young people [14].

### Pulmonary Hypertension

Pulmonary hypertension can be associated with many childhood chronic conditions, including congenital heart disease, rheumatologic disorders, primary pulmonary disorders, and prematurity. Pulmonary hypertension is associated with an increased risk of a variety of postoperative complications [3], but the best method of mitigating these is unknown. Patients with known pulmonary hypertension who are managed by a multidisciplinary team should ideally be evaluated by their treating team prior to surgery, with recommendations documented. Their baseline medication regimen should be well documented, as should their response to vasodilators if known [12].

### Chronic Tracheostomy and Mechanical Ventilation

The adult patient who has been dependent on tracheostomy with or without mechanical ventilation since childhood should be followed by a multidisciplinary pulmonary team, and have clear pre-existing documentation of issues important to the operative team. This is, however, difficult to find in the adult setting [15], and patients who have been stable for many years are still frequently followed by pediatric programs and occasionally have been lost to follow-up. The preoperative consultation may be an opportunity to refer patients to age-appropriate pulmonary care.

Whether the patient is followed by a trach/vent team or not, it is important for the preoperative evaluator to document their level of respiratory support, size and type of supportive devices, and airway clearance regimen. The reason for dependence on mechanical ventilation should be clarified (patients with primary neuromuscular disorders having very different risks from patients with primary parenchymal lung disease). Any past postoperative complications should also be discussed. The preoperative documentation of pulmonary support must include size and type of tracheostomy tube, baseline day and nighttime level of respiratory support (capped tube, speaking valve, heat moisture exchanger, supplemental oxygen, mechanical ventilation including mode and levels). The frequency of tracheostomy changes, difficulties with changes, and timing of last change are also important to the anesthesia and postoperative team. Related medications (nebulizer treatments, inhalers, and secretion management medications) and airway clearance regimen (frequency and settings of cough assist, percussive vest, or chest physiotherapy) must be documented. As for any patient with a disability affecting communication, the evaluator should establish what methods of communication the patient typically uses and ensure that any needed devices or support will be available.

### Restrictive Lung Disease

Restrictive lung disease is a sequela of many chronic childhood conditions, including cerebral palsy, neuromuscular disorders, and genetic disorders. It is frequently accompanied by disorders of airway clearance. In the pediatric setting, patients with restrictive lung disease have presented high risk for postoperative complications [4]; in the adult setting, restrictive lung disease has been associated with longer postoperative need for mechanical ventilation and hospital stays [16]. No studies have been performed to guide recommendations for decreasing complication rates for these patients. However, it is reasonable to suggest that particular attention should be paid to preoperative pulmonary optimization and postoperative pulmonary toilet in this setting.

## Hematologic Conditions

### Sickle Cell Anemia

A hematologist should be consulted whenever surgery is planned for a patient with sickle cell anemia. Sickle cell disease increases the risk of poor outcomes during surgery, and patient should be carefully evaluated and monitored before, during, and after surgery. Transfusion to a hemoglobin goal of at least 10 g/dL preoperatively for any procedure involving general anesthesia has been demonstrated to reduce postoperative complications [17].

Anesthesia and surgical procedures can be complicated by sickling of red blood cells, by the longstanding complications of sickle cell disease, and by the medications used to treat both pain and the underlying disease. The evaluator should document known complications of sickle cell disease for the convenience of the surgical team, particularly including asplenia (present almost universally), history of pulmonary infarctions, renal insufficiency and concentrating deficits, and any prior strokes. The frequency of prior transfusions should be discussed, and the operative team should be made aware of any prior difficulties obtaining crossmatched blood. A clear overview of outpatient pain management, both daily and with pain crises, should be provided in order to help plan for anesthesia and postoperative analgesia [17].

### Bleeding Disorders

Appropriate perioperative management of a bleeding disorder is clearly critical, and should include replacement of specific deficient factors, guidelines for transfusion, and other considerations which vary depending on type of surgery and specific bleeding disorder. The National Hemophilia Foundation has a comprehensive set of guidelines regarding perioperative management of patients with bleeding disorders tailored to specific bleeding disorder and procedure, found at hemophilia.org/healthcare-professionals/guidelines-on-care/masac-documents. These should be reviewed by the operative team in conjunction with hematology consultation.

## Endocrinology

### Diabetes

Both type 1 and type 2 diabetes can be of childhood onset. Complications and insulin deficiency are frequently earlier and more severe in childhood-onset type 2 diabetes than that which develops later in life. A preoperative consultation should include an overview of known complications and recommendations for perioperative medication management. For those patients treated with insulin, any bolus insulin (i.e., fast-acting/mealtime insulin) should be withheld on the morning of surgery. Recommendations vary regarding management of basal insulin; this should likely be decreased at least somewhat on the morning of (or night before) surgery. A decrease of 25–50% is probably reasonable for most patients [18].

For patients on continuous subcutaneous insulin infusion (CSII, insulin pump), it is frequently possible to continue CSII throughout elective (non-emergent) surgery and any subsequent hospital stay. However, the inpatient team must be prepared to manage this, and consultation with an endocrinologist with experience in CSII should be obtained. Of note, devices allowing for continuously adjusting (partial closed-loop) CSII are increasingly used, and changes in insulin needs and sensitivity during surgery and hospitalization may make these devices less effective. Recommendations from the patient's outpatient endocrinology team and the inpatient endocrinology or glucose management consultation service should be closely followed [19].

The preoperative consultant should document any known complications of diabetes, particularly renal, cardiovascular, and neurologic, and be aware that peripheral neuropathy is sometimes accompanied by unrecognized autonomic neuropathy that can complicate anesthesia. The most recent hemoglobin A1c should be documented, and an updated level should be checked if the most recent available test is more than 3 months old. Elective surgery would ideally be postponed if A1c is greater than 8%, and glucose should be maintained at <250 mg/dL immediately prior to nonemergent surgery.

### Adrenal Insufficiency

Adrenal insufficiency can occur in a variety of childhood-onset chronic conditions. Primary (Addison's disease), central, and iatrogenic adrenal insufficiency must all be considered. For patients who were receiving exogenous corticosteroids over the very long term (many years), stress-dosing for surgery can be considered even if the patient has been off of steroids for the months preceding the surgery. In the general population, topical or inhaled corticosteroids are not considered an indication for stress-dosing, but some conditions are managed with very high doses of topical or inhaled corticosteroids, and adrenal insufficiency should be considered for these patients.

Stress-dosing should be individualized to the severity and duration of the physiologic stressor; minor surgeries require lower doses than those that are major or prolonged. Endocrine society guidelines recommend 25–75 mg hydrocortisone daily for 24–48 h for minor to moderate surgical stressors, and for major surgical stressors 100 mg IV hydrocortisone followed by a continuous infusion of 200 mg hydrocortisone per 24 h, continued until the patient is hemodynamically stable and tolerating oral intake [20]. Lower doses may be adequate for patients with secondary adrenal insufficiency [21]. Of note, this dosing strategy differs significantly from typical pediatric dosing, which is based on body surface area, and a decreased dose could be considered for unusually small patients in consultation with an endocrinologist.

## Hypopituitarism

A variety of genetic and childhood conditions (e.g., septo-optic dysplasia, non-accidental trauma, and pituitary adenoma) can result in the deficiency of multiple pituitary hormones, causing any combination of adrenal insufficiency, hypothyroidism, hypogonadism, diabetes insipidus, and growth hormone deficiency. For those affected patients who have entered adulthood, the necessary replacement doses have generally been well-defined for years. However, upon hospitalization or the physiologic stress of surgery, the inability to respond appropriately to changes in intake, output, and physiologic stress become important [20].

The preoperative consultant should carefully document all known pituitary hormone deficiencies, the established plan for adjustment if any, and recommendations for specific monitoring. Every affected patient would, ideally, have a regularly-updated stress or hospitalization plan from their managing endocrinologist [20]. For those patients who are expected to have difficulty with fluid balance (diabetes insipidus, adrenal insufficiency), the surgical team should be alerted to the need for more careful monitoring and to any recommendations regarding intraoperative fluid management. Patients with adrenal or growth hormone deficiency should be monitored for abnormalities in glucose metabolism. Rarely, surgical stress can unmask mild deficiencies in pituitary hormones that are not significant in the absence of marked physiologic stress, so the known presence of one pituitary hormone deficiency should prompt investigation for other deficiencies in a patient whose recovery is not proceeding as expected.

## Developmental/Behavioral Conditions

The patient with intellectual or developmental disability is at particular risk pre- and postoperatively due to difficulties interacting with the healthcare system at large. These patients are frequently better served from a behavioral standpoint in a pediatric hospital, but as they are also at high risk of adult-onset comorbidities, operative procedures will frequently be undertaken in an adult healthcare system. However, consultation with pediatric resources including child life specialists and behavior therapists is invaluable for this group if available.

For a planned hospitalization or surgery, a behavior plan should ideally be developed well ahead of time in conjunction with the patient, family members, their outpatient team, and if possible, with the consultation of child life or behavioral specialists. If this has not been performed prior to the preoperative evaluation, the evaluator should review prior difficulties with hospitalizations, known behavioral triggers, and useful strategies for behavior management or de-escalation with the family. Many patients with developmental disabilities have great difficulty with recovery from surgical procedures, given their attendant pain and alterations in normal routine, and this should be considered carefully when planning for surgery. Unit nursing and leadership is ideally involved in the development and implementation of behavior management plans pre- and postoperatively.

## Genetic Conditions

A rapidly increasing number of children with genetic conditions are surviving into adulthood and given the advent of widely-available whole exome and whole genome sequencing, more adults with developmental disabilities are having genetic causes for their underlying syndromes identified. This poses a difficult challenge for the preoperative evaluator; we are unlikely to be familiar with the growing number of genetic syndromes our patients may be diagnosed with, but we nevertheless need to identify the operative risks they may pose.

For more common genetic conditions (e.g., trisomy 21, neurofibromatosis, and 22q deletion syndrome), evaluation and management guidelines may be available, although adult recommendations sometimes must be extrapolated from pediatric guidelines [22–24]. However, most conditions do not have this type of reference material available. Online Mendelian Inheritance in Man (omim.org), the National Organization for Rare Disorders (rarediseases.org), and the Vademecum Metabolicum (vademetab.org) provide useful and frequently updated online references for rare genetic and metabolic diseases.

## Conditions Affecting Multiple Organ Systems

Many pediatric conditions, as discussed above, can have simultaneous effects on multiple organ systems. The non-expert provider may be familiar with some of the most frequent of these manifestations, but as the complexity and rarity of a condition increases, the risk of missed preoperative conditions increases. The below case and discussion exemplify one such possibility and provide suggestions for avoiding such situations.

### Case Vignette

A 35-year-old man with a history of trisomy 21 presented to an adult institution for the correction of a longstanding ventricular septal defect (VSD). He was diagnosed in utero with a large VSD and had been medically managed. For the previous several months, he had reported worsening symptoms of congestive heart failure which had progressed to three pillow orthopnea. His initial preoperative encounter was notable for mild tachycardia which was presumed to be physiologic. He had not experienced cough, hemoptysis, or weight loss. He had occasional loose stools and some palpitations, all felt to be related to his heart failure, and was otherwise well with a preserved functional capacity of >6 METs. He was therefore cleared for the operating room.

In the operating room, he received intravenous glycopyrrolate in anticipation of anesthesia induction and subsequently rapidly developed fever to 40° C, hypertension with systolic blood pressures above 200 mmHg and diastolic blood pressures above 100 mmHg, and tachycardia to the 180 s. Ice packs, cool lactated ringers, and acetaminophen were used to lower his temperature. Esmolol and labetalol were used to control his heart rate. There were no clinical findings consistent with malignant hyperthermia. Thyroid storm was suspected and confirmed when a serum TSH returned undetectable with profound elevation in T3 and free T4. With continued supportive care, the patient's vitals normalized. The operative case was postponed.

### Discussion

Trisomy 21 is associated with various endocrinopathies including hyperthyroidism [25]. The above case demonstrates the possibility of mildly symptomatic or sub-clinical hyperthyroidism being mistaken for complications of congenital heart disease and resulting in the life-threatening condition of thyroid storm, which can be triggered by host of factors, including anesthesia. A preoperative assessment of potential endocrinopathies associated with specific chronic illnesses of childhood is routinely practiced at many pediatric institutions [26]. Failure to do so can result in both clinical complications for patients as well as delayed procedures and increased health systems costs. Situations such as the one described above demonstrate the importance of preoperative consultation with experts in underlying conditions, whether within the institution performing the procedure or at an outside pediatric center.

## Systems Considerations

### Patients of Unusual Size

In both adult and pediatric hospitals, patients of unusual size for their population pose unique and potentially critical challenges to the system. Pediatric hospitals frequently have difficulty providing equipment for the morbidly obese teenager; similarly, adult hospitals often do not have appropriately sized equipment for the 40-year patient with dwarfism.

The consultant should, if possible, document the size of medical equipment previously used for a pediatric-sized adult patient, including endotracheal or tracheostomy tube, indwelling catheters, central lines, and similar devices. If these have not been previously needed, an estimate of the required endotracheal tube size can be provided based on the patient's size. If time allows, the consultant can play an important role in ensuring that the adult facility has access to appropriately sized equipment for both planned procedures and potential necessary unplanned interventions to avoid detrimental delays in the delivery of care or use of inappropriately-sized devices in emergent situations.

## Legal Decision-Making

Many, although far from all, complex childhood conditions are accompanied by varying degrees of intellectual disability. Adult institutions frequently struggle with the legalities surrounding consent for operative procedures, either attempting to obtain consent from a third party when a patient does retain decision-making capacity (e.g., a patient with cerebral palsy who relies on a communication device but whose cognitive function is intact) or failing to obtain consent from the appropriate party when a legal guardian has been appointed by the courts. If this is not already clear in the chart or provided records, the preoperative care team should not hesitate to involve departmental social workers or case managers to help clarify issues surrounding consent.

## Risk Calculators

Although no validated risk calculators specific to any of the populations discussed above exist, calculators targeted more broadly towards the general population can be used to give a lower-end risk assessment. The Revised Cardiac Risk Index can be used to estimate the cardiac risk of a procedure, and the NSQIP has an online risk estimator (riskcalculator.facs.org) that gives a graphical presentation of a variety of surgical risks which can be used to facilitate discussion with patients and caregivers [27].

## References

1. Maxwell BG, Wong JK, Lobato RL. Perioperative morbidity and mortality after noncardiac surgery in young adults with congenital or early acquired heart disease: a retrospective cohort analysis of the National Surgical Quality Improvement Program database. Am Surg. 2014;80(4):321–6.
2. Wazeka AN, DiMaio MF, Boachie-Adjei O. Outcome of pediatric patients with severe restrictive lung disease following reconstructive spine surgery. Spine (Phila Pa 1976). 2004;29(5):528–34; discussion 535.
3. Ramakrishna G, et al. Impact of pulmonary hypertension on the outcomes of noncardiac surgery: predictors of perioperative morbidity and mortality. J Am Coll Cardiol. 2005;45(10):1691–9.
4. Payo J, et al. Severe restrictive lung disease and vertebral surgery in a pediatric population. Eur Spine J. 2009;18(12):1905–10.
5. Dindo D, et al. Obesity in general elective surgery. Lancet. 2003;361(9374):2032–5.
6. Wilson RJ, et al. Impaired functional capacity is associated with all-cause mortality after major elective intra-abdominal surgery. Br J Anaesth. 2010;105(3):297–303.
7. Ito H, et al. Comprehensive risk analysis of postoperative complications in patients with rheumatoid arthritis for the 2020 update of the Japan College of Rheumatology clinical practice guidelines for the management of rheumatoid arthritis. Mod Rheumatol. 2022;32(2):296–306.
8. Birnkrant DJ, et al. American College of Chest Physicians consensus statement on the respiratory and related management of patients with Duchenne muscular dystrophy undergoing anesthesia or sedation. Chest. 2007;132(6):1977–86.
9. Spurney CF, et al. Current state of cardiac troponin testing in Duchenne muscular dystrophy cardiomyopathy: review and recommendations from the Parent Project Muscular Dystrophy expert panel. Open Heart. 2021;8(1):e001592.
10. Stout KK, et al. 2018 AHA/ACC guideline for the management of adults with congenital heart disease: a report of the American College of Cardiology/American Heart Association task force on clinical practice guidelines. Circulation. 2019;139(14):e698–800.
11. Fleisher LA, et al. 2014 ACC/AHA guideline on perioperative cardiovascular evaluation and management of patients undergoing noncardiac surgery: a report of the American College of Cardiology/American Heart Association task force on practice guidelines. Circulation. 2014;130(24):e278–333.

12. Smetana GW. Preoperative pulmonary evaluation. N Engl J Med. 1999;340(12):937–44.
13. Smetana GW, et al. Preoperative pulmonary risk stratification for noncardiothoracic surgery: systematic review for the American College of Physicians. Ann Intern Med. 2006;144(8):581–95.
14. Cullen KA, et al. e-Cigarette use among youth in the United States, 2019. JAMA. 2019;322(21):2095–103.
15. Cheng PC, Panitch HB, Hansen-Flaschen J. Transition of patients with neuromuscular disease and chronic ventilator-dependent respiratory failure from pediatric to adult pulmonary care. Paediatr Respir Rev. 2020;33:3–8.
16. Fujii M, Nishina D, Bessho R. Preoperative assessment of pulmonary function tests and outcomes after cardiac surgery. Heart Surg Forum. 2020;23(2):E245–9.
17. Yawn BP, et al. Management of sickle cell disease: summary of the 2014 evidence-based report by expert panel members. JAMA. 2014;312(10):1033–48.
18. Simha V, Shah P. Perioperative glucose control in patients with diabetes undergoing elective surgery. JAMA. 2019;321(4):399–400.
19. Partridge H, et al. Clinical recommendations in the management of the patient with type 1 diabetes on insulin pump therapy in the perioperative period: a primer for the anaesthetist. Br J Anaesth. 2016;116(1):18–26.
20. Fleseriu M, et al. Hormonal replacement in hypopituitarism in adults: an Endocrine Society clinical practice guideline. J Clin Endocrinol Metabol. 2016;101(11):3888–921.
21. Bornstein SR, et al. Diagnosis and treatment of primary adrenal insufficiency: an Endocrine Society clinical practice guideline. J Clin Endocrinol Metabol. 2016;101(2):364–89.
22. Antonarakis SE, et al. Down syndrome. Nat Rev Dis Primers. 2020;6(1):9–9.
23. Stewart DR, et al. Care of adults with neurofibromatosis type 1: a clinical practice resource of the American College of Medical Genetics and Genomics (ACMG). Genet Med. 2018;20(7):671–82.
24. McDonald-McGinn DM, et al. 22q11.2 deletion syndrome. Nat Rev Dis Primers. 2015;1:15071.
25. Whooten R, Schmitt J, Schwartz A. Endocrine manifestations of Down syndrome. Curr Opin Endocrinol Diabetes Obes. 2018;25(1):61–6.
26. Park JT, Lim HK, Park JH, Lee KH. Thyroid storm during induction of anesthesia. Korean J Anesthesiol. 2012;63(5):477–8.
27. Lee TH, et al. Derivation and prospective validation of a simple index for prediction of cardiac risk of major noncardiac surgery. Circulation. 1999;100(10):1043–9.

# Patient Safety for Hospitalized Young Adults and Adults with Chronic Childhood Conditions

# 48

Francis Coyne, Ashley Marie Jenkins, and Amanda Paige Laprime

## Abbreviations

| | |
|---|---|
| CCC | Chronic childhood conditions |
| I/DD | Intellectual and developmental disability |

## Introduction

The incidence of hospitalizations for adults with chronic childhood conditions (CCC), as well as intellectual/developmental disabilities (I/DD), continues to rise [1–3]. Almost all of these hospitalizations occur in adult hospitals [4]. Hospital-based care involves the complex interplay between the patient, their family and caregivers, healthcare team, the hospital environment and resources, and organizational conditions. For adults with CCCs, the patient's life course, disease trajectory, and past experiences with healthcare (especially hospitalizations) is an added layer of complexity that impacts the hospital experience [5, 6]. Many people who have a chronic condition and/or disability have a history of trauma associated with healthcare use that can have an adverse effect on behavior. This trauma could be related to experiences with critical illness and intensive care unit stay [7]; interpersonal bias and stigma directed at chronic conditions, race, and/or disability [8, 9]; etc. Ultimately, adults with CCCs and I/DD will have both overlapping and distinct needs during hospitalization compared to other adult populations to ensure quality, safe, and equitable healthcare.

There is a strong support for patient-, provider-, and system-level interventions that prevent adverse events, increase patient and staff safety during hospitalization, and improve overall patient experience with hospitalization, particularly for vulnerable populations like adults with CCCs and/or I/DD. The most common patient safety issues for adults with CCCs and I/DD are missed or delayed diagnoses; challenges delivering age-, developmental-, or condition-appropriate care; inappropriate use of pharmacotherapy for behavioral crises; and patient or staff harm [6, 10–15]. We consider hospitalization a multi-phase process such as (1) Pre-Admission (before a patient ever arrives), (2) Admission and Acute Care Phase, and (3) Discharge Planning and Transition to Home (or other long-term care setting). Drawing from the Systems Engineering

F. Coyne · A. M. Jenkins (✉)
Department of Medicine, University of Rochester School of Medicine and Dentistry, Rochester, NY, USA

Department of Pediatrics, University of Rochester School of Medicine and Dentistry, Rochester, NY, USA
e-mail: ashley_jenkins@urmc.rochester.edu

A. P. Laprime
Department of Pediatrics, University of Rochester School of Medicine and Dentistry, Rochester, NY, USA


A. A. Kuo et al. (eds.), *Care of Adults with Chronic Childhood Conditions*,
https://doi.org/10.1007/978-3-031-54281-7_48

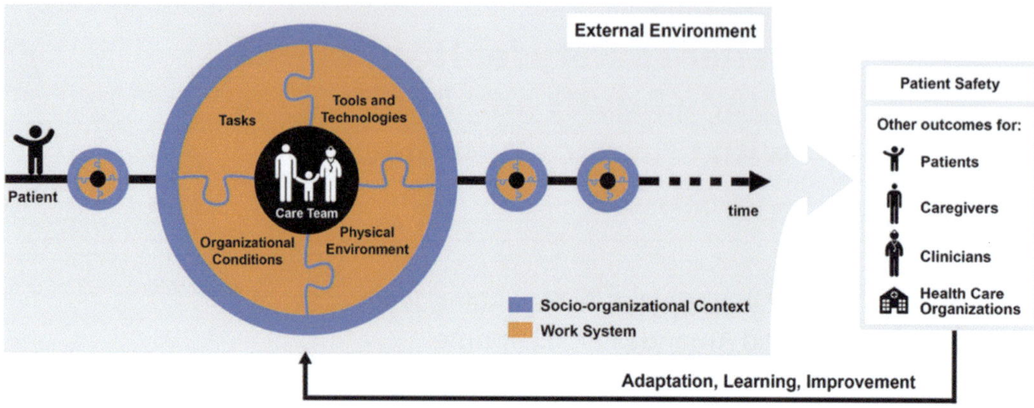


**Fig. 48.1** SEIPS 3.0 on the sociotechnical systems approach to patient journey and patient safety. [Printed with permission from the authors. (Citation: 1. Carayon P, Wooldridge A, Hoonakker P, Hundt AS, Kelly MM. SEIPS 3.0: Human-centered design of the patient journey for patient safety. *Applied Ergonomics*. 2020;84:103033. doi: https://doi.org/10.1016/j.apergo.2019.103033)]

Initiative for Patient Safety model (SEIPS, see Fig. 48.1) [6], we discuss how health systems and healthcare teams can intervene to promote patient safety for hospitalized adults with CCC and I/DD in an adult hospital setting. Each phase of the admission process is organized by the core SEIPs model components: (1) organizational model conditions, (2) environment, (3) tools, (4) tasks, and (5) people. We emphasize implementation of structural system-level supports as these tend to be more reliable and sustainable as compared to interventions that focus on people. We expect that many of the proposed interventions may also be applicable to other patient populations (e.g., patients at risk for delirium, patients with cognitive impairment or dementia) during hospitalization as well.

Our authorship team includes an internal medicine and pediatrics trained primary care physician for adults with CCCs and I/DD (FC), an internal medicine and pediatrics trained hospitalist and health systems researcher (AJ), and a doctoral-level behavior analyst who is an expert in crisis care and systems analysis for individuals with autism spectrum disorders and I/DD who experience overutilization of psychiatric and hospital services (AL). We have worked to cite available literature and resources. For example, much of the behavioral intervention development we describe pull from evidence in other fields (e.g., applied behavior analysis, autism research, safety and workplace violence). Yet, due to the current lack of evidence-based interventions in the space of hospital-based care for adults with CCCs and/or I/DD, much of this chapter's content is based on our own experiences as providers, health system improvers, researchers, and patient advocates.

## Case Study

We use a patient case created from a combination of patient experiences to illustrate challenges that arise during hospitalization and potential solutions. Leslie Mansfield is a 22-year-old woman with trisomy 21, intellectual disability, autism spectrum disorder, common variable immunodeficiency, tetralogy of Fallot with atrioventricular canal defect status post repair complicated by post-operative stroke with subsequent development of a seizure disorder. She lives in a group home, though spends time on the weekends with her mother and father through the support of private duty nursing. Her parents are her court-appointed guardians and are very much involved (e.g., attend all her medical appointments). She is frequently admitted to the hospital for pneumonia due to poor airway clearance in the setting of her immunodeficiency.

Her hospitalizations are marked by behavioral decompensations with violent outbursts and attempts at absconding. She has particular difficulty with the loud noises. Her risk for behavioral decompensation has frequently led to delays in her care as noted in the following examples: it (1) will often refuse to allow nursing to place intravenous lines for medication administration; (2) requires sedation for all imaging studies; and (3) requires general anesthesia for any medical procedure.

## Pre-Admission

### Organizational Conditions

#### Shared Understanding of Local Context

Before a patient is even admitted, a health system and its leadership should ask the following questions related to hospital care of AYA with CCC and I/DD:

- Who are the primary collaborators and specialists that can inform system-level supports (e.g., is child life needed or should a pediatric specialty counterpart be involved; are other specialists integral to the care team such as neurology, sleep medicine, or psychiatry?)
- What workflows are in place to proactively assess and prepare for a patient's medical/behavioral/mental health challenges (e.g., order sets and patient flow algorithms)?
- What documentation standards have been developed to ensure clear communication and information sharing across the care team (e.g., safety or care plans)?
- Has adequate training been provided on the care of patients with I/DD and the related behavioral or mental health challenges that can ensue during a hospitalization?
- What supports are in place should a patient experience a crisis (e.g., Behavioral Emergency Response Team, Psychiatry responses, Hospital Security)?

#### Situational Awareness

Hospital situational awareness for the identification and mitigation of risks inherent to caring for higher risk populations is essential for patient safety. Adults with CCCs or I/DD may have a higher risk for either clinical or behavioral decompensation. For example, Leslie is both at higher risk for acute respiratory failure as well as behavioral outbursts and self-injury. As will be discussed under *PREADMISSION: Tools*, screening tools embedded in the electronic health record can identify patients at risk. These real-time data can be leveraged by hospital units and systems to ensure appropriate staffing and resources.

Healthcare continues to become increasingly specialized. Just as an adult with a stroke or myocardial infarction should go to specific stroke or cardiac centers, an adult with a CCC may require care at a specific hospital. Leslie, for example, would benefit from hospitalization where there is access to pulmonology, infectious disease, and critical care subspecialties that are experienced with CCCs.

### Environment

There are physical and operational components that guide the way a healthcare system creates structure for supporting their patients. In this section, we will focus on the environmental variables to address as a system. While these may not be all-inclusive, we have highlighted those that we feel are most pertinent, and also the easiest for a hospital team to accomplish when planning for a complex admission. Hospitalists may participate in advocacy or committees that address areas such as workplace safety, informatics, etc. We recommend leveraging these roles to advocate for system-wide solutions for the system-level supports defined below.

#### Visitation

We recommend removing fixed visiting time restrictions for family, caregivers, and close friends of patients with an I/DD [16, 17]. In certain circumstances, residential and/or group home staff may serve in this role as well. This general approach permits people to be with the person with an I/DD as much as they wish. This has many added benefits for the patient, including greater understanding of the patient's particular needs, patient advocacy, and providing support during a time of stress. Leslie, for example, does not speak during hospitalization unless a known caregiver is present. Having a caregiver at the bedside can provide clinicians and staff with vital information real-time and thereby reduces the likelihood of clinical risks.

### Bedside Support

Hospitals should have mechanisms that allow family and/or caregiver support for patients with an I/DD for up to 24/7 coverage. These mechanisms might include having a bedside convertible chair-to-bed available and ability to tele-video with the patient. Leslie's parents and group home caregivers, for example, would alternate who was present at the bedside during a hospitalization. This would facilitate communication about clinical progress and new symptoms, as well as help with patient coping. When a patient's supports are not available during a hospital stay, consider in-person or telemonitoring support staff who can provide 1:1 safety checks, engage with the patient, and work to support the patient through acute stressors and prevent agitation.

## Tools

### Sensory-Friendly Hospital Rooms

A consideration for supporting the I/DD population during hospitalization is the development of sensory friendly hospital rooms [18]. Ideally, these are identified rooms where items may be quickly removed based on the individual needs of the patient. For example, patients with an I/DD like Leslie may become overwhelmed with numerous objects and clutter, harsh lighting, and repeated noises (e.g., beeping from a machine). If a patient has a behavioral health challenge that results in the destruction of property, removing any unnecessary items from rooms is a safety priority. When done reactively, the time and cost to a hospital trying to quickly dismantle a room is significant. Consider creating rooms that can be efficiently and effectively "turned-over." This will save time, money, and ensure a safer environment for patients.

### Screening Tools, Processes, and Order Sets

Embedded screening tools can facilitate providers quickly and proactively accessing medical or behavioral health collaborators. For example, the addition of a behavior screening tool can quickly identify patients at risk for a behavioral crisis during an admission. In these situations, a positive screen for behavioral events (Table 48.1) would have a linked aggression order set (Fig. 48.2) [19]. This order set could include protective equipment, medications, behavior plans, and consultation from behavioral health providers. Depending on the system needs and resources, similar tools could be used for CCCs. For example, should Leslie be admitted for a primarily cardiac reason, this may require consultation from adult congenital heart disease. A screening process by the admitting physician could help identify this need, which would allow for quicker and efficient collaboration, optimization of care, and ultimately implementation of best practice interventions.

## People

### Trained Employees

Though adults with an I/DD are more frequently admitted to the hospital than their neurotypical counterparts, they meet significant barriers to their care [2, 3]. Common themes include poor communication with patients and their family [17], as well as poor provider confidence and

**Table 48.1** Example questions that can be asked of the patient or patient's guardian

| |
|---|
| What is the best way to communicate with the patient? |
| What are calming strategies for the patient? |
| Does that patient have a history of inflicting harm to others or themselves? |
| Does the patient have a history of acting out behaviorally? (Examples: hitting, kicking, tantruming, throwing items or objects, refusal, elopement, yelling) |

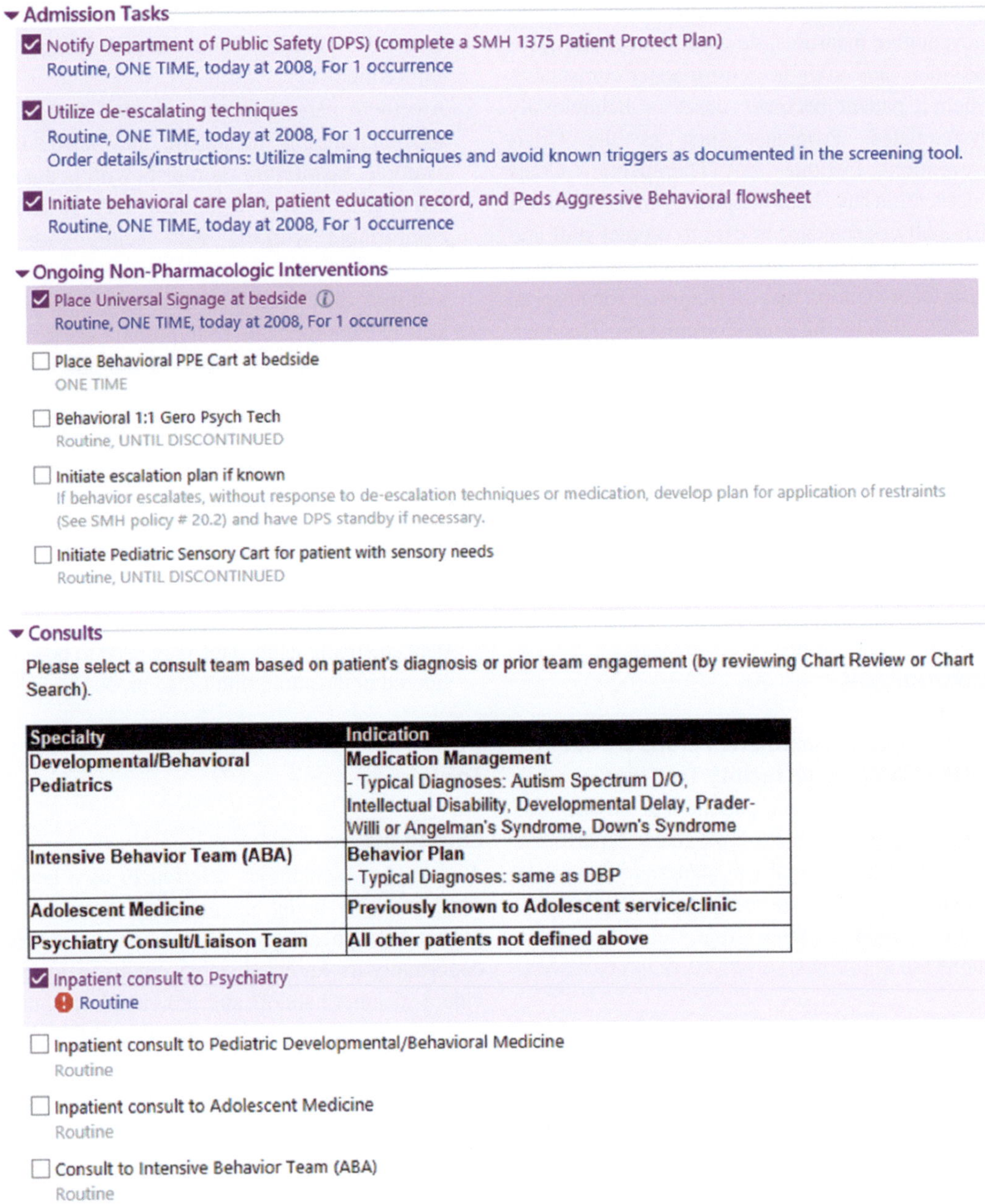

**Admission Tasks**

- [x] Notify Department of Public Safety (DPS) (complete a SMH 1375 Patient Protect Plan)
  Routine, ONE TIME, today at 2008, For 1 occurrence
- [x] Utilize de-escalating techniques
  Routine, ONE TIME, today at 2008, For 1 occurrence
  Order details/instructions: Utilize calming techniques and avoid known triggers as documented in the screening tool.
- [x] Initiate behavioral care plan, patient education record, and Peds Aggressive Behavioral flowsheet
  Routine, ONE TIME, today at 2008, For 1 occurrence

**Ongoing Non-Pharmacologic Interventions**

- [x] Place Universal Signage at bedside
  Routine, ONE TIME, today at 2008, For 1 occurrence
- [ ] Place Behavioral PPE Cart at bedside
  ONE TIME
- [ ] Behavioral 1:1 Gero Psych Tech
  Routine, UNTIL DISCONTINUED
- [ ] Initiate escalation plan if known
  If behavior escalates, without response to de-escalation techniques or medication, develop plan for application of restraints (See SMH policy # 20.2) and have DPS standby if necessary.
- [ ] Initiate Pediatric Sensory Cart for patient with sensory needs
  Routine, UNTIL DISCONTINUED

**Consults**

Please select a consult team based on patient's diagnosis or prior team engagement (by reviewing Chart Review or Chart Search).

| Specialty | Indication |
|---|---|
| **Developmental/Behavioral Pediatrics** | **Medication Management**<br>- Typical Diagnoses: Autism Spectrum D/O, Intellectual Disability, Developmental Delay, Prader-Willi or Angelman's Syndrome, Down's Syndrome |
| **Intensive Behavior Team (ABA)** | **Behavior Plan**<br>- Typical Diagnoses: same as DBP |
| **Adolescent Medicine** | **Previously known to Adolescent service/clinic** |
| **Psychiatry Consult/Liaison Team** | **All other patients not defined above** |

- [x] Inpatient consult to Psychiatry
  Routine
- [ ] Inpatient consult to Pediatric Developmental/Behavioral Medicine
  Routine
- [ ] Inpatient consult to Adolescent Medicine
  Routine
- [ ] Consult to Intensive Behavior Team (ABA)
  Routine

**Fig. 48.2** Example order set components for risk for inpatient behavioral aggression

knowledge about adults with CCCs and I/DD [20, 21], Ancillary support is beneficial for ameliorating some of these issues that arise for adults with an I/DD. Furthermore, this support may be expected by patients and their families as it is more often provided in the pediatric care setting. Examples include employees who can develop and implement social stories or other visual supports, as well as services such as child life and music therapy to help patients cope with the hospital setting and medical interventions. Interventions or presence of staff members who can provide developmentally appropriate support can decrease the need of pharmacotherapy for procedures such as lab draws. In addition to these preventative measures, de-escalation training for providers and staff is helpful in circumstances when a patient becomes upset or behaviorally dysregulated. Programs such as the Crisis Prevention Institute or Therapeutic Crisis Intervention have been adopted by many hospitals nationally as standard of care to protect staff and patients. In the near future, the implementation of these interventions may be required for hospital accreditation by the Joint Commission. The presence of appropriately trained staff to provide these supports can make the difference between a patient like Leslie having episodes of self-harm or staff injury-potentially prolonging hospitalization and leading to other adverse events and having her acute issue addressed without complication.

## Admission

### Environment

#### Emergency Department Versus Direct Admit Versus Interfacility Transfer

In many scenarios, the patient will be admitted after being triaged in the emergency department. In some cases, especially at quaternary hospitals, patients may be transferred from another hospital or direct admission from clinic. Helpful considerations are as follows:

1. Is there specialty care required for this patient? If so, is it something readily available in the hospital? For example, the clinical and procedural expertise Leslie might need when acutely ill could range from a relatively simple admission for pneumonia to something more complex like heart failure with underlying congenital heart disease.
2. Is the patient known to the hospital and if so, has this patient been admitted to a particular unit where they are familiar with staff (and vice versa)?
3. Are there any behavioral concerns? If so, does the hospital have experience and/or tools managing behavioral concerns?
4. Does this patient have a care plan or a key medical provider who helps direct the treatment plan during hospitalization? If so, should they be notified and talked prior to admission?
5. Are there particular units or staff that have specific training the patient may need? For example, respiratory therapists with pediatric training in airway clearance may be more comfortable working with adults with I/DD. Airway clearance and respiratory support will look different for an individual with poor airway clearance due to hypotonia associated with trisomy 21 compared to an adult with cystic fibrosis.
6. What is this patient's risk of clinical deterioration during their hospitalization? Many patients with severe neurologic impairment may not be candidates for non-invasive positive pressure ventilation due to poor tolerance should their respiratory status decline. These patients may also have difficult airways and require an experienced airway team. This may need to be considered in the admission triage process.

### Tools

#### Care Plans

A care plan (sometimes referred to as a health passport) is a living document that follows a patient across healthcare settings and provides an opportunity for knowledgeable caregivers to provide a succinct handoff and individualized guidance about their patients to other healthcare providers. It is an evidence-based tool with data showing improvement in quality care delivery such as decreasing in unnecessary emergency department utilization, hospital length of stay, and healthcare costs [22]. It has been used frequently in some health systems to help optimize the care of complex patients, including those with CCC and I/DD, as they are often transitioning between health systems and hospital types (e.g., pediatric and adult) [23–25]. While there is no standard on the development of a care plan [26], there are specific components to look for that can be helpful in caring for a hospitalization patient.

In the acute care setting (i.e., urgent care, emergency department, and inpatient settings), care plans help contextualize common medical complaints for a patient, provide initial management suggestions, provide situational awareness regarding a patient's risk of clinical or behavioral deterioration, and care team connections. Our example care plan for Leslie (in Table 48.2) underlines a few key hospital care elements. First, she has repeatedly grown multi-drug-resistant *Pseudomonas aeruginosa* in their sputum. There is a recommendation that initial antimicrobials should include anti-pseudomonal coverage. Second, the care plan highlights behavioral management techniques that Leslie needs sedation and/or general anesthesia for imaging and procedures. Last, the presence of information on who has decision-making capacity is included. Identifying if a patient has decision-making capacity is an especially important component of care plans for adults with I/DD.

**Table 48.2** Care plan for Leslie

| | |
|---|---|
| **Summary statement**<br>Leslie Mansfield is a 22 year old woman with a history of trisomy 21 complicated by hypotonia with poor airway clearance, intellectual disability, autism spectrum disorder, CVID, and tetralogy of Fallot with AVCD s/p repair | |
| The following is the patient's care team. Please contact the patient's primary care physician if any changes are made<br>• Dr. Wilson, primary care physician<br>• Dr. Jones, pediatric cardiology<br>• Dr. Smith, psychologist<br>• Dr. Wiley, psychiatrist | |
| **Clinical pearls**<br>Leslie common presents with aspiration pneumonias. She has grown MDR Pseudomonas, thus would recommend anti-pseudomonal antibiotics on presentation | **Special circumstances**<br>Legal guardians/ decision makers: Mom (Sue) and dad (Joe) are legal guardians<br>Patient lives in a group home located at 1234 Fairpoint Dr. (Phone 288-9909), though parents attend all medical appointments are very involved |
| **Baseline exam**<br>Generally is withdrawn and shy in new clinical settings<br>Has a III/VI systolic murmur at the LSB, at baseline does not have crackles or peripheral edema | **Behavior**<br>Struggles with the hospital setting and is particularly sensitive to loud noises. Would recommend private room if possible<br>Responds positively to proactive warning and preparation for medical procedures, e.g. "I am going to hold your right hand to look for a vein" |
| **Communication**<br>Understands simple language. Will respond yes/ no to questions. May not respond during times of stress | **Other**<br>Leslie usually needs sedation for imaging studies<br>For painful procedures, she generally needs general anesthesia |

## Medical Orders for Scope of Treatment (MOLST) or Other Advanced Care Planning Documents

Similar to any hospitalized adult patient, goals of care are important to assess (and reassess depending on clinical scenario). Particularly for those patients who have a guardian and live in a group home or long-term care facility or lack capacity to make their own healthcare decisions and have a health proxy, admitting providers should clarify goals of care and code status on admission. Need for hospitalization often marks a new acute problem or acute decompensation of a chronic problem. For these reasons, it may be appropriate, depending on the severity and type of acute illness, to readdress these goals of care during hospitalization. It is also important to understand the process of changing code status or goals of care for those patients with I/DD and/or a guardian. For example, in New York state, there is a very specific process set in the Health Care Decisions Act that includes assessment by a provider of the Office of People with Developmental Disabilities and court approval of a change in code status or goals of care [27]. Therefore, it is important to proactively discuss and review goals of care with patients with I/DD and their families.

## Medications and Supplies

Medication safety is of particular importance to the care of adults with CCCs. These adults often have complicated medication regimens and sometimes do not reach their full growth potential, with weights <40 kg. In the latter circumstance, both provider and pharmacy expertise are needed to evaluate if, and when, weight-based dosing is appropriate. This may be the standard already for medications like enoxaparin for venous thromboembolism prophylaxis or antibiotics. However, less common is weight-based adult dosing for medications such as opiates, benzodiazepines, and acetaminophen. Additionally, adult hospitals, especially those without an integrated pediatric hospital or unit, will need to consider having the following supplies (and others) available in pediatric sizing:

- Endotracheal tubes
- Phlebotomy expertise
- Gastric and gastro-jejunal tubes
- Endoscopy equipment
- Bronchoscopy equipment

## Tasks

### Screening for Adaptations or Challenges during the Admission

#### Environmental Adaptations

As previously mentioned, numerous components of the inpatient environment as well as the course of an admission can be challenging for a patient with complex needs. The admitting nurse should work with the patient and/or caregivers to identify environmental barriers to accessing care. This can include the sensory environment, dietary concerns, challenging interventions, sleep or feeding issues, or any other identified areas of preference or challenge. This information should be documentation and a means for communication that can and cannot be accommodated and should be clearly communicated to the patient and/or caregiver.

#### Mental or Behavioral Health Needs

While not all patients with CCC or an I/DD may have a mental or behavioral health need, we know that those with I/DD are more likely to experience comorbidities as compared to their neurotypical peers. As such, an effort to screen and mitigate challenges would be beneficial. This screening can be accomplished in a variety of ways. As described previously, screening can be accomplished in a short, efficient manner (refer Table 48.1 for an example aggression screening tool) and allows the team to proactively implement interventions-through an order set (see Fig. 48.2), for example, to reduce the probability of a crisis occurring. This will help prevent patient and staff injury and mitigate the need for restrictive interventions (i.e., restraints or intramuscular injections). Once implemented consistently as part of admission workflows, a positive screen should be tied to proactive measures, inclusive of but not limited to an order set for PRNs, behavioral consultation (if available), and should trigger other measures reviewed further down in this section.

Upon admitting a patient who has screened positive for a potential crisis event, we would recommend first and foremost notifying your hospital department of public safety or security. The purpose of this is to ensure that they know who the patient is, and what challenges the unit may encounter during an admission. Next, we would immediately recommend that the care team should be made aware of calming techniques or known triggers for the patient. Posting sensitive and thoughtful signs outside the room indicating who may be vulnerable to challenging behavior helps others on the care team be aware of the risk. Lastly, a consultation for providers (psychiatric, behavioral, and psychological) who can create an individual behavior or safety plan should occur within the first 24–48 h.

## People

### Consultations

Additional consultative resources can be highly beneficial in care for behaviorally acute patients with I/DD. It is important for providers to be aware that different providers can provide support to help pre-actively manage individuals who screen positive for challenging behaviors.

Examples include but would not be limited to psychiatry, psychologists, mental health counselors, behavior analyses/specialists, or providers knowledgeable in the care of adults with I/DD. It is highly recommended to order these services, proactively, to allow for assessment and intervention to occur in lieu of a challenging event. The role of consultation should be to proactively help plan for this patient, as well as respond to acute events.

## Patient Communication

Find the best way to communicate with the patient, their family, and other caregivers. Not everyone is able to communicate verbally, so use photos, signs, symbols, and pictures alongside speech. The patient and their family/caregivers are experts. They can help interpret behaviors and signs that may indicate pain or distress or identify high pain tolerances in the patient. Patients may also commonly use communication assistance devices at home that are not readily available in the hospital setting. Every attempt should be made to ensure patients have access to these devices to maximize their ability to communicate.

## Healthcare Team Providers and Staff

*Diagnostic Uncertainty:* Beware of missing serious illness. This is of particular concern for patients with learning disabilities and I/DD who may not be able to communicate symptoms effectively. There may also be unanticipated sequelae because of their underlying CCC. In short, do not ignore medical symptoms by seeing them as part of the person's disability or chronic condition. For new signs and symptoms, acting quickly helps to maintain patient safety and avoid complications. Consider using the Noncommunication Children's Pain Scale or the CHARGE Non-Vocal Pain Assessment as tools for assessing individuals who do not accurately report pain or are nonverbal [28, 29]. Unrecognized and subsequently untreated pain can lead to behavioral decompensation in patients with an I/DD [30–32].

**Table 48.3** Proactive and reactive responses to mitigating challenging behaviors

| General proactive interventions | Responding to challenging behaviors |
|---|---|
| Remove known triggers | Minimize and simplify language |
| Establish predictable routines | Ensure only one person is talking at a time |
| Provide warning prior to interventions or transitions | Tell the patient what to do (instead of what not to do) |
| Identify best ways for communication to patients and vice versa | Refrain from discussing the behavior or event immediately during or following the event |
| Use visual supports to supplement verbal information | Debrief with the patient and staff to create a plan for moving forward |
| Offer choices | Honor all reasonable requests |
| Modify expectations | Provide physical distance and space |
| Identify a support person | |
| Develop rapport and build trust | |
| Allow for extended process time | |

*Behavioral Management Strategies:* To ensure behavioral safety for patients with a known history of aggression or other challenging behaviors, there are general proactive and reactive strategies that can be used (see Table 48.3). Proactive strategies aim to prevent behavioral decompensation. Reactive strategies are employed when varying levels of behavioral decompensation have already occurred. In Table 48.4, we show an example behavioral plan of our case patient Leslie that shows patient-specific proactive and reactive behavioral management strategies.

**Table 48.4** Acute inpatient behavioral plan for Leslie

<table>
<tr><td colspan="2">Proactive engagement<br>– Work with Leslie's parents and group home to ensure bedside support<br>– Praise for making a choice: "That's a good decision Leslie!"<br>– Throughout your shift, ensure that there are no items left out that could potentially be thrown. Neutrally put them away in the cabinet. "I'm just straightening up"<br>– Use a visual schedule for any medical procedures and identify a motivating reward for completing the intervention<br>– Keep busy throughout the day with a visual schedule showing progression of events<br>– Do not provide reprimands. (Examples: "We don't do that," "That's not ok," etc.)</td></tr>
<tr><td colspan="2">Step 1: Response to agitation</td></tr>
<tr><td>What Leslie Looks Like:<br>When upset, Leslie starts to pace around the room, she may yell, throw items, and pound surfaces</td><td>How to respond:<br>1. Offer a distracting activity (puzzles, TV, iPad, snack)<br>2. Use a soft calm voice to validate her feelings<br>3. Give her space and refrain from too much talking<br>4. Offer first line PRN</td></tr>
<tr><td colspan="2">Step 2: Response to more dangerous behaviors</td></tr>
<tr><td>What Leslie Looks Like:<br>At the height of her agitation Leslie may hit, destroy objects in the room, or attempt to elope into the hallway while yelling</td><td>Staff response:<br>1. Move away from Leslie to the door<br>2. Encourage her to make a safe choice: "We need to make a good decision, do you want to sit in your orange chair or your bed?" continue until she calms or escalates further<br>3. Praise for choice-making then follow strategies below<br>If at any point Leslie poses a safety threat to herself or others (hits you, rushes to the door, destroys an object that poses a safety threat) use the least restrictive means to maintain safety. This may include restraints at the discretion of the nursing team/attending. Notify security at the start of the episode</td></tr>
</table>

## Discharge

Transitioning out of the hospital to home or another facility from a hospitalization is a high-risk time period. This is especially true for those patients that (1) have a longer length of stay (>1 week), (2) are more complex (3 or more chronic conditions), and/or (3) live in long-term care or a group home setting [33–36].

## Environment

Transitions tend to be more difficult for complex patients as well as those with an I/DD. Having less overall stimulation on the day of discharge (e.g., no lab draws or room changes) and known caregivers present are two proactive strategies that can foster a calmer environment, enable patient coping skills, and potentially decrease risk of adverse behavioral and safety events.

## Tools

### Behavioral and Care Plans

Has a behavior or care plan been created, or have there been any changes or updates to an existing plan? It is important to make sure that there is consistency across existing documents, which is a challenge for more complex patients with more frequent healthcare utilization. Changes should be communicated not only with the patient, but also with their caregiver or guardian (if indicated), primary care physician, potentially any specialists, and their long-term care site (if indicated).

### Medical Orders for Scope of Treatment (MOLST) and other Advanced Care Planning Documents

Make sure any forms are updated if there are changes to goals of care or intervention preferences. These updated forms should then travel with the patient. Follow guidance and legislation from the state of discharge (and state where patient will be transitioning to if different) to ensure rules are followed (e.g., if code status is a separate form and original must travel with the patient to be valid). Have there been any changes in decision-making? Like any other patient, assessing someone's capacity to consent to treatment is time and topic dependent. All of these steps are especially important if the patient has an I/DD and has a guardian or healthcare proxy who makes medical decisions.

## Tasks

### Discharge Planning

We strongly recommend having pre-discharge and discharge inter-disciplinary collaborative meetings as they are invaluable to ensure a safe discharge plan. The function of such meetings is to ensure adequate medical follow-up, clear communication of medication and management changes, provision and delivery of medical supplies prior to discharge, and clear communication amongst healthcare team members. Consider if Leslie, our patient with trisomy 21 and poor airway clearance, was diagnosed with obstructive sleep apnea during her admission, the impact of a new need for CPAP would impact her discharge planning and potentially disposition, as some group homes are not equipped to provide care for patients needing CPAP. Sometimes, care limitations (e.g., not being able to use prescribed CPAP) in the group home setting are acceptable to the patient and/or their caregivers in order to keep the patient in their long-term home that they know and with people who love and care for them.

Addressing this new need earlier can identify if the facility is able to handle this new requirement, has the necessary equipment and staff, etc. If the group home does not, this also allows time for the patient, care team, family/guardian, and home jointly decide about goals and if a change in living situation to allow for CPAP outweighs the risk of not using CPAP. With more complex patients like this, there are frequently unanticipated issues that arise as discharge nears that could unnecessarily prolong hospitalization and risk of safety events.

Hospital discharge also allows for refinement of a patient's inpatient care recommendations across both medical and behavioral domains.

## People

Adults with CCCs or an I/DD will often have multiple people who need, at a minimum, to be notified of potential discharge. Many should contribute to discharge planning. As noted under Discharge Planning, having an inter-disciplinary meeting prior to discharge can not only help care coordination but also help avoid adverse events. For Leslie, ensuring that the following people are notified of her pending discharge and given the opportunity to voice questions or concerns would be important:

- Parents
- Primary care physician
- Specialty consultants for active issues
- Outpatient care manager or case worker if indicated
- Long-term care facility or group home representative (ideally at least medical liaison or RN level) if indicated

Notification should leverage digital forms of communication, ideally through the electronic health record. This has the added benefit of being able to reference tools and documentation in the patient's chart.

## Conclusion

There are specific patient safety that hospitals and providers need to address when an adult with a CCC or an I/DD is hospitalized. Interventions target these populations, though, can have benefit for other adult populations seen in the hospital. We recommend hospitals take a structured approach, such as through use of the SEIPS model, to identify existing and needed organizational and physical environment conditions, as well as personnel and training, to optimize patient care for these high-risk and increasingly prevalent hospitalized patient populations.

## References

1. Dunbar P, Hall M, Gay JC, Hoover C, Markham JL, Bettenhausen JL, et al. Hospital readmission of adolescents and young adults with complex chronic disease. JAMA Netw Open. 2019;2(7):e197613.
2. Lindgren S, Lauer E, Momany E, Cope T, Royer J, Cogan L, et al. Disability, hospital care, and cost: utilization of emergency and inpatient care by a cohort of children with intellectual and developmental disabilities. J Pediatr. 2021;229:259–66.
3. Phillips KG, Wishengrad JS, Houtenville AJ. Ambulatory care sensitive conditions among all-payer claimants with intellectual and developmental disabilities. Am J Intellect Dev Disabil. 2021;126(3):203–15.
4. Jenkins AM, Berry JG, Perrin JM, Kuhlthau K, Hall M, Dunbar P, et al. What types of hospitals do adolescents and young adults with complex chronic conditions use? Acad Pediatr. 2021;22(6):1033–40. https://www.sciencedirect.com/science/article/pii/S1876285921006380.
5. Jenkins AM, Burns D, Horick R, Spicer B, Vaughn LM, Woodward J. Adolescents and young adults with spina bifida transitioning to adulthood: a comprehensive community-based needs assessment. Acad Pediatr. 2021;21(5):858–67.
6. Carayon P, Wooldridge A, Hoonakker P, Hundt AS, Kelly MM. SEIPSs 3.0: Human-centered design of the patient journey for patient safety. Appl Ergon. 2020;84:103033.
7. Franks ZM, Alcock JA, Lam T, Haines KJ, Arora N, Ramanan M. Physical restraints and post-traumatic stress disorder in survivors of critical illness. A systematic review and meta-analysis. Annals Am Thorac Soc. 2021;18(4):689–97.
8. Whetten K, Reif S, Whetten R, Murphy-McMillan LK. Trauma, mental health, distrust, and stigma among HIV-positive persons: implications for effective care. Psychosom Med. 2008;70(5):531–8.
9. Bulgin D, Tanabe P, Jenerette C. Stigma of sickle cell disease: a systematic review. Issues Ment Health Nurs. 2018;39(8):675–86.
10. Flood B. Safety of people with intellectual disabilities in hospital. What can the hospital pharmacist do to improve quality of care? Pharmacy (Basel). 2017;5(3):44.
11. Hughes RB, Robinson-Whelen S, Goe R, Schwartz M, Cesal L, Garner KB, et al. "I really want people to use our work to be safe"…using participatory research to develop a safety intervention for adults with intellectual disability. J Intellect Disabil. 2020;24(3):309–25.
12. Louch G, Albutt A, Harlow-Trigg J, Moore S, Smyth K, Ramsey L, et al. Exploring patient safety outcomes for people with learning disabilities in acute hospital settings: a scoping review. BMJ Open. 2021;11(5):e047102.
13. Tuffrey-Wijne I, Goulding L, Gordon V, Abraham E, Giatras N, Edwards C, et al. The challenges in monitoring and preventing patient safety incidents for people with intellectual disabilities in NHS acute hospitals: evidence from a mixed-methods study. BMC Health Serv Res. 2014;14(1):1–13.
14. Mimmo L, Harrison R, Travaglia J, Hu N, Woolfenden S. Inequities in quality and safety outcomes for hospitalized children with intellectual disability. Dev Med Child Neurol. 2022;64(3):314–22.
15. Mimmo L, Woolfenden S, Travaglia J, Harrison R. Creating equitable healthcare quality and safety for children with intellectual disability in hospital. Child Care Health Dev. 2020;46(5):644–9.
16. Holderle KE, Poleshuck E, Rosenberg T, Pulcino T. Integrated behavioral health in primary care for adults with complex childhood onset medical and developmental diagnoses. J Clin Psychol Med Settings. 2021;29:586. https://doi.org/10.1007/s10880-021-09798-w.
17. Charles ML. Communication experiences of family caregivers of hospitalized adults with intellectual and developmental disabilities—a qualitative study. Nurs Open. 2020;7(6):1725–34.
18. Press Story: Autism-friendly emergency room [Internet]. DCC Design Group. 2020. https://www.dccdesigngroup.com/press-story-autism-friendly-emergency-room/. Accessed 21 May 2022.
19. Scotto Rosato N, Correll CU, Pappadopulos E, Chait A, Crystal S, Jensen PS, et al. Treatment of maladaptive aggression in youth: CERT guidelines II. Treatments and ongoing management. Pediatrics. 2012;129(6):e1577–86.
20. Hunt S, Sharma N. Pediatric to adult-care transitions in childhood-onset chronic disease: hospitalist perspectives: pediatric to adult-care transitions. J Hosp Med. 2013;8(11):627–30.
21. Okumura MJ, Heisler M, Davis MM, Cabana MD, Demonner S, Kerr EA. Comfort of general internists and general pediatricians in providing care for young adults with chronic illnesses of childhood. J Gen Intern Med. 2008;23(10):1621–7.
22. Theodorou ME, Henschen BL, Chapman M. The comprehensive care plan: a patient-centered, multidisciplinary communication tool for frequently hospitalized patients. Jt Comm J Qual Patient Saf. 2020;46(4):217–26.
23. Broder-Fingert S, Shui A, Ferrone C, Iannuzzi D, Cheng ER, Giauque A, et al. A pilot study of autism-specific care plans during hospital admission. Pediatrics. 2016;137(Suppl 2):S196–204.
24. Fraze TK, Beidler LB, Briggs ADM, Colla CH. Translating evidence into practice: ACOs' use of care plans for patients with complex health needs. J Gen Intern Med. 2021;36(1):147–53.
25. Welch-Coltrane JL, Wachnik AA, Adams MCB, Avants CR, Blumstein HA, Brooks AK, et al. Implementation of individualized pain care plans decreases length of stay and hospital admission rates for high utilizing adults with sickle cell disease. Pain Med. 2021;22(8):1743–52.

26. Lunsky Y. Hospital passports require standardisation to improve patient safety and person-centred care for those with intellectual disability. Evid Based Nurs. 2018;21(2):56.
27. Health Care Decisions [Internet]. Office for people with developmental disabilities. https://opwdd.ny.gov/providers/health-care-decisions. Accessed 21 May 2022.
28. Murgia M, Izzo R, Bettinelli A, Di Maggio C, De Angelis M, Mangone M, et al. Validity and reliability of Italian version of the Non-Communicating Children's Pain Checklist: revised version. Eur J Phys Rehabil Med. 2019;55(1):89–94. https://www.minervamedica.it/index2.php?show=R33Y2019N01A0089.
29. Behavior and Pain Assessment | Charge Syndrome Foundation [Internet]. Charge Syndrome Foundation | A better world for people with CHARGE Syndrome. https://www.chargesyndrome.org/. Accessed 21 May 2022.
30. Baldridge KH, Andrasik F. Pain assessment in people with intellectual or developmental disabilities. AJN Am J Nurs. 2010;110(12):28–35.
31. Hauer J, Houtrow AJ, Section on Hospice and Palliative Medicine COCWD, Feudtner C, Klein S, Klick J, et al. Pain assessment and treatment in children with significant impairment of the central nervous system. Pediatrics. 2017;139(6):e20171002.
32. McGuire BE, Kennedy S. Pain in people with an intellectual disability. Curr Opin Psychiatry. 2013;26(3):270–5.
33. Forster AJ, Murff HJ, Peterson JF, Gandhi TK, Bates DW. The incidence and severity of adverse events affecting patients after discharge from the hospital. Ann Intern Med. 2003;138(3):161.
34. Complexity of Care Post-Discharge. Hospital Quality Institute. https://www.hqinstitute.org/post/complexity-care-post-discharge. Accessed 21 May 2022.
35. Kahn KL. Optimizing patients' vital interests post-discharge. J Gen Intern Med. 2017;32(1):14–6.
36. Kripalani S, LeFevre F, Phillips CO, Williams MV, Basaviah P, Baker DW. Deficits in communication and information transfer between hospital-based and primary care physicians: implications for patient safety and continuity of care. JAMA. 2007;297(8):831.

# Institutional Considerations for Transitions of Care

49

Jamie Prevedel Bowen, Ronald J. Williams, and Niraj Sharma

In hospital medicine, the term "transition of care" often refers to the transition of care for a patient between different medical settings, i.e., inpatient care to outpatient. However, the process of transferring patients with chronic medical conditions from pediatric to adult care can also be referred to "transition of care" or "health care transition." This process can be challenging for some patients, particularly if institutional policies are not in place, providers are not well-versed in the issues associated with transition, or if structural factors such as health insurance access lead to delayed or suboptimal transfer to adult care. In this chapter, we explore the impact of structural or organizational barriers to health care transition on patient outcomes.

J. Prevedel Bowen (✉)
Department of Internal Medicine, Intermountain Health, Utah Valley Hospital, Provo, UT, USA
e-mail: jamie.prevedelbowen@imail.org

R. J. Williams
Department of Pediatrics and Internal Medicine, Penn State Health Hershey Medical Center and Children's Hospital, Hershey, PA, USA
e-mail: rwilliams@pennstatehealth.psu.edu

N. Sharma
Department of Medicine, Brigham and Women's Hospital, Boston, MA, USA

Department of Pediatrics, Boston Children's Hospital, Boston, MA, USA

Harvard Medical School, Boston, MA, USA
e-mail: nsharma@bwh.harvard.edu

## Case

An 18-year-old male with a history of chronic lung disease presents to the emergency department with fever and worsening shortness of breath. He had been prescribed antibiotics 3 days ago by an urgent care physician which he had been taking as directed, but despite the antibiotics, he continued to have fever. He is tachypneic with a respiratory rate of 36. A chest X-ray shows a left lower lobe infiltrate, and the emergency physician decides to have the patient admitted for a pneumonia because the patient had failed outpatient therapy. The patient's primary care physician (PCP) is a pediatrician, and he has a pediatric pulmonologist (although he hasn't seen him in several years). When the pediatric pulmonologist is called, they refuse admission stating he is now 18 and should be seen by adult doctors. When the adult pulmonology service is called, they state he should be admitted to pediatrics since he still has a pediatrician as the PCP and has been followed by pediatric pulmonology.

The above scenario is common, playing out in emergency departments in hospitals across the country. The pediatric pulmonology physician loosely refers to a perceived policy that seems reasonable: the patient is now technically an adult so should be seen by adult physicians. Perhaps, there is an actual formal policy at this institution that provider transfer should happen when patients become adults; perhaps, there is


A. A. Kuo et al. (eds.), *Care of Adults with Chronic Childhood Conditions*,
https://doi.org/10.1007/978-3-031-54281-7_49

not. Having a formal policy is a good place to start, and it is endorsed by the Maternal and Child Health Bureau's Center for Health Care Transition Improvement (also known as Got Transition). However, even if there is a formal policy in place, the fact that this patient should be admitted is not clear to the physicians involved in this case. In addition, the transition of a patient from pediatric to adult care needs to start prior to the patient's turning 18, so that scenarios like this do not occur.

Developing a process for transitioning from pediatric to adult care for patients, caregivers, and adult and pediatric providers is very important for optimal health care, especially for those with chronic health care needs. Many young adults have "fallen through the cracks" because they did not get proper follow-up as they aged out of their pediatric specialists. Pediatric specialists vary in their practices of seeing patients as they become adults. Some prefer to have their patients begin seeing adult specialists during their teenage years while others may continue to treat them into their mid-twenties or even later. This individualization of care is supported by the American Academy of Pediatrics (AAP) [1]. Transition process education is important for pediatric hospital systems to provide, so their patients can maintain their health as they move to adult care. It is equally important for adult hospital systems as those patients who have not been properly transitioned, as shown in the case vignette, often present in crisis and transitioning to adult specialty care in the hospital while acutely ill can be challenging for the patients, their families, and their health care providers.

Transition is best for the patient and family when done in the outpatient setting but it can happen in the inpatient setting. This may be more challenging if the patient and family are facing an acute illness. Furthermore, there may be challenges in obtaining medical records from the patient's prior specialists, limited time for medical decisions and communication, and a lack of communication from the pediatric provider to the new consultant. Having a guideline or a process for when the need for inpatient transition of care occurs can provide a valuable service to the patient as well as the medical team and hospital.

Transition of care from pediatrics to adult medicine can take place in many models, such as institutions with a children's hospital within an adult hospital, others with separate adult and children's hospitals connected by a bridge/same campus, and adult and children's hospitals separated by distance. With planning, motivation, and institutional endorsement, processes for transition of care for patients can improve patient care in all of these settings.

## How to Establish an Institutional Transition of Care Process Guideline

Several steps can be considered in establishing a guideline: understanding the structure of the health system, identifying key stakeholders, defining the overall aims and goals for the transition guideline, and determining patient and provider education needs.

### Define the Existing Health System Structure

As a first step to establishing a transition process, it is important to understand how the health system is organized. Organization goes beyond the mere structures delineated above, such as whether the children's and adult hospitals are connected physically. Whether or not pediatric and adult specialists communicate, whether health care transition policies exist and are followed, and whether resources are allocated to support the transition process are all factors that contribute to successful transitions in institutions. Answering these questions and conducting an inventory and needs assessment for each primary care and specialty division will help determine the next steps. A Strengths, Weaknesses, Opportunities, Threats [2] (SWOT) analysis can help organize a strategy for developing an institutional transition process.

## Identify Key Stakeholders

A transition process champion should be found at the outset as this person can lead the project effort. While this individual could be a physician, it does not have to be. In many cases, a social worker is often the transition champion in an institution. Finding supportive key stakeholders is also crucial for the success of any project. These stakeholders must have the power to make decisions about resources (e.g., personnel, space, and supplies) and must be supportive of the cause. Likely, key stakeholders include the chairs of the departments of pediatrics and medicine, financial administrative leads of pediatrics and medicine, nursing administration, social work, child life specialists, medical trainees, and patient (adolescent) and caregiver representatives.

## Aims, Goals, and Measurement

Once the stakeholders have been identified, it will be important to gather the individuals to determine what the aim and goals are of a program. Inpatient transition policies need to consider opportunities for improvement in patient care, communication, patient safety, and expectations when transitioning from pediatric inpatient care to adult inpatient care, and hospitalist and specialist concerns. Consider what value may be added by implementing a transition of care guideline.

At the same time, determine how success will be measured and define what a successful transition means. Examples can include establishing a comprehensive transition document in the medical record, finding an adult specialist, documenting a follow-up appointment, or measuring improved satisfaction with communication by patient and members of the medical team.

## Education of Patients and Providers

The education of patients and providers needs to be considered and built into the transition process. For patients, a general education curriculum should be developed to teach the skills individuals need to take control of their health care to prepare for transition and transfer. Topics include how to make an appointment, refill a medication, learn their personal medical history, and understanding their medical insurance. Other considerations include disease-specific education for patients, including the impact of their disease on their education, career, reproductive choices, and future care needs. This should be delivered in a developmentally appropriate fashion as some patients will become fully independent adults and have significant ownership of their medical care while others will need ongoing support from family or guardians.

Education is also needed for pediatric and adult specialists. This will include topics in patient care, such as strategies to communicate with young adults, as well as the logistics of coordinating care between the two services.

## Implementing the Transition Policy

Although an institution may adopt a health care transition policy, the implementation of the policy mostly occurs through a stepwise process, often in divisions or units in which multiple champions already exist. It is often advantageous for these "early adopters" to implement a process first, as more challenges often arise with the first implementations of new processes due to people's natural resistance to change. However, once processes have been successfully implemented in one or a few units, implementing these processes in other units is often easier and faster.

## Process Development and Patient Education

Process development should happen with all stakeholders. This could mean across specialties resulting in meetings between adult specialists and analogous pediatric specialists (e.g., adult cardiology and pediatric cardiology). This could also mean across disciplines, meaning meetings with physicians, nurses, social workers, care coordinators, and child life specialists. Engaging as many stakeholders as possible will lead to a smoother implementation of processes.

Patient education materials should be developed as part of the process development in order to communicate to patients what is expected in an optimal health care transition from pediatrics to adult medicine. This is often the last step in the process development because all groups have to agree on what will be shared with patients.

## Documentation and Electronic Health Records

Prior to the advent of electronic health records, a comprehensive summary paper document was often prepared by the pediatric specialty team to inform their adult colleagues of the major past medical events and ongoing issues for each patient. With EHRs, it is easier for new physicians to find records in one location; however, a summary document could still be useful to assist in the transfer of care between pediatrics and adult medicine. This summary could refer to dates of major events and interventions (as opposed to reproducing past reports as was done previously) and anticipated future needs. If the transfer is occurring within entities that share an EHR system, the summary could be relatively brief.

An important consideration is where the document will be located within the EHR system. Simply entering a note as one would do for any visit does not guarantee that it will be able to be found easily for reference. Part of the development process should include consideration for any modifications to the EHR that could facilitate awareness that a health care transition summary is available for the patient and where to find it.

## Pediatric to Adult Handoffs (Transfers of Care)

In general, patients are more likely to follow through with a visit to a new adult provider if that individual has been recommended by their pediatric provider. In addition, the adult provider may be more likely to accept the patient with the outreach of a physician who knows the patient [3].

It would be ideal if an adult provider is able to come to the pediatric transition visit (last pediatric visit) for a "warm handoff". However, with the rise in the use of virtual visits, it may be possible to have this handoff occur virtually for accepting adult specialist. The website www.gottransition.org now has a toolkit resource to guide this virtual transition visit [4]. The American College of Physicians (ACP) also has transition education materials available [5]. Transition of care has been designated as an important area of high value care by the ACP.

## Timing of Transfer

Hospital logistics and availability of specialists may dictate some of the specialty-specific transition ages. Some adult specialists are constrained to only seeing hospitalized patients beginning at age 18, where other specialists may be comfortable treating adolescent patients with specific conditions (for example, it is a mutual decision between patients and hematologists when to transition, and generally patients transition to adult specialist care in their mid-teenage years). However, at this same institution, all patients admitted to a pediatric care area with endocrine conditions are cared by pediatric endocrinology (this includes patients up to 21). While working toward a unified approach to transition and a health-system wide guideline (policy), it is very important to have clear communication about each specialty to avoid delays and miscommunications in care.

## Coordination

Transition education and coordination is the best way to ensure optimal care of young adults with chronic medical conditions. Local hospital resources need to be considered when determining who will be responsible for carrying out this work. Social workers and child life can be excellent team members while primary care doctors and the primary specialist can often play a role but may be limited due to time constraints, especially if the transition happens while patient is hospitalized. Some hospitalist groups assign "primary hospitalists" or "primary intensivists" to patients with chronic medical conditions requiring frequent or high-acuity hospitalizations and these individuals may also know the transition needs of the patient.

## Process Assessment

Periodic follow-up by the transition process champion is essential to ensure that the momentum of the process implementation continues. Utilizing the measurements that were determined earlier will allow for the process to be evaluated. This can be an opportunity to utilize quality improvement methodology to assess if any step of the process needs to be adjusted.

## References

1. Hardin AP, Hackell JM, Committee on Practice and Ambulatory Medicine, Simon GR, Boudreau ADA, Baker CN, et al. Age limit of pediatrics. Pediatrics. 2017;140(3):e20172151.
2. Teoli D, Sanvictores T, An J. SWOT analysis. In: StatPearls. Treasure Island (FL): StatPearls Publishing; 2022. http://www.ncbi.nlm.nih.gov/books/NBK537302/.
3. White P, Cuomo C, Johnson-Hooper T, Robbins B, Harwood C, McManus P. Adult provider willingness to accept young adults into their practice: results from three integrated delivery systems. Gottransitionorg. 2022. https://gottransition.org/resource/?adult-provider-willingness-accept-ya-practice.
4. White P, Greenberg A. Telehealth toolkit for a joint visit with pediatric and adult health care clinicians and transferring young adults. 2022. https://gottransition.org/resource/?telehealth-toolkit-joint-visit-pediatric-adult-clinicians>.
5. Acponline.org. Pediatric to Adult Care Transitions Initiative. 2022. https://www.acponline.org/clinical-information/high-value-care/resources-for-clinicians/pediatric-to-adult-care-transitions-initiative.

# Inpatient Care of Adults with Conditions of Childhood

# 50

Brian Herbst, Rachel Peterson, Jennifer Sun, and Niraj Sharma

## Cases

### Case Study 1

A 26-year-old male with congenital muscular dystrophy mutation, restrictive lung disease, mild left ventricular dysfunction, adrenal insufficiency, and developmental disability was admitted with fever, cough, and weakness secondary to right lower lobe pneumonia on chest X-ray. Approximately, 4 days after admission, the patient developed intermittent tachycardia to HR in 160 s of unknown etiology, with subsequent evaluation demonstrating changes in his EKG with new ST elevation in V2, worsening ST elevation in V4 and V5 and T-wave inversions in T4 and T5. High sensitivity troponin was obtained and elevated at 16,991 ng/L (nL <14 ng/L). Pro-BNP was also elevated at 1802 pg/mL (nL <25 pg/mL). Urgent transthoracic echocardiogram (TTE) demonstrated globally decreased left ventricular function from normal prior TTE 4 months ago. The patient was well-appearing, but after discussion with an Internal Medicine provider, a Rapid Response Team evaluation was called for ICU evaluation, given his history of developmental delay and inability to accurately describe his current symptoms. Of note, the ST-elevation MI team at the partnering adult hospital was paged to discuss management, but did not return their pages to discuss the case further. In discussion with the ICU and Cardiology team,

Brian Herbst and Rachel Peterson contributed equally to the development of this chapter.

B. Herbst · R. Peterson
Department of Pediatrics, Cincinnati Children's Hospital Medical Center, Cincinnati, OH, USA

Department of Internal Medicine, University of Cincinnati, Cincinnati, USA
e-mail: Brian.herbst@cchmc.org; rachel.peterson@cchmc.org

J. Sun (✉)
Department of Internal Medicine, Hospital of the University of Pennsylvania, Philadelphia, PA, USA

Department of Pediatrics, Children's Hospital of Philadelphia, Philadelphia, PA, USA
e-mail: sunjk@chop.edu

N. Sharma
Department of Medicine, Brigham and Women's Hospital, Boston, MA, USA

Department of Pediatrics, Boston Children's Hospital, Boston, MA, USA

Harvard Medical School, Boston, MA, USA
e-mail: nsharma@bwh.harvard.edu


A. A. Kuo et al. (eds.), *Care of Adults with Chronic Childhood Conditions*,
https://doi.org/10.1007/978-3-031-54281-7_50

it was decided to transfer the patient to the cardiovascular ICU for further management. Ultimately, the patient's troponins peaked at around 20,000, with stable cardiac function and no evidence of cardiovascular shock. The patient was diuresed with improvement. It was felt that the patient's presentation was related to myocarditis in combination with his underlying muscular dystrophy.

**Case Study 2**
A 25-year-old male with history of ornithine transcarbamylase (OTC) deficiency, developmental delay, autism, and intermittent explosive disorder was admitted for vomiting, lethargy, and anorexia secondary to gastroenteritis, with resultant hyperammonemia secondary to his OTC deficiency. The patient was admitted to an adult hospital with an ammonia level of 312 and was given an initial IV fluid bolus and started on LR. Attempts to contact Genetics for further recommendations were delayed. When Genetics was contacted, the ammonia level of the patient had increased to 372. Recommendations were made to start IV arginine hydrochloride, IV sodium phenylacetate–sodium benzoate, and oral citrulline. Unfortunately, IV sodium phenylacetate–sodium benzoate was not carried at the pharmacy, and in conjunction with the local pediatric hospital, this medication was obtained via rush order. At this point, the ammonia level of the patient had peaked to 406 and then subsequently improved once IV infusions were started. On HD #2, the patient was noted to have behavioral agitation, becoming aggressive with staff, and pulling at IV lines. Nursing was experiencing difficulties, keeping the patient on IV infusions. Security was called due to aggression, and the patient was placed in restraints. Ultimately, psychiatry was consulted and started the patient on medications for agitation management, and the patient was discharged home after an additional 5 days of admission.

## Case Discussion

The cases above highlight the challenges that certain patient populations can create for healthcare systems. In the first case, the patient was adult-aged who developed a problem not often encountered in the pediatric setting—massive troponin elevation with concerning EKG findings. Recognition and identification of features suggesting ischemic coronary disease, infrequently encountered in the pediatric system, was delayed, and systems barriers (i.e., activation of the STEMI team for consideration of PCI) was also a barrier. In the second case, the management of a more typical and life-threatening pediatric condition rarely seen in adult patients was delayed due to unfamiliarity with the management of his condition, the delay in contacting the pediatric expert in this area for recommendations (and by extension, the lack of treatment protocols that would have been useful), as well as the absence of pharmaceuticals required for the treatment of the patient's condition. Furthermore, the management of behavioral disturbances frequently seen in children and adolescents with developmental delay or autism posed a particular challenge, as escalation to security and restraints is not the treatment of choice for this sort of behavioral escalation [1].

While the end result in each case did not result in patient harm per se, the potential for harm existed. Strategies to mitigate these harms are essential for healthcare systems, but incredibly challenging for conditions not frequently encountered and for which solutions may not be easy. Furthermore, situations like the above result in delays in the delivery of appropriate care, whether they be related to lack of access to appropriate adult medicine related issues or because transfer of care is delayed. These issues pose increased costs to the healthcare system and more opportunity for adverse outcomes.

## Background

### The Scope of the Issue

#### A Growing Population
Advances in pediatric care have provided opportunities for patients with conditions of childhood to age into adulthood [2]. There is a growing number of adult-aged patients being admitted to children's hospitals (see Fig. 50.1) [3].

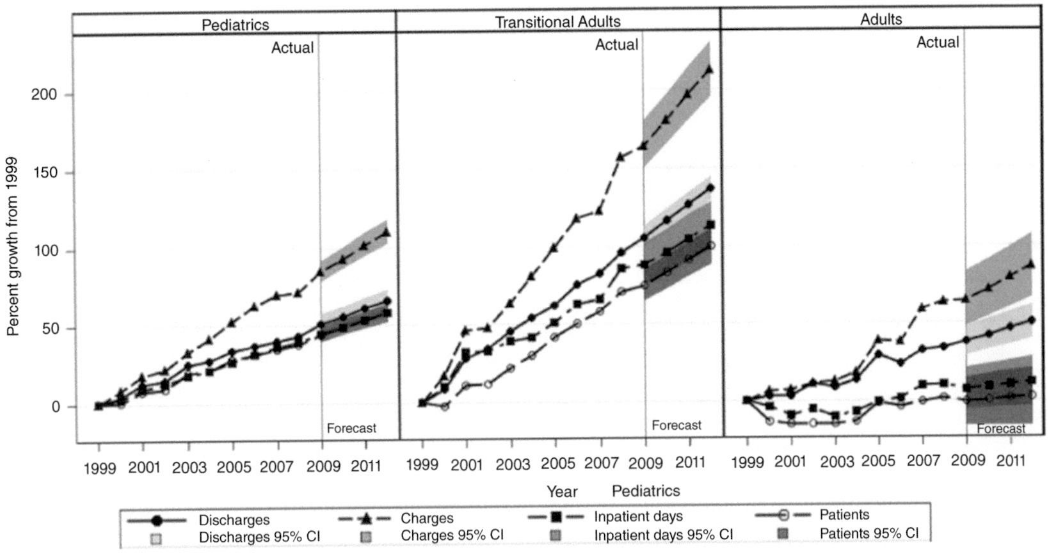


**Fig. 50.1** Increase in adults treated at children's hospitals, 1999–2012, according to age group [7]. Review of patients admitted to pediatric hospitals outlines that certain populations are having rising admissions to pediatric hospitals, whereas others are transitioning into adult care (or at least out of pediatric care) for their inpatient needs

Historically, these pediatric conditions were primarily managed by pediatricians. The subpopulations of aging patients are now developing chronic conditions more commonly seen in adult medicine. Neither pediatricians nor internists feel completely comfortable caring for these patients [4–6].

These adults, often with more complex conditions, are more likely to utilize an increasing amount of medical resources [8, 9]. Costs associated with these admissions are rising [7]. While their numbers are not large, comparatively, to the children admitted to pediatric hospitals, these adults do constitute a high-risk population [10]. The great variability in the transition of care for this growing population is leaving many children's hospitals with adults in their service [11]. Consensus guidelines by major medical societies do not specify inpatient care transitions for these youth when considering the move from pediatric to adult hospitals [12].

## Specific Populations

Some of these patients continue to be seen at pediatric hospitals because their primary conditions are childhood in onset (e.g., congenital heart disease, neurodevelopmental disabilities). Others are growing because pediatric-based management has been shown to have better outcomes (e.g., hematologic malignancy [13, 14], specialized surgical interventions) and have the potential to improve the financial outcomes of pediatric hospitals.

Specific populations, such as patients with cystic fibrosis, have demonstrated better pediatric-to-adult transition rates as part of initiatives brought forward by foundations aimed at the improvement of their care [15]. Other subpopulations, such as sickle cell disease, might experience quicker but less consistent and thorough transition [16]. Some of this is thought to be related to organizational and funding initiatives moving transition efforts forward. Different diagnoses have varying levels of support on a national level, which can impact the outcomes of pediatric to adult transition (see Fig. 50.2).

Patients with neurodevelopmental disabilities encompass a unique population as some of their care may be mirror pediatric-based care, regardless of their age. These patients may also not have designated specialists on the adult side (i.e., neurodevelopmental pediatricians) who feel comfortable to safely accepting them into care. Many adult-trained physicians report discomfort in car-

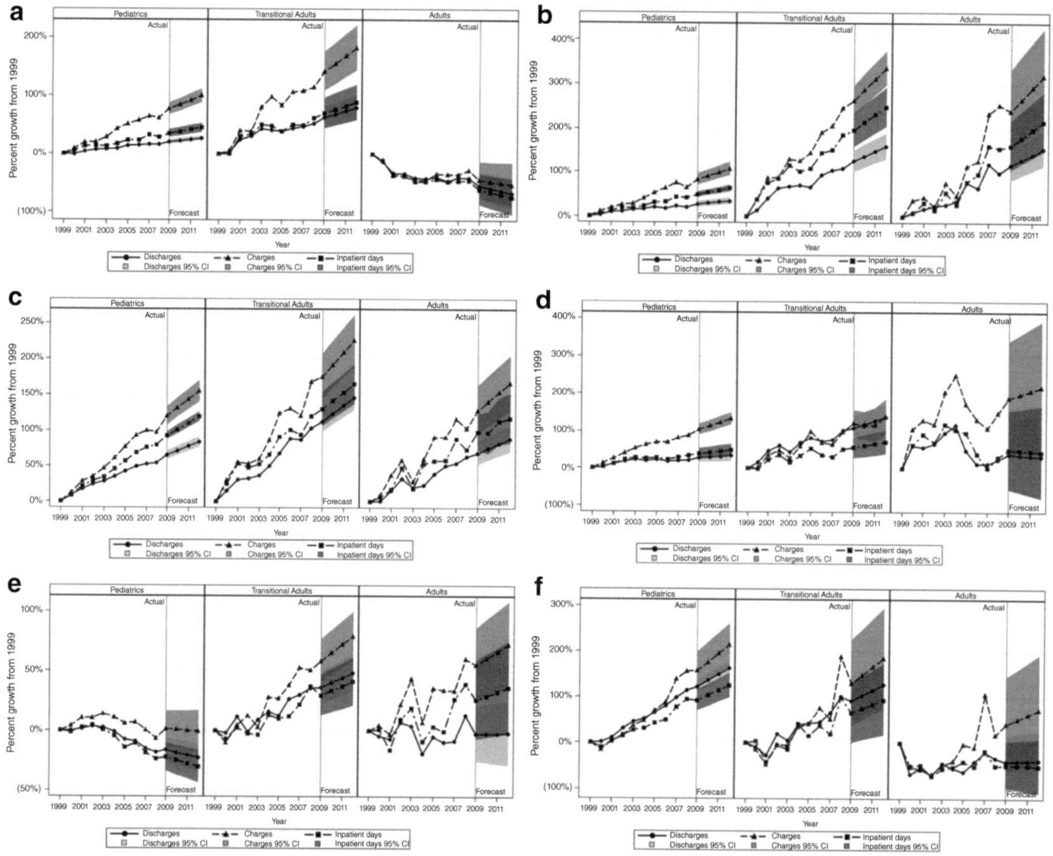

**Fig. 50.2** Percentage growth in the numbers of adults treated at children's hospitals, 1999–2012, according to age group and disease [7]. Disease populations by panels include (with confidence intervals) (**a**) cystic fibrosis; (**b**) malignant neoplasms; (**c**) congenital heart disease; (**d**) sickle cell disease; (**e**) cerebral palsy; (**f**) epilepsy

ing for this population as a result of minimal training surrounding their care [17]. Considerations around guardianship and healthcare proxy are also important to weigh in this population. Another component of consideration in this category is patient size. Many adult healthcare facilities do not have the appropriately sized equipment or nursing staff trained to navigate care for a patient <30 kg, if they do not otherwise provide pediatric care.

Another important consideration is those in the "adult survivorship" category [3]. Issues related to survivorship include healthcare access and follow-up, later effects of treatments, secondary cancers, and quality of life. These patients may have received the majority of their initial care in pediatric institutions, and ownership and monitoring of their care during survivorship may then occur in adult realms [18].

## Consult Service Characteristics—What Do Consult Services Provide?[1]

### Whole Person Quality Care

As previously discussed, bridging the divide between pediatric- and adult-based care requires specialized expertise around both pediatric and adult issues. Med-Peds or Family Medicine-trained providers may have had experience caring for both age spectrums and thus might be more comfortable with patients who bridge both arenas. Of the dozen children's hospitals that

[1]The following characteristics stem from work that has been done and manuscript is under review, led by Dr. Rachel Peterson and Dr. Ashley Jenkins, based on a mixed methods study of inpatient adult services in pediatric hospitals nationwide.

have adult consult services, all of them have a majority of their staffing performed by Med-Peds trained physicians and may also provide support at their collaborating adult institutions [19, 20]. Awareness of the congenital issues carried by these patients as well as the impending and possible adult focused ailments is required in providing care that looks at the whole care.

Whole person care takes into consideration the childhood conditions as well as the potential developing adult-related conditions. These services can also connect experts from both arenas (for instance, congenital heart surgeons and stroke expertise) and advocate for patients to get optimal care regardless of the hospital setting they might be residing in.

## Navigating Health Systems

Increasingly, healthcare systems are recognized as complex entities, both in design and delivery of care [21]. Each healthcare system has nuances in how their system works. In addition, there are drastic differences in how systems work to deliver care in pediatric medicine compared to adult medicine. For patients, navigating these systems can be a frustrating experience. For providers, who may be presumed as adept at navigating these complex systems, many of the same challenges are encountered. This may further be exacerbated by the system in which a provider practices.

Considerations around navigating health systems can include the following:

- For a patient receiving the majority of care in the pediatric setting, if an adult provider is needed, how will their pediatric providers assist in providing a referral?
- Do they have specific recommendations for providers or are their providers that they know and trust?
- Will they know the logistics on how to assist scheduling an appointment for their patient, or even be able to provide a scheduling number?
- For adult providers caring for a patient with a pediatric condition, who might they turn to if questions arise for their patient's specific pediatric condition, particularly if this is the only patient with this condition?
- For patients with chronic technology dependence, can their physician's office accommodate a motorized scooter, or a ventilator?

While unlikely to solve many of these aforementioned challenges, having providers adept at navigating pediatric and adult systems can be helpful to patients, families, providers, and to the systems they work in. While the inpatient setting is not the ideal time to transition care, providing education, expectations, contact information, and coordination and communication of care can help set the framework for a successful transition. It also facilitates navigation of complex situations that might otherwise become barriers to care. Discharge planners caring for this population need greater familiarity with methods to communicate with caregivers, as well as alternative discharge support options for caregivers who co-reside with the patient [22]. Such improvement in adult discharge planning quality has been associated with lower rates of 30-day hospital readmissions [23, 24].

For issues where primary or specialty providers may not have time to effectively communicate in the outpatient setting, [25] having a team be able to discuss these issues, set expectations, and coordinate with existing teams and providers can be particularly valuable.

## Economies of Scale

While most would identify that those with adult conditions and of adult age should be seen by adult clinicians, the nuances of particular childhood conditions necessitate consideration of best location. For instance, with rising numbers of adult aged patients with congenital heart disease, there has been a concurrent rise in proportions of surgeries in pediatric hospitals for adult aged patients (from 2.5 to 3.6% over 8 years) [26]. These patients may have higher costs, higher resource utilization, and higher morbidity and mortality overall. When thinking about best location of treatment, utilizing highly trained specialists has been shown to improve outcomes. However, location of treatment can also impact mortality of adults, and familiarity with adult conditions may be a part of this [27]. As health systems and patients consider the best location of treatment, it is also important they consider the involved specialists needed and where the final treatment and recovery occurs. Alternatively, if tools and teams are not present in the adult system at the time that healthcare utilization is required, one-time visits for adults in pediatric healthcare centers may be necessary to help provide coordination of care.

## Patient Safety Considerations

Preparation for medical situations that may impact patient care is paramount. The development of processes and protocols can assist in navigating some of these difficult situations. For issues that may not be commonplace in a particular practice setting (i.e., acute coronary syndrome or illicit substance use by patients or family members in a pediatric hospital, management of once-fatal or life-limiting illnesses now progressing into adulthood, or even fall risk in the inpatient setting) [28], having access to providers familiar with up-to-date practices assist with difficult cases or situations is pivotal. Identifying the means to obtain input specialist providers is critical. Hospitals should also work on building systems to anticipate needs and provide care that is necessary.

For example, in a free-standing children's hospital, partnering with a nearby adult institution to provide telehealth consultation (including establishing a streamlined credentialing process for physicians to provide this care and ensuring the ability of these providers to access medical records) or establishing a streamlined transfer process can greatly help with reducing delays in care and mitigating possible adverse outcomes that may result from unpreparedness in these situations.

Certain situations necessitating important medical decisions can also be assisted by having a transition team involved. For example, it is far less common for considerations like advanced directives or code consideration to be considered in the pediatric setting [29], yet discussion about the expectations and wishes are essential. Furthermore, many pediatric providers may be uncomfortable or unfamiliar with assessment of medical decision-making capacity, which is far more frequently encountered in the adult setting. Similarly, patient- and family-centered rounds is a more pediatric-specific practice. For patients with developmental delay, shared decision-making with family and patient involvement has become more the norm. Family involvement in these shared decisions may not be as familiar to adult-trained providers. Without involvement of families, rapport building may be impaired. Having providers adept at these communication practices can help provide more comprehensive, complete, and cooperative care.

In addition to medical knowledge gaps, providers caring for patients with pediatric conditions may benefit from having awareness of specific logistical or physical considerations to improve the care of these patients. Physical plant issues such as availability of proper bed sizes, bed lifts, and adequate staffing to care for patients requiring more attention may be limited. Having properly sized and compatible supplies such as urinary catheters, suction catheters, and feeding tube adapters and pumps may present another challenge. Certain medications may be used more exclusively in pediatric or adult medicine and availability of these might impact a patient's care in one system or another. If care is reliant upon or must be provided at another partnering site, delineating how to best coordinate transfers between partnering institutions and providers is equally important. If, for example, the partnering institution is located several miles away, establishing a process by which supply or medication acquisition, or transportation of patients, is required. Identifying resources to mitigate these challenges and impacts to patients is essential for providing comprehensive care.

"An ounce of prevention is worth a pound of cure." The ability of health systems to identify at-risk patient populations, while incredibly challenging, can provide great benefit to the patients served and teams caring for those patients.

Institutionally, understanding the priorities of unique patient populations is a necessary start. For example, is it a focus of the institution to recruit patients with congenital heart disease, or grow the adolescent and young adult oncology population? If so, anticipating specific needs and building areas of expertise (i.e., surgical, procedural, subspecialty requirements) can assist with initial stages of planning. For higher-risk patient populations that currently exist, creating a system to track and monitor these patients, their activities (i.e., admissions, rapid response/code events, transfers) and their outcomes can also help future planning. In the inpatient setting, quickly identifying deterioration in these patients and addressing mitigation and management strategies is vital. At Cincinnati Children's Hospital Medical Center, the National Early Warning Score (NEWS) system for admitted patients aged 21 years and older allowed for patient scores to be used during institutional safety huddles to predict deterioration and mitigation strategies for patients at risk [30].

Not all complications can be anticipated in every patient. Having clear pathways to get at "cures" for issues is essential. Communication and coordination between caregivers, providers, and health systems is required to address unforeseen issues when they arise. Having proper stakeholder involvement (allied health, physicians, information services, etc.) with clear means of communicating, reporting, and tracking of issues when they arise should be a requisite component of building a care system. Having robust support and expertise in quality improvement to identify issues, develop mitigation strategies, implement these strategies, and evaluate for effectiveness is also invaluable to this process.

### Support for Transitions of Care

Inpatient transition services may not be able to fully bridge the divide between pediatric and adult care for a patient, but they can help facilitate smooth transition in the outpatient setting. Young adults often under-utilize healthcare resources as a result of decreasing apparent needs and increasing autonomy of care. Even adults with intellectual disabilities may not visit their pediatrician as often, and at times, a hospitalization for an acute illness offers an opportunity for intervention and redirection for these patients.

Inpatient adult services can improve communication between adult and pediatric providers and help clarify "gray" areas. They may facilitate advanced care planning and communicate between medical teams and families. At last, coordination with "next steps" might be taken during a hospitalization and help patients and families understand where they should go the next time they need care for a condition (i.e., adult specialists) or for acute care needs (i.e., adult hospital). They can also create guidelines for patients that help clarify where best care can be given. Transition Care Plans are a common tool used in outpatient transition clinics for these patients. Inpatient guidelines can be incorporated into those Care Plans to help facilitate continued good care regardless of the hospital the patient might present to.

## Additional Considerations When Setting Up Inpatient Services for Adults with Conditions of Childhood

### Stakeholder Engagement

When planning to build a service or planning to care for this unique patient population, it is important to assess the local needs of your institution, and based on those needs, identify who the key stakeholders are. Some stakeholders may be within the larger institutional structure if recruitment and care for certain adult patients is a larger institutional priority but will also include division directors or clinicians in specialized clinical care programs, or specific groups of providers with a particular area of expertise. While there may be overlap with the above individuals, finding advocates supportive of the needs, missions, and growth opportunities for these patient populations can assist with advancing these goals, and may also include representatives from organizational patient safety groups, other business administrators, as well as nursing and other allied health professionals who will be responsible for supporting these patient groups. It is worth emphasizing that incorporating nursing and other allied health professionals is essential to supporting any adult program since this group often serves as the first point of patient contact. Additionally, patient and family advocates can also be key in building a program, as input from patients and families can oftentimes provide the most illustrative examples of strategies that work well, or that may require further improvements.

## Population Identification

In identifying the adult population with childhood conditions that might be present, leaders should look to see what areas of specialty their institution seeks to fill. Having access to certain pediatric or adult-congenital surgical specialists (i.e., adult congenital heart surgery, neuro-oncologic surgery) or programs aimed at adolescent and young adult populations (i.e., AYA hematologic–oncologic malignancies) might influence the numbers of patients seen at each institution. Monitoring the numbers in these populations, as well as hospital leadership growth plans around these populations, is important in providing proactive care aimed at appropriate adult management. Inpatient leads of adult services can also consider database monitoring to capture and track adult aged patients served in pediatric hospitals, in an effort to monitor outcomes. Whereas pediatric systems collate data in the Pediatric Health Information System database, adult care in the US health system is fragmented and continuity monitoring is difficult. Creation of databases can help with this newer area of medicine and will hopefully enable improved scholarly output and effective care in the future.

## Identification of Points of Service Integration

Integration of providers or systems for small patient populations, or populations that may be encountered less frequently, may be a challenge for health systems. Committees and engaged groups consisting of providers and individuals who will be involved with the care of these patient populations is a necessary step. Planning and reliance on existing infrastructure can serve as a means to mitigate some of these challenges. For example, existing safety reporting systems can be used to generate feedback on incidents from providers, to identify safety risks and common themes surrounding those incidents, and to develop strategies of mitigation. Having individuals responsible for taking ownership in reviewing and acting upon these reports is also necessary; ideally, these individuals will be champions of the cause of caring for these specific adult populations. For systems that conduct regular safety huddles, having an adult-specific provider or reporting structure specifically for adult patients can bring necessary attention to high-risk patients who require more consideration and coordination to provide safe care.

Some health systems may also rely on patient and family advocacy groups. These teams provide valuable feedback from patients and families about their experiences. Having "champions of care" or providers with adult-specific expertise and interest leading these initiatives is also important to creating, building, and modifying systems to make them successful in the mission of caring for select adult populations. These champions might help with the creation of institutional policies, identifying and mitigating system risks, and assisting in developing and maintaining a complex system of patient care. Individuals and teams with relationships with other systems help bridge gaps in care and facilitate transitions between healthcare systems which can help set the foundation for a successful program.

## Administrative Considerations

Creating a system to care for adult patient populations requires providers with expertise in adult-specific care, as well as individuals responsible for the oversight of the program. Creating, sustaining, and improving such a system can be complex, and require resources from a financial and personnel standpoint. When considering care for adults, if current infrastructure in a healthcare system cannot support aspects of adult-specific care (i.e., cardiac catheterization, endoscopy, or other procedures more common in pediatric or adults; pediatric- or adult-specific supplies; or specialists to provide specific aspects of adult care such as inpatient consultation or outpatient follow up), partnering with a regional institution or institutions is necessary.

Decisions about personnel are equally important in providing direct care for patients. Providers should have some degree of expertise and comfort with the patient population served. For physician coverage, volume of patients served should be a consideration in order to create a model of coverage with adequate staffing.

Leaders and administration should consider several questions when creating these systems of coverage:

- Will it be incumbent on providers who may be seeing patients already working on an inpatient service or in an outpatient clinic to see consults?
- Will patient volume allow for a dedicated consult or co-management service, or an inpatient service who admits adults?
- Is there a larger institutional priority to care for certain patient populations, and if so, ways to integrate physicians into this care model (i.e., Med-Peds trained Oncology hospitalists)?
- If dually trained providers (i.e., Med-Peds or Family Medicine) are employed, it is important to think about how providers might maintain competency.
- If an adult care program is housed at a Pediatric hospital, will they be required to still care for adults in other care locations or institutions?
- If providers do work in separate care locations or institutions, delineation of salary/compensation, credentialing, benefits, and complex scheduling requirements that may result from this split in employment or time must be considered and may result in complex contractual agreements between institutions.

While the discussion often focuses on physicians, equal consideration should be given to nursing and allied health professional staffing as well:

- Do these individuals have the training and expertise to care for this specific patient population?
- What will be required to maintain competency in their niche area?
- What is the exact number of healthcare professionals required to care for patients around the clock on the inpatient setting?

Financial viability for a service is an important consideration. This impacts how a service is structured or staffed. Financial support may include institutional support if certain patient populations (i.e., congenital cardiac or adult congenital diseases, complex care patients, etc.) are a priority. For a consulting service, determining volume and anticipated revenue can be difficult, but approximations can help determine sufficient and reasonable staffing models.

Billing for patient care also impacts financial viability. Billing for an internal medicine consult in a pediatric hospital can be straightforward but justifying the billing for an adult with pediatric medical complexity in an adult hospital may be less straightforward and require alternative care model with corresponding documentation to support. Infrastructure should track adult volumes, billing data, and other metrics should be considered when administering a program to help inform potential changes and improvements.

## Conclusion

Inpatient services aimed at the care of adults with conditions of childhood are relatively new. They support the growing population of these patients.

Inpatient services have varying structures and methods, but all aim to build bridges to appropriately support the unique subpopulations in the health system communities that they reside in.

## References


1. Allen DE, de Nesnera A, Moreau MA, Barrnett RJ. Seclusion and restraint use in children and adults: differences between age groups. J Psychosoc Nurs Ment Health Serv. 2014;52(3):20–5.
2. Vaks Y, Bensen R, Steidtmann D, et al. Better health, less spending: redesigning the transition from pediatric to adult healthcare for youth with chronic illness. Healthc (Amst). 2016;4(1):57–68.
3. Goodman DM, Mendez E, Throop C, Ogata ES. Adult survivors of pediatric illness: the impact on pediatric hospitals. Pediatrics. 2002;110(3):583–9.
4. Okumura MJ, Heisler M, Davis MM, Cabana MD, Demonner S, Kerr EA. Comfort of general internists and general pediatricians in providing care for young adults with chronic illnesses of childhood. J Gen Intern Med. 2008;23(10):1621–7.
5. Hunt S, Sharma N. Pediatric to adult-care transitions in childhood-onset chronic disease: hospitalist perspectives. J Hosp Med. 2013;8(11):627–30.
6. Reiss JG, Gibson RW, Walker LR. Health care transition: youth, family, and provider perspectives. Pediatrics. 2005;115(1):112–20.
7. Goodman DM, Hall M, Levin A, et al. Adults with chronic health conditions originating in childhood: inpatient experience in children's hospitals. Pediatrics. 2011;128(1):5–13.
8. Berry JG, Hall M, Hall DE, et al. Inpatient growth and resource use in 28 children's hospitals: a longitudinal, multi-institutional study. JAMA Pediatr. 2013;167(2):170–7.
9. Blaskowitz MG, Hernandez B, Scott PW. Predictors of emergency room and hospital utilization among adults with intellectual and developmental disabilities (IDD). Intellect Dev Disabil. 2019;57(2):127–45.
10. Edwards JD, Houtrow AJ, Vasilevskis EE, Dudley RA, Okumura MJ. Multi-institutional profile of adults admitted to pediatric intensive care units. JAMA Pediatr. 2013;167(5):436–43.
11. Coller RJ, Ahrens S, Ehlenbach ML, et al. Transitioning from general pediatric to adult-oriented inpatient care: National Survey of US Children's hospitals. J Hosp Med. 2018;13(1):13–20.
12. American Academy of Pediatrics, American Academy of Family Physicians, American College of Physicians-American Society of Internal Medicine. A consensus statement on health care transitions for young adults with special health care needs. Pediatrics. 2002;110(Supplement 3):1304–6.
13. de Bont JM, Van Der Holt B, Dekker AW, van der Does-van den Berg A, Sonneveld P, Pieters R. Significant difference in outcome for adolescents with acute lymphoblastic leukemia treated on pediatric vs adult protocols in The Netherlands. Leukemia. 2004;18(12):2032–5.
14. Schafer ES, Hunger SP. Optimal therapy for acute lymphoblastic leukemia in adolescents and young adults. Nat Rev Clin Oncol. 2011;8(7):417–24.
15. Tuchman LK, Schwartz LA, Sawicki GS, Britto MT. Cystic fibrosis and transition to adult medical care. Pediatrics. 2010;125(3):566–73.
16. Viola A, Porter J, Shipman J, Brooks E, Valrie C. A scoping review of transition interventions for young adults with sickle cell disease. Pediatr Blood Cancer. 2021;68(9):e29135.
17. Peter NG, Forke CM, Ginsburg KR, Schwarz DF. Transition from pediatric to adult care: internists' perspectives. Pediatrics. 2009;123(2):417–23.
18. Schwartz LA, Hamilton JL, Brumley LD, et al. Development and content validation of the transition readiness inventory item Pool for adolescent and young adult survivors of childhood cancer. J Pediatr Psychol. 2017;42(9):983–94.
19. Stehouwer N, Sawaya A, Shaniuk P, White P. Consultation needs for young adults with intellectual and developmental disabilities admitted to an adult tertiary care hospital: implications for inpatient practice. J Pediatr Nurs. 2021;60:288–92.
20. Lonquich B, Woo J, Stutz M, Agnihotri N, Kuo A. The frontier of transition medicine: a unique inpatient model for transitions of care. J Hosp Med. 2018;13:69–70.
21. Lipsitz LA. Understanding health care as a complex system: the foundation for unintended consequences. JAMA. 2012;308(3):243–4.
22. Dunbar P, Hall M, Gay JC, et al. Hospital readmission of adolescents and young adults with complex chronic disease. JAMA Netw Open. 2019;2(7):e197613.
23. Henke RM, Karaca Z, Jackson P, Marder WD, Wong HS. Discharge planning and hospital readmissions. Med Care Res Rev. 2017;74(3):345–68.
24. Jack BW, Chetty VK, Anthony D, et al. A reengineered hospital discharge program to decrease rehospitalization: a randomized trial. Ann Intern Med. 2009;150(3):178–87.
25. Scal P. Transition for youth with chronic conditions: primary care physicians' approaches. Pediatrics. 2002;110(6 Pt 2):1315–21.
26. Kim YY, Gauvreau K, Bacha EA, Landzberg MJ, Benavidez OJ. Resource use among adult congenital heart surgery admissions in pediatric hospitals: risk factors for high resource utilization and association with inpatient death. Circ Cardiovasc Qual Outcomes. 2011;4(6):634–9.
27. Kogon BE, Plattner C, Leong T, et al. Adult congenital heart surgery: adult or pediatric facility? Adult or pediatric surgeon? Ann Thorac Surg. 2009;87(3):833–40.

28. Jamerson PA, Graf E, Messmer PR, et al. Inpatient falls in freestanding children's hospitals. Pediatr Nurs. 2014;40(3):127–35.
29. Sanderson A, Hall AM, Wolfe J. Advance care discussions: pediatric clinician preparedness and practices. J Pain Symptom Manag. 2016;51(3):520–8.
30. Conway-Habes EE, Herbst BF, Herbst LA, et al. Using quality improvement to introduce and standardize the National Early Warning Score (NEWS) for adult inpatients at a children's hospital. Hosp Pediatr. 2017;7(3):156–63.

# Contact with Primary Care Providers

# 51

Susan Hunt and Jenn Azen

## Introduction

Medical advances in care for childhood conditions have resulted in rising numbers of young adults with these chronic conditions, who are shown to have high hospital utilization and costs compared to their peers, both as children and adults [1, 2]. Increased demands on the time of primary care physicians, increasing complexity of inpatient care due to robust use of home health for minor issues, and the growth of hospital medicine-focused physicians mean that the majority of hospitalized patients are no longer cared for by their primary care physician while being inpatient. Particularly in adult-centered settings, the proportion of patients cared for by hospitalists has steadily increased over the last two decades, with nearly 60% of hospitalized adults now cared for by these specialty providers, followed by general internists about 25% of the time and PCPs less than 15% of the time [3, 4]. Overall, inpatient outcomes between those cared for by hospitalists or PCPs are not different, aside from a slightly shorter length of stay in patients on hospitalist services; patient satisfaction with care is also similar [5, 6]. Regardless of these data, patients, especially those with complex medical needs, value the involvement of their trusted PCPs in their inpatient care [7]. Although communication studies have not shown differences in readmission rates or mortality, research has focused on general populations and mainly on communication at the time of discharge, whereas more longitudinal communication may be more appropriate for complex patients [8, 9]. Primary care providers also express frustration with changes made during inpatient stays and confusion about responsibility for follow-up of studies and labs ordered during a hospitalization that do not take into account their input and knowledge of the patient [10, 11]. Finally, communication partnering with primary care providers throughout the hospital stay is a positive step for all parties.

## Determine PCP Status

Establishing whom the adult with chronic childhood conditions considers their primary care provider (PCP) is the first step in communication. Many adults with chronic childhood conditions have already transferred to an adult-oriented provider or may have a PCP with both adult and

S. Hunt (✉)
Departments of General Internal Medicine and Pediatric Medicine, University of Washington Medical Center and Seattle Children's Hospital, Seattle, WA, USA
e-mail: hunts1@uw.edu

J. Azen
Department of General Internal Medicine, University of Washington Medical Center, Seattle, WA, USA
e-mail: azen@uw.edu


A. A. Kuo et al. (eds.), *Care of Adults with Chronic Childhood Conditions*,
https://doi.org/10.1007/978-3-031-54281-7_51

pediatric expertise, such as a family medicine or dual-trained Medicine-Pediatrics provider, and will continue with this well-established provider through their adult years. While transition from pediatric-centered to adult-centered outpatient care is recommended between ages 18–21, a large retrospective health plan survey showed that many young adults are transferred later than age 21 and therefore young adults close to transition age may still view their pediatrician as their PCP [12]. Discontinuity of primary care is a significant concern for young adults with complex needs and gaps often occur at the time of transfer from a pediatric to an adult-oriented PCP; the above survey showed a median gap of over a year and a half between last pediatric PCP visit and first adult PCP visit [12]. Disjointed care can also result from retirement of a prior provider or loss to follow-up brought on by insurance changes or moves.

While transition from pediatric to adult care is ideally completed in the outpatient setting, for young adults who do not have an identified PCP or are in need of transition to a new provider, the inpatient stay presents an opportunity to identify someone appropriate for continuing care. Discussing the patient's conditions and specific medical needs with the new provider or their medical team prior to discharge, at the time of referral, is especially important for adults with chronic childhood conditions to ensure that the needed services are available prior to their first new PCP visit. For example, adults with cerebral palsy or spina bifida who are wheelchair users need a clinic that has rooms and scales that can accommodate them. Providing the admission note or discharge summary is important but not sufficient; two-way communication is ideal to confirm that needs can be met.

Once the PCP, or future PCP, has been identified, determining which aspects of care they manage is the next step. Adults with complex needs may seek care from a combination of specialists in conjunction with their PCP; for example, a young adult with neurogenic bladder who uses straight catheterization may have her catheter supplies written by her urologist, but seek treatment for standard UTIs from her PCP. Pediatric care for complex illness is often more subspecialty-driven than in adult care, so for patients who are transferring, or have recently transferred, to adult providers, discussing the expected shift of their "medical home" to primary care can ease tensions with new providers and prevent delays in meeting care needs [13, 14]. Many issues which may have required prolonged admission in a pediatric hospital can shift to outpatient management earlier with strong adult outpatient care, such as home IV antibiotics for cystic fibrosis exacerbations. Items that are often shifted from pediatric subspecialty care to PCPs in adult care include treatment for issues more common in adults, such as hypertension and family planning, as well as paperwork, nutrition support, and majority of prescription refills. In communicating with inpatient providers, PCPs desire clarity on specific roles and responsibilities following discharge [10, 11].

## Communication Method

Preferred communication method may vary between providers, but methods that offer opportunity for two-way discussion between the inpatient provider and PCP should be prioritized. Traditionally, a phone conversation is the most efficient and effective mode of communication with a PCP, but the rapid growth of shared electronic medical records has also allowed for efficient discontinuous communication that can adapt to busy provider schedules while still allowing provider dialogue [15]. Communication preferences can vary among PCPs and initial outreach should establish the preferred method. If phone calling is pursued, reaching out early in the day allows the most opportunity for connection. As PCPs are often difficult to reach directly when seeing clinic patients, leaving a detailed message with the provider team includes specific questions and a direct number or pager can increase the efficiency of a return call during a break in their day. Hospital systems may employ standardized outreach to remove the initial contact burden from inpatient physicians, increasing successful contacts [16]. When secure email is available, this can be a reasonable alternative, but many providers will not regularly check this during their workday and nonsecure servers should not be used due to the need to protect patient information. Faxed communications are often lost among the increasing amounts of paperwork in primary care offices, leading to a considerable delay in communication.

## Early Communication

As young adults with chronic childhood conditions move to adult care, their PCP typically becomes their most visited medical provider and the knowledge of baseline needs and health provides valuable insight to inpatient care. Contacting the PCP within 24 h of admission can provide background for baseline level of health, recent medication adjustments, or other events that led to the admission [17]. Early communication can also help establish availability of outpatient services which may help shape initial care recommendations and result in shorter hospital stays, particularly in adults with significant medical complexity and technology dependence. For instance, a patient with quadriplegia on mechanical ventilation who presents with new fever and initial workup showing a sacral wound and chest X-ray with pulmonary infiltrate. Early discussion with the PCP reveals that the wound is recently worsening, whereas the pulmonary infiltrate is chronic and he did not have any pulmonary symptoms prior to presentation, narrowing the differential and allowing targeted antibiotics for the wound. Furthermore, the PCP relates that the patient can receive IV antibiotics and wound care in his home environment since he lives in a group home with 24-h nursing care, thus shortening his inpatient stay by days through a brief initial conversation. Early communication with the PCP can also build trust between inpatient providers, who are typically new to the patient, and the patient by assuring them their medical context is appreciated.

## Collaborative Care Planning

In addition to medical background, patients with significant mental health or behavioral concerns benefit from inpatient behavioral care planning with the PCP, particularly those with intellectual and developmental disabilities who can have distress in unfamiliar situations resulting in behavioral issues and resistance to care [18].

Direct communication can help develop strategies for least restrictive methods of behavioral management that ease patient comfort and safety, such as having parent or caregiver stay with the patient, how patient prefers explanations of care, and clustering of interventions.

Understanding limitations of outpatient follow-up that contribute to admissions and may be addressed during the acute hospital stay is another benefit of early and ongoing PCP communication. Expediting evaluations or studies that are complicated to obtain as an outpatient or adjacent to the reason for admission, can improve care and prevent recurrent admissions for unaddressed needs. The outpatient environment is a more complex landscape for medically complex young adults, many of whom require wheelchair transport and caregiver support to complete diagnostic testing [19]. A urinary tract infection in a patient with a chronic indwelling catheter for neurogenic bladder, for example, may be related to a chronic issue with sediment or stones that could be assessed during admission, rather than awaiting scheduling of follow-up imaging, often weeks after discharge. Patients with intellectual disability may require sedation for procedures; if a sedated procedure is planned during the current hospitalization, coordination of other needed painful procedures such as blood draws or imaging during that event can reduce anesthesia events for the patient and advance needed workup for the PCP. Similarly, studies such as a 24-h urine collection and timed lab or imaging studies that require fasting or special preparation (such as bowel prep) can be completed seamlessly in the hospital, but require significant coordination in the outpatient setting. Such consolidation of care is commonly accommodated in a pediatric care setting, but less often used in adult settings.

Inpatient stays also present an opportunity to access ancillary services that are sparser in the outpatient realm, such as wound care, nutrition, and physical and occupational therapy consultations. Primary care providers may be limited in their ability to fully evaluate wounds in the office if they have difficulty with physically transferring adults with physical disabilities, such as cerebral palsy. Nutritional assessments are more limited in adult outpatient care due to insurance limitations on coverage and outpatient providers may have less experience with the concurrent complexity of chronic illness or special situations such as supplemental formulas or tube feeding. Physical and occupational therapy can be particularly important for patients with baseline limitations which may be contributing to hospital admission, such as improperly fitted orthotics leading to wounds. Discussing utility of engaging these services with the PCP can set patients and their outpatient team up for success as they progress toward discharge.

## Discharge Preparation

Communication surrounding discharge is essential for successful transition to outpatient care and adults with chronic childhood conditions may have special situations that require additional planning.

When formulating a final medication and treatment regimen, it is important to consider the home environment of the medically complex young adult. Most young adults with chronic childhood disease live and manage their care independently, but may still need special attention with regard to medication adjustments and treatment schedules during discharge planning. Reviewing a typical daily schedule is essential in developing a medication schedule that will work with the patient's unique sleep cycle, work schedule, and school schedule [20, 21]. Many young adults struggle with complex medication schedules which can lead to nonadherence and recurrent admissions [22]. PCPs will need updates about medication timing to appropriately manage care, including lab draws for drug levels, such as immunosuppressive trough testing in transplant patients.

Adults who have significant physical disability or concurrent intellectual disability may have specialized home situations such as family caregiving support, in-home nurse delegated care, or a formal supported living situation such as an adult family home placement [23]. Discharge plans should include the home care team to ensure caregiver comfort and availability to comply with any changes in home treatment or procedures as availability of nurse-delegated caregivers may be limited and new procedures, such as new subcutaneous injections for insulin or anticoagulation, may require additional training. Patients in fully supported situations with 24-h nursing assistance may have fewer limitations; however, these situations may require additional paperwork including resumption of home care and equipment orders or updating medical and/or behavioral care plans. Any changes to such orders should be discussed with the PCP in a way that allows questions and closed-loop communication on any further steps that must be completed as an outpatient, including who will confirm changes or orders that will not be completed until after the patient arrives home. Young adults in extended schooling and day programs may also require paperwork for administering medications at school; ensuring the PCP is aware of any new needs can avoid missed doses.

Any discharge that involves controlled substances, such as opiates, should ensure that the amounts, discharge prescriptions, and follow-up plan are clearly discussed with the PCP prior to returning home. These medications are highly regulated in the outpatient setting and understanding home supply and next appointment with prescribing doctor is essential to avoid lapses in the prescription and provide consistent care between the inpatient and outpatient settings.

Adults with chronic childhood conditions who have technological dependence, such as feeding by tube, respiratory equipment such as suction, oxygen, or ventilation support (noninvasive or via tracheostomy), or mobility devices, should have their equipment needs reviewed and communicated to the PCP at the time of discharge. Technology-dependent adults are a small subset of all those with childhood conditions, but are disproportionately represented in hospitalized populations; surveys indicate children with these levels of complexity frequently experience challenges after hospital discharge related to their technology and medication needs [24]. Proactively addressing these needs with the PCP can help reduce caregiver strain, but the complexity of the discharge itself sometimes limits inpatient physician outreach [25]. Home equipment can be challenging to obtain as an outpatient due to regulations and required documentation, an area that inpatient therapy consults may be held expedite.

## Conclusion

Adults with chronic conditions since childhood are a high-risk population both during hospitalization and following discharge. Early and longitudinal involvement of continuity primary care providers through closed-loop communication provides insight into inpatient management and helps smooth transition to outpatient care on discharge. Inpatient providers should be aware of discharge location and equipment needs to facilitate outpatient transition.

## References


1. Berry JG, Poduri A, Bonkowsky JL, Zhou J, Graham DA, Welch C, Putney H, Srivastava R. Trends in resource utilization by children with neurological impairment in the United States inpatient health care system: a repeat cross-sectional study. PLoS Med. 2012;9(1):e1001158.
2. O'Leary JM, Siddiqi OK, de Ferranti S, Landzberg MJ, Opotowsky AR. The changing demographics of congenital heart disease hospitalizations in the United States, 1998 through 2010. JAMA. 2013;309(10):984–6.
3. Linenauer PK, Rothberg MB, Pekow PS, Kenwood C, Benjamin EM, Auerback AD. Outcomes of care by hospitalists, general internists, and family physicians. N Engl J Med. 2007;357:2589–600.
4. Stevens JP, Nyweide DJ, Maresh S, Hatfield LA, Howell MD, Landon BE. Comparison of hospital resource use and outcomes among hospitalists, primary care physicians, and other generalists. JAMA Intern Med. 2017;177(12):1781–7.
5. Okumura MJ, Campbell AD, Nasr SZ, Davis MM. Inpatient health care use among adult survivors of chronic childhood illnesses in the United States. Arch Pediatr Adolesc Med. 2006;160:1054–60.
6. Seiler A, Visintainder P, Brzostek R, Ehresman M, Benjamin E, Whitcomb W, Rothberg MB. Patient satisfaction with hospital care provided by hospitalists and primary care physicians. J Hosp Med. 2012;7(2):131–6.
7. Rieger EY, Kuschner JNS, Sriram V, Klein A, Wiklund LO, Meltzer DO, Tang JW. Primary care physician involvement during hospitalisation: a qualitative analysis of perspectives from frequently hospitalized patients. BMJ Open. 2021;11(12):e05378.
8. Bell CM, Schnipper JL, Auerback AD, Kaboli PJ, Wetterneck TB, Gonzales DV, Arora VM, Zhang JX, Meltzer DO. Association of communication between hospital-based physicians and primary care providers with patient outcomes. J Gen Intern Med. 2009;24(3):381–6.
9. Oduyebo I, Lehmann CU, Pollack CE, Durkin N, Miller JD, Mandell S, Ardolino M, Deutschendorf A, Brotman DJ. Association of self-reported hospital discharge handoffs with 30-day readmissions. JAMA Intern Med. 2013;173(8):624–9.
10. Jones CD, Vu MB, O'Donnell CM, Anderson ME, Patel S, Wald HL, Coleman EA, DeWalt DA. A failure to communicate: a qualitative exploration of care coordination between hospitalists and primary care providers around patient hospitalizations. J Gen Intern Med. 2015;30(4):417–24.
11. Solan LG, Sherman SN, DeBlasio D, Simmons JM. Communication challenges: a qualitative look at the relationship between pediatric hospitalists and primary care providers. Acad Pediatr. 2016;16(5):453–9.
12. Wisk LE, Finkelstein JA, Sawicki GS. Predictors of timing of transfer from pediatric-to adult-focused primary care. JAMA Pediatr. 2015;169(6):e150951.
13. Gray W, Dorriz P, Kim H, Zupanc M, Grant K, Weiss M. Adult provider perspectives on transition and transfer to adult care: a multi-specialty, multi-institutional exploration. J Pediatr Nurs. 2021;59:173–80.
14. Antonelli RC, Tille C, Freeman LC. Enhanced collaboration between primary and subspecialty care providers for children and youth with special health care needs. http://gucchd.georgetown.edu/commcan.html.
15. Munchof A, Gruber R, Lane KA, Bo N, Rattray NA. Beyond discharge summaries: communication

preferences in care transitions between hospitalists and primary care providers using electronic medical records. J Gen Intern Med. 2020;35(6):1789–96.
16. Enzinger L, Dumanoir P, Boussat B, Couturier P, Francois P. Direct phone communication to primary care physician to plan discharge from hospital: feasibility and benefits. BMC Health Serv Res. 2021;21(1):1352.
17. Zackoff MW, Graham C, Warrick D, Pulda K, Gosdin C, Simpson B, Marischen J, Bunch P, Vossmeyer M, Mussman GM. Increasing PCP and hospital medicine physician verbal communication during hospital admissions. Hosp Pediatr. 2018;8(4):220–6.
18. Stehouwer N, Sawaya A, Shaniuk P, White P. Consultation needs for young adults with intellectual and developmental disabilities admitted to an adult tertiary care hospital: implications for inpatient practice. Pediatr Nurs. 2021;60:288–92.
19. Langmaid L, Ratner L, Huysman C, Curran S, Uluer A. Supporting the medically fragile: individualized approach to empowering young adults with chronic disease during the COVID-19 pandemic. J Adolesc Health. 2020;67(3):453–5.
20. Leppin AL, Montori VM, Gionfriddo R. Minimally disruptive medicine: a pragmatically comprehensive model for delivering care to patients with multiple chronic conditions. Healthcare (Basel). 2015;3(1):50–63.
21. Dunbar P, Hall M, Gay J, Hoover C, Markam JL, Bettenhausen JL, Perrin JM, Kuhlthau KA, Crossman M, Garrity B, Berry JG. Hospital readmission of adolescents and young adults with complex chronic disease. JAMA Netw Open. 2019;2(7):e197613.
22. Leppin AL, Gionfriddo MR, Kessler M, Pablo Brito J, Mair FS, Gallacher K, Wang Z, Erwin PJ, Sylvester T, Boehmer K, Ting HH, Murad MH, Shippee ND, Montori VM. Preventing 30-day hospital readmission: a systematic review and meta-analysis of randomized trials. JAMA Intern Med. 2014;174(7):1095–107.
23. Woodman AC, Mailick MR, Anderson KA, Esbensen AJ. Residential transitions among adults with intellectual disability across 20 years. Am J Intellect Dev Disabil. 2014;119(6):496–515.
24. Musial A, Butts B, Loechtenfeldt A, Herrmann LE, Schmidlin E, Kelley J, Hail T, White CM, Thomson J. Challenges following hospital discharge for children with medical complexity. Hosp Pediatr. 2020;10(6):531–6.
25. Rush M, Herrera N, Melwani A. Discharge communication practices for children with medical complexity: a retrospective chart review. Hosp Pediatr. 2020;10(8):651–6.

# Care in the Emergency Department

52

Colby Feeney, Niraj Sharma, and Priya Jain

## Case

Alex is a 19-year-old male with X-linked adrenoleukodystrophy who presents to your emergency department (ED) with a new oxygen requirement and increased secretions. He is nonverbal and has limited ability to communicate or move his face or body. He arrives with his mother, who is his full-time caregiver. He has a tracheostomy and typically only uses a heat moisture exchanger. He is now requiring 4 L of oxygen per minute to maintain oxygen saturations >90%. The patient's mother explains that she has been suctioning thick, white secretions from his tracheostomy every 30–60 min over the last 24 h. He is tolerating both feeds and medications through his gastrostomy tube. Height and weight are not obtained as the patient is in a wheelchair and unable to stand on the scale. Prior bed weight is 45 kg.

## Epidemiology

Young adults use acute care services, including the emergency department, more frequently, than children or older adults [1]. There are many reasons why young adults may prefer to use acute care services over routine care. Young adults may not have a primary care doctor or may have fallen out of care completely. It is estimated that following the Affordable Care Act in 2010, only about half of young adults sought routine care [2]. When they do become ill, young adults are left seeking care at urgent care clinics or EDs. Early adulthood is also a time of changing financial support, and with that, they often experience lapses in health insurance. Young adults may be between jobs or currently employed without the benefit of health insurance. Key ages that youths age out of Medicaid (19 years old) or coverage under their parental caregivers (26 years old) are often unanticipated by patients and unaddressed proactively by the healthcare team or family. In fact, young adults are the most likely age group to be uninsured, with up to one third lacking insurance [3]. Lack of health insurance coverage

C. Feeney (✉)
Duke University Hospital, Durham, NC, USA

Departments of Medicine and Pediatrics, Duke University School of Medicine, Durham, NC, USA
e-mail: colby.feeney@duke.edu

N. Sharma
Department of Medicine, Brigham and Women's Hospital, Boston, MA, USA

Department of Pediatrics, Boston Children's Hospital, Boston, MA, USA

Harvard Medical School, Boston, MA, USA
e-mail: nsharma@bwh.harvard.edu

P. Jain
Department of Pediatrics, Ann and Robert H. Lurie Children's Hospital of Chicago, Chicago, IL, USA

Northwestern University Feinberg School of Medicine, Chicago, IL, USA
e-mail: pgjain@luriechildrens.org


A. A. Kuo et al. (eds.), *Care of Adults with Chronic Childhood Conditions*,
https://doi.org/10.1007/978-3-031-54281-7_52

results in young adults seeking acute care services when they are ill.

Similarly, children with medical complexity use emergency services more than their peers, accounting for up to 20% of emergency visits at some pediatric EDs. When they do present to the ED, they have a higher odd of being admitted to the hospital and to the intensive care unit (ICU) [4]. Young adult patients with chronic pediatric disorders are unique in that they may choose to present to either pediatric or adult EDs. These patients may account for almost half of the adults seen in a pediatric emergency room [5]. Patients who are younger, have technology-dependence, and have multiple complex chronic conditions are more likely to seek care in pediatric EDs [6]. When transitional-aged patients present for care at pediatric EDs, they almost always undergo diagnostic procedures and are twice as likely to be admitted and 4.5 times more likely to require ICU admission compared to other pediatric patients [5].

More than 90% of visits of transitional-aged patients occur in general EDs. Interestingly, patients are admitted at similar rates, regardless of the type of ED from which they receive care [6]. The patient described in the case, Alex, would be more likely to present to a pediatric ED given his age, tracheostomy-dependence, and having multiple chronic conditions. Emergency providers may not be well-versed in X-linked leukodystrophy, especially if at a general ED. However, they still need to understand the special considerations when caring for young adults with chronic childhood disease.

## Triage Special Considerations

Adult patients with chronic childhood conditions have a number of special considerations that should be acknowledged at the time of triage. First, it is important to note if the patient's weight and size are more consistent with adult sizing or pediatric sizing. For those patients who are pediatric-sized, it is crucial to determine if size- or age-based norms for vital signs are more appropriate. For example, an adult-aged patient who is child-sized due to short stature skeletal dysplasia should still be expected to have age-appropriate blood pressure, while an adult-aged patient who is child-sized due to their underlying chromosomal disorder may be more likely to have size-appropriate blood pressure. Given these disease-specific considerations, it is often helpful for triaging providers to compare current vital signs to prior measurements and to take current vital signs in context with the clinical presentation. Additionally, it is important to remember that subtle vital sign changes may be the only indicator that the patient is acutely ill, particularly in those patients who cannot communicate due to significant neurologic insult or those who are technology-dependent.

Triaging providers should take special note of even subtle mental status or behavioral changes from baseline that are reported by the patient or caregiver. Similar to vital sign changes, these alterations from baseline that are noted by a caretaker who knows the patient well may be the only signal that the patient is feeling pain or ill. Triaging providers should also be aware of the presence of indwelling medical equipment including central lines, ventriculoperitoneal shunts, or other tubes and lines that place the patient at increased risk for infection, including sepsis [7].

Finally, it is imperative that medical providers be aware that because of their underlying medical conditions, patients with chronic childhood conditions may be at higher risk for complications and significant acute events as compared to healthy patients of the same age. For example, young adult patients (ages 25–35) with achondroplasia have a 10 times higher risk of heart disease-related mortality as compared to the general population [8], while patients with nephrotic syndrome have an 8 times higher risk of venous thromboembolism as compared to an age- and sex-matched general population [9].

By understanding how to appropriately interpret a patient's vital signs, being aware of how the patient's current presentation differs from their baseline, and taking into consideration any risk factors the patient may have due to their medical history and indwelling medical equipment, these adult patients with chronic childhood conditions can be appropriately triaged, their level of illness quickly recognized, and high-quality care delivered in a timely fashion.

## Care Plans

A care plan is an individualized plan created to meet a patient's acute or chronic needs. It can be a useful tool for both pediatric and adult patients and is typically created for patients with high utilization, complex medical or social needs, or need for intricate care coordination. Applying care plans in the ED has been shown to reduce ED visits of patients with high utilization [10] and may improve patient and staff satisfaction [11] and patient's self-management of their disease [12].

Care plans can be extremely useful for young adults with complex diseases. For example, for patients with sickle cell disease presenting to the ED with pain, a care plan may outline initial opioid dosing, adjuvant pain medications to be used, and recommendations on starting doses on patient-controlled analgesia (PCA) pumps. For a patient with a metabolic disorder presenting to the ED with vomiting or lethargy, a care plan may outline specific laboratory diagnostics and immediate interventions to be taken to prevent worsening metabolic crisis.

In Alex's case, an individualized care plan may include home respiratory settings, information about previous infections to guide antibiotic therapy, or even a more nuanced approach to how the patient typically presents with recurrent tracheitis or pneumonia. Review of the care plan should be incorporated into taking a patient's history. Instead of having to review a lengthy chart of all previous hospitalizations, it provides a succinct summary and plan based on prior encounters. For rare diseases, it may communicate the special needs of the patient to the provider who otherwise may be unfamiliar with them.

Care plans should serve as guides rather than strict prescriptions for care. Clinicians should use their own clinical judgment to deviate from the care plan when needed. However, the majority of the time, care plans will be helpful road maps for clinicians. We have also found it to be a useful communication tool, providing information that caregivers may not be able to easily recall. It can also help to build trust that a patient will receive a certain approach to their care, no matter the provider. In this way, patients and caregivers may be more satisfied with their care when they receive a standardized, yet individualized, approach consistently across multiple encounters. In our experience, care plans can help to reduce anxiety of the patient or caregiver regarding whether they will receive the care they need. Finally, providing a copy of the care plan to the patient in order to make it available across health systems may aid future providers who are unfamiliar with the patient.

## Location of care

After initial triage and the medical screening exam are completed , the next decision is whether the patient should continue to be cared for in the general ED or would be better served in a dedicated pediatric specialty center. This decision should ideally be made in conjunction with the patient's caregiver and consider a number of factors.

The first consideration is if the current facility has the medical providers and the equipment required to adequately care for the patient. Medical providers, including nurses, respiratory therapists, mid-level providers, and physicians, should be trained to not only provide medical care, but also to perform any necessary diagnostic studies and/or procedures for the chronically ill patient. Particularly in situations in which the patient is pediatric-sized or has physical limitations, appropriately sized and specialized equipment may be required and should be readily available.

If the decision is made to care for the patient in the general ED, determining where to admit the patient should they require it, warrants special consideration. Similar to the ED, the inpatient unit must have the appropriate staff and equipment to care for the patient.

When considering disposition from the ED, the needs and desires of the patient and any caretakers of these adults with chronic childhood conditions should be taken into account. On one hand, the patient or their caretaker may already be set up with home health and/or medical equipment and may have the skill set to manage a significant level of care at home. For example, they may already have home monitors, home oxygen, a home ventilator, tube feeds, central lines, and/or access to IV medications. On the other hand, the patient or their caretaker may also have exhausted their capabilities at home—whether in terms of equipment or their ability to keep up with care needs. Providers should recognize the importance of respite for caretakers, taking this into consideration if the needs of the patient are too great for the caretaker at that particular time. For Alex, his caregiver has already been using home equipment to suction the airways and started supplemental oxygen, but he now needs inpatient care for additional respiratory support.

As with all patients seen in the ED, adults with chronic childhood conditions should be discharged with appropriate follow up—whether that be with their primary care physician or subspecialists, either adult or pediatric. Following an ED visit, it is ideal to have the patient follow up with providers who are familiar with their care. Although patients may benefit from eventual transition to adult care services, the transfer itself should be done at a time of medical stability.

## References

1. Fortuna RJ, Robbins BW, Mani N, Halterman JS. Dependence on emergency care among young adults in the United States. J Gen Intern Med. 2010;25(7):663–9.
2. Wong CA, Ford CA, French B, Rubin DM. Changes in young adult primary care under the affordable care act. Am J Public Health. 2015;105(Suppl 5):S680–5.
3. Callahan ST, Cooper WO. Uninsurance and health care access among young adults in the United States. Pediatrics. 2005;116(1):88–95.
4. O'Mahony L, O'Mahony DS, Simon TD, Neff J, Klein EJ, Quan L. Medical complexity and pediatric emergency department and inpatient utilization. Pediatrics. 2013;131(2):e559–65.
5. McDonnell WM, Kocolas I, Roosevelt GE, Yetman AT. Pediatric emergency department use by adults with chronic pediatric disorders. Arch Pediatr Adolesc Med. 2010;164(6):572–6.
6. Murtagh Kurowski E, Byczkowski T, Grupp-Phelan JM. Comparison of emergency care delivered to children and young adults with complex chronic conditions between pediatric and general emergency departments. Acad Emerg Med. 2014;21(7):778–84.
7. Shah S, Smith M, Zaoutis T. Devise-related infections in children. Pediatr Clin N Am. 2005;52(4):1189–208.
8. Wynn J, King TM, Gambello MJ, Waller DK, Hecht JT. Mortality in achondroplasia study: a 42-year follow-up. Am J Med Genet. 2007;143A(21):2502–11.
9. Anderson F Jr, Wheeler H, Goldberg R, Hosmer D, Patwardhan N, Jovanovic B, Forcier A, Dalen J. A population-based perspective of the hospital incidence and case-fatality rates of deep vein thrombosis and pulmonary embolism. The Worcester DVT study. Arch Intern Med. 1991;151(5):933–8.
10. Pope D, Fernandes CMB, Bouthillette F, Etherington J. Frequent users of the emergency department: a program to improve care and reduce visits. CMAJ. 2000;162:1017–20.
11. Pugh L, Duffy L, Stauss M. Patient care plans: an innovative approach to superusers in the emergency department. J Emerg Nurs. 2010;36(4):344–6.
12. Coulter A, Entwistle VA, Eccles A, Ryan S, Shepperd S, Perera R. Personalised care planning for adults with chronic or long-term health conditions. Cochrane Database Syst Rev. 2015;2015(3):CD010523.

# 53 In-Hospital Rapid Responses and Clinical Emergencies

Clement Lee and Niraj Sharma

## General Overview

Occasionally, adult patients are admitted to a children's hospital, either for a chronic childhood disease being managed by pediatricians or in special circumstances like the COVID-19 pandemic that resulted in a shortage of adult hospital beds. Such patients are at risk of in-hospital adult medical emergencies that can be unfamiliar to the unprepared pediatric hospitalist. Successful triage and treatment of these critical problems require certain unique hospital processes to be thoughtfully organized ahead of time.

On a systemic level, most pediatric hospitals do not have the appropriate staffing for adult medical emergencies requiring immediate procedural intervention. For instance, large ischemic strokes may require a neuro-interventional radiologist for thrombectomy and acute coronary syndromes may require an adult interventional cardiologist for stent deployment. Pediatric hospitals treating adult patients should liaise with partner adult hospitals to determine the appropriate teams or personnel to contact should such needs arise. In addition, pediatric hospital pharmacies may lack adult medications (e.g., nitroglycerin) or only carry doses used in pediatrics (e.g., lower doses of epinephrine), so these gaps must be addressed before emergencies occur. Development of specific pathways to address these issues may be beneficial in streamlining care in the event of a medical emergency.

## Acute Ischemic Stroke

Strokes and stroke preparedness are becoming more salient in many children's hospitals. Although not a common occurrence, in-hospital strokes are increasingly described. Historically, there were major delays in stroke diagnosis, with the median time from symptom onset to diagnosis being over 20 hours [1]. In one major academic pediatric hospital's experience, 56 "code stroke" alerts were activated in a span of 5 years, with 45% of the final diagnoses being either a hemorrhagic or ischemic stroke [2]. In another study from the same hospital, 1 in 4 stroke alerts activated in the emergency department resulted in a diagnosis of a stroke [3].

The presence of a protocol for acute strokes may decrease the time to diagnosis for patients and potentially improve outcomes by increasing eligibility for reperfusion therapies. The implementation of stroke protocols in two

C. Lee
Departments of Medicine and Pediatrics, Newton-Wellesley Hospital, Newton, MA, USA

N. Sharma (✉)
Department of Medicine, Brigham and Women's Hospital, Boston, MA, USA

Department of Pediatrics, Boston Children's Hospital, Boston, MA, USA

Harvard Medical School, Boston, MA, USA
e-mail: nsharma@bwh.harvard.edu


A. A. Kuo et al. (eds.), *Care of Adults with Chronic Childhood Conditions*,
https://doi.org/10.1007/978-3-031-54281-7_53

separate networks of children's hospitals was associated with mean times to diagnosis (79 min and 165 min) that were shorter than times reported in literature [3, 4]. After the implementation of a stroke alert system at another children's hospital, the median time to diagnosis was halved from 196 to 82 minutes [1]. A separate study showed no decrease in time to diagnosis after the implementation of a stroke alert system, but inclusion criteria allowed for enrollment of patients with symptoms lasting up to 14 days [5]. These data underscore the potential importance of establishing a "code stroke" pathway in pediatric hospitals, with some evidence that such a pathway can expedite care for patients with an acute stroke.

Recognition of strokes in children and adults is similar, with focal neurologic deficits being the most common presenting symptoms. Limb weakness, sensory deficits, and dysarthria appear to be common symptoms in children experiencing strokes [1]. However, headaches, which are commonly seen in children with strokes (30–40% of cases), may be less prevalent in adults with strokes [6]. A neurologic exam should be performed and documented specifically using the National Institutes of Health Stroke Scale (NIHSS), which exists in different formats for pediatric (age 2–17) and adult patients (age ≥18). Fleeting symptoms or physical exam findings should not reassure physicians, as a transient ischemic attack (TIA) can present with a stuttering course yet portend an imminent acute ischemic stroke (AIS).

The diagnosis of a stroke requires the presence of clinical symptoms in combination with abnormal neuroimaging. If a stroke is suspected, emergent computed tomography (CT) imaging of the head should be performed to exclude an intracranial hemorrhage [7]. The next imaging of choice is usually magnetic resonance imaging (MRI) along with diffusion-weighted imaging (DWI) to assess for ischemia and resultant cytotoxic death leading to abnormal water diffusion in the brain. Additional imaging to assess the patency of intra- and extracranial arteries is often performed, depending on the clinical background and risk factors of the patient. If an emergent MRI cannot be obtained but the patient is stable, options include transferring the patient to an adult hospital with MRI capabilities or empirically managing an ischemic stroke under the guidance of a neurologist.

In adult acute ischemic stroke (AIS) occurring within 4.5 hours of symptom onset, thrombolysis has become standard of care [7]. However, the benefit of thrombolysis is less clear in children. In the experience of one academic hospital, none of the 25 pediatric strokes in a 5-year period were treated with thrombolysis or thrombectomy [2]. Fewer than 10% of pediatric strokes diagnosed in the emergency department were treated with thrombolysis or thrombectomy in another study [3]. In very young children under age 2, thrombolysis is contraindicated due to the lack of safety data on thrombolytic agents and ambiguity in the time of symptom onset [8]. These data demonstrate that pediatricians are probably unfamiliar with thrombolysis and should discuss cases of AIS with an adult neurologist to elucidate candidacy for thrombolysis and/or thrombectomy and inform decisions to transport the patient to an adult hospital.

In addition to thrombolysis or thrombectomy, empiric therapy for AIS may also involve an antiplatelet agent such as aspirin. If brain hemorrhage has been definitively excluded, aspirin at the dose of 300 mg per day can be started [7]. Functional outcomes after a stroke are improved with careful regulation of electrolytes and vital signs. With any facial weakness, there is the risk of involvement of cranial nerves IX and X, so it is prudent to institute nil per os (NPO) status until safe swallowing can be demonstrated. Ultimately, transport to an adult hospital is probably beneficial in most cases where feasible, as management of an adult stroke patient on a dedicated stroke unit has been associated with improved mortality [9].

## Acute Coronary Syndrome

Chest pain is not an uncommon symptom in the pediatric hospital, accounting for up to 1% of pediatric emergency department visits [10].

However, only 1–5% of chest pain in the pediatric population is attributed to cardiac ischemia [11]. Conversely, the probability of an acute coronary syndrome (ACS) is higher in adults presenting with chest pain, with a reported prevalence of up to 10% in certain age groups [12]. Accordingly, chest pain in a patient of adult age presenting to a pediatric hospital deserves special consideration, especially because up to 18% of these visits ultimately result in a diagnosis of cardiac chest pain and 5% may require emergent percutaneous coronary intervention [13]. Alarmingly, one study performed at two pediatric hospitals noted that only 69% of eligible adults received aspirin, an electrocardiogram (EKG) was performed within American Heart Association (AHA)-recommended time intervals less than half of the time, and perhaps most worrisome, only 5% of patients were transferred to an adult hospital within the recommended door-in-door-out time [13].

In the adult patient presenting with chest pain, as in children, evaluation begins with obtaining a history and performing a physical exam. Older adults and women are more likely to present with non-classic features such as shortness of breath and diaphoresis [14]. There is a lower threshold for cardiac evaluation in adult patients due to the higher prevalence of ischemic cardiac disease; such evaluation generally includes performing an EKG and measuring cardiac enzymes. In contrast to the undefined reference intervals for high-sensitivity troponins in the pediatric population, normal ranges for troponins are well-described in adult patients and the measurement of troponins is recommended in the setting of adults presenting with chest pain that could be cardiac in nature [14, 15]. Protocols for obtaining an EKG likely depend on the institution (e.g., physician-obtained vs. technician-obtained), but the general position of lead placement and interpretation of results are similar in children and adults.

The pattern of chest pain, presence of troponin elevation, and type of EKG changes allow for classification of the chest pain syndrome into noncardiac chest pain, stable angina, or ACS. ACS can be further subdivided into unstable angina, non-ST-elevation myocardial infarction (NSTEMI), or ST-elevation myocardial infarction (STEMI), though the adult patient likely needs to be transported to an adult hospital with catherization capabilities for further management regardless of the type of ACS. T-wave inversions (TWI) deserve special mention, as they can be a normal finding in children before adolescence but are rarely normal in the adult patient and may represent prior or ongoing cardiac ischemia.

After confirmation of ACS, priority should be given to transferring the patient to an adult hospital, especially one that has capability to perform percutaneous coronary intervention (PCI), a standard of care for ACS. Prior to transfer, high-dose aspirin (325 mg) can be started, along with nitroglycerin for symptom relief if there is ongoing chest pain. A second antiplatelet agent (e.g., clopidogrel, ticagrelor, or prasugrel) may likely need to be given, but this is often at the discretion of the cardiologist. An anticoagulant in the form of heparin is often started simultaneously, bolused at a dose of 60 units/kg and followed by a continuous infusion at 12 units/kg, with the goal of reaching a partial thromboplastin time (PTT) of 50–70 seconds. If the EKG shows signs of a right-sided myocardial infarction, fluid administration to help with the patient's right ventricular preload may be helpful. A right-sided myocardial infarction is suspected if ST elevations are seen in an inferior distribution, with the ST elevation higher in lead III than in lead II; it is confirmed if right-sided EKG leads capture an ST elevation in the fourth right-sided lead ("V4R").

Paralleling the literature on adult ischemic strokes, it is recommended that adult patients with ACS are admitted to a specialized adult cardiac unit [16]. Superior clinical outcomes in this setting probably reflect a heightened ability to recognize the complications of myocardial infarction, stricter adherence to heparin target doses, and increased referrals for cardiac rehabilitation upon hospital discharge. It is thus critically important that every attempt be made to quickly triage such patients and organize for their transfer to centers where favorable cardiac outcomes may be maximized.

Some additional considerations for certain adults who are transferred to an adult hospital bear mentioning. In patients with chronic childhood illnesses, growth failure is common, and the sizing of endotracheal (ET) tubes may be inappropriately large in an adult hospital. It may be prudent to collaborate with both pediatric and adult anesthesiologists before initiating transfer to ensure that an ET tube of appropriate size is available. Many chronic childhood diseases are also comorbid with intellectual disability; proceduralists should be aware of and comfortable with the nuances of obtaining informed consent in this special population. Finally, childhood illness often makes diagnosing underlying pathologies more complex. Providers of adult patients may need to consider pediatric diseases that are uncommon in their clinical practice. For instance, ACS could be due to radiation cardiotoxicity in a childhood cancer survivor, and AIS could be related to moyamoya disease in those with trisomy 21.

## Prophylaxis of Venous Thromboembolism

Hospitalized adults undergoing medical or surgical treatment are routinely prescribed mechanical or pharmacologic prophylaxis for the prevention of venous thromboembolism (VTE). Thromboembolic events are less common in the pediatric population, but evolving data show that the prevalence is rising in children, with a recent increase of as much as 10% per year [17]. Adolescents seem to be at particular risk due to risk factors such as obesity that they share with adult patients [18]. This worrisome trend calls for pediatric providers to consider VTE prophylaxis in adolescents and adults hospitalized in the pediatric hospital.

In general, risk factors for acute deep venous thrombosis (DVT) or pulmonary embolism (PE) are similar for children as well as adults. Various studies have identified risk factors that include acute conditions (e.g. trauma, infection, central venous catheters), chronic conditions (e.g. obesity, inflammatory bowel disease, acquired or inherited thrombophilia, estrogen-containing contraceptives, malignancy), and historical factors (personal history of VTE) [17, 19]. Risk factors identified in a minority of studies include glucocorticoid use, sickle cell disease, low Glasgow Coma Scale (GCS) score, the use of inotropes, and hyperosmolar therapy. One major difference between hospitalized children and adults is that the former tend to be more mobile, though this is not universal. Some pediatric guidelines suggest that mobile patients do not require VTE prophylaxis [17]. Additionally, the number one risk factor for VTE in children is the presence of a central venous catheter, which is not the case in adults; this may explain why infants, who often require venous catheterization in the setting of prematurity, are a high-risk population [17, 18].

Routine thromboprophylaxis in children appears feasible and safe. In a major academic children's hospital that initiated an algorithm for risk-based thromboprophylaxis, none of the patients enrolled experienced any bleeding [19]. The most commonly recommended mechanical methods of thromboprophylaxis are pneumatic compression boots and graduated compression stockings; the former is preferred, given data in the adult stroke population on superior efficacy [20, 21]. In children with the highest risk of VTE, pharmacologic prophylaxis in the form of unfractionated or low-molecular-weight heparin (LMWH) may be used, as in adults. Dosing varies and is based on the agent used, the age of the patient, and the patient's body mass index (BMI).

Whether thromboprophylaxis in children leads to reduced mortality or morbidity from VTE is currently uncertain. There have been no randomized controlled trials examining this question in the pediatric population, and due to the overall low prevalence of such events, thousands of children will need to be randomized for a trial to be powered adequately [17]. However, there is general agreement among pediatric specialists that high-risk patients should receive VTE prophylaxis while awaiting high-quality evidence to inform this decision. In one survey, up to half of pediatric hospitals have guidelines for thromboprophylaxis in their patients; most do not support universal prophylaxis but adopt a more risk-based approach [22]. Consensus guidelines should be written with consideration of local VTE risk factors and preferably within committees including pediatric hospitalists, critical care specialists, hematologists, nurses, and pharmacists.

## References


1. Harrar DB, Salussolia CL, Kapur K, Danehy A, Kleinman ME, Mannix R, et al. A stroke alert protocol decreases the time to diagnosis of brain attack symptoms in a pediatric emergency department. J Pediatr. 2020;216:136–141.e6.
2. Barry M, Le TM, Gindville MC, Jordan LC. In-hospital pediatric stroke alert activation. Pediatr Neurol. 2018;88:31–5.
3. Ladner TR, Mahdi J, Gindville MC, Gordon A, Harris ZL, Crossman K, et al. Pediatric acute stroke protocol activation in a children's hospital emergency department. Stroke. 2015;46(8):2328–31.
4. Tabone L, Mediamolle N, Bellesme C, Lesage F, Grevent D, Ozanne A, et al. Regional pediatric acute stroke protocol: initial experience during 3 years and 13 recanalization treatments in children. Stroke. 2017;48(8):2278–81.
5. Shack M, Andrade A, Shah-Basak PP, Shroff M, Moharir M, Yau I, et al. A pediatric institutional acute stroke protocol improves timely access to stroke treatment. Dev Med Child Neurol. 2017;59(1):31–7.
6. Evans RW, Mitsias PD. Headache at onset of acute cerebral ischemia. Headache J Head Face Pain. 2009;49(6):902–8.
7. Powers WJ, Rabinstein AA, Ackerson T, Adeoye OM, Bambakidis NC, Becker K, et al. Guidelines for the early management of patients with acute ischemic stroke: 2019 update to the 2018 guidelines for the early management of acute ischemic stroke: a guideline for healthcare professionals from the American Heart Association/American Stroke Association. Stroke. 2019;50(12):211. https://doi.org/10.1161/STR.0000000000000211.
8. Elbers J, Wainwright MS, Amlie-Lefond C. The pediatric stroke code: early management of the child with stroke. J Pediatr. 2015;167(1):19–24.e4.
9. Warner JJ, Harrington RA, Sacco RL, Elkind MSV. Guidelines for the early management of patients with acute ischemic stroke: 2019 update to the 2018 guidelines for the early management of acute ischemic stroke. Stroke. 2019;50(12):3331–2.
10. Selbst SM. Approach to the child with chest pain. Pediatr Clin N Am. 2010;57(6):1221–34.
11. Drossner DM, Hirsh DA, Sturm JJ, Mahle WT, Goo DJ, Massey R, et al. Cardiac disease in pediatric patients presenting to a pediatric ED with chest pain. Am J Emerg Med. 2011;29(6):632–8.
12. Hsia RY, Hale Z, Tabas JA. A national study of the prevalence of life-threatening diagnoses in patients with chest pain. JAMA Intern Med. 2016;176(7):1029.
13. Sacks JH, Flueckiger PB, Spandorfer PR, Mahle WT, Costello BE. Adult chest pain in the pediatric emergency department: treatment and timeliness from door in to door out. Pediatr Emerg Care. 2017;33(11):740–4.
14. Gulati M, Levy PD, Mukherjee D, Amsterdam E, Bhatt DL, Birtcher KK, et al. 2021 AHA/ACC/ASE/CHEST/SAEM/SCCT/SCMR guideline for the evaluation and diagnosis of chest pain: a report of the American College of Cardiology/American Heart Association Joint Committee on Clinical Practice Guidelines. Circulation. 2021;144(22):1029. https://doi.org/10.1161/CIR.0000000000001029.
15. Clerico A, Aimo A, Cantinotti M. High-sensitivity cardiac troponins in pediatric population. Clin Chem Lab Med (CCLM). 2022;60(1):18–32.
16. Antman EM, Anbe DT, Armstrong PW, Bates ER, Green LA, Hand M, et al. ACC/AHA guidelines for the management of patients with ST-elevation myocardial infarction—executive summary. J Am Coll Cardiol. 2004;44(3):671–719.
17. Faustino EVS, Raffini LJ. Prevention of hospital-acquired venous thromboembolism in children: a review of published guidelines. Front Pediatr. 2017;5:9. https://doi.org/10.3389/fped.2017.00009/full.
18. Andrew M, David M, Adams M, et al. Venous thromboembolic complications (VTE) in children: first analyses of the Canadian Registry of VTE. Blood. 1994;83(5):1251–7.
19. Raffini L, Trimarchi T, Beliveau J, Davis D. Thromboprophylaxis in a pediatric hospital: a patient-safety and quality-improvement initiative. Pediatrics. 2011;127(5):e1326–32.
20. Dennis M, Sandercock P, Reid J, et al. Effectiveness of intermittent pneumatic compression in reduction of risk of deep vein thrombosis in patients who have had a stroke (CLOTS 3): a multicentre randomised controlled trial. Lancet. 2013;382(9891):516–24.
21. Dennis M, Sandercock PA, Reid J, et al. Effectiveness of thigh-length graduated compression stockings to reduce the risk of deep vein thrombosis after stroke (CLOTS trial 1): a multicentre, randomised controlled trial. Lancet. 2009;373(9679):1958–65.
22. Badawy SM, Rychlik K, Sharathkumar AA. Current practice of pharmacological thromboprophylaxis for prevention of venous thromboembolism in hospitalized children: a survey of pediatric hemostasis and thrombosis experts in North America. J Pediatr Hematol Oncol. 2016;38(4):301–7.

# 54 Considerations for Hospitalized Adults with Chronic Childhood Conditions

Madeline Eckenrode and Nicole Oakman

## Introduction

The experience of caring for a hospitalized adult with a chronic condition since childhood can vary widely depending on the patient's age, disease process, age of diagnosis, social support, and physical and cognitive abilities. These are just a few of the many factors that impact inpatient hospitalization of adults with chronic diseases since childhood. Unfortunately, many inpatient settings are not well-equipped to care for these adults. While the national conversation surrounding transition has been growing in recent years, transition programs and discussions of transition of children to adult care often fail to consider the inpatient setting [1].

Data on the pediatric conditions that adult providers may encounter during an inpatient stay are sparse. Despite this, we know that there are tens of thousands of admissions per year of adults with complex conditions since childhood [2]. The most commonly addressed conditions in the literature include cystic fibrosis, type I diabetes, inflammatory bowel disease, spina bifida, and sickle cell disease [3]. Patients with cerebral palsy (CP) also represent a growing group of adult patients. One recent study found that adults with CP access emergency healthcare resulting in admission much more often than pediatric patients with CP and that their length of stay is significantly longer [4].

We also know that a significant number of adult patients will be hospitalized in pediatric centers. In 2011, a study revealed that there were 59,974 adult or transitional patients discharged 119,573 times from 30 children's hospitals surveyed (2.8% of the total number of patients) [5]. Adult hospitalizations are one of the fastest growing categories in pediatric centers. Pediatric providers should therefore be aware of adult-specific concerns, such as prophylaxis for venous thromboembolism and consent.

As more patients with chronic diseases transition to adult care settings, adult providers must be prepared to treat common conditions they may be unaccustomed to witnessing. They also need to consider challenges or barriers to care that are commonly considered by pediatric providers, such as a need for a caregiver at the bedside, size of devices for smaller patients such as masks for noninvasive ventilation, and sensory consider-

Madeline Eckenrode and Nicole Oakman contributed equally with all other contributors.

M. Eckenrode (✉)
Departments of Internal Medicine and Pediatrics, University of Alabama—Birmingham, Birmingham, AL, USA
e-mail: meckenrode@uabmc.edu

N. Oakman
Division of Internal Medicine and Pediatrics, Department of Pediatrics, University of Texas Southwestern Medical Center, Dallas, TX, USA
e-mail: Nicole.oakman@UTSouthwestern.edu


A. A. Kuo et al. (eds.), *Care of Adults with Chronic Childhood Conditions*,
https://doi.org/10.1007/978-3-031-54281-7_54

ations for patients with autism, among other issues. This chapter will address these commonly overlooked challenges in the hospital setting, with a goal of guiding hospital medicine providers towards optimal management of these issues.

## Need for Caregiver Support While Inpatient

Hospital visitation policies between adult and pediatric hospitals often vary significantly. During the COVID-19 pandemic, this has been especially true, as some hospitals placed extreme limitations on visitors. Even during pre-pandemic times, visitation policies at adult hospitals, especially, could be strict, often limiting visitors to certain hours. In critical care settings, this is even more common [6].

This can be extremely detrimental for young adult patients with medical complexity, especially those who are nonverbal and who have cognitive deficits. Visitation policies that are not family-friendly are one of the barriers preventing families and patients from transitioning to adult care. Patients' families express fear that when their child is alone, particularly in a post-procedural setting like the PACU, adverse events may occur [7]. These fears are not unfounded, as many adult providers are less experienced in caring for young adults with medical complexity and may not recognize communication challenges that are often present in this patient population. In pediatrics, it is sometimes taken for granted that parents and guardians are the experts when it comes to their children. Unfortunately, this core value is less recognized in the adult setting [8]. Allowing caregivers access to patients at every reasonable step of their hospital journey is critical for patient safety. This is something that should be addressed at a hospital-wide level.

Communication is not the only arena in which caregivers provide critical support. Making sure that patients receive correct medications, are able to complete their typical personal care regimens (such as intermittent catheterization), assuring that their pain is recognized, and being able to alert care providers to changes in patient conditions are all extremely important [9].

## Difficulty in Obtaining Vital Signs

Obtaining vital signs in patients who are not able to communicate verbally and who may have difficulty controlling their movements can be a formidable task, especially for nursing staff who are not familiar with caring patients with significant disability. Tachycardia and hypertension can sometimes be rationalized as related to a lack of cooperation. While this may be true, adult inpatient providers should be aware that a change in vital signs, particularly tachycardia, is often a sign of pain or distress in a nonverbal patient [10].

If at all possible, inpatient providers should know a patient's baseline vital signs. Vital signs taken at the patient's home or in an outpatient setting are very helpful as a comparator. Additionally, speaking with the nursing staff about the circumstances in which the vital signs were measured can also be helpful. Patients with significant upper extremity spasticity may have pain or discomfort when their arms are extended to take blood pressure, for instance, thus confounding the measurements.

Although continuous vital sign monitoring can be expensive, unavailable, or irritating to patients with developmental disabilities, at times it may be necessary in order to measure heart rate and oxygen saturation in a way that is less disruptive to the patient. If a patient with significant intellectual disability can tolerate monitoring, the continuous measurements can be used to determine whether the patient is only tachycardic when a member of the care team is engaging with him or her, or whether the tachycardia is more continuous, suggesting something like pain, sepsis, etc.

## Medical Device Management in the Inpatient Setting

Implanted medical devices are becoming more common. The devices we commonly associate with the adult population, such as artificial joints, valves, pacemakers, implantable cardioverter defibrillators (ICDs), and spinal cord stimulators, are less frequent in young adults. More common devices include vagus nerve stimulators (VNS) for refractory seizures, insulin pumps for type I diabetes, and intrathecal baclofen pumps for patients with severe spasticity [11]. Asking about implanted medical devices is often part of routine admission screening performed by nurses, but some evidence suggests that devices are often missed and that clinicians are unaware of patients' devices [12].

For patients with a baclofen pump, asking the patient and/or the caregiver about the last time the pump was refilled is helpful. Typically, the pumps are refilled every 1–6 months. While inpatient, the patient may require a refill, which is usually done by anesthesia, neurosurgery, or physical medicine and rehab medical providers. Asking about when a baclofen pump is due to be refilled will help avoid baclofen withdrawal and patient discomfort. Patients with baclofen pumps can usually have magnetic resonance imaging (MRI) performed, but the pump will temporarily turn off during the MRI. After the MRI, it should automatically turn back on, but this may require additional assessment.

For patients with vagus nerve stimulators, the major safety concern in a hospital setting is during MRI. Some MRIs may be safely performed, but consulting with the implanting physician and/or the device manufacturer may be required in order to determine the safety of specific MRI testing. Radiation therapy may also pose a risk, so if a patient is admitted to an inpatient service and is about to receive radiation, a discussion should be made with the neurologist overseeing the VNS about the long-term effects of the radiation therapy on the device effectiveness. Extracorporeal shockwave lithotripsy can also damage the VNS.

As insulin pumps become more common, adult providers and hospitals are gaining more experience with their use in the inpatient setting. By 2018, 30–40% of patients with type I diabetes were using insulin pumps [13], and this number is only growing. Ideally, patients and/or caregivers who are cognitively and physically able to manage their pump during hospitalization should be allowed to do so. This solidifies good habits that are being practiced outside the hospital and also improves glycemic control while patients are hospitalized [14]. For this to happen safely and effectively, hospital staff will need to communicate about the device name, insulin bolus rate, and be aware of common concerns with insulin pumps (such as the kinking of device tubing). If changes need to be made, the care team should discuss these with the patient.

## Device Sizes

Young adults with complex conditions are more likely than their age-matched peers to be underweight. At times, these young adults are extremely underweight [15]. In the pediatric hospital setting, weight and patient-size are considered at every level of care delivery—bed size/type, medication dosing, intravenous (IV) diameter, tube sizes (for nasogastric tube [NG], etc.), and mask size (for noninvasive ventilation). Unfortunately, in the adult acute-care setting, the patient's physical size is not always accounted for in the same way.

While many hospitals are working to make accommodations for the comfort and safety of obese patients, smaller patients, especially those who have physical limitations such as scoliosis and contractures, are often not easily accommodated. Adult hospitals may not stock very small face masks for noninvasive ventilation, small-bore needles for starting IV lines, and small intubation supplies (small blades, tubes). To address this, acute care hospitals could consider collaborations with suppliers or other institutions to ensure that appropriately sized equipment for very small individuals are available and that staff members know how to access these items.

## Hydrocephalus and Shunt

While adult patients without medically complex conditions of childhood may develop hydrocephalus and require central nervous system (CNS) shunt placement, the prevalence of shunted hydrocephalus is more common in patients with chronic childhood conditions. These patients often have a history of extreme prematurity and intraventricular hemorrhage (IVH), CNS malignancy, congenital/genetic forms of hydrocephalus, and spina bifida.

Caring for patients with shunts (most commonly ventriculoperitoneal shunts) requires special knowledge. Complications with shunts, such as infection and mechanical shunt obstruction, are common [16]. It is important for adult providers to be aware of the symptoms that can indicate a shunt malfunction. These can be very subtle, especially in patients who are nonverbal. As in many cases, the parents and/or caregivers of these patients are often the experts. Asking patients and caregivers what the symptoms were of the last shunt malfunction (if any) is a good first step. These may include classic symptoms of increased intracranial pressure, such as headache and vomiting, but can also include symptoms such as fatigue, sleep apnea, difficulty swallowing, and voice changes [17].

Once there is concern for shunt malfunction, consultation with neurosurgery providers is often the best next step. They may recommend additional imaging and determine whether it is necessary to obtain cerebral spinal fluid (CSF) from the shunt to evaluate for infection [17]. Aspiration of CSF from the shunt is not recommended without consultation from a neurosurgeon. Additionally, lumbar puncture in patients with CNS shunts is not recommended without the guidance of a neurosurgical consultant.

## Sensory Considerations

We often associate sensory processing disorders with autism, and indeed, sensory processing issues are a hallmark of autism. However, patients with other conditions, such as cerebral palsy and genetic conditions such as Trisomy 21, may also have sensory processing disorders [18]. The number of patients with these conditions who are becoming adults is increasing, and so addressing sensory processing disorders while patients are in the inpatient setting is advised [19]. Patients with sensory processing problems often have difficulty with new situations from a sensory perspective. Loud sounds (such as beeps from a medication pump), rough or sticky textures (bandages, hospital linen, etc.), and procedures (NG tube placement, IV placement, etc.) can all be very disruptive for these patients. In turn, these problems can lead to decreased cooperation, vital sign abnormalities, and disruptions to the plan of care.

At least one pediatric hospital has developed a pathway to address sensory issues of hospitalized patients. The effort included stakeholder discussions. Parents and patients were asked to identify the most challenging aspects of their hospital experience from a sensory perspective. Staff members were educated about sensory issues and were asked to identify patients who might benefit from the sensory pathway. Finally, patients who were placed on the pathway were assessed by child life, provided with toolkits specific to their sensory need (noise-canceling headphones for patients with auditory sensitivities, for instance), and provided with storyboards particular to their hospitalization experience [18].

Ideally, this level of personalization would be available to all patients regardless of the setting. Adult hospital providers should be aware of sensory issues and advocate for patients to have access to simple, low-cost interventions to help ameliorate them.

## Inpatient Imaging Considerations

Timing of imaging procedures must be carefully considered in most patients with marked intellectual and/or physical disability. These patients may require advanced planning in order for a successful imaging study to be executed [20]. Scans that require patients to be still for prolonged periods of time, such as MRIs, may require sedation. This can require communication with anesthesia teams and advanced planning.

Awareness of the hospital's procedure for adults who require anesthesia for imaging tests is critical. If there is no protocol in place for these situations, it may be beneficial to gather stakeholders from various groups (anesthesia, radiology, critical care medicine, hospital medicine) in order to put protocols into place for patients who may need anesthesia to complete an imaging study.

Airway evaluation and postoperative care are also important components of this planning process. It is more common for adults with developmental delay to experience hypoxemia during and after receiving anesthesia [21]. This may result in a need for increased monitoring.

Other considerations include decreased awareness of anesthesia reactions (because of incomplete histories and patients who are unable to give their own histories) and medical conditions that can make anesthesia administration more complex (such as congenital cardiac defects) [21].

## Pain Assessment and Management in Intellectually Disabled Patients

For patients with intellectual disability or developmental delays, assessing and managing pain during hospitalization may have additional challenges. In particular, for patients who are nonverbal, pain is not easily assessed with traditional methods. Caregivers familiar with the patient may be particularly useful in interpreting a patient's facial expressions or utilizing nonverbal cues to assess the patient's level of pain [22]. This reinforces the need for familiar caregivers to be present at the bedside at all hours. If a caregiver is not available, alternative pain scales based on a patient's behaviors and facial expressions may be utilized, such as the Pediatric Pain Profile (PPP), Noncommunicating Children's Pain Checklist (NCCPC), and Revised Faces Legs Activity Cry Consolability Scale (r-FLACC) [23]. The physical exam is important to help localize the etiology of the pain, including performing an unclothed exam and observing for consistent reproduction of pain symptoms with examination of one area [24]. Nonopioid analgesics such as acetaminophen or nonsteroidal anti-inflammatory drugs (NSAIDs) may be preferred initial therapy in these patients given their increased risk for somnolence with opioids [24].

## Venipuncture and Intravenous Line Placement

For adult patients with chronic childhood conditions, venipuncture and similar minor procedures may lead to heightened anxiety related to prior experiences in childhood [25]. Child life specialists are often readily available in children's hospitals to help prepare patients in a developmentally appropriate manner for intravenous (IV) line placement or venipuncture. These resources may not be easily accessed in the adult setting. In pediatric settings, it is also commonplace to reduce the frequency of venipuncture and to limit lab collection to only necessary studies. For example, for a patient with several pending consults who are likely to request additional labs, a pediatric provider may withhold ordering nonurgent studies until all consultants have submitted their recommendations so that they can be collected simultaneously. While there is overall a movement towards the reduction of unnecessary labs in adult hospital medicine [26], this discrepancy in hospital culture between pediatric and adult settings should be kept in mind particularly for patients accustomed to the pediatric hospital setting, patients with intellectual disability, and those who express anxiety regarding venipuncture. In addition, use of topical anesthetics such as lidocaine or distraction techniques prior to minor procedures may help improve cooperation and success in these patients [27].

## Fluid Management

In the pediatric setting, a patient's weight determines the rate of fluid administration. In the adult setting, there are often standard orders or order sets when IV fluids are being ordered that do not consider a patient's weight. Fluid rates of 100 or 120 milliliters per hour are commonly used. For some smaller patients, these fluid rates may be too rapid for their size. As previously discussed, malnutrition is very common in this patient population [28]. Excessive administration of fluids can lead to pulmonary edema and ileus, worsen acute kidney injury, cause edema in dependent areas increasing risk for pressure injuries, and prolong length of hospitalization due to the need for diuresis, among many other negative sequelae [29]. Similar to other conditions that predispose patients to volume overload, such as congestive heart failure and cirrhosis, adult providers may need to use fluids judiciously in smaller patients. Providers can also calculate the patient's maintenance fluid rate based on weight to avoid fluid overload.

In the United States, no clear guidelines are in place regarding fluid administration. In the United Kingdom (UK), National Institute for Health and Care Excellence (NICE) guidelines were originally published in 2013 to help adult providers consider individual patient factors such as weight and patients' nutritional status when prescribing fluids [30]. The guidelines were updated in 2017 and reviewed in 2020. The NICE algorithms are detailed and could be a helpful resource for individualizing fluids therapy, especially in medically complex young adults.

## Bowel Programs/Management of Constipation

Constipation management is critical in patients with medical complexity, especially in patients who have neurogenic bowel issues, are nonverbal, and who are not ambulatory. Constipation may lead to hospitalization due to discomfort, urinary tract infections, stercoral colitis, and fecal impaction [31]. In addition to the aforementioned issues, constipation can cause behavioral issues, aggression, and self-harm. A Canadian study found that adults with cognitive disability were 7.9 times more likely to be admitted with a problem stemming from constipation than age-matched peers [32].

When patients are admitted to the hospital, inpatient providers should clarify their home bowel regimen. Given that many laxatives are over-the-counter and administered as needed, they may not appear on a formal medication reconciliation list. This often necessitates more direct questioning about medications used for constipation. Similarly, patients may receive interventions such as soap suds enemas that also may not be easily discoverable through an electronic medical record.

It is also important to discuss the success of the bowel regimen, as an inpatient hospitalization (especially if it's related to sequelae of constipation) can be an excellent time to modify or formalize the bowel regimen and for caregiver education. If nutrition support services are available in the hospital, a consultation with a dietitian may be helpful for some patients. The role of nutrition in constipation is well-known, and studies have shown that caregivers of people with disabilities often have a below average knowledge of nutrition [33].

## Weight-Based Dosing and Medication Formulation

Both pediatric and adult providers should be aware of a patient's weight when prescribing medications. Pediatric providers should be wary of utilizing weight-based dosing for adult-sized patients, as this may easily exceed the recommended daily dose. Conversely, underweight patients admitted to adult settings may require weight-based dosing for common medications. Close collaboration with pharmacists is needed to determine if weight-based dosing for enteral or intravenous medications such as antibiotics, narcotics, or anti-seizure medications should be considered [34].

Hospital providers should also consider the route and method of administration when discharging a patient home, including the increased cost of many liquid formulations and potential impracticality of acquiring and administering a large volume of liquid medications [35]. Alternatives to liquid formulations for patients with gastrostomy tubes such as capsules or tablets that can be crushed may be better alternatives to liquid formulations [35].

## Venous Thromboembolism (VTE) Prophylaxis

While consideration of venous thromboembolism (VTE) prophylaxis is commonplace in patients admitted to adult hospitals, use of VTE prophylaxis is less common in pediatric hospitals [36, 37]. Risk scores such as the Padua prediction score [38] or IMPROVE score [39] can help determine the appropriateness and necessity of VTE prophylaxis in adults [40] (Table 54.1). Patients with low-risk scores likely do not require any VTE prophylaxis, while those with high risk may warrant mechanical and/or pharmacologic thromboprophylaxis [40] (Table 54.2). While pharmacologic prophylaxis is preferred for most high-risk patients at low risk of bleeding, current guidelines recommend utilization of mechanical prophylaxis such as intermittent pneumatic compression devices or graduated compression stockings in patients at high risk who have contraindications to pharmacologic prophylaxis [41]. Options for pharmacologic prophylaxis include low molecular weight heparin (LMWH) and low-dose unfractionated heparin [37, 40, 41]. Of note for pediatric providers, weight-based dosing is not typically utilized for adult patients with a normal body mass index (BMI), and the

**Table 54.1** Risk assessment models for venous thromboembolism (VTE) in adult patients

| Padua Prediction Score | | International Medical Prevention Registry on Venous Thromboembolism (IMPROVE-VTE) Score | |
|---|---|---|---|
| Active cancer[a] | 3 | Previous VTE | 3 |
| Previous venous thromboembolism[b] | 3 | Known thrombophilia | 2 |
| Reduced mobility[c] | 3 | Lower limb paralysis | 2 |
| Known thrombophilic condition[d] | 3 | Cancer | 2 |
| Recent (δ1 month) trauma and/or surgery | 2 | Immobilization ε7 days[e] | 1 |
| Elderly age (ε70 years) | 1 | ICU/CCU stay[f] | 1 |
| Heart and/or respiratory failure | 1 | Age >60 years | 1 |
| Acute myocardial infarction or ischemic stroke | 1 | | |
| Acute infection and/or rheumatologic disorder | 1 | | |
| Obesity (BMI ε 30) | 1 | | |
| Ongoing hormonal treatment | 1 | | |

[a] Patients with local or distant metastases and/or receiving chemotherapy or radiation in the past 6 months
[b] Superficial vein thrombosis excluded
[c] Bedrest with bathroom privileges (due to patient limitations or physician orders) for at least 3 days
[d] Known defects of antithrombin, protein C or S, factor V leiden, G20210A prothrombin mutation, antiphospholipid syndrome
[e] Immobilized ε7 days before or after hospitalization
[f] Intensive care unit (ICU) and coronary care unit (CCU)

**Table 54.2** Venous thromboembolism (VTE) risk assessment scoring and suggested intervention

| Padua Prediction Score | | | International Medical Prevention Registry on Venous Thromboembolism (IMPROVE-VTE) Score | | |
|---|---|---|---|---|---|
| Score | Risk assessment | Intervention | Score | Risk | Intervention |
| 0–3 low risk | 0.3% 90-day risk symptomatic VTE | No intervention. Encourage mobilization | 0–2 low risk | 0.4–1% 3-month VTE risk | No intervention. Encourage mobilization |
| ε4 high risk | 11% 90-day risk symptomatic VTE | Assess bleeding risk and consider pharmacologic VTE prophylaxis | ε3 high risk | >1.7% 3-month VTE risk | Assess bleeding risk and consider pharmacologic VTE prophylaxis |

majority of patients require only once daily dosing. In general, serum monitoring of anti-Xa levels is not typically utilized with adult dosing of LMWH [37, 41].

## Independent or Shared Decision-Making/Consent

Assessment of capacity can be challenging for patients with intellectual or physical disability. Similar to patients with altered mental status, assessment of capacity will depend on the patient's understanding of the decision, appreciation of the potential consequences, and ability to communicate a choice [42]. While involvement of a patient's caregiver is often necessary to facilitate medical decision-making, there may be instances where a patient with an intellectual disability can consent for simple interventions [42]. However, patients with mild intellectual disability may be misinterpreted as having decision-making capacity when they lack a clear understanding of the questions being asked, so additional care should be taken to ensure adequate comprehension by the patient. It is reasonable to involve ethics, psychiatry, or social work when the identity or role of the surrogate decision-maker is unclear. Of note, young adult patients with childhood chronic conditions who are developmentally normal may desire to involve their family in the decision-making process regardless of their ability to consent. It is important to offer patients an opportunity to include family and caregivers in important conversations about treatment and prognosis according to their preferences.

## Trainee Education

Many internal medicine trainees report discomfort with caring for adult patients with a history of childhood chronic conditions [43]. Similarly, pediatric providers express a lack of confidence in caring for patients over age 18 with certain conditions [44]. The inpatient setting provides an important opportunity for trainees to gain additional experience in caring for these patients. Therefore, it is important that both adult and pediatric physicians are adequately equipped to manage patients with chronic childhood conditions in order to educate trainees about their care [45].

## Transitions at Discharge

Patients with chronic childhood conditions undergoing transition to adult care may require additional counseling and discharge support. Hospitalization highlights an opportunity to discuss important aspects of chronic care that can have long-term impacts on a patient's health and wellness [46]. For patients nearing 18 years of age who are newly diagnosed with a chronic condition during a pediatric hospitalization, the primary and consulting teams may consider discussions with the patient and family regarding referral to an adult subspecialty clinic as opposed to referral to a pediatric clinic for further care given the patient's age at the time of diagnosis. In addition, for patients admitted to an adult facility who are still seeing their pediatric providers, the inpatient team may offer referrals to adult primary care and specialists to help facilitate the patient's transition based on the patient and family's preferences.

Hospitalization may also be an opportunity to explicitly discuss aspects of the transition that may not have been emphasized in the outpatient setting. For example, many patients with chronic conditions are accustomed to the subspecialty service acting as the primary team during hospitalization. However, this is much less common in the adult setting where patients are often admitted to a hospitalist or general medicine service with the option to consult a subspecialty team. Infrastructure and research to support inpatient transitions is lacking [45–47]. Explicit discussion about the similarities and differences between adult and pediatric care environments may provide greater context to help patients transitioning to adult care [46].

## Conclusion

To date, the focus on transition care for young adults with medical complexity and medical conditions since childhood has mainly been as it relates to the outpatient setting. However, more young adults in this population are being hospitalized every year in both adult and pediatric facilities. Unfortunately, there is a dearth of evidence-based information regarding how to best care for this patient population. Patients and families sense the unpreparedness of most institutions for this transition.

Hospital providers should focus on the ways in which this patient population is unique, including differences in physical size, sensory processing, cognitive or intellectual disability, family and caregiver involvement, and special needs as they relate to medical devices and medication and fluid dosing and administration. With a coordinated effort between hospital administration, nursing staff, pharmacists, and physicians, we can work together to ensure the safe and appropriate care of adults with medical conditions of childhood.

## References


1. Coller RJ, Ehlenbach ML, Shadman KA, Ahrens S, Larocque A, Sheehy A, et al. Transitioning from general pediatric to adult-oriented inpatient care: national survey of US children's hospitals. J Hosp Med. 2018;13(1):13–20.
2. Okumura MJ, Campbell AD, Nasr SZ, Davis MM. Inpatient health care use among adult survivors of chronic childhood illnesses in the United States. Arch Pediatr Adolesc Med. 2006;160(10):1054–60.
3. Dunbar P, Garrity B, Berry JG, Hall M, Markham JL, Bettenhausen JL, et al. Hospital readmission of adolescents and young adults with complex chronic disease. JAMA Netw Open. 2019;2(7):e197613.
4. Morgan P, Enticott J, Nikam R, Tracy J. Profile of hospital admissions for adults with cerebral palsy: a retrospective cohort study. Dev Med Child Neurol. 2020;62(8):939–45.
5. Goodman DM, Levin A, Hall M, Watson RS, Williams RG, Shah SS, et al. Adults with chronic health conditions originating in childhood: inpatient experience in children's hospitals. Pediatrics. 2011;128(1):5–13.
6. Liu V, Read JL, Scruth E, Cheng E. Visitation policies and practices in US ICUs. Crit Care. 2013;17(2):R71.
7. Berkowitz S, Lang P. Transitioning patients with complex health care needs to adult practices: theory versus reality. Pediatrics. 2020;145(6):e20193943.
8. Davidson JE, Powers K, Hedayat KM, Tieszen M, Kon AA, Shepard E, et al. Clinical practice guidelines for support of the family in the patient-centered intensive care unit: American College of Critical Care Medicine Task Force 2004–2005. Crit Care Med. 2007;35:605.
9. Charles ML. Communication experiences of family caregivers of hospitalized adults with intellectual and developmental disabilities—A qualitative study. Nurs Open. 2020;7(6):1725–34.
10. Kildal E, Stadskleiv K, Boysen ES, Øderud T, Dahl I-L, Seeberg TM, et al. Increased heart rate functions as a signal of acute distress in non-communicating persons with intellectual disability. Sci Rep. 2021;11(1):1–8.
11. Saulino M, Ivanhoe CB, McGuire JR, Ridley B, Shilt JS, Boster AL. Best practices for intrathecal baclofen therapy: patient selection. Neuromodulation. 2016;19(6):607–15.
12. Harman MK. 3.1.9. Medical device failure—implant retrieval, evaluation, and failure analysis. In: Wagner WR, Sakiyama-Elbert SE, Zhang G, Yaszemski MJ, editors. Biomaterials science, 4th ed. Academic Press; 2020. p. 1485–1495.
13. Umpierrez GE, Klonoff DC. Diabetes technology update: use of insulin pumps and continuous glucose monitoring in the hospital. Diabetes care 2018;41:1579-1589. Diabetes Care. 2019;42(4):E66–E7.
14. Yeh T, Yeung M, Mendelsohn Curanaj FA. Managing patients with insulin pumps and continuous glucose monitors in the hospital: to wear or not to wear. Curr Diab Rep. 2021;21(2):7.
15. Patusco R, Matarese L, Ziegler J. Body composition in adults with intellectual disabilities: implications for practice. Health Promot Pract. 2018;19(6):884–95.
16. Conforto A, Wagner J. Management of increased intracranial pressure and intracranial shunts. Roberts and Hedges' clinical procedures in emergency medicine and acute care. 7th ed. Elsevier; 2019. p. 1243–1257.
17. Paff M, Alexandru-Abrams D, Muhonen M, Loudon W. Ventriculoperitoneal shunt complications: a review. Interdiscip Neurosurg Adv Techn Case Manag. 2018;13:66–70.
18. Gupta N, Kong M, Brown C, Deneke J, Maha J. Utilization of a novel pathway in a tertiary pediatric hospital to meet the sensory needs of acutely ill pediatric patients. Front Pediatr. 2019;7:367.
19. Carter J, Broder-Fingert S, Neumeyer A, Giauque A, Kao A, Iyasere C. Brief report: meeting the needs of medically hospitalized adults with autism: a provider and patient toolkit. J Autism Dev Disord. 2017;47:1510–29.
20. Perry H, Eisenberg RL, Swedeen ST, Snell AM, Siewert B, Kruskal JB. Improving imaging care for

diverse, marginalized, and vulnerable patient populations. Radiographics. 2018;38(5):1833–44.

21. Chaudhary K, Bagharwal P, Wadhawan S. Anesthesia for intellectually disabled. J Anaesthesiol Clin Pharmacol. 2017;33(4):432–40.
22. Findlay L, Williams ACC, Baum S, Scior K. Caregiver experiences of supporting adults with intellectual disabilities in pain. J Appl Res Intellect Disabil. 2015;28(2):111–20.
23. Barney CCA, Randi D, Defrin R, Genik LM, McGuire BE, Symons FJ. Challenges in pain assessment and management among individuals with intellectual and developmental disabilities. Pain Rep. 2020;5(4):e821.
24. Hauer J, Houtrow AJ. Pain assessment and treatment in children with significant impairment of the central nervous system. Pediatrics. 2017;139(6):e20171002.
25. Turkel S, Pao M. Late consequences of chronic pediatric illness. Psychiatr Clin North Am. 2007;30(4):819–35.
26. Bulger J, Nickel W, Messler J, Goldstein J, O'Callaghan J, Auron M, et al. Choosing wisely in adult hospital medicine: five opportunities for improved healthcare value. J Hosp Med. 2013;8(9):486–92.
27. Slifer KJ, Hankinson JC, Zettler MA, Hendricks MC, Ward CM, Reesman J, et al. Distraction, exposure therapy, counterconditioning, and topical anesthetic for acute pain management during needle sticks in children with intellectual and developmental disabilities. Clin Pediatr. 2011;50(8):688–97.
28. Humphries K, Traci MA, Seekins T. Nutrition and adults with intellectual or developmental disabilities: systematic literature review results. Intellect Dev Disabil. 2009;47(3):163–85.
29. Sansom LT, Duggleby L. Intravenous fluid prescribing: improving prescribing practices and documentation in line with NICE CG174 guidance. BMJ Qual Improv Rep. 2014;3(1):u205899.w2409.
30. Padhi S, Bullock I, Li L, Stroud M. Intravenous fluid therapy for adults in hospital: summary of NICE guidance. BMJ. 2013;347:f7073.
31. Robertson J, Baines S, Emerson E, Hatton C. Constipation management in people with intellectual disability: a systematic review. J Appl Res Intellect Disabil. 2018;31(5):709–24.
32. Balogh R, Brownell M, Ouellette-Kuntz H, Colantonio A. Hospitalisation rates for ambulatory care sensitive conditions for persons with and without an intellectual disability—a population perspective. J Intellect Disabil Res. 2010;54(9):820–32.
33. van Timmeren EA, van der Putten AAJ, van Schrojenstein Lantman-de Valk HMJ, van der Schans CP, Waninge A. Prevalence of reported physical health problems in people with severe or profound intellectual and motor disabilities: a cross-sectional study of medical records and care plans. J Intellect Disabil Res. 2016;60(11):1109–18.
34. Pan SD, Zhu LL, Chen M, Xia P, Zhou Q. Weight-based dosing in medication use: what should we know? Patient Prefer Adherence. 2020:549.
35. Williams NT. Medication administration through enteral feeding tubes. Am J Health Syst Pharm. 2008;65(24):2347–57.
36. Raffini L, Davis D, Trimarchi T, Beliveau J. Thromboprophylaxis in a pediatric hospital: a patient-safety and quality-improvement initiative. Pediatrics. 2011;127(5):e1326–32.
37. Sharma M, Carpenter SL. Thromboprophylaxis in a pediatric hospital. Curr Probl Pediatr Adolesc Health Care. 2013;43(7):178.
38. Barbar S, Noventa F, Rossetto V, Ferrari A, Brandolin B, Perlati M, et al. A risk assessment model for the identification of hospitalized medical patients at risk for venous thromboembolism: the Padua prediction score. J Thromb Haemost. 2010;8(11):2450.
39. Spyropoulos AC, Anderson FA, FitzGerald G, Decousus H, Pini M, Chong BH, et al. Predictive and associative models to identify hospitalized medical patients at risk for VTE. Chest. 2011;140(3):706–14.
40. Skeik N, Westergard E. Recommendations for VTE prophylaxis in medically ill patients. Ann Vasc Dis. 2020;13(1):38–44.
41. Kahn SR, Lim W, Dunn AS, Cushman M, Dentali F, Akl EA, et al. Prevention of VTE in nonsurgical patients: antithrombotic therapy and prevention of thrombosis, 9th ed: American College of Chest Physicians Evidence-Based Clinical Practice Guidelines. Chest. 2012;141(2 Suppl):e195S–226S.
42. Fisher KM, Bhattacharya A, Orkin FK, Green MJ, Chinchilli VM. Proxy healthcare decision-making for persons with intellectual disability: perspectives of residential-agency directors. Am J Intellect Dev Disabil. 2009;114(6):401–10.
43. White PH, Cooley WC. Supporting the health care transition from adolescence to adulthood in the medical home. Pediatrics. 2018;142(5):e20182587.
44. Okumura MJ, Cabana MD, Heisler M, Davis MM, Kerr EA, Demonner S. Comfort of general internists and general pediatricians in providing care for young adults with chronic illnesses of childhood. J Gen Intern Med. 2008;23(10):1621–7.
45. Hunt S, Sharma N. Pediatric to adult-care transitions in childhood-onset chronic disease: hospitalist perspectives. J Hosp Med. 2013;8(11):627–30.
46. Dwyer-Matzky K, Blatt A, Asselin BL, Wood DL. Lack of preparedness for pediatric to adult-oriented health care transition in hospitalized adolescents and young adults. Acad Pediatr. 2018;18(1):102–10.
47. Coller RJ, Ahrens S, Ehlenbach ML, Shadman KA, Mathur M, Caldera K, et al. Priorities and outcomes for youth-adult transitions in hospital care: perspectives of inpatient clinical leaders at US children's hospitals. Hosp Pediatr. 2020;10(9):774–82.

# Part IX

# Sociolegal Aspects of Young Adult Care

# Assessing and Enhancing Psychosocial Functioning

# 55

Daniel J. Coletti and Naomi Kane

## Psychosocial Development and Young Adults with Chronic Childhood Conditions

Young adults with chronic childhood conditions (YACCC) face the same developmental milestones as unaffected peers, and the PCP assesses social development as part of comprehensive care [1]. Some social milestones have clear chronological markers, such as the age-related transfer of decisional capacity from guardian-to-patient at age 18, transitional dates in educational programming (starting college, aging out of special education services), and workforce entry. Most social milestones are processes that emerge over time, however, and are better defined by the *development* of peer and collegial social networks, *growth* towards independence from guardians and the family, and the *emergence* of gender and sexual identity and an interest in intimate relationships. Adolescents with chronic medical conditions also transition into young adulthood coping with the social effects (or late effects) of childhood disease and its treatment [2]. When treatment has required extended school absences, or when motor or communication deficits impair the quantity and quality of peer relationships, illness can *delay* the attainment of social skills and milestones [3]. Conversely, illness can *accelerate* social development—either positively (e.g., when experience interacting with medical providers enhances a patient's abilities to communicate with adults) or in a maladaptive way, when poor social adjustment and self-image fuels experimentation with risky health behaviors (such as substance use) [4]. Finally, social competence and support influence the ways in which young adults handle illness-related stressors. Social skills and well-developed social networks buffer the demands of managing a chronic medical condition, particularly when support from family and peers is perceived conjointly [5–7]. An extensive body of research has identified relationships between social connectedness and enhanced psychological wellbeing [8, 9]. Enhanced social functioning can protect against premature mortality in adulthood [10, 11], perhaps by influencing the inflammatory process [12]. These findings underscore the importance of attending to this aspect of patient functioning early in life for subsequent wellbeing across the lifespan.

Although social impairments in YACCC should not be assumed, it is important to consider the types of problems they are likely to experi-

D. J. Coletti (✉)
Division of General Internal Medicine, Northwell Health, Great Neck, NY, USA
e-mail: dcoletti@northwell.edu

N. Kane
Women's Health Clinic, Department of Psychiatry, VA Ann Arbor Healthcare System, University of Michigan Medical School, Ann Arbor, MI, USA


A. A. Kuo et al. (eds.), *Care of Adults with Chronic Childhood Conditions*,
https://doi.org/10.1007/978-3-031-54281-7_55

ence. The increased caregiving supports that YACCC require during childhood place them at heightened risk of developing dependency on caregivers in adulthood and experiencing social exclusion [13]. YACCC may find that a disproportionate number of their interactions as children and adolescents were with adults rather than similarly aged peers, and less peer contact meant fewer opportunities to develop social skills [14]. In addition, they were more likely to have faced bullying and ostracism from peer groups [15].

Impaired social functioning appears to increase the risk of illness-related distress and physical symptoms [16]. Although relations between illness severity and psychosocial functioning are complex and not always linear, the extent of social isolation may depend on illness severity [17]. For example, patients with moderate levels of illness severity appear to be at greater risk of problems in social functioning. Individuals with mild illness severity—or those with severe illness who are provided supports to help overcome social challenges—show less impact on social development [18]. The likelihood of developing social problems includes the degree to which the condition is visibly recognizable [19] and if the condition involves the central nervous system and impacts motor development [20–23]. The association between degree of motor impairment and psychosocial functioning is more equivocal [24]. In fact, some researchers identify a "disability paradox" or counterintuitive associations between *greater* impairment and *higher* levels of psychosocial satisfaction [25]. Therefore, chronic health conditions may foster resilience as well as vulnerability.

Despite common perceptions that illness-related delays in social development might protect from experimentation with risky substances, YACCC may in fact be more likely than their peers to smoke cigarettes daily, endorse marijuana use, and perform antisocial behaviors (e.g., fighting, vandalism, fire-setting, etc.) [26]. For example, a study of young adults (ages 19–21) with congenital heart defects found that half endorsed alcohol consumption (including binge drinking) in the prior month [27]. Adolescents with chronic conditions are at least as likely as their peers to engage in sexual intercourse or risky sexual behaviors [28, 29]. Moreover, young people with chronic conditions may be more prone to adverse outcomes associated with behavioral experimentation [30]. For example, poor outcomes are identified when patients with childhood asthma smoke tobacco, increasing risk for adult respiratory dysfunction [31]; when unplanned pregnancy creates risks for the young woman and to fetal health [32–34]; and when young persons who are immunosuppressed engage in unprotected sex, they are at an elevated risk of developing STIs [35]. Finally, caution is urged in assuming that pediatric practitioners have adequately screened and addressed these social-mediated risky health behaviors (smoking, alcohol use, sex education) in adolescence, as significant barriers to evaluation in pediatric practice persist [36].

Social problems are also more likely to occur in the presence of socioeconomic or environmental challenges. Patients must often manage a medical condition and its treatment with limited language proficiency [37], low health-care-related skills, inadequate housing, unemployment or low income, or unsafe residential environments [18]. Strong associations between socioeconomic indicators and health status were identified across studies in a recent literature review of research in chronic kidney disease [38]. Finally, socioeconomic indicators, such as parent level of education, can influence the transition process when families lack knowledge and skills to assist their adolescent in preparing for adult-oriented medical care [39].

Perhaps the most significant negative impact on YACCC's social functioning occurs when integrated special education programming services end. Significant declines in social activity and perceived social wellbeing are often observed in young adults when support services end (typically at age 21). Young adults who require high levels of support can experience feelings of loneliness and greater social isolation when they leave school [40]. Forming a social network of peers with similar support needs or experience of illness can enhance social maturity and resiliency [20].

Potential accelerators of perceived social isolation are embedded in the healthcare transition process itself. YACCC often lack the skills to navigate a complex healthcare system with greater independence and less familial involvement [41]. Transition readiness improves over time, but knowledge and self-management skills remain low [42]. Adult transition narratives have common themes of confusion about relationships with providers and feelings of alienation, with patients perceiving the adult healthcare environment to be significantly less engaging and person-centered than pediatric care [43, 44]. A successful healthcare transition may minimize these risks and augment self-efficacy, independence, responsibility, and self-sufficiency [45]. A person-centered approach during the transition process involves understanding the young patient's world, by conveying interest in the patient's social functioning and observing the ways in which the patient interacts with others.

## Assessment of Social Functioning in YACCC

The variable effects of chronic conditions on social functioning underscore the need for individualized assessment of each of the following: the patient's relationship to their illness, the type and severity of functional impairment, the impact of the illness on social wellbeing, and the ways existing social supports facilitate or hinder wellbeing. To identify key areas for investigation, adolescent specialists have described a "Psychosocial Systems Review" where domains to assess correspond to the acronym HEEADSSS (**H**ome environment, **E**ducation and employment, **E**ating, peer-related **A**ctivities, **D**rugs, **S**exuality, **S**uicide/depression, and **S**afety from injury and violence) [46].

A fourth "S" might include "**S**ocial Media" involvement. Even prior to the COVID-19 pandemic, it was estimated that up to 83% of young people aged 18–29 had some online presence, and research suggested that increased social media use in adolescence may be associated with poorer psychosocial functioning [47, 48]. The pandemic has profoundly impacted the nature of social interactions among all youth, including more use of screens and virtually mediated interaction [49]. Participation in social media sites can have enormous positive and negative effects on social wellbeing [50], and emerging evidence suggests that chronic illness-related social media interactions are increasing [51]. Although the ultimate impact of the pandemic on YACCC remains to be ascertained, changes in social interaction including use of electronic/virtual communication modalities are likely to present with both challenges to psychosocial functioning and opportunities for enhancing connectedness for YACCC [52].

Optimal assessment integrates both formal (e.g., questionnaires, interviews, etc.) and informal (semi-structured questioning and observation) strategies to assess the social functioning of YACCC. Screening also facilitates improved communication about psychosocial functioning among providers, patients, and family [53]. Although screening for problems with psychological and behavioral functioning is now broadly implemented, identifying social problems is rarely identified as an active problem [54] or a reason for referral to behavioral health services [55], despite its critical relationship to psychological wellbeing.

Screening and brief counseling for depression and alcohol misuse are United States Preventive Services Task Force (USPSTF) recommendations in the general population [56, 57]. However, calls for comparable guidelines in young adults have yet to be articulated and evidence supporting universal screening for illicit substance use in adults or in adolescents has yet to be confirmed [58, 59]. Given the overlap between social functioning, mood problems, and risky health behaviors, supplementing screening of these domains with a review of social competence, activities, and support can enhance broader psychosocial screening and provide context and solutions for identified difficulties.

Choosing appropriate standardized screening tools can be daunting. There are options for implementing universal screening strategies of substance and alcohol use, including the 4-item

CAGE [60] used for lifetime drinking patterns, the 10-item Alcohol Use Disorders Identification Test (AUDIT) focused on current drinking problems [61], and subsets of the AUDIT designed to be rapid screenings (e.g., the reduced 3-item AUDIT-C used to screen based on consumption) [62, 63]. For illicit substance use disorders, the Drug Abuse Screening Test (DAST) [64] is a 28-item survey (with a more commonly used 10-item version) [65] that assesses the impact of substance use on functioning. A single-item from the DAST—*"How many times in the past year have you used an illegal drug or used a prescription medication for nonmedical reasons?"* was identified in a recent report as a highly sensitive (100%) and specific (73.5%) screen for drug use disorder in a large primary care trial [66].

Standardized assessment of social functioning is typically part of more extensive psychosocial assessment. Questionnaire-based psychosocial assessments typically used in clinical research, such as the Medical Outcomes Study Health Survey [67], the Social Adjustment Scale [68], and the Social Adaptation Evaluation scale [69], were identified in one primary-care study as strategies identified by patients as acceptable for real-world self-report assessment [70]. However, each of these measures takes time and requires relatively high levels of patient literacy, and administration can impact patient workflow in busy practices. The broadly disseminated Patient Health Questionnaire (PHQ) [71] has items tapping social concomitants of depression (e.g., "little interest or pleasure in doing things"; "Feeling…as you have let your family down") and depression-related functional impairment, but is an inadequate screener for social functioning or distress.

For providers who collaborate with behavioral health professionals and implement comprehensive questionnaire assessment, the Adult Behavior Checklist [72] is a developmental extension of its widely used pediatric counterpart, the Child Behavior Checklist. The ABCL has both parent and Adult Self-Report forms and contains 137 items pertaining to youth problems, some of which tap social competence and functioning. Similarly, the Behavioral Assessment System for Children (second edition) [73] has normative data up to age 21 and includes parent-report data on constructs such social skills and adaptive behavior. The Patient-Reported Outcomes Measurement Information System (PROMIS) is a comprehensive set of larger "item banks" tapping a conceptually integrated "domain framework," with smaller breakout subscales tackling multiple areas of patient functioning [74]. The PROMIS Social Health and Social Function domains include subscales assessing patient satisfaction with "Participation in Social Roles" (work, household responsibilities, routines, etc.) and "Participation in Discretionary Activities" (e.g., leisure activities, enjoyable activities with friends, etc.). Items are scored and compared with a normative database.

Many self-report questionnaires tend to skew towards assessing functioning within the normative ranges of social and behavioral development. For YACCC with known impairments in adaptive and intellectual functioning and/or with communication delays, parent/caregiver reports are paramount. An alternative assessment for social problems would be the Aberrant Behavior Checklist [75], a 58-item caregiver report of socially mediated behavioral problems such as lethargy/social withdrawal, stereotypic behaviors, hyperactivity, and inappropriate speech.

Screening for socially mediated problems should of course consider the social context of the screening itself—for example, *when* the screening was completed (at home, in the office), *how* it was completed (on paper, via physician or medical assistant interview, alone at home on a tablet computer,), and *who* completed the assessment (patient, parent, case manager, etc.). These factors influence responses to social items more than other areas of functioning. Social desirability bias, the attempt to present oneself more favorably, should be considered during interpretation. Incorporating review of patient forms and questionnaires can be time-consuming, though best practice for standardized screening suggests that it is important to review the respondent's answers prior to or during the appointment—perhaps with a medical assistant, nurse, or extender flagging items above a threshold value. Prereview can synthesize key findings, provide focus for further investigation, and engage the patient who appreciates that you are responding to their concerns. For example, noting a flagged response to an item on the YABCL assessing grades in school can be a jumping-off point to expand into a more in-depth review of health-related barriers in the classroom (e.g., insulin administration, use of PRN medication), future career goals, and social functioning in general outside the home.

In addition to questionnaire-based assessment, much can be learned by attending to patients' verbal and nonverbal communication to detect problems in social functioning. The degree of apparent patient comfort within the medical encounter can hold clues to a patient's social functioning in other settings. Observing whether the patient can make and sustain eye contact, engage in reciprocal interactions, and respond to questions (particularly open-ended questions) may suggest social competence or difficulties in similarly structured environments. During telehealth encounters, it may be helpful to ask about how activity and social connectedness have been influenced by social distancing or remote learning [76]. Young adults typically will involve their caregivers in some way during a visit; noting the degree to which children expect parents to provide verbal reports to their medical providers may shed light on problems with independent functioning, social initiation, and family dynamics. For private conversations involving sexual activity and substance use, utilize questions that easily permit positive responses and that open the door to voluntary and authentic disclosure (e.g., *"How many times have you tried smoking cigarettes?"*; *"Tell me about the drugs that you've tried…"*). Ask patients about sensitive topics such as sexual matters in open-ended ways that allow a broad range of options including alternative identities, behaviors, and lifestyles, or lack of sexual activity, which can be equally uncomfortable to disclose (*"Are you currently dating or are you having sex with anybody?"*; *"Are you attracted to men, or women, or both?"*). Particularly with YACCC, variable development may make it necessary to assess multiple informants about social functioning. For example, YACCC may be more likely to present with uneven social development and more severe problems in one area than another. Therefore, obtaining a questionnaire from a vocational therapist in a special education program and then comparing it to a parent's report of the patient's social skills may identify areas of discrepancy across the home, work, and school environments. In addition, primary care providers should be mindful of the risk for diagnostic overshadowing [77, 78]. This term was originally used to describe the tendency of physicians to misattribute the behavioral difficulties of people with intellectual disabilities to (more stable) cognitive deficits rather than to (potentially treatable) psychiatric conditions. More broadly defined and applied to the area of social functioning is the aspect that providers should be cautious about making assumptions about social competence, leisure interests, and supports based on initial presentation or on features of the illness. For example, diagnostic overshadowing might be at play if we were to assume that patients with intellectual disabilities fail to perceive subtle bullying or fail to communicate in a medical encounter because they lack communication skills, when in fact they are socially anxious.

## Ways Primary Care Providers Can Promote Young Patients' Social Functioning

Cross-validating sources and seeking additional information from a standardized screening or questionnaire with interview probes enhance the treatment validity of the assessment [79] by tying the content of the assessment to specific goals for interventions. Perhaps the most valuable thing a primary care provider can do to intervene in a young person's social development is to ask and assess about their parents and family, their school and/or work life, and about their friends and partners. Asking a patient, *"How do you explain your (illness, medical condition) to other people?,"* can open the door for more information about the patient's social adaptation to their condition and whether they perceive support from their social environment. At the practice level, screening and assessment procedures are best integrated along the lines of the Screening, Brief Intervention, and Referral to Treatment (SBIRT) model for alcohol and substance use problems [80], in which universal screening identifies at-risk patients and subsequent assessment and treatment is triaged according to level of risk. SBIRT models have been implemented in adult and adolescent primary care settings [81, 82] and have shown to be effective, particularly in reducing problem of alcohol use [83]. SBIRT processes rely on the therapeutic impact of brief interventions occurring in the medical setting and provides clear criteria and mechanisms for referring within or outside the practice for behavioral health or substance abuse services.

Communicating with patients about their social world might incorporate the tenets of Motivational Interviewing (MI) [84], now widely used to negotiate behavior change and reduce high-risk patient behaviors. Although a complete primer on MI is beyond the scope of this chapter, interventions using this approach take a nonconfrontational, person-centered stance to address patient ambivalence and resistance to making change or addressing problems. Key MI strategies include active listening techniques to elicit *patient-generated* motivations for making behavior change. Although proven effective in medical settings for a variety of health behaviors [85], MI has not been examined to promote social competence and support per se. One might speculate, however, that a therapeutic approach characterized by supportive but nondirective engagement, active listening, and support for positive change, might effectively address social problems and reduce gaps between patients' functional status and goals they have for themselves in areas such as school, home, friends, and the workplace. For example, one possible goal of a brief intervention using MI techniques might involve identifying "making more friends in my day program" as an important goal for a 20-year-old male patient with spina bifida and social anxiety. Active listening would identify specific people, behavioral settings, supportive adults, and potential barriers to attaining this goal as part of a behavioral plan, perhaps with family or day program personnel assistance.

Additional assistance for patients with problems involving social isolation or impaired social functioning would ideally be implemented in concert with behavioral health professionals integrated into your practice through an integrative team, a colocated professional, or by collaborating with trusted community partners. Promising evidence exists for psychological interventions reinforcing social skills when these treatments teach effective communication techniques and are of adequate intensity and duration (>6 sessions over >3 months) [86]. In addition, effective group therapy has been developed targeting psychoeducation about illness [82, 87], group training in coping skills with managing illness-related exchange of information, improving social competence, and learning positive self-talk [83, 88]. Finally, an emerging body of literature supports the effectiveness of professionally moderated social support interventions provided over the internet [89, 90].

In the absence of formalized treatment programs for YACCC in your community, an optimal referral to a behavioral health professional (BHP) should involve collaboratively engaging the BHP in recreating some of the best practices identified in laboratory settings. For example, providing information to the therapist about the young person's medical status—and what you have learned about his/her social adjustment—can help a BHP develop a treatment plan that fosters optimal physical functioning as well as psychological wellbeing. For example, to help a 22-year-old female with adolescent Type 2 diabetes and social anxiety, sharing details about the patient's illness regimen with the therapist can help him/her develop a treatment based on both regimen-specific needs (e.g., understanding when diabetes tasks might interfere with social interactions) and evidence-based psychological strategies. When evidence-based practices are unclear for optimizing social functioning, asking specific questions and making clear requests of the professional can improve the quality of the consultation as well as the intervention that the patient receives. It might be particularly advantageous to identify behavioral health supports within school and day habilitation programs to work collaboratively in key environments where social processes unfold. Finally, becoming aware of the social activities sponsored by local disease-specific organizations, as well as local youth groups, sports clubs, theater and music associations, and church-based organizations, can promote social functioning with like-minded individuals in meaningful ways [91].

## Concluding Comments

Primary care providers have a unique opportunity to keep YACCCs on track in all areas of functioning and to help them establish themselves in the world of interpersonal interactions and meaningful relationships. Consider ways to incorporate questions about social competence, activities, and perceived support into normative practice screening procedures. Evaluate features of the medical conditions that are most likely to impair social functioning such as central nervous system involvement, motor and communication impairments, facial anomalies, and the severity of the condition. When problems in social functioning are pronounced, impairing, and might be amenable to intervention, engage behavioral health partners and community/social service agencies in collaborative care. Increasing comfort and expertise with engaging young patients around their social functioning can transform the healthcare transition process of a YACCC from one characterized by fear and alienation to an opportunity to promote mature adult interactions from within the medical encounter to the patient's social world (Tables 55.1 and 55.2).

**Table 55.1** Screening measures

| ***Alcohol and substance use*** | | |
|---|---|---|
| **Measure** | **Purpose** | **Description** |
| CAGE Questionnaire (Ewing 1984) | Lifetime drinking patterns | 4-questions are asked to help provider diagnose problematic alcohol use: "Have you felt you should *cut down* on your drinking?" "Have people *annoyed* you by criticizing your drinking?" "Have you ever felt bad or *guilty* about your drinking?" "Have you ever had a drink first thing in the morning to steady your nerves or get rid of a hangover (*eye opener*)?" |
| Alcohol Use Disorder Identification Test (AUDIT; Saunders et al. 1993) | Problematic alcohol use screen | *10-item* self-report questionnaire that assesses problematic alcohol use across several domains: alcohol consumption, drinking-related behavior, and problems related to alcohol use. Scores range from 0 to 40, with scores of 8 or more indicative of problematic alcohol use. Also, available as a brief screening instrument (AUDIT-C; Bush et al. 1998) |
| Drug Abuse Screening Test (DAST; Bohn et al. 1991) | Influence of drug use on functioning | Clinician-administered or self-report *28-item* questionnaire with yes/no responses that assesses the impact of drug use, excluding alcohol and tobacco, on health, withdrawal, and family functioning. Also, available as a briefer 10-item version (DAST-10; Bohn et al. 2011), with scores of 3 or greater requiring further assessment |
| ***Quality of life and social functioning*** | | |
| **Measure** | **Purpose** | **Description** |
| Medical Outcomes Study Health Survey (SF-36; Ware and Sherbourne 1992) | General health status | Self-report *36-item* questionnaire measuring health functioning across eight domains including limitations in social and physical functioning, pain, general wellbeing, and energy/fatigue level |
| Social Adjustment Scale (SAS-SR; Weissman and Bothwell 1976) | Social functioning | *42-item* self-report questionnaire evaluating an individual's level of satisfaction and role performance within social interactions in major domains of functioning including work/school, leisure, and family. Also, available as a screener and short form |

(continued)

**Table 55.2** (continued)

| | | |
|---|---|---|
| Social Adaptation Self-evaluation Scale (SASS; Bosc 2000) | Social functioning in depression | *21-item* self-report measure assessing interest in initiating and maintaining social activities in patients with depression. Perceptions of social environment are sensitive to change with treatment for depression |
| ***Behavioral functioning*** | | |
| Adult Behavior Checklist (ABCL) and Adult Self-Report (Achenbach and Rescorla 2003) | Social competence and behavioral functioning | Comprehensive measure of adaptive/social competence and behavioral functioning; parallel measures for self and parent/partner report |
| Aberrant Behavior Checklist (ABC; Aman et al. 1985) | Socially influenced behavioral problems for individuals with cognitive/adaptive impairments | *58-item* informant and/or caregiver report of socially mediated behavioral problems such as lethargy/social withdrawal; stereotypic behaviors; hyperactivity; and inappropriate speech among individuals 18–30 |

**Table 55.2** Techniques to enhance the social functioning of YACCC

| Strategy | Description | Rationale |
|---|---|---|
| Facilitated communicating about illness | *"How do you explain your (illness, medical condition) to other people?" How does it get in the way of what you want to do?"* | Help patient articulate their relationship with their illness in the context of their social identity<br>Explore patient's perceptions of social support from peers, family, employers, etc. |
| Screening, Brief Intervention, and Referral to Treatment, (SBIRT; Gryczynski et al. 2011) | Universal screening; brief targeted interventions to address problem behavior; referral to community-based treatment for patients with clinical levels of misuse | Provide education about the impact of alcohol and drug on physical functioning and illness status, resulting influence on adaptive functioning<br>Explore risks and benefits of continued drug use on condition<br>Focus on developing patient goals for healthy behavior and assistance obtaining behavioral health intervention |
| Motivational Interviewing (Miller and Rollnick 2023) | Foster social behavior change by providing information and support using an empathetic, nonconfrontational approach | Engages patient to create socially relevant goals (e.g., to participate in youth group/club, make friends other YACCC, etc.)<br>Help patient articulate and resolve ambivalence about change, focus conversation on areas according to patient priorities<br>Support and problem-solve practical changes the patient can make |
| Collaborating with Behavioral Health Professionals (BHP) | Provide information about medical status to BHP; cocreate behavioral goals that foster both social and physical functioning | Help BHP integrate special healthcare needs into a treatment plan that is manageable within medical limitations; share in assessment of outcomes of treatment; and maintain ongoing communication with the BHP |

## References


1. Geist R, Grdisa V, Otley A. Psychosocial issues in the child with chronic conditions. Best Pract Res Clin Gastroenterol. 2003;17(2):141–52.
2. Evan EE, Zeltzer LK. Psychosocial dimensions of cancer in adolescents and young adults. Cancer. 2006;107(7 Suppl):1663–71.
3. Runions KC, Vithiatharan R, Hancock K, Lin A, Brennan-Jones CG, Gray C, Payne D. Chronic health conditions, mental health and the school: a narrative review. Health Educ J. 2020;79(4):471–83.

4. Zbikowski SM, Klesges RC, Robinson LA, Alfano CM. Risk factors for smoking among adolescents with asthma. J Adolesc Health. 2002;30(4):279–87.
5. Compas BE, Jaser SS, Dunn MJ, Rodriguez EM. Coping with chronic illness in childhood and adolescence. Annu Rev Clin Psychol. 2012;8:455.
6. Kyngäs H. Support network of adolescents with chronic disease: adolescents' perspective. Nurs Health Sci. 2004;6(4):287–93.
7. Oris L, Seiffge-Krenke I, Moons P, et al. Parental and peer support in adolescents with a chronic condition: a typological approach and developmental implications. J Behav Med. 2016;39(1):107–19.
8. Jose PE, Ryan N, Pryor J. Does social connectedness promote a greater sense of Well-being in adolescence over time? J Res Adolesc. 2012;22(2):235–51.
9. Kearns A, Whitley E, Tannahill C, Ellaway A. Loneliness, social relations and health and well-being in deprived communities. Psychol Health Med. 2015;20(3):332–44.
10. Steptoe A, Shankar A, Demakakos P, Wardle J. Social isolation, loneliness, and all-cause mortality in older men and women. Proc Natl Acad Sci U S A. 2013;110(15):5797–801.
11. Berkman LF, Syme SL. Social networks, host resistance, and mortality: a nine-year follow-up study of Alameda County residents. Am J Epidemiol. 1979;109(2):186–204.
12. Uchino BN, Trettevik R, de Grey RGK, Cronan S, Hogan J, Baucom BR. Social support, social integration, and inflammatory cytokines: a meta-analysis. Health Psychol. 2018;37(5):462.
13. Morris J. Social exclusion and young disabled people with high levels of support needs. Crit Soc Policy. 2001;21(2):161–83.
14. Reiter-Purtill J, Waller J, Noll R. Empirical and theoretical perspectives on the peer relationships of children with chronic conditions. In: Roberts M, Steele R, editors. Handbook of pediatric psychology. 4th ed. New York: Guilford Press; 2009.
15. Twyman KA, Saylor CF, Saia D, Macias MM, Taylor LA, Spratt E. Bullying and ostracism experiences in children with special health care needs. J Dev Behav Pediatr. 2010;31(1):1–8.
16. Husson O, Zebrack BJ, Aguilar C, Hayes-Lattin B, Cole S. Cancer in adolescents and young adults: who remains at risk of poor social functioning over time? Cancer. 2017;123(14):2743–51.
17. Vanhalst J, Rassart J, Luyckx K, et al. Trajectories of loneliness in adolescents with congenital heart disease: associations with depressive symptoms and perceived health. J Adolesc Health. 2013;53(3):342–9.
18. Perrin JM, MacLean WE, Perrin EC. Parental perceptions of health status and psychologic adjustment of children with asthma. Pediatrics. 1989;83(1):26–30.
19. Van Cleave J, Davis MM. Bullying and peer victimization among children with special health care needs. Pediatrics. 2006;118(4):e1212–9.
20. Nassau JH, Drotar D. Social competence among children with central nervous system-related chronic health conditions: a review. J Pediatr Psychol. 1997;22(6):771–93.
21. Rantanen K, Eriksson K, Nieminen P. Social competence in children with epilepsy—a review. Epilepsy Behav. 2012;24(3):295–303.
22. Gebauer-Bukurov K, Markovic J, Sekulic S, Bozic K. Social competence among well-functioning adolescents with epilepsy. Epilepsy Behav. 2015;42:54–60.
23. Yeates KO, Bigler ED, Gerhardt CA, et al. Theoretical approaches to understanding social function in childhood brain insults: toward the integration of social neuroscience and developmental psychology. In: Anderson V, Beauchamp MH, editors. Developmental social neuroscience and childhood brain insult: theory and practice. New York: Guilford Press; 2012.
24. Livingston MH, Rosenbaum PL, Russell DJ, Palisano RJ. Quality of life among adolescents with cerebral palsy: what does the literature tell us? Dev Med Child Neurol. 2007;49(3):225–31.
25. Albrecht GL, Devlieger PJ. The disability paradox: high quality of life against all odds. Soc Sci Med. 1999;48(8):977–88.
26. Suris J-C, Michaud P-A, Akre C, Sawyer SM. Health risk behaviors in adolescents with chronic conditions. Pediatrics. 2008;122(5):e1113–8.
27. Reid GJ, Irvine MJ, McCrindle BW, et al. Prevalence and correlates of successful transfer from pediatric to adult health care among a cohort of young adults with complex congenital heart defects. Pediatrics. 2004;113(3):e197–205.
28. Suris J-C, Parera N. Sex, drugs and chronic illness: health behaviours among chronically ill youth. Eur J Public Health. 2005;15(5):484–8.
29. Britto MT, Garrett JM, Dugliss MA, et al. Risky behavior in teens with cystic fibrosis or sickle cell disease: a multicenter study. Pediatrics. 1998;101(2):250–6.
30. Sawyer SM, Drew S, Yeo MS, Britto MT. Adolescents with a chronic condition: challenges living, challenges treating. Lancet. 2007;369(9571):1481–9.
31. Aanerud M, Carsin A-E, Sunyer J, et al. Interaction between asthma and smoking increases the risk of adult airway obstruction. Eur Respir J. 2015;45(3):635–43.
32. Hargrove A, Penny D, Sawyer S. Sexual and reproductive health in young people with congenital heart disease: a systematic review of the literature. Pediatr Cardiol. 2005;26(6):805–11.
33. Cardenas DD, Topolski TD, White CJ, McLaughlin JF, Walker WO. Sexual functioning in adolescents and young adults with spina bifida. Arch Phys Med Rehabil. 2008;89(1):31–5.
34. Kakleas K, Kandyla B, Karayianni C, Karavanaki K. Psychosocial problems in adolescents with type 1 diabetes mellitus. Diabetes Metab. 2009;35(5):339–50.
35. Orlicka K, Barnes E, Culver EL. Prevention of infection caused by immunosuppressive drugs in gastroenterology. Ther Adv Chronic Dis. 2013;4(4):167–85.
36. Henry-Reid LM, O'Connor KG, Klein JD, Cooper E, Flynn P, Futterman DC. Current pediatrician prac-

tices in identifying high-risk behaviors of adolescents. Pediatrics. 2010;125(4):e741–7.

37. Eneriz-Wiemer M, Sanders LM, Barr DA, Mendoza FS. Parental limited English proficiency and health outcomes for children with special health care needs: a systematic review. Acad Pediatr. 2014;14(2):128–36.
38. Vart P, Gansevoort RT, Joosten MM, Bultmann U, Reijneveld SA. Socioeconomic disparities in chronic kidney disease: a systematic review and meta-analysis. Am J Prev Med. 2015;48(5):580–92.
39. Knapp C, Huang IC, Hinojosa M, Baker K, Sloyer P. Assessing the congruence of transition preparedness as reported by parents and their adolescents with special health care needs. Matern Child Health J. 2013;17(2):352–8.
40. Ng S, Dinesh S, Tay S, Lee E. Decreased access to health care and social isolation among young adults with cerebral palsy after leaving school. J Orthop Surg. 2003;11(1):80.
41. Bonnie RJ, Stroud C, Breiner H. Investing in the health and well-being of young adults. Washington, DC: National Academy of Sciences; 2015.
42. Uzark K, Yu S, Lowery R, Afton K, Yetman AT, Cramer J, Rudd N, Cohen S, Gongwer R, Gurvitz M. Transition readiness in teens and young adults with congenital heart disease: can we make a difference? J Pediatr. 2020;221:201–6.
43. Fegran L, Hall EO, Uhrenfeldt L, Aagaard H, Ludvigsen MS. Adolescents' and young adults' transition experiences when transferring from paediatric to adult care: a qualitative metasynthesis. Int J Nurs Stud. 2014;51(1):123–35.
44. Reiss JG, Gibson RW, Walker LR. Health care transition: youth, family, and provider perspectives. Pediatrics. 2005;115(1):112–20.
45. Sawin KJ, Rauen K, Bartelt T, et al. Transitioning adolescents and young adults with spina bifida to adult healthcare: initial findings from a model program. Rehabil Nurs. 2015;40(1):3–11.
46. Goldenring JM, Rosen DS. Getting into adolescent heads: an essential update. Contemp Pediatr. 2004;21(1):64–92.
47. Duggan M, Brenner J. The demographics of social media users, 2012. vol. 14: Pew Research Center's Internet & American Life Project Washington, DC; 2013.
48. Puukko K, Hietajärvi L, Maksniemi E, Alho K, Salmela-Aro K. Social media use and depressive symptoms—a longitudinal study from early to late adolescence. Int J Environ Res Public Health. 2020;17(16):5921.
49. Fernandes B, Biswas UN, Mansukhani RT, Casarín AV, Essau CA. The impact of COVID-19 lockdown on internet use and escapism in adolescents. Rev psicol clín con niños adolesc. 2020;7(3):59–65.
50. Best P, Manktelow R, Taylor B. Online communication, social media and adolescent wellbeing: a systematic narrative review. Child Youth Serv Rev. 2014;41:27–36.
51. Greene JA, Choudhry NK, Kilabuk E, Shrank WH. Online social networking by patients with diabetes: a qualitative evaluation of communication with Facebook. J Gen Intern Med. 2011;26(3):287–92.
52. Serlachius A, Badawy SM, Thabrew H. Psychosocial challenges and opportunities for youth with chronic health conditions during the COVID-19 pandemic. JMIR Pediatr Parent. 2020;3(2):e23057.
53. Hayutin LG, Reed-Knight B, Blount RL, Lewis J, McCormick ML. Increasing parent-pediatrician communication about children's psychosocial problems. J Pediatr Psychol. 2009;34(10):1155–64.
54. Rosendal M, Vedsted P, Christensen KS, Moth G. Psychological and social problems in primary care patients—general practitioners' assessment and classification. Scand J Prim Health Care. 2013;31(1):43–9.
55. Linton JC. Psychological assessment in primary care. In: Hass LJ, editor. Handbook of primary care psychology. New York: Oxford University Press; 2004.
56. Moyer VA. Screening and behavioral counseling interventions in primary care to reduce alcohol misuse: U.S. preventive services task force recommendation statement. Ann Intern Med. 2013;159(3):210–8.
57. Siu AL, Bibbins-Domingo K, Grossman DC, et al. Screening for depression in adults: US preventive services task force recommendation statement. JAMA. 2016;315(4):380–7.
58. Saitz R, Palfai TP, Cheng DM, et al. Screening and brief intervention for drug use in primary care: the ASPIRE randomized clinical trial. JAMA. 2014;312(5):502–13.
59. Moyer VA. Primary care behavioral interventions to reduce illicit drug and nonmedical pharmaceutical use in children and adolescents: U.S. preventive services task force recommendation statement interventions to reduce drug use in children and adolescents. Ann Intern Med. 2014;160(9):634–9.
60. Ewing JA. Detecting alcoholism: the CAGE questionnaire. JAMA. 1984;252(14):1905–7.
61. Saunders JB, Aasland OG, Babor TF, De la Fuente JR, Grant M. Development of the alcohol use disorders identification test (AUDIT): WHO collaborative project on early detection of persons with harmful alcohol consumption-II. Addiction. 1993;88(6):791–804.
62. Gomez A, Conde A, Santana J, Jorrin A. Diagnostic usefulness of brief versions of Alcohol Use Disorders Identification Test (AUDIT) for detecting hazardous drinkers in primary care settings. J Stud Alcohol. 2005;66(2):305–8.
63. Bush K, Kivlahan DR, McDonell MB, Fihn SD, Bradley KA. The AUDIT alcohol consumption questions (AUDIT-C): an effective brief screening test for problem drinking. Ambulatory Care Quality Improvement Project (ACQUIP). Alcohol use disorders identification test. Arch Intern Med. 1998;158(16):1789–95.
64. Yudko E, Lozhkina O, Fouts A. A comprehensive review of the psychometric properties of the Drug Abuse Screening Test. J Subst Abus Treat. 2007;32(2):189–98.

65. Bohn M, Babor T, Kranzler H. Validity of the Drug Abuse Screening Test (DAST-10) in inpatient substance abusers. Problems of Drug Dependence. 1991;119:233–5.
66. Smith PC, Schmidt SM, Allensworth-Davies D, Saitz R. A single-question screening test for drug use in primary care. Arch Intern Med. 2010;170(13):1155–60.
67. Ware JE Jr, Sherbourne CD. The MOS 36-item short-form health survey (SF-36). I. Conceptual framework and item selection. Med Care. 1992;30(6):473–83.
68. Weissman MM, Bothwell S. Assessment of social adjustment by patient self-report. Arch Gen Psychiatry. 1976;33(9):1111.
69. Bosc M. Assessment of social functioning in depression. Compr Psychiatry. 2000;41(1):63–9.
70. Weissman MM, Olfson M, Gameroff MJ, Feder A, Fuentes M. A comparison of three scales for assessing social functioning in primary care. Am J Psychiatry. 2001;158:460.
71. Kroenke K, Spitzer RL, Williams JB. The Phq-9. J Gen Intern Med. 2001;16(9):606–13.
72. Achenbach T, Rescorla LA. Manual for the ASEBA adult forms and profiles. Burlington: Research Center for Children and Families, University of Vermont; 2003.
73. Reynolds CR, Kamphaus RW. BASC-2 behavioral assessment system for children manual. Circle Pines: AGS Publishing; 2004.
74. Northwestern University. PROMIS [Internet]. HealthMeasures. [cited 2022 Oct 25]. https://www.healthmeasures.net/explore-measurement-systems/promis.
75. Aman MG, Singh NN, Stewart AW, Field CJ. The aberrant behavior checklist: a behavior rating scale for the assessment of treatment effects. Am J Ment Defic. 1985;89(5):485–91.
76. Curfman A, McSwain SD, Chuo J, Yeager-McSwain B, Schinasi DA, Marcin J, Herendeen N, Chung SL, Rheuban K, Olson CA. Pediatric telehealth in the COVID-19 pandemic era and beyond. Pediatrics. 2021;148(3):e2020047795.
77. Happell B, Ewart SB, Bocking J, Platania-Phung C, Stanton R. 'That red flag on your file': misinterpreting physical symptoms as mental illness. J Clin Nurs. 2016;25(19–20):2933–42.
78. Reiss S, Levitan GW, Szyszko J. Emotional disturbance and mental retardation: diagnostic overshadowing. Am J Ment Defic. 1982;86(6):567–74.
79. Hayes SC, Nelson RO, Jarrett RB. The treatment utility of assessment: a functional approach to evaluating assessment quality. Am Psychol. 1987;42(11):963.
80. Muench J, Jarvis K, Gray M, et al. Implementing a team-based SBIRT model in primary care clinics. J Subst Abus. 2015;20(2):106–12.
81. Gryczynski J, Mitchell SG, Peterson TR, Gonzales A, Moseley A, Schwartz RP. The relationship between services delivered and substance use outcomes in New Mexico's screening, brief intervention, referral and treatment (SBIRT) initiative. Drug Alcohol Depend. 2011;118(2):152–7.
82. Ozechowski TJ, Becker SJ, Hogue A. SBIRT-A: adapting SBIRT to maximize developmental fit for adolescents in primary care. J Subst Abus Treat. 2016;62:28–37.
83. Tanner-Smith EE, Parr NJ, Schweer-Collins M, Saitz R. Effects of brief substance use interventions delivered in general medical settings: a systematic review and meta-analysis. Addiction. 2022;117(4):877–89.
84. Miller WR, Rollnick S. Motivational interviewing: helping people change and grow. United States: Guilford Publications; 2023.
85. Lundahl B, Moleni T, Burke BL, et al. Motivational interviewing in medical care settings: a systematic review and meta-analysis of randomized controlled trials. Patient Educ Couns. 2013;93(2):157–68.
86. Sansom-Daly UM, Peate M, Wakefield CE, Bryant RA, Cohn RJ. A systematic review of psychological interventions for adolescents and young adults living with chronic illness. Health Psychol. 2012;31(3):380–93.
87. Roberts CS, Piper L, Denny J, Cuddeback G. A support group intervention to facilitate young adults' adjustment to cancer. Health Soc Work. 1997;22(2):133–41.
88. Scholten L, Willemen AM, Last BF, et al. Efficacy of psychosocial group intervention for children with chronic illness and their parents. Pediatrics. 2013;131(4):e1196–203.
89. Stewart M, Letourneau N, Masuda JR, Anderson S, McGhan S. Impacts of online peer support for children with asthma and allergies: "it just helps you every time you can't breathe well". J Pediatr Nurs. 2013;28(5):439–52.
90. Maurice-Stam H, Scholten L, de Gee EA, et al. Feasibility of an online cognitive behavioral-based group intervention for adolescents treated for cancer: a pilot study. J Psychosoc Oncol. 2014;32(3):310–21.
91. Suris J-C, Michaud P-A, Viner R. The adolescent with a chronic condition. Part I: developmental issues. Arch Dis Child. 2004;89(10):938–42.

# 56 Adherence and Self-management

Gregory S. Sawicki

## Overview

Advances in medical care have led to an increasing number of adolescents and young adults (AYA) surviving into adulthood with childhood-onset chronic health conditions. Examples of such conditions include asthma, cystic fibrosis, diabetes, human immunodeficiency virus (HIV), inflammatory bowel disease, sickle cell disease, chronic renal disease, and cerebral palsy. As AYA with a range of diagnoses transition from pediatric to adult-focused healthcare systems, developing strategies to maintain health outcomes during this period is critical [1]. A key driver for maintaining optimal outcomes is adherence to recommended care therapies and condition-specific management plans. However, for AYA, particularly those with complex chronic health conditions, adherence to a daily regimen is a challenge. Therapeutic regimens are often complex, multifaceted, and time-consuming to administer. Chronic health conditions often progress during adolescence and early adulthood, so the need to maintain prescribed regimens increases at a very time of life when youths are vulnerable from a physiologic perspective. Additionally, normal adolescent development, including a desire for independence from caregivers, can hinder appropriate adherence behaviors and disease self-management. Illness perceptions and beliefs are being established during this period, and struggles with parents and caregivers over roles and responsibilities can negatively influence adherence behaviors. Therefore, improving adherence is a key part of transitional care. This chapter reviews the clinical approach to adherence for AYA with chronic health conditions, including the recognition of distinct patterns of adherence behaviors, outlines barriers to optimal adherence, and suggests strategies to improve adherence in this high-risk population.

## Defining Adherence Behaviors

Broadly defined, adherence to medical therapies is the extent to which an individual completes a mutually agreed upon treatment plan. "Adherence" and "disease self-management" are sometimes used as interchangeable terms to describe an individual patient's behavior related to maintaining a chronic therapeutic regimen [2]. Unlike the term "compliance," which indicates a unidirectional directive in which an individual receives a treatment plan or prescription from a healthcare provider, the term "adherence" encompasses a shared decision-making approach to therapies in which both the individual and their healthcare provider have provided input into the

G. S. Sawicki (✉)
Division of Pulmonary Medicine, Boston Children's Hospital, Harvard Medical School, Boston, MA, USA
e-mail: Gregory.sawicki@childrens.harvard.edu


A. A. Kuo et al. (eds.), *Care of Adults with Chronic Childhood Conditions*,
https://doi.org/10.1007/978-3-031-54281-7_56

therapeutic regimen. Therefore, labeling health behavior as "noncompliance" suggests that the individual is solely responsible for the failure to complete a therapeutic plan, whereas "nonadherence" implicates challenges for an individual, their support network, and their healthcare providers and system.

Although nonadherence is a common occurrence among AYA with chronic health conditions, an understanding of the type of nonadherence behaviors is important to develop appropriate individualized interventions. An individual may exhibit *unwitting* nonadherence in which they do not realize that they are failing at maintaining a prescribed treatment plan. An example of unwitting nonadherence is an adolescent with asthma who uses their controller medication once daily instead of twice daily as prescribed. They may not understand the prescription directions, or may have been misinformed, but they do not realize that they are not following a prescribed plan. A second type of nonadherence behavior is *erratic*, in which an individual has periods of good adherence interspersed with periods of nonadherence. Such an individual likely understands and agrees with therapy, but has difficulty consistently maintaining their regimen. An example of erratic nonadherence is a young adult with cystic fibrosis who is able to complete all recommended therapies during the week, but on weekends often neglects his therapies as his schedule differs during those days. Similarly, a transplant patient may not consistently take oral antirejection medication on a daily schedule. Erratic nonadherence generally results from lack of structure, forgetfulness, or competing priorities, which may be variable. A third type of nonadherence is *intentional*, in which an individual understands one's treatment plan but chooses not to follow it. For instance, an adolescent with diabetes may not use insulin during every meal or snack or a young adult with inflammatory bowel disease may avoid her anti-inflammatories on a regular basis. Such intentional nonadherence often results from anger at a health condition, health system, or caregivers, or may be due to underlying depression or other mental health comorbidities common with chronic illness. Similarly, such behaviors may be due to the avoidance of side effects or a desire to remain "normal" in the eyes of peers by not disclosing an illness. Finally, *rationalized* nonadherence occurs when an individual deliberately alters or discontinues therapy, often without consulting with their healthcare team. This type of behavior may result if an individual does not believe that they need a particular therapy or they feel no immediate benefit from a therapy. For instance, an individual with epilepsy may perceive no immediate benefit symptomatically from a daily medication, or a person with asthma may not notice any difference after several weeks of not taking a daily inhaler. For AYA, such rationalized behavior is quite common and may indicate a desire for risk taking, or similar to intentional nonadherence, be a manifestation of anger, depression, or misinformation.

When approaching nonadherence, therefore, a clinician needs to evaluate the type of behavior that each individual is exhibiting and use that information and assessment to guide intervention plans.

## Assessing Adherence: Measurement Tools

It is important for clinicians to obtain measurement data to help assess adherence among their patients. Biomarkers, such as serum drug levels, would appear to be the best measure of adherence, but are only routinely available for certain classes of medications. For most therapies, there is no "gold standard" for adherence measurement, and types of measures vary depending on therapies prescribed. It is clear, however, that self-report and caregiver report of adherence are inadequate. Multiple studies have shown that self-report is subjective and overestimates true adherence behaviors when compared to direct observation, monitoring, or other measurement methods [3]. This does not mean that clinicians should not ask subjectively about nonadherence during routine clinical care; rather, they should carefully phrase questions about adherence to

**Table 56.1** Measuring adherence

| Measurement tool | Example | Advantages | Disadvantages |
|---|---|---|---|
| Prescription refill history | Medication possession ratio (MPR)<br>Number of refills<br>Proportion of days covered (PDC) | Identify what medications an individual has obtained as opposed to what is prescribed<br>Allows for evaluation of adherence over a longer time period without need for individual input/recall | Only measures dispensing of medication<br>Not always clear exactly what has been prescribed<br>Does not account for "overfilling" of a prescription<br>May not correlate with written treatment plans<br>May not account for changing treatments over time |
| Electronic monitors | Metered-dose inhaler counters<br>Continuous glucose monitors<br>CPAP monitors | Continuous, long-term, real-time measures<br>More objective than diaries or self-report<br>Can identify a spectrum of issues<br>Underdosing<br>Delayed dosing<br>Drug "holidays"<br>"White-coat" adherence | Device malfunction/Technology failure<br>Recording events that did not occur or failure to record events that did occur<br>Cost<br>Privacy concerns |

*CPAP* continuous positive airway pressure

allow an individual to report their challenges. Asking "do you take medication X?" sets up a response that will lead to overreporting, whereas framing a question "over the past week, how often did you miss taking medication X?" may elicit more accurate self-report.

Ideally, a clinician has access to additional objective measures of adherence. Various measurement tools exist, including data from prescription refills and electronic monitors [4]. Each of these tools has advantages and disadvantages as outlined in Table 56.1. Access to such measurements may be limited to research studies, but increasingly, electronic medical records have improved capabilities for such data to be captured in the context of routine chronic disease case management. With such data becoming more available, clinician training on how to communicate adherence data to individuals is also critical. Accurate, yet practical measures of adherence that provide real-time data are essential to provide patients, families, and their care team useful information to guide interventions if needed, and these measures need to be aligned with efficacious adherence interventions. Several monitoring devices are on the market or in development and are increasingly acceptable in our society as we become more "quantified," yet there is little evidence that this big data approach has improved health [5]. Online data platforms in which individuals with a chronic illness interact with the healthcare system present a viable opportunity for both adherence measurement and intervention designs. There is also an increasing desire for cell phone applications to be tailored to the chronic illness experience, include multiple functions, and facilitate coordination and communication, yet be low burden and customizable [6]. Currently, there is still a need for technology-based systems that integrate adherence and clinical data with decision support and also provide a platform for coordinating and executing effective adherence promotion interventions. Such technology also needs to be created in a practical and feasible manner to enable wider spread dissemination.

## Barriers and Facilitators of Adherence

Adherence behaviors are affected by multiple factors stemming from (1) individuals, (2) families, (3) health systems, and (4) communities [2].

For many chronic health conditions, treatment complexity is an important barrier to adherence, and the degree of complexity may be associated with differing rates of adherence. In cystic fibrosis, for example, adherence rates vary between types of treatments, with higher rates of adherence with oral medications, lower rates with nebulized therapy, exercise and physiotherapy, and nutritional care [7]. Broadly, treatment complexity can lead to time trade-offs based on other competing priorities, particularly those that allow a youth to engage in "normal" developmentally appropriate activities with their peers. Other key barriers include immediate time pressures, lack of time to complete therapies, uncertain schedules, and forgetfulness, either accidental or purposeful. Many youth may avoid therapies in favor of other activities and may skip therapies in order to be "normal." Finally, for many youth a barrier to adherence is a lack of perceived consequences, specifically not seeing an impact on one's health right away after skipping treatments or medications.

Conversely, key motivators for adherence behaviors for AYA include developing trusting relationships with clinicians, being treated as an adult, and early and repeated practice and skill building. Therefore, effective healthcare for AYA needs to address the developmental progression from adolescence to young adulthood. In childhood, self-management of a chronic disease generally rests in the hands of the parents. At school age, optimally there should be an initiation of the transition to a shared model based on partial self-management, and in adolescence, there should be an increasing assertion of independence on the part of the teenager. The gradual immersion into independent self-management needs to be tracked by clinicians throughout adolescence, and parental support needs to be augmented. Encouragement of this progression into adulthood should be the cornerstone for programs to enhance adolescent disease knowledge, skills, and self-management. Additional facilitators such as improved communication and engagement of social support have been identified in multiple studies of adherence interventions [8].

## Strategies to Improve Adherence

Interventions to improve adherence often are multicomponent and may be costly, labor-intensive, and complex [9, 10]. However, there are relatively straightforward interventions that clinicians in practice can use to address nonadherence among individuals. One mnemonic that has been developed is "SIMPLE": Simplifying regimen characteristics; Imparting knowledge; Modifying patient beliefs; Patient communication; Leaving the bias; and Evaluating adherence [11]. Examples of behavioral intervention strategies aligned with these strategies are shown in Table 56.2 [11].

Adherence interventions can also be embedded into the Chronic Care Model (CCM), a framework with documented success for improving chronic illness care that can be used to incorporate the patient, caregiver, and healthcare system in designing interventions [12]. In this model, focusing on self-management support, delivery system design, decision support, and clinical information systems is proposed to facilitate the development of systems in which informed, activated patients work collaboratively

**Table 56.2** Strategies to improve adherence

| "SIMPLE" strategies | Behavioral approaches |
|---|---|
| Simplifying the regimen | Creating reminders<br>Promoting self-monitoring<br>Tailoring the regimen<br>Developing contingencies and rewards |
| Imparting knowledge | Improving health education<br>Assessing health literacy |
| Modifying beliefs | Health and behavioral feedback/coaching<br>Cognitive behavioral therapy<br>Motivational interviewing |
| Patient communication | Problem solving<br>Family therapy<br>Social support |
| Leaving the bias | Addressing mental health<br>Assessing individual barriers<br>Assessing type of adherence behavior |
| Evaluating adherence | Asking open-ended questions<br>Electronic monitors<br>Pharmacy refill data |

Adapted from [11]

with prepared, proactive care teams. In a review of the evidence for the CCM, 32 of 39 studies examined found that interventions based on the CCM components improved at least 1 process or outcome measure when utilized for patients with diabetes [13]. Application of the CCM has demonstrated improvements in adherence in individuals with either diabetes or asthma [14, 15].

A clinician needs to evaluate the multiple factors affecting adherence for an individual patient. In this way, addressing nonadherence is a part of routine personalized medical care. Identifying the type of nonadherence for an individual, including a recognition and understanding of individual barriers, can guide an appropriate intervention strategy. As an example, for those with unwitting nonadherence, efforts to improve knowledge of the condition and its treatments could be the cornerstone for adherence interventions. An adolescent who only uses their asthma controller medication when they are feeling unwell could be educated about the chronicity of airway inflammation even in the absence of symptoms. In this type of case, the lack of immediate perceived benefits to chronic therapies also needs to be discussed as part of an adherence intervention approach. Similarly, reminder systems may provide a structure for those with unwitting nonadherence. Automated reminders such as mobile text messages align with the self-management support component of the CCM and have led to improvements in adherence behaviors in varied populations, including individuals with asthma, diabetes, and HIV [16–18]. Messaging interventions can be designed as one-way or two-way, enabling communication between an individual and the healthcare system. Small studies of adolescents with asthma showed high satisfaction with tailored, individual messaging reminders targeting self-management [19]. However, these interventions alone, particularly in a complex therapeutic regimen for a youth with a chronic health condition, likely would not lead to dramatic changes if not accompanied by a greater understanding of the global context of an individual's day-to-day needs. For those with rationalized nonadherence, particularly those who identify time as a key barrier, reminders likely would not help as much. Interventions to address time pressures and competing priorities would be an appropriate strategy. Interventions would require more than simply reducing the number of prescribed therapies or shortening the actual administration of medications. Discussions would need to identify the reason that time is an issue and likely address the overall place of therapies in the context of an individual's other daily routines. Examining family relationships, focusing on problem-solving skills, are robust targets for adherence interventions. Such interventions might best be implemented using techniques such as motivational interviewing [20].

Across all types of adherence interventions, developing a strong relationship with the clinical care team, particularly with respect to communication and respect, is a key driver of improved adherence. Recent opportunities for improving such interactions have entered the realm of health information technology. For example, a cell phone support program for teenagers and young adults with CF was designed to provide CF information and social support [21]. Such technologies are likely to enhance existing care models and allow for innovative adherence interventions outside routine clinical visits. However, such programs would still need to promote structured knowledge, support, and shared decision-making while enabling youth to develop effective communication with their treating clinicians.

Since poor communication with clinicians has been associated with lower levels of adherence [8], enhancing communication efforts may lead to adherence improvements. One way to support communication is providing feedback on adherence data to clinical care teams. Such feedback can enhance patient-provider communication, alert clinicians to lapses in adherence in periods between routine clinical visits, and therefore align with the decision support and clinical information system components of the CCM. Feedback of adherence data to patients combined with counseling to overcome adherence barriers is increasingly being evaluated in other chronic health conditions (e.g., asthma, transplant, heart failure, hypertension, sickle cell disease) and has been shown to be superior to usual care or counseling alone in improving medication adherence [22–26]. Offering objective feedback of behaviors can be eye-opening for patients and, if provided in a supportive, patient-centered conversation, can encourage patients to play a more informed and activated role in their care.

## Conclusion

In summary, youth transitioning from pediatric to adult-focused care, particularly those with chronic health conditions, may struggle with adherence to recommended therapies and care plans. Clinicians need to be able to identify nonadherence and differentiate the type of nonadherence behaviors that an individual patient may exhibit. They should also work with patients to identify their unique barriers and possible strategies to improve adherence. Interventions to improve adherence need to be multifaceted, incorporating an understanding of barriers and behaviors. Technology, including monitoring and reminders, clearly has a role in adherence promotion, but needs to ultimately be coupled with personalized approaches tailored to the challenges facing each individual patient.

## References

1. American Academy of Pediatrics, American Academy of Family Physicians, American College of Physicians, Transitions Clinical Report Authoring Group, Cooley WC, Sagerman PJ. Supporting the health care transition from adolescence to adulthood in the medical home. Pediatrics. 2011;128(1):182–200.
2. Modi AC, Pai AL, Hommel KA, Hood KK, Cortina S, Hilliard ME, Guilfoyle SM, Gray WN, Drotar D. Pediatric self-management: a framework for research, practice, and policy. Pediatrics. 2012;129(2):e473–85.
3. Stirratt MJ, Dunbar-Jacob J, Crane HM, Simoni JM, Czajkowski S, Hilliard ME, et al. Self-report measures of medication adherence behavior: recommendations on optimal use. Transl Behav Med. 2015;5(4):470–82.
4. Ingerski LM, Hente EA, Modi AC, Hommel KA. Electronic measurement of medication adherence in pediatric chronic illness: a review of measures. J Pediatr. 2011;159(4):528–34.
5. Almalki M, Gray K, Sanchez FM. The use of self-quantification systems for personal health information: big data management activities and prospects. Health Inf Sci Syst. 2015;3(Suppl 1):S1.
6. Hilliard ME, Hahn A, Ridge AK, Eakin MN, Riekert KA. User preferences and design recommendations for an mHealth app to promote cystic fibrosis self-management. JMIR Mhealth Uhealth. 2014;2(4):e44.
7. Zindani GN, Streetman DD, Streetman DS, Nasr SZ. Adherence to treatment in children and adolescent patients with cystic fibrosis. J Adolesc Health. 2006;38(1):13–7.
8. Ratanawongsa N, Karter AJ, Parker MM, Lyles CR, Heisler M, Moffet HH, et al. Communication and medication refill adherence: the Diabetes Study of Northern California. JAMA Intern Med. 2013;173(3):210–8.
9. Nieuwlaat R, Wilczynski N, Navarro T, Hobson N, Jeffery R, Keepanasseril A, et al. Interventions for enhancing medication adherence. Cochrane Database Syst Rev. 2014;20(11):CD000011.
10. Kahana S, Drotar D, Frazier T. Meta-analysis of psychological interventions to promote adherence to treatment in pediatric chronic health conditions. J Pediatr Psychol. 2008;33(6):590–611.
11. Atreja A, Bellam N, Levy SR. Strategies to enhance patient adherence: making it simple. MedGenMed. 2005;7(1):4.
12. Coleman K, Austin BT, Brach C, Wagner EH. Evidence on the chronic care model in the new millennium. Health Aff (Millwood). 2009;28(1):75–85.
13. Bodenheimer T, Wagner EH, Grumbach K. Improving primary care for patients with chronic illness: the chronic care model, part 2. JAMA. 2002;288(15):1909–14.
14. Mackey K, Parchman ML, Leykum LK, Lanham HJ, Noel PH, Zeber JE. Impact of the chronic care model on medication adherence when patients perceive cost as a barrier. Prim Care Diabetes. 2012;6(2):137–42.
15. Moullec G, Gour-Provencal G, Bacon SL, Campbell TS, Lavoie KL. Efficacy of interventions to improve adherence to inhaled corticosteroids in adult asthmatics: impact of using components of the chronic care model. Respir Med. 2012;106(9):1211–25.
16. Hamine S, Gerth-Guyette E, Faulx D, Green BB, Ginsburg AS. Impact of mHealth chronic disease management on treatment adherence and patient outcomes: a systematic review. J Med Internet Res. 2015;17(2):e52.
17. Fischer HH, Moore SL, Ginosar D, Davidson AJ, Rice-Peterson CM, Durfee MJ, et al. Care by cell phone: text messaging for chronic disease management. Am J Manag Care. 2012;18(2):e42–7.
18. de Jongh T, Gurol-Urganci I, Vodopivec-Jamsek V, Car J, Atun R. Mobile phone messaging for facilitating self-management of long-term illnesses. Cochrane Database Syst Rev. 2012;12:CD007459.
19. Britto MT, Munafo JK, Schoettker PJ, Vockell AL, Wimberg JA, Yi MS. Pilot and feasibility test of adolescent-controlled text messaging reminders. Clin Pediatr (Phila). 2012;51(2):114–21.

20. Spoelstra SL, Schueller M, Hilton M, Ridenour K. Interventions combining motivational interviewing and cognitive behaviour to promote medication adherence: a literature review. J Clin Nurs. 2015;24(9–10):1163–73.
21. Marciel KK, Saiman L, Quittell LM, Dawkins K, Quittner AL. Cell phone intervention to improve adherence: cystic fibrosis care team, patient, and parent perspectives. Pediatr Pulmonol. 2010;45(2):157–64.
22. Creary SE, Gladwin MT, Byrne M, Hildesheim M, Krishnamurti L. A pilot study of electronic directly observed therapy to improve hydroxyurea adherence in pediatric patients with sickle-cell disease. Pediatr Blood Cancer. 2014;61(6):1068–73.
23. Foster JM, Usherwood T, Smith L, Sawyer SM, Xuan W, Rand CS, et al. Inhaler reminders improve adherence with controller treatment in primary care patients with asthma. J Allergy Clin Immunol. 2014;134(6):1260–8.
24. Wu JR, Corley DJ, Lennie TA, Moser DK. Effect of a medication-taking behavior feedback theory-based intervention on outcomes in patients with heart failure. J Card Fail. 2012;18(1):1–9.
25. Russell C, Conn V, Ashbaugh C, Madsen R, Wakefield M, Webb A, et al. Taking immunosuppressive medications effectively (TIMELink): a pilot randomized controlled trial in adult kidney transplant recipients. Clin Transplant. 2011;25(6):864–70.
26. Ruppar TM. Randomized pilot study of a behavioral feedback intervention to improve medication adherence in older adults with hypertension. J Cardiovasc Nurs. 2010;25(6):470–9.

# 57 Education

Kitty O'Hare, Alice A. Kuo, and Niraj Sharma

## Introduction

Americans who obtain more education after high school have a higher likelihood of earning more, leading healthier lives, and living longer. In general, about 75% of high school graduates go on to obtain some form of postsecondary education, and 66% enroll in college. However, for graduates with a chronic childhood condition, the rates are lower. For example, for students on the autism spectrum, only 36% attended any type of postsecondary education [1].

Postsecondary education can include 2-year college, 4-year college, or vocational, business, or technical school. For some, 2-year college is their sole postsecondary experience; for others, attending 2-year college first before transferring to a 4-year college to graduate offers the opportunity to save some money or obtain general education units in a less competitive environment.

Vocational education is education that prepares people to work in a trade, in a craft, as a technician, or in support roles in professions such as engineering, accountancy, nursing, medicine, architecture, or law. Craft vocations are usually based on manual or practical activities and are traditionally related to a specific trade or occupation, such as culinary arts, hospitality management, or fire science. Vocational education is sometimes referred to as career education or technical education.

More and more young adults with chronic childhood conditions (YACCC) and youth with intellectual disabilities/developmental disabilities (ID/DD) are pursuing postsecondary educational opportunities. As a result, internists and family medicine providers as well as pediatricians are likely to encounter concerns about educational attainment. YACCCs have lower rates of educational attainment than do their peers without chronic medical conditions. Having a coexisting mental health condition, as well as a physical condition, has particular effects on educational success. YACCCs who do not graduate from high school are less likely to be employed and more likely to receive financial assistance.

K. O'Hare (✉)
Duke Primary Care, Durham, NC, USA

Department of Medicine, Duke University School of Medicine, Durham, NC, USA
e-mail: frances.ohare@duke.edu

A. A. Kuo
Division of Medicine-Pediatrics and Preventive Medicine, University of California, Los Angeles, CA, USA
e-mail: AKuo@mednet.ucla.edu

N. Sharma
Department of Medicine, Brigham and Women's Hospital, Boston, MA, USA

Department of Pediatrics, Boston Children's Hospital, Boston, MA, USA

Harvard Medical School, Boston, MA, USA
e-mail: nsharma@bwh.harvard.edu


A. A. Kuo et al. (eds.), *Care of Adults with Chronic Childhood Conditions*,
https://doi.org/10.1007/978-3-031-54281-7_57

**Table 57.1** Definitions

| | |
|---|---|
| Rehabilitation Act (Rehab Act) | Prohibits discrimination on the basis of disability in programs run by federal agencies; programs that receive federal financial assistance; in federal employment; and in the employment practices of federal contractors |
| 504 Plan | Ensures that students with a disability receive reasonable accommodations in their primary or secondary education<br>Used for students who need accommodations for equal access to their learning environment, but who do not require the specialized instruction stipulated by an individualized education plan (IEP) |
| Individuals with Disabilities Education Act (IDEA) | Stipulates that children and youth with disabilities must be provided with a free, appropriate public education in the least restrictive environment<br>The law allows for early intervention services for children aged 0–2 years, and special education services for children and youth aged 3–21 years |
| Individualized Education Plan (IEP) | A plan or program that ensures that students with a disability receive specialized instruction in their primary or secondary education |
| Transition Plan | Under the IDEA, students with an IEP must have a personalized transition plan by age 16 years<br>Must incorporate the student's strengths, preferences, and interests<br>Geared toward developing functional skills for work and for community life |
| Americans with Disabilities Act (ADA) | Stipulates that public accommodations, including private schools, may not discriminate on the basis of disability<br>Certain physical modifications are necessary to make buildings and public spaces accessible<br>Services must also be provided to individuals with visual or hearing impairments |
| Accommodations | Modifications that allow a student to learn and demonstrate learning without the interference of their disability |
| Family Educational Rights and Privacy Act (FERPA) | Protects the privacy of student records<br>At the level of primary and secondary education, FERPA (rather than HIPAA) applies to immunization records, school nurse records, and special education records |
| Higher Education Opportunity Act | Provides some federal financial aid for some students with ID/DD pursuing postsecondary education<br>Creates and expands college level programs for students with ID/DD |

*HIPAA* health insurance portability and accountability act, *ID/DD* intellectual disabilities/developmental disabilities

Beginning with the Rehabilitation Act of 1973 [2], and then with the Individuals with Disabilities Education Act of 1975 [3] and the Americans with Disabilities Act of 1990, [4] educational opportunities for youth with chronic medical conditions and disabilities have expanded rapidly (Table 57.1). Now all primary and secondary students are entitled to supports that optimize their educational experiences when compared with their nondisabled peers. These supports can include testing accommodations, human aides, assignment accommodations, materials/technical adaptations, and physical adaptations.

## Preparing for Postsecondary Education

While college students are afforded some legal protections, they do not have the same entitlements as primary and secondary (K-12) students; special education plans do not extend beyond high school. The burden is on the student to identify themselves to the college as needing accommodation and to work with the college to determine whether the college can provide reasonable accommodations. Added to the challenge is that, in most states, students aged 18 or older are legal adults; they must advocate for themselves without the direct intervention of parents or other family members. Nevertheless, colleges can provide a number of accommodations, from note-taking services to extended time for tests. Responsibility for providing accommodations may be divided among multiple college offices. Most colleges do not have a systematic way to identify YACCCs on their campuses. Students typically must initiate the disclosure of a chronic condition and advocate for their needs. Although the federal government does not mandate accommodating students with disabilities on college campuses, most institutions of higher learning

**Table 57.2** College resources for students with disabilities

| |
|---|
| *Student health* |
| This office varies in scope from school to school. Some larger institutions have a health service that is staffed 24/7 by physicians and nurses, with some primary and specialty care available. Other institutions may have a physician or nurse practitioner available for urgent care needs. Some student health services are staffed only by a nurse for limited hours. It is important for YACCCs to ask about the scope of the student health service prior to enrolling in college |
| *Disability services* |
| This is the office that manages accommodations, ranging from physical access, to low vision and hard-of-hearing services, to learning disabilities. If a student will require accommodation for any reason, then they must notify the disability services office at the time of enrollment |
| *Dean of students* |
| This is the office that is often involved if a student withdraws due to medical concerns, either temporarily or permanently. YACCCs should inquire about school policies regarding withdrawals prior to enrollment |
| *Student life* |
| This is the office that, in many schools, trains resident advisors and manages student housing. YACCCs may interact with this office if their condition is disclosed to their resident advisor or if their condition will impact their housing services |

have Offices for Students with Disabilities (Table 57.2), which can coordinate services and provide accommodations such as longer time on tests or a quieter location to take tests; note-taking services; transportation; audiovisual (AV) equipment for the visually or hearing impaired; video conferencing; or arrangements for testing accommodations for major standardized tests. These services are completely voluntary and require the student to self-identify and seek them out.

## Chronic Disease Management in the College Setting

### Healthcare Access

As YACCCs begin to consider different options for postsecondary education, a discussion with their healthcare provider could be useful. In particular, health insurance status is an important consideration. The Affordable Care Act (ACA) [5] allows for children to stay on their parents' health insurance until age 26-years, provided that parents have health insurance in the first place. However, for parents who are self-employed, uninsured, or have insurance in which the premiums to add dependents are too costly to afford, YACCCs may lose their health insurance upon reaching adulthood. If these YACCCs are considering postsecondary education, then a 4-year college may be the best option, given that most universities provide relatively affordable student health insurance. YACCCs opting to attend vocational school or 2-year college may end up uninsured, which for those with chronic medical conditions may be a challenging situation. YACCCs and their families should be counseled on the importance of maintaining health insurance through the college years. Students do need to compare what is offered through their college versus the benefits on their parents' insurance plan. If the student is attending an out-of-state school, then they should be especially vigilant about what services are covered near their school. In recent years, telehealth has become more widely available, which supports YACCs in obtaining care at a distance from their college campus. However, YACCs should seek guidance on insurance coverage for telehealth services, also any legal restrictions to the scope of services, such as seeking care across state lines.

The ACA expands Medicaid eligibility for individuals with disabilities in states that chose to implement the Medicaid expansion. Because some people may be reluctant to self-identify as having a disability, it is important for YACCCs seeking insurance coverage with Medicaid to understand that answering the disability screening questions can affect the contents of their benefits package. States must provide information to applicants and beneficiaries about the different Medicaid coverage groups and associated benefit packages so that people can make an informed decision about whether to seek coverage in a disability-related group with a benefits package that may better meet their needs. The online version of the single streamlined application contains two questions designed to identify people with disabilities: applicants are asked whether they have a physical disability or mental health condition that limits their ability to work, attend school, or take care of their daily needs; and whether they need help with activities of daily living (such as bathing, dressing, and using the bathroom) or live in a medical facility or nursing home. For YACCCs seeking Medicaid coverage with the intention of attending postsecondary education, accommodations for the health condition or disability should qualify them under the first question.

States generally must provide Medicaid to people who receive Supplemental Security Income (SSI) benefits [6]. To be eligible for SSI, beneficiaries must have low incomes, limited assets, and a significant disability that impairs their ability to work at a substantial gainful level. States also have the option to provide Medicaid to certain other related groups, including people with disabilities whose income exceeds the SSI limits, but is still below the federal poverty level (FPL, $11,670 per year for an individual in 2014) [7]. In some situations, making parents aware of these benefits and guidelines can help them determine how to structure their family's financial assets so that the YACCC can qualify and obtain health insurance and financial assistance in the long term.

Additional planning for healthcare access may be necessary depending on supplementary activities such as semester abroad, work-study, internships, and athletics. Providers can encourage YACCS to consider the intersection of healthcare with their postsecondary educational goals.

## General Healthcare

During the college exploration and admission process, YACCCs can explore the health services available at the schools they are considering. Based on the availability of care at the school, YACCCs and their healthcare teams can negotiate how care will be provided during the college years. One area of anxiety for many YACCCs is how to reach their provider with questions or urgent care needs. Providers can share the options available through their practice, whether an online patient portal, email, text messaging, or even virtual consultations. Providers should discuss their expectations regarding visit frequency, particularly in regard to medication refills. Most YACCCs prefer to coordinate appointments during school vacations. Assessment of a YACCC's ability to describe their health conditions, name their allergies, name their medications, fill a prescription, and name the common side effects of their medication should be a routine part of office visits. Providers also play a role in coaching YACCs about the functionality of patient portals, which offer the opportunity of viewing historical medical records in addition to active problem lists, medication lists, and immunization records. Some YACCs may permit a parent or other trusted caregiver to interface with their patient portal as a proxy, for assistance in navigating healthcare needs. Providers should counsel YACCs about their proxy options, with special discussion of protected information categories such as reproductive health and mental health.

Every pediatric practice has its own transfer policy. Some practices continue to see their YACCCs until they graduate college; others encourage their patients to transfer to adult providers at age 18 years. It is important for practices to be transparent about their policies and to notify patients, in advance, when they will need to transfer care, especially if a care transfer is expected before or during the college experience. If the practice is not transparent, then parents or the YACCC should ask what the transfer policy is. The transfer policy should be posted where all patients can see it, including the office website and waiting area. Frontline staff should be trained in the specifics of the policy. Pediatric providers should give specific recommendations for finding an adult healthcare team.

## Mental Health

Mental health concerns are very common among college students, from attention deficit/hyperactivity disorder (ADHD) to depression and anxiety. Some students enter college with a preexisting mental health concern, while others will develop a mental health problem after starting postsecondary school. Just as with physical health services, mental health services vary from college to college. Students should be encouraged to explore the options for services at their school, particularly counseling/psychotherapy versus medication management. Prescribers of mental health-related medication need to assess the student's understanding of its side effects and its potential impact on college habits, including alcohol use. Students and families should inquire if the college student health office will continue to prescribe medications. If not, prescribers should be clear about their expectations regarding frequency of office visits and management of refills. Diversion of mental health medications is unfortunately common on college campuses; prescribers should be very clear about the consequences of improper medication use. In some cases, routine drug testing is carried out for young adults with ADHD on stimulant medications with each set of refills because of the high diversion potential of these medications.

## Confidentiality

YACCCs may be nervous about sharing their health information. However, selective sharing is an important part of safety planning. Selective sharing of information is particularly valuable for YACCCs who are living on campus. While Student Health or Disability Services may be aware of students' medical needs, these offices generally are not available during off hours or weekends/holidays. YACCCs should be encouraged to disclose their condition to someone in proximity to their residential environment, such as the dorm resident advisor, or a roommate. In the classroom, some selective sharing is necessary to ensure that students get appropriate accommodations. For example, professors need to be aware of accommodations needed for visual impairment or hearing impairment. However, professors do not need to know extensive details of a student's health history. Students should know that the Family Educational Rights and Privacy Act (FERPA) [8] prevents colleges from disclosing educational records, including student health information, to third parties.

Routine office visits provide an opportunity for YACCCs to practice selective sharing. YACCCs should have the opportunity to spend a portion of each office visit alone with their provider, to develop some trust in sharing confidential information. YACCCs can sign a release for the practice to share health information with student health services, or vice versa. The provider and the youth can discuss which information is most important for the college to have.

## Emergency Planning

Many YACCCs will experience a medical emergency while on campus. With advanced preparation, emergency management can proceed much more smoothly. Prior to coming to campus, YACCCs and their families should decide who the best emergency contact is. YACCCs should also identity a healthcare proxy (HCP) who is authorized to make health decisions if the student becomes incapacitated. No-cost state-specific HCP forms are available online. There is some provision in FERPA to allow notification of a student's family in case of emergency, even if the student has not identified a specific HCP.

A portable healthcare summary is a useful tool for communicating with hospitals and emergency responders. These allow first responders to triage appropriately and in a timely fashion based on the YACCC's situation. Examples of portable healthcare summaries are available online through the American Academy of Pediatrics and the Center for Health Care Transition Improvement (Got Transition; www.gottransition.org). If saved as a portable document file (PDF), the summary can be easily available via a cell phone, tablet, or encrypted portable flash drive. A variety of apps are available to organize health information on a phone, tablet, or other device. Given the sensitive nature of the information, ensuring that an electronic device is properly encrypted could be an important consideration.

Medical alert bracelets, smart watches, or similar identifiers are helpful for first responders. YACCCs can find a variety of styles online. Healthcare providers can encourage YACCCs to introduce themselves to student health when they arrive on campus. Even if the student does not plan to utilize student health services on a regular basis, the student health service should still be aware of how to respond if the student experiences a medical emergency. In particular, student health should know how to contact the YACCC's primary care physician and specialists.

## Wellness

Like all college students, YACCCs need to learn how to incorporate wellness into their daily routine. Regular exercise is important for all college students; healthcare providers can stress the benefits of exercise for specific chronic conditions. Guidance on nutrition is also essential, given the variety of options available on most college campuses. Adequate sleep is being appreciated more and more as an important component of overall wellness. YACCCs can be counseled on the effects of sleep deprivation on their specific condition. Finally, stress management is an essential component of wellness and most college campuses offer some stress management services through psychological counseling or the Office of Student Life.

## Social Life

College is often a time of exploration and of testing limits. Most YACCCs report that their provider did not discuss the impact of nicotine, alcohol, cannabis, and other substances on their health. It is important for healthcare providers to demonstrate their openness to discussing challenging topics such as substance use. Healthcare providers can counsel YACCCs on how tobacco, alcohol, marijuana, and other drugs can impact their particular chronic condition. Medication interactions with substances are a common concern. Complete abstinence from tobacco products (including cigarettes, e-cigarettes, chewing tobacco, and hookah) is the best approach, though providers should also offer cessation materials when needed.

YACCCs may need assistance in identifying sexual health services. While many college campuses offer contraception, emergency contraception, and testing for sexually transmitted infections, these supports are not universal. Many female YACCCs have not been counseled about the impact of pregnancy or of hormonal birth control on their health condition. Young women may be unaware of the impact that pregnancy can have on their health. Healthcare providers should demonstrate openness to questions about contraception and pregnancy. Long-acting reversible contraception (LARC) is a reasonable choice for female YACCCs during their postsecondary education period.

## Postsecondary Education for People with Intellectual Disabilities/Developmental Disabilities

Students with I/DD also benefit from postsecondary educational experiences. According to national surveys, youths with I/DD value their college experiences as opportunities to interact with same-age peers, as well as to develop independent living skills. Youths with I/DD who receive postsecondary educational services are more likely to sustain paid employment. This can lead to improved quality of life. Postsecondary education is a time for youths to explore their self-identity. Some students may have strong feelings about the labels applied to them as they enroll in services.

Whether or not young adults with I/DD are able to attend some postsecondary education is often dependent on their adaptive skills (i.e., practical, everyday skills needed to function and meet the demands of one's environment, including the skills necessary to effectively and independently take care of oneself and to interact with other people). If young adults with I/DD are planning to go away to college, a discussion about the ability to function independently could be valuable for the young adult and his/her parents. Often, it is not the academic work that proves to be challenging for the young adult with I/DD, but navigating adult social situations that can ultimately lead to the young adult leaving school and moving back home. Parents should be aware of this possibility and be prepared to consider postsecondary opportunities closer to home, with the ability for the young adult to be with trusted friends and family members more frequently. Many community colleges offer flexible, local postsecondary opportunities that meet the needs of youth with I/DD.

A variety of postsecondary education options are available to youth with I/DD. Vocational or working-training programs can offer young adults with I/DD practical education while preparing them to enter the workforce in a supported environment. Often times, programs such as these offer a wide variety of job opportunities that can be tailored to the interests of the young adult. The young adult works part time and still receives some training or education for new jobs, with coaching or mentoring included. A recent movement has been to shift from a readiness model (train and place) to a support model (place and train) so that the YACCC with an I/DD can have work that is customized and yet still meets the needs of an employer.

## Conclusion

Postsecondary education should be encouraged in YACCCs with or without I/DD. A primary care provider can counsel on appropriate placement and health insurance considerations ("Appendix"). In addition, emergency plans, healthcare proxies, and confidentiality are issues that should be discussed and planned appropriately with the help of a primary care provider.

## Appendix

### Resources

- Disability.gov: https://www.dol.gov/agencies/odep/topics
- Champaloux SW, Young DR. Childhood chronic health conditions and educational attainment: a social ecological approach. J Adol Health. 2015;56:98–105.
- Maslow GR, Haydon A, Ford CA, Halpern CT. Young adult outcomes of children growing up with chronic illness: an analysis of the National Longitudinal Study of Adolescent Health. Arch Pediatr Adolesc Med. 2011;165:256–61.
- Ip W, Yang S, Parker J, et al. Assessment of prevalence of adolescent patient portal account access by guardians. JAMA Netw Open. 2021;4(9):e2124733.
- HEATH Resource Center at the National Youth Transitions Center, Graduate School of Education and Human Development, The George Washington University. https://www.heath.gwu.edu/transitioning-high-school-college-spotlight-section-504#:~:text=Under%20Section%20504%2C%20colleges%20are,subjected%20to%20undue%20financial%20hardship
- Got Transition: www.gottransition.org.
- Lemly DC, Lawlor K, Scherer EA, Kelemen S, Weitzman ER. College health service capacity to support youth with chronic medical conditions. Pediatrics. 2014;134(5):885–91.
- Think College: www.thinkcollege.net.
- American Academy of Pediatrics Emergency Information Form. https://www.acep.org/by-medical-focus/pediatrics/medical-forms/emergency-information-form-for-children-with-special-health-care-needs/.

## References

1. Roux A, Rast J, Rava J, Anderson K, Shattuck P. National Autism Indicators report: transition into young adulthood. Drexel: Drexel Autism Institute, Drexel University; 2015.
2. U.S Equal Employee Opportunity Commission. The Rehabilitation Act of 1973 [Internet]. US EEOC. 1973 [cited 2022 Oct 11]. https://www.eeoc.gov/statutes/rehabilitation-act-1973.
3. Individuals with Disabilities Education Act (IDEA). Individuals with Disabilities Education Act (IDEA) [Internet]. Individuals with Disabilities Education Act. [cited 2022 Oct 11]. https://sites.ed.gov/idea/.
4. US Department of Justice Civil Rights Division. ADA.gov homepage [Internet]. ADA.gov. [cited 2022 Oct 11]. https://www.ada.gov/.
5. Individuals with Disabilities Education Act (IDEA). Affordable Care Act [Internet]. [cited 2022 Oct 11].

https://www.hhs.gov/healthcare/about-the-aca/index.html.

6. Social Security Administration. Supplemental Security Income (SSI) Benefits [Internet]. [cited 2022 Oct 11]. https://www.ssa.gov/benefits/ssi/.
7. US Department of Health and Human Services, Office of the Assistant Secretary for Planning and Evaluation (ASPE). Poverty guidelines [Internet]. ASPE. [cited 2022 Oct 15]. https://aspe.hhs.gov/topics/poverty-economic-mobility/poverty-guidelines.
8. US Department of Education. Family Educational Rights and Privacy Act (FERPA) [Internet]. US Department of Education (ED); 2021 [cited 2022 Oct 15]. https://www2.ed.gov/policy/gen/guid/fpco/ferpa/index.html.

# 58 Employment

Emily Nations Bufkin, Carlie Stein, and Alice A. Kuo

## Case Presentation

Nigel is 16 yo with Trisomy 21, hypothyroidism, and ADHD who is presenting to the clinic for his yearly physical. From a medical standpoint, his pre-visit labs show well-controlled hypothyroidism on his current dose of levothyroxine and no signs of iron deficiency. There are no behavioral concerns. He follows biannually with an optometrist, and there are no current vision or hearing concerns. Nigel is currently enrolled in his local public school's special education program, which has been great for Nigel's socialization and has allowed his mother to return to work full-time. He proudly tells you he will graduate when he is 21 and that he wants to start a job right after graduation like his classmate did last year. His mother reports that they will be discussing postgraduation plans at his upcoming annual IEP meeting and inquires about any additional resources you would recommend regarding finding suitable employment for Nigel.

## Introduction

Employment for adults fulfills many needs. The first and foremost is a paycheck—an ability to have some financial independence, whether for pocket money or complete living expenses. However, having a job also anchor's one's identity and can influence quality of life. Being successfully employed can give purpose and build self-esteem in one's life. More practically, paying into the US Social Security system for 40 quarters (10 years) makes an adult eligible to draw upon the Social Security system as a senior citizen and also be eligible for Medicare. Numerous national employers provide medical insurance for full or part-time employment, which can enhance healthcare access and alleviate the financial burden of medical expenses.

For young adults with chronic childhood conditions (YACCC) with intellectual/developmental disabilities (I/DD), the road to employment can be arduous, depending on the level of cognitive impairment. Many young adults with disabilities have the option to remain public school students until the year they turn 21. These extra years of schooling can focus on academic supports or vocational training. In every high school

E. N. Bufkin (✉)
Division of Internal Medicine-Pediatrics, Department of Internal Medicine, University of Texas Southwestern Medical Center, Dallas, TX, USA
e-mail: emily.bufkin@utsouthwestern.edu

C. Stein
Department of Medicine, UAB School of Medicine, Birmingham, AL, USA
e-mail: chstein@uabmc.edu

A. A. Kuo
Division of Medicine-Pediatrics and Preventive Medicine, University of California, Los Angeles, CA, USA
e-mail: akuo@mednet.ucla.edu


A. A. Kuo et al. (eds.), *Care of Adults with Chronic Childhood Conditions*,
https://doi.org/10.1007/978-3-031-54281-7_58

year, during their Individualized Education Plan (IEP) meeting, some level of transition planning should have occurred, focusing on what the student was going to do once he finished his school experience. Typically, options range from going on to college, into a job training program, to a vocational support environment, or to an adult day program focused on recreation.

For those young adults interested in obtaining employment, whether full- or part-time, it is essential that they connect with their local vocational rehabilitation (VR) program. VR services are offered to people who have "barriers to employment." Those barriers can be anything from a physical disability, visual impairment, or psychiatric conditions. VR programs are funded by both federal and state governments and administered by states to help people with disabilities obtain gainful employment. VR programs have their origins in the rehabilitation for disabled World War I veterans. The Rehabilitation Act of 1973 (the "Rehab Act") is the legal basis for today's VR system and shifted the focus in vocational services for people with I/DD through its emphasis on services and individualized plans for employment [1]. In addition, Employment First is a national movement that promotes integrated employment as the primary and preferred outcome for people with I/DD and establishes that the default setting of services should be a presumption of ability [2]. Integrated employment is defined as "full or part-time work for which an individual is (a) compensated at or above minimum wage and comparable to the customary rate paid by the employer to employees without disabilities performing similar duties and with similar training and experience; (b) receiving the same level of benefits provided to other employees without disabilities in similar positions; (c) at a location where the employee interacts with other individuals without disabilities; and (d) presented opportunities for advancement similar to other employees without disabilities in similar positions" [2].

VR services can provide a bridge as high school students prepare to leave school and enter the workforce; however, the involvement of VR during the special education transition process has been rare. Although VR primarily provides services for working-age adults, due to recent shifts in federal funding toward transition-age services, VR should be increasingly involved with younger adults just entering the workforce for the first time.

The Workforce Innovation and Opportunity Act (WIOA) was signed in July 2014 as an amendment to the Rehabilitation Act of 1973. It required VR agencies to set aside 15% of federal funds for "pre-employment transition services" for students with disabilities who may be eligible for VR services. This act requires states to strategically coordinate the needs of employers and individuals. A feature of this act includes American job centers with youth programs located in specific locations that provide school tutoring, counseling, job training, education, and employment resources for in-school youth aged 14–21 and out-of-school youth aged 16–24. Core services, including job search, job placement, and assessment of skills and needs, are available to all individuals who are of 18 years of age and older with or without a disability. Find a local American Job Center (AJC) here: https://www.careeronestop.org/LocalHelp/local-help.aspx.

## Transition from Education to Employment

High school students with a disability can receive in-school supports through special education, as mandated by the Individuals with Disabilities Education Act [3]. When a high school student is 16 or older, a transition plan should be developed that specifies the supports needed to get a job, continue postsecondary education, and/or live independently. If the immediate goal after high school is to get a job, then special education services could include vocational education (including part-time employment during high school), career counseling, life skills, and transportation training.

The challenge for many young adults with disability is that there is no entitlement for services in adulthood. After exiting the public K-12 school system, young adults and their families must apply for services from a myriad of adult-serving public systems. Young adults with a documented intellectual disability may have an easier time qualifying for services; however, many young adults with a developmental disability without an intellectual disability (such as autism) may need significant support to function in the workplace.

## Eligibility for Vocational Rehabilitation Services

All individuals with disabilities are eligible for VR services. Specifically, this includes a person:

1. Who has a physical or mental impairment;
2. Whose impairment substantially interferes with the ability to get a job;
3. Whose impairment requires VR services to prepare for secure, retain, or regain employment; and.
4. Who intends to achieve an employment outcome.

The federal Rehabilitation Act specifies that VR should operate with the presumption that the person can achieve employment through VR services [1]. If it is decided that a person cannot benefit from VR services, there must be clear and convincing evidence as to why. Additionally, a person eligible for Social Security Income (SSI) benefits is also automatically presumed eligible for VR services [4]. Importantly, a patient does not need to be on SSI or SSDI to be eligible for VR services.

## Vocational Rehabilitation Services

VR services can assist clients with resume writing, interview skills, job trials, volunteer opportunities, job coaching, and job placement. They can also pay for job-required training, including certifications or college degrees. In some cases, if someone has a physical disability that requires an accessible vehicle to get to and from work, VR services may pay for modifications to a vehicle already owned by the client to make it accessible. A more complete list of VR service categories is provided in Table 58.1 [5].

VR services also have Benefits Counselors who can guide young adults through the confusing maze of eligibility for government benefits, such as Supplemental Security Income (SSI) and Medicaid, while earning a paycheck. These professionals can be accessed through the Ticket to Work helpline. These professionals can explain programs that will allow them to save their income while not losing their benefits [6]. Notably, these programs include Plan to Achieve Self-Support (PASS) and Achieving a Better Life Experience (ABLE) accounts. PASS accounts allow qualifying individuals to use their income or property to reach a work goal, such as setting aside funding to return to school or complete specialized training to obtain a job that will earn enough to reduce or eliminate the need for benefits provided under SSI [7]. ABLE accounts are tax-advantaged savings accounts for YACCC in which the account's assets can be used to cover qualified expenses up to a certain amount before SSI benefits are impacted [8]. A patient facing financial toolkit was released by the Leadership for the Employment and Economic Advancement of People with Disabilities (LEAD) Center in August 2021. This resource provides helpful information on the core topics of preparing for, starting, maintaining, changing or losing, and retiring from a job [9].

Another service VR can help with is for the legal rights of employees with disabilities. Many adults are unsure of their legal rights under the Americans with Disabilities Act (ADA) which protects individuals with disabilities against discrimination in employment [10]. Prospective employers are not allowed to ask an applicant if she has any disabilities or medical conditions. They are allowed to ask, "With proper accommodations, are you able to fulfill the duties of this job?" VR can direct applicants on how to answer interview questions and protect themselves from discrimination.

**Table 58.1** Vocational rehabilitation service categories and definitions

| Assessment |
|---|
| Assessment means services and activities used to determine an individual's eligibility for VR services, to prioritize level of employment needs, and/or to determine the nature and scope of VR services to be included in the IPE |
| Assessment services might include |
| • Trial work experiences and extended evaluation |
| • Psychological assessments |
| • Dental and medical exams |
| • Assessments of personality, interests, interpersonal skills, intelligence and related functional capacities, educational achievements, work experience, vocational aptitudes, personal and social adjustments, and employment opportunities of the individual |
| VR Counseling and Guidance |
| VR counseling and guidance provides information and support services to assist people in making informed choices about employment |
| Job Placement Services |
| Job placement assistance is a referral to a specific job resulting in an interview, whether or not the individual obtained the job |
| Job Search Assistance |
| Job search activities support and assist an individual in searching an appropriate job. Job search assistance may include helping in resume preparation, identifying appropriate job opportunities, developing interview skills, and contacting businesses |
| Information and Referral |
| Information and referrals to other agencies are provided for services that are not available through the VR program |
| On-the-Job Supports (Supported Employment) |
| Ongoing support services and other appropriate services are needed to support and maintain an individual with a most significant disability in supported employment for a period of time generally not to exceed 18 months. Such services, such as job coaching, are for individuals who have supported employment and long-term supports identified on their IPE. For example, an employee may need support in understanding job tasks or workplace rules, or learning how to navigate to/from work or within the workplace |
| Job Readiness Training |
| Training provided to prepare an individual for the world of work (e.g., appropriate work behaviors, getting to work on time, appropriate dress and grooming, increasing productivity) |
| Diagnosis and Treatment of Impairments |
| VR services will pay for diagnosis and treatment of the listed physical and mental impairments, if and only if other sources of funding (i.e., grant funding) cannot be secured, and if the physical or mental impairment negatively affects ability to work. Services include, but are not limited to: |
| • Diagnosis and treatment for mental and emotional disorders by licensed providers |
| • Nursing services |
| • Prescription of eyeglasses and visual services |
| • Physical, occupational, and speech or hearing therapy |
| • Mental health services |
| • Other medical or medically related rehabilitation services |
| On-the-Job Supports, Short Term |
| Services provided to support a person in maintaining their job once he or she is employed. Such services include short-term job coaching for persons who do not have a supported employment goal in their IPE |

Reprinted with permission from Roux AM, Rast JE, Anderson KA, Shattuck PT. National Autism Indicators Report: Vocational Rehabilitation. Philadelphia, PA: Life Course Outcomes Research Program, A.J. Drexel Autism Institute, Drexel University; 2016
*VR* vocational rehabilitation, *IPE* individual plan for employment

## Vocational Rehabilitation Service Use and Outcomes

Few studies have been published in the traditional research literature about the use of VR services and outcomes. However, the 2016 National Autism Indicators Report produced by researchers at Drexel University focused on VR and examined service use and outcomes using administrative data from the Rehabilitation Services

Administration for the federal fiscal year 2014 [5]. Their key findings included the following:

- Overall, 80% of those who got a job were employed part-time with median weekly earnings of $160. Earnings were slightly higher for those who were employed without supports and lower for those in supported employment.
- The most common job type was office and administrative support. About 1 in 4 people worked in an office job.
- The employment rates following VR services were comparable for those with autism (60%), intellectual disability (55%), and other disabilities (56%). A lower percentage with autism had supported employment compared to those with ID.
- The rate of working part-time was the same for those with autism and those with ID: nearly 90%.
- Those with autism were more likely to work in office jobs compared to their peers who received VR services. Working in food service or cleaning jobs was less likely compared to those with ID.

Individuals who receive job placement services with VR are more likely to exit VR with employment [11–15]. Job placement services are the most predictive of a positive employment outcome in VR.

## Job Training or Placement

Besides VR, individual agencies may provide job training or job placement services. Companies like Goodwill Industries and Salvation Army are some of the larger, more established organizations in the country, but each state has many options. Young adults can find a list of providers through their state agency on disability, either for intellectual/developmental disabilities or the department of aging and physical disabilities.

Two models of job training/placement are worth mentioning, especially as programs are moving toward a support model (place, then train) as opposed to a readiness model (train, then place).

### Project SEARCH

Project SEARCH was developed at Cincinnati Children's Hospital [16] and has been disseminated internationally with strong program fidelity to replicate impressive outcomes. The primary goal of SEARCH is to obtain competitive employment opportunities for people with disabilities. More information about Project SEARCH and its model is available at: www.projectsearch.us.

### TEACCH Autism Program

A second model of supported employment was developed in 1972 at the University of North Carolina, called the TEACCH Autism Program [17]. In an effort to provide each individual with ASD the greatest chance of obtaining and maintaining successful competitive employment, the TEACCH ® Supported Employment Program has developed four models of support: One-to-One Placement, Mobile Crew, Group Shared Support Site, and Standard Placement. More information about the TEACCH model is available at: https://teacch.com/.

### The Arc

Several nonprofits offer employment support including the Arc [18]. The Arc Employment Support Program offers several resources, including:

1. Detailed assessment of workspace.
2. Disability awareness and bias training.
3. Connecting employers to the untapped disability labor pool.
4. Supports for new hires.
5. Achieving a cultural and financial return on investment.

More information about the Arc Employment support program is at https://thearc.org/our-initiatives/employment/employment-services/.

## Family Medical Leave

As adults with chronic diseases or disabilities enter the workforce, they need to know about and understand the Family Medical Leave Act (FMLA) [19]. FMLA is federal protection against termination from employment for missing work due to a disclosed medical condition. Once an adult has accepted employment. It is suggested he talks with his Human Resources department about completing FMLA paperwork. This entails his physician attesting to the diagnosis and giving an estimate of the amount of time the employee may need to miss work over the course of the year. FMLA protection is effective for up to 12 weeks per year. There are some exclusions to FMLA protections, particularly around the length of employment and the size of the business. It is advised to learn more about FMLA at the Department of Labor Website at https://www.dol.gov/agencies/whd/fmla/forms.

## Implications of COVID-19 on the Workplace for YACCC

The COVID-19 pandemic had a significant impact on multiple facets of daily life, but perhaps, its most significant and likely longest-lasting impact had been on the workplace. The pandemic called into question the need for physical presence in the workplace. Out of necessity, employers were forced to consider remote work options and to invest in the infrastructure to sustain them. McKinsey Global Institute modeled the future of work following the COVID-19 pandemic utilizing a database of eight countries comprising 62% of the global gross domestic product [20]. The following conclusions were drawn about the post-pandemic workplace and workforce: (1) Remote work will continue, although less robustly than at the height of the pandemic; (2) Adoption of automation/artificial intelligence will be accelerated, and; (3) Job growth is limited in low-wage occupations. Remote work has both pros and cons for YACCC. Working remotely may allow YACCC with rigid inflexibilities to retain employment due to less need for soft skills—such as emotional intelligence and adaptability—required to thrive in the workplace. However, a blended workplace utilizing both in-office and remote workers may also disadvantage YACCC, who need in-job supports due to the lack of supervision or mentoring by those whose positions allow them to work from home. Faster adoption of automation/artificial intelligence will impact jobs with high physical proximity requirements. This will eliminate positions for YACCC who are more likely to do well in these roles. Finally, the mix of occupations is expected to shift post-pandemic with little projected growth in low-wage occupations, with jobs in food service, customer sales, service roles, and less-skilled office support roles expected to be most negatively impacted. Displaced workers will likely need to acquire new skill sets to shift occupations in higher-wage brackets. This underscores the importance for YACCC to utilize VR services and for employers to use support models to train the workforce they need post-pandemic.

## References

1. US Equal Employment Opportunity Commission. The Rehabilitation Act of 1973 [Internet]. US EEOC. https://www.eeoc.gov/statutes/rehabilitation-act-1973. Accessed 16 Oct 2022.
2. US Department of Labor. Employment First | U.S. Department of Labor [Internet]. https://www.dol.gov/agencies/odep/initiatives/employment-first. Accessed 16 Oct 2022.
3. Individuals with Disabilities Education Act (IDEA). Individuals with Disabilities Education Act (IDEA) [Internet]. Individuals with Disabilities Education Act. https://sites.ed.gov/idea/. Accessed 16 Oct 2022.
4. Assessment for Determining Eligibility and Priority for Services [Internet]. Title 34 Ch. III § 361.42 Jul 1, 2006. https://www.govinfo.gov/content/pkg/CFR-2006-title34-vol2/pdf/CFR-2006-title34-vol2-sec361-42.pdf.
5. Roux AM, Rast J, Anderson K, Shattuck P. National Autism Indicators Report: Vocational Rehabilitation.

6. Social Security Administration. Contact—Ticket to Work—Social Security [Internet]. https://choosework.ssa.gov/contact/. Accessed 16 Oct 2022.
7. ORDP.OPDR. Plan to Achieve Self-Support (PASS) [Internet]. https://www.ssa.gov/disabilityresearch/wi/pass.htm. Accessed 16 Oct 2022.
8. Achieving A Better Life Experience Act (ABLE) National Resource Center [Internet]. ABLE National Resource Center. https://www.ablenrc.org/. Accessed 16 Oct 2022.
9. US Department of Labor Employee Benefits Security Administration. Secure Your Financial Future A Toolkit for Individuals with Disabilities [Internet]. https://www.dol.gov/agencies/ebsa/secure-your-financial-future. Accessed 16 Oct 2022.
10. US Department of Labor. Americans with Disabilities Act. Americans with Disabilities Act | U.S. Department of Labor [Internet]. https://www.dol.gov/general/topic/disability/ada. Accessed 16 Oct 2022.
11. Chen JL, Sung C, Pi S. Vocational rehabilitation service patterns and outcomes for individuals with autism of different ages. J Autism Dev Disord. 2015;45(9):3015–29.
12. Schaller J, Yang NK. Competitive employment for people with autism correlates of successful closure in competitive and supported employment. Rehabil Couns Bull. 2005;49(1):4–16.
13. Lawer L, Brusilovskiy E, Salzer MS, Mandell DS. Use of vocational rehabilitative services among adults with autism. J Autism Dev Disord. 2009;39(3):487–94.
14. Butterworth J, Migliore A, Timmons J. Services and outcomes for transition age young adults with autism spectrum disorders: secondary analysis of the NLTS2 and RSA 911. Boston: University of Massachusetts Boston; 2010. https://mchtraining.net/media/research/documents/finalreports/butterworth_r40_mc_22646_final_report.pdf.
15. Alsaman MA, Lee C-L. Employment outcomes of youth with disabilities in vocational rehabilitation. A multilevel analysis of RSA-911 data. Rehabil Couns Bull. 2016;60(2):98–107.
16. Cincinnati Children's Hospital Medical Center. Project SEARCH. Educating people with disabilities. http://www.projectsearch.us/OurPROGRAM/ProgramModel.aspx. Accessed 16 Oct 2022.
17. University of North Carolina. TEACCH Autism Program. TEACCH® Supported Employment Program. http://teacch.com/clinical-services/supported-employment-1/introduction-to-models-ofsup port. Accessed 22 Oct 2022.
18. The Arc. [Internet]. https://thearc.org/. Accessed 22 Oct 2022.
19. US Department of Labor. Wage and Hour Division. Family and Medical Leave Act. [Internet]. https://www.dol.gov/agencies/whd/fmla. Accessed 22 Oct 2022.
20. McKinsey Global Institute. The Future of Work after COVID-19. [Internet]. https://www.mckinsey.com/featured-insights/future-of-work/the-future-of-work-after-covid-19. Accessed 22 Oct 2022.

# Independent Living 59

David E. DeLaet and Cory Ellen Nourie

## Introduction

This chapter will focus on challenges faced by young adults from vulnerable populations as they attempt to transition to an independent living environment as well as existing programs and legislation that can help young adults address these obstacles. Vulnerable populations to be considered include young adults with chronic childhood conditions (YACCC), those with learning and developmental disabilities, individuals with mental health conditions, and those emerging from the foster care system.

## Vulnerable Populations and Scope of the Problem

As has been highlighted throughout this text, advances in medicine over the last several decades have resulted in a significant increase in the population of YACCC. For example, from the period 1979 to 2017, the median age at death among Blacks with sickle cell disease in the United States increased from 28 to 43 years [1]. Likewise, the median predicted age of survival for patients with cystic fibrosis has risen from approximately 30 years of age among those born between 1989 and 1993 to 50 years among those born between 2016 and 2020 [2]. Similar trends of improved survival have been seen for pediatric and adolescent patients diagnosed with malignancies and congenital heart disease [3, 4]. This diverse and growing population of YACCC represents a group of patients for whom the transition period from adolescence to young adulthood can be particularly difficult.

Another population for whom this transition can be challenging includes those patients with intellectual disability, developmental delay, or mental health illness. Recent estimates suggest a prevalence of intellectual disability of 14.0 people per thousand and of developmental delay of 30.8 people per thousand among children aged 13–17 years [5]. Further, data from the 2020 National Survey on Drug Use and Health revealed a past-year prevalence of any mental illness of 30.6% and of serious mental illness of 9.7% among young adults aged 18–25 years [6].

Lastly, those young adults transitioning from foster care are also susceptible to the obstacles inherent to this period of transition. According to the most recently available data from the Adoption and Foster Care Analysis and Reporting System (AFCARS), there were an estimated

D. E. DeLaet (✉)
Department of Medicine, University of Cincinnati College of Medicine, Cincinnati, OH, USA
e-mail: delaetde@ucmail.uc.edu

C. E. Nourie
Division of Developmental Disabilities Services, Delaware Department of Health and Social Services, Woodbrook Professional Center, Dover, DE, USA
e-mail: cory.nourie@delaware.gov


A. A. Kuo et al. (eds.), *Care of Adults with Chronic Childhood Conditions*,
https://doi.org/10.1007/978-3-031-54281-7_59

407,493 children in foster care on September 30, 2020. Of those, 87,250 were between the ages of 14 and 18 years and an additional 7000 between 19 and 20 years [7]. Though a few states define the legal age of majority as 19 or even 21 years of age, most states recognize 18 years as the age of majority. It is this legal definition by states that largely dictates when a young adult will age out of the foster care system. During fiscal year (FY) 2020, an estimated 16,445 young adults in the United States were thus emancipated [7].

## Transition to Independent Living Among Young Adults

Multiple surveys have demonstrated that the transition to independent living can be difficult for many young adults. According to analysis of the Current Population Survey data, 47% of 18–29-year-olds in the United States were living with a parent as of February 2020; this number is even more pronounced among racial/ethnic minorities, with 55% of Latinx and 50% of Black young adults living with a parent [8]. Among adults aged 18–24 years, 67% still receive financial support from their parents and 63% still live in a parental home [8, 9]. Further, young adults also continue to rely on their parents for emotional support and guidance, with degree of dependence perhaps influenced by race and ethnicity. A 2001 survey of 300 subjects of 18–22 years of age suggested that Black and Latinx young adults were more reliant on caregivers for direction and nurturing than White counterparts [10]. While this period of transition appears to be difficult for many young adults, it would be anticipated to be even more challenging for the susceptible populations previously described.

## Independent Living Issues for Young Adults with Chronic Medical and Mental Health Conditions and Disabilities

Adolescents and young adults with chronic medical conditions and disabilities, intellectual disabilities, developmental disabilities, and mental health disease are likely to face many obstacles as they attempt to transition towards independent living. Similar to their peers in the general population, adolescents and young adults with disabilities rely on their parents for financial support during this period of transition. In fact, many of these young adults are more likely than their peers to remain in the family home as they complete secondary education or vocational training [11]. However, families with children with disabilities are significantly more likely to suffer financial hardship, and this may limit available resources for continued support [12]. Such financial hardship is further aggravated by limited employment opportunities for these young adults: 21% of people with disabilities as compared to 59% of those who do not have disabilities are working [13]. The majority of these unemployed disabled individuals would like to be working [14]. The independence of many disabled adults is also limited by inadequate transportation [15, 16]. These obstacles may lead to increased emotional stressors on these individuals. As compared with their peers in the general population, individuals with disabilities are twice as likely to be worried about not being able to care for themselves or being a burden to their families [16].

The successful transition to a minimally restrictive living environment may be particularly problematic for those individuals with intellectual disabilities and mental health diseases. The Community Mental Health Centers Act of 1963 initiated the era of community mental health and deinstitutionalization practices in the United States [17]. Over the subsequent decades, the result was a dramatic decrease in the number of individuals with mental illness who were institutionalized in state mental hospitals [18]. Legislative efforts have been made to assure adequate housing opportunities for the mentally disabled such as the Fair Housing Act of 1968, which prohibits discrimination in the sale, rental, and financing of dwellings, and in other housing-related transactions, based on race, color, national origin, religion, sex, familial status, and disability [19]. Despite such legislation, access to adequate community alternatives to hospitalization has not kept pace with such deinstitutionalization. For example, options for out-of-home placement, such as small group homes, for disabled individuals are limited [20]. As a likely consequence of these policy changes, recent estimates have suggested that approximately 75% of adults with intellectual or developmental disabilities live with an aging parent or caregiver [20].

As another example of inadequate access to mental health resources, research has demonstrated that the majority of adolescents who receive publicly funded mental health services do not continue to receive such services as young adults, with this being more notable among minority groups [21, 22]. This lack of service support is underscored by the high rate of unemployment, poverty, substance abuse, criminal activity, and homelessness exhibited by these young adults with mental health conditions [23, 24]. These coexisting social conditions contribute to the challenges experienced by this transitioning demographic.

Given these difficulties with transition, it is important for young adults from susceptible populations and their families to be aware of available resources that might assure a better transition experience. From the standpoint of financial assistance, patients and their families should inquire about eligibility for Supplemental Security Income (SSI) and Social Security Disability Insurance (SSDI) through the United States Social Security Administration [25]. Though many patients may have already been receiving benefits through SSI prior to the age of 18 years, eligibility standards for adults are not identical to those for individuals less than 18 years of age; as such, patients may no longer qualify for assistance [25]. For planning purposes, it is therefore critical to clarify eligibility well in advance of reaching the age of majority. Additionally, some states provide additional cash subsidies to children and adults with intellectual and developmental disabilities living in the family home, though this support varies greatly from state to state [26].

For the large majority of unemployed individuals with disabilities who want to work, it is important that they be familiar with programs and legislation that support this goal. Historically, SSI has had employment and income restrictions; such restrictions often served as disincentives to becoming self-supportive through work [27]. The Center for Medicare and Medicaid Services "Ticket to Work and Work Incentives Improvement Act of 1999" was enacted to allow patients to work while continuing to receive SSI and the associated Medicaid benefits [28]. Despite such initiatives, a large percentage of individuals receiving SSI remain unemployed [29]. It is essential then that these individuals understand their protected rights for employment under the 1990 Americans with Disabilities Act (ADA), which states that "no covered entity shall discriminate against a qualified individual on the basis of disability in regard to job application procedures, the hiring, advancement, or discharge of employees, employee compensation, job training, and other terms, conditions, and privileges of employment" [30]. It would also be beneficial that these young adults are made aware of the federally supported state vocational rehabilitation programs that can assist youth with disabilities in vocational education and supported employment services and that such information be provided well before 18 years of age [31]. Benefits counselors at these vocational rehabilitation programs can additionally help guide young adults regarding their eligibility for the aforementioned SSI and SSDI benefits and the related "Ticket to Work" program as well as assist with issues pertaining to legal rights of employees with disabilities.

Patients with physical or developmental disabilities should be familiar with provisions of the ADA in terms of being able to secure independent housing. The law allows individuals, at their own cost, "to make reasonable structural modifications to units and public/common areas in a dwelling when those modifications may be necessary for a person with a disability to have full enjoyment of a dwelling" [32]. They should also explore with a social worker or other support providers in the local community the availability of family support services such as respite services for families, home health attendant or homemaker services, assistive technology and environmental modification, adaptive medical equipment, transportation services, as well as respite services and counseling services for caretakers [26].

Additionally, young adults with physical, mental, or developmental disabilities might benefit from involvement with one or more of several available community resources in addressing concerns about independence. Examples of such community resources include, but are not limited to, the vocational rehabilitation programs previously discussed as well as Centers for Independent Living, Aging and Disability Resource Centers, Assistive Technology Resource Centers, and state agencies for individuals with intellectual or developmental disabilities.

Centers for Independent Living are consumer-controlled, community-based, cross-disability, nonresidential, private, and nonprofit agencies that are designed and operated within local communities by individuals with disabilities and that provide an array of independent living services, including the core services of information and referral, independent living skills training, peer support, and individual and systems advocacy [33]. Similarly, patients with mental health disorders should be, where available, referred to community-based transition programs. There are several examples of the success of such programs, which provide patients with services including individualized counseling, vocational training, and educational support [34, 35].

Young adults with chronic physical conditions or disabilities should register with their state's office of aging and/or physical disabilities (the name of the agency will vary from state to state). Every state has an Aging and Disability Resource Center run by this agency. By connecting with an Aging and Disability Resource Center, clients can engage in person-centered counseling to discuss their specific needs for supports to live independently. Depending on funding, waivers, and insurance, some people are eligible for home healthcare attendants, nurses, aides, or funding to pay a private caregiver of her choice [36].

Living on one's own may be full of challenges for the adult with physical or intellectual disabilities. Oftentimes, the young adult and his or her family may worry about physical accessibility, safety, and the ability to handle functional needs. Every state has Assistive Technology Resource Centers, where residents can meet with an assistive technology (AT) specialist to discuss needs and then be given a device to take home for a free trial, typically for 2 weeks. Once an individual knows if a device meets his or her needs, the AT specialist can recommend places to purchase the item. The assistive technology options can range from simple items, such as a doorknob lever, to more complex items, such as a communication device. Access to such devices often affords an individual with a disability greater ability to live in a more independent, less restrictive environment.

Those young adults with intellectual or developmental disabilities should register with their state agency for individuals with intellectual or developmental disabilities (the name of the agency will vary from state to state), found through their Department of Health and Human Services. Types of residential supports vary among states, but the state agency provides funds to the individual service providers. Adults can live in a variety of settings, from totally independent with no care giving needs to a community group home with staff members who assist with activities of daily living to an institutional facility or nursing home with around-the-clock care. As there are substantial waitlists/registries for access to residential programs in every state, adults with disabilities and their caregivers should register as soon as possible.

## Independent Living Issues for Young Adults Emerging from the Foster Care System

Young adults who are "aging out" of the foster care system may find this period of transition particularly daunting. As compared to peers among the general population, youths in the foster care system tend to have a higher prevalence of physical, developmental, and mental health illness and disabilities as well as higher rates of alcohol and drug abuse [37–39]. Further, given the instability of their social and family relationships, youth emerging from foster care are less likely to have available to them a sustained support network [40, 41]. As previously described, minorities may be even more susceptible to the absence of ongoing family support systems as they transition to adulthood, and minorities tend to be relatively overrepresented among youths in the foster care system, with the 2020 AFCARS data revealing that 43% were non-Latinx Whites as compared to 23% Black and 22% Latinx [7].

Existing data confirm that young adults who have recently emancipated from the foster care system are a vulnerable population with poor social status. A survey of 100 young adults who had been out of the foster care system for at least 6 months yielded many concerning findings. Of those surveyed, 26% reported not having steady employment since leaving care, and 41% indicated that they did not have enough money to cover living expenses; 24% had dealt drugs and 11% had exchanged sex for money. Additionally, 41% admitted to having legal issues and 7% reported having been incarcerated, while 2% admitted to being homeless at some point since emancipation [41].

There are many barriers to a successful transition for young adults leaving foster care. Importantly, many young adults leaving foster care cite that, while they had received independent living services training, very few actually receive concrete assistance for independence. For example, it has been demonstrated that less than 70% of individuals identified having a place to live and 50% noted having less than $250 at time of discharge from foster care [41]. This situation might be aggravated by the fact that very few emancipating young adults had regular, if any, contact with their case worker in their final year in the system [41]. Additionally, as discussed previously, the failure of many of these young adults to establish reliable family and social relationships contributes to difficulty with the transition period. Difficulty placing older children in permanent homes from the foster care system contributes to this problem. During FY2020, the mean age of adoption was 6.5 years of age, with only 8.2% of the 57,881 adopted at age of 14 years or older [7]. Many surveyed foster system case workers, in fact, have the perception that older youth are unlikely to be placed [42].

In an effort to diminish these problems in transition, federal legislation has been enacted over the years to fund independent living programs. The first such piece of legislation was the 1986 Independent Living Initiative, which amended the Title IV-E Social Security Act in order to establish the distribution of federal funding to states for independent living programs. The focus of these programs was on education and employment assistance, training in daily living skills, individual and group counseling, integration and coordination of services, and a transitional independent living plan for each participant [43]. Given the continued hardships of many emancipated young adults, the Foster Care Independence Act of 1999 was passed and so created the John Chafee Foster Care Independence Program, which not only doubled federal funding for state independent living programs, but, in part, also allowed for funds to be used for housing and allowed for vouchers for postsecondary education and training [44]. In some states, such as California and Illinois, there has been an increased emphasis by the courts that foster care agencies and minors preparing for emancipation demonstrate that they have met specific requirements and developed plans for independent living that would increase the success of transitioning out of the foster care system [45]. As an important part of this process, as early as age 14 years and continuing through the age of 21 years, foster youth should establish regular contact with the Independent Living Coordinator for their state.

There are data to support the effectiveness of such legislation. One survey of 100 subjects revealed that young adults who had received more independent living training and services prior to discharge were less likely to report legal trouble, felt better prepared to live on their own, and were more satisfied with their current living arrangements [41]. An additional survey of 479 young adults formerly in the foster care system demonstrated that those who had received better independent living preparation had a decreased risk for drug dependency [46].

While such programs have improved outcomes, there has been more recent emphasis on the continued need to enhance social support for these young adults, suggesting that the ideal scenario would be concurrent efforts to establish stable relationships with at least one adult while providing independent living services and training [45]. An obvious opportunity for providing such a relationship would be through legal adoption. Though this has long been considered an unlikely option for older youths, recent data have suggested more significant success in finding permanent families for these adolescents, often through existing relationships [47]. In cases where this is not possible, emphasizing the benefit of having a non-kin mentor is critical. One recent survey of 339 foster youths approaching 18 years of age revealed that 62% revealed the presence of a non-kin mentor relationship, many of which were established through formal care systems, including adults that work in child welfare, education, and mental health systems. Of note, minorities were less likely than Whites to identify the presence of a mentor, making this perhaps an even greater challenge among these subpopulations [48]. There are examples of successful programs in several cities and states that have focused on the development of such relationships, with an important component being the involvement of the youth in the process of identifying such mentors [45].

## Conclusion

Young adults with chronic childhood conditions, learning and developmental disabilities, mental health conditions, and those emerging from the foster care system comprise a diverse population that faces numerous barriers to a successful transition to independent living. However, there are a large number of existing programs, legislation, and community resources that can aid these vulnerable young adults in overcoming these barriers ("Appendix"). Adult medical providers should be familiar with these resources to assure that their young adult patients achieve their maximum level of independent functioning and are able to live in as minimally restrictive of a living environment as possible.

## Appendix

### Resources

- Titles I and V of the Americans with Disabilities (ADA) Act of 1990: https://www.eeoc.gov/laws/statutes/ada.cfm
- Fair Housing Act—Equal Opportunity for All: https://www.hud.gov/sites/documents/FHEO_BOOKLET_ENG.PDF
- U.S. Social Security Administration Red Book—Overview of Disability Programs: https://www.ssa.gov/pubs/EN-64-030.pdf
- Independent Living Research Utilization Directory of Centers for Independent Living: http://www.ilru.org/projects/cil-net/cil-center-and-association-directory
- National Organization on Disability: https://www.nod.org
- Find a Local Aging and Disability Resource Center: https://acl.gov/programs/aging-and-disability-networks/aging-and-disability-resource-centers
- John H. Chafee Foster Care Independence Program: http://www.acf.hhs.gov/programs/cb/resource/chafee-foster-care-program

## References

1. Payne AB, Mehal JM, Chapman C, Haberling DL, Richardson LC, Bean CJ, et al. Trends in sickle cell disease-related mortality in the United States, 1979–2017. Ann Emerg Med. 2020;76(3S):S28–36.
2. Cystic Fibrosis Foundation. Cystic Fibrosis Foundation Patient Registry. 2020 Annual data report. Bethesda, MA. © 2021; Sep 2021. https://www.cff.org/sites/default/files/2021-11/Patient-Registry-Annual-Data-Report.pdf. Accessed 18 Feb 2022.
3. Howlader N, Noone AM, Krapcho M, Miller D, Brest A, Yu M, et al. (eds). SEER cancer statistics review, 1975–2018, National Cancer Institute. Bethesda, MD, based on November 2020 SEER data submission; Apr 2021. https://seer.cancer.gov/csr/1975_2018. Accessed 18 Feb 2022.
4. Mandalenakis Z, Giang KW, Eriksson P, Liden H, Synnergren M, Walhander H, Fedchenko M, Rosengren A, Delborg M. Survival in children with congenital heart disease: have we reached a peak at 97%? J Am Heart Assoc. 2020;9(22):e017704.
5. Zablotsky B, Black LI, Blumberg SJ. Estimated prevalence a of children with diagnosed developmental

disabilities in the United States, 2014–2016. NCHS Data Brief. 2017;291:1–8.
6. National Institute of Mental Health. Mental Illness. Washington, DC: United States Department of Health and Human Services, National Institute of Mental Health; 2022. https://www.nimh.nih.gov/health/statistics/mental-illness. Accessed 18 Feb 2022.
7. U.S. Department of Health and Human Services. The AFCARS report: preliminary FY 2020 estimates as of October 4, 2021—No. 28. Washington, DC: DHHS; 2021. https://www.acf.hhs.gov/sites/default/files/documents/cb/afcarsreport28.pdf. Accessed 18 Feb 2022.
8. Pew Research Center. A majority of young adults in the U.S. live with their parents for the first time since the great depression. 2020. https://www.pewresearch.org/fact-tank/2020/09/04/a-majority-of-young-adults-in-the-u-s-live-with-their-parents-for-the-first-time-since-the-great-depression/ft_2020-09-04_livingwithparents_03. Accessed 19 Feb 2022.
9. McNair K. Nearly 30% of millennials still receive financial support from their parents. 2021. https://www.magnifymoney.com/blog/news/parental-financial-support-survey. Accessed 19 Feb 2022.
10. Gnaulati E, Heine BJ. Separation-individuation in late adolescence: an investigation of gender and ethnic differences. J Psychol. 2001;135(1):59–70.
11. Easter Seals. Life disparities for adults living with disabilities and their families. Disabled World 2010. www.disabled-world.com/disability/life-disparities.php. Accessed 19 Feb 2022.
12. Parish SL, Rose RA, Grinstein-Weiss M, Richman EL, Andrews ME. Material hardship in U.S. families raising children with disabilities. Except Child. 2008;75(1):71–92.
13. The Kessler Foundation/National Organization on Disability. 2010 survey of employment of Americans with disabilities. 2010. https://www.nod.org/wp-content/uploads/06d_2010_employment_survey_final_report-2.pdf. Accessed 19 Feb 2022.
14. Blomquist KB. Health, education, work, and independence of young adults with disabilities. Orthop Nurs. 2006;25(3):168–86.
15. Wasfi R, Steinmetz-Wood M, Levinson D. Measuring the transportation needs of people with developmental disabilities: a means to social inclusion. Disable Health. 2017;10(2):356–60.
16. National Organization on Disability. Harris survey of Americans with disabilities. Washington, DC: National Organization on Disability; 2004. https://mobilitylab.org/wp-content/uploads/2017/07/NationalOrganizationonDisabilityHarrisSurvey.htm. Accessed 20 Feb 2022.
17. Rochefort DA. Origins of the "third psychiatric revolution": the community mental health centers act of 1963. J Health Polit Policy Law. 1984;9(1):1–30.
18. Lamb HR, Bachrach LL. Some perspectives on deinstitutionalization. Psychiatr Serv. 2001;52(8):1039–45.
19. U.S. Department of Justice. The Fair Housing Act. 2022. https://www.justice.gov/crt/fair-housing-act-1. Accessed 20 Feb 2022.
20. Friedman C. There's no place like home: a national study of how people with intellectual and/or developmental disabilities and their families choose to live. Washington, DC and Towson MD: The Arc of the United States and the Council on Quality and Leadership; 2019. https://futureplanning.thearc.org/assets/CFP_Housing_Survey_Technical_Report-80e6eb718c816d07a15a9972df06a6e73b1393d5b56ae145acc058fce243cd93.pdf. Accessed 20 Feb 2022.
21. Davis M, Sondheimer DL. State child mental health efforts to support youth in transition to adulthood. J Behav Health Serv Res. 2005;32(1):27–42.
22. Abraczinskas M, Bory C, Plant R. Predictors of behavioral health service utilization in a Medicaid enrolled sample of emerging adults. Child Youth Serv Rev. 2020;108:104611.
23. Davis M, Vander Stoep A. The transition to adulthood for youth who have serious emotional disturbance: developmental transition and young adult outcomes. J Ment Health Adm. 1997;24(4):400–27.
24. Vander Stoep A, Beresford S, Weiss NS, McKnight B, Cauce AM, Cohen P. Community-based study of the transition to adulthood for adolescents with psychiatric disorder. Am J Epidemiol. 2000;152(4):352–62.
25. U.S. Social Security Administration. Red book: overview of our disability programs. Washington, DC: U.S. Social Security Administration; 2020. https://www.ssa.gov/pubs/EN-64-030.pdf. Accessed 20 Feb 2022.
26. Rizzolo MC, Hemp R, Braddock D, Schindler A. Family support services for persons with intellectual and developmental disabilities: recent national trends. Intellect Dev Disabil. 2009;47(2):152–5.
27. Parsons DO. The decline in male labor force participation. J Pol Econ. 1980;88(1):117–34.
28. U.S. Department of Health and Human Services. HHS historical highlights. Washington, DC: U.S. DHHS; 2021. http://www.hhs.gov/about/historical-highlights/index.html. Accessed 20 Feb 2022.
29. Liu S, Stapleton DC. Longitudinal statistics on work activity and use of employment supports for new social security disability insurance beneficiaries. Soc Secur Bull. 2011;71(3):35. https://www.ssa.gov/policy/docs/ssb/v71n3/v71n3p35.html.
30. U.S. Equal Employment Opportunity Commission. Titles I and V of the Americans with disabilities act of 1990 (ADA). Washington, DC: The U.S. Equal Employment Opportunity Commission; 1990. https://www.eeoc.gov/laws/statutes/ada.cfm. Accessed 20 Feb 2022.
31. American Academy of Pediatrics. Committee on children with disabilities and committee on adolescence. Transition of care provided for adolescents with special health care needs. Pediatrics. 1996;98(6):1203–6.
32. U.S. Department of Justice and the U.S. Department of Housing and Urban Development. Joint

Statement on the Department of Housing and Urban Development and the Department of Justice: Reasonable Accommodations Under the Fair Housing Act. Washington, DC: The U.S. Department of Justice and the U.S. Department of Housing and Urban Development. 2004. https://www.justice.gov/crt/us-department-housing-and-urban-development. Accessed 20 Feb 2022.
33. National Council on Independent Living. About independent living. Washington, DC: National Council on Independent Living; 2022. http://www.ncil.org/about/aboutil. Accessed 20 Feb 2022.
34. Bullis M, Moran T, Benz MR, Todis B, Johnson MD. Description and evaluation of the Aries project: achieving rehabilitation, individualized education, and employment success for adolescents with emotional disturbance. Career Dev Except Individ. 2002;25(1):41–58.
35. Baker AJL, Olsen D, Mincer C. The WAY to work: an independent living/aftercare program for high risk youth. Washington, DC: Child Welfare of American League Press; 2000.
36. U.S. Department of Health and Human Services, Administration for Community Living and Center for Medicare and Medicaid Services. No wrong door. Washington, DC: US DHHS, Administration for Community Living; 2017. https://nwd.acl.gov/index.html. Accessed 21 Feb 2022.
37. American Institutes for Research. Young adults formerly in foster care: challenges and solutions. Arlington, VA; 2022. https://youth.gov/youth-briefs/foster-care-youth-brief/challenges. Accessed 21 Feb 2022.
38. Ahrens KR, Garrison MM, Courtney ME. Health outcomes in young adults form foster care and economically diverse backgrounds. Pediatrics. 2014;134(6):1067–74.
39. Havlicek J, Garcia A, Smith DC. Mental health and substance use disorders among foster youth transitioning to adulthood: past research and future directions. Child Youth Serv Rev. 2013;35(1):194–203.
40. Courtney ME, Piliavin I, Grogan-Kaylor A. Foster youth transition to adulthood: a longitudinal view of youth leaving care. Child Welfare. 2001;80(6):685.
41. Reilly T. Transition from care: status and outcomes of youth who age out of foster care. Child Welfare. 2003;82(6):727–46.
42. Avery RJ. Perceptions and practice: agency efforts for the hardest-to-place children. Child Youth Serv Rev. 2000;22(6):399–420.
43. Collins ME. Transition to adulthood for vulnerable youths. Soc Serv Rev. 2001;75(2):271–91.
44. Fernandes AL. CRS report for congress. Child Welfare: the Chafee Foster care Independence Program (CFCIP). Washington, DC: Congressional Research Service, Library of Congress. Order Code RS22501; 2007. https://digital.library.unt.edu/ark:/67531/metadc810626/m1/1. Accessed 21 Feb 2022.
45. Bussiere A. Adoption and foster care: permanence for older foster youth. Fam Court Rev. 2006;44(2):231–43.
46. White CR, O'Brien K, White J, Pecora PJ, Phillips CM. Alcohol and drug use among alumni of foster care: decreasing dependency through improvement of foster care experiences. J Behav Health Serv Res. 2007;35(4):419–34.
47. Avery RJ. An examination of theory and promising practice for achieving permanency for teens before they age out of foster care. Child Youth Serv Rev. 2009;32(3):399–408.
48. Munson MR, McMillen JC. Non-kin natural mentors in the lives of older youths in foster care. J Behav Health Serv Res. 2008;35(4):454–68.

# Decision-Making and Guardianship

# 60

John C. Berens, Jennifer H. Chuang, and Jane Subak Kennedy

## The Healthcare Provider's Role in Medical Decision-Making

The role of a healthcare provider sometimes includes an assessment of a patient's capacity to make medical decisions. Though often used interchangeably, the terms competency and capacity are not equivalent. Competency refers to a static legal determination, and any person consenting to medical care must be competent to do so. In this regard, the competent person should be able to: (1) understand the potential benefits, risks, and alternatives involved in a specific treatment or procedure; (2) make the healthcare decision on his/her own behalf; and (3) communicate that healthcare decision to any other person. A person may be competent to make some healthcare decisions but not others. Capacity refers to a clinical assessment of decision-making ability at the time of the assessment, so lack of capacity may be transient and due to reversible conditions such as an altered level of consciousness (hypoglycemia, medication, or substance toxicity), delirium due to any number of causes, or a mental health concern. To this end, a capacity assessment made the previous day may not apply to the present day.

There are several circumstances where a healthcare provider may need to perform a capacity evaluation. Sometimes, evaluation of a person's capacity to give informed consent can be an urgent question, such as during an acute psychiatric crisis or other significant change in mental status. Other times, a parent or caregiver may express concerns that their adult child or loved one with a cognitive disability does not have the capacity to make medical decisions (or will not be expected to once they become an adult).

During a capacity assessment, the healthcare provider should consider the following four legally relevant areas: (1) the ability to communicate a choice; (2) the ability to understand relevant information about their condition and treatment; (3) the ability to appreciate how that information applies to their own situation and the consequences of treatment options (including no treatment); and (4) the ability to reason with that information [1–3]. There are currently no formal guidelines from professional societies to assess a patient's capacity. Resources and tools are available to assist providers to assess their patients'

J. C. Berens (✉)
Department of Medicine, Section of Transition Medicine, Baylor College of Medicine, Houston, TX, USA
e-mail: john.berens@bcm.edu

J. H. Chuang
Craig-Dalsimer Division of Adolescent Medicine, Children's Hospital of Philadelphia, Philadelphia, PA, USA

J. S. Kennedy
Department of Social Work and Family Services, Children's Hospital of Philadelphia, Philadelphia, PA, USA


A. A. Kuo et al. (eds.), *Care of Adults with Chronic Childhood Conditions*,
https://doi.org/10.1007/978-3-031-54281-7_60

capacity [1–3]. Below are examples of questions that may be used:

1. To assess the ability to communicate a choice:
   - We have discussed a lot of information about your condition. Have you decided which medical option is best for you right now?
2. To assess the ability to understand relevant information about their condition and treatment:
   - What is your understanding of your condition? What are the options for your condition? What are the risks and benefits of the treatment options? What are the risks and benefits if nothing is done?
3. To assess the ability to appreciate how that information applies to their own situation and the consequences of treatment options:
   - Why do you think your doctor has recommended this specific test or treatment for you? Do you think that treatment is the best treatment for you? Why or why not? What do you think will happen if you accept this treatment? What do you think will happen if you do not accept this treatment?
4. To assess the ability to reason with the information regarding the patient's condition, situation, and treatment options:
   - What factors are most important to you in deciding about your options? How are you balancing the pluses and minuses of the treatments? What do you think will happen to you now? How did you decide to accept or reject the recommended treatment? What makes one option better than another option?

The practitioner should keep in mind that decision-making capacity is not equivalent to agreeing with the practitioner's recommendation. The patient may make a decision that will result in greater harm or potentially death, but the patient may still have capacity to make the decision if the above four criteria were met. If decision-making capacity is not present, the next question is whether this finding is the result of a fluctuating condition.

In the case of an acute psychiatric emergency, the patient may not have the capacity to refuse the recommended treatment. If the patient is 18 years or older, then one may petition for emergency psychiatric hospitalization for the patient. After the initial emergency psychiatric hold, a judge may determine whether the patient needs civil commitment to be held in a hospital beyond the emergency period. Some states allow a commitment for assisted outpatient treatment. The details of involuntary commitment for psychiatric emergencies vary from state to state [4, 5].

In the case of a nonpsychiatric, temporary lack of capacity (e.g., delirium, intoxication), the decision-making responsibility would transfer to a previously appointed surrogate, such as a medial power of attorney or someone previously designated in an advanced directive or living will. If such a person has not been previously identified, then the usual recourse is to contact family members. There is variation between states in terms of the priority order in which the family members are approached. In emergency cases in which no surrogate is available, physicians can provide treatment under the premise that a reasonable person would have consented to the given care.

If the lack of decision-making capacity is due to an underlying condition that is not reasonably expected to improve (e.g., intellectual disability, progressive neurologic disease), the immediate medical decision would also go to the next-of-kin as described above. While there may be a previously designated surrogate decision-maker in this case as well, this requires that the person previously had capacity to make such a decision; in the case of more severe cognitive disability, this is likely not an option. The remainder of this chapter will focus on the available options and approach for healthcare providers addressing a static lack of medical decision-making capacity due to a chronic underlying condition.

Decisions regarding guardianship and medical decision-making capacity can be lengthy and emotional. The healthcare provider is in a key role to facilitate discussions with the patient and family regarding these decisions in a proactive and thoughtful manner, ideally before the patient turns 18-years-old. Allowing the patient and family the time and space to process these important decisions in advance may ease concerns that may otherwise arise in the event of an emergency.

## The Competence Model and Guardianship

Historically, the medical field has used the competence model in their approach to medical decision-making. Put simply, it states that if a person is determined to lack capacity, then a substitute decision-maker must step in. While real life may not be so black and white, this philosophy does tend to create a binary where a person either has or does not have autonomy as a function of their capacity, or lack thereof. If the person lacking capacity has a previously identified surrogate decision-maker, this model is logical since it fulfils previously made self-identified wishes. Typically, public or personal safety is used to justify the use of other uses of substituted decision-making, such as in an acute psychiatric emergency. In the case of a static lack of capacity (e.g., cognitive disability), the competence model then leads to the need for a long-term substituted decision-maker, typically interpreted to be a guardianship. In some states, "conservatorship" is used instead of adult guardianship, but the terms mean roughly the same thing. For the rest of this chapter, we will use the term "guardianship" to refer to adult guardianships and conservatorships.

Guardianship may be granted over all aspects of an individual's life ("total") or restricted to specific areas ("partial"). If a court appoints someone to take care of financial matters, that person is usually called a "conservator of the estate," while a person in charge of medical and personal decisions is a "conservator of the person." The same person can be appointed to take both roles. Conservators of any kind are supervised by and held accountable to a court.

The process for establishing guardianship may proceed when an individual turns 18 and assumes legal responsibility for their decisions instead of the parent or previous legal guardian. If there are concerns that the individual is incapable of handling medical and financial manners, then the parent or previous legal guardian may wish to consider petitioning for guardianship.

Guardianship is a legal process whereby the court appoints a guardian to make legal decisions on the individual's behalf, including medical decision-making [6]. The guardian may be a parent, other family member, a friend, or a court-appointed public or private entity. The process of applying for guardianship varies from state to state (Table 60.1). The procedure includes a court petition filed by the potential guardian that typically includes a description of the physical and mental condition of the patient and any functional limitations. The healthcare provider may be asked to provide an evaluation of the patient's capabilities and limitations [6, 7]. An annual court review and assessment will monitor the need to continue the guardianship, and the individual's rights may be reinstated if the patient gains (or reestablishes) capacity, though this process can be complex.

It is important to note that, while the appointed guardian should take into account the wishes and

**Table 60.1** Steps on establishing guardianship (details vary state by state)

| Establishing adult guardianship |
|---|
| 1. The guardian applicant determines that the adult-aged individual may not have the capacity to fully make his or her own decisions |
| 2. The guardian applicant completes a court petition or application for legal guardianship of the adult individual |
| 3. The individual should have a medical and psychological evaluation to determine his or her capabilities and limitations that would affect their ongoing capacity to make decisions |
| 4. The guardian applicant is required to give notice of the application to the individual in question and attend a hearing before a judge, which the individual is allowed (but not required) to attend |
| 5. Consultation with a lawyer by the guardian applicant is often recommended to facilitate the guardianship process |

desires of the individual, the guardian has the ultimate say on all authorized decisions. Additionally, healthcare providers should know and counsel parties seeking guardianship that obtaining guardianship typically removes a person's rights as a citizen, such as the ability of an individual to possess a driver's license, own or possess a firearm, marry, vote, file lawsuits, and buy or sell property.

Lastly, it is important to distinguish assent from consent. Assent is the agreement expressed by the individual if they are not able to legally consent. Healthcare providers should attempt to obtain assent whenever possible, such as in research studies, medication administration, and surgical procedures. Information should be given to the patient in an easily understood manner to optimize comprehension.

## Supported Decision-Making

The competence model has come under scrutiny over the past 1–2 decades. The UN Convention on the Rights of Persons with Disabilities issued Article 12 in 2006 that recommended a new paradigm whereby a person retains autonomy irrespective of their decision-making capacity and advocates moving exclusively to a model of supported decision-making [8]. With this approach, a person receives any additional support that may be needed in order to make a decision, as opposed to assigning a substitute decision-maker if they lack capacity to make decisions independently. This approach has its critics, and there are concerns that this recommendation, if fully employed, could actually lead to a decrease in the rights of persons with disabilities; specifically, there would be no justification for involuntary admission (e.g., for a psychiatry emergency), guardianship in any circumstance, or diversion from the criminal justice system [9]. There are other potential harms to persons with disabilities in an exclusively supported decision-making model as highlighed in Scholten and Gather (2018), [10] who advocate for a hybrid approach that appeals both to the principles of autonomy and of well-being.

With this being said, it is important to note that both civil rights and disability advocacy groups (see below) are strong advocates in moving away from the competence model and toward supported decision-making—motivated especially by the loss of legal/civil rights during the guardianship process, as highlighted above. Practically speaking, supported decision-making allows an individual to officially designate another person(s) to help them make choices about their life that can include anything from managing finances to healthcare decisions. The designation does not remove any rights, nor does it remove a person's autonomy, though they may relinquish control of a given decision to their designee if desired.

Laws regarding supported or shared decision-making vary state by state; state-specific information can be found at the National Resource Center for Supported Decision-Making (www.supporteddecisionmaking.org) [11]. As an example, supported decision-making has been formally recognized in the state of Texas under the "Supported Decision-Making Agreement Act" passed in 2015. It allows a "process of supporting and accommodating an adult with a disability to enable the adult to make life decisions, including decisions related to where the adult wants to live, the services, supports, and medical care the adult wants to receive, whom the adult wants to live with, and where the adult wants to work, without impeding the self-determination of the adult" [12]. Further information about supported decision-making for patients and families can be found at the American Civil Liberties Union (ACLU) Disability Rights Program (www.aclu.org/disability) [13] or Quality Trust for Individuals with Disabilities (www.dcquality-trust.org) [14].

## Other Variations or Alternatives to Guardianship

There are other options to consider, depending on the state, to support individuals with disabilities instead of full guardianship—particularly if the state of residence does not have laws formally recognizing supported decision-making. In all cases, it is imperative to take the least intrusive measures on the individual's autonomy when considering the possibilities. Some of these options are listed below; it is important to note that several of them require capacity to understand the agreement at the time of signing, so may not be appropriate for some people with more severe cognitive disabilities:

- *A guardian of the estate*: a person who is responsible for the individual's finances.
- *Limited/partial guardianship*: limits substituted decision-making to certain discrete areas, such as medical decision-making.
- *Temporary guardianship*: limits decision-making to a guardian for a defined period of time.
- *Joint bank accounts*: a joint account may allow the guardian to monitor spending activity on the account, or the guardian and adult-aged patient may choose to have a joint account where both signatures are needed for transaction activity.
- *Advanced directives/living will*: while these terms are sometimes used interchangeably to designate specific instructions of an individual's wishes regarding advanced or end-of-life medical care, "advanced directives" is a slightly broader term that may include instructions for a medical power of attorney (see below).
- *Representative payee*: a person who manages funds received by government agencies, such as Social Security.
- *Power of attorney*: typically refers to a person granted legal authority to make financial decisions on another's behalf in the event that the individual is unable to do so.
- *Medical power of attorney/healthcare proxy*: grants a person legal authority to make decisions on another's behalf in the event that the individual is unable to do so. A person filling this role may not have specific written wishes, but is a substituted decision-maker based on what they believe the individual would want (see "advanced directives" above).
- *Appointment of a Community Advocate*: allows an agent to advocate on the individual's behalf with administrative and government agencies.
- *A Trust*: to place funds and other assets in the control of a trustee. Access to these funds by the patient would need to be coordinated with the trustee.

## Medical Decision-Making and Long-Term Care Planning

Long-term care planning refers to making future plans for an individual's finances, living situation, etc. and is especially important for individuals with disabilities who rely on others for daily support [15]. Identifying alternative supports for decision-making is an important part of this planning. For adults with disabilities who have an appointed guardian, it can be a lengthy court process to determine who obtains legal authority of the individual in the event of their guardian's death if it is not specifically spelled out in the guardian's estate planning. Without legal documentation, the individual may be placed with child or adult protective services or the court may place them with another family member, which may or may not have been the intent of the deceased guardian. Understandably, these situations can be emotionally challenging and potentially traumatic for the individual as well as the family. Thus, it is incredibly important to discuss long-term care planning with the caregivers of individuals with disabilities, particularly if they are legal guardians. In addition to appointing legal authority to an alternative guardian, estate planning should include distribution of financial assets (even if the sum is modest) to avoid lengthy proceedings for banks to release funds. Depending on the age of the individual, the caregiver may consider putting the inheritance in a trust until they reach an age or maturity that is deemed appropriate.

## Appendix

### Resources

- American Civil Liberties Union: ACLU Supported Decision-Making Resource Library. www.aclu.org/supported-decision-making-resource-library.

- The Arc: for people with intellectual and developmental disabilities. www.thearc.org.
- Department of Developmental Services: offices available in each state.
- National Resource Center for Supported Decision-Making. www.supporteddecision-making.org
- National Center for Medical-Legal Partnership. medical-legalpartnership.org.
- National Guardianship Association. www.guardianship.org.

## References

1. Tunzi M. Can the patient decide? Evaluating patient capacity in practice. Am Fam Physician. 2001;64:299–306.
2. Grisso T, Appelbaum PS. Assessing competence to consent to treatment: a guide for physicians and other health professionals. New York: Oxford University Press; 1998.
3. Appelbaum PS. Assessment of patients' competence to consent to treatment. N Engl J Med. 2007;357:1834–40.
4. American Bar Association. Guardianship Law and Practice. http://www.americanbar.org/groups/law_aging/resources/guardianship_law_practice.html. Accessed 22 Oct 2022.
5. National Alliance on Mental Illness. https://www.nami.org/. Accessed 22 Oct 2022.
6. National Guardianship Association. http://www.guardianship.org/. Accessed 22 Oct 2022.
7. National Disability Rights Network. http://www.ndrn.org/. Accessed 22 Oct 2022.
8. United Nations Convention on the Rights of Persons with Disabilities Article 12. https://www.un.org/development/desa/disabilities/convention-on-the-rights-of-persons-with-disabilities/article-12-equal-recognition-before-the-law.html. Accessed 22 Oct 2022.
9. Freeman MC, Kolappa K, de Almeida JMC, Kleinman A, Makhashvili N, Phakathi S, et al. Reversing hard won victories in the name of human rights: a critique of the General Comment on Article 12 of the UN Convention on the Rights of Persons with Disabilitie. Lancet Psychiatry. 2015;2:844–50.
10. Scholten M, Gather J. Adverse consequences of article 12 of the UN Convention on the Rights of Persons with Disabilities for persons with mental disabilities and an alternative way forward. J Med Ethics. 2018;44:226–33.
11. National Resource Center for Supported Decision-Making. https://supporteddecisionmaking.org. Accessed 22 Oct 2022.
12. Bechyne G. Supported decision-making agreements in Texas. https://epj.us/article/19112.pdf. Accessed 22 Oct 2022.
13. American Civil Liberties Union (ACLU) Disability Rights Program. www.aclu.org/disability. Accessed 22 Oct 2022.
14. Quality Trust for Individuals with Disabilities. http://dcqualitytrust.org. Accessed 22 Oct 2022.
15. McCallion P, Nickle T. Individuals with developmental disabilities and their caregivers. J Gerontol Soc Work. 2008;50(sup1):243–66.

# Access to Health Insurance

# 61

Beth Sufian, James Passamano, and Amy Sopchak

## Introduction

Adults with chronic illness must have some form of health insurance coverage to help them pay for the medical care and the medications needed to treat their disease. When young adults transition to adult care, their ability to access insurance coverage often changes, and changes in coverage often affect access medical care. Transitioning adults may have fewer options accessing health insurance than children.

This chapter will provide an overview of the laws and programs that provide health insurance options for young adults with chronic illness transitioning to adult care.

Some options include eligibility for Social Security benefits that include Medicaid or Medicare coverage, coverage offered by state government programs, employer-sponsored group coverage, or a health insurance plan that can be purchased from a Health Insurance Exchange operated by the federal or a state government. Also, this chapter will explain situations that will allow health insurance coverage to be extended to a disabled dependent child.

The information in this chapter is general in nature and is not intended as legal advice. Laws frequently change and consequently the information contained in this chapter is subject to change without notice. A person with a legal question should consult an attorney.

B. Sufian (✉) · J. Passamano · A. Sopchak
CF Social Security Project, Sufian and Passamano, L.L.P., Houston, TX, USA
e-mail: bsufian@sufianpassamano.com; Jpassamano@sufianpassamano.com; asopchak@sufianpassamano.com

## Social Security Benefits

### Overview

The Social Security Administration (SSA) administers two programs for disabled individuals that provide health benefit coverage. The two programs are easily confused, but it is important to understand their differences.

***Social Security Disability Insurance (SSDI)*** provides a monthly cash benefit and *Medicare* coverage. To be eligible to receive SSDI, the applicant must meet both work history requirements and medical requirements. A person who has never worked or who has not worked the requisite amount is not eligible for SSDI benefits. Medicare coverage for those who are eligible for SSDI begins 24 months after the beneficiary begins receiving the monthly cash benefit.

***Supplemental Security Income (SSI)*** provides a monthly cash benefit and *Medicaid* coverage. An applicant must meet both Social Security Administration's income and resource require-


A. A. Kuo et al. (eds.), *Care of Adults with Chronic Childhood Conditions*,
https://doi.org/10.1007/978-3-031-54281-7_61

ments and medical requirements to be eligible for SSI benefits. Eligibility for the Medicaid coverage associated with SSI begins after the Social Security Administration approves an application for SSI benefits.

## Social Security Medical Criteria

A diagnosis of a chronic illness alone does not make a person eligible for Social Security benefits. A person applying for SSDI or SSI benefits must meet the medical criteria specified in the Social Security regulations. Both SSI and SSDI use the same medical criteria for eligibility. Social Security often calls the medical criteria "The Social Security Listing".

The Social Security medical listings at www.ssa.gov for children and adults may be found in a publication known as the Social Security Blue Book. The Blue Book lists the criteria for each disability and the evidence necessary to meet the criteria. The SSA medical listing for children is often different from the medical listing for adults with the same condition. Consequently, when a person transitions to adult care, the medical eligibility criteria for Social Security benefits may be different from the pediatric criteria.

Children receiving SSI benefits will have their eligibility reviewed by Social Security when they reach age 18. During an 18-year-old review, Social Security uses the adult eligibility standards. SSA may find that the beneficiary does not meet the adult eligibility criteria, even though the beneficiary received benefits throughout childhood. However, a beneficiary who does not meet one of the listed eligibility criteria still has an opportunity to show that the condition is as severe as one of the listed criteria.

## Social Security and Medical Records

SSA medical eligibility determinations are based on medical evidence. The principal form of evidence are medical records from the treating physician. Social Security looks to the records for the clinical indications and test results specified in the Social Security listing for the condition. If the medical evidence supports a finding that the condition is at least as severe as a listed medical criterion, then the applicant may be found to be disabled.

Typically, Social Security considers medical records from 12 months prior to the application date because Social Security considers the applicant's medical condition in the prior 12 months as relevant to the current disability status. In some circumstances, however, Social Security needs medical records for more than 12 months.

Social Security will request medical records from medical providers, but records often do not arrive in the applicant's Social Security file. For this reason, many advocates suggest that the applicant provides medical records to Social Security themselves to assure that the records are available when the determination is made. The applicant should also keep a copy of the medical records.

A letter from the treating physician can help Social Security understand how the applicant meets the medical criteria. The most helpful letters are consistent with the medical records and quantify the limitations the person experiences in daily life compared to a person without the condition. The letter can be submitted with the SSA application.

## Social Security Disability Insurance (SSDI) [1]

### Who is Eligible for SSDI Benefits?

Social Security Disability Insurance (SSDI) is a program that provides a monthly cash benefit and Medicare coverage. Medicare coverage begins 29 months after the disability onset date determined by the Social Security Administration.

Often parents of transitioning young adults mistakenly believe their child can apply for SSDI benefits. If the child has not worked or has not worked the required amount, then the child is not eligible for SSDI benefits even if the child meets the Social Security medical eligibly criteria. A person who has never worked or has not worked the required amount will not be eligible for SSDI benefits because the person has not made the required contributions to the Social Security system from payroll withholdings.

To be eligible for SSDI benefits, a person must have participated in the workforce for the required amount of time, made the minimum contribution to the Social Security system, and must meet the Social Security medical requirements.

Also, the individual cannot be engaged in substantial gainful activity when applying for SSDI benefits. Generally, working more than 20 h per week or earning more than $1350 (in 2022) is considered a substantial gainful activity. Uncompensated activities, such as enrollment in an educational program or substantial volunteer activity, may also be considered to determine if the applicant is engaged in substantial gainful activity. A person working more than part-time or earning more than $1350 per month is considered to be engaged in substantial gainful activity. A person engaged in substantial gainful activity is not eligible for SSDI benefits. It is important to note that the earning limit may change every year.

A person who is self-employed is subject to a different earning limit when assessing substantial gainful activity for SSDI benefits. A person should contact Social Security for more information on work limits for self-employment.

An individual's monthly SSDI cash benefit is determined by the amount of contribution the individual has made to the Social Security system during their work history. SSDI cash benefits begin five full months after the disability onset date determined by the Social Security Administration. Therefore, it is important to apply for SSDI as soon as possible after becoming unable to work due to a disability. There is no exception to the five-month waiting period, so each applicant should plan for the time when work income has ended and the cash benefits have not yet begun.

### Appealing a Denial of SSDI Benefits

A claimant may file an appeal when an initial application is denied. Filing an appeal allows the applicant to accrue benefits while the appeal pends. If the appeal is successful, the beneficiary may receive the benefits that accrued while the appeal pended. Filing a second claim rather than filing an appeal on the first claim will cut off the opportunity to receive benefits that accrued while the first claim was pending.

**Example:** Jack's application for SSDI benefits is denied. Jack has 60 days to appeal the denial. Jack's appeal is resolved in his favor 10 months after he filed his initial application. Jack receives five months of back benefits. Jack does not receive 10 months of back benefits because there is a waiting period during the first five full months after the disability onset date.

### Medicare Eligibility for SSDI Beneficiaries

In addition to the monthly cash benefit, an SSDI beneficiary will become eligible for Medicare coverage. Medicare coverage begins 24 months after the beneficiary receives the first monthly cash benefit payment. The combination of the five-month waiting period for the monthly cash benefit payment and the 24-month Medicare waiting period means that Medicare benefits begin 29 months after the disability onset date determined by the Social Security Administration. An SSDI beneficiary will need to plan for health benefit coverage during the 29-month period waiting for Medicare to prevent a lapse of coverage. Some individuals may have more options than others, but common options are COBRA continuation of employer-sponsored coverage, Affordable Care Act coverage, and enrollment in expanded Medicaid where available.

## Supplemental Security Income (SSI) [2]

### Who is Eligible for SSI Benefits?

SSI eligibility requires meeting both the household income and asset criteria and meeting the medical criteria. Three common situations are:

- A child under the age of 18 who meets medical criteria and whose parents' income and assets do not exceed the resource limits.

- -An adult who has not worked or who has not worked enough to receive SSDI and who meets the medical criteria and whose own income and assets do not exceed the resource limits.
- An adult who has worked enough to receive SSDI, but the monthly SSDI cash benefit and any other income is less than the monthly SSI benefit amount in their State.

### Benefit Review at Age 18

A child receiving SSI will have a benefit review when the child reaches the age of 18 years. During an 18-year-old-review, Social Security assesses whether the young adult still meets the household income and asset criteria and the medical criteria. The SSA evaluates whether the beneficiary's own income and assets meet the financial criteria and whether the beneficiary's condition meets the medical criteria for an adult with the disabling condition. If Social Security determines that the 18-year-old beneficiary is no longer eligible for SSI benefits, the beneficiary may appeal that determination.

An appeal cannot be taken more than 60 days after an unfavorable 18-year-old-review, but when the appeal is filed within 60 days, it has an important impact on benefits. A beneficiary who files an appeal within 10 days after an unfavorable determination of an 18-year-old-review may be able to retain the SSI monthly cash benefit and Medicaid coverage while the appeal is pending. However, if the appeal is filed more than 10 days after the unfavorable determination, Social Security will suspend all benefits while the appeal pends, including the Medicaid coverage. If the appeal is ultimately unsuccessful, the SSI benefits will terminate.

### SSI Issues Specific to Transitioning Adults

When a child under the age of 18 and living with their parents applies for SSI, Social Security will count the income and assets of the applicant's parents to determine if the applicant meets the financial criteria. When counting the income and assets of an adult SSI applicant, Social Security will count the applicant's own income and assets to determine if the applicant meets the SSA income and asset criteria. Therefore, a child who was not eligible for SSI before age 18 may become eligible for SSI after reaching age 18 if his own income and assets meet the Social Security eligibility criteria.

Social Security will not count the income and assets of the parents of an adult even if the adult continues to live in the parents' home. However, Social Security will likely consider the value of any free room and board when calculating the monthly cash benefit and may reduce the amount of the benefit. However, if the adult applying for SSI has a valid written agreement obligating the applicant to pay a fair share of household expenses, then Social Security should not reduce the SSI benefit amount. Such written agreements are submitted to Social Security with the application for benefits. The written agreement must contain specific language in order for the agreement to be valid. An applicant for benefits can inquire about the elements of a valid loan agreement with the Social Security Administration.

## SSI Benefits and Medicaid Coverage

In addition to the monthly cash benefit, SSI beneficiaries receive Medicaid health benefits. SSI is a federal Social Security program, and the monthly cash benefit is administered by the federal government. Medicaid, however, is a joint federal and state program. Each state administers its own Medicaid program, so the way that an SSI beneficiary is enrolled in Medicaid depends on the state where the beneficiary resides.

Most States and the District of Columbia allow the Social Security Administration to determine Medicaid eligibility for SSI beneficiaries and enroll them directly into the State Medicaid program without any further action by the beneficiary. When a person living in one of these 35 jurisdictions is approved for SSI, they will be automatically enrolled in Medicaid. These jurisdictions are: The District of Columbia, Alabama, Arizona, Arkansas, California, Colorado, Delaware, Florida, Georgia, Indiana, Iowa, Kentucky, Louisiana, Maine, Maryland,

Massachusetts, Michigan, Mississippi, Montana, New Jersey, New Mexico, New York, North Carolina, Ohio, Pennsylvania, Rhode Island, South Carolina, South Dakota, Tennessee, Texas, Vermont, Washington, West Virginia, Wisconsin, and Wyoming.

Seven states make their own Medicaid eligibility decisions, but use the same income, resource, and disability criteria that Social Security uses for the SSI program. When a person living in one of these States is approved for SSI, the beneficiary is not automatically enrolled in Medicaid, but is required to file a separate Medicaid enrollment application. Because these states use the same eligibility criteria as the Social Security Administration, each person approved for SSI by Social Security should also be approved by the State Medicaid program when they present a separate application for enrollment. These states are Alaska, Idaho, Kansas, Nebraska, Nevada, Oregon, and Utah.

Nine states have Medicaid eligibility criteria that are more restrictive than SSI's criteria. These states require both a separate application for Medicaid and additional evidence of eligibility. However, the federal government limits how restrictive the states can be when screening SSI recipients for Medicaid eligibility. These states are Connecticut, Hawaii, Illinois, Minnesota, Missouri, New Hampshire, North Dakota, Oklahoma, and Virginia.

## Eligible for Both SSDI and SSI

Some young adults with chronic illness may have worked a short time before becoming unable to continue work. These young adults may have contributed the minimum amount to the Social Security system to be an insured person for SSDI. Yet, because their total contribution is near the minimum required amount, the monthly cash benefit due is relatively small. Consequently, a person may be eligible for SSDI, but their monthly SSDI cash benefit and other income is still low enough to also be eligible for SSI. These individuals are often called "Dual Eligible". Although they are eligible for both, the SSI monthly benefit is reduced by the amount of the monthly SSDI benefit received.

**Example**: If Isabella is eligible to receive an SSDI benefit of $200 per month and if the maximum SSI benefit in her state is $794 per month, then the amount of her SSI benefit would be $794 – $200 = $594.

Dual eligible beneficiaries are eligible for both Medicaid and Medicare. Medicare will be the primary benefit and Medicaid will be secondary if there is no other health coverage.

## Coverage Under the Affordable Care Act [3]

### Expanded Medicaid Under the Affordable Care Act

The Affordable Care Act (ACA) expanded Medicaid benefits to low-income adults who meet certain low income and asset criteria. Generally, expanded Medicaid coverage is available to individuals between the ages of 18 and 65 years and with resources not exceeding 138% of the federal poverty level applicable for the size of the individual's household.

The Medicaid expansion was intended to be mandatory under the Affordable Care Act statute. However, the United States Supreme Court held that Congress could not mandate states to expand their Medicaid programs to nondisabled low-income adults. The Supreme Court held that the ACA's expansion of Medicaid is voluntary, not mandatory. By the end of 2021, 38 states and the District of Columbia had voluntarily adopted a Medicaid expansion program under the ACA. Twelve states have not yet adopted the expansion. The states that have not adopted an ACA Medicaid expansion program are Alabama, Florida, Georgia, Kansas, Mississippi, North Carolina, South Carolina, South Dakota, Tennessee, Texas, Wisconsin, and Wyoming.

A transitioning adult who lives in one of the 38 expansion states (or in the District of Columbia) may apply for Medicaid coverage even if the person is not eligible for SSI benefits and regardless of disability status. However, in the 12 states that have not expanded Medicaid, the only way for a disabled adult to enroll in Medicaid is to apply and be approved for SSI benefits.

Some states that have not expanded their Medicaid program under the ACA have adopted special programs (known as Section 1115 Waiver Programs) that allow the state to operate their Medicaid programs in ways not otherwise allowed under federal law. These waiver programs may provide a pathway to Medicaid coverage for adults in the absence of ACA expansion. However, waiver programs usually have restrictions and requirements for participation, such as work requirements, that transitioning adults with a chronic illness are unlikely to meet.

## Affordable Care Act Insurance Market Reforms

The Affordable Care Act enacted several insurance market reforms to protect consumers and make health insurance coverage more accessible.

### Prohibition on Preexisting Condition Exclusions

Prior to the adoption of the Affordable Care Act, preexisting condition exclusions were common and excluded coverage for claims related to a condition that was treated or diagnosed before enrollment in a health benefit plan.

The Affordable Care Act now prohibits preexisting condition exclusions in health insurance policies sold in the United States. Insurance companies can no longer exclude a person from coverage or deny enrollment in a health benefit plan because of a preexisting condition.

### Limiting Age Not Less than 26 Years

The Affordable Care Act prohibits insurance companies from imposing a limiting age less than 26 years for dependent coverage under a health benefit plan. This means that a person enrolled as a dependent child on their parent's health benefit plan may remain as a covered dependent until the age of 26 years. The covered dependent may be married and remain a covered dependent on their parent's health insurance policy.

The dependent child can be employed and remains covered dependent on their parent's health insurance policy. A dependent child does not need to be a full-time student in order to continue coverage until age 26. There is no requirement that the dependent be receiving Social Security benefits to continue as a covered dependent on their parent's health insurance policy until the age 26. Age is the governing factor.

### No Caps on Coverage

The Affordable Care Act prohibits individual and group health plans from placing a lifetime limit on the aggregate dollar value of coverage that will be provided to a plan beneficiary. Since January 2014, insurers have been prohibited from placing annual limits on overall plan coverage, such as a lifetime cap on benefits.

### Essential Covered Services

The ACA specifies ten categories of essential covered services that all ACA plans must cover. All plans offered in an ACA Health Insurance Exchange must cover these essential health benefits:

- Ambulatory patient services
- Emergency services
- Hospitalization
- Pregnancy, maternity, and newborn care
- Mental health and substance use disorder services, including behavioral health treatment
- Prescription drugs
- Rehabilitative and habilitative services and devices
- Laboratory services
- Preventive and wellness services and chronic disease management
- Pediatric services (including oral and vision care for children)

An ACA plan must include all of these as covered services and cannot exclude any of these services from the plan of coverage. While these categories of coverage are required, they may be subject to deductibles, co-pay requirements, or limits on the amount of the service.

One important difference between adult coverage and pediatric coverage under ACA plans includes dental and vision coverage. Dental and vision coverage are part of essential *pediatric* health benefits, but dental and vision coverage are *not* essential covered services for adults. A person covered under an ACA plan who is transitioning from pediatric care to adult care will find that dental and vision coverage are not required categories for adult coverage under an ACA policy.

## Health Insurance Exchanges

A Health Insurance Exchange is a government-operated insurance marketplace for ACA compliant plans that is accessed through the internet. There is a federal Health Insurance Exchange operated by the U.S. Department of Health and Human services, and several State health insurance exchanges operated by some States. Health Insurance exchanges offer all the plans available in the state where the applicant resides and certifies that the plans comply with the ACA requirements.

The health insurance plans offered on an exchange are operated by private insurance companies. The government does not operate the health insurance plans, it simply provides the marketplace and assures that the plans offered comply with ACA regulations. The federal Health Insurance Exchange can be found at www.healthcare.gov. Several states operate their own Healthcare Exchange.

A person is not required to purchase a health insurance plan through a health insurance exchange. However, there are two important advantages of using a health insurance exchange to purchase a plan of coverage.

First, the Health Insurance Exchange certifies that the plans offered comply with the ACA.

Second, subsidies that lower the cost of coverage are available if the coverage is purchased through a Healthcare Exchange. The Health Insurance Exchanges have an income and family size calculator that determines the amount of premium subsidy available to an individual or family if the coverage is purchased on the Healthcare Exchange.

## Enrolling in an ACA Plan

### Open Enrollment Period for ACA Plans

Open enrollment for ACA plans occurs once each year. Usually, the open enrollment period begins in November and ends in December, with coverage becoming effective in January. The specific dates for the annual open enrollment period are determined each year. For example, in 2021 the open enrollment period was adjusted to provide a greater opportunity for individuals and families affected by the COVID19 pandemic to enroll in ACA coverage. The open enrollment dates for the current year can be found on the www.Healthcare.gov website operated by the U.S. Department of Health and Human Services. Open enrollment is the primary opportunity to enroll in ACA coverage.

### Special Enrollment Period for ACA Plans [4]

If an individual or family did not enroll in ACA coverage during the open enrollment period, they may qualify for a special enrollment period. Applicants may qualify for a special enrollment if they lost other coverage or experienced a qualifying event after the end of the open enrollment period.

#### Loss or Change in Other Coverage

A person applying for ACA coverage may qualify for a special enrollment period if they (or anyone in the applicant's household) experienced a loss of or change in qualifying health coverage after the open enrollment period ended. A person can also qualify for special enrollment if they expect to lose coverage within the next 60 days. The special enrollment period during which a person may enroll is 60 days beginning on the day the other coverage ends. Changes in coverage that may qualify for a special enrollment period include:

- Loss of employer-sponsored coverage
- Loss of individual health coverage
- Loss of eligibility for Medicaid or CHIP
- Loss of eligibility for Medicare; or
- Loss of coverage based on a family member's coverage, such as dependent coverage

Special Enrollment is also available if the person applying for coverage (or anyone in their household) gained access to an individual coverage health reimbursement arrangement after open enrollment. A health reimbursement arrangement is an employee benefit where the employer offers to pay all or part of an employee's health insurance expense.

### Changes in Household Membership

A person may also qualify for a special enrollment period if the composition of their household changed in the past 60 days. Changes in household that may qualify for a special enrollment period include:

- Marriage
- Divorce or separation that results in a loss of coverage
- Death of a family member that results in a loss of coverage; or
- Birth, adoption, or placement of a child

### Changes in Place of Residence

A person may also qualify for a special enrollment period if their place of residence changed in the past 60 days. Changes in place of residence that may qualify for a special enrollment period include:

- Moving to a different ZIP code or county
- Moving to the United States from a foreign country or a US territory
- Moving to or from the place where the applicant attends school
- Moving to or from the place where the applicant both lives and works for seasonal employment; or
- Moving to or from a shelter or other transitional housing

It is important to note that visiting a place without changing residence does not qualify for a special enrollment period.

### Other Life Changes

Changes in other life circumstances may qualify for a special enrollment period, such as starting or ending service as AmeriCorps, VISTA, or NCCC volunteer. The rules for special enrollments may be expanded from time-to-time for extraordinary events, such as the COVID19 pandemic.

## Short-term Policies

A word of caution is appropriate regarding Short-term policies. In August 2018, a change in regulations permitted the sale of short-term, limited-duration health insurance plans. These short-term plans are not required to comply with federal market requirements governing individual health insurance coverage. Transitioning adults should understand that short-term policies are not governed by the ACA and lack the ACA consumer protections.

Because short-term plans are not governed by the ACA, these plans can deny coverage or charge higher prices to people with preexisting conditions. These short-term plans usually exclude benefits for preexisting conditions. Short-term plans may exclude some or most of the essential health benefits required in ACA-regulated plans.

The stated purpose of short-term plans was to create "more affordable options" with a lower premium cost. However, lower premium costs and less regulatory requirements typically mean that the policy has fewer benefits and less coverage than ACA plans. Short-term plans tend to have high premiums relative to the value of the benefits received.

Short-term plans are not likely to meet the needs of a person with a chronic condition with ongoing healthcare needs. It is important for individuals selecting health insurance coverage to understand that ACA-regulated insurance plans and short-term insurance plans are different insurance products with markedly different scopes of coverage and benefits. Some individuals are attracted to the lower monthly premium cost of short-term plans compared to ACA-regulated plans without understanding that the short-term plans lack the essential covered services of ACA plans and lack the consumer protections provided in ACA plans.

## State Programs

### Children with Special Healthcare Needs Program [5]

Children with Special Healthcare Needs (CSHCN) are state programs that offer health insurance to children with specific medical conditions. CSHCN programs have income eligibility limits that are less restrictive than Medicaid. Each State CSHCN program varies regarding age limitations. CSHCN may provide insurance coverage to some transitioning young adults with chronic illness.

### State Children's Health Insurance Program (SCHIP) [6]

State Children's Health Insurance Programs (SCHIP) provides Medicaid coverage to children who live in households that exceed the income limits for Medicaid enrollment, but are still within the income limits set by the SCHIP program. SCHIP coverage is limited to children under the age of 18, and in some states under the age of 19.

When a SCHIP participant reaches the limiting age, the participant will need to transition to other coverage. Transitioning young adults should understand when their SCHIP eligibility ends and make a plan to replace SCHIP to avoid any gap in health benefit coverage.

### Continued Coverage for Children Incapable of Self Support

Because of the ACA reforms, children may remain a covered dependent until age 26 years. Some states have adopted laws that allow dependent child coverage to extend beyond age 26. Each such state law has its own terms and conditions, but generally these laws require health insurers to continue coverage for children with a mental or physical disability if the child is incapable of self-support because of the disability.

Generally, these laws require the child to either live with the covered parent or be dependent on care regularly provided by the covered parent. The continuation of coverage lasts while the parent remains covered and while the child remains incapable of self-support. If the employer contributes to premium payments for dependents, the employer will typically be required to continue to do so for disabled child coverage.

**Example:** Amy is covered under her mother's employer-sponsored health plan. Amy's mother contributes $100 toward the premium and her employer pays the other $400. Amy reaches the policy's limiting age of 26 years. Amy's treating physician certifies in writing that Amy is incapable of self-support due to her medical condition. Amy's enrollment is extended beyond the limiting age and she continues coverage as a disabled dependent child. The employer continues to contribute $400 of the premium costs.

Disabled child continuation of coverage is not automatic. The covered parent must apply for the continuation of coverage for the dependent child. The application process depends on the requirement of state law and terms of each insurance policy, but generally the steps include:

- Obtaining the application form from the employer or the health insurance company before the dependent child reaches the limiting age on the policy. Many insurance companies have the forms available online and some still use paper forms that must be specifically requested.

- Obtaining a certification from the treating physician that the dependent child is incapable of self-support due to one's medical condition. This certification must be in writing and often has to be made on the insurance company's standard form.
- Responding to requests for information from the insurance company about the dependent child's income earned from work and other activities, if any.
- Responding to the insurance company's recertification, which may occur annually or from time-to-time as permitted by the policy or the state law.

Disabled child continuation of coverage is intended to benefit individuals who cannot care for or support themselves. "Incapable of self-support" does not mean that the disabled child cannot have any income. It means that the amount the disabled child is capable of earning, if any, is insufficient to support the child. Most state laws do not specify the amount of income a child can earn from work activity and still be considered incapable of self-support. Typically, this determination is made by the insurance company. If the disabled child has earnings deemed sufficient for self-support, then the disabled child coverage will end. Once it ends, there may not be an opportunity to restore the coverage if the disabled child again becomes incapable of self-support.

## COBRA Continuation of Benefits [7]

### COBRA Overview

Transitioning young adults may be able to extend employer-sponsored health benefit coverage under a federal law known as the Consolidated Omnibus Budget Reconciliation Act of 1985 (COBRA). The federal COBRA law requires employers with 20 or more employees to offer continuation of health insurance coverage to employees, their spouses, former spouses, and dependent children when group health coverage would otherwise be lost due to certain qualifying events. The length of continuation depends on the qualifying event. The different qualifying events and the length of the continuation period are listed below:

| COBRA qualifying event | Maximum continuation period |
|---|---|
| – Termination, resignation, or layoff | 18 months |
| – Death of policyholder | 36 months |
| – Divorce or separation from policyholder | 36 months |
| – Adult becomes eligible for SSDI benefits | 29 months |
| – Child reaches a limiting age under the policy | 36 months |

### Covered Employers

The federal COBRA statute applies to employers with 20 or more employees. The federal COBRA statute does not apply to plans sponsored by the Federal Government, by churches, or certain church-related organizations.

Some states have adopted laws similar to the federal law that apply to employers with fewer than 20 employees. These state laws are often referred to as mini-COBRA or State COBRA laws.

### COBRA Election

The federal COBRA law requires employers to offer employees the opportunity to elect COBRA continuation of coverage when a qualifying event occurs. Employers must give eligible employees at least 60 days to elect continued coverage. The 60-days begins on the date the employer gives the employee the election notice or the date the employee would lose coverage, whichever date is later. The coverage received under COBRA is the same plan of benefits available to current employees, but the employer may change or discontinue the plan of benefits available to all employees during the COBRA continuation period.

## COBRA Insurance Premiums

COBRA continuation coverage is often more expensive than the amount that active employees are required to pay for group health coverage because employers often pay part of the cost of employees' coverage. An employee or dependent who elects COBRA coverage is obligated to pay the full cost of the premium, even if the employer paid all or part of the premium before the qualifying event. In addition to the full premium of COBRA coverage, the person electing COBRA may be required to pay an administrative fee, but the amount paid for COBRA continuation cannot be more than 102% of the full monthly premium.

## COBRA May End Before the Maximum Continuation Period

COBRA coverage ends when the applicable continuation period expires or when:

- Premiums are not paid in full and on time
- The employer ceases to maintain any group health plan
- A qualified beneficiary begins coverage under another group health plan after electing continuation coverage
- A qualified beneficiary becomes entitled to Medicare benefits after electing continuation coverage; or
- A qualified beneficiary engages in conduct that would justify the plan in terminating coverage (such as fraud)

## Additional Resources

1. To obtain each state's Department of Insurance contact information go to: https://content.naic.org/state-insurance-departments
2. The Social Security Administration's website has information on the different SSA programs and application procedures at: www.ssa.gov
3. To apply for Social Security benefits call SSA at 1-800-772-1213. Applications may also be completed online at www.ssa.gov or at a local Social Security office but only for those applying for Social Security Disability Insurance benefits.
4. A list of the SSA medical criteria can be found at: www.ssa.gov/disability/professionals/bluebook
5. For a list of Medicaid eligibility income guidelines by state visit: http://www.statehealthfacts.org/comparetable.jsp?ind=203&cat=4
6. For more information about each state's SCHIP program please visit: http://www.insurekidsnow.gov
7. The Department of Labor has information on COBRA at: https://www.dol.gov/sites/dolgov/files/ebsa/about-ebsa/our-activities/resource-center/faqs/cobra-continuation-health-coverage-consumer.pdf

## References


1. 42 U.S.C. §421(a)(1): Disability determinations. https://www.govinfo.gov/content/pkg/USCODE-2020-title42/pdf/USCODE-2020-title42-chap7-subchapII-sec421.pdf. Accessed 15 Apr 2022.
2. 42 U.S.C. §1382: Supplemental security income. https://www.govinfo.gov/content/pkg/USCODE-2020-title42/pdf/USCODE-2020-title42-chap7-subchapXVI.pdf. Accessed 15 Apr 2022.
3. 42 U.S. Code § 1396a: Expansion of Medicaid. https://www.govinfo.gov/content/pkg/USCODE-2020-title42/pdf/USCODE-2020-title42-chap7-subchapXIX.pdf. Accessed 15 Apr 2022.
4. 45 C.F.R. § 155.420—Special enrollment periods. https://www.govinfo.gov/content/pkg/CFR-2020-title45-vol2/pdf/CFR-2020-title45-vol2-sec155-420.pdf. Accessed 15 Apr 2022.
5. 42 U.S.C. §12311: Children with special health-care needs program general contents. https://www.govinfo.gov/content/pkg/USCODE-2020-title42/pdf/USCODE-2020-title42-chap7-subchapXIX.pdf. Accessed 15 Apr 2022.
6. 42 U.S.C. §1397aa: State Children's Health Insurance Program. https://www.govinfo.gov/content/pkg/USCODE-2020-title42/pdf/USCODE-2020-title42-chap7-subchapXXI.pdf. Accessed 15 Apr 2022.
7. 26 C.F.R. § 54.4980B-4: COBRA qualifying events. https://www.govinfo.gov/content/pkg/CFR-2021-title26-vol19/pdf/CFR-2021-title26-vol19-sec54-4980B-4.pdf. Accessed 15 Apr 2022.

# Index





A. A. Kuo et al. (eds.), *Care of Adults with Chronic Childhood Conditions*,
https://doi.org/10.1007/978-3-031-54281-7

**B**

## D



## E

## N

U



V



W



X



Y

MIX
Papier aus verantwortungsvollen Quellen
Paper from responsible sources
FSC® C105338

If you have any concerns about our products,
you can contact us on
**ProductSafety@springernature.com**

In case Publisher is established outside the EU,
the EU authorized representative is:
**Springer Nature Customer Service Center GmbH**
**Europaplatz 3, 69115 Heidelberg, Germany**

Printed by Libri Plureos GmbH
in Hamburg, Germany